COMPUTED TOMOGRAPHY
AND MAGNETIC RESONANCE IMAGING
OF THE WHOLE BODY

VOLUME TWO

COMPUTED TOMOGRAPHY AND MAGNETIC RESONANCE IMAGING OF THE WHOLE BODY

JOHN R. HAAGA, M.D.

Professor and Chairman, Department of Radiology
Case Western Reserve University School of Medicine
Director, Division of Diagnostic Radiology
Head, Section of Computed Tomography
University Hospitals of Cleveland
Cleveland, Ohio

CHARLES F. LANZIERI, M.D.

Associate Professor, Department of Radiology
Case Western Reserve University School of Medicine
Director, Division of Neuroradiology
University Hospitals of Cleveland
Cleveland, Ohio

DAVID J. SARTORIS, M.D.

Professor
Department of Radiology, Musculoskeletal Section
University of California School of Medicine
Chief, Quantitative Bone Densitometry
Department of Radiology
University of California–San Diego Medical Center
San Diego, California

ELIAS A. ZERHOUNI, M.D.

Professor and Director, Thoracic Imaging and MRI
Department of Radiology
The Johns Hopkins Medical Institutions
Baltimore, Maryland

THIRD EDITION

with 4082 illustrations

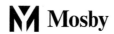 Mosby

St. Louis   Baltimore   Berlin   Boston   Carlsbad   Chicago   London   Madrid
Naples   New York   Philadelphia   Sydney   Tokyo   Toronto

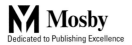
Mosby
Dedicated to Publishing Excellence

Editor: Susan M. Gay
Developmental Editor: Emma D. Underdown
Project Manager: Linda Clarke
Project Supervisor: Allan S. Kleinberg
Cover Designer: Sheilah Barrett
Manufacturing Supervisor: Theresa Fuchs

THIRD EDITION

Copyright © 1994 by Mosby-Year Book, Inc.
Previous editions copyrighted 1988, 1983

Printed in the United States of America
Composition by The Clarinda Company, Inc.
Printing/binding by Maple Vail-York

Mosby-Year Book, Inc.
11830 Westline Industrial Drive
St. Louis, Missouri 63146

Library of Congress Cataloging-in-Publication Data

Computed tomography and magnetic resonance imaging of the whole body /
   edited by John R. Haaga . . . [et al.].—3rd ed.
      p.   cm.
   Previous eds. published under title: Computed tomography of the
whole body.
   Includes bibliographical references and index.
   ISBN 0-8016-7057-8 (v. 1)
   1. Tomography.   I. Haaga, John R. (John Robert), 1945-   .
RC78.7.T6C6425   1994
616.07′54—dc20   94-16745
                                                            CIP

95 96 97 98 / 9 8 7 6 5 4 3 2

CONTRIBUTORS

JAMES J. ABRAHAMS, M.D.

Associate Professor
Department of Radiology
Yale University School of Medicine;
Attending Physician
Department of Diagnostic Radiology
Yale-New Haven Medical Center
New Haven, Connecticut

RICHARD L. BARON, M.D.

Professor and Co-Director, Abdominal Imaging
Professor of Radiology
University of Pittsburgh School of Medicine;
Director, Body Computed Tomography
Department of Radiology
Presbyterian-University Hospital
Pittsburgh, Pennsylvania

ERROL M. BELLON, M.D.

Professor
Department of Radiology
Case Western Reserve University;
Director
Department of Radiology
MetroHealth Medical Center
Cleveland, Ohio

JAVIER BELTRAN, M.D.

Associate Professor
Department of Radiology
New York University Medical Center;
Chairman
Department of Radiology
Hospital for Joint Diseases Orthopedic Institute
New York, New York

SUSAN BLASER, M.D., FRCPC

Assistant Professor
Department of Radiology
University of Toronto School of Medicine;
Staff Neuroradiologist
Division of Neuroradiology
The Hospital for Sick Children
Toronto, Ontario, Canada

MARTHA BROGAN, M.D.

Staff Radiologist
Department of Radiology
Grant Medical Center
Columbus, Ohio

DONALD W. CHAKERES, M.D.

Professor
Department of Radiology
Ohio State University College of Medicine;
Head of Neuroradiology and Clinical MRI
Department of Radiology
Ohio State University Hospitals
Columbus, Ohio

ROBERT J. CHURCHILL, M.D.

Professor and Chairman
Department of Radiology
University of Missouri School of Medicine;
Department of Radiology
University of Missouri Hospital and Clinics
Columbia, Missouri

RICHARD H. COHAN, M.D.

Associate Professor
Department of Radiology
University of Michigan School of Medicine;
Department of Radiology
University of Michigan Medical Center
Ann Arbor, Michigan

ALAN M. COHEN, M.D.

Professor and Chief
University of Texas—Houston
Health Science Center
Department of Radiology
Houston, Texas

DEWEY J. CONCES, JR., M.D.

Professor
Department of Radiology
University of Indiana School of Medicine;
Department of Radiology
Indiana University Hospital
Indianapolis, Indiana

HUGH D. CURTIN, M.D.

Professor
Department of Radiology
University of Pittsburgh Medical Center;
Director
Department of Radiology
Eye and Ear Institute
Pittsburgh, Pennsylvania

MURRAY K. DALINKA, M.D.

Professor
Department of Radiology
Hospital of the University of Pennsylvania
Philadelphia, Pennsylvania

MONY J. DE LEON, B.A., M.A., ED.D.

Associate Professor and
Director, Neuroimaging Laboratory
Department of Psychiatry
New York University Medical Center
New York, New York

PEDRO J. DIAZ, PH.D.

Assistant Professor
Departments of Biomedical Engineering and Radiology
Case Western Reserve University;
Department of Radiology
MetroHealth Medical Center
Cleveland, Ohio

N. REED DUNNICK, M.D.

Professor and Chairman
Department of Radiology
University of Michigan Medical Center
Ann Arbor, Michigan

CHARLES R. FITZ, M.D.

Professor
Department of Radiology
University of Pittsburgh School of Medicine;
Head of Neuroradiology
Department of Radiology
Children's Hospital of Pittsburgh
Pittsburgh, Pennsylvania

AMILCARE GENTILI, M.D.

Assistant Professor
Department of Radiology
Case Western Reserve University
Department of Radiology
University Hospitals of Cleveland
Cleveland, Ohio

AJAX E. GEORGE, M.D.

Professor
Department of Radiology
New York University School of Medicine;
Senior Neuroradiologist
Department of Radiology/Neuroradiology
New York University Medical Center
New York, New York

KATHRYN GRUMBACH, M.D.

Associate Professor
Department of Radiology
University of Maryland School of Medicine;
Attending Radiologist
Department of Radiology
University of Maryland Medical Center
Baltimore, Maryland

E. MARK HAACKE, PH.D.

Professor
Department of Radiology
Mallinckrodt Institute of Radiology
Washington University School of Medicine
St. Louis, Missouri

DEREK HARWOOD-NASH, MB, CHB, FRCPC

Professor
Department of Radiology
University of Toronto School of Medicine;
Head, MRI Centre
Department of Radiology
The Hospital for Sick Children
Toronto, Ontario, Canada

ROBERT R. HATTERY, M.D.

Professor
Department of Radiology
Mayo Medical School;
Consultant in Diagnostic Radiology
Mayo Clinic and Mayo Foundation
Rochester, Minnesota

TAMARA MINER HAYGOOD, M.D., PH.D.

Assistant Professor
Department of Radiology
The Bowman Gray School of Medicine
Winston-Salem, North Carolina

THOMAS E. HERBENER, M.D.

Assistant Professor
Department of Radiology
Case Western Reserve University;
Assistant Professor
Department of Radiology
University Hospitals of Cleveland
Cleveland, Ohio

LEO HOCHHAUSER, M.D., FRCPC

Assistant Professor
Department of Radiology
State University of New York Health Science Center
Syracuse, New York

ROY A. HOLLIDAY, M.D.

Assistant Professor
Department of Radiology
New York University School of Medicine;
Director, Head and Neck Radiology
Department of Radiology
New York University Medical Center
New York, New York

DAVID S. JACOBS, M.D.

Staff Radiologist
Hillcrest Radiology Associates
Mayfield Heights, Ohio

STEPHEN A. KIEFFER, M.D.

Professor and Chairman
Department of Radiology
State University of New York Health Sciences Center;
Chief
Department of Radiology
University Hospital
Syracuse, New York

J. BRUCE KNEELAND, M.D.

Associate Professor
Department of Radiology
Hospital of the University of Pennsylvania
Philadelphia, Pennsylvania

JANET E. KUHLMAN, M.D.

Associate Professor and Director of Chest Radiology
Department of Radiology
The Johns Hopkins Medical Institutions
Baltimore, Maryland

FRED J. LAINE, M.D.

Assistant Professor and Clinical Director of MR
Department of Radiology
Medical College of Virginia Hospitals
Richmond, Virginia

BARTON LANE, M.D.

Associate Professor
Department of Radiology
Stanford University Medical Center
Stanford, California

ERROL LEVINE, M.D., PH.D., FACR, FRCR

Professor and Head, Sections of Computed Body Tomography,
Magnetic Resonance Imaging, and Uroradiology
Department of Diagnostic Radiology
University of Kansas Medical Center
Kansas City, Kansas

JAMES M. LIEBERMAN, M.D.

Assistant Professor
Department of Radiology
Case Western Reserve University;
Staff Radiologist
Department of Radiology
University Hospital
Cleveland, Ohio

WEILI LIN, PH.D.

Assistant Professor
Department of Radiology
Washington University School of Medicine
St. Louis, Missouri

NEAL MANDELL, M.D.

Instructor
Department of Radiology
Yale University School of Medicine
New Haven, Connecticut

JAMES V. MANZIONE, M.D.

Fellow, Interventional Radiology
Department of Radiology
State University of New York Health Science Center
Syracuse, New York

THERESA C. McLOUD, M.D.

Associate Professor
Department of Radiology
Harvard University Medical School;
Chief of Thoracic Radiology
Department of Radiology
Massachusetts General Hospital
Boston, Massachusetts

RHONDA McDOWELL, M.D.

Resident
Department of Radiology
Case Western Reserve University
Cleveland, Ohio

ALEC J. MEGIBOW, M.D.

Professor
Department of Radiology
New York University School of Medicine;
Director, Abdominal Imaging
Department of Radiology
New York University Medical Center
New York, New York

FLORO MIRALDI, M.D., SC.D.

Professor
Department of Biomedical Engineering
Associate Professor
Department of Radiology
Case Western Reserve University School of Medicine;
Director, Division of Nuclear Radiology and PET Facility
University Hospitals of Cleveland
Cleveland, Ohio

STUART C. MORRISON, M.B., CH.B., M.R.C.P.

Associate Professor
Department of Radiology
Case Western Reserve University School of Medicine;
Associate Professor
Department of Radiology
University Hospitals of Cleveland
Cleveland, Ohio

MARK D. MURPHEY, M.D.

Associate Professor and Chief, Musculoskeletal Section
Department of Radiologic Pathology
Armed Forces Institute of Pathology
Washington, D.C.

M. HOSSAIN NAHEEDY, M.D.

Associate Professor
Department of Radiology
Case Western Reserve University School of Medicine;
Director, Radiology Service
Wade Park Veterans Administration Medical Center
Cleveland, Ohio

ERIC K. OUTWATER, M.D.

Assistant Professor
Department of Radiology
Thomas Jefferson University School of Medicine;
Assistant Professor
Department of Radiology
Thomas Jefferson University Hospital
Philadelphia, Pennsylvania

KATHLEEN GALLAGHER OXNER, M.D.

Staff Radiologist
Greenville Radiology, P.A.
Greenville, South Carolina

LARRY B. POE, M.D.

Assistant Professor
Department of Radiology
State University of New York Health Science Center
Syracuse, New York

CATHRYN POWERS, M.D.

Clinical Assistant Professor
Department of Radiology
University of Florida College of Medicine
Gainesville, Florida;
Associate Radiologist
Radiology Associates of Ocala, P.A.
Ocala, Florida

MICHAEL P. RECHT, M.D.

Cleveland Clinic
Cleveland, Ohio

DEBORAH L. REEDE, M.D.

Vice Chairman
Department of Radiology
Long Island College Hospital;
Adjunct Associate Professor
Department of Radiology
New York University Medical Center;
Associate Professor
State University of New York Health Science Center
Brooklyn, New York

PABLO R. ROS, M.D., FACR

Professor and Director, Division of Abdominal Imaging and MRI
Department of Radiology
University of Florida College of Medicine
Gainesville, Florida

MARK E. SCHWEITZER, M.D.

Assistant Professor of Radiology
Department of Radiology
Thomas Jefferson University School of Medicine;
Department of Radiology
Thomas Jefferson University Hospital
Philadelphia, Pennsylvania

HERVEY D. SEGALL, M.D.

Professor and Director of Neuroradiology
Department of Radiology
University of Southern California School of Medicine
Los Angeles, California

STEVEN SHANKMAN, M.D.

Assistant Professor
Department of Radiology
New York University School of Medicine;
Director of Residency Training
Department of Radiology
The Hospital for Joint Diseases
New York, New York

PATRICK F. SHEEDY II, M.D.

Professor
Department of Radiology
Mayo Medical School;
Department of Radiology
Mayo Clinic and Mayo Foundation;
Department of Radiology
Saint Marys Hospital and Rochester Methodist Hospital
Rochester, Minnesota

ALISON S. SMITH, M.D.

Assistant Professor
Department of Radiology
Case Western Reserve University School of Medicine;
Staff
Department of Radiology
University Hospitals of Cleveland
Cleveland, Ohio

JOHN E. SUNDERLAND, M.D.

Resident
Department of Radiology
Mallinckrodt Institute of Radiology
Washington University School of Medicine;
Resident
Department of Diagnostic Radiology
Barnes Hospital
St. Louis, Missouri

STEPHEN W. TAMARKIN, M.D.

Instructor
Department of Radiology
Case Western Reserve University School of Medicine;
Body Imaging Fellow
Department of Radiology
University Hospitals of Cleveland
Cleveland, Ohio

ROBERT W. TARR, M.D.

Assistant Professor
Department of Radiology
Case Western Reserve University School of Medicine;
Assistant Professor
Department of Radiology
University Hospitals of Cleveland
Cleveland, Ohio

ROBERT D. TARVER, M.D.

Professor
Department of Radiology
Indiana University School of Medicine;
Professor and Director, Chest Imaging
Department of Radiology
Wishard Memorial Hospital
Indianapolis, Indiana

JAMES W. WALSH, M.D.

Professor
Department of Radiology
University of Minnesota School of Medicine
Minneapolis, Minnesota

JOHN J. WASENKO, M.D.

Assistant Professor
Department of Radiology
State University of New York Health Sciences Center
Syracuse, New York

TIMOTHY J. WELCH, M.D.

Consultant
Department of Diagnostic Radiology
Mayo Clinic
Rochester, Minnesota

ERNEST J. WIESEN, E.E.

Assistant Professor
Department of Radiology
Case Western Reserve University School of Medicine;
Radiological Physicist
Department of Radiology
MetroHealth Medical Center
Cleveland, Ohio

CHI-SHING ZEE, M.D.

Associate Professor
Department of Radiology
University of Southern California School of Medicine;
Staff
Department of Radiology
Los Angeles County/University of Southern California Medical
Center
Los Angeles, California

Dedication

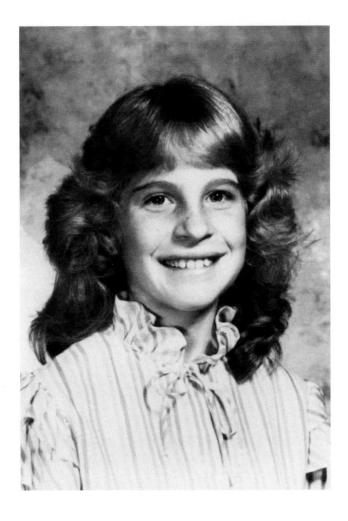

This book is dedicated to Elizabeth E. Haaga, daughter of John and Ellen Haaga, who was born on August 19, 1972, and died December 9, 1985. Beth had a disseminated neuroblastoma, which was diagnosed in 1984. She was treated with a bone marrow transplant and died from graft versus host disease and infection. As her parents, we loved her dearly and cherish the memory of her early years when she was well. After the onset of her illness, we came to know that her gentle and loving nature was accompanied by a remarkably strong character. She endured her pain and suffering without bitterness and never sought to hurt those who loved her. Indeed, most incredulously, she tried to lessen our emotional pain even while enduring her physical discomforts. Many authors have marveled at the qualities of children, and although Beth's short life and premature death have left us saddened beyond comprehension, her remarkable courage and sweetness have given us a lasting pride and respect. We remember her lovingly.

This book is dedicated in memorium to Precy Grepo and Barbara Sartoris, both of whom excelled at life's most important responsibility, motherhood, and whose final earthly days were rendered less painful by cross-sectional imaging technology.

PREFACE TO THIRD EDITION

This new book, *CT and MRI of the Whole Body*, was written to replace the second edition of *CT of the Whole Body*. We had not considered writing such a comprehensive book about CT and MRI before now because we believed the science of MRI was advancing so quickly that an integrated, complete text was not possible. Knowing that the technology for both of these fields has now stabilized and considerable experience has been accumulated, we are comfortable putting this book together. Fortunately we were able to solicit the support of the many knowledgeable contributors who made this large work possible.

This book is unique in that it is one of the few books available that covers all aspects of CT and MRI in the major areas of the body. While we have tried to be comprehensive in our coverage, the desire and requirement to have a book of manageable size did force some limitation of coverage. We are confident that our excellent contributors have accomplished these goals within the scope and depth of their work.

The organization of the book is similar to its predecessors. The chapters on the brain cover the various disease processes in the different anatomic areas. The chapters covering the chest are divided into different regions as well as disease processes. The abdominal chapters discuss anatomic topics or related pathologic processes. The musculoskeletal section has been significantly expanded and includes chapters of various anatomic areas. There is a large chapter on interventional procedures, which covers very specific information about instruments, organ systems, and specific techniques.

Finally, we believe this book will be very helpful to our radiology colleagues who are being pressured by the current trends in medicine. With the sweeping changes that are occurring in medicine, radiologists and other subspecialists are confronted with two diverging agendas and directions. On one hand, the government and patients are demanding a continuation of the remarkably high technology diagnostic tests that require subspecialization to ensure appropriate outcomes and utilization. On the other hand, the managed health care systems and the primary care orientation are forcing physicians and radiologists into providing a more generally oriented type of care. We believe that this book can be a useful reference source because it is very broad in its coverage of topics and yet very comprehensive in its depth.

JOHN R. HAAGA
CHARLES F. LANZIERI
DAVID J. SARTORIS
ELIAS A. ZERHOUNI

PREFACE TO FIRST EDITION

Since the introduction of computed tomography (CT) in 1974, there has been a remarkable revolution in the medical treatment of patients. The clinical use of CT has had a broad positive impact on patient management. Literally thousands of patients have been saved or their quality of life improved as a result of the expeditious and accurate diagnosis provided by CT. This improvement in diagnosis and management has occurred in all medical subspecialties, including neurological, pulmonary, cardiac, gastrointestinal, genitourinary, and neuromuscular medicine. Aside from the imaging advantages provided, the role of CT in planning and performing interventional procedures is now recognized. It is the most accurate method for guiding procedures to obtain cytological, histological, or bacteriological specimens and for performing a variety of therapeutic procedures.

The evolution and refinement of CT equipment have been as remarkable as the development of patient diagnosis. When we wrote our first book on CT, the scanning unit used was a 2-minute translate-rotate system. At the time of our second book the 18-second translate-rotate scanning unit was in general use. Currently standard units in radiological practice are third and fourth generation scanners with scan times of less than 5 seconds. All modern systems are more reliable than the earlier generations of equipment. The contrast and spatial resolution of these systems are in the range of 0.5% and less than 1 mm, respectively. The sophistication of the computer programs that aid in the diagnosis is also remarkable. There are now programs for three-dimensional reconstructions, quantitation of blood flow, determination of organ volume, longitudinal scans (Scoutview, Deltaview, Synerview, and Topogram), and even triangulation programs for performing percutaneous biopsy procedures.

CT units are now being installed in virtually every hospital of more than 200 beds throughout the United States. Most radiologists using these units are generalists who scan all portions of the anatomy. Because of the dissemination of this equipment and its use in general diagnosis, there exists a significant need for a general and complete textbook to cover all aspects of CT scanning. Our book in intended to partially supplement the knowledge of this group of physicians. We have attempted to completely and succinctly cover all portions of CT scanning to provide a complete general reference text. In planning the book, we chose to include the contributions of a large number of talented academicians with expertise different from and more complete than our own in their selected areas. By including contributors from outside our own department, we have been able to produce an in-depth textbook that combines the academic strengths of numerous individuals and departments.

The book is divided into chapters according to the organ systems, except for some special chapters on abscesses and interventional procedures. In each of the chapters the authors have organized the material into broad categories, such as congenital, benign, or neoplastic disease. Each author has tried to cover the major disease processes in each of the general categories in which CT diagnosis is applicable. Specific technical details, including the method of scanning, contrast material, collimation, and slice thickness, are covered in each chapter. The interventional chapter extensively covers the various biopsy and therapeutic procedures in all the organ systems. Finally, the last chapter presents an up-to-the-minute coverage of current and recent developments in the CT literature and also provides extensive information about nuclear magnetic resonance (NMR) imaging. At this time we have had moderate experience with the NMR superconducting magnetic device produced by the Technicare Corporation and have formulated some initial opinions as to its role relative to CT and other imaging modalities. A concise discussion of the physics of NMR and a current clinical status report of the new modality are provided.

We would like to thank all those people who have worked so diligently and faithfully for the preparation of this book. First, we are very grateful to our many contributors. For photography work, we are deeply indebted to Mr. Joseph P. Molter. For secretarial and organizational skills, we are indebted especially to Mrs. Mary Ann Reid and Mrs. Rayna Lipscomb. The editorial skills of Ms. B. Hami were invaluable in preparing the manuscript. Our extremely competent technical staff included Mr. Joseph Agee, Ms. Ginger Haddad, Mrs. E. Martinelle, Mr. Mark Clampett, Mrs. Mary Kralik, and numerous others.

Finally, we are, of course, very appreciative of the support, patience, and encouragement of our wonderful families. In the Haaga family this includes Ellen, Elizabeth, Matthew, and Timothy, who provided the positive motivation and support for this book. Warm gratitude for unswerving support is also due to Rose, Sue, Lisa, Chris, Katie, Mary, and John Alfidi.

JOHN R. HAAGA
RALPH J. ALFIDI

CONTENTS

PART VI

IMAGING OF THE ABDOMEN AND PELVIS

28

The Gastrointestinal Tract

ALEC J. MEGIBOW

Initial clinical use of computed tomography (CT) in the luminal gastrointestinal tract focused on the ability to recognize a thickened bowel wall. The appearances of a variety of entities were described, and several clinical applications were forecast.[80] CT has become an established procedure in a variety of common gastrointestinal disorders. Two basic factors have increased its use. First is the increasing availability of CT to patients because of a growing number of units, increasing use of magnetic resonance imaging (MRI) for neuromuscular disease, and improved patient throughout afforded by modern-day equipment. Second, because CT visualizes the endoluminal, intramural, and perienteric components of disease processes, it provides sufficient diagnostic specificity and the ability to make therapeutic decisions rapidly. The indication for CT depends on the clinical condition of the patient. If the history suggests mucosal processes, barium studies or endoscopic evaluation is an appropriate first choice; however, when diseases are suspected in which the extraluminal extension of disease may be more critical than the changes along the mucosal surface, CT assumes a frontline role.

This chapter evaluates the role of CT in a variety of disorders involving the gastrointestinal tract and details those applications in which CT has begun to emerge as the primary radiological imaging modality.

TECHNIQUES
Conventional techniques

Successful performance and interpretation of CT examination of the gastrointestinal tract requires adequate bowel opacification as well as distention of that portion of the alimentary tract being analyzed.[8] This is achieved by the use of orally administered contrast material, which is given before and during the examination. Oral contrast material has two purposes in body CT: (1) to identify a given bowel loop and differentiate it from an adjacent or pathological mass (unopacified bowel loops are still a major source of error in the interpreta-

tion of body CT images) and (2) to distend that bowel loop to evaluate true thickness of the wall (Fig. 28-1).

Two types of positive oral contrast materials are used in body CT: dilute barium suspensions and dilute solutions of water-soluble contrast material.[99] In our practice, we prefer the oral barium suspensions for routine CT, reserving the water-soluble agents for special cases. We believe that there is better patient acceptance with the oral barium agents and that the mucosal detail, particularly in the small bowel, is superior.[90] These agents are available as approximately 1% to 2% suspensions of barium sulfate. They are successful in opacifying the gastrointestinal tract because agents are added to the barium to maintain them in suspension at low concentrations. This avoids problems with flocculation. Ball and associates[7] have shown barium suspensions to be stable at low gastric pH, whereas water-soluble solutions may precipitate.

We use water-soluble contrast agents as a 2% solution in specific instances. These include trauma patients, patients with suspected gastrointestinal perforation, patients who are recently or immediately preoperative, and patients in whom a percutaneous CT-guided interventional procedure (either needle biopsy or abscess drainage) is being performed.

The protocol for contrast administration should ensure uniform opacification of the entire alimentary canal. Patients are instructed to come to the department approximately 30 to 60 minutes before their examination to guarantee successful bowel opacification. At our institution, we require the patient to drink between four and six 7-ounce cups of contrast agent before the examination. We ask the patient to consume the entire volume at a steady rate of approximately one cup every 10 minutes.

Immediately before scanning and just before the patient lies on the scan table, a final cup of oral contrast agent is given that serves to opacify the stomach, duodenum, and proximal jejunum. This cup is given regard-

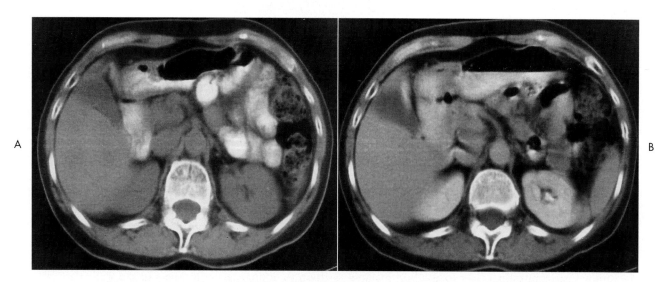

Fig. 28-1. A, Noncontrast CT scan through upper abdomen. Excellent opacification of duodenum and proximal small bowel noted. **B,** Same patient approximately 5 minutes later during contrast-enhanced scan. The stomach remains filled, but contrast in the duodenum an jejunum is dilated and washed out. (From Megibow AJ, Balthazar EJ: *CT of the gastrointestinal tract,* St. Louis, 1986, CV Mosby.)

less of the amount of contrast agent the patient has consumed. We have found that the proximal portion of the gastrointestinal tract is the most difficult segment in which to maintain dense opacification. This is due to the dilutional effect of the large amount of water transported into the duodenal lumen when the stomach is filled, resulting in diminished contrast density in the proximal small bowel. This is overcome by flooding the segment immediately before the examination. When the study is performed both without and with contrast material, more oral medium should be administered before the second run through the abdomen to avoid the possibility of dilution of the contrast material in the jejunum.

We do not routinely attempt to opacify the colon on our CT examinations. Many centers give oral contrast agents the night before an examination to opacify the sigmoid colon.[36] We have found, however, that this delayed opacification often results in dense opacity of the contrast material, causing streak artifacts. We believe that we can adequately identify the sigmoid colon in a sufficient number of cases because of its fecal and air content to avoid having to give contrast agents the night before. If the purpose of the examination requires colonic opacification, however, particularly in cases of staging pelvic neoplasms, we ask the patient to prepare the colon the night before. We then insufflate air at the time of the CT scan; in this fashion, we believe we can optimally evaluate the pelvic colon. We use delayed opacification techniques in assessing early postoperative complications,

particularly anastomotic leaks, in patients who have had colorectal surgery (Fig. 28-2).

We routinely use 0.1 mg of intravenous glucagon during all of our abdominal CT examinations. We find that the hypotonia produced by this agent improves the scan quality as a result of diminution of peristalsis. Using 0.1 mg of glucagon is a minimal increase in cost; in cases in which the colon is to be insufflated, we use 0.5 mg of intravenous glucagon to reduce cramping and facilitate retention.

Several situations may require modifications in the contrast regimen. In recently postoperative patients, transit time may be prolonged; therefore more time should be allowed for contrast dispersion through the small bowel. Similarly a medication history is useful in identifying those patients in whom intestinal transit time may be affected. Finally, if equipment problems occur during the day and the scanner "goes down" for a period of time, the patients who drank oral contrast agents earlier may have to take more in an attempt to reopacify the proximal small bowel into the colon; mistakes can be made if the patient is not asked to drink again and refill the small bowel (Fig. 28-3).

In many clinical situations, the radiologist is pressured to scan the patient quickly either because the machine time is limited or an emergency situation is present. In such cases, rigid adherence to a reliable bowel opacification protocol and confidence in the ability to opacify small bowel loops are necessary. If the scan is rushed, it

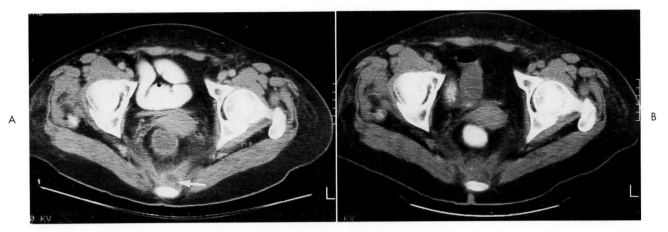

Fig. 28-2. Delayed opacification for pelvic abscess. **A,** CT scan in a patient who recently underwent an abdominal sacral resection for rectal carcinoma. Presacral abscess *(arrow)* is seen. What is the status of anastomosis? **B,** Same patient rescanned within 5 hours. The rectum is well filled. There is no evidence of contrast extravasation either in the soft tissues or into the abscess.

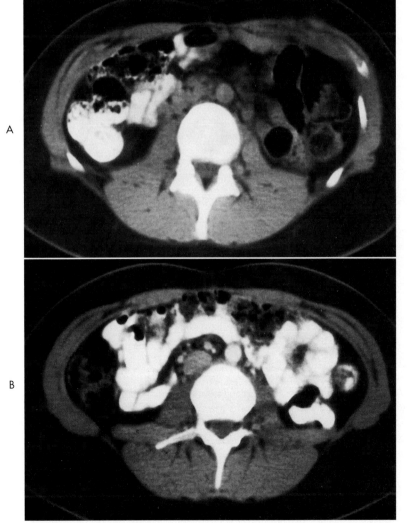

Fig. 28-3. Unopacified bowel loops simulating retroperitoneal lymphoma. **A,** Scan in 32-year-old woman with Hodgkin's disease interpreted as retroperitoneal adenopathy. Note lack of small bowel filling and predominance of colonic opacification. Scheduling delays and emergencies delayed her actual examination for 4 hours after she drank an oral contrast agent. **B,** Repeat scan after proper timing of contrast administration. Normal retroperitoneum is evident.

is likely that the patient will have to return for extra delayed cuts, or mistakes in interpretation may be made.

Alternative techniques

Since 1983, we have used air insufflation of the colon and effervescent gas distention of the stomach to study gastrointestinal pathology. Negative contrast heightens appreciation of the bowel wall and enhances recognition of subtle pathologic changes.[74] Air-contrast techniques provide reliable distention of the viscus and help demarcate it from adjacent structures. Unsuspected pathological conditions may be detected at the time of CT that can lead to more directed radiological studies.

Air insufflation of the stomach is achieved by substituting a dose of gas-forming crystals for the final cup of positive contrast agent. At our institution, this is done

at the time when the patient has lain on the table, the scout image has been obtained, and the setup is in place for intravenous contrast administration; in other words, immediately preceding the beginning of scanning. At that time, we ask the patient to consume one packet of E-Z-GAS, dissolved in approximately 7 oz of water. This immediately distends the stomach, and the gaseous distention is maintained through the cuts of the upper abdomen. The large volume of water provides distention and negative contrast for the dependent fundus.

If the colon is to be insufflated, this is done at the end of the examination. Patient positioning depends on the area of the colon to be studied. We have found that by placing patients prone, we achieved superior distention in the pelvic sigmoid and rectum because of its posterior position. Therefore our pelvic CT scans are

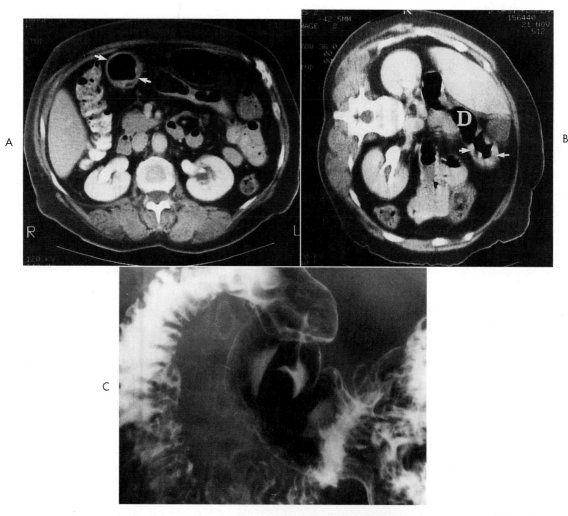

Fig. 28-4. Positional change improves diagnostic ability on CT. **A,** Suspicion of antral thickening *(arrow).* **B,** Scan through antrum in left-side-down decubitus position. Thick folds are confined in the prepyloric antrum *(arrow)* D, Duodenal bulb. **C,** Spot film from gastrointestinal series revealing hypertrophic antral gastritis. CT was the first examination in this patient with nonspecific abdominal pain.

done with the patient in the prone position.[93] If we are evaluating pathological change in the right colon, a left-side-down decubitus view may be useful in attempting to distend the cecal area. Conversely, if the left side of the colon is being evaluated, the opposite decubitus position is appropriate. In conventional fluoroscopic examination of the gastrointestinal tract, different portions of the alimentary canal require alteration in position to eliminate superimposition and to distend the area in question maximally. This is true in CT examination of the gastrointestinal tract as well; the slight amount of extra time necessary to rescan the patient in optimized position defines more precisely the nature of pathological processes in different segments of the gastrointestinal tract (Fig. 28-4). Specific uses of positional changes are illustrated in appropriate sections in this chapter.

Literature has accumulated on the use of water as a contrast agent for gastrointestinal CT.[4] Water has several advantages over gas. These include the ability to see the thickness of the intestinal wall of clinical window and level settings and lack of necessity of positional change to distend varying portions of the alimentary canal.[57,58] We have begun using water routinely in examining the pancreas because water elegantly outlines the duodenum. The disadvantages of water include slightly decreased conspicuity of lesions and patient discomfort related to distention.

PRINCIPLES OF DIAGNOSIS

The first findings of pathological change in the gastrointestinal tract recognized on CT were those in which visible wall thickening could be identified. Initial reports claimed excellent sensitivity in identifying an abnormally thickened intestinal wall but commented on a relative lack of specificity in distinguishing inflammatory from neoplastic processes.[35] As overall system resolution has improved and radiologists have learned sophisticated methods for administering intravenous contrast material, we have been able to improve both sensitivity in the detection of lesions and specificity because of our ability not only to see thickness of the wall, but also to analyze the components of the wall in the area of pathological thickening.

When approaching gastrointestinal CT, first identify pathological areas of wall thickening, then systematically analyze the luminal surface, the appearance of the wall, the appearance of the serosa, and finally the nature of any change within the local perienteric fat. A combination of these factors enables us to construct a differential diagnosis of gastrointestinal lesions. During the discussions of specific disease entities, when appropriate, we highlight those features in the radiological appearance of the lesion and surrounding structures that have differential diagnostic significance.

STOMACH

The primary indication for CT evaluation of gastric diseases is in the detection and staging of gastric neoplasms. Occasionally, serendipitous findings of gastric disease are encountered on routine CT scans. CT is not indicated for the adjunctive evaluation of inflammatory diseases.

Anatomy

The stomach is readily recognizable on CT examinations of the upper abdomen. Several normal anatomical features of the stomach must be remembered when interpreting CT examinations (Fig. 28-5). Using air-contrast techniques, features of the normal wall can be recognized. Normal areas of wall thickening include the insertion of the gastrohepatic ligament at the esophagogastric (EG) junction and the pyloric canal. Anatomical wall thickening in these areas can be confirmed by change of patient positioning and by overdistention with positive or negative contrast material. The pyloric canal is often seen with the lumen running centrally between the two bundles of thickened muscle. This causes little problem in differential diagnosis. At the EG junction, there is a more complex anatomy, and differential diagnosis of anatomical as opposed to pathological wall thickening may be more difficult. Marks and colleagues[86] have shown thickening in 38% of normal patients in this region. Identification of the fissure at the ligamentum venosum at the same level as the thickening helps in the differential diagnosis. Scanning the patient in the prone position after gas distention is a useful method of further evaluating this region.

The relationship of the stomach with its mesenteric attachments must be thoroughly understood. Gastric neoplasms extend locally across these peritoneal reflections, and major lymph node groups are located here as well. The lesser omentum originates from the fissure of the ligamentum venosum and fans along the lesser curvature from the EG junction to its free edge, the hepatoduodenal ligament. Within the lesser omentum, lymph nodes, the coronary vein, and occasionally the left gastric artery are seen.[6] The supramesocolic portion of the greater omentum originates along the greater curvature aspect of the stomach, sweeping from the gastrosplenic ligament—its most posterior extension—to the right side of the abdomen. This ligament contains gastroepiploic vessels and greater curvature lymph nodes. It inserts along the upper portion of the transverse colon, fusing with the pancreatic reflection of the transverse mesocolon (Fig. 28-6). The lymph node drainage of the stomach has been traditionally subdivided into four classic zones:[32] the paracardiac, subpyloric, gastroepiploic, and splenic hilar. Because of connecting intramural lymphatics, one often cannot predict the precise drainage pat-

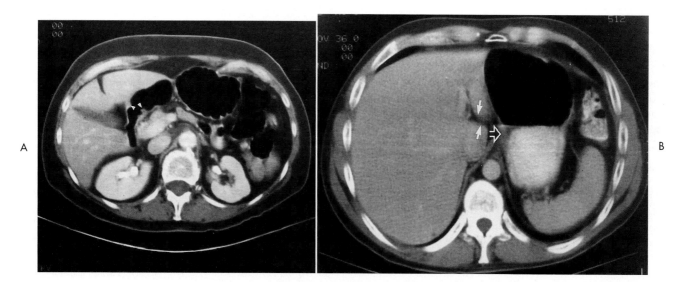

Fig. 28-5. Air-contrast CT anatomy of the stomach. **A,** Distal stomach. The antrum is featureless compared with the cardia. The pyloric canal is seen in the open position *(arrow).* Distally the duodenal bulb and proximal sweep can be easily recognized. **B,** Esophagogastric junction. Minimal thickening is noted along lesser curvature aspect of the stomach *(open arrow).* Note the relation to the fissure of the ligamentum venosum *(closed arrow).* This thickening is an anatomical variant reflecting ligamentous attachments of the lesser omentum into the stomach.

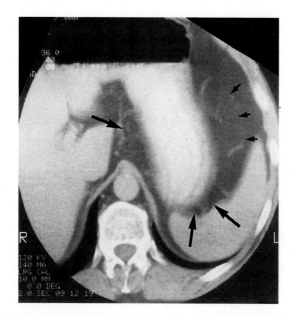

Fig. 28-6. Ligamentous attachments of the stomach. Loops of the gastroepiploic vessels can be seen coursing in the fibrofatty tissue of the greater omentum *(small arrows).* The most posterior portion is the gastrosplenic ligament *(large arrows).* Left gastric artery branches are seen in the lesser omentum *(single arrow).* (From Megibow AJ, Balthazar EJ: *CT of the gastrointestinal tract,* St. Louis, 1986, CV Mosby.)

terns of gastric neoplasms in these zones The Japanese Research Society for Gastric Cancer has developed a more complex but clinically useful classification. They divide the nodes into intramural, intermediary, and extramural groups. The intermediary nodes (corresponding to the four zones of Coller) consist of four major drainage pathways that deposit into the extramural system—these extramural nodes are located adjacent to the major arteries.[79] Applications of this staging system in gastric carcinoma are discussed later.

Non-neoplastic disease

Gastritis. Inflammatory disease of the stomach is not a primary indication for CT. Diffuse wall thickening with preservation of the mucosal pattern may be detected, signifying gastritis. It is helpful to realize that the visualization of the normal rugal pattern as seen by air contrast helps in differentiating wall thickening from gastritis as opposed to wall thickening from neoplastic disease (hypertrophic gastritis). It is important to observe the smoothly lobulated, clearly defined folds in the proximal stomach.[45] Other forms of hypertrophic gastritis, such as Zollinger-Ellison syndrome, may show evidence of pancreatic mass or liver metastases, suggesting the diagnosis of metastatic pancreatic islet cell tumor. Focal non-neoplastic masses may be seen in surrounding benign ulcers (ulcer mounds) (Fig. 28-7). Using dynamic

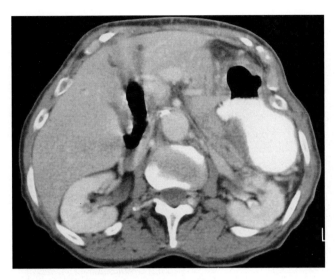

Fig. 28-7. Gastric ulcer with benign mass. The ulcer crater is filled with barium. Note the low attenuation within the thickened gastric wall. The appearance results from edema, as opposed to tumor infiltration.

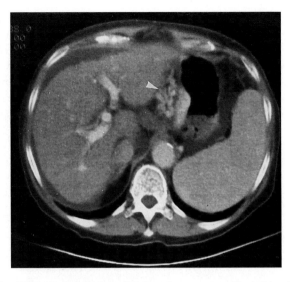

Fig. 28-8. Gastric varices. Bright enhancement afforded by dynamic CT reveals varices in the lesser omentum *(arrowhead)*. The patient has class IV primary biliary cirrhosis.

incremental bolus contrast enhancement, one can recognize the low attenuation in the mass representing edema as opposed to solid tumor tissue. *H. pylori* gastritis has been described as giving a similar appearance to carcinoma; however, contrast enhancement was not carefully controlled in this report.[122] In acquired immunodeficiency syndrome (AIDS) patients, gastritis may yield a similar appearance. This is most typically due to a combination of cryptosporidia and cytomegalovirus infiltrating the distal stomach.[116]

Gastric varices. CT has been shown to be sensitive to the presence of varices. In conventional barium studies, varices may be confused with rugal folds or polypoid tumor masses. In a reported series of 13 patients with proven gastric varices, diagnostic features could be defined in 11, including (1) well-defined clusters of tubular soft tissue densities within the posterior and posteromedial wall of the stomach, (2) tubular structures running along the circumference of the gastric fundus, (3) significant enhancement of the previously mentioned abnormalities equal to that of a normal vessel, and (4) intra-abdominal collateral venous channels indicative of portal hypertension (Fig. 28-8). The gastrohepatic ligament should be carefully inspected. In the same study, only 7 of 13 patients had diagnostic features on barium studies compatible with gastric varices.[17] In analyzing patients with gastric varices, it is apparent that only a small percentage of lesions abut the luminal surface of the stomach, explaining why CT is more sensitive. Varices are best studied with bolus/rapid contrast infusion and bolus and dynamic sequential scanning.

Gastric carcinoma

The primary role of CT in evaluation of gastric disorders is in the detection and staging of gastric carcinoma. Early reports suggested that CT could adequately and accurately stage cases of gastric carcinoma and prevent unnecessary surgery from being performed in a majority of cases.[102] In our experience, surgeons are unwilling to defer a potentially palliative operation based on radiographic examination. What is clear, however, is that CT can show sites of disease not detected at the time of original laparotomy. This obviously depends on the extent of the surgical procedure performed at an individual institution. At our institution, most gastric carcinoma is treated with palliative subtotal gastrectomy. During this procedure, median suprapancreatic nodes and nodes in the hepatoduodenal ligament and the retroperitoneum are removed. These sites have been shown to be common sources of local regional failure in gastric carcinoma patients.[62] Perhaps further use of CT in these patients may help segregate patient groups from whom more aggressive and radical surgery may be beneficial from those in whom less aggressive palliative surgery is indicated.

To evaluate the patient with gastric cancer fully, it is necessary to evaluate not only the tumor within the gastric wall, but also areas in which the tumor spread is most likely. This includes the liver; local extension into the pancreas, liver, and mesocolon; local and distant lymph node metastases; and the peritoneal cavity. We analyze these features of gastric carcinoma separately in the following discussion.

Gastric wall. The normal gastric wall should be

no thicker than 2 to 3 mm on CT scans. The true thickness of the wall is most easily appreciated by routine use of gas effervescent distention (Fig. 28-9).[65] If one uses water distention, the wall may appear somewhat thicker. The proximal stomach should have a symmetrical distribution of rugal folds when visualized in cross section. These two features are lost in the presence of abnormality.

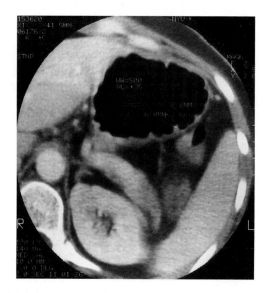

Fig. 28-9. Normal gastric wall. The wall is no thicker than 2.2 mm. Rugal folds are symmetrically seen surrounding the circumference (compare with Fig. 28-5). (From Megibow AJ, Balthazar EJ: *CT of the gastrointestinal tract*, St. Louis, 1986, CV Mosby.)

Gastric carcinoma produces focal thickening of the gastric wall. The basic CT appearances are focal, sessile, lobulated polypoid tumors as opposed to infiltrating (linitis plastica) lesions. The polypoid tumors tend to be seen more commonly in the proximal stomach, as opposed to the infiltrating tumors, which may diffusely involve the stomach or the distal antral segments (Fig. 28-10). By using water distention and dynamic scanning, small ulcerated lesions can be demonstrated.[100] An interesting feature of the infiltrating tumors is their bright enhancement on dynamic CT scanning (Fig. 28-11). This feature has allowed us to detect infiltrating tumors when the wall is less than 1 cm thick. In retrospective analysis of our own case material, the average thickness of the wall was considerably less than in other reported series.[5]

In analysis of 32 patients with infiltrating gastric carcinoma, the wall thickness measures between 10 and 19 mm in 21, greater than 20 mm in 5, and less than 10 mm in 6. In all cases of suspicious wall thickening, change in patient's position to distend optimally the proximal (prone) or distal (left-side-down decubitus) should be obtained (Fig. 28-12). Calcification in mucinous carcinomas of the stomach may be more readily detected with CT than by plain radiography. Use of negative contrast techniques aids in their recognition.[70]

Lymphadenopathy. Detection of lymphadenopathy requires knowledge of the distribution of gastric nodes. These include the lesser omentum, the greater omentum, splenic hilum, and the subpyloric regions (intermediary nodes) (Fig. 28-13). Recognition of local ad-

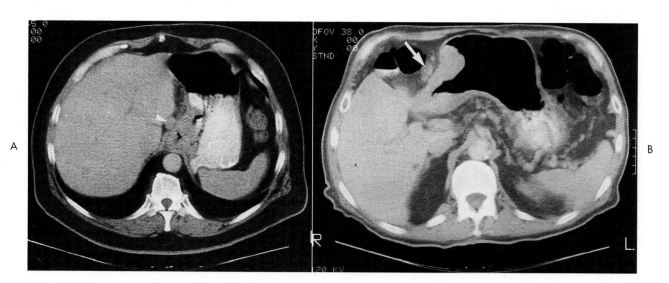

Fig. 28-10. Typical CT appearances of gastric carcinoma. **A,** Polypoid, lobulated tumor at esophagogastric junction with extension into distal esophgus. Note the enlarged lymph node in the lesser omentum *(arrowhead)*. **B,** Infiltrating antral carcinoma. Marked wall thickening is present. Local adenopathy is seen in the gastrocolic ligament *(arrow)*.

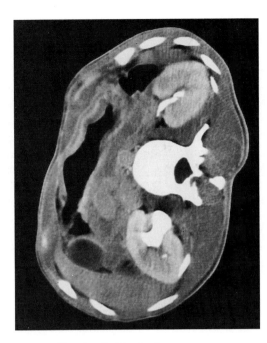

Fig. 28-11. Infiltrating linitis plastica tumor as seen on a right lateral decubitus position. The mucosal features are absent. Note the dense enhancement of the gastric wall, which aids in the identification of linitis plastica lesions.

enopathy has less significance than does adenopathy in secondary sites (extramural nodes) because these nodes are often removed at the time of the original gastrectomy whether visibly diseased or not. It must be stressed that the involved nodes may be at sites distant from the primary lesion in the stomach.[48] This reflects the complex intramural lymphatic communications within the stomach, leading to a lack of predictability as to which nodes will be involved. Detection of disease in these extramural nodes has greater prognostic significance than disease in intermediary nodes. Therefore close inspection of the celiac axis, root of the mesentery, and hepatoduodenal ligament is essential. In a cooperative study from Japan, CT was able to help correctly predict metastatic disease in 86% of involved nodes. A mass, such as lymphadenopathy, is more predictive of metastatic disease (96%) than is solitary lymphadenopathy (48%). Nodes less than 5 mm were involved by metastases in 17%, nodes 6 to 15 mm were involved in 50%, and those greater than 16 mm were involved in 77%.[67] Lymph nodes containing metastatic tumor did not enhance during dynamic scanning. In a study of 75 patients, CT demonstrated a 67% sensitivity and 61% specificity in the evaluation of locoregional lymphadenopathy.[118] CT accuracy in detecting secondary nodes that may not be removed at the time of original laparotomy is higher than for local nodes. Residual disease in these nodes is responsible for significant locoregional failures.[62]

Direct extension. The reflections of the lesser omentum allow gastric lesions to extend directly across this peritoneal reflection and invade the liver. It may be difficult in given cases to determine whether the liver is secondarily involved or primarily involved by tumor. The

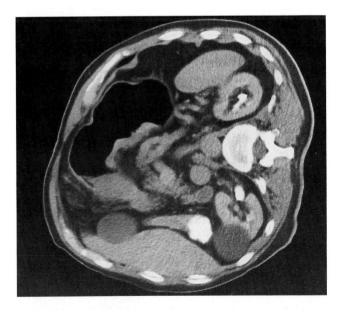

Fig. 28-12. Minimal wall thickening is seen along the lesser curvature. The thickness is approximately 8 mm. Even though this is less than reported wall thickness in gastric cancer, the tumor is obvious on the air-contrast CT scan and augmented by decubitus positioning.

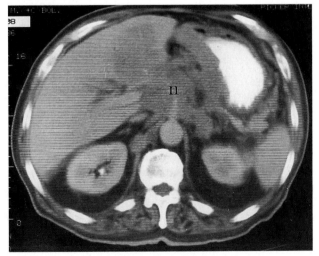

Fig. 28-13. Gastric carcinoma (adenopathy). Enlarged nodes (*n*) are seen in the celiac axis (intermediary) group. Liver metastases are present as well.

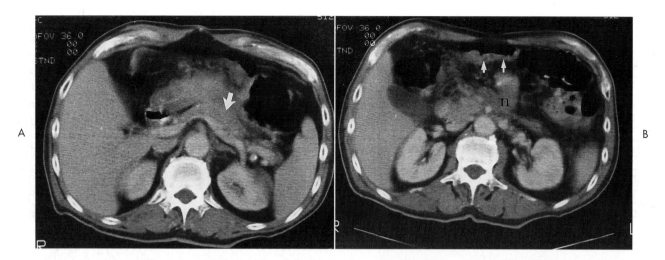

Fig. 28-14. Gastric carcinoma (direct extension). **A,** Loss of fat plane between tumor and body of pancreas is present, comparable with direct extension into the gland *(arrow)*. **B,** Scan on same patient reveals soft tissue mass along inferior portion of transverse mesocolon *(arrows)*. Adenopathy *(n)* is present in the root of the mesentery.

reflections of the gastrocolic ligament provide pathways for direct invasion of the pancreas or transverse colon. Pancreatic involvement may be difficult to predict on CT because of the lack of fat, and clear margins in the lesser sac may not be present even if the pancreas is not invaded (Fig. 28-14). In large studies, the detection of pancreatic invasion had a false-positive rate of 5% to 26% and a false-negative rate of 8% to 12%.[3,118] A significant number of patients in which CT suggested pancreatic invasion were found to have inflammatory disease simulating invasion. Accuracy of hepatic invasion has been reported as high as 100% by Dehn and coworkers.[38]

Endoscopic ultrasonography offers superb resolution of lesions and local adenopathy. Although operator dependent and requiring endoscopic assistance, this technique can evaluate the lumen, the wall, and surrounding adenopathy. Several centers now rely on results from this procedure to select patients for esophagogastrectomy or palliative laser therapy.[20] In advanced cases, needle biopsy can be used to establish the diagnosis.[21]

Distant metastases. Gastric carcinoma may metastasize widely through both arterial and venous pathways. Liver metastases are commonly seen. Dynamic sequential scanning is recommended for the routine evaluation of hepatic metastases.[1] In comparative studies of CT in the detection of laparotomy-proven liver metastases, sensitivity rates varied between 29% and 67%, and specificities varied between 96% and 98%.[64,118]

Peritoneal implants may be more difficult to detect, but with routine use of 2-second scanners with a 512 × 512 display matrix, peritoneal nodules become more readily apparent (Fig. 28-15).

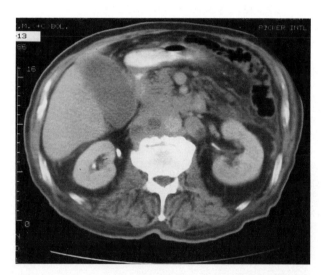

Fig. 28-15. Peritoneal seeding of gastric carcinoma. Extensive seeding of gastric carcinoma in gastrocolic ligament in patient with gastric carcinoma. The findings include thickening of fascial planes and reticular density in the fat. Retroperitoneal nodes are present.

New studies on the accuracy of CT in the high-resolution era have not been published. Most published series mix experience of case material on earlier generations of equipment with patients studied on new scanners. Despite this, the overall accuracy in prediction of gastric carcinoma is in the 90% range. As subtler findings of peritoneal implantation and lymph node discrimination in the lesser omentum become more reliably de-

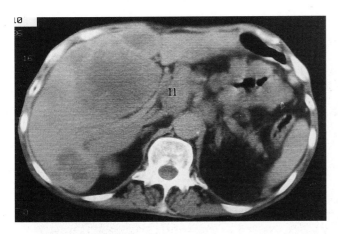

Fig. 28-16. Follow-up gastric carcinoma. The remnant is encased in recurrent tumor. Large hepatic metastases are seen. Adenopathy is present in the lesser omentum *(n)*.

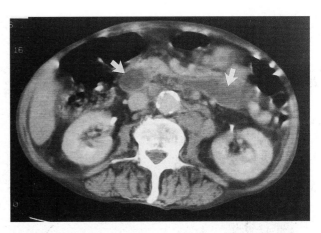

Fig. 28-17. Afferent loop obstruction in current gastric carcinoma. The dilated afferent loop is easily recognized surrounding the head of the pancreas *(arrows)*. Note retroperitoneal adenopathy below the left renal artery.

tectable and as better contrast resolution in the liver with more dynamic scanning becomes more routine, the accuracy in the initial staging of gastric carcinoma should improve.

Follow-up in gastric carcinoma. CT is ideally suited in the follow-up of gastric carcinoma, particularly because measurable sites of disease are often left behind at the initial laparotomy. The progression of liver metastases and nodal disease is readily followed on the postoperative scan.[104] By using air contrast in the gastric remnant, the anastomoses are elegantly evaluated, providing a mechanism for the evaluation of local progression of disease (Fig. 28-16). Other complications, such as afferent loop obstruction, have been described and have the characteristic CT appearance[52] (Fig. 28-17).

Other gastric neoplasms

Primary tumors. A variety of other neoplastic conditions may be imaged by CT. Tumors in this group include leiomyoma, lipoma, neurogenic tumors, aberrant pancreas tumors, and duplication cysts and lipoma.[91,120] Leiomyomas are well-circumscribed, soft tissue density, round masses located anywhere in the stomach. Their homogenous appearance is helpful in suggesting benign disease.[95] Leiomyosarcomas are larger lesions, generally greater than 5 cm in diameter. They have a heterogeneous appearance reflecting large areas of necrosis.[29] Leiomyosarcomas grow exophytically, which makes CT particularly suitable to their evaluation.[23] They can behave similarly to a primary adenocarcinoma of the stomach—they can invade locally and metastasize widely in the peritoneal cavity[28] (Fig. 28-18). Gastric lymphoma can be confused with adenocarcinoma, but more often

it produces greater thickening of the wall with a homogeneous overall attenuation. Gastric lymphoma minimally enhances after intravenous contrast administration. Gastric lymphoma may involve the stomach diffusely, it may produce thickened, scalloped folds with variable degrees of wall thickening and with less symmetry than that of hypertrophic gastritis (Fig. 28-19). It may be seen as a focal polypoid mass. These masses may extend exophytically to invade the pancreas or other local structures. The presence of diffuse retroperitoneal and mesenteric adenopathy may be more suggestive that the gastric lesion could be a lymphoma rather than carcinoma; however, adenocarcinoma of the stomach may occur with diffuse retroperitoneal and mesenteric adenopathy simulating gastric lymphoma.[25,92]

In patients being staged for lymphoma (particularly non-Hodgkin's varieties) elsewhere in the abdomen, always assess for the presence of gastrointestinal involvement. The stomach is the most common site. When gastric lymphoma is known, CT is requested to evaluate whether the disease is isolated to the stomach or whether the stomach is a part of systemic lymphoma. Survival rates for isolated gastric lymphoma, even with local adenopathy, is excellent, with 5-year survival rates approaching 82%[83] (Fig. 28-20).

Metastases to the stomach. A variety of neoplasms may metastasize to the stomach, including carcinoma of the lung, carcinoma of the breast, melanoma, and Kaposi's sarcoma.[82] Tumors from the pancreas, colon, or gallbladder may extend directly into the stomach. Hematogenous metastases from carcinoma of the breast are a common cause of linitis plastica.[34] On CT, the enhanced, thickened wall typical of primary gastric carcinoma may be seen (Fig. 28-21).

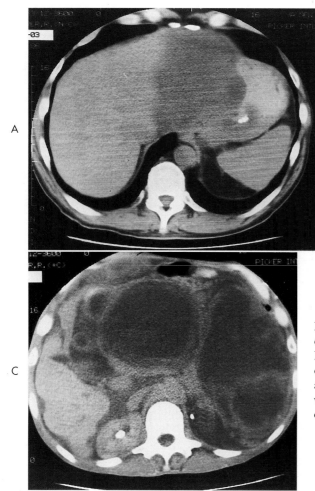

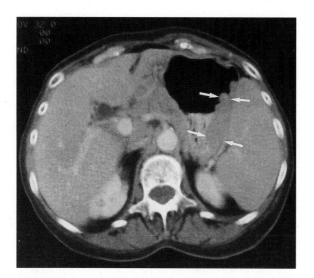

Fig. 28-18. Gastric leiomyosarcoma. **A,** Exophytic mass crosses the lesser omentum to invade the left lobe of the liver. **B,** Scan inferiorly reveals large, lobulated inhomogeneous mass characteristic of leiomyosarcoma. **C,** Same patient 1 year after attempted surgical resection. The bulk of the primary tumor was resected; however, extensive peritoneal dissemination occurred.

DUODENUM

CT evaluation of the duodenum is generally requested to characterize further abnormalities found in gastrointestinal series. The most useful clinically applicable role of CT in evaluation of the duodenum is in the differentiation of primary duodenal pathology from invasion of the duodenum by extrinsic spread of disease from one of the many anatomical structures with which it interfaces, particularly the kidney, pancreas, and retroperitoneum. CT has been shown to be useful in the evaluation of duodenal trauma and detects signs of duodenal rupture earlier than does plain film.[75] In cases of blunt abdominal trauma, the duodenum should be carefully inspected for increased density representing a periduodenal hematoma (Fig. 28-22). Occasionally a penetrating duodenal ulcer into the bed of the pancreas can simulate a primary mass in the pancreas[85] (Fig. 28-23).

Duodenal neoplasms

A variety of duodenal neoplasms have been imaged by CT.[41] The CT appearances can be correlated

Fig. 28-19. Gastric lymphoma. The wall is thickened and homogeneous in attenuation. Splenomegaly is present.

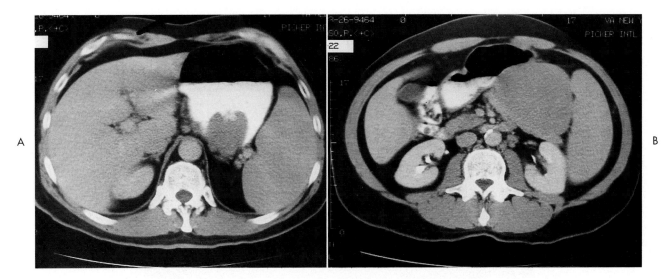

Fig. 28-20. Exophytic gastric lymphoma. **A,** Intramural, ulcerated mass is present along the greater curvature of stomach. **B,** Caudal scan reveals large exophytic left upper quadrant mass. Note the homogeneity typical of lymphoma (compare with Fig. 28-15).

with malignant potential.[77] Duodenal adenocarcinomas appear similar to adenocarcinomas elsewhere in the gastrointestinal tract. A focal area of thickening of the duodenal lumen, often with proximal obstruction, is detected. Ampullary neoplasms infiltrate the papilla of Vater and may produce obstructive jaundice, usually in association with pancreatic duct dilatation. It is important to observe the duodenum in all patients being scanned for obstructive jaundice in whom no mass is seen within the pancreas. Often, better definition of the periampullary region is obtainable when the patient is placed in a left-side-down decubitus position and given an effervescent agent. Intravenous glucagon, 0.1 mg, should be administered concurrently. This is equivalent to CT hypotonic duodenography and allows for evaluation of ampullary and periampullary abnormalities (Fig. 28-24).

Other duodenal neoplasms, such as lymphoma and smooth muscle tumors, thicken the wall to a greater degree than does primary adenocarcinoma. Tumors with a predilection for exophytic growth, such as leiomyosarcoma, are particularly well suited to CT imaging (Fig. 28-25).

Another group in whom CT plays a role in differential diagnosis is patients with duodenal obstruction, which may often be predicted by the CT examination. This group includes patients with retroperitoneal metastases encasing the duodenum, patients with pancreatitis in which the duodenum is enveloped in a pancreatic exudate (Fig. 28-26), and patients after aortic aneurysm sur-

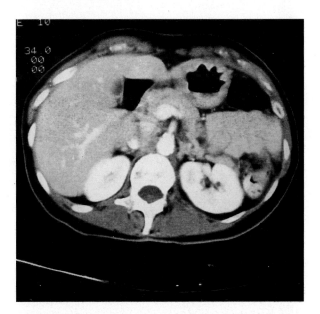

Fig. 28-21. Breast carcinoma metastatic to the stomach. Although the fold pattern is preserved, there is prominent enhancement of the gastric wall. Deep biopsy revealed lobulated adenocarcinoma in the gastric submucosa, consistent with a breast primary.

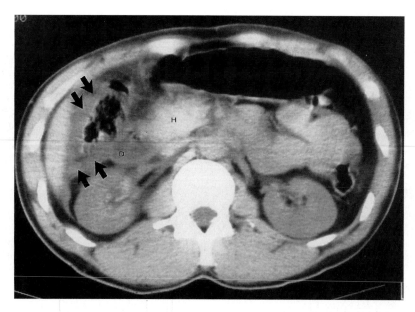

Fig. 28-22. Periduodenal hematoma. Noncontrast CT scan in a patient after a motorcycle accident reveals high-density mass *(H)* adjacent to the duodenum *(D)*. Ascites is noted in the peritoneal cavity *(arrows)*. (Courtesy of Dr. S. Toder, Orange, NJ. From Megibow AJ, Balthazar EJ: *Computed tomography of the GI tract*, St. Louis, 1986, CV Mosby.)

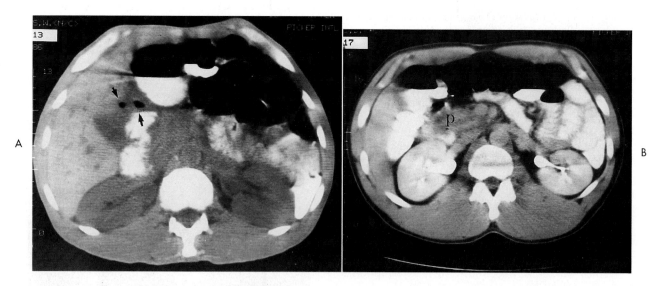

Fig. 28-23. Penetrating duodenal ulcer. **A,** Ectopic gas is noted adjacent to the duodenal bulb *(arrows)*. **B,** Scan slightly caudal reveals an enlarged pancreatic head *(p)*. Pancreatitis as a result of penetrating ulcers was found.

gery in whom a relative duodenal ileus may be present. In this last group, CT is able to evaluate the proximal suture line, diagnosing abscess or hematoma.

SMALL BOWEL

A wide variety of small bowel abnormalities have been visualized on CT scans. Analysis of small bowel diseases requires meticulous bowel opacification to prevent misinterpretation of nondistended loops for pathological masses. The presence of disease is recognized by abnormal thickness of the intestinal wall. One should also, however, observe the character of the mucosal surface, the enhancement patterns of the wall, and changes in the perienteric tissues.[71]

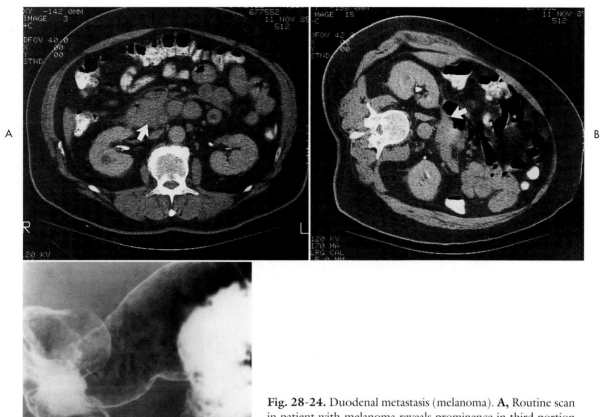

Fig. 28-24. Duodenal metastasis (melanoma). **A,** Routine scan in patient with melanoma reveals prominence in third portion of duodenum *(arrow)*. **B,** Patient placed in left-side-down position, given oral effervescent and 0.1 mg of intravenous glucagon. Lobulated density noted along lateral wall of duodenum *(arrow)*. **C,** Spot film from gastrointestinal series.

Non-neoplastic small bowel disorders

Non-neoplastic disorders of the small bowel in which CT provides clinically useful information include those disorders related to the blood supply of the small bowel (the arterial supply or small vessels in the wall or venous drainage) and disorders in patients with prior inflammatory disease of the small bowel, specifically regional enteritis. We first examine the spectrum of vascular-induced disease within the small bowel.

Ischemia. Ischemic disease of the small bowel is usually not associated with major vessel occlusion but is rather the result of low flow states from a variety of conditions. Rarely, one can see thrombus in a mesenteric ves-

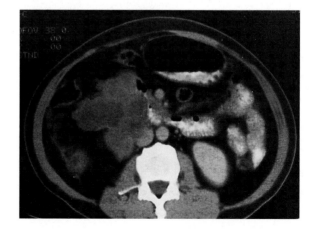

Fig. 28-25. Leiomyosarcoma in the duodenum. A bulky exophytic mass extends from the lateral portion of the duodenal sweep. The appearance is typical of leiomyosarcoma.

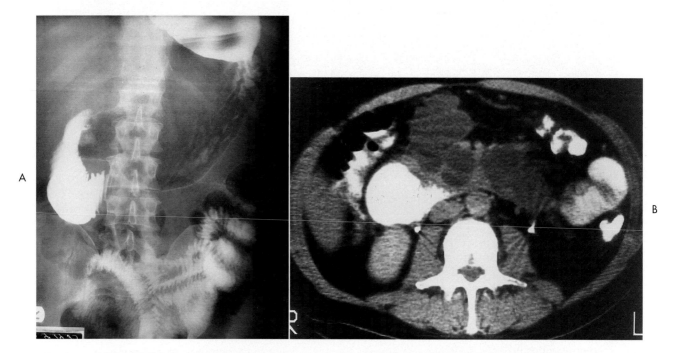

Fig. 28-26. Duodenal obstruction from acute pancreatitis. **A,** Film from gastrointestinal series reveals obstruction of the third portion of the duodenum. The findings are nonspecific. **B,** CT reveals pancreatitis-related exudate encasing the duodenum. (From Megibow AJ, Balthazar EJ: *CT of the gastrointestinal tract,* St. Louis, 1986, CV Mosby.)

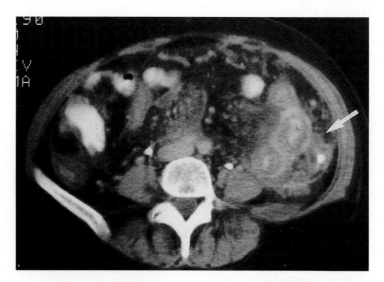

Fig. 28-27. Small bowel ischemia from acute pancreatitis. Thickened loops of jejunum are seen in the left upper quadrant. Note the target appearances. Relative mesenteric ischemia secondary to fulminant acute pancreatitis is responsible for the CT appearance. (From Megibow AJ, Balthazar EJ: *CT of the gastrointestinal tract,* St. Louis, 1986, CV Mosby.)

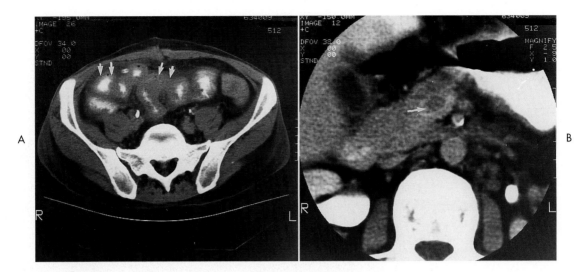

Fig. 28-28. Diffuse bowel wall thickening from superior mesenteric vein thrombosis. **A,** Multiple thickened loops of small bowel are seen in a patient 1 week after terminal ileal resection for Crohn's disease. **B,** Magnified view from dynamic CT revealed thrombosis in the superior mesenteric vein. Symptoms resolved following anticoagulation. (From Megibow AJ, Balthazar EJ: *CT of the gastrointestinal tract*, St. Louis, 1986, CV Mosby.)

sel; usually, one recognizes ischemic change by the presence of localized submucosal edema. Bowel wall edema presents as circumferential thickening of the affected loop demonstrating a hyperdense serosa, relatively hypoattenuating submucosa, and mucosal hyperemia. This has been termed a "target" appearance (Fig. 28-27). This finding is nonspecific except that one can confidently state that the wall thickening is not due to neoplasm. When there is diffuse thickening of small bowel loops displaying the target sign, particularly in the appropriate clinical setting, CT may be useful to rule out superior mesenteric venous thrombosis. Dynamic scanning with intravenous contrast administration may reveal a filling defect in the superior mesenteric vein as well as diffuse bowel wall edema associated with this state[108] (Fig. 28-28).

The differentiation between ischemia and infarction may be impossible unless secondary signs are present.[115] The presence of pneumatosis intestinalis must raise the suspicion of bowel infarction. Pneumatosis intestinalis may be seen in two forms. Most cases are benign and may be idiopathic or associated with systemic diseases, particularly collagen-vascular disease. Pneumatosis may arise as a result of bowel infarction. In these cases, a thin stripe of subserosal air is seen. Many of these patients have associated ascites. The finding may be subtle and require lung windows to differentiate the wall from the intraluminal and intraluminal air.[33] The finding of small bowel ischemia includes demonstration of thrombus within the superior mesenteric artery, intralu-

minal gas within the bowel wall or portal venous system, focal bowel wall thickening, and hyperemia of the bowel wall (Fig. 28-29).

Intestinal vasculitides. The CT appearance of small intestinal vasculitis reveals a focal segment of thickened bowel with a target appearance reflecting edema. This appearance is nonspecific with respect to origin; clinical history is necessary for a specific diagnosis. Radiation enteritis is a prototypical disease resulting from abnormalities of small vessels. In radiation enteritis, the mucosal folds appears thickened and crowded, and linear streaks of increased density in the mesentery (edema) are seen[46] (Fig. 28-30). Dynamic scanning reveals a hyperdense wall with a low attenuation region within the bowel wall. Other vasculitides include systematic lupus erythematosus, polyarteritis, drug-induced vasculitis (Fig. 28-31), and amyloidosis (Fig. 28-32). Intestinal ischemia also results from strangulating intestinal obstruction. Recognition of this complication in patients with bowel obstruction makes CT especially useful in this clinical setting.

Intramural hemorrhage. Intramural hemorrhage within the small bowel is usually secondary to anticoagulation therapy but may also be seen in bleeding disorders or trauma. Hemorrhage results in thickened small bowel loops with high-density material within the wall of the bowel (Fig. 28-33). Ascites may be present, and at times fluid levels within the high-density ascites may result from the presence of blood within the peritoneal cavity. In patients with blunt abdominal trauma,

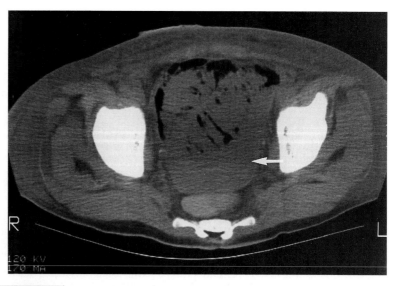

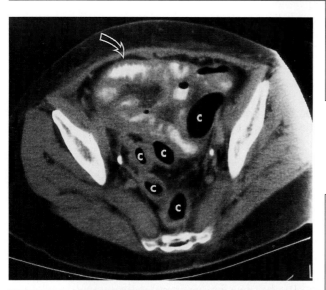

Fig. 28-29. Bowel infarction with pneumatosis. Curvilinear gas collections are seen along the serosa of the distal ileum. Ascites is seen in the pelvis. Marked bowel infarction secondary to unrelieved closed loop obstruction was present at surgery. (From Megibow AJ, Balthazar EJ: *CT of the gastrointestinal tract*, St. Louis, 1986, CV Mosby.)

Fig. 28-30. Radiation enteritis. Thickened wall in the small bowel loops *(arrow)* and colon *(c)* results from small vessel fibrosis (induced by radiation) in the wall of the intestine. (From Megibow AJ, Balthazar EJ: *CT of the gastrointestinal tract*, St. Louis, 1986, CV Mosby.)

Fig. 28-31. Intramural hemorrhage. **A,** CT scan through left lower quadrant in a patient with Henoch-Schönlein purpura. High-density fluid surrounds narrowed jejunal loops. Reactive changes are seen in the mesentery. **B,** Film from small bowel series reveals localized narrowing in region of intramural hemorrhage.

A
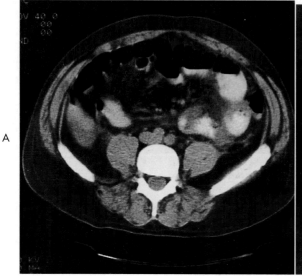
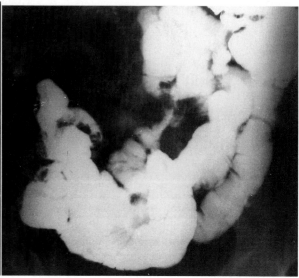
B

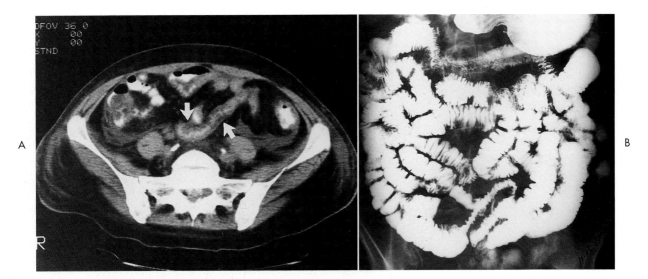

Fig. 28-32. Amyloidosis (infiltration of small bowel). **A,** CT scan through lower abdomen reveals narrowed loop of ileum with a low-density wall *(arrows)*. Ascites is present in the peritoneal cavity. **B,** Small bowel series reveals area of submucosal narrowing with mild proximal dilatation. Amyloidosis was proved by rectal biopsy.

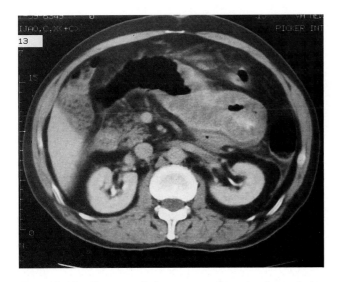

Fig. 28-33. Intramural hematoma from anticoagulation therapy. The patient was on warfarin (Coumadin) therapy for atrial fibrillation. Jejunal hematoma and mild reaction in the lateroconal fascia are present.

small bowel laceration may go undiagnosed. In a review of 24 patients with bowel injury seen on CT, 15 patients underwent surgery. Bowel injury was confirmed in 14. Nine patients with bowel wall hematomas were successfully managed conservatively.[18] The CT findings included ectopic intraperitoneal or extraperitoneal gas, extravasated oral contrast material, and focal thickening of the abdominal wall with adjacent mesenteric hematomas.

Small bowel obstruction. CT is a clinically useful diagnostic tool in the evaluation of patients with small bowel obstruction. CT is able to diagnose accurately the presence of obstruction, predict the cause in close to 80% of patients, and offer information concerning the presence or absence of strangulation.[51,89] CT is particularly useful in cancer patients in whom the differentiation between adhesive obstruction versus peritoneal carcinomatosis determines therapy.

Bowel obstruction is recognized by the presence of a change in caliber between the prestenotic and poststenotic loops of bowel. When this is observed, a systematic inspection of the course of the bowel is necessary to localize the point(s) of obstruction. This is more readily apparent if one examines the study from the rectum in an orad fashion. Once the point is detected, careful analysis of the appearance of the loop and the presence of abnormality in the perienteric tissue are necessary to determine the cause (Fig. 28-34). Adhesions are suspected when no surrounding masses are visualized in the surrounding mesentery or fat. Peritoneal implants are recognized as nodules or loculated fluid collections. Careful inspection of the serosal surfaces of obstructed loops and a systematic search of the peritoneal cavity are necessary to make the diagnosis. Mesenteric changes indicative of strangulating obstruction should be observed. Furthermore, intravenous contrast material and dynamic scanning are essential to detect changes in the intestinal wall indicative of strangulation. Closed-loop obstruc-

Fig. 28-34. Small bowel obstruction. **A,** Dilated contrast-filled loops of jejunum are seen entering the pelvis. **B,** Collapsed loops of distal ileum are noted. The large loops filled with air and fluid are actually jejunal; note the adjacent collapsed colon. No mass is seen at the transition point; the cause is presumed to be adhesions (confirmed at laparotomy).

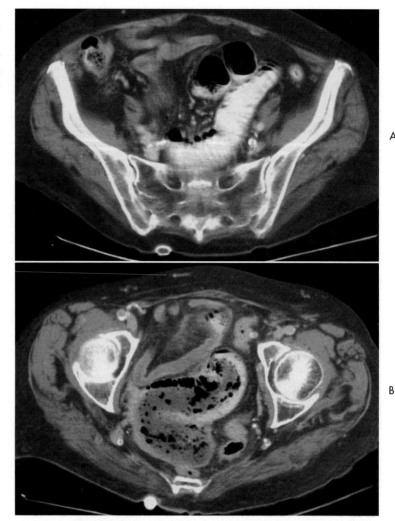

tions lead to strangulation and bowel infarction if undiagnosed. Visualization of a focal region of thickened, hyperdense bowel wall, local ascites, loss of mesenteric borders, and a U-shaped configuration are characteristic of this condition (Fig. 28-35). CT can lead to early diagnosis and prevent gangrenous complications by displaying the need for immediate surgery.[9,10]

Primary inflammatory disease

Primary inflammatory disease of the small bowel may be imaged by CT, but specific diagnosis is made by mucosal changes seen on barium studies or direct biopsy. Ancillary findings, such as local adenopathy or streaking in the perivisceral fat, aid in differential diagnosis.[84] The changes in the adjacent fat may range from a poorly defined cloudy haze, representing mild lymphedema or phlegmon, to a well-defined perivisceral fluid collection or abscess. Loculated fluid and well-defined thick reticu-

lar changes within the peritoneal cavity suggest accompanying peritonitis.

Primary infectious disease of the small bowel. We have seen increasing evidence of infectious enteritis caused in a large part by the AIDS epidemic.[88] Unusual organisms have been found in these patients.[61] Small bowel enteritis, secondary to *Cryptosporidia* and *Isospora belli* disease, produces CT features including diffuse small bowel dilatation with fluid-filled loops and marked intraluminal hypersecretion (Fig. 28-36). In many cases, there is concomitant involvement of the duodenum and gastric antrum. In many AIDS patients, multiple infections are present, and the duodenum and small bowel may be involved with cryptosporidia, whereas the stomach and esophagus may harbor cytomegalovirus.

Mycobacterial infections have increased in this population as well. *Mycobacterium tuberculosis* is recognized by the predilection of mesenteric and peripancre-

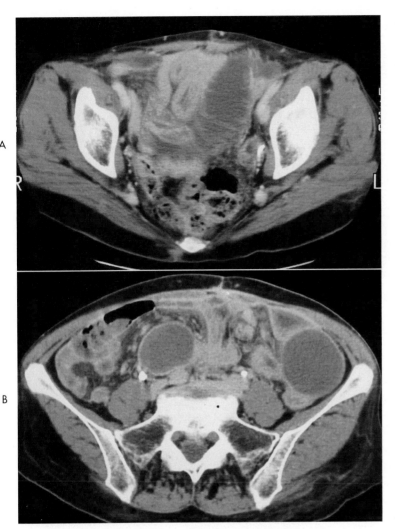

Fig. 28-35. Bowel obstruction from peritoneal carcinomatosis (ovarian carcinoma). **A,** Dilated small bowel is seen with collapsed ileum diagnostic of obstruction. **B,** Multiple peritoneal nodules can be seen associated with thickened, collapsed loops at multiple levels, allowing distinction between adhesions and neoplastic implants.

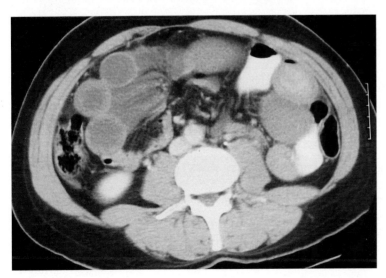

Fig. 28-36. Closed-loop obstruction. Dilated loops of ileum demonstrating a radial configuration are seen. The wall is thickened. There is fluid in the mesentery. A collapsed loop of ileum is also present in the image. This constellation of findings indicates complicated intestinal obstruction mitigating immediate surgery.

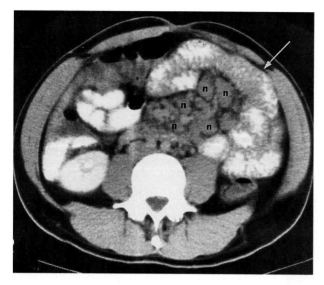

Fig. 28-37. *M. avium-intracellulare* infection in small bowel in an AIDS patient. Multiple enlarged mesenteric lymph nodes (*n*) are seen. The mucosal folds in the small bowel are prominent (*arrow*). This has been described as the pseudo-Whipple appearance. (From Megibow AJ, Balthazar EJ: *CT of the gastrointestinal tract,* St. Louis, 1986, CV Mosby.)

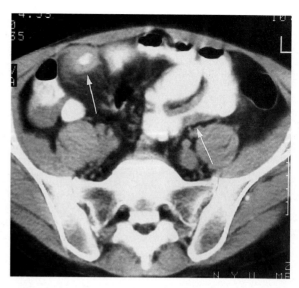

Fig. 28-38. Crohn's disease in the small bowel. Thickening in the terminal ileum is seen. Another lesion separated by normal intervening bowel is seen (a skip lesion) (*arrow*). (From Megibow AJ, Balthazar EJ: *CT of the gastrointestinal tract,* St. Louis, 1986, CV Mosby.)

atic lymphadenopathy associated with splenomegaly. In these patients, when intestinal involvement is present, the disease is most easily recognized in the distal ileum. Associated low-attenuation adenopathy is present as well.[11] Infections with *M. avium–intracellulare* result in diffuse thickening of mucosal folds of the proximal small bowel folds and mesenteric adenopathy[105] (Fig. 28-37). In one fourth to one third of cases, the adenopathy has peculiar low density (almost water-density appearance) simulating findings of Whipple's disease.[124]

CT is not indicated for evaluation of patients with known infections (unless one is looking for other complications of the disease). These diseases are seen in patients with confusing clinical symptoms in whom CT is requested to sort out multiple diagnostic possibilities. In this context, we have seen patients with *Salmonella,* *Yersinia,* and even ileal diverticulitis imaged. Specific diagnosis requires appropriate culture.

Regional enteritis (Crohn's disease)

CT evaluation of patients with Crohn's disease is useful because the process is transmural, and there are frequently associated changes within the intestinal wall and local mesentary. The extraluminal features may be seen to greater advantage than on barium studies. CT is of greatest use in the evaluation abscesses and fistulae.[47]

The findings of Crohn's disease on CT have been well documented. Skip areas may be seen (Fig. 28-38).

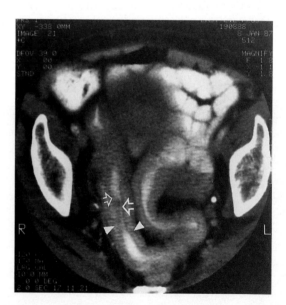

Fig. 28-39. Crohn's disease (double halo appearance). A long segment of distal ileum is diseased. The contrast-filled lumen is bordered by a fine rim of low attenuation (*open arrows*). An enhancing region within the muscular coat is appreciated (*arrowheads*).

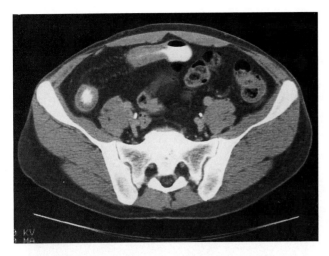

Fig. 28-40. Crohn's disease (mesenteric fat proliferation). Extensive fatty proliferation is present in the mesentery adjacent to a long segment of involved distal ileum.

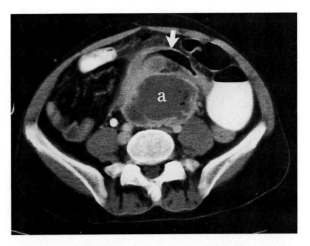

Fig. 28-41. Mesenteric abscess from Crohn's disease. A mass with an enhanced rim and fluid and air contrast is seen within the lower mesentery *(a)*. The diseases loop is seen immediately adjacent to the abscess *(arrow)*.

Marked narrowing of distal ileum—the string sign—has been described on CT.[113] In many cases, a target appearance may be visualized[49,55] (Fig. 28-39). The pathophysiology of the target sign in Crohn's disease is similar to other entities in that it represents submucosal edema. The target sign was originally described as pathognomonic of Crohn's disease; we have seen it in patients with radiation enteritis; patients with mesenteric venous thrombosis; and even in patients with acute pancreatitis, graft-versus-host disease, and vascular compromised loops of obstructed bowel. Jones and colleagues[73] reported this finding to represent submucosal fat deposition in patients with chronic disease.

CT is of greatest use in the documentation of the extraluminal manifestations of regional enteritis, including visualization of adjacent abscess and fistulous tracts. As the inflammatory process extends transmurally, there is hypertrophy and a mass-like configuration in the mesenteric fat, "creeping fat," or sclerolipomatosis (Fig. 28-40). This "creeping fat" may result in separation of the loops as seen on barium studies. Local mesenteric adenopathy may be present as well between these separated loops. Depending on the activity of the disease, the local fat may be bland or may have areas of poorly defined increased density, representing phlegmon or localized lymphedema. In advanced cases, abscess formation is seen, and this is identified as a fluid collection in the mesentery subtending the inflamed loops of bowel. The rim is hyperemic and densely enhanced on dynamic scanning (Fig. 28-41).

Fistula formation is a common complication of Crohn's disease. Although the tract itself may not be ac-

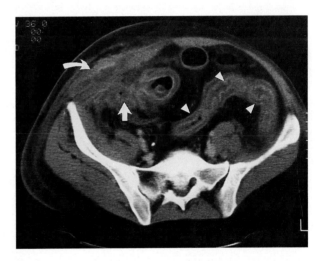

Fig. 28-42. Severe ileocolitis with fistulization into the body wall. CT in a patient with severe Crohn's disease. Note double halo appearance in colon *(arrowheads)* and terminal ileal region *(straight arrow)*. Extraluminal gas is seen in an abscess with penetration into the anterior abdominal wall *(curved arrow)*.

curately mapped, extraluminal gas collections and spike-like projections of soft tissue density into the local mesentery signal the presence of fistulae on sinus tracts. When these findings are present, barium studies are necessary to map the precise localization of the tracts (Fig. 28-42).[126] Secondary signs in adjacent involved viscera aid in the recognition of fistula.[98]

CT can also be used to guide interventional procedures, such as abscess drainage. In contrast to other bowel diseases in which surgical intervention and resection are the procedures of choice, in Crohn's disease patients, efforts to avoid surgery are mandated making the role of percutaneous drainage essential. Several studies have documented this clinical utility.[26,109]

Neoplasms. Primary neoplasms of the small bowel include adenocarcinomas, lymphoma, carcinoid tumors, and intramural tumors. CT helps to evaluate and demonstrate the tumor mass and reveals sites of spread; lymph nodes, other viscera, omentum and peritoneal surfaces, bones, lungs, and mediastinum.

Features diagnostic of small-bowel tumors include mass, focal areas of wall thickening, ulceration and dilatation of the contrast-filled lumen, and obstruction either from mass or intussusception.[40]

The CT appearance of intussusception has been

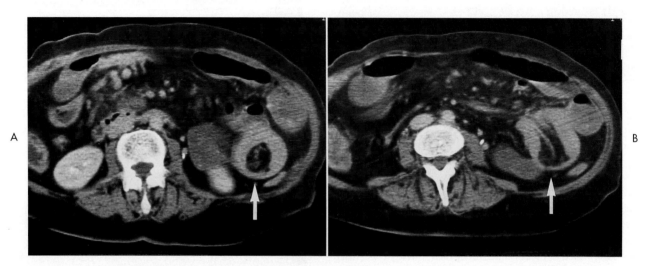

Fig. 28-43. Nonobstructing intussusception in sprue. **A,** The eccentrically located fat of the intussusception is seen surrounded by contrast-filled intussusception. **B,** In longitudinal section, the mesenteric vasculature can be seen entering the intussusception.

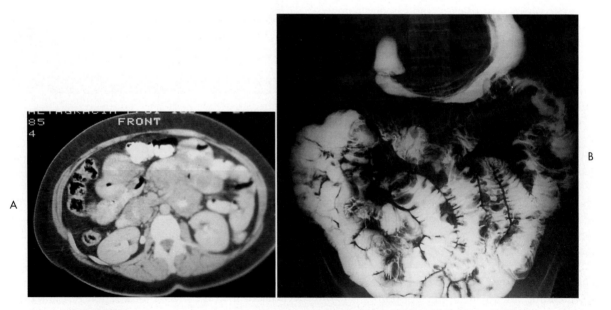

Fig. 28-44. Diffuse small bowel involvement in non-Hodgkin's lymphoma. **A,** Multiple thick-walled loops of small bowel are seen. **B,** Small bowel series reveals separated loops in left upper quadrant and multiple nodules in the remaining ileum. (Courtesy of Dr. S. Hilton, New York, NY.)

well described.[37,97] The characteristic findings include the central loop of soft tissue density defined by eccentric fat, which represents the mesenteric fat of the intussusceptum, which is in turn completely surrounded within the intussuscipiens. This appearance is characteristic throughout all segments of the intestinal tract. Most cases in adults are due to tumor, however nonobstructive intussusception may occasionally be appreciated in patients with sprue (Fig. 28-43).

Lymphoma. Lymphomas of the small bowel are important to recognize because their presence changes the staging of a given patient. They are more frequently seen in patients with non-Hodgkin's lymphoma (Fig. 28-44). In our original series of the CT evaluation of gastrointestinal lymphoma, fewer than half of the patients with gastrointestinal lesions were symptomatic in relation to the intestinal tract.[92] Therefore it becomes important to evaluate carefully all of the small bowel to visualize potential deposits of lymphoma. A variety of appearances are possible, including excavated masses, segmental infiltration, mesenteric masses invading bowel loops, and thickened nodular folds. Recognition of these changes is important in the "staging" of these patients because of the predilection of the lymphoma to undergo rapid necrosis on therapy. Mesenteric adenopathy is invariably seen in non-AIDS patients, but is rare in patients with AIDS-related lymphoma.[121]

Adenocarcinoma. Adenocarcinoma arising primarily in the small intestine is an unusual occurrence. In contrast to lymphoma, the proximal small bowel is more frequently involved than the ileum. As with gastric or colorectal adenocarcinoma, small intestinal tumors may arise de novo as polypoid masses or annular stenosing lesions or may evolve from villous tumors. The second and third duodenal segments are a site favored by villous tumors, and in this location they may compromise the papilla of Vater and cause biliary or pancreatic duct obstruction. The lesions can be identified as focal masses thickening the bowel wall and compromising the lumen either concentrically or asymmetrically. In comparison with lymphoma, the tumors are more likely to be solitary and to involve a shorter segment of bowel. The lesions are usually heterogeneous in tissue density and enhance moderately with intravenous contrast administration. The liver, peritoneal surfaces, and ovaries are favorite sites of secondary involvement. Associated bulky adenopathy is less commonly seen than in lymphoma, although lymphatic metastases are found at surgery in up to 60% of cases (Fig. 28-45).

Carcinoid. Carcinoid tumors are the most common primary neoplasms of the small intestine. Generally the tumor mass itself is not visualized on the CT scan (Fig. 28-46). Characteristic desmoplastic changes in the mesentery are seen (Fig. 28-47). In these cases, angu-

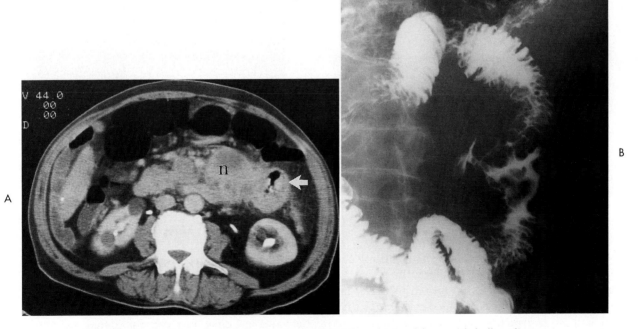

Fig. 28-45. Small bowel adenocarcinoma. **A,** A thickened jejunal loop with bulky adjacent adenopathy *(n)* is seen. **B,** Spot film from a small bowel series reveals ulcerated neoplasm with mesenteric sinus tract. Surgery confirmed unresectable primary adenocarcinoma in the small bowel.

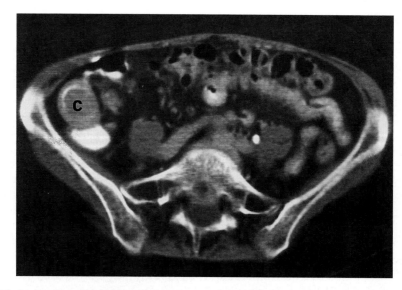

Fig. 28-46. Carcinoid distal ileum. An intramural, homogeneous soft tissue mass *(c)* is seen in the right lower quadrant. Note the narrowing of the contrast-filled lumen. Visualization of the primary carcinoid tumor is unusual. (From Megibow AJ, Balthazar EJ: *CT of the gastrointestinal tract,* St. Louis, 1986, CV Mosby.)

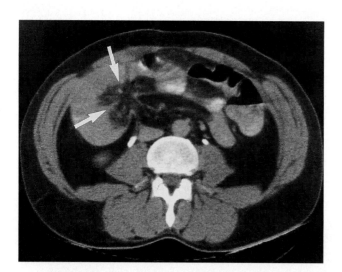

Fig. 28-47. Mesenteric changes (carcinoid). Stellate, centripetally oriented, thickened mesenteric vessels are seen subtending a dilated, "kinked" loop of distal ileum. The primary tumor is not visualized. (From Megibow AJ, Balthazar EJ: *CT of the gastrointestinal tract,* St. Louis, 1986, CV Mosby.)

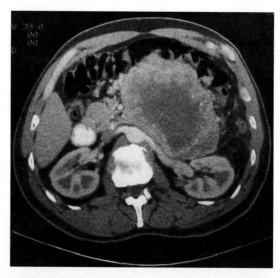

Fig. 28-48. Leiomyosarcoma (small bowel). The large mass in the mesentery has a complex appearance with a highly vascularized outer rim of enhancing tissue and an unenhanced low-density necrotic center. The finding is typical of leiomyosarcoma anywhere in the gastrointestinal tract.

lated bowel loops associated with a stellate radiating pattern of mesenteric nodular-vascular bundles are present.[30] Dystrophic calcification related to tumor necrosis in local lymph nodes as well as liver metastases has been described. In patients with carcinoid tumors, the hypervascular hepatic metastases may best be visualized on noncontrast scans as opposed to dynamic-enhanced scans.[22]

Other primary neoplasms, such as leiomyoma and leiomyosarcoma, may be encountered. As elsewhere in the gastrointestinal tract, size and homogeneity help differentiate benign from malignant lesions[87] (Fig. 28-48).

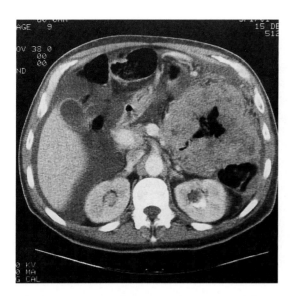

Fig. 28-49. Metastatic melanoma to the jejunum. A large mass is present in the left upper quadrant. Centrally an irregular air-filled cavity is present, indicating ulceration. The inhomogeneous appearance reflects the sarcomatous nature of the lesion.

Metastatic disease. Metastases to the small bowel can occur secondary to intraperitoneal seeding, hematogenous seeding, or direct extension from adjacent masses. The CT appearance reflects these pathological mechanisms. Intraperitoneal seeding is most often secondary to primary tumors of the ovary, breast, or gastrointestinal tract, including intestinal sarcomas. In these cases, the serosal deposits appear as localized areas of loculated ascites or soft tissue masses. Reticular changes within the greater omentum are indicative of "caking," a sign of peritoneal carcinomatosis.[125]

Hematogenous spread occurs in patients with melanoma, breast carcinoma, lung carcinoma, or Kaposi's sarcoma. These lesions appear as discrete masses but may become large and extensively ulcerated (Fig. 28-49). Multiple lesions and a clinical history of previous primary suggest the diagnosis of metastatic disease.[76]

Direct invasion from contiguous extra-alimentary structures may also involve the small bowel. Pancreatic colonic and renal carcinoma may invade the duodenum or transverse mesocolon; pelvic malignancies may grow directly to involve small bowel loops.

COLON

As clinical experience with CT increases, applications in colonic disease are becoming more frequent. The optimal evaluation of the colon requires some modifications of technique, described earlier in this chapter. Sufficient cleansing to remove fecal material and luminal distention state to evaluate the true thickness of the wall

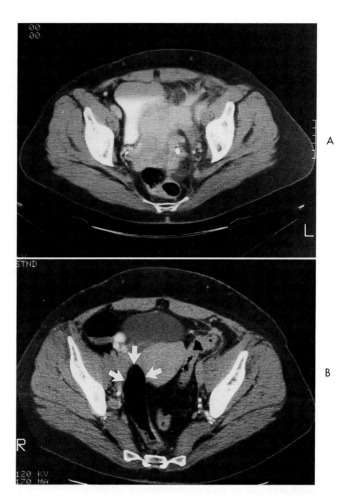

Fig. 28-50. Air-contrast colon. **A,** Patient with diverticulitis and questionable adnexal mass. Air was not administered into the colon because the patient had significant fever and elevated white blood cell count. **B,** Scan several days later after resolution of clinical symptoms. Air insufflation of the colon reveals the mass was collapsed sigmoid *(arrow)*. Notice the intimate relation of the sigmoid to the broad ligament, making colonic opacification mandatory in evaluating the female pelvis.

are necessary. At our institution, we use air insufflation as the method of choice for colonic distention. Not only does this method mark the colon so it is not confused with pathological masses (Fig. 28-50), but also it allows accurate evaluation of the thickness of the wall. The average thickness of the colon wall should not exceed 3 mm,[42,43] although in clinical practice this is rarely measured. When the colon is air distended, the only region with any perceptible wall is the rectum; often the wall of the remaining colon is not seen at all. Some advocate rectally administered water to produce negative contrast. Although this method certainly provides excellent evaluation of the colonic wall, patient tolerance is considerably less and administration slightly more awkward.

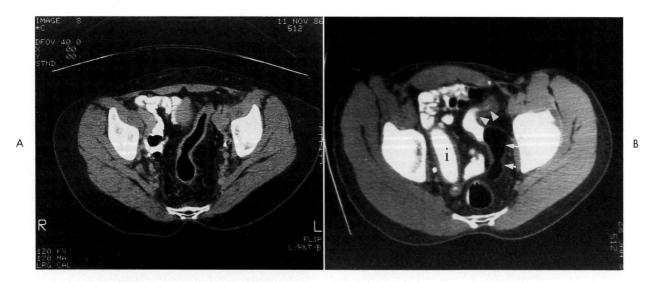

Fig. 28-51. Colitis. **A,** Crohn's disease. The wall of the sigmoid is markedly thickened. Proliferation of perirectal and pericolic fat is present. **B,** Ulcerative colitis. The rectal wall is thickened; the wall of the sigmoid is thickened as well *(arrows).* Note the low-density region paralleling the contrast-filled lumen *(arrowheads).* Backwash ileitis is present *(i).*

Our indications for colonic insufflation include staging of colorectal neoplasms, patients in whom inflammatory bowel disease is suspected, and staging gynecological neoplasms. In patients with inflammatory bowel disease, air is not insufflated if the patients are septic or have a significantly elevated white blood cell count.

Inflammatory diseases

Colitis. CT is of limited use in the evaluation of colitis. There is a wide overlap in the CT appearance of all types of colitides (Fig. 28-51). CT findings in patients with colitis include a variably thickened wall (mean 7.8 mm)[23] and hypertrophy of the pericolic fat. In patients with acute symptoms, increased density in the pericolic fat is seen.

Gore and associates[56] described the double halo or target sign in patients with ulcerative colitis, but we have seen it in patients with Crohn's disease, ulcerative colitis, radiation colitis, and neutropenic colitis[123] and in AIDS patients with cytomegalovirus colitis (Fig. 28-52). This finding therefore has little differential diagnostic significance but does allow one to predict that the thickened wall is due to inflammatory disease as opposed to neoplasm. As in the small intestine, this target appearance usually reflects acute inflammation within submucosa or in rare cases submucosal fat deposition.

Occasionally, patients with vague clinical symptoms are diagnosed from the CT scan as having colitis. This is a frequent occurrence in patients with pseudomembranous colitis.[44,54] Up to 10% of these pa-

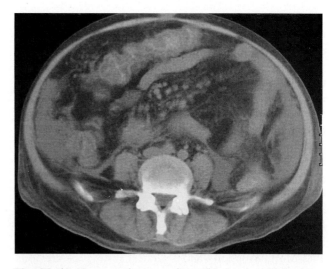

Fig. 28-52. Cytomegalovirus colitis. CT scan in AIDS patient reveals thickened low attenuation transverse colon and ascending colon. Ascites is present. The findings in this patient population are compatible with cytomegalovirus colitis.

tients present with a fever and no associated diarrhea; therefore CT is often requested as an initial examination. Marked dilatation of the colonic lumen is noted with thickening of the wall. Dynamic scanning aids in visualization of the target sign. In advanced cases, thickening of the fascial planes and pericolic gutters and sigmoid mesocolon may be seen as a nonspecific response to a contiguous inflammatory process.[94] Once the history of

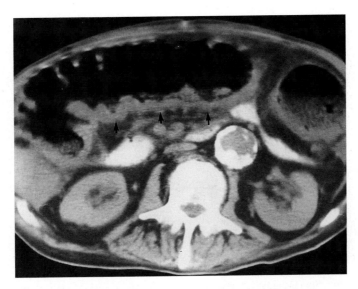

Fig. 28-53. Pseudomembranous colitis. The colon is dilated and thick walled. Transverse haustral markings are seen. Reactive ascites in the paracolic gutter is present. (From Megibow AJ, Balthazar EJ: *CT of the gastrointestinal tract,* St. Louis, 1986, CV Mosby.)

antibiotic use is elicited, endoscopic verification of pseudomembranes and documentation of elevated *Clostridium difficile* titers are necessary to confirm the diagnosis and institute therapy (Fig. 28-53).

Indications for CT scanning in patients with colonic Crohn's disease are similar to those for small intestinal disease. In addition, CT has a primary role in the evaluation of patients with perianal disease. Because of the extensive fistulization and abscess formation, conventional radiological examinations are impossible, and physical examination may be performed only under general anesthesia. The cross-sectional view available from CT allows detection of abscesses and their relation to the levator sling. These relations dictate the type and extent of surgical debridement.[126]

Appendicitis. CT has become a frontline radiographic procedure in the evaluation of patients with clinically unclear cases of right lower quadrant inflammatory disease. We have demonstrated appendicitis with and without abscess, cecal diverticulitis, and even infections such as *Salmonella* and *Yersinia* on the CT examination.

The emerging usefulness of CT in appendicitis reflects the parallel development of CT technology and its clinical application. In a study published in 1986, CT demonstrated right lower quadrant pathology in 92% of patients and was specific for appendicitis in 79%. Findings included pericecal inflammation in 58%, abscess in 55%, appendicolith in 23%, and an abnormal appendix in 18%. The disease is manifested within the appendix, and the periappendiceal fat may be infiltrated with phlegmon or abscess, but in many cases of uncomplicated ap-

pendicitis, the fat is spared (Fig. 28-54). With improved CT technology, particularly the ability to examine regions of interest with thin collimation (5 mm sections), we have been able to image the abnormal appendix in 82% of cases. Conspicuity is further improved by bolus administration of iodinated contrast material.[14]

In reviewing 100 cases of appendicitis studied by CT, we were able to diagnose the condition with specificity and sensitivity in the range of 93% to 95%. In this series, only 20% had an abscess. In these cases, the appendix may be ruptured and not recognized by the surgeon.[12] This reflects the fact that the anatomical alteration in appendicitis is more often restricted to the appendix itself, and one requires more sophisticated imaging technology to visualize these changes.

Cecal diverticulitis may have findings identical to appendicitis. If a normal appendix can be visualized on the CT scan, the diagnosis of cecal diverticulitis becomes more likely. Cecal diverticulitis results in phlegmon, in most cases manifested as poorly defined areas of increased density in the pericecal fat (Fig. 28-55). Occasionally an abscess secondary to cecal diverticulitis may be present; in those cases, distinction from appendicitis is impossible, although not clinically relevant.[13] When there is no defined abscess, the differentiation of cecal diverticulitis and appendicitis is significant because in the former, the treatment of choice is antibiotic therapy as opposed to surgery for appendicitis. Clinical evidence suggests that treatment of periappendiceal abscesses with percutaneous catheter drainage may obviate the need for surgery.[19] Percutaneous drainage of large abscess collec-

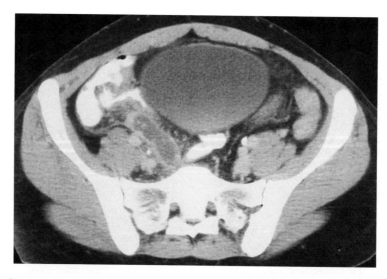

Fig. 28-54. Acute appendicitis. CT image through the right lower quadrant reveals a dilated, thick-walled tubular appendix. There is minimal periappendiceal inflammatory reaction. Note the excellent filling of distal ileum and cecum, establishing the diagnosis.

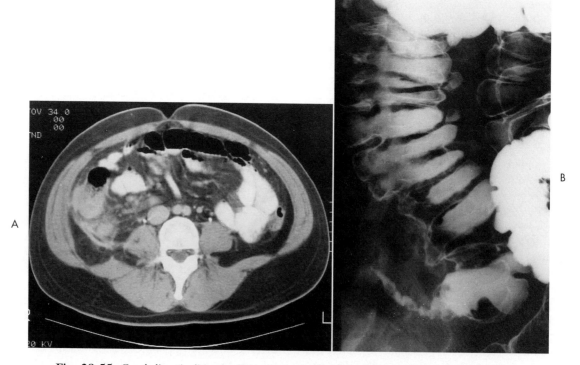

Fig. 28-55. Cecal diverticulitis. **A,** CT scan through right lower quadrant in a patient with fever and right lower quadrant pain. No fluid collections were seen; rather phlegmon was present. **B,** Spot film from barium edema reveals submucosal mass effect on ascending colon. The appendix fills. The patient was treated successfully with antibiotics. No surgery was performed.

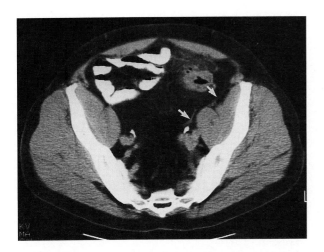

Fig. 28-56. Acute diverticulitis. The wall of the sigmoid colon is thickened. Air within diverticula is seen. Localized increased density in the pericolic fat is appreciated. There is visualization of the insertion of the sigmoid mesocolon along the pelvic sidewall *(arrows)*.

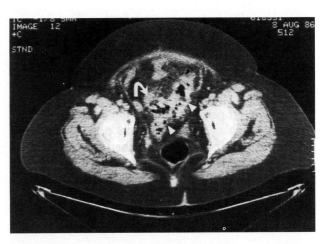

Fig. 28-57. Pericolic abscess (diverticulitis). Diverticula are present in a thickened colon. Fluid collection *(arrowheads)* emanates from the colon *(curved arrow)*. On higher cuts, a large abscess could be seen.

tions in debilitated patients may reduce time in the operating room and may limit the extent of resection; however, in our hands, most cases of right lower quadrant pericolic abscesses are treated surgically.

Diverticulitis. CT has revolutionized the diagnosis and evaluation of patients with acute diverticulitis.[2] Because the disease is truly a pericolic pathological process rather than disease of the colonic lumen, CT is ideally suited in the evaluation of this entity.[101] Once again, as in patients with appendicitis, the major role of CT has been in the identification of those patients with abscess. Often the clinical symptoms cannot distinguish between these two groups.

The CT findings in acute diverticulitis were documented by Hulnick and colleagues.[69] These include increased density in the pericolic fat, thickening of the wall, and presence of diverticula. The most significant finding is in the are of increased density in the pericolic fat. It has been reported that the colonic wall is less than 3 mm in patients with symptoms of diverticulitis (Fig. 28-56). In the mild cases, only a cloudy haze of increased density is seen around the bowel wall. There may be thickening of the lateral conal fascia and the attachments of the sigmoid mesocolon along the left lateral pelvic sidewall as a nonspecific response of a contiguous inflammatory reaction. As the severity increases, progressive intensity of the pericolic reaction may be observed leading to phlegmon (Fig. 28-56). In more severe cases, actual well-defined linear reticular densities within the fat may be seen associated with fluid collections (Fig. 28-56). These fluid collections adjacent to a loop of bowel represent abscesses. Abscesses may appear as bland fluid collections, masses with air fluid levels within, or complex masses filled with debris. Rarely a localized perforation is manifested as extraluminal air collections and associated phlegmon (Fig. 28-57). In our experience, the presence of an abscess in a patient with diverticulitis means that the patient requires surgery after stabilization with intravenous antibiotics.

When an abscess is associated with a poorly defined fluid collection and marked increased density in the pericolic fat, localized peritonitis is often found at surgery. When this constellation of findings is present, our surgeons take these patients immediately to surgery and drain the abdominal cavity. This is accompanied by a resection of the perforated segment with mucous fistula and proximal colostomy (a two-stage procedure).

The role of CT to aid in percutaneous drainage of pericolic abscesses is becoming more clearly defined. Percutaneous techniques may be instituted for preoperative abscess drainage. This allows the surgeon to create a primary anastomosis because the inflammatory exudate has been removed from the operative field (Fig. 28-58). Studies have shown that percutaneous drainage of diverticular abscesses under CT guidance reduces surgical morbidity and aids in the performance of a one-stage resection with primary anastomosis.[110] We believe that any patient with a diverticular abscess requires surgical treatment and resection of the diseased portion of the colon. A successful and complete drainage of a peridiverticular abscess is not an alternative to surgical therapy but rather a procedure that, it is hoped, will make the definitive surgical procedure simpler and safer and decrease surgical morbidity.

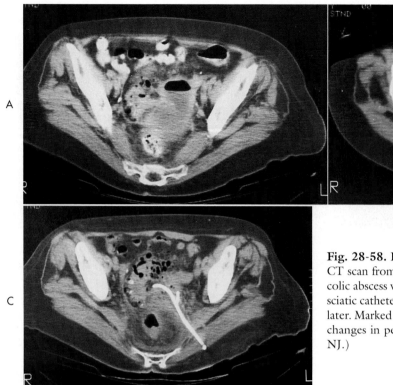

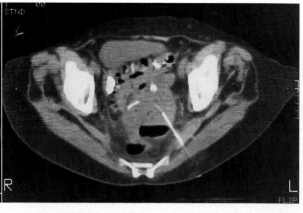

Fig. 28-58. Diverticulitis (preoperative abscess drainage). **A,** CT scan from patient with acute diverticulitis and large pericolic abscess with air-fluid level. **B,** Prone scan following transsciatic catheter placement for abscess drainage. **C,** Scan 3 days later. Marked resolution of abscess with residual phlegmonous changes in pericolic fat. (Courtesy of Dr. S. Toder, Orange, NJ.)

In comparing contrast enema and CT, we found that although the contrast enema may be equal or slightly superior in its ability to discriminate the origin of a pericolic abscess,[72] i.e., whether due to diverticulitis or a perforated neoplasm, we have been constantly impressed by the relative inability of the contrast enema to document the presence of pericolic abscess and understage the true extent of inflammatory process. Publications highlight the superiority of CT to conventional contrast studies in the diagnosis of diverticulitis. In a series of 29 patients, CT was shown to have a 93% sensitivity for the diagnosis of diverticulitis compared with an 80% sensitivity for enema.[27] In a series reported in a clinical journal, CT correctly diagnosed 10 of 10 abscesses, whereas only 3 of 8 abscesses were correctly diagnosed by enema.[81] In that same series, 12 of 13 fistulae were diagnosed by CT, whereas only 2 of 8 were diagnosed by enema. CT may be superior to barium studies in the detection of colovesical fistula (Fig. 28-59). In a series of 20 patients, CT was able to document fistulae in 100%; in the same population, barium enema was positive in 20%, cystography in 50%, and cystoscopy in 20%.[53]

Diverticulitis may occur anywhere in the colon. Right-sided diverticulitis may be impossible to distinguish from appendicitis, especially when the abnormal appendix cannot be visualized.[111] Differential diagnosis in diverticulitis includes Crohn's disease and perforated carcinoma. Crohn's disease may be indistinguishable from diverticulitis because of the transmural inflammatory process with pericolic reaction. Often the associated changes in the bowel wall, such as thickening with a double halo sign, are present to help differentiate between the two entities. The detection of perforated neoplasm as the underlying cause of pericolic inflammatory process is a difficult imaging question. In our experience, the degree of wall thickening in diverticulitis is generally less than that in patients with a perforated neoplasm.[68] On rare instances, one may misinterpret a focally thickened wall in diverticulitis for a neoplasm, particularly in patients with a history of multiple clinical attacks. We have not yet overlooked a neoplasm by performing CT alone. In those cases in which the wall is focally thickened, either a contrast enema or endoscopic evaluation is necessary to exclude tumor. In clinical practice, this problem may arise in approximately 11% of patients.[16] In day-to-day practice, this differentiation is not important in that patients with abscesses are operated on, and the diagnosis is established at laparotomy. In 5% of cases, the surgeon suspects carcinoma on palpation. The pathologist is not able to exclude carcinoma until the specimen is examined histologically.

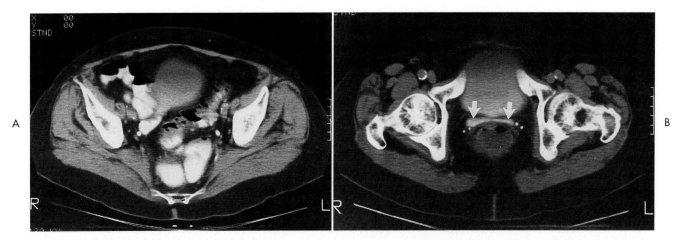

Fig. 28-59. Colovaginal fistula (diverticulitis). **A,** Changes of diverticulosis in sigmoid colon. **B,** Scan through lower pelvis reveals oral contrast material within vagina, diagnostic of colovaginal fistula.

Neoplasms

CT has become part of our routine preoperative evaluation of patients with colorectal neoplasms. This is because CT can not only stage local extent of neoplasm, but also it can detect liver metastases and other extrahepatic foci of disease. CT can also evaluate the urinary tract as to the number of ureters and their course and any unsuspected ureteral complications. Thus in a single examination, we can obviate the need for traditional preoperative assessment, which has included liver spleen scan and intravenous urography. If the patient had an endoscopic diagnosis of colonic carcinoma made, CT is adequate to show the position in relation to the tumor within the colon. This is aided by use of air or water insufflation, which distends the colon.

Freeny and coworkers[50] compared the success of CT in staging colonic carcinoma in comparison to the Duke's system. Although CT demonstrated 85% of the primary tumors, it is unable to categorize the lesions successfully in terms of the Duke's staging system. Compared with Duke's classification, CT correctly staged 47.5% of patients. In the cases incorrectly staged, the tumor was upstaged in 16.7% of cases and downstaged in 83.3% of the cases. Poor results were also found in the exact correlation of local lymphadenopathy with a sensitivity of 25.9% and a positive predictive value of 77%. Balthazar and associates[15] reported similar results in a series of 90 patients. In this group of patients, the accuracy of CT was considerably improved in more advanced lesions.[15] Colorectal carcinoma appears as a focal area of thickening of the bowel wall.[119] As opposed to wall thickening seen in non-neoplastic diseases, the luminal surface appears irregular and lobulated; occasionally, ul-

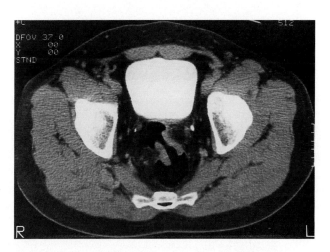

Fig. 28-60. Carcinoma (rectosigmoid). An "applecore" lesion is easily recognized on the air study. Notice streaking in pericolic fat and poor serosal margination, signs of a transmural lesion. Preoperative CT can evaluate the liver and kidneys and show the number and position of the ureters, thereby obviating the need for further preoperative workup.

ceration can be recognized. The target appearance is absent. When present, the "applecore" appearance of some tumors can be appreciated, particularly when the air insufflation technique is used (Fig. 28-60). In other cases, intraluminal polypoid masses are seen.

The adjacent pericolic fat should appear homogeneously low attenuating. Tumor extension appears as spike-like densities protruding from the lesion or reticular linear streaks in the pericolic fat. Our experience is equivalent to Freeny's; despite the use of thin sections, unless there is blatant violation of the pericolic fat, we cannot definitively state whether a lesion is confined to the wall or is extended into the pericolic fat (Fig. 28-61).

Complications of carcinoma of the colon include intussusception, obstruction, and perforation. These are readily detected on CT. Colonic carcinoma may perforate locally or disseminate widely through the peritoneal

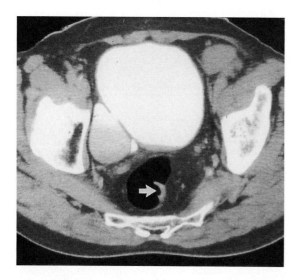

Fig. 28-61. Small rectal carcinoma seen via air-contrast technique. Despite the small size and apparent lack of serosal penetration, this lesion histologically is a Duke's c, poorly differentiated tumor. CT is unreliable in attempting to "stage" colonic adenocarcinoma preoperatively.

cavity. As stated in the previous section on diverticulitis, when a soft tissue mass predominates a pericolic inflammatory response, the possibility of an underlying perforated neoplasm must be ruled out. In our series of 24 patients with perforated colorectal neoplasms, the diagnosis was often unsuspected on barium examination. We have seen no case in which the neoplasm was unrecognized in the setting of pericolid inflammation, although false-positive cases from chronic diverticulitis may be encountered. CT has aided in the interpretation of equivocal barium studies (Fig. 28-62). When the mass effect is less pronounced than the submucosal infiltration of the wall, CT may be helpful in detecting the full extent of the neoplasm (Fig. 28-63).

There are ongoing evaluations of endorectal ultrasound and endorectal MRI in the preoperative staging of these tumors. These techniques can exquisitely demonstrate the layers of the bowel wall and precisely document the degree of transmural penetration. Adaptation of these technologies within an individual department depends on the treatment philosophies within an individual institution or practice.

Metastatic disease occurs hematogenously, by direct extension, or by lymphatic extension. Hematogenous metastases are most often seen in the liver; however, we have seen colon carcinoma metastases to the lung, body wall, and even to the renal pelvis and ureters. Local extension of colon carcinoma into adjacent bowel loops with either obstruction or fistualization is well described. This is most often seen in transverse co-

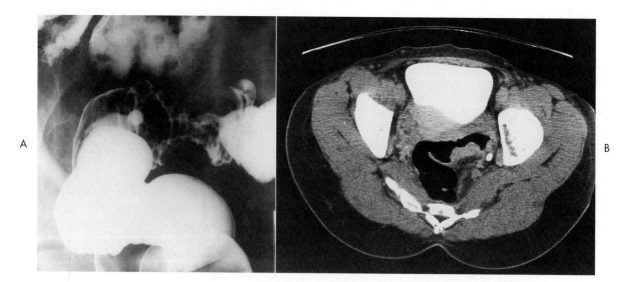

Fig. 28-62. Carcinoma versus inflammation. **A,** Barium enema spot in a 39-year-old patient with change in bowel habits. An asymmetrical mass effect is noted along the mesenteric border. The folds appear thickened but regular. Inflammatory versus neoplasm? **B,** Air-contrast CT reveals extensive well-defined soft tissue mass consistent with colon carcinoma. At surgery, adenocarcinoma of sigmoid was found.

lon carcinoma with extension into the stomach, producing gastrocolic fistualization. CT is able to document this on serial slices by visualizing the primary tumor and following it into the transverse mesocolon directly into the stomach.

Careful evaluation of the pericolic vessels allows one to track the major regional node groups draining the colon. Although epicolic nodes are of less importance, mesenteric nodes have predictable locations based on the visualization of the primary neoplasm.[60] Identification of these nodes is important for the operating surgeon and in preoperative or adjuvant therapy planning.

Follow-up studies in patients having undergone surgical resection of colorectal carcinoma are perhaps more useful than preoperative evaluation.[117] Clearly the perineum and lower pelvis after abdominal perineal resection previously could not be examined by any other technique.[41,62,107] Follow-up studies in these patients reveal small deposits of tumor along the perineal crease that can grow locally and extensively (see Fig. 28-65). These can be subsequently confirmed by needle biopsy and irradiated either externally or with direct implantation into the tumor mass.[24] In these patients, it is of critical importance to ensure good bowel opacification because small bowel loops can herniate between the bladder into the rectal fossa and, unless filled, can simulate recurrent tumor (Fig. 28-64).

Postoperative scarring and fibrosis may simulate recurrent tumor in this area. It is therefore critical to get a baseline CT scan approximately 3 months after abdominal perineal resection if these patients are to be followed radiographically[78] (Fig. 28-65). Several groups are investigating the potential value of MRI in an effort to distinguish fibrosis from active tumor. The recurrence may appear as a complex mass, often as a low-density center with high-density rim. Biopsy of both areas of the mass must be performed to obtain adequate proof of recurrent tumors.[17]

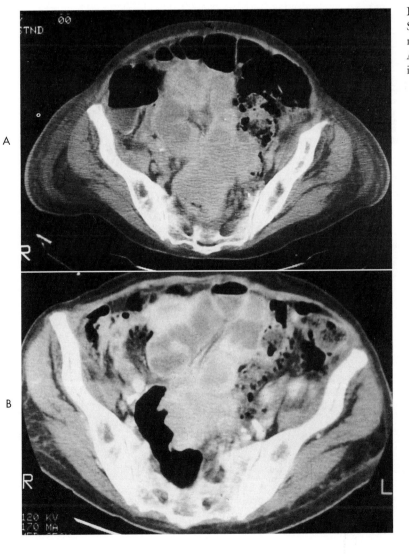

A

B

Fig. 28-63. Unusual primary colon carcinoma. **A,** Scan through pelvis reveals a large central pelvic mass thought to represent a gynecological lesion. **B,** After air insufflation, the relation of the mass growing from the colon lumen could be appreciated.

CT is also useful in evaluating anastomotic recurrence from colorectal carcinoma.[59] Often, these occur beyond the reach of the endoscope in the serosa. When the type of surgery performed is known, the patient can be optimally positioned, and thin sections can be obtained through the area of anastomosis to reveal the presence of tumor. Thus, if the patient had a low anterior resection, scanning in the prone position with air insufflation optimally distends the anastomotic segment (Fig. 28-66). If the patient has had a right hemicolectomy, the patient may be scanned in the supine position because air rises to the anteriorly located anastomosis (Fig. 28-67). The anastomosis is a frequent site of recurrence and should be included in all follow-up CT scans. Extension from the serosa into the body wall across the transverse mesocolon into the duodenum and the kidney has been shown on CT scan. CT is an elegant method for mapping the extent of recurrence in these patients.

Other colonic neoplasms. Lymphoma of the colon is generally differentiated from primary adenocarcinoma because it tends to thicken the wall to a much greater degree than primary carcinoma (Fig. 28-68). Often, walls as thick as 4 cm can be seen in patients with lymphoma. Furthermore, the appearance is that of a homogeneous mass. In our experience, lymphoma is rarely isolated to the colon but is found as a part of a systemic disease. As in other patients, the gastrointestinal lymphoma patients with histiocytic lymphoma and non-Hodgkin's disease are more likely to have colonic involvement than are patients with Hodgkin's disease. In patients with AIDS, colonic lymphoma is far more common than in the general population. The masses are generally not associated with adenopathy. An unusual, unique form of the disease occurs in the anal canal and return of these patients (Fig. 28-68, C). In these cases, bulky masses fill the entire lower pelvis. The diagnosis of lymphoma should be suspected in any AIDS patients with a large perirectal mass.

Metastatic disease to the colon. The colon may be affected by metastatic disease, as direct extension from the pelvic primary (Fig. 28-69), by pelvic hematogenous dissemination from tumors (particularly from lung and breast carcinoma), or by serosal implantation by a peritoneal dissemination tumor. All of these different processes have distinct appearance on CT scans. This appears as focal areas of wall thickening often associated with dis-

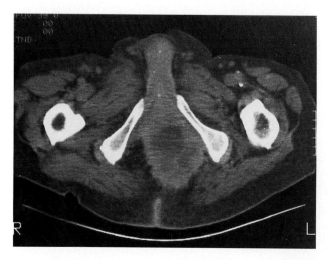

Fig. 28-64. Perineal recurrence of rectal carcinoma following abdominoperineal resection with extension into the pelvic sidewall.

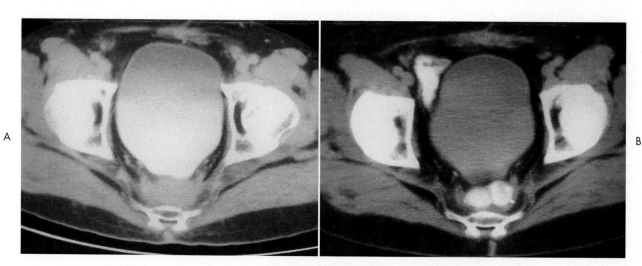

Fig. 28-65. Pseudomass in rectal fossa owing to unopacified small bowel. **A,** Scan in patient following abdominoperineal resection reveals apparent retrovesical mass. **B,** Delayed scan reveals oral contrast material opacifying pelvic loops.

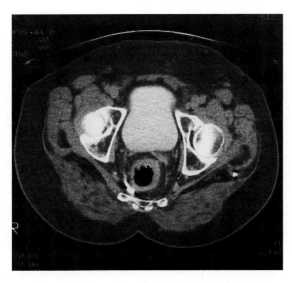

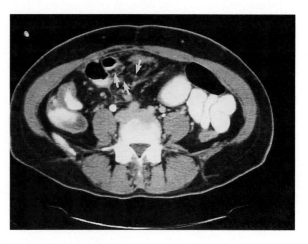

Fig. 28-66. Anastomotic recurrence following low anterior resection. Scanning in prone position after air insufflation allows detailed evaluation of anastomotic segment. The thickened wall contained tumor.

Fig. 28-67. Anastomotic recurrence (right hemicolectomy). Although the anastomotic region is normal, there are discrete peritoneal foci of tumor studding the local fat *(arrow)*.

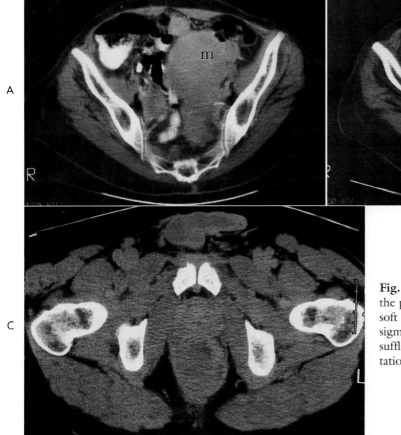

Fig. 28-68. Colonic lymphoma. **A,** Scan through the pelvis in patient with lymphoma reveals pelvic soft tissue mass *(m)*. **B,** Massive thickening of the sigmoid colon is seen accounting for mass. Air insufflation identifies the lumen. **C,** Typical presentation of anorectal lymphoma in AIDS patient.

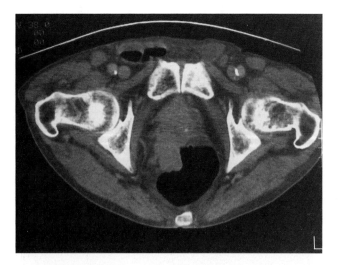

Fig. 28-69. Carcinoma of prostate invading rectum.

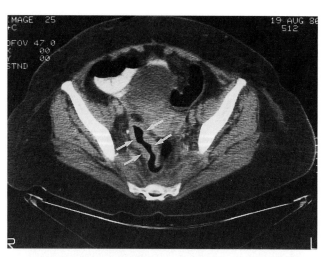

Fig. 28-71. Linitis plastica lesion in sigmoid *(arrow)*. Biopsy revealed submucosal infiltration with breast carcinoma.

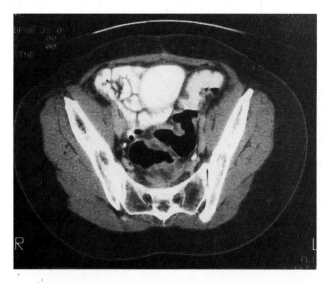

Fig. 28-70. Serosal implantation along sigmoid in patient undergoing therapy for carcinoma of the ovary.

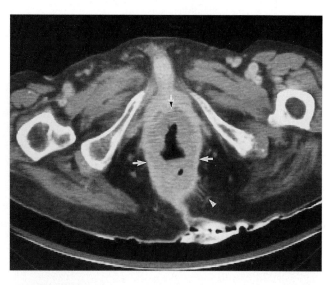

Fig. 28-72. Squamous cell carcinoma of anal canal. The lesion is low attenuation and infiltrating. Note the extension into the perirectal fat and skin.

crete collection of ascitic fluid. Omental implants may also involve the serosa of the transverse colon, producing focal thickening in areas of contract with the mass (Fig. 28-70). Hematogenous disease to the colon has been seen simulating a linitis plastica appearance. On CT, this appears as a thickened colonic wall over a long segment (Fig. 28-71). There may be relative bowel obstruction. We have seen similar cases of metastases to the anal canal hematogenously disseminated from carcinoma of the stomach.

Tumors of the anal canal. A variety of neoplasms are unique to the anal canal. The most common includes squamous cell carcinomas of the anal glands. These are generally large masses that displace the anal canal eccentrically or infiltrate the perianal tissues.[31] Their extension within the perineum is well documented by CT (Fig. 28-72). The lymph node drainage is different from colorectal tumors. It is important to inspect the deep femoral nodes and inguinal nodes for these other primary sources of metastases. Other tumors of the anal canal include giant condyloma (Buschke-Lowenstein tumor) and Paget's disease. We have seen cases of Burkitt's lymphoma of the anal canal in patients with AIDS. These are small masses having nondescript radiographic appearance, but the possibility of a lymphoma should be considered when evaluating AIDS patients, particularly those with perineal masses.

REFERENCES

1. Alpern MB, et al: Focal hepatic masses and fatty infiltration of the liver detected by enhanced dynamic CT. *Radiology* 158:45-49, 1986.
2. Ambrosetti P, et al: Incidence, outcome, and proposed management of isolated abscesses complicating acute left-sided colonic diverticulitis. A prospective study of 140 patients. *Dis Colon Rectum* 35:1072-1076, 1992.
3. Andaker L, Morales O, Hojer H, et al: Evaluation of preoperative computed tomography in gastric malignancy. *Surgery* 109:132-135, 1991.
4. Baert AL, Roex L, Marchal G, et al: Computed tomography of the stomach with water as an oral contrast agent: technique and preliminary results. *J Comput Assist Tomogr* 13:633-636, 1989.
5. Balfe DM, Koehler RE, Karstedt N: Computed tomography of gastric neoplasms. *Radiology* 140:431-436, 1981.
6. Balfe DM, et al: Gastrohepatic ligament: normal and pathologic CT anatomy. *Radiology* 150:485-490, 1984.
7. Ball DS, et al: Contrast medium precipitation during abdominal CT. *Radiology* 158:258-260, 1986.
8. Balthazar EJ: CT of the gastrointestinal tract. Principles of interpretation. *AJR* 156:23-29, 1991
9. Balthazar EJ, Bauman JS, Megibow AJ: CT diagnosis of closed loop obstruction. *J Comput Assist Tomogr* 9:953-955, 1985.
10. Balthazar EJ, Birnbaum BA, Megibow AJ, et al: Closed-loop and strangulating intestinal obstruction: CT signs. *Radiology* 185:769-775, 1992.
11. Balthazar EJ, Gordon RB, Hulnick DH: Ileocecal tuberculosis: CT and radiological evaluation. *AJR* 154:499-502, 1991.
12. Balthazar EJ, Megibow AJ, Siegel S, Birnbaum BA: Appendicitis: prospective evaluation with high resolution CT. *Radiology* 180:21-24, 1991.
13. Balthazar EJ, Megibow AJ, Gordon RB, Hulnick DH: Cecal diverticulitis: evaluation with CT. *Radiology* 162:79-81, 1987.
14. Balthazar EJ, Megibow AJ, Gordon RB, et al: CT of the normal and abnormal appendix. *J Comput Assist Tomogr* 12:595, 1988.
15. Balthazar EJ, Megibow AJ, Hulnick D, Naidich DP: Carcinoma of the colon: detection and preoperative staging by CT. *AJR* 150:301-306, 1988.
16. Balthazar EJ, Megibow A, Schinella RA, Gordon R: Limitations in the CT diagnosis of acute diverticulitis: comparison of CT, contrast enema, and pathologic findings in 16 patients. *AJR* 154:281-285, 1990.
17. Balthazar EJ, et al: Computed tomographic recognition of gastric varices. *AJR* 142:1121-1125, 1984.
18. Balthazar EJ, et al: Computed tomography of intramural intestinal hemorrhage and bowel ischemia. *J Comput Assist Tomogr* 11:67-72, 1987.
19. Barakos JA, et al: CT in the management of periappendiceal abscess. *AJR* 1161-1164, 1986.
20. Botet JF, Lightdale CJ, Zauber AG, et al: Preoperative staging of gastric cancer: comparison of endoscopic US and dynamic CT. *Radiology* 181:426-432, 1991.
21. Bree RL, McGough MF, Schwab RE: CT or US-guided fine needle aspiration biopsy in gastric neoplasms. *J Comput Assist Tomogr* 15:565-569, 1991.
22. Bressler EL, et al: Hypervascular hepatic metastases: CT evaluation. *Radiology* 162:49-53, 1987.
23. Bruneton JN, Caramella E, Cazenave P, et al: Gastric leiomyosarcoma. Comparative value of barium examinations, ultrasonography and CT scans. *Eur J Radiol* 7:160-162, 1987.
24. Butch RJ, et al: Presacral masses after abdominanoperineal resection for colo-rectal carcinoma: the need for needle biopsy. *AJR* 144:309-312, 1985.
25. Buy JN, Moss AA: Computed tomography of gastric lymphoma. *AJR* 138:859-865, 1982.
26. Casola G, van Sonnenberg E, Neff CC, et al: Abscesses in Crohn disease: percutaneous drainage. *Radiology* 163:19-22, 1987.
27. Cho KC, Morehouse HT, Alterman DD, Thornhill BA: Sigmoid diverticulitis: diagnostic role of CT—comparison with barium enema studies. *Radiology* 176:111-115, 1990.
28. Choi BY, Lee WWJ, Chi JG, et al: CT manifestations of peritoneal leiomyosarcomatosis. *AJR* 155:799-803, 1990.
29. Clark RA, Alexander ES: Computed tomography of gastrointestinal leiomyosarcoma. *Gastrointest Radiol* 7:1127-1129, 1982.
30. Cockey BM, et al: Computed tomography of abdominal carcinoid tumors. *J Comput Assist Tomogr* 9:30-42, 1985.
31. Cohan RH, et al: Computed tomography of epithelial neoplasms of the anal canal. *AJR* 145:569-572, 1985.
32. Coller FN, Kay EB, McIntyre RS: Regional lymphatic metastases of carcinoma of the stomach. *Arch Surg* 43:748-761, 1941.
33. Connor R, et al: Pneumatosis intestinalis: role of computed tomography in diagnosis and management. *J Comput Assist Tomogr* 8:269-275, 1984.
34. Cormier J, Jeffrey T, Welch J: Linitis plastica caused by metastatic lobulated carcinoma of the breast. *Mayo Clin Proc* 55:747-753, 1980.
35. Coscina WF, Arger PH, Levine MS, et al: Gastrointestinal tract focal mass lesions: role of CT and barium evaluations. *Radiology* 158:581-587, 1986.
36. Cranston PE: Technical note: colon opacification by oral water soluble contrast medium administration the night prior to CT examination. *J Comput Assist Tomogr* 6:413-415, 1982.
37. Curcio CM, et al: Computed tomography of entero-enteric intussusception. *J Comput Assist Tomogr* 6:969-974, 1982.
38. Dehn TCB, et al: The preoperative assessment of advanced gastric cancer by computed tomography. *Br J Surg* 71:413-417, 1984.
39. Deutch SJ, Sandler MA, Alpern MB: Abdominal lymphadenopathy in benign diseases: CT detection. *Radiology* 163:335-338, 1987.
40. Dudiak KM, Johnson CD, Stephens DH: Primary tumors of the small intestine: CT evaluation. *AJR* 152:995-998, 1989.
41. Farah MC, et al: Doudenal neoplasms: role of CT. *Radiology* 162:839-843, 1987.
42. Fisher JK: Normal colon wall thickness on CT. *Radiology* 145:415-418, 1982.
43. Fisher JK: Abnormal colonic wall thickening on computed tomography. *J Comput Assist Tomogr* 7:90-97, 1983.
44. Fishman EK, Kavuru M, Jones B, et al: Pseudomembranous colitis: CT evaluation of 26 cases. *Radiology* 180:57-61, 1991.
45. Fishman EK, et al: Menetrier disease: case report. *J Comput Assist Tomogr* 7:143-145, 1983.
46. Fishman EK, et al: Computed tomographic diagnosis of radiation ileitis. *Gastrointest Radiol* 9:149-152, 1984.
47. Fishman EK, et al: CT evaluation of Crohn's disease: effect on patient management. *AJR* 148:525-530, 1987.
48. Fly OA, Waugh JM, Dockerty MB: Splenic hilar nodal involvement in carcinoma of the distal part of the stomach. *Cancer* 9:459-462, 1956.
49. Frager DH, Goldman M, Beneventano T: Computed tomography in Crohn's disease. *J Comput Assist Tomogr* 7:819-824, 1983.
50. Freeny PC, et al: Colorectal carcinoma, evaluation with CT: preoperative staging and detection of postoperative recurrence. *Radiology* 158:347-353, 1986.

51. Fukuya T, Hawes DR, Lu CC, et al: CT diagnosis of small bowel obstruction: efficacy in 60 patients. *AJR* 158:765-769, 1992.
52. Gale ME, et al: CT appearance of afferent loop obstruction. *AJR* 138:105-108, 1982.
53. Goldman SM, et al: CT demonstration of colovesical fistulae secondary to diverticulitis. *J Comput Assist Tomogr* 8:462-468, 1984.
54. Goodman PC, Federle MP: Pseudomembraneous colitis. *J Comput Assist Tomogr* 4:403-404, 1980.
55. Gore RM: Cross-sectional imaging of inflammatory bowel disease. *Radiol Clin North Am* 25:115-131, 1987.
56. Gore RM, et al: CT findings in ulcerative, granulomatous and indeterminate colitis. *AJR* 143:403-405, 1980.
57. Gossios KJ, et al: Use of water or air as oral contrast media for computed tomographic study of the gastric wall: comparison of the two techniques. *Gastrointest Radiol* 16:293-297, 1991.
58. Gossios KJ, et al: Water as contrast medium for computed tomography study of colonic wall lesions. *Gastrointest Radiol* 17:125-128, 1992.
59. Grabbe E, Winkler R: Local recurrence after sphincter saving resection for rectal and rectosigmoid carcinoma: value of various diagnostic methods. *Radiology* 155:305-310, 1985.
60. Granfield CA, et al: Regional lymph node metastases in carcinoma of the left side of the colon and rectum: CT demonstration. *AJR* 15:757-761, 1992.
61. Greyson-Fleg RT, Jones B, Fishman EK, et al: Computed tomography findings in gastrointestinal involvement by opportunistic organisms in acquired immune deficiency syndrome. *J Comput Assist Tomogr* 10:175-181, 1986.
62. Gunderson LL, Sosin H: Adenocarcinoma of the stomach: areas of failure in a reoperation series (second or symptomatic look). Clinicopathologic correlations and implications for adjuvant therapy. *Intro J Radiat Oncol Biol Phys* 8:1-11, 1982.
63. Hachigian MP, Honickman S, Eisenstat TE, et al: Computed tomography in the initial management of acute left-sided diverticulitis. *Dis Colon Rectum* 35:1123-1129, 1992.
64. Halvorsen RA Jr, Thompson WM: Computed tomographic staging of gastrointestinal tract malignancies. Part I. Esophagus and stomach. *Invest Radiol* 22:2-16, 1987.
65. Hammerman AM, Mirowitz SA, Susman N: The gastric air-fluid sign: aid in CT assessment of gastric wall thickening. *Gastrointest Radiol* 14:109-112, 1989.
66. Heiken JP, Forde KA, Gold RP: Computed tomography as a definitive method for diagnosing gastrointestinal lipomas. *Radiology* 142:409-414, 1982.
67. Hori S, Tsuda K, Murayama S, et al: CT of gastric carcinoma: preliminary results with a new scanning technique. *Radiographics* 12:257-268, 1992.
68. Hulnick DH, Megibow AJ, Balthazar EJ, et al: Perforated colorectal neoplasms: correlation of clinical, contrast enema and CT examination. *Radiology* 164:611-615, 1987.
69. Hulnick DH, et al: Computed tomography in the diagnosis of diverticulitis. *Radiology* 152:491-495, 1984.
70. Hwang HY, Choi BI, Han JK, et al: Calcified gastric carcinoma: CT findings. *Gastrointest Radiol* 17:311-315, 1992.
71. James S, Balfe DM, Lee JK, Picus D: Small-bowel disease: categorization by CT examination. *AJR* 148:863-868, 1987.
72. Johnson CD, Baker ME, Rice RP, et al: Diagnosis of acute colonic diverticulitis: comparison of barium enema and CT. *AJR* 148:541-546, 1987.
73. Jones B, Fishman EK, Hamilton SR, et al: Submucosal accumulation of fat in inflammatory bowel disease: CT/pathologic correlation. *J Comput Assist Tomogr* 10:759-763, 1986.
74. Karantanas AH, Tsianos EB, Kontogiannis DS, et al: CT demonstration of normal gastric wall thickness: the value of adminis-

75. tering gas-producing and paralytic agents. *Comput Med Imaging Graph* 12:333-337, 1988.
75. Karnaze GC, et al: Computed tomography in duodenal rupture due to blunt abdominal trauma. *J Comput Assist Tomogr* 5:267-269, 1981.
76. Kawashima A, Fishman EK, Kuhlman JE, Schuchter LM: CT of malignant melanoma: patterns of small bowel and mesenteric involvement. *J Comput Assist Tomogr* 15:570-574 1991.
77. Kazerooni EA, Quint LE, Francis IR: Duodenal neoplasms: predictive value of CT for determining malignancy and tumor resectability. *AJR* 159:303-307, 1992.
78. Kelvin FM, et al: The pelvis after surgery for rectal carcinoma: serial CT observations with emphasis on non-neoplastic features. *AJR* 41:959-964, 1983.
79. Komaki S: Gastric carcinoma. In Meyers MA, editor: *Computed tomography of the gastrointestinal tract,* New York, 1986, Springer-Verlag.
80. Kressel HY, et al: Computed tomography in the evaluation of disorders affecting the alimentary tract. *Radiology* 129:451-454, 1978.
81. Labs JD, Sarr MG, Fishman EK, et al: Complications of acute diverticulitis of the colon: improved early diagnosis with computerized tomography. *Am J Surg* 155:331-336, 1988.
82. Leibman AJ, Gold BM: Gastric manifestations of autoimmune deficiency syndrome-related Kaposi's sarcoma on computed tomography. *J Comput Assist Tomogr* 10:85-88, 1986.
83. Lewin KJ, Ranchod M, Dorfman RE: Lymphoma of the gastrointestinal tract. *Cancer* 42:693-707, 1978.
84. Lubat E, Balthazar EJ: The current role of computerized tomography in inflammatory disease of the bowel. *Am J Gastroenterol* 83:107-113, 1988.
85. Madrazo BC, et al: Computed tomographic findings in penetrating peptic ulcer. *Radiology* 153:757-754, 1984.
86. Marks W, et al: Esophageal region: a source of confusion on CT. *AJR* 140:359-362, 1981.
87. McLeod AJ, Zornoza J, Shirkhoda A: Leiomyosarcoma: computed tomographic findings. *Radiology* 152:133-136, 1984.
88. Megibow AJ, Balthazar EJ, Hulnick DH: Radiology of non-neoplastic gastrointestinal disorders in acquired immune deficiency syndrome. *Semin Roentgenol* 22:31-41, 1987.
89. Megibow AJ, Balthazar EJ, Cho KC, et al: Bowel obstruction: evaluation with CT. *Radiology* 180:313-318, 1991.
90. Megibow AJ, Bosniak MA: Dilute barium solution as a contrast agent for abdominal CT scanning. *AJR* 134:1273-1274, 1980.
91. Megibow AJ, et al: CT diagnosis of gastrointestinal lipomas. *AJR* 133:743-745, 1979.
92. Megibow AJ, et al: Computed tomography of gastrointestinal lymphoma. *AJR* 141:541-543, 1983.
93. Megibow AJ, et al: Air opacification of the colon as an adjunct in CT evaluation of the pelvis. *J Comput Assist Tomogr* 8:997-800, 1984.
94. Megibow AJ, et al: Pseudomembraneous colitis: diagnosis by computed tomography. *J Comput Assist Tomogr* 8:281-283, 1984.
95. Megibow AJ, et al: CT of leiomyomas and leiomyosarcomas. *AJR* 144:727-733, 1985.
96. Merine D, Fishman EK, Jones B: CT of the small bowel and mesentery. *Radiol Clin North Am* 27:707-715, 1989.
97. Merine D, Fishman EK, Jones B, Siegelman SS: Enteroenteric intussusception: CT findings in nine patients. *AJR* 148:1129-1132, 1987.
98. Merine D, Fishman EK, Kuhlman JE, et al: Bladder involvement in Crohn disease: role of CT in detection and evaluation. *J Comput Assist Tomogr* 13:90-93, 1989.

99. Miller DG, et al: Gastrograffin vs. dilute barium for colonic CT examinations: a blind, randomized study. *J Comput Assist Tomogr* 9:451-453, 1982.

100. Minami M, Kawauchi N, Itai Y, et al: Gastric tumors: radiologic-pathologic correlation and accuracy of T staging with dynamic CT. *Radiology* 185:173-178, 1992.

101. Morris J, Stellato TA, Lieberman J, Haaga JR: The utility of computed tomography in colonic diverticulitis. *Ann Surg* 204:128-132, 1986.

102. Moss AA, et al: Gastric adenocarcinoma: a comparison of the accuracy and economics of staging by computed tomography and surgery. *Gastroenterology* 80:45-50, 1981.

103. Mueller PR, Ferrucci JT, Harbin WP, et al: Appearance of lymphomatous involvement of the mesentery by ultrasound and body computed tomography: the "sandwich" sign. *Radiology* 134:467-473, 1980.

104. Mullin D, Shirkhoda A: CT after gastrectomy for gastric carcinoma. *J Comput Assist Tomogr* 9:30-33, 1985.

105. Nyberg DA, et al: Abdominal CT findings of disseminated Mycobacterium avium intracellulare in AIDS. *AJR* 145:297-299, 1985.

106. Picus D, et al: Computed tomography of abdominal carcinoid tumors. *AJR* 143:581-584, 1984.

107. Reznek RH, et al: The appearance on computed tomography after abdomino-perineal resection for carcinoma of the rectum: comparison between normal appearances and those of recurrence. *Br J Radiol* 56:237-240, 1983.

108. Rosen A, et al: Mesenteric vein thrombosis: CT identification. *AJR* 143:83-86, 1984.

109. Safrit HD, Mauro MA, Jaques PF: Percutaneous abscess drainage in Crohn's disease. *AJR* 148:859-862, 1987.

110. Sanai S, et al: Percutaneous drainage of diverticular abscess. *Arch Surg* 121:675-678, 1986.

111. Scatarige JC, Fishman EK, Crist DW, et al: Diverticulitis of the right colon: CT observations. *AJR* 148:737-739, 1987.

112. Scatarige JC, et al: Gastric leiomyosarcomas: CT observations. *J Comput Assist Tomogr* 9:320-327, 1985.

113. Schner MJ, Weiner SN: The "string sign" on computerized tomography. *Gastrointest Radiol* 7:43-46, 1982.

114. Silverman PM, Baker ME, Cooper C, Kelvin FM: Computed tomography of mesenteric disease. *Radiographics* 7:309-320, 1987.

115. Smerud MJ, Johnson CD, Stephens DH: Diagnosis of bowel infarction: a comparison of plain films and CT scans in 23 cases. *AJR* 154:99-103, 1990.

116. Soulen RC, et al: Cryptosporidiosis of the gastric antrum: detection using CT. *Radiology* 159:705-706, 1986.

117. Sugarbaker PH, Gianola FJ, Dwyer A, Neuman NR: A simplified plan for follow-up of patients with colon and rectal cancer supported by prospective studies of laboratory and radiologic test results. *Surgery* 102:79-87, 1987.

118. Sussman SK, Halvorsen RA, Ilescas FF, et al: Gastric adenocarcinoma: CT versus surgical staging. *Radiology* 167:335-340, 1988.

119. Thoeni RF: Colorectal cancer: cross-sectional imaging for staging of primary tumor and detection of local recurrence. *AJR* 156:909-915, 1991.

120. Thornhill BA, Cho KC, Morehouse HT: Gastric duplication associated with pulmonary sequestration: CT manifestations. *AJR* 1338:1168-1171, 1982.

121. Townsend RR: CT of AIDS related lymphoma. *AJR* 156:969-974, 1991.

122. Urban BA, Fishman EK, Hruban RH: Helicobacter pylori gastritis mimicking gastric carcinoma at CT evaluation. *Radiology* 179:689-691, 1991.

123. Vas WG, Seelig R, Mahanta B, et al: Neutropenic colitis: evaluation with computed tomography. *J Comput Assist Tomogr* 12:211-215, 1988.

124. Vincent ME, Robbins AH: Mycobacterium avium intracellulare complex enteritis: pseudo Whipple's disease in AIDS. *AJR* 144:921-922, 1985.

125. Walkey MM, Friedman AC, Sohotra P, Radecki PD: CT manifestations of peritoneal carcinomatosis. *AJR* 150:1035-1041, 1988.

126. Yousem DM, Fishman EK, Jones B: Crohn disease: perirectal and perianal findings at CT. *Radiology* 167:331-334, 1988.

29

Hepatic Mass Lesions

CATHRYN POWERS
PABLO R. ROS

Hepatic masses can be classified in the following categories: primary benign neoplasms, primary malignant neoplasms, secondary malignant liver neoplasms, and infectious lesions. Primary hepatic neoplasms may arise from each one of the cellular components of the liver: hepatocytes, biliary epithelium, and mesenchymal tissues, which explains the varied gamut of liver tumors.[46] In this chapter, discussion of primary benign and malignant liver lesions is followed by a review of secondary malignant neoplasms and infectious lesions. The chapter is completed with our practical approach to the differential diagnosis of liver masses.

Computed tomography (CT) has assumed a primary role in the evaluation of hepatic masses. Magnetic resonance (MR) imaging is often used to further characterize a mass found by CT or ultrasound and may be helpful in formulating a more specific differential diagnosis. The development of tissue-specific MR imaging contrast agents holds promise for further increases in the sensitivity and specificity of MR imaging.

BENIGN LIVER NEOPLASMS
Hemangioma

A hemangioma is a benign tumor composed microscopically of multiple vascular channels lined by a single layer of endothelial cells supported by thin septa of fibrous stroma. Hemangioma is grossly solitary, well circumscribed, and blood-filled, ranging in size from a few millimeters to larger than 20 cm.[46] It is classically considered a solitary lesion in 90% of cases. However, with the increased use of imaging, there is mounting evidence that the number of multiple hemangiomas is higher than 10% and above, likely 30%. When larger than 10 cm, a hemangioma is defined by convention as giant. On cut-section, areas of fibrosis are almost always present, with cystic zones and areas of necrosis often but less frequently seen.[122,214]

Hemangioma is the most common benign liver tumor, with an incidence ranging from 0.4% to 20%, the latter figure the result of a prospective autopsy series that performed a dedicated search for this lesion.[122] Occurring primarily in women, hemangioma may be present at any age. The vast majority are clinically silent because of their small size but may become symptomatic when large or compressing adjacent structures, only then becoming a surgical lesion primarily to relieve pain. The remote chance of rupture does not usually constitute an indication for surgery.

On unenhanced CT scans, hemangioma appears as a low-attenuation mass having lobulated, well-defined borders. Calcification may be present in up to 20% of cases, either amorphous or in the form of phleboliths.[211] Following intravenous (IV) contrast administration, large feeding vessels cause peripheral enhancement with centripetal fill-in of the lesion within 15 minutes[73,74] (Fig. 29-1, A). While small (less than 2 cm) lesions may show complete enhancement, the large tumors may have central nonenhancing zones that are due to fibrosis and hemorrhage[224] (Figs. 29-1, A, 29-2). The centripetal enhancement may be demonstrated by dynamic scanning at the same level through the lesion at 30-second intervals for the first few minutes, followed by longer intervals up until 20 minutes or if completely opacified, sooner. Centripetal filling alone is not a characteristic sign of hemangioma because all benign and malignant liver tumors, except for FNH, may have peripheral vascular supply and thus enhancement. The peripheral filling coupled with the delayed filling and persistence of enhancement constitute the diagnostic triad of hemangiomas by single-level dynamic CT. However, this technique has been largely replaced by the increased specificity of MR with IV contrast in the evaluation of a suspected hemangioma.[96,278]

MR imaging is used for the evaluation of a suspected hemangioma because of the hemangioma's characteristic appearance as a result of the slow blood flow

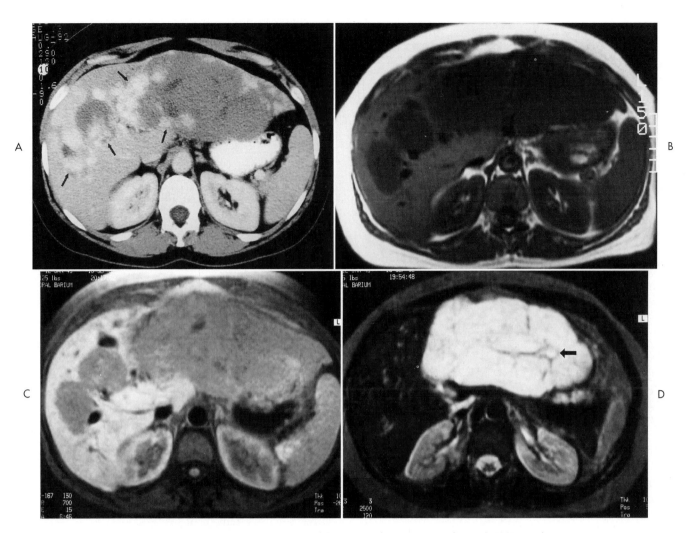

Fig. 29-1. Hemangiomas in a 43-year-old woman. **A,** Contrast-enhanced CT scan demonstrates peripheral enhancement of several hemangiomas *(arrows)*. A giant hemangioma occupies much of the left lobe. **B,** The T1-weighted image (TR 300/TE 12) demonstrates a large hypointense mass of the left lobe and two smaller hemangiomas of the right lobe. **C,** Fat-suppression T1-weighted image (TR 700/TE 15) shows the lesions to be of decreased signal intensity relative to normal liver. **D,** T2-weighted image (TR 2500/TE 120) through the center of the giant hemangioma shows the significant hyperintensity to the liver. A central scar is present with cystic change *(arrow)*.

through the vascular channels of the lesion. On T1-weighted (T1W) images, hemangioma is hypointense to the surrounding hepatic parenchyma with smooth, well-defined, often lobulated margins (Figs. 29-1, *B*, 29-3, *A*). On T2-weighted (T2W) images, it becomes significantly hyperintense to normal liver, increasing in relative signal intensity to the liver with increasing TE[110,111,235] (Figs. 29-1, *C*, 29-3, *B*). Spin-echo pulse sequences of TR 2000 msec with increasing TE from 60 to 180 msec are often used. A double-echo technique of TE 60 and 120 msec, in our experience, has been useful for suspected hemangioma evaluations while minimizing the

length of the examination. The diagnosis of hemangioma by MR imaging rests not only in the signal characteristics but also in morphological features such as sharp and geographic margins, lack of peripheral halo in T2W images, lack of deformity of the liver surface in the majority of cases, superficial location, and lack of displacement of the hepatic vessels surrounding the lesion.

Dynamic gradient-echo MR imaging, after the IV injection of gadopentetate dimeglumine, is useful in increasing the specificity of MR imaging for the study of hemangiomas.[96,278] Gradient-echo T1W FLASH images are obtained before contrast at the level that best dem-

A   B

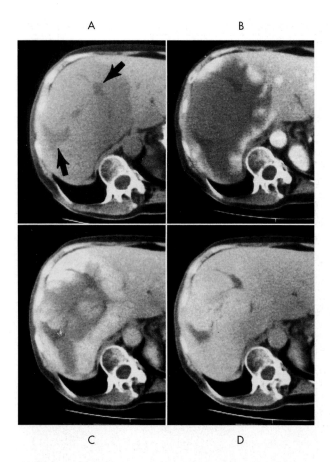

C   D

Fig. 29-2. Large hemangioma with unenhancing central fibrotic scar. **A,** Unenhanced CT scan shows the large lesion, hypodense relative to normal liver, containing areas *(arrows)* of very low attenuation. **B-D,** Contrast-enhanced scans obtained at early *(B)*, middle *(C)*, and late *(D)* stages of contrast enhancement show the internal fibrotic components to remain unenhanced.

onstrates the lesion on the spin-echo images. Repeated FLASH images are then obtained at that level after the injection of gadopentetate dimeglumine (0.05 mmol/ kg). Peripheral enhancement with centripetal fill-in similar to that demonstrated by CT is observed (Figs. 29-3, C, 29-3, D). Central areas lacking enhancement, especially in large tumors, correspond to areas of fibrosis that appear as low attenuation on CT.[38] These fibrotic areas will appear hypointense on T2W images, which may be helpful in making the distinction between a large heterogeneous hemangioma (containing areas of fibrosis) from that of a necrotic tumor, such as hepatocellular carcinoma (HCC) or metastasis, having hyperintense necrotic areas on T2W images. Dynamic Gd-DTPA-enhanced MR imaging is often useful for distinguishing hypervascular metastases from hemangioma; this may not be possible simply with spin-echo imaging.[96]

Focal nodular hyperplasia (FNH)

Focal nodular hyperplasia (FNH) is a benign tumor-like condition comprised of a central fibrous scar surrounded by nodules of hyperplastic hepatocytes and small bile ductules.[46] Vessels are prominent throughout the lesion but are most abundant in the fibrous scar. FNH is believed to be a hyperplastic response to an underlying arteriovenous malformation.[263] Grossly, FNH is well circumscribed, usually solitary (95%); it is often present on the liver surface, or it may be pedunculated. Although sharply marginated, there is no capsule. The majority of lesions are smaller than 5 cm, having a mean diameter of 3 cm at discovery. However, occasionally FNH may replace an entire lobe of the liver, being called lobar FNH.[46]

FNH is the second most common benign tumor of the liver, representing 8% of primary hepatic tumors.[46] It is more common in women and has been associated with oral contraceptive use (although not as frequently as with hepatocellular adenoma).[39] It is predominantly discovered in the third to fifth decades of life as an incidental finding during imaging, surgery, or autopsy, with fewer than one third of cases being discovered because of clinical symptoms such as epigastric or right upper quadrant pain due to compression by large FNHs.

FNH appears on unenhanced CT scans as a homogeneous, low attenuation mass, often with a central low-density area representing the central scar (Fig. 29-4, A). After IV contrast injection, the tumor becomes isodense to slightly hyperdense with normal liver while the central scar may remain of low attenuation[152,270] (Fig. 29-4, B). If a low-density central scar is not present to help identify the lesion on contrast-enhanced scans, the tumor may only produce a bulge or deformity of the liver if peripherally located.[217] On delayed images, there is accumulation of contrast within the scar. This sign has been described as highly indicative of FNH.[152]

FNH is typically isointense to liver on unenhanced T1W MR images (Fig. 29-4, C), becoming slightly hyperintense to isointense on T2W images (Fig. 29-4, E). The central scar when apparent is usually hypointense on T1W images and hyperintense on T2W images.[138,158,219,258] After IV gadopentetate dimeglumine administration, there is enhancement of the central scar because of its excellent vascularity.[249] A high degree of enhancement during early imaging in the arterial phase was noted using turbo FLASH imaging after the bolus IV injection of gadolinium tetraazacyclododecane tetraacetic acid (DOTA).[154] Intravenous superparamagnetic iron oxide (SPIO) particles should be phagocytosed by FNH similar to normal liver because it contains Kupffer cells and has an excellent vascular supply; our preliminary experience confirms this.[46,94]

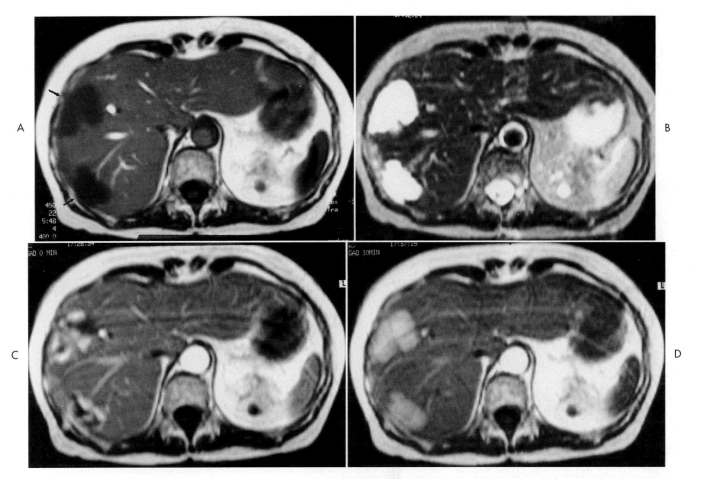

Fig. 29-3. Hemangiomas in a 63-year-old woman. **A,** T1-weighted image (TR 450/TE 22) shows two hypointense, well-defined lobulated peripheral lesions *(arrows)* of the right lobe of the liver. **B,** T2-weighted image (TR 2200/TE 120) demonstrates the lesions to have very high signal intensity relative to the liver. **C,** T1-weighted image (TR 300/TE 22) obtained within 2 minutes after IV Gd-DTPA shows enhancement of the lesions, beginning peripherally. **D,** T1-weighted image (TR 253/TE 22) obtained within 10 minutes after IV Gd-DTPA demonstrates uniform and persistent enhancement of the lesions.

Hepatocellular adenoma (HCA)

Hepatocellular adenoma (HCA) is a benign lesion consisting of hepatocytes arranged in cords that occasionally form bile.[46] Although known to contain Kupffer cells, it lacks portal tracts, hepatic veins, and biliary canaliculi.[89] Fat and glycogen-rich hepatocytes are often present. Grossly, HCA is usually single, 8 to 10 cm in diameter at discovery, with pedunculation present in 10% of cases.[46] A capsule containing large vessels is frequently present. On cut-section, the tumor often contains areas of hemorrhage or infarction, with internal hemorrhage being one of its hallmarks. Rupture of an adenoma may occur, resulting in hemoperitoneum. Rarely, multiple adenomas may be seen, usually involving both hepatic lobes; this is termed *multiple hepatocellular adenomatosis.*[35,147]

The majority of HCA are found in women of childbearing age using oral contraceptives with an estimated overall incidence of 4/100,000 users.[39,208] When the tumor is large, upper abdominal pain may lead to discovery of HCA. The potential for rupture of this benign tumor results in its consideration as a surgical lesion.

HCA appears as a low-attenuation mass on unenhanced CT because of the fat and glycogen contained within the tumor.[152,270] However, areas of increased density that correlate with fresh hemorrhage may be seen. After IV contrast administration, enhancement of the peripheral vessels occurs early with a centripetal en-

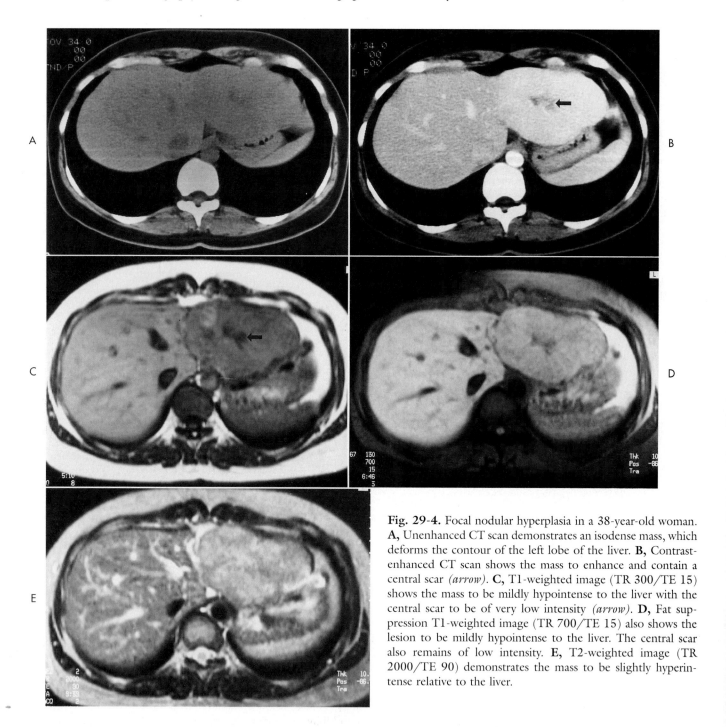

Fig. 29-4. Focal nodular hyperplasia in a 38-year-old woman. **A,** Unenhanced CT scan demonstrates an isodense mass, which deforms the contour of the left lobe of the liver. **B,** Contrast-enhanced CT scan shows the mass to enhance and contain a central scar *(arrow)*. **C,** T1-weighted image (TR 300/TE 15) shows the mass to be mildly hypointense to the liver with the central scar to be of very low intensity *(arrow)*. **D,** Fat suppression T1-weighted image (TR 700/TE 15) also shows the lesion to be mildly hypointense to the liver. The central scar also remains of low intensity. **E,** T2-weighted image (TR 2000/TE 90) demonstrates the mass to be slightly hyperintense relative to the liver.

hancement pattern somewhat similar to hemangioma.[152] (Figs. 29-4, *A*, 29-6, *A*). However, unlike that seen with hemangioma, contrast enhancement does not persist on later scans, because of arteriovenous shunting present in HCA.[211]

On T1W MR images, areas of mildly increased signal intensity may be demonstrated because of the presence of fat and hemorrhage in HCA[81,171,183,210,219] (Figs. 29-5, *B*, 29-6, *B*). The T2W imaging appearance is variable, having hypointense, isointense, and hyperintense areas, depending upon the nature of the lesion and the stage of hemorrhage (Figs. 29-5, *D*, 29-6, *C*). The heterogeneous appearance on both T1W and T2W images makes distinction from HCC difficult. The capsule appears as a hypointense rim surrounding the tumor and may contain large vessels.[81,210] The use of MR imaging

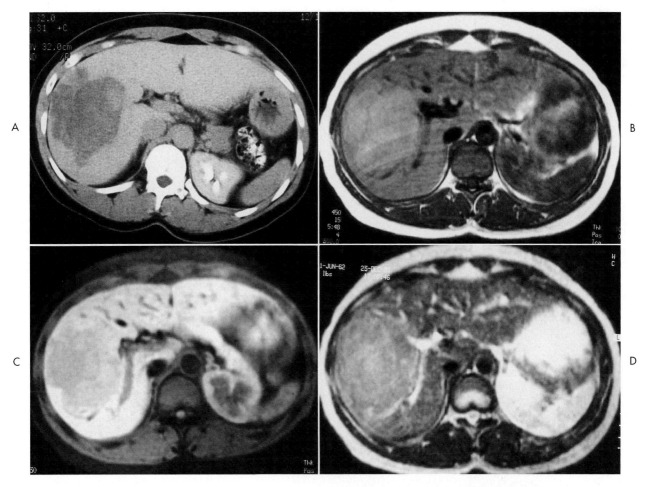

Fig. 29-5. Hepatocellular adenoma in a 29-year-old woman. **A,** Contrast-enhanced CT scan demonstrates a large mass of mixed attenuation in the right lobe of the liver. **B,** T1-weighted image (TR 450/TE 15) shows the mass to have slightly increased signal intensity relative to the liver. **C,** Fat-suppression T1-weighted image (TR 550/TE 15) now shows the lesion to be lower in signal intensity relative to the liver. This indicates the mass to have a fatty composition. **D,** T2-weighted image (TR 2000/TE 90) shows the mass to be slightly hyperintense relative to the liver.

contrast material has not been reported. Our experience with SPIO in a single case showed little uptake in a large tumor probably because of its poor vascularity.[210]

Nodular regenerative hyperplasia (NRH)

Nodular regenerative hyperplasia (NRH) of the liver is defined as diffuse, multiple regenerative nodules not associated with fibrosis.[239] The nodules consist of cells resembling normal hepatocytes. The absence of fibrosis is an important distinction between NRH and regenerating nodules of cirrhosis.[243] Multiple diffuse bulging nodules are present on the liver surface, varying in size from a few millimeters to several centimeters in diameter.

NRH is also referred to as nodular transformation of the liver, diffuse nodular hyperplasia, and noncirrhotic nodulation.[46] It is a rare condition that is discovered incidentally or during the evaluation of portal hypertension. Several drugs, including steroids and antineoplastic medications, as well as multiple systemic conditions, including myeloproliferative, lymphoproliferative, immunologic and collagen vascular disorders, have been associated with NRH.[49,177,243,264] It is the leading cause of noncirrhotic portal hypertension in the West. Complications include esophageal varices and ascites.[168]

The CT appearance of NRH may range from that of a normal liver to that of focal liver nodules of varied but predominantly low attenuation.[49] Hemorrhage may

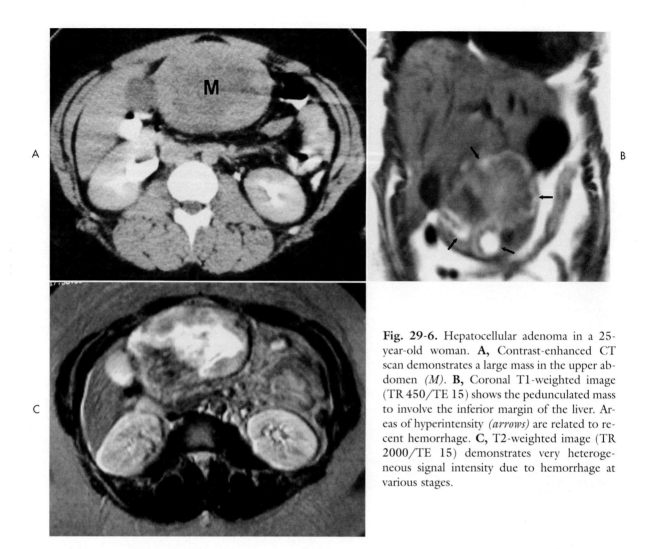

Fig. 29-6. Hepatocellular adenoma in a 25-year-old woman. **A,** Contrast-enhanced CT scan demonstrates a large mass in the upper abdomen *(M)*. **B,** Coronal T1-weighted image (TR 450/TE 15) shows the pedunculated mass to involve the inferior margin of the liver. Areas of hyperintensity *(arrows)* are related to recent hemorrhage. **C,** T2-weighted image (TR 2000/TE 15) demonstrates very heterogeneous signal intensity due to hemorrhage at various stages.

occur, resulting in a complex mass of mixed density. The MR imaging appearance has not been reported.

Adenomatous hyperplastic nodule (AHN)

Adenomatous hyperplastic nodule (AHN), also referred to as adenomatoid hyperplasia and macroregenerative nodule, is a benign but premalignant lesion that appears in cirrhotic livers. Larger than other regenerative nodules of the cirrhotic liver, it has also been called macroregenerative nodule. Histologically, it contains portal tracts and bile ducts but has no capsule.[46]

The conventional CT findings of AHN of a low attenuation nodule are indistinguishable from small HCC. However, CT arterial portography is useful because AHN is not demonstrated (because of the existence of portal blood flow to the lesion), while HCC is demonstrated as a low-attenuation lesion because of a lack of portal flow.[157] The use of CTAP for this differentiation is limited, however, as a result of its invasive nature.

MR imaging is also useful for distinguishing AHN from HCC.[156] On T1W imaging, AHN is hyperintense, while T2W imaging demonstrates a hypointense nodule[109,156,186] (Fig. 29-7). This is in contrast to the T2W imaging appearance of HCC of a hyperintense nodule. The finding of a "nodule within a nodule" on gradient-echo and T2W images consisting of a large low-intensity nodule containing a smaller nodule of isointensity or hyperintensity relative to liver has been shown to indicate a small HCC developing within a hyperplastic nodule.[163]

Lipomatous tumors

Benign hepatic tumors consisting of fat cells may be seen in rare cases. These include lipoma, hibernoma, and mixed tumors such as angiomyolipomas (fat and blood vessels), myelolipoma (fat and hematopoietic tissue), and angiomyelolipoma (fat, blood vessels, and hematopoietic tissue).[87] Hepatic lipomatous tumors usually are round, well-defined, solitary lesions that occur in a noncirrhotic liver.[88] Their microscopic appearance is

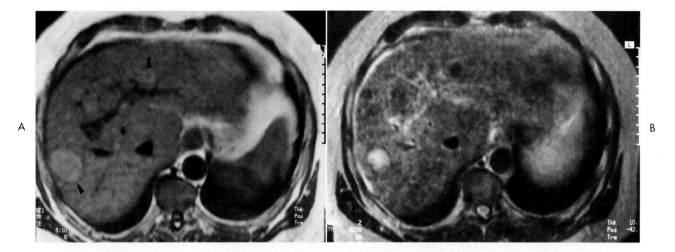

Fig. 29-7. Adenomatous hyperplastic nodules in a man with hepatocellular carcinoma. **A,** T1-weighted image (TR 300/TE 15) shows a small hyperintense nodule of the left lobe of the liver *(arrow)* and a larger hypertense nodule of the right lobe of the liver *(arrowhead)*. **B,** T2-weighted image (TR 2000/TE 90) demonstrates the adenomatous hyperplastic nodule of the left lobe of the liver to be of low signal intensity, while the hepatocellular carcinoma of the right lobe of the liver is of high signal intensity.

similar to that seen in lipomatous lesions of soft tissues.[46]

Hepatic lipomatous tumors may occur in approximately 10% of patients with tuberous sclerosis and renal angiolipomas[206] (Fig. 29-8). However, solitary liver lipomas may be present without other lesions (Fig. 29-9). Most are found incidentally and are asymptomatic but may occasionally bleed, causing abdominal pain.

Benign lipomatous tumors of the liver have the characteristic appearance on CT scans of a lesion composed of radiolucent fat[22,206] (Figs. 29-8, 29-9). In a reported case of the MR findings of a hepatic lipoma, the lesion appeared homogeneous and well defined, with similar signal intensity as retroperitoneal fat on all pulse sequences, with a lesion/fat ratio of 1[22] (Fig. 29-9, *B*).

Infantile hemangioendothelioma (IHE)

Infantile hemangioendothelioma (IHE) is a benign vascular tumor consisting of vascular channels formed by proliferating endothelial cells. Usually made up of multiple spongy nodules varying in diameter from a few millimeters to 15 cm or more, a solitary lesion is a less common variant.[160] Nodules may become fibrotic with age.[217]

Microscopically, IHE consists of a proliferation of vascular channels with an endothelial cell lining. Areas of hemorrhage, thrombosis, fibrosis, and calcification are common. Cavernous areas are also seen.[46]

IHEs are the most common liver tumor during the first 6 months of life; ninety percent of them are discovered during that period. IHE accounts for 12% of all childhood hepatic tumors, with females being affected more often than males.[53] Hepatomegaly, congestive heart failure in up to 25% of cases, thrombocytopenia due to trapping of platelets by the tumor, and occasional rupture with hemoperitoneum may be seen.[26,139] Cutaneous hemangiomas may be associated with the multinodular form of IHE (occurring in up to 40% of patients) and may involve other organs.[46] Although IHE may grow to a large size with resulting hemodynamic compromise, spontaneous involution will occur with time if the child survives.[194]

IHE demonstrates an appearance similar to that of hemangioma on CT.[146] On precontrast scans, IHE appears as a well-defined mass that may contain calcifications (Fig. 29-10, *A*). After IV contrast administration, peripheral enhancement occurs (Fig. 29-10, *B*). On delayed CT scans, a variable degree of centripetal enhancement is seen with prolonged and persistent contrast enhancement similar to that seen with hemangioma.[125]

MR imaging of IHE demonstrates a heterogeneous appearance on both T1W and T2W images because of the presence of hemorrhage, necrosis, and fibrosis (Fig. 29-11). The vascular nature of the lesion produces various degrees of hyperintensity on T2W images similar to that of hemangioma.[125]

Mesenchymal hamartoma

Mesenchymal hamartoma is a benign cystic developmental lesion consisting of gelatinous mesenchymal tissue with cyst formation and remnants of normal he-

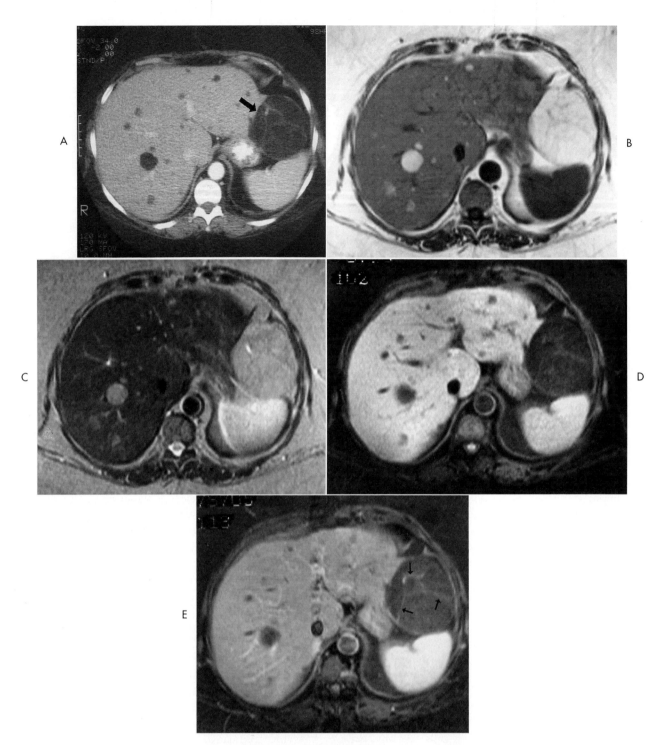

Fig. 29-8. Woman with tuberous sclerosis having angiomyolipomas of the liver and kidneys. **A,** Contrast-enhanced CT scan demonstrates multiple lipomatous lesions of the liver having fat attenuation. A large pedunculated angiomyolipoma *(arrow)* is present in the lateral segment of the left lobe of the liver. **B,** T1-weighted image (TR 300/TE 15) demonstrates the multiple lipomatous tumors of the liver to be of increased signal intensity similar to that of the subcutaneous and retroperitoneal fat. Fibrous septa of the angiomyolipoma of the left lobe of the liver have low signal intensity. **C,** T2-weighted image (TR 2400/TE 90) shows the lesions to continue to have signal intensity similar to that of other fatty areas. **D,** Fat-suppression T1-weighted image (TR 800/TE 15) demonstrates the fatty lesions to be of low signal intensity similar to that of other fatty areas. **E,** Fat-suppression T1-weighted image (TR 800/TE 15) obtained after IV Gd-DTPA demonstrates mild enhancement of the septa *(arrows)* of the angiomyolipoma of the left lobe of the liver, similar to that seen on CT.

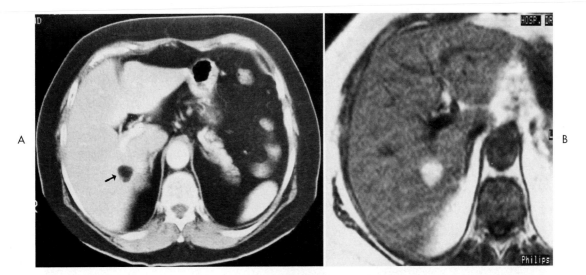

Fig. 29-9. Lipoma of the liver. **A,** Contrast-enhanced CT scan demonstrates a lesion of low attenuation *(arrow),* with similar attenuation to subcutaneous and retroperitoneal fat. **B,** T1-weighted image demonstrates the lesion to have high signal intensity similar to other fatty areas. (Permission from Marti-Bonmati L, Menor F, Vizcaino J, et al: Lipoma of the liver: US, CT and MRI appearance. *Gastrointest Radiol* 14:155-157, 1989.)

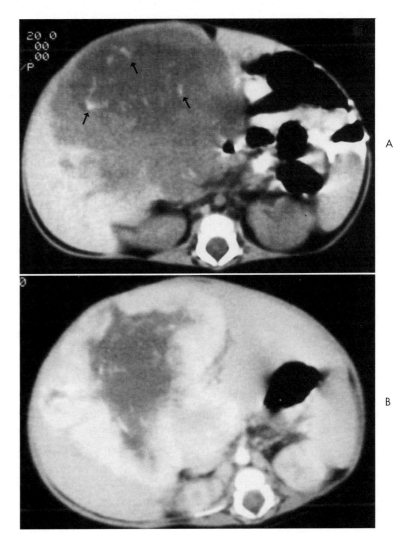

Fig. 29-10. Infantile hemangioendothelioma in a 1-month-old boy. **A,** Unenhanced CT scan shows a large mass of the liver containing calcifications *(arrows).* **B,** Contrast-enhanced CT scan shows the enhancement to begin in the periphery similar to that seen with hemangioma.

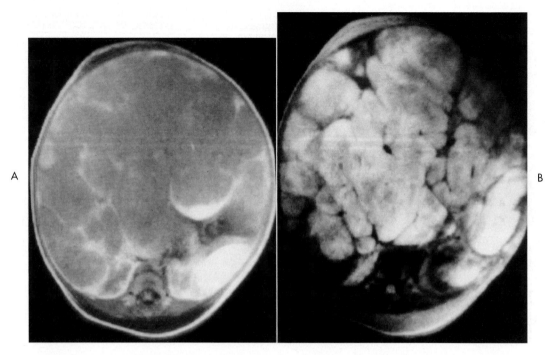

Fig. 29-11. Infantile hemangioendothelioma in a female infant. **A,** T1-weighted image obtained with the patient in the decubitus position reveals a large, multinodular lesion of heterogeneous signal intensity of the liver that fills the abdomen. **B,** T2-weighted image shows that the lesion has predominately high signal intensity due to its vascular nature.

patic parenchyma.[52,242] It is large, usually 15 cm or more in diameter at diagnosis, with cysts present in 80% of cases.[105] It is a well-defined tumor that may be encapsulated or pedunculated.[213] On cut-section, mesenchymal hamartoma may have either mesenchymal predominance (solid appearance) or cystic predominance (multiloculated cystic masses). Microscopically, it consists of cysts, remnants of portal triads, hepatocytes, and fluid-filled mesenchyme.

Mesenchymal hamartoma is uncommon and accounts for only 8% of all childhood liver masses.[105] The majority of cases are found by age 3, with a slight male predominance.[242] Although usually slow, progressive, painless abdominal enlargement is seen, occasionally rapid enlargement may result from rapid fluid accumulation in the cysts. Mass effect from the bulky tumor may cause respiratory distress and lower extremity edema.[245] Extensive surgery is not necessary because mesenchymal hamartoma is not a neoplasm but a failure of normal development; simple excision, marsupialization, or incisional drainage may be all that is required for treatment.[213]

Mesenchymal hamartoma appears as a well-defined mass with central areas of low density and internal septa on CT scans (Fig. 29-12, *A*). Both solid and cystic areas are seen.[213,234]

The MR appearance of mesenchymal hamartoma is dependent on its mesenchymal (stromal) or cystic predominance. Lesions of mesenchymal predominance have lower intensity than normal liver on T1W images because of their fibrotic tissue content. Cystic predominant lesions are of variable intensity on T1W images and significantly hyperintense on T2W images because of cyst contents (Figs. 29-12, *B* and *C*). Multiple septa are best seen on T2W imaging, which demonstrates the complex nature of the cystic mass.[188]

Simple hepatic cysts

A simple hepatic cyst, or bile duct cyst, is defined as a solitary, unilocular cyst with a lining composed of a single layer of cuboidal bile duct epithelium.[46] Its wall is a thin (less than 1-mm thickness) layer of fibrous tissue, surrounded by normal hepatic parenchyma. Although the simple hepatic cyst is thought to be of congenital, developmental origin, usually it is discovered in the adult.[144]

Simple hepatic cysts have an incidence ranging from 1% to 14% in autopsy series, with a tendency to occur more frequently in women than in men by a 5:1 ratio.[46] They are usually found incidentally but may cause mass effect, resulting in abdominal pain or jaundice.[221] If symptomatic, surgical excision or percutaneous aspira-

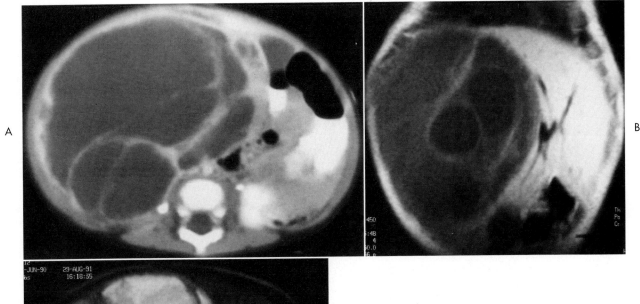

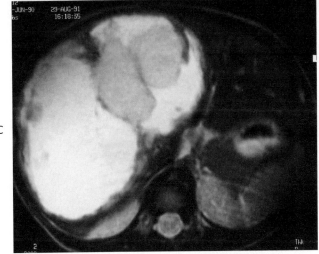

Fig. 29-12. Mesenchymal hamartoma in a 14-month-old boy. **A,** Contrast-enhanced CT scan shows a large cystic mass of the liver with several locules of fluid separated by septa. **B,** Coronal T1-weighted image (TR 450/TE 15) shows the predominately cystic mass to be composed of slightly hyperintense proteinacious fluid with locules of lower-intensity fluid. **C,** T2-weighted image (TR 2000/TE 90) demonstrates the hyperintense mass to contain several low-signal intensity septations that surround locules of lower-intensity fluid.

tion with alcohol sclerotherapy may be helpful.[11,118,144,221]

A simple hepatic cyst appears on CT scans as a well-defined intrahepatic mass having water attenuation, a round or oval shape, smooth thin walls, no internal structures, and no enhancement after IV contrast administration.[9,176] Usually solitary and peripheral, they may be multiple and occur more centrally. When more than 10 cysts are present, a polycystic disease should be considered.[24] Cysts that become complicated by hemorrhage or infection may have septations and internal debris, as well as wall enhancement.

MR imaging of simple hepatic cysts demonstrates hypointensity on T1W images and hyperintensity on T2W images.[275] It may be difficult to differentiate a cyst from hemangioma without the use of IV gadopentetate dimeglumine.

Congenital hepatic fibrosis and polycystic liver disease

Congenital hepatic fibrosis and polycystic liver disease are part of the spectrum of fibropolycystic disease of the liver. Congenital hepatic fibrosis is characterized by periductal fibrosis and aberrant bile duct proliferation.[46] Typically, the cysts of congenital hepatic fibrosis are only visible with magnification. However, numerous large and small cysts, which are pathologically identical to simple or bile duct cysts, are present with fibrosis in the polycystic liver disease variant. In polycystic liver and/or kidney disease, the liver, which surrounds the cysts, is not normal and frequently contains von Meyenburg's complexes and increased fibrous tissue. Hepatic involvement occurs in approximately 30% to 40% of patients with autosomal dominant (adult) polycystic kidney disease.[118] Occasionally, hepatic cysts oc-

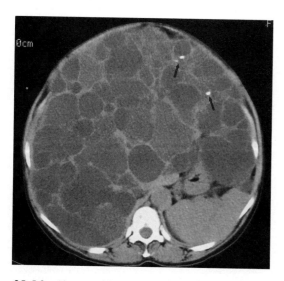

Fig. 29-13. 60-year-old woman with polycystic kidney and liver disease. Noncontrast CT scan demonstrates multiple cysts of varying attenuation involving the liver. A few calcifications *(arrows)* of the cyst walls are present.

cur without radiologically evident renal cysts; approximately 70% of patients with polycystic liver disease also have autosomal dominant polycystic kidney disease.[24]

Most patients with congenital hepatic fibrosis present in childhood with complications of portal hypertension such as bleeding varices.[124] In patients with polycystic disease, lesions are often found incidentally on imaging studies.

CT demonstrates multiple cysts of the liver and may reveal calcification of the cyst walls (Figs. 29-13, 29-14, *A*). Hemorrhage into cysts may occur, as in the kidneys; this results in increased attenuation of the cyst contents.[24,140,176] Contrast enhancement of the cysts should not occur unless they become complicated by infection.

MR imaging demonstrates the simple, noncomplicated cysts to have decreased signal intensity on T1W images and increased signal intensity on T2W images (Figs. 29-14, *B*, 29-14, *C*). Calcification of cyst walls may be difficult to detect as areas of signal void. When complicated by hemorrhage, varying signal intensity on all

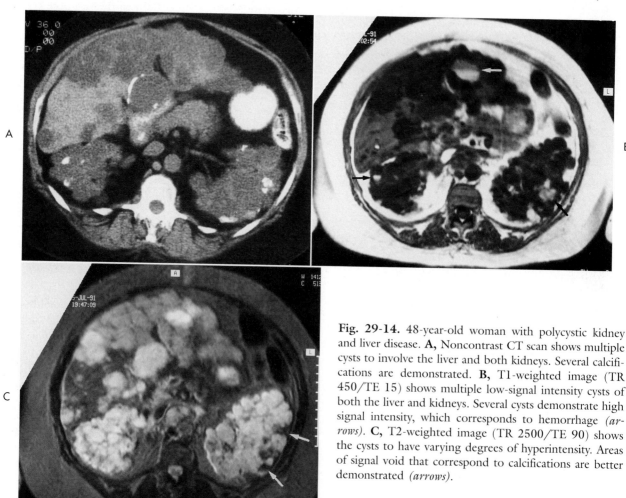

Fig. 29-14. 48-year-old woman with polycystic kidney and liver disease. **A,** Noncontrast CT scan shows multiple cysts to involve the liver and both kidneys. Several calcifications are demonstrated. **B,** T1-weighted image (TR 450/TE 15) shows multiple low-signal intensity cysts of both the liver and kidneys. Several cysts demonstrate high signal intensity, which corresponds to hemorrhage *(arrows).* **C,** T2-weighted image (TR 2500/TE 90) shows the cysts to have varying degrees of hyperintensity. Areas of signal void that correspond to calcifications are better demonstrated *(arrows).*

pulse sequences that depends on the age of the bleeding episode may be seen.[272]

MALIGNANT HEPATIC TUMORS

Hepatocellular carcinoma (HCC)

The most common primary malignant hepatic tumor and one of the most common malignancies in the world, hepatocellular carcinoma (HCC) is composed of malignant hepatic cells that mimic normal hepatocytes.[46] It is often difficult to distinguish microscopically the cells of HCC from normal hepatocytes and/or hepatocellular adenoma; this affects the accuracy of cytologic needle aspiration biopsy.[182] The malignant hepatocytes may be so well differentiated in some tumors as to even produce bile, which is found in the tumor cells and in biliary canaliculi. Fat and glycogen are often present in the cytoplasm of HCC hepatocytes. Several growth patterns occur, the most frequent being the trabecular pattern, which may give the tumor a pseudoglandular or acinar pattern. When the trabeculae grow together, a solid pattern is produced.

Grossly, three major patterns of growth are seen: large solitary mass, nodular or multifocal masses, and diffuse or cirrhotomimetic HCC. A gross variant of the solitary form, encapsulated HCC, may have an improved prognosis because of easier resectability.[72,215] In all forms of growth, HCC is a soft tumor with frequent necrosis and hemorrhage as a result of its lack of stroma. Vascular invasion of portal and hepatic veins is common, while biliary invasion is uncommon.[244]

The incidence of HCC is highest in subSaharan Africa and Asia, with its peak incidence in Japan.[174,178] In the high incidence areas, presentation is often at a young age (30 to 45 years) and men are affected eight times more frequently than women. The primary etiologic factors in these areas are hepatitis B virus and aflatoxin exposure. HCC is aggressive in these patients and may present with both rupture of the liver and hemoperitoneum.

In the Western hemisphere, where HCC occurs at a lower rate, the usual age of presentation is 70 to 80 years with a male to female ratio of 2.5 : 1.[174] Most patients have underlying cirrhosis due to alcohol abuse, hemochromatosis, or toxin exposure, with hepatitis B virus becoming increasingly responsible, especially in younger patients. Symptoms are insidious in onset and include malaise, fever, and abdominal pain. Jaundice is rare, and liver function tests may be normal except for elevation of alpha-fetoprotein level. Paraneoplastic syndromes may occur; these include erythrocytosis, hypercalcemia, hypoglycemia, hypercholesterolemia, and hirsutism.

Unenhanced CT demonstrates HCC usually as a large, hypodense mass, often with central areas of low attenuation representing areas of necrosis. However, occasionally the tumor may be isodense to the liver on unenhanced CT scans.[132,247] Calcification may rarely be present.[133,247] In North American and European patients, cirrhosis (60%) or hemochromatosis (20%) is often seen in the remainder of the liver[72] (Fig. 29-15). After IV contrast administration, the nonnecrotic areas of the tumor may enhance and appear hyperdense[72] (Fig. 29-16). If a capsule is present, it will appear as an en-

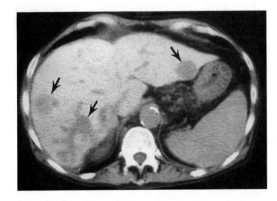

Fig. 29-15. Hemochromatosis with multifocal hepatocellular carcinoma. Unenhanced CT scan demonstrates multiple masses of low attenuation relative to the overall increased density of the liver as a result of the high levels of iron in the liver. The lesion of the posterior segment of the right lobe has portal-vein invasion, which causes the venous dilatation peripheral to the lesion.

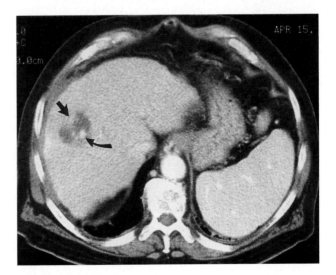

Fig. 29-16. 70-year-old man with hepatocellular carcinoma in a cirrhotic liver. Contrast-enhanced CT scan demonstrates a predominately low attenuation mass with enhancement of the nonnecrotic area of the tumor *(straight arrow).* An enhancing vessel *(curved arrow)* is well demonstrated on this dynamic bolus-enhanced scan. A rim of ascites is present.

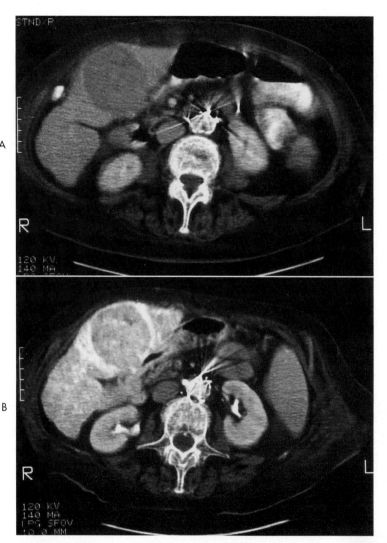

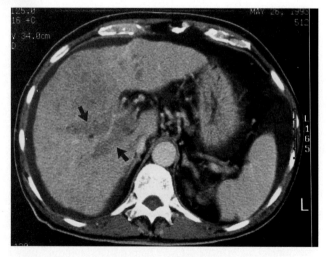

Fig. 29-17. Encapsulated hepatocellular carcinoma in a cirrhotic liver. **A,** Contrast-enhanced CT scan demonstrates the well-defined low-attenuation mass, which deforms the liver contour. **B,** CT scan performed during hepatic-arterial injection of contrast better demonstrates the enhancing rim.

hancing rim around the tumor[215] (Fig. 29-17). In the solid histologic forms of HCC, the density of the lesion may be similar to that of the surrounding liver, with detection depending on changes in the liver contour. Low attenuation persists in areas of necrosis and fat.[133,279] Vascular invasion of venous structures including portal veins, hepatic veins, and inferior vena cava may be seen after contrast administration[153,167,244] (Figs. 29-18, 29-19). Intra-arterial CT portography, CT after iodized oil (Lipiodol) injection, and intra-operative ultrasound have been shown to be more sensitive than IV bolus dynamic CT for the detection of HCC smaller than 3 cm.[246] However, contrast-enhanced CT has been shown to be more accurate than abdominal sonography for identifying and staging HCC.[167] Intraperitoneal rupture of HCC may be demonstrated by CT as high-density blood adjacent to a peripheral mass and may be predicted to occur in patients with very large peripheral tumors with extrahepatic protrusion[121] (Fig. 29-20).

Fig. 29-18. 70-year-old man with cirrhosis and diffuse hepatocellular carcinoma. Contrast-enhanced CT scan demonstrates the diffuse low density of the cirrhotomimetic hepatocellular carcinoma. There is extensive portal vein thrombosis *(arrows).* Ascites and multiple venous collaterals are present.

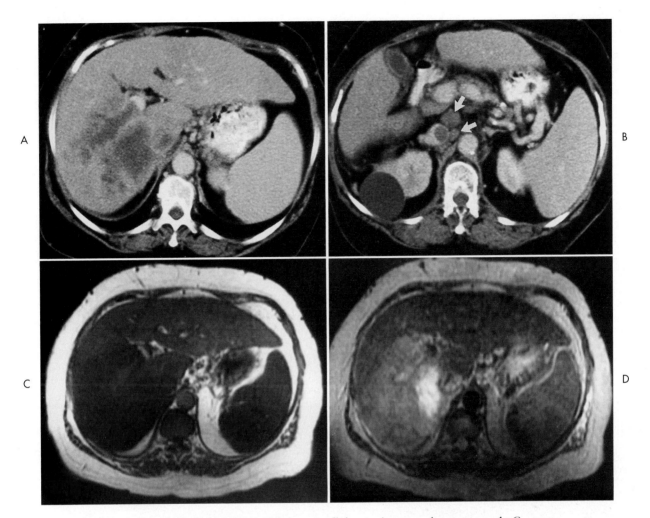

Fig. 29-19. 63-year-old woman with hepatocellular carcinoma and metastases. **A,** Contrast-enhanced CT scan demonstrates a large mixed attenuation mass of the posterior segment of the right lobe of the liver with thrombus involving the right portal vein and IVC. **B,** At a more caudal level to A, lymphadenopathy *(arrows)* is demonstrated with extension of the IVC thrombus. There are multiple venous collaterals present. Incidentally noted is a large right renal cyst and gallbladder-wall thickening. **C,** T1-weighted image (TR 350/TE 20) shows the large hypointense mass. There is slightly higher signal in the right portal vein and IVC. **D,** T2-weighted image (TR 2500/TE 80) demonstrates the mass to be moderately to significantly hyperintense relative to the remainder of the liver. Abnormal signal intensity is again noted of the right portal vein and IVC.

MR imaging of HCC reveals a variable appearance on T1W images depending on the degree of fatty change, internal fibrosis, hemorrhage, and dominant histologic pattern[55,113,219] (Figs. 29-19, *C,* 29-21, *A*). T2W imaging usually shows HCC as hyperintense relative to liver, with higher intensity seen in areas of necrosis (Figs. 29-19, *D,* 29-21, *B,* 29-22). The encapsulated form of HCC often has a thin, low signal rim on T1W images that represents the tumor capsule. This capsule appears on T2W images as a double layer of inner low

signal and outer high signal in approximately one half of encapsulated HCC, with the inner layer representing fibrous tissue and the outer layer consisting of compressed vessels and bile ducts.[113]

Gradient-echo MR imaging and other flow techniques are sensitive for the detection of hepatic and perihepatic vascular invasion.[185] Contrast-enhanced MR imaging of HCC may reveal variable enhancement of the lesion after IV gadolinium because of its hypervascular nature.[187,278] Intravenous SPIO, a reticuloendothelial

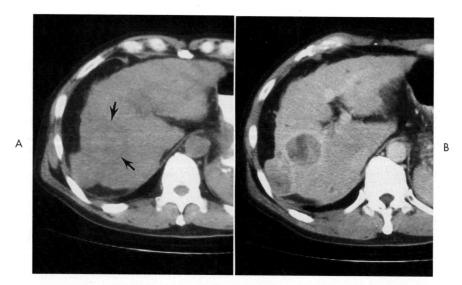

Fig. 29-20. Multifocal hepatocellular carcinoma in a cirrhotic liver as a result of chronic active hepatitis B. **A,** Unenhanced CT scan shows two low-density lesions in the right lobe of the liver, one protruding from the liver margin and the other defined by a slightly hypodense peripheral rim *(arrows).* **B,** Contrast-enhanced CT scan shows peripheral rim enhancement and heterogeneous internal density. The protruding lesion is at increased risk for rupture.

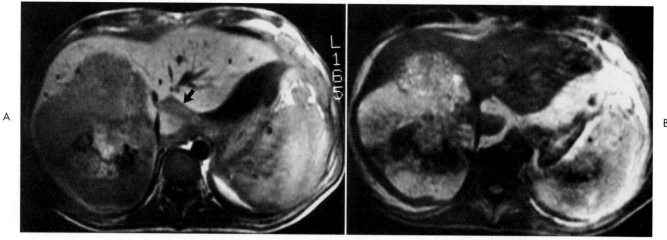

Fig. 29-21. Hepatocellular carcinoma in a 46-year-old man. **A,** Fat-suppression T1-weighted image (TR 550/TE 20) demonstrates the large mass to be predominately hypointense with central hemorrhage of mixed signal intensity. Regional extension of tumor is present *(arrow).* **B,** T2-weighted image (TR 2500/TE 80) reveals the heterogeneous hyperintense mass with low signal intensity in the region of hemorrhage, indicating the presence of hemosiderin. The ascitic fluid is of higher signal intensity than is the area of regional spread.

contrast material, increases the sensitivity of MR imaging by decreasing the signal of normal parenchyma[64] (Fig. 29-22).

Fibrolamellar carcinoma (FLC)

Fibrolamellar carcinoma (FLC) is a slow-growing malignant tumor of hepatocellular origin that arises in a noncirrhotic liver. Composed of neoplastic hepatocytes separated into cords by lamellar fibrous strands, these lesions have a distinctive histologic pattern with eosinophilic malignant hepatocytes that contain prominent nuclei.[46,47,207] The alpha-fetoprotein body inclusions that are usually seen in HCC are not present in FLC. A fibrous central scar may be seen in larger lesions.[46]

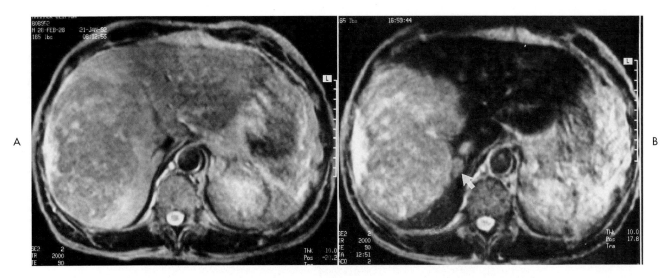

Fig. 29-22. Hepatocellular carcinoma in a 63-year-old man with cirrhosis. **A,** T1-weighted image (TR 2000/TE 90) demonstrates ascites and heterogeneous slightly increased signal intensity involving the right lobe of the liver. **B,** T2-weighted image (TR 2000/TE 90) post-IV SPIO shows the large mass to be defined as increased signal intensity while the liver demonstrates decreased signal intensity. A satellite lesion is now demonstrated *(arrow)*.

Grossly, FLC usually arises in a normal liver; only 20% of patients have cirrhosis.[207] Satellite lesions are often seen. FLC may be similar in appearance to FNH because both tumors may have central scars and multiple fibrous septa. Hemorrhage and necrosis are rarely seen in FLC.

Usually occurring in adolescents and adults younger than 40 years of age without cirrhosis, FLC has no sex predilection.[207] The mean survival is much better than that of HCC, 45 to 60 months compared with only 6 months, and FLC has a higher likelihood of cure (40%) if the lesion is surgically resected.[16] Most patients with FLC present with pain, malaise, and weight loss. Jaundice may occur if occasional biliary tree invasion is present. In two thirds of patients with FLC, a palpable mass is found.[69] Alphafetoprotein levels are most commonly normal.

Unenhanced CT demonstrates FLC as a well-defined low-attenuation mass.[69,79] The central scar appears of lower attenuation. Calcifications may be present within the scar in a stellate pattern. After IV contrast administration, there is enhancement of the tumor because of its hypervascularity[69,79] (Fig. 29-23, *A*).

MR imaging of FLC shows it to be isointense relative to normal liver on T1W images[158,254] (Fig. 29-23, *B*). On T2W images, it remains isointense to slightly hyperintense, occasionally hypointense, relative to liver (Fig. 29-23, *C*). The central scar remains hypointense on T1W and T2W images because of its fibrous nature. This

hypointensity of the central scar of FLC may be useful in differentiating this lesion from FNH with its hyperintense central scar.[253]

Intrahepatic cholangiocarcinoma (I-CAC)

Intrahepatic cholangiocarcinoma (I-CAC) is an adenocarcinoma that originates in the small intrahepatic ducts and represents approximately 10% of all cholangiocarcinomas.[46,127,170] Grossly, these tumors are typically large firm masses with a large amount of fibrous tissue. Rarely do they contain internal necrosis or hemorrhage.[212] Mucin and calcification are often demonstrated microscopically, and desmoplastic reaction is often prominent.

The second most common primary hepatic malignancy in adults, I-CAC is usually found in the seventh decade of life, with a slight male predominance.[46] Symptoms are often vague until the tumor has reached a large size, causing abdominal pain and a palpable mass. Jaundice is rarely a presenting symptom in I-CAC as it arises in the peripheral biliary ducts.

On unenhanced CT scans, I-CAC usually has the appearance of a homogeneous, hyperdense mass.[32,108,112,252] Mild diffuse centripetal enhancement is often seen after IV contrast administration, with persistent small low-attenuation areas representing internal fibrosis. Satellite nodules and tumor extension through the hepatic capsule with invasion of adjacent organs may be present. Encasement of large vascular structures such

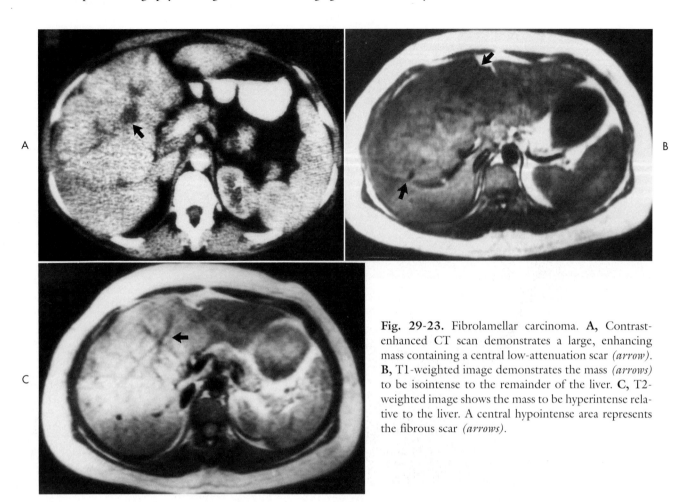

Fig. 29-23. Fibrolamellar carcinoma. **A,** Contrast-enhanced CT scan demonstrates a large, enhancing mass containing a central low-attenuation scar *(arrow).* **B,** T1-weighted image demonstrates the mass *(arrows)* to be isointense to the remainder of the liver. **C,** T2-weighted image shows the mass to be hyperintense relative to the liver. A central hypointense area represents the fibrous scar *(arrows).*

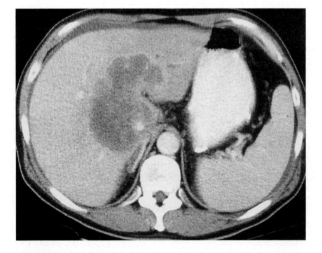

Fig. 29-24. Intrahepatic cholangiocarcinoma in a 45-year-old man. Contrast-enhanced CT scan demonstrates a large central, predominately hypointense mass with peripheral enhancement. The lobulated mass encases the IVC, which remains patent.

as portal and hepatic veins is often present but usually without tumor thrombus (Figs. 29-24, 29-25, *A*).

MR imaging demonstrates I-CAC as a large central mass with irregular borders, hypointense on T1W imaging and hyperintense on T2W imaging relative to liver[60,209] (Figs. 29-25, *B*, 29-25, *C*). Small satellite nodules may be seen. Large central areas of fibrosis in the mass cause hypointensity on T2W images and an overall heterogeneous appearance. The periphery of I-CAC is more hyperintense than its center on T2W images, suggesting the presence of a central scar. Progressive, concentric enhancement is often seen after IV gadopentetate dimeglumine administration (Fig. 29-25, *B*). This centripetal enhancement pattern spares central areas of fibrosis and reflects the presence of viable peripheral tumor. The typical finding of vascular encasement without tumor thrombus seen in I-CAC is well demonstrated by gradient-echo images and MR angiography.[209]

Biliary cystadenoma and cystadenocarcinoma

Two forms of a spectrum of disease, biliary cystadenoma and cystadenocarcinoma are rare tumors. They

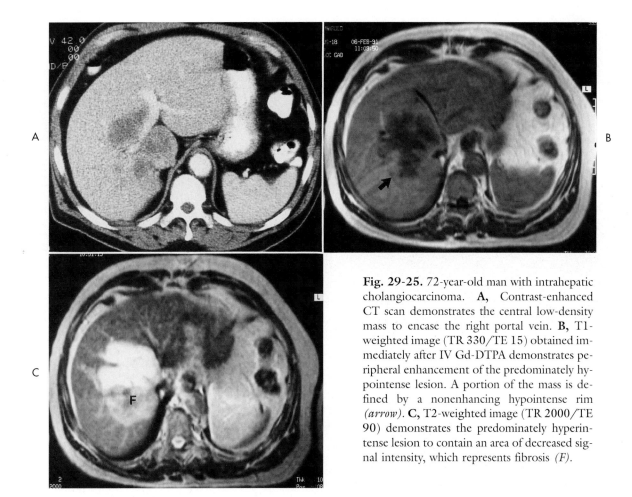

Fig. 29-25. 72-year-old man with intrahepatic cholangiocarcinoma. **A,** Contrast-enhanced CT scan demonstrates the central low-density mass to encase the right portal vein. **B,** T1-weighted image (TR 330/TE 15) obtained immediately after IV Gd-DTPA demonstrates peripheral enhancement of the predominately hypointense lesion. A portion of the mass is defined by a nonenhancing hypointense rim *(arrow)*. **C,** T2-weighted image (TR 2000/TE 90) demonstrates the predominately hyperintense lesion to contain an area of decreased signal intensity, which represents fibrosis *(F)*.

represent only 5% of all intrahepatic cysts of bile duct origin, with the overwhelming majority of cases corresponding to the bile duct or simple cysts.[176] Cystadenocarcinoma is the overtly malignant form of the disease, while cystadenoma has a high propensity for recurrence and malignant transformation.[107,271] The tumors occur most often in middle-aged women and are likely congenital in origin because of the presence of aberrant bile ducts.[46] Though the tumors are most commonly mucinous, a serous variety is recognized. These tumors contain locules that are lined by columnar, cuboidal, or flattened epithelium. Papillary areas and polypoid projections are often present. Focal calcification within the well-formed wall is occasionally seen. Biliary-type epithelium overlies a compact mesenchymal stroma in the cystadenoma, while malignant epithelial cells line the cysts of cystadenocarcinoma.

Grossly, the tumor is usually solitary but is often large, measuring up to 30 cm in diameter.[46] Multiple communicating locules of varying size are contained within the tumor and have a predominately smooth lining with papillary excrescences and mural nodules pro-

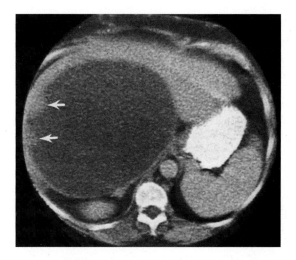

Fig. 29-26. Biliary cystadenocarcinoma. Contrast-enhanced CT scan demonstrates this large cystic mass of the liver to contain mural nodules *(arrows)*, distinguishing it from a large simple cyst.

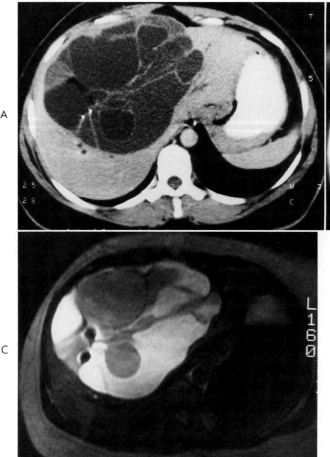

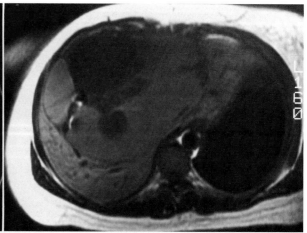

Fig. 29-27. 37-year-old woman with recurrent biliary cystadenoma. **A,** Contrast-enhanced CT scan shows the large, predominately cystic attenuation, multiloculated intrahepatic lesion to contain several surgical clips from a previous resection. **B,** T1-weighted image (TR 500/TE 20) shows the mass to be composed of multiple locules of variable low-signal intensity relative to the remainder of the liver. **C,** T2-weighted image (TR 2200/TR 80) shows the mass to consist of varied signal, predominately hyperintense as a result of the protein content of the locules.

jecting from the cyst wall. There is no consistent distinction grossly between the benign and malignant forms of the disease.

On CT scans, both cystadenoma and cystadenocarcinoma are seen as large, low-attenuation intrahepatic masses, often with thick, irregular walls[4,37,130] (Figs. 29-26, 29-27, *A*). Although cystadenocarcinomas tend to have more solid components and are more irregular than cystadenomas, these signs are not reliable. The presence of adenopathy or metastatic disease is most indicative of cystadenocarcinoma.

MR imaging shows the multiple locules of cystadenoma or cystadenocarcinoma to be of variable signal intensity on T1W and T2W imaging, depending on the protein content or presence of hemorrhage within the locules.[191,210] Septations are seen as low-intensity bands[123] (Figs. 29-27, *B*, 29-27, *C*).

Angiosarcoma

Angiosarcoma of the liver is a tumor that consists of malignant endothelial lining cells, occurring primarily in adults exposed to chemical agents and radiation.[46,112,129] The malignant endothelial cells line vascular channels of sizes that vary from cavernous to capillary, which attempt to form sinusoids. When associated with thorium dioxide (thorotrast) exposure, the thorotrast particles may be found within the malignant endothelial cells. Grossly, most angiosarcomas are multiple and contain internal hemorrhage.[129] When it appears as a large single mass, it often has cystic areas of bloody debris and does not have a capsule. Concurrent cirrhosis is common.

A rare neoplasm that is 30 times less common than HCC, angiosarcoma occurs most commonly in men in the seventh decade of life.[102] It is associated with previous exposure to radiation, thorotrast, or toxins such as polyvinyl chloride (PVC), arsenics, and steroids; it has also been associated with hemochromatosis. Patients may present with weakness, weight loss, abdominal pain, ascites, and hepatomegaly. Platelet segregation in a large angiosarcoma may cause thrombocytopenia. Rupture with hemoperitoneum may rarely occur.[103,145]

On unenhanced CT, single or multiple hypodense masses may be seen except for slightly hyperdense nod-

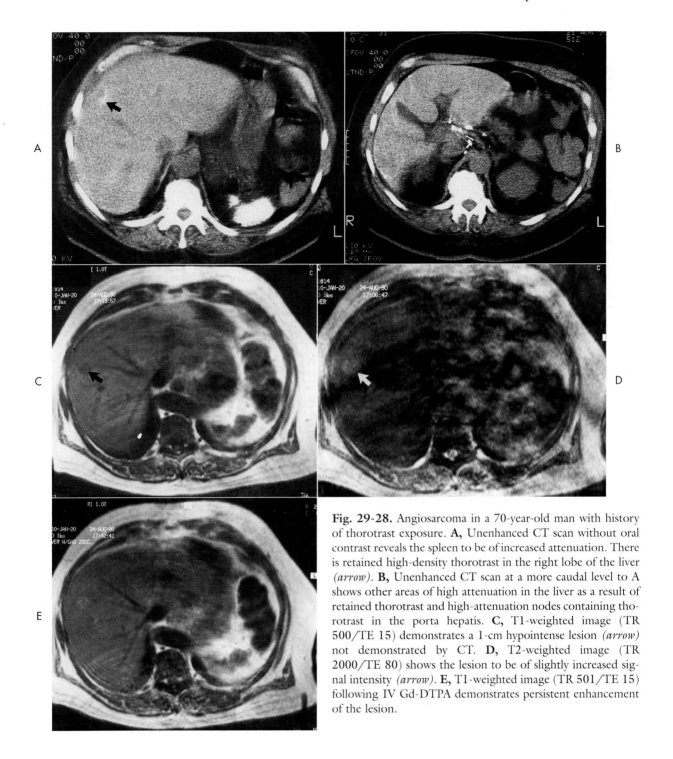

Fig. 29-28. Angiosarcoma in a 70-year-old man with history of thorotrast exposure. **A,** Unenhanced CT scan without oral contrast reveals the spleen to be of increased attenuation. There is retained high-density thorotrast in the right lobe of the liver *(arrow)*. **B,** Unenhanced CT scan at a more caudal level to A shows other areas of high attenuation in the liver as a result of retained thorotrast and high-attenuation nodes containing thorotrast in the porta hepatis. **C,** T1-weighted image (TR 500/TE 15) demonstrates a 1-cm hypointense lesion *(arrow)* not demonstrated by CT. **D,** T2-weighted image (TR 2000/TE 80) shows the lesion to be of slightly increased signal intensity *(arrow)*. **E,** T1-weighted image (TR 501/TE 15) following IV Gd-DTPA demonstrates persistent enhancement of the lesion.

ules seen with recent hemorrhage.[141,232] After IV contrast administration, a centripetal enhancement pattern similar to that seen with hemangioma has been reported.[232] When related to thorotrast exposure, the reticular pattern of thorotrast deposition may be well seen in the liver, with significantly increased density in the spleen and lymph nodes (Figs. 29-28, *A,* 29-28, *B*). If

rupture occurs, hemoperitoneum may be demonstrated.[149] In our experience, circumferential displacement of thorotrast in the periphery of a nodule is a characteristic finding of angiosarcoma. The MR imaging appearance of angiosarcoma is limited.[209] In our experience, angiosarcoma appears as a hypointense mass relative to liver on T1W imaging, and it is hyperintense on T2W imaging (Figs. 29-28, *C*, 29-28, *D*). Peripheral rim enhancement is present after the administration of IV gadolinium, with persistent enhancement, seen in delayed images that may mimic the appearance of hemangioma (Fig. 29-28, *E*). The presence of thorotrast is not detectable by MR imaging.

Epithelioid hemangioendothelioma (EHE)

Epithelioid hemangioendothelioma (EHE) is a very rare malignant neoplasm of the liver and is of vascular origin.[46] EHE develops in adults and should not be confused with infantile hemangioendothelioma, which occurs in young children. These tumors are often multiple, consisting of neoplastic cells that infiltrate the sinusoids, hepatic veins, and portal vein branches. Although usually an incidental finding, EHE may occasionally cause jaundice, hepatic failure, and rupture with hemoperitoneum.[106] It is more common in women than men. The prognosis of EHE is more favorable than that of angiosarcoma, with extrahepatic metastases occurring in only one third of reported cases. Metastatic or synchronous lesions may also be found in the lungs and soft tissues.

Epithelioid hemangioendothelioma appears on unenhanced CT as multiple peripheral nodules that coalesce to form large confluent low-attenuation masses.[166,199,256] Peripheral portions of the mass become isodense relative to liver after IV contrast administration, thus making identification of the extent of the lesion less sensitive than on the unenhanced scan. The lesions often cause capsular retraction or flattening and may contain calcifications. A peripheral hypodense hypovascular rim and venous invasion may be seen after contrast administration.

MR imaging of epithelioid hemangioendothelioma accurately depicts the extent of the lesions.[166,256] Variable signal intensity, predominantly low to isointense relative to liver, has been described on T1W images. On T2W images, the lesions are of heterogeneous increased signal intensity. On both T1W and T2W images, peripheral low signal intensity rims are often seen. After IV Gd-DTPA administration, concentric layers of alternating signal intensity are seen with an outer, nonenhancing hypointense rim that corresponds with the hypovascular, hypodense rim seen on contrast-enhanced CT. Capsular retraction or flattening over the multiple peripheral nodules, which coalesce into confluent masses, is shown by MR similar to that seen by CT.

Mesenchymal sarcoma

Tumors that arise in the mesenchymal elements of the liver are very rare. These include angiomyosarcoma, leiomyosarcoma, fibrous sarcoma, malignant fibrous histiocytoma, and rhabdomyosarcoma.[42,66,150]

These mesenchymal sarcomas usually appear as large, solitary masses that may be smoothly lobulated and contain fibrous septa, often with central necrosis and hemorrhage.

CT usually demonstrates primary hepatic sarcoma as a large, noncalcified, low-attenuation homogeneous mass on unenhanced scans. After IV contrast administration, there is inhomogeneous peripheral enhancement. The MR imaging appearance is nonspecific, with the mass having low signal intensity relative to liver on T1W imaging and increased signal intensity on T2W imaging.[209]

Hepatoblastoma

Hepatoblastoma, the most common primary liver neoplasm of childhood, is a malignant neoplasm of hepatocyte origin that often contains mesenchymal tissues.[104] It is classified histologically as epithelial or mixed (epithelial-mesenchymal).[46] Epithelial hepatoblastoma is composed of malignant fetal and/or embryonal hepatocytes. The mixed hepatoblastoma consists of both an epithelial (hepatocyte) component and a mesenchymal component composed of primitive mesenchymal tissue and osteoid material and/or cartilage.[265] This histologic classification is useful for predicting clinical outcome. The epithelial type, especially that with a fetal hepatocyte predominance, has the best prognosis.[93,265] Tumors with the embryonal epithelial cell type have a poor prognosis. A rare anaplastic form of hepatoblastoma has the poorest prognosis of all types.[46]

Grossly, hepatoblastoma is usually a large, solitary well-circumscribed mass with a nodular or lobulated surface. In 20% of cases, it may be multifocal.[46] Epithelial hepatoblastomas are homogeneous internally, while mixed hepatoblastomas with osteoid and cartilage may have large calcifications, fibrotic bands, and an overall heterogeneous appearance.[265]

Hepatoblastoma usually is found in the first 3 years of life; it has a peak incidence between 18 and 24 months of age. However, it may be present at birth or may develop in adolescents and young adults.[93] It is more frequent in males than females. The child with hepatoblastoma may present with abdominal swelling, often with anorexia or weight loss. The serum alpha-fetoprotein level is usually significantly elevated. Metastatic disease to the lungs is often present at diagnosis.[48]

Hepatoblastoma appears on unenhanced CT scans as a large, solid, low-attenuation mass that may contain calcifications.[48] Bands of fibrosis, when present, may cause a lobulated pattern. Calcification is most extensive in the mixed form of hepatoblastoma. Following IV contrast administration, there may be extensive enhancement because of the tumor's hypervascular nature. Vascular invasion may be present (Fig. 29-29, *A*).

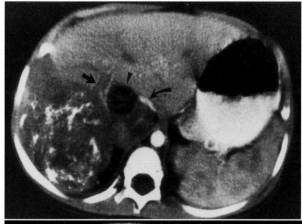

A

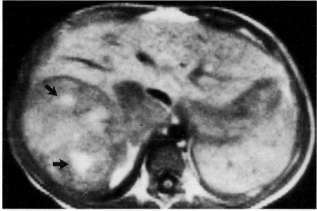

B

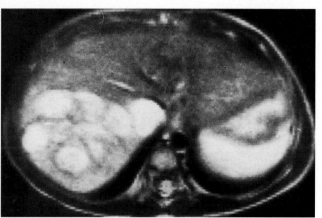

C

Fig. 29-29. Hepatoblastoma, mixed type. **A,** Dynamic contrast-enhanced CT scan shows a large mass of the right lobe of the liver of predominately low attenuation and containing multiple calcifications. There is right portal vein invasion *(straight arrow).* A cystic area of necrosis is present *(arrowhead).* The IVC *(curved arrow)* is compressed by a portion of the mass. **B,** T1-weighted image shows the mass to be of predominately hypointense signal with areas of increased signal intensity that represent hemorrhage *(arrows).* **C,** T2-weighted image demonstrates the lesion to have increased signal intensity with hypointense bands that represent fibrous septations.

MR imaging demonstrates hepatoblastoma to be hypointense relative to liver on T1W imaging and hyperintense on T2W imaging[21] (Figs. 29-29, *B,* 29-29, *C*). Fibrotic septa, when present, appear as low-signal–intensity bands on T2W images. Vascular invasion when present is well demonstrated by gradient-echo imaging or MR angiography.

Undifferentiated embryonal sarcoma (UES)

Undifferentiated embryonal sarcoma (UES) is a malignant tumor that is the fourth most common hepatic neoplasm of childhood, after hepatoblastoma, IHE, and HCC.[241] It consists of primitive, undifferentiated spindle cells resembling primitive (embryonal) cells with frequent mitoses and a myxoid stroma. Grossly, UES is a large, usually solitary mass having well-defined margins with an occasional pseudocapsule. Internally, it has cystic areas of varying sizes that contain necrotic debris, hemorrhage, blood, and/or gelatinous material.[101,241] Predominantly cystic tumors are more common than solid tumors.

UES usually occurs in older children, 6 to 10 years of age, with 90% of cases under the age of 15. UES occurs with almost equal frequency in males and females.[241] Presenting symptoms are usually a painful ab-

dominal mass, with fever, jaundice, weight loss, and gastrointestinal complaints less common. Serum alpha-fetoprotein levels are usually not elevated.

On CT, UES appears as a low-attenuation mass that may have a cystic or heterogeneous appearance, depending on the degree of necrosis and hemorrhage present[216] (Fig. 29-30, *A*). Septa and solid portions of the tumor appear as dense bands within the cystic tumor. If a pseudocapsule is present, it may appear as a thin rim of dense tissue that surrounds the predominantly cystic mass.

The MR imaging appearance of UES has not been reported. In our experience, UES appears as a predominantly hypointense mass relative to liver on T1W imaging with areas of high signal intensity, corresponding to areas of recent hemorrhage (Fig. 29-30, *B*). The mass is significantly hyperintense relative to liver on T2W imaging, reflecting the predominantly cystic nature of the lesion (Fig. 29-30, *C*). Internal debris and septations are well shown on T2W images.

Lymphoma

Hepatic lymphoma is seen as a secondary tumor in both Hodgkin's disease and nonHodgkin's lymphoma. Rarely, it may be a primary lesion, almost always

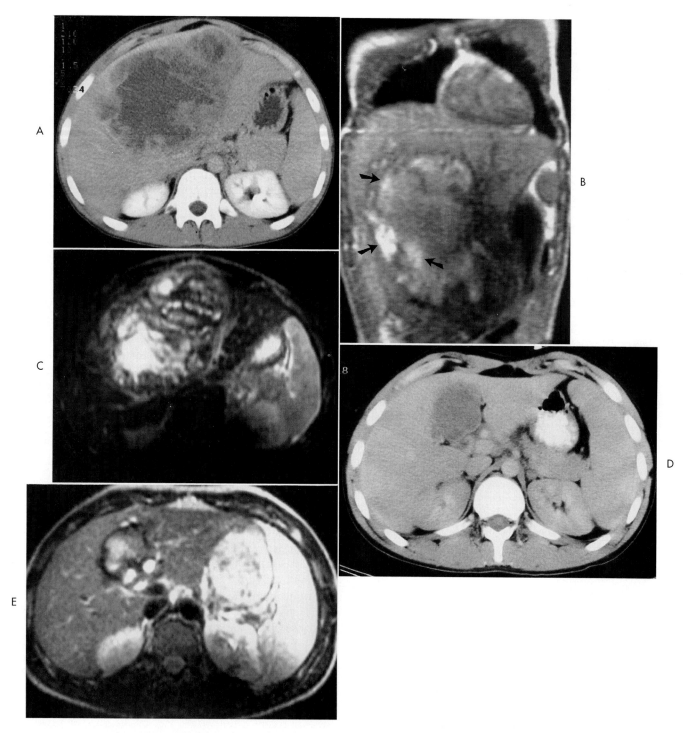

Fig. 29-30. Undifferential embryonal sarcoma in a 15-year-old male. **A,** Contrast-enhanced CT scan demonstrates a very large, central, predominately low attenuation mass having a very heterogeneous appearance. **B,** Coronal T1-weighted image (TR 400/TE 12) demonstrates the large mass to have areas of high signal intensity, corresponding to hemorrhage *(arrows)*. **C,** T2-weighted image (TR 2000/TE 90) shows the mass to be of predominately very high signal intensity. **D,** Following chemotherapy, this contrast-enhanced CT scan demonstrates a significant reduction in the size of the mass. **E,** T2-weighted image (TR 2200/TE 80) following chemotherapy shows the mass to continue to be of mixed signal intensity. The hypointense rim, which represents a pseudocapsule, is demonstrated as low signal intensity. Following the excellent response to chemotherapy, the mass was successfully resected.

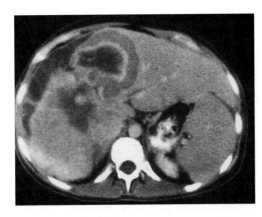

Fig. 29-31. Primary hepatic lymphoma. The contrast-enhanced CT scan shows a large mass of varying attenuation, with contrast enhancement of the tumor lining the necrotic central component. The outer zone of hypovascular tumor remains relatively unenhanced.

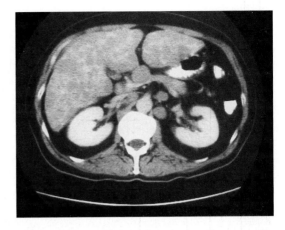

Fig. 29-33. Diffuse infiltrative lymphoma. Contrast-enhanced CT scan demonstrates diffuse involvement of the liver. Lymphadenopathy is present.

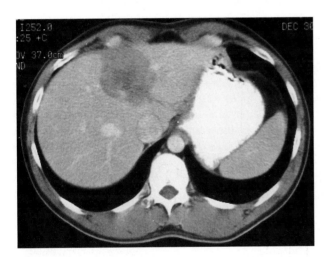

Fig. 29-32. 34-year-old man with nonHodgkin's lymphoma. Contrast-enhanced CT scan demonstrates a focal mass of low attenuation that extended into the portal region on more caudal images.

of the nonHodgkin's large cell type.[220] Grossly, nodular and diffuse forms of hepatic lymphoma may occur. Secondary hepatic lymphoma of Hodgkin's disease occurs more often as diffuse miliary lesions than as focal masses. Hodgkin's disease of the liver is almost always associated with splenic involvement, with the likelihood of hepatic involvement increased when splenic involvement is extensive.[91,30] In both Hodgkin's disease and non-Hodgkin's lymphoma, the portal area is typically initially involved because this is the region where lymphatic tissue of the liver is present.

While primary hepatic lymphoma was previously found most commonly in middle-aged white men, today it is found with increasing frequency in patients who are immunocompromised, such as organ transplant recipients or patients with acquired immunodeficiency syndrome (AIDS).[231] The liver may or may not be enlarged, and patients may present with right upper quadrant pain or a tender mass of the upper abdomen.[20]

CT reveals primary and secondary lymphoma as low attenuation masses of the liver, often large and well circumscribed.[231] Focal solitary or multiple masses may be seen (Figs. 29-31, 29-32). Diffuse infiltration may or may not cause hepatomegaly and may be difficult to distinguish from normal liver tissue (Fig. 29-33). While the specificity of CT for lymphoma of the liver is almost 90%, the sensitivity only approaches 60%, mainly because of the difficulty in detection of the infiltrative form of hepatic lymphoma.[34,280]

MR imaging demonstrates focal masses of hepatic lymphoma to be of low signal intensity relative to liver on T1W imaging and of high signal intensity relative to liver on T2W imaging.[269] The diffuse infiltrative form of hepatic lymphoma cannot be reliably detected by MR imaging any better than by CT.

Metastatic disease

Hepatic metastatic disease is the most common malignancy of the noncirrhotic liver, surpassed in incidence of focal lesions only by hemangioma, focal fatty change, and simple cysts. Metastases occur 30 times more commonly than other malignancies in the noncirrhotic liver. However, in the cirrhotic liver HCC remains about nine times more common than metastatic disease.[161] Malignant tumors metastasize to the liver from almost all primary sites, most frequently from carcinomas of the GI tract (most commonly colon, rectum, stomach, and pancreas), lung, and breast.[56] Hepatic metastases may vary in size, consistency, uniformity of growth, response of surrounding tissue, and vascularity.[56,57] Lesions may be infiltrative, expansive or miliary. The primary source of metastasis and the mode of spread influence all of these factors. Individual metastatic liver lesions may differ greatly in appearance in the same patient because of variations in cellular differentiation, fibrosis, necrosis, hemorrhage, and blood supply. This is most common in the vascular metastatic tumors of renal cell carcinoma, carcinoid, choriocarcinoma, and some types of lung cancer. A zone of venous stasis may be observed surrounding a metastatic lesion, extending up to 1 cm, in approximately 25% of patients.[56,57] The zone is uniformly circumferential and either all or none of the metastatic lesions have this finding in a given patient. Seen most commonly with lung cancer and least commonly with colon carcinoma, it has important implications for imaging.

Tumor thrombi that occlude the portal and/or hepatic veins may be seen in approximately 7% to 15% of patients with hepatic metastatic disease.[56,57] When the large portal veins are penetrated, metastases disseminate throughout peripheral portal branches. When the hepatic veins are penetrated, pulmonary metastases may result. The vascular supply of liver metastases is almost entirely from the hepatic artery.[1] Although hepatic metastases from gastrointestinal tract neoplasms originally derive their blood supply from the portal vein, it progressively becomes arterial. However, if therapeutic arterial ligation is performed, the blood supply may revert to the portal vein.

Metastases may develop calcification that is detectable by CT scanning in the presence of mucin, necrosis, and phosphatase activity. This is most commonly seen in metastases of mucinous adenocarcinomas of the colon, pancreas, and stomach.

The most common cause of malignant focal liver lesions, metastases outnumber primary malignant tumors in the noncirrhotic liver 18 to 1. The liver is second only to regional lymph nodes as a site of metastatic disease. Approximately 25% to 50% of all patients who die of malignant disease have metastatic disease of the liver at autopsy. The most common primary neoplasms to cause hepatic metastases are colon (42%), stomach (23%), pancreas (21%), breast (14%), and lung (13%). A silent primary neoplasm with hepatic metastasis is most often found to be a result of pancreatic, stomach, or lung carcinomas. The highest percentage of liver metastases occur in primary carcinomas of the gallbladder, pancreas, colon, and breast, while the lowest occurs in prostate carcinoma.[56,57]

In patients who died with metastatic disease of the liver, approximately 50% had signs or symptoms of liver disease. Hepatomegaly (31%) is the most common finding, followed by ascites (18%) and jaundice (14.5%). Liver function tests are very poor for the detection of hepatic metastatic disease, with normal results in 25% to 50% of patients with metastases. They may be abnormal because of parenchymal replacement by tumor, biliary ductal obstruction, chemotherapy, or hepatotoxicity. Therefore, radiologic imaging has become essential in the evaluation of hepatic metastatic disease.[85,266,273]

Diagnostic challenges in the radiologic evaluation of metastatic disease include staging and follow-up in patients with a known malignancy, and the evaluation of resectability in patients with solitary or few metastases. Dynamic sequential CT during the bolus administration of IV water-soluble iodinated contrast material has gained widespread acceptance as the primary modality in the staging and follow-up of metastatic disease. This technique uses the attenuation difference between the enhancement of the vascular space (injection phase) and normal extravascular tissue (redistribution phase) of the liver parenchyma. The liver must be scanned within 2 minutes of the bolus administration of IV contrast material so that the lesion which is usually hypovascular relative to the liver parenchyma will be displayed as a low-attenuation focus.

Paushter and co-workers found that the bolus technique was superior to the bolus-plus-drip-infusion technique for the detection of metastases.[195] This latter technique results in scanning the liver during the equilibrium phase when the intravascular and interstitial concentrations of contrast material have equilibrated and decline equally, yielding less difference in attenuation between low-attenuation lesions and normal liver than the single-bolus technique.

Although various authors are in agreement in principle, the optimal technique for bolus-enhanced dynamic hepatic CT remains a focus of controversy.* Comparisons made between uniphasic and biphasic IV contrast bolus injection techniques show the uniphasic bolus injection to produce superior hepatic enhancement.[71,80] Single bolus injection rates of 3.0 and 4.5 ml/second have been shown to produce higher CT hepatic contrast enhancement than that reported previously with other techniques.[98]

Bernadino and co-workers have shown that delayed CT scanning performed 4 to 6 hours after the IV bolus injection of a 60-g dose of iodinated contrast material led to increased lesion detection when compared with conventional dynamic bolus-enhanced hepatic CT scanning.[17] The delayed CT scanning technique is based on the normal hepatobiliary secretion of 1% to 2% of the

---

*References 13, 44, 45, 67, 181, 260, 261.

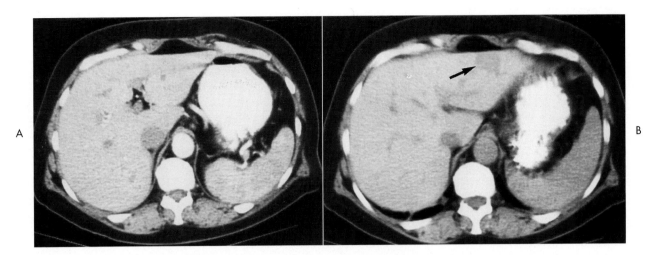

Fig. 29-34. Metastatic breast carcinoma in a middle-aged woman. **A,** Contrast-enhanced CT scan was negative for metastatic disease. **B,** Four-hour delayed CT scan demonstrates hepatic parenchymal enhancement with a low-attenuation lesion *(arrow)* of the left lobe now revealed.

iodine dose, which results in a 20 Housfield unit (HU) difference in liver density between precontrast scans and those obtained 4 to 6 hours later. Iodine secretion is not naturally present in focal benign or malignant hepatic lesions not containing hepatocytes. Therefore, this technique results in lower attenuation of the lesion compared with the increased attenuation of the adjacent liver (Fig. 29-34). However, if liver function is abnormal as in the setting of biliary obstruction or diffuse hepatic disease, this technique may be less successful.

Other IV contrast techniques not in clinical use but undergoing investigation include perfluorooctylbromide (PFOB) and iodized oil emulsion (EOE-13).[29,159,164,165,205] Although both appear to have increased sensitivity for the detection of hepatic metastases, their use may be limited by their side effects.

CT arterial portography (CTAP) and CT arteriography (CTA) are invasive techniques developed to improve lesion detection by maximizing the contrast enhancement difference between normal hepatic parenchyma, which receives approximately 75% to 80% of its blood supply from the portal vein, and hepatic neoplasms, which receive their blood supply from the hepatic artery. CTA of the liver is performed by scanning the liver during iodinated contrast injection of the hepatic or celiac artery, resulting in increased attenuation of focal lesions and improving the detection rate when compared with IV bolus-enhanced dynamic CT.[76] Continuous CT angiography is a technique that obtains 10 to 18 images at each contiguous section level of the liver during the injection of 10 to 20 cc of iodinated contrast material into the hepatic artery. This technique, when compared with biphasic IV bolus-enhanced CT, has been shown to

have higher sensitivity (98%) and accuracy (81%) when correlated with surgical and intraoperative ultrasound findings.[189] However, CTA is limited in patients with anomalous hepatic arterial supply and altered hepatic hemodynamics, producing homogeneous contrast enhancement in only about two thirds of patients.[75]

CTAP is performed during injection of iodinated contrast material through a catheter placed in the superior mesenteric artery, resulting in low attenuation in hepatic lesions as a result of their predominately arterial blood supply while the portal venous return homogeneously enhances the normal hepatic parenchyma (Fig. 29-35). This technique has gained widespread acceptance as the most sensitive preoperative method of detecting liver metastases, with its superiority being manifest in the detection of lesions less than 1 cm in diameter.[8,99,180] It has also been shown to be useful in determining the segmental location (as described by Couinaud) of lesions for surgical planning.[179] However, a significant false-positive rate due to benign lesions and perfusion variations in normal hepatic parenchyma persists. Peterson and co-workers, correlating CTAP results in 60 patients with pathologic, surgical, and intraoperative ultrasound findings, sought to reduce the false-positive rate by characterizing benign perfusion defects.[196] Peripheral wedge-shaped and flat perfusion defects were found to be almost always benign. Benign perfusion defects were identified in two characteristic locations: in the anteromedial aspect of the medial segment adjacent to the intersegmental fissure, and within the posterior, peripheral aspect of the medial segment, immediately anterior to the porta hepatis.

MR imaging is often used for staging and

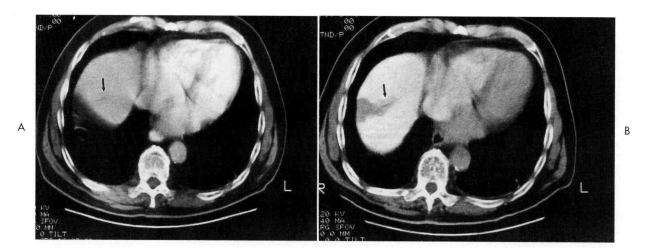

Fig. 29-35. Metastatic adenocarcinoma of the colon. **A,** Contrast-enhanced CT scan suggests a lesion *(arrow)* of the dome of the liver. **B,** CTAP scan demonstrates a low-attenuation lesion with a perfusion defect extending from the lesion *(arrow)* to the periphery of the liver.

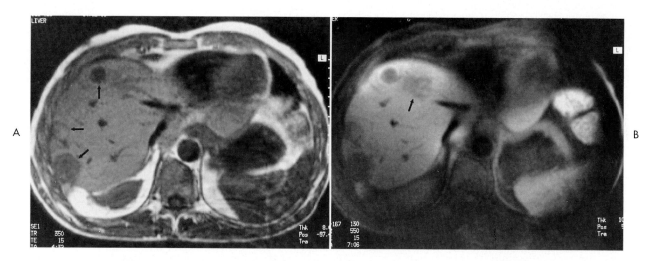

Fig. 29-36. Metastases of colorectal adenocarcinoma. **A,** Conventional T1-weighted image (TR 350/TE 15) demonstrates three focal liver lesions *(arrows)* of varying signal intensity. **B,** Fat-suppression T1-weighted image (TR 550/TE 15) reveals an additional lesion *(arrow)*, seen only retrospectively on the conventional T1-weighted image.

follow-up of metastatic disease when a contraindication to iodinated contrast administration exists such as in patients with a history of serious contrast reaction.[204] It is also often used for further characterization of lesions suspected to represent fatty change and hemangioma rather than metastases.[58] MR imaging, with its superb sensitivity for lesion detection and excellent depiction of vascular anatomy, is well suited as a noninvasive method in the determination of lesion resectability. Although initial reports suggested MR has increased sensitivity for the de-

tection of metastatic disease to the liver, spin-echo MR imaging and dynamic contrast-enhanced CT are now considered by many to have similar overall sensitivity rates approaching 90% in the evaluation of hepatic metastases.[99,237] Fat-suppression techniques and the development of contrast agents that are reticuloendothelial system-directed (such as superparamagnetic iron oxide) and hepatobiliary-specific (such as manganese-DPDP) appear to produce increased sensitivity for the detection of liver metastases by MR imaging, resulting in the po-

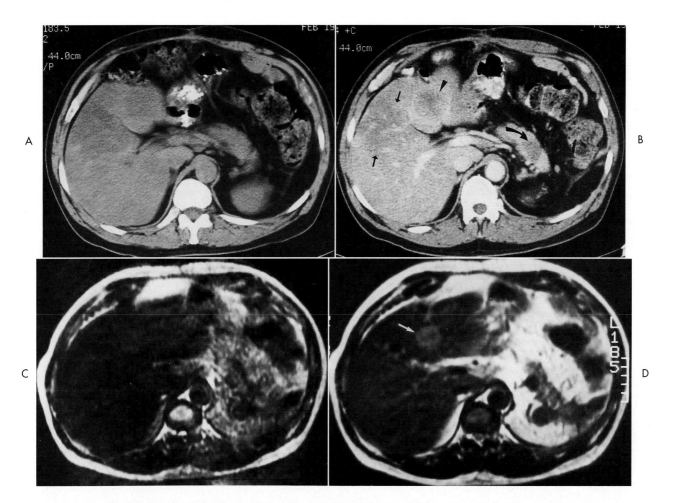

Fig. 29-37. 57-year-old man with metastatic islet cell tumor of the pancreas. **A,** Noncontrast CT scan demonstrates several low-attenuation areas of the right lobe of the liver. **B,** Contrast-enhanced CT scan demonstrates one area of low attenuation to represent fatty infiltration *(straight arrows),* while enhancement of a hypervascular metastatic lesion is noted *(arrowhead).* The islet cell tumor of the pancreas is also demonstrated *(curved arrow).* **C,** Conventional T2-weighted image (TR 2500/TE 90; acquisition time 10 min, 50 sec) demonstrates prominent ghosting artifacts because of respiratory motion. **D,** Fast spin-echo T2-weighted image (TR 6000/TE 102; acquisition time 4 min, 48 sec) confirms the presence of the lesion *(arrow)* suspected by CT.

tential for MR to become the most sensitive noninvasive method of detecting hepatic metastases[64,77,97,143,236] (Fig. 29-36).

On CT scans, metastatic lesions may be hyperdense, isodense, hypodense, hypodense with peripheral enhancement, cystic, complex, calcified, or diffusely infiltrative. The CT appearance is dependent on tumor size, vascularity, hemorrhage, and necrosis, as well as the type of IV contrast bolus and timing of scanning.[10,14,68,78,240]

Hyperdense metastases usually are hypervascular in nature, resulting from primary neoplasms such as melanoma, carcinoid, renal cell carcinoma, pancreatic is-

let cell tumor, choriocarcinoma, pheochromocytoma, and thyroid carcinoma (Fig. 29-37). Breast and bronchogenic carcinoma may also occasionally result in hypervascular metastases (Fig. 29-38). During contrast-enhanced CT scanning, the lesions may become isodense to the normal hepatic parenchyma; therefore, precontrast scans have been recommended before contrast is given[27] (Fig. 29-39).

Some metastases may have a cystic appearance, with an attenuation of less than 20 HU. These "cystic" lesions may be seen with adenocarcinomas such as mucinous carcinoma of the colon and cystadenocarcinoma of the ovary (Fig. 29-40). Other neoplasms having rapid

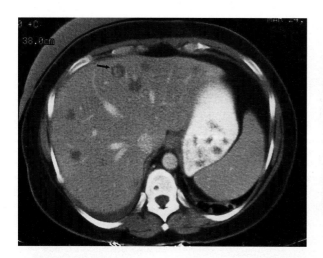

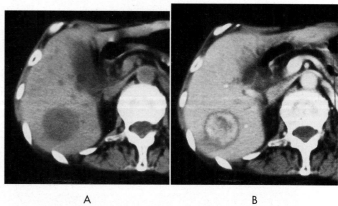

Fig. 29-38. Metastatic breast carcinoma in a 44-year-old woman. Contrast-enhanced CT scan demonstrates several low-attenuation lesions of the liver, one showing central enhancement *(arrow)*, indicating a hypervascular nature.

Fig. 29-39. Hypervascular leiomyosarcoma metastases. **A,** Unenhanced CT scan demonstrates a large low-attenuation mass. **B,** Contrast-enhanced CT scan demonstrates central enhancement with a circumferential unenhancing peripheral rim.

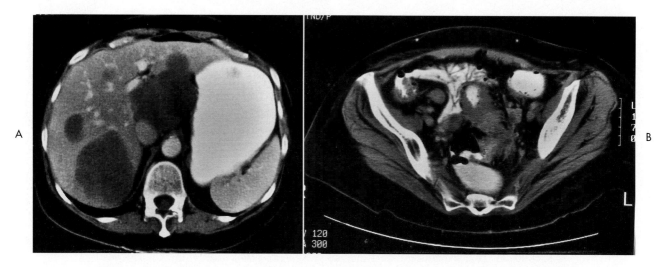

Fig. 29-40. 56-year-old woman with mucinous carcinoma of the sigmoid colon and "cystic" metastases. **A,** Contrast-enhanced CT scan demonstrates multiple low-attenuation lesions of the liver having a cystic appearance. **B,** A large mass of the sigmoid colon is demonstrated with evidence of regional spread.

growth leading to necrosis and a cystic appearance include sarcoma, melanoma, carcinoid, and lung carcinoma. Occasionally, a fluid-debris level may be present[277] (Fig. 29-41).

The majority of liver metastases are hypodense relative to normal liver. Because these lesions are usually hypovascular, the administration of IV contrast material increases the density difference between the lesion and the normal parenchyma. Centrally, low attenuation may be marked if associated with central necrosis or cystic

change (Fig. 29-42). Rim enhancement representing the vascularized viable tumor periphery may be seen (Fig. 29-43). The borders of metastases may be sharply defined, ill-defined, or nodular, and their shape may be ovoid, round, or irregular (Figs. 29-44, 29-45). Calcifications, when present, are well displayed by CT, better when unenhanced[18,225] (Fig. 29-46). Portal vein invasion is best displayed after IV contrast administration (Fig. 29-47).

The T1 and T2 relaxation times of liver metasta-

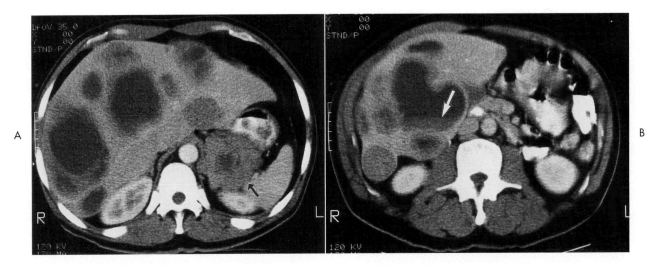

Fig. 29-41. Gastric leiomyosarcoma with cystic metastases. **A,** Contrast-enhanced CT scan demonstrates multiple masses of the liver, with several having very low attenuation centers. A portion of the gastric mass *(arrow)* is shown. **B,** Several centimeters caudal to A, a fluid-debris level *(arrow)* is present in a very large metastatic liver lesion.

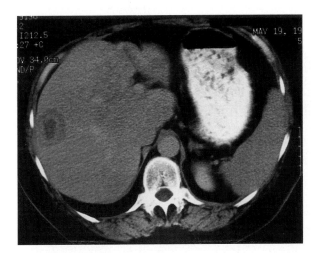

Fig. 29-42. 54-year-old woman with metastatic breast carcinoma. Contrast-enhanced CT scan shows a metastatic lesion having very low attenuation centrally, suggesting necrosis.

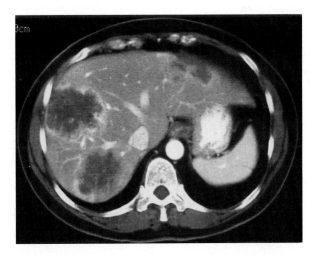

Fig. 29-43. Metastatic breast carcinoma in a 60-year-old woman with fatty infiltration of the liver. Contrast-enhanced CT scan demonstrates rim enhancement of several metastases representing the vascularized viable tumor periphery. Diffuse low attenuation of the liver is due to fatty infiltration as a result of chemotherapy.

ses vary greatly depending on the primary tumor and on the degree of necrosis, hemorrhage, and vascularity. However, the T1 and T2 relaxation times of metastases are longer than those of normal liver and usually shorter than those of simple cysts and hemangiomas, except in some hypervascular metastases.* With the use of Gd-DTPA, hypervascular metastases can be distinguished from hemangioma because of the specific persistence of contrast enhancement in hemangioma. Six major mor-

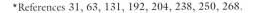

*References 31, 63, 131, 192, 204, 238, 250, 268.

phologic patterns of liver metastases on MR imaging have been described.

Metastatic liver lesions may appear as low-signal–intensity masses containing a distinct central region of even lower signal intensity on T1W imaging because of their long T1 relaxation time (Fig. 29-48). This pattern is often seen with larger lesions and those that undergo necrosis. However, metastases containing mucin, fat,

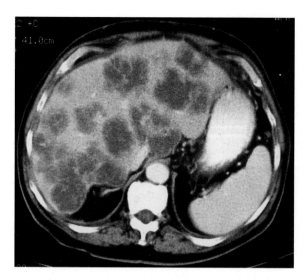

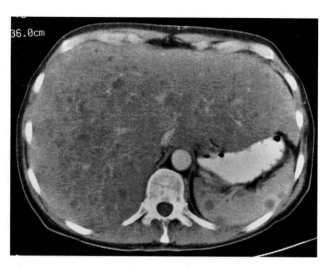

Fig. 29-44. 66-year-old man with metastatic colon carcinoma. Contrast-enhanced CT scan demonstrates multiple metastases having various borders and shapes. A mild degree of rim enhancement is present.

Fig. 29-45. Metastatic melanoma in a 66-year-old woman. Contrast-enhanced CT scan reveals diffuse infiltration of the liver with several focal lesions also shown in the spleen.

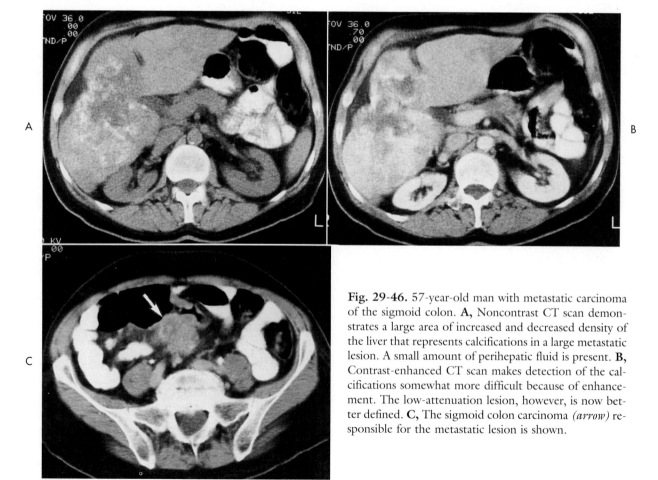

Fig. 29-46. 57-year-old man with metastatic carcinoma of the sigmoid colon. **A,** Noncontrast CT scan demonstrates a large area of increased and decreased density of the liver that represents calcifications in a large metastatic lesion. A small amount of perihepatic fluid is present. **B,** Contrast-enhanced CT scan makes detection of the calcifications somewhat more difficult because of enhancement. The low-attenuation lesion, however, is now better defined. **C,** The sigmoid colon carcinoma *(arrow)* responsible for the metastatic lesion is shown.

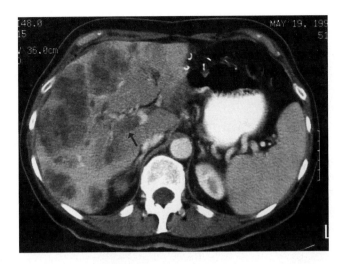

Fig. 29-47. 68-year-old man with extensive gastric adenocarcinoma metastases and portal vein thrombosis. Contrast-enhanced CT scan shows multiple low-attenuation masses of the liver with thrombus present in the right portal vein *(arrow)*. Surgical clips are present related to previous partial gastrectomy.

hemorrhage, or melanin may have a relatively high signal intensity on T1W images.[274]

Some metastatic lesions appear on T2W imaging to have a central rounded area of high signal intensity surrounded by a rim of somewhat weaker signal intensity. This pattern is also commonly seen in large lesions and those that contain necrosis[137,190,274] (Fig. 29-48, C).

Other metastases have variable increased signal intensity on T2W images with inhomogeneous and featureless contents (Fig. 29-49). These amorphous lesions have outer margins that tend to be round and indistinct.[274]

A pattern described as that often seen with colorectal metastases, a rim or "halo" of distinct high-signal intensity varies in thickness from 2 to 10 mm and encircles a lesion of somewhat lower signal intensity on T2W imaging (Fig. 29-50). The lower signal intensity may represent the presence of fibrosis, coagulative necrosis, or mucin. The halo likely is a manifestation of greater water content than the adjacent normal liver parenchyma. Although it has been proposed to represent

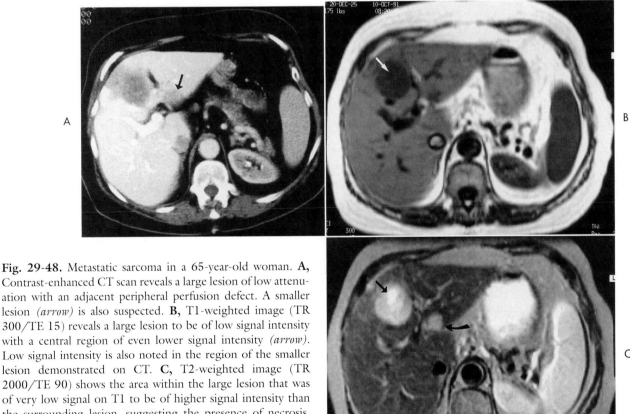

Fig. 29-48. Metastatic sarcoma in a 65-year-old woman. **A,** Contrast-enhanced CT scan reveals a large lesion of low attenuation with an adjacent peripheral perfusion defect. A smaller lesion *(arrow)* is also suspected. **B,** T1-weighted image (TR 300/TE 15) reveals a large lesion to be of low signal intensity with a central region of even lower signal intensity *(arrow)*. Low signal intensity is also noted in the region of the smaller lesion demonstrated on CT. **C,** T2-weighted image (TR 2000/TE 90) shows the area within the large lesion that was of very low signal on T1 to be of higher signal intensity than the surrounding lesion, suggesting the presence of necrosis. The smaller lesion *(curved arrow)* now appears more rounded than it did on the T1-weighted image.

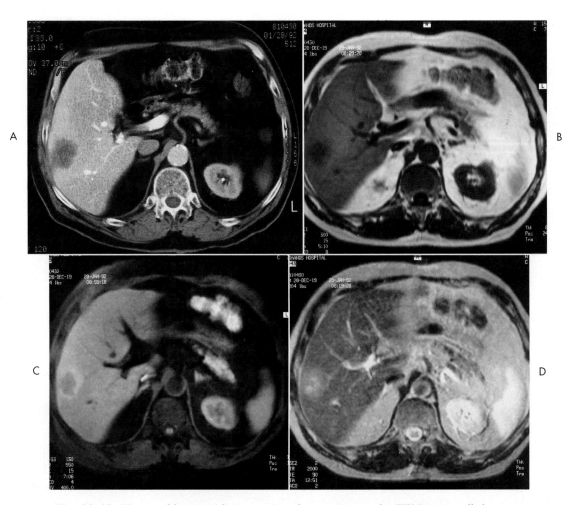

Fig. 29-49. 72-year-old man with metastatic colon carcinoma. **A,** CTAP scan well demonstrates a low-attenuation metastasis of the right lobe of the liver. **B,** T1-weighted image (TR 300/TE 15) shows the low-signal–intensity lesion to be ill-defined. **C,** Fat-suppression T1-weighted image (TR 550/TE 15) shows the mass to be better defined with slightly higher signal intensity of the periphery. **D,** T2-weighted image (TR 2000/TE 90) shows variable increased signal intensity of the lesion with an overall rounded shape but indistinct margins.

peritumoral edema incited by tumor cell infiltration, it more likely represents viable tumor and should be considered when estimating tumor volume and planning resection.[137,190,274]

Hepatic metastatic lesions having smooth, sharply defined borders and being round or elliptical with very high signal intensity on T2W imaging have been described as having a "light bulb" appearance (Fig. 29-51). This may be due to complete tumor necrosis and liquefaction or hypervascularity and has been noted in cystic neoplasms and metastases from primaries such as pheochromocytoma, carcinoid, and islet cell tumor.[84,137,190,274]

Some metastases may change in both size and shape with different pulse sequences. This may be due

to peritumoral edema, which is caused by tumor compromise of the circulation of the more peripheral tissues[274] (Figs. 29-48, *B,* 29-48, *C*).

INFECTIOUS LESIONS
Bacterial (pyogenic) liver abscess

Bacterial abscess of the liver may develop from several routes, most commonly today via the biliary tree, because of ascending cholangitis from benign or malignant biliary obstruction.[6,120] Other sources include portal vein or superior mesenteric vein phlebitis related to appendicitis, diverticulitis, pancreatitis, or other gastrointestinal (GI) infectious source; arterial septicemia as a result of endocarditis, pneumonitis, or osteomyelitis; direct extension from contiguous organs such as perforated

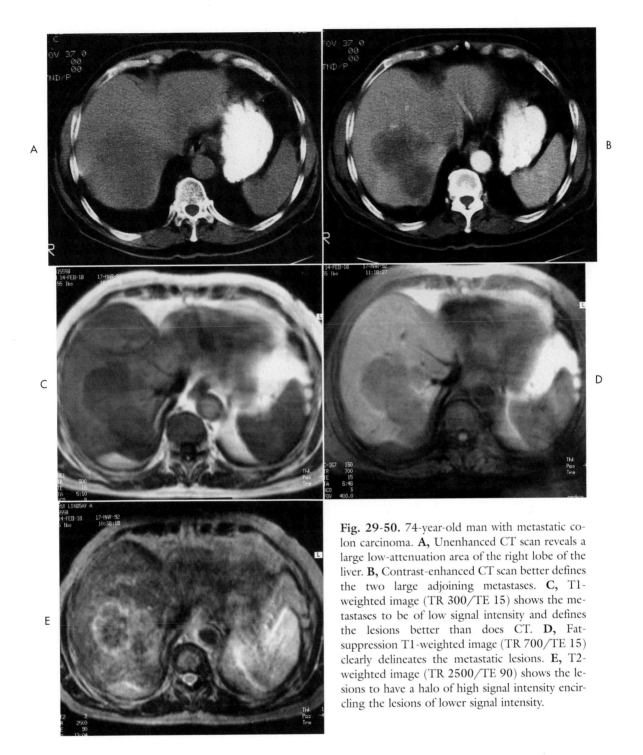

Fig. 29-50. 74-year-old man with metastatic colon carcinoma. **A,** Unenhanced CT scan reveals a large low-attenuation area of the right lobe of the liver. **B,** Contrast-enhanced CT scan better defines the two large adjoining metastases. **C,** T1-weighted image (TR 300/TE 15) shows the metastases to be of low signal intensity and defines the lesions better than does CT. **D,** Fat-suppression T1-weighted image (TR 700/TE 15) clearly delineates the metastatic lesions. **E,** T2-weighted image (TR 2500/TE 90) shows the lesions to have a halo of high signal intensity encircling the lesions of lower signal intensity.

ulcer, pneumonia, or pyelonephritis; post-traumatic; and iatrogenic causes. In patients with diabetes mellitus, a cryptogenic abscess may occur with no identifiable source. Metastases may also become infected.*

*References 5, 6, 33, 41, 120, 162, 173, 233.

Anaerobic or mixed anaerobic and aerobic organisms account for the majority of bacterial liver abscesses. Facultative gram-negative enteric bacilli, anaerobic gram-negative bacilli, and microaerophilic streptococci are often the responsible organisms. In adults, *Escherichia coli* is most commonly isolated, while staphylococcus is most often isolated from pediatric liver abscesses.[25]

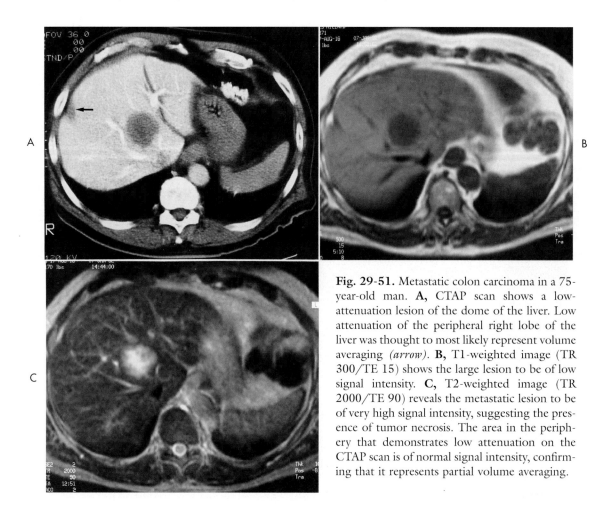

Fig. 29-51. Metastatic colon carcinoma in a 75-year-old man. **A,** CTAP scan shows a low-attenuation lesion of the dome of the liver. Low attenuation of the peripheral right lobe of the liver was thought to most likely represent volume averaging (*arrow*). **B,** T1-weighted image (TR 300/TE 15) shows the large lesion to be of low signal intensity. **C,** T2-weighted image (TR 2000/TE 90) reveals the metastatic lesion to be of very high signal intensity, suggesting the presence of tumor necrosis. The area in the periphery that demonstrates low attenuation on the CTAP scan is of normal signal intensity, confirming that it represents partial volume averaging.

While the incidence of pyogenic abscesses has decreased in the United States, in this country these abscesses do remain the most common infectious lesion of the liver. Individuals between 40 and 60 years of age are most often affected with a slight female predominance. Tender hepatomegaly, fever, malaise, rigors, weight loss, and nausea and vomiting are the most common signs and symptoms of pyogenic liver abscess. Leukocytosis, elevated serum alkaline phosphatase, hypoalbuminemia, and prolonged prothrombin time are the most common laboratory findings.[25,51,198]

Abscesses that are of biliary origin are most often multiple, involving both hepatic lobes in 90% of cases. Abscesses from portal vein sources are often solitary, with 65% occurring in the right lobe, 12% in the left lobe, and 23% in both lobes. This distribution has been attributed to the pattern of mesenteric blood flow in the portal vein.[198]

Treatment of pyogenic liver abscess includes elimination of the abscess as well as the source of infection. Therapeutic options for abscess treatment include surgical drainage, antibiotics alone, percutaneous aspiration with antibiotics, or percutaneous catheter drainage with antibiotics.* Complications of pyogenic liver abscess include septic shock, secondary infection to other organs, perforation with peritonitis, and fistula formation.

CT has greater than 90% sensitivity for the detection of hepatic abscesses, which appear as low-attenuation, rounded masses on both noncontrast and contrast-enhanced scans[95] (Figs. 29-52, 29-53). The attenuation range between 0 and 45 HU overlaps with that of other lesions such as cysts, bilomas, and neoplasms. However, most abscesses have an enhancing peripheral rim or capsule. Although usually sharply defined, some abscesses have a lobulated contour and circumferential "transition zones" of intermediate attenuation.[155] The "cluster" sign may also be seen, with small, less than 2-cm–diameter lesions clustering together with apparent coalescence into a large abscess[114] (Fig. 29-54). These described findings are nonspecific, with aspiration required for diagnosis. Gas bubbles or an air-fluid level are

*References 5, 19, 25, 33, 54, 62, 115, 134, 173, 197.

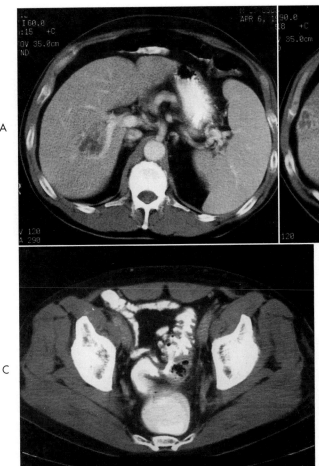

Fig. 29-52. 67-year-old man with pyogenic abscesses resulting from diverticulitis. A, Contrast-enhanced CT scan reveals a low-attenuation lesion near the right portal vein with mild peripheral enhancement. B, A second, more peripheral lesion is also present in the right lobe of the liver, also having enhancement. C, A diverticular abscess was revealed in the pelvis as the source of the abscesses.

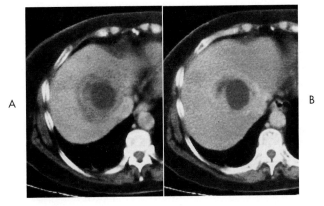

Fig. 29-53. Pyogenic abscess. A, Unenhanced CT scan shows a zone of intermediate densities that surrounds the central low-attenuation cavity. B, Contrast-enhanced CT scan reveals the hyperemic peripheral zone to enhance.

specific signs but are present in less than 20% of cases[95] (Fig. 29-55). The presence of an air-fluid or fluid-debris level may indicate the formation of an enteric communication with the abscess.

MR imaging of pyogenic liver abscess is nonspecific with hypointensity on T1W images and hyperintensity on T2W images relative to liver as in other focal hepatic lesions.[262] The abscess cavity may be homogeneous or heterogeneous, depending on its contents and degree of necrosis and debris. The capsule may appear as a low-intensity rim. After IV Gd-DTPA administration, rapid enhancement of the abscess wall is followed by a slower increase in signal intensity centrally.[227,267]

Fungal abscesses

Candidiasis, the most frequent systemic fungal infection in immunocompromised patients, is becoming more common with the increase in incidence of the acquired immunodeficiency syndrome (AIDS) and with bone marrow transplantation, chemotherapy, and radia-

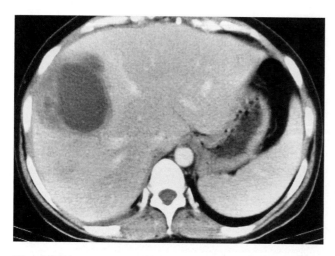

Fig. 29-54. Pyogenic abscess. Contrast-enhanced CT scan demonstrates the "cluster" sign with two small lesions adjacent to the large central cavity.

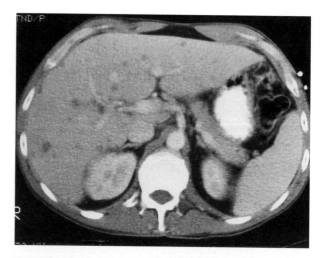

Fig. 29-56. Immunocompromised man with leukemia having hepatic candidiasis. Contrast-enhanced CT scan demonstrates multiple low-attenuation foci of the liver.

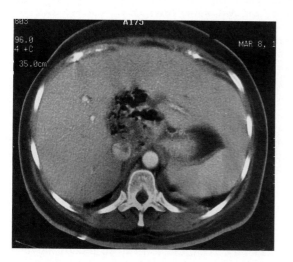

Fig. 29-55. Gram-negative pyogenic abscess of unknown etiology in a 52-year-old woman with diabetes. Contrast-enhanced CT scan demonstrates multiple air-fluid levels in this large central hepatic abscess.

tion therapy. At autopsy, hepatic candidiasis is found in up to 70% of acute leukemia patients and in 50% of patients with lymphoma. Concurrent splenic involvement is most common, often termed *hepatosplenic candidiasis.* Detection may be difficult as blood cultures are positive in only 50% of patients.[70,90,248] Although aspiration for culture and diagnosis may be needed, treatment usually is by antifungal therapy alone without percutaneous drainage.

The most common appearance of hepatic candidiasis on CT scans is that of multiple small round areas of decreased attenuation that may require both precon-

trast and postcontrast scans to visualize (Fig. 29-56). On noncontrast scans, areas of scattered increased density that represent calcification may be seen. Periportal fibrosis appearing as increased attenuation may also be present.[15,229,230]

MR imaging of Candida microabscesses of the liver and spleen has been reported to show multiple small lesions of intermediate signal intensity on T1W images and increased signal intensity on T2W images relative to liver. However, in this case report of a patient with increased iron deposition in the liver and spleen related to multiple blood transfusions, the decreased signal intensity of the liver and spleen improved the contrast resolution of the candidal microabscesses.[36]

Amebic abscess

Amebiasis occurs most often in tropical or subtropical zones of the world, but it is seen more commonly in the United States as a result of travel and migration, and in institutionalized patients and homosexuals.[203] Caused by the protozoan parasite *Entamoeba histolytica,* amebic liver abscess is the most common extraintestinal manifestation of amebiasis.[92,117,128,203,228] Amebic liver abscesses result when the parasite crosses the colonic mucosa and enters the portal circulation (most common route) or lymphatics, or directly extends into the liver from the hepatic flexure.[92,198]

The cavitary amebic abscess occurs as liver tissue is focally destroyed. Initially, the lesion contains necrotic tissue including the viable organism. As the lesion becomes larger, central cavitation is apparent, and the active organism lies within the necrotic tissue lining the cavity. Surrounding this layer is an inflammatory zone of hepatic parenchyma being invaded by the organisms. Centrally, the cavity is often filled by a thick fluid that resembles "anchovy paste." Frequently solitary, the abscess is most commonly located in the right lobe. This is related to the venous drainage from the usually infected right colon, via the superior mesenteric vein to the portal vein, preferentially flowing into the right lobe of the liver.[198] Complications include rupture of the abscess through the diaphragm into the pleural space or lung or into the pericardium or peritoneum.[117,198,228]

Serologic testing is often useful for the detection of amebiasis.[92,128,203] However, percutaneous aspiration is occasionally needed for diagnosis. Biopsy of the abscess wall, which contains the living parasite, is more likely to be diagnostic than is aspiration of the thick reddish-brown "anchovy paste" fluid, which may or may not be present. Percutaneous drainage may be helpful if usually successful medical therapy should fail.[201,222,255,257]

On CT scans, amebic abscesses of the liver appear as low-attenuation lesions, with the density of a lesion dependent on its stage of development and internal contents.[95,200] Lesions that are early in development may have an appearance similar to those of solid tumors, while older abscesses are more cystic in appearance. If multiple, lesions may have differing appearances as a result of different stages of development. The zone of inflammation, of variable thickness and density, is isodense to hypodense on unenhanced CT scans and usually enhances after contrast administration. A thin outer rim of lower attenuation may surround the enhancing layer, giving the lesion a target appearance, and defines the outer boundary of the inflamed hepatic parenchyma (Fig. 29-57).

On T1W and T2W MR images, amebic abscesses have a well-defined appearance with rims of varying signal intensity[59,202] (Fig. 29-58, A, and B). On T1W images, the central cavity is usually of decreased signal intensity relative to normal liver. The central cavity has increased signal intensity on T2W images and often is surrounded by a ring of higher signal intensity that corresponds to the reactive zone. Adjacent high-signal intensity on T2W images is suspected to represent segmental edema. After Gd-DTPA administration, the hyperemic reactive zone demonstrates enhancement similar to that seen with contrast-enhanced CT (Fig. 29-58, D). MR imaging after successful medical therapy shows a reduction in the signal intensity of the hyperintense area that surrounded the abscess cavity on T2W images.

Echinococcal disease

Hydatid disease of the liver, caused by the larvae of a tapeworm, has two different forms. The cystic form, caused by *Echinococcus granulosus*, is more common, occurring in Mediterranean countries, South America, Australia, and New Zealand. The alveolar form, caused by

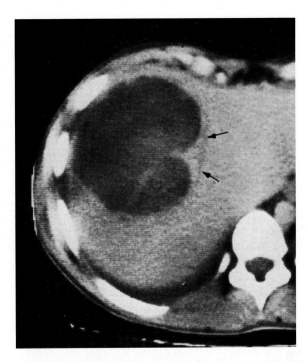

Fig. 29-57. Amebic abscess. Contrast-enhanced CT scan shows the peripheral low-attenuation rim *(arrows)* to define the outer limit of the inflammatory wall. An internal septum is present in the large, low-attenuation central cavity.

Echinococcus multilocularis (alveolaris), is found in central Europe, the Soviet Union, and other areas of the northern hemisphere, including Alaska.[135]

In echinococcal disease caused by *E. granulosus,* the dog is usually the definitive host with sheep being the most common intermediate hosts. In some areas, about 50% of dogs and up to 90% of sheep and cattle may be infected. When material contaminated by dog feces containing eggs of the parasite is ingested, humans may become intermediate hosts. The eggs hatch within the intestinal tract of the host and penetrate the intestinal mucosa, entering the lymphatics and portal venous system. Most are then filtered by the liver and lungs, thus accounting for the high rate of cyst development in the liver (up to 75% of cases) and lungs.

The cysts, which may be solitary or multiple, grow slowly to reach a large size. The wall of the cyst contains three layers: the pericyst, the outer layer formed by the reactive tissue of the host organ; the endocyst, the inner germinal layer containing the growing parasite; and the ectocyst, the intermediate layer consisting of a proteinaceous membrane. Daughter cysts may develop within the parent cyst as a result of fragmentation of the germinal layer. Brood capsules, also produced by the germinal layer, give rise to scolices, which are infectious miniature tapeworms. When brood capsules and scolices separate

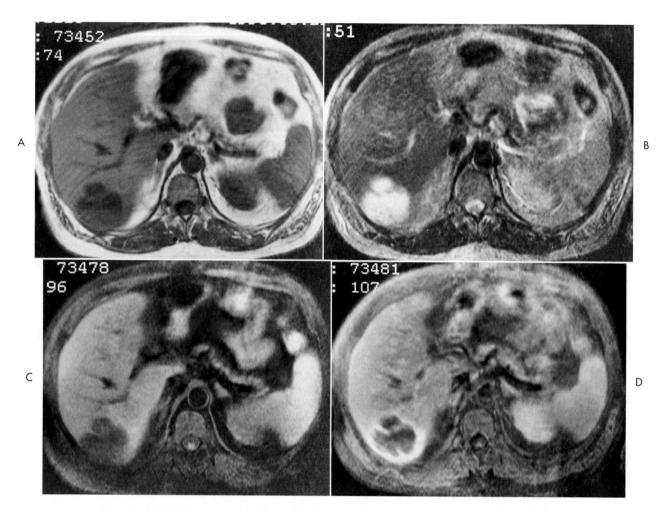

Fig. 29-58. 60-year-old man with amebic liver abscess. **A,** T1-weighted image (TR 300/TE 15) demonstrates a lobulated, low-signal–intensity lesion of the posterior segment of the right lobe of the liver. **B,** T2-weighted image (TR 2400/TE 90) demonstrates the lesion to be of high signal intensity relative to the liver. The internal septa are of low signal intensity. **C,** Fat-suppression T1-weighted image (TR 800/TE 15) demonstrates the lesion to continue to be of low signal intensity. **D,** Fat-suppression T1-weighted image (TR 800/TE 15) after IV Gd-DTPA demonstrates enhancement of the rim and internal septa.

from the germinal layer, debris termed "hydatid sand" that falls to the dependent portion of the cyst is formed. Calcification of the ectocyst alone may occur, and when the parasite dies, the true cyst wall (both ectocyst and endocyst) may also calcify or may separate from the pericyst.[43,135,175]

Hydatid cysts of the liver are often asymptomatic for many years, becoming painful only after reaching a very large size.[86] Often they are discovered incidentally during radiologic imaging performed for other reasons. The majority of complications of hydatid cysts are related to rupture of the cysts into surrounding structures such as the biliary tree, pleura, or peritoneum.[23,142] If peritoneal rupture or spillage during surgical excision occurs,

a serious anaphylactic reaction may result. Serologic testing for echinococcal disease is positive in more than 80% of patients with hepatic lesions.[86] Treatment includes medical antiparasitic drug therapy and surgical removal.[12,136] Several reports describe successful percutaneous drainage.* Medical therapy before drainage is advocated to reduce the risk of anaphylactic reaction in case of accidental spillage.

Echinoccocal cyst of the liver appears on CT scans as a well-defined, round or oval cystic mass of the liver having a density near that of water[2,119,176,193,226] (Fig. 29-59). Daughter cysts, indicating viability, give the le-

*References 3, 28, 65, 83, 126, 172, 223.

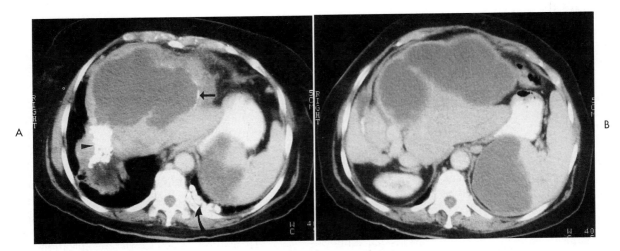

Fig. 29-59. 77-year-old woman with echinococcal cysts of the liver and spleen. **A,** Contrast-enhanced CT scan shows a large cyst of the liver with calcification of the cyst wall *(straight arrow)*. An area of dense calcification *(arrowhead)* is related to a previous resection. Involvement of the spleen is present. Calcification in the left lung base *(curved arrow)* is related to prior involvement of the pleural space. **B,** Several centimeters more caudal to A, additional cysts involving the liver, as well as the large splenic cyst, are shown.

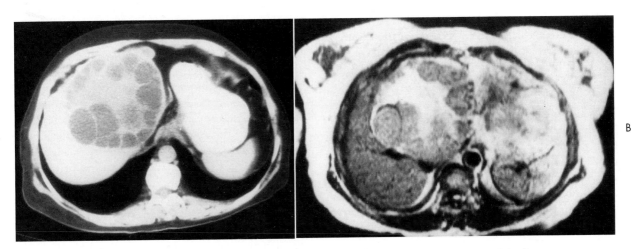

Fig. 29-60. Echinococcal cyst. **A,** Contrast-enhanced CT scan shows a large cyst of the liver that contains multiple daughter cysts, which indicate viability. **B,** T2-weighted image demonstrates the low-signal–intensity rim that corresponds to the collagen-rich pericyst. The daughter cysts are shown to be slightly hyperintense relative to the liver but hypointense relative to the very high signal intensity of the internal hydatid fluid.

sion a multilocular appearance (Fig. 29-60, *A*). The outer wall may appear as a rim of tissue outlined peripherally by a line of slightly lower attenuation, or it may contain calcification. However, extensive calcification usually indicates that the lesion is no longer viable. When detached from the pericyst, the true cyst wall may appear as a thin, wavy membrane within the fluid-filled cyst.[2] After IV contrast administration, the hyperemic ectocyst may slightly enhance.

Hydatid cysts are of decreased signal intensity on T1W MR images and increased signal intensity on T2W images relative to normal liver.[100,151,259,276] A low-signal intensity rim, best seen on T2W images, corresponds to the collagen-rich pericyst surrounding the cyst. The internal architecture is well demonstrated by MR imaging, with the daughter cysts being hypointense to isointense on T1W imaging, and isointense on T2W imaging relative to the hyperintense hydatid fluid and sand of the mother cyst (Fig. 29-60, *B*). The floating membranes seen in a cyst undergoing degeneration appear as low-intensity structures. Intraparenchymal rupture of the wall appears as a defect in the low-intensity rim.[148,259] Calcifications, when present, are not as well demonstrated by MR imaging as by CT but may produce signal void when thick.

The alveolar form of echinococcal disease is distinct from the cystic form in several aspects.[251] The main definitive host is the fox, with small rodents being the usual intermediate hosts. Humans become infected by ingestion of contaminated materials or by direct contact with infected foxes. This disease, in contrast to the expansile cysts of *E. granulosus,* is characterized by the formation of one or more infiltrative liver lesions that stimulate a granulomatous reaction. Internal necrosis, cavitation, and calcification may be seen within the lesion. The CT and MR imaging appearance of the predominately solid lesion of *E. multilocularis* is indistinguishable from that of primary or secondary malignant liver neoplasms.[40,50,226] Atrophy of a lobe or segment of the liver may occur when the lesion is located centrally in the liver.[218] Serologic testing and percutaneous biopsy may be useful for diagnosis when alveolar echinococcal disease is suspected. It should be included in the differential of hepatic lesions in patients who live in or have traveled to endemic regions of the world.

Schistosomiasis

Schistosomiasis is a common parasitic infection with a prevalence of 70% in endemic areas and 10% of patients in these areas developing hepatosplenic involvement.[184] *Schistosoma japonicum* occurs in coastal areas of China, Japan, Formosa, and the Philippines. *S. mansoni* is found in parts of Africa, in the Middle East, and West Indies, and in the northern regions of South America. *S. haematobium* occurs in North Africa, the Mediterranean, and southwest Asia.

The larvae are shed by snails, the intermediate host, into fresh water where human infection occurs when the parasite penetrates skin or mucous membranes. The schistosomes migrate via venules and lymphatics, reaching the heart and then passing through the pulmonary circulation. All die except those that reach the mesenteric circulation, maturing within the intrahepatic portal venous system. A granulomatous reaction to the ova occurs; this leads to periportal fibrosis and may result in portal hypertension. The incidence of hepatocellular carcinoma is increased. The life cycle of the blood fluke is completed after the mature female worm, which has lived with the male in the portal vein for 10 to 15 years, swims to reach the venules of the urinary bladder *(S. haematobium)* or gut *(S. mansoni and S. japonicum)* to lay its eggs. The eggs then pass through the wall of the bladder or intestine to be excreted via urine or feces to infect snails.

On CT scans, peripheral hepatic septal or capsular calcification is characteristic of *S. japonicum* infection.[7,169] Gross pseudoseptations with geographic bands of calcification and notches of the liver margin are also noted. Septal, capsular, and amorphous enhancement may be seen after IV contrast administration.[169] Periportal low-density areas may be apparent. *S. mansoni* infection appears as round, low-attenuation foci with linear branching low-attenuation fibrotic bands engulfing the portal tracts. These bands occasionally show enhancement after IV contrast administration but do not usually calcify.[61]

MR features of schistosomiasis infection include the morphologic changes and associated findings of portal hypertension. The regions of calcification and fibrosis may be demonstrated as curvilinear areas of low signal intensity.

PRACTICAL APPROACH TO HEPATIC MASSES

Advances in radiologic imaging have led to the detection of additional and smaller hepatic lesions. The detection of lesions smaller than 15 mm may be problematic because of their uncertain clinical significance. A single small (≤1.5 cm) lesion was benign in 65% of patients, and two to four small lesions were benign in 59% of cases in a study using CT.[116] As the number of lesions increased, or with the presence of an additional large lesion, there was an increase in the likelihood of malignancy. Even when an extrahepatic malignancy was present, 51% of these small lesions proved to be benign. In patients with dominant metastases who are under consideration for hepatic resection, the possibility that other smaller lesions may be benign must be considered.

A systematic approach to the differential diagnosis of hepatic mass lesions should include both clinical information as well as imaging appearance. Clinically, most important are the age and sex of the patient and whether an extrahepatic malignancy, cirrhosis, infection, or immunocompromise is present. In adults younger than 40 years of age, hemangioma, metastases, FLC, FNH, and HCA are seen. In patients over 50 years of age, hemangioma, metastases, HCC, I-CAC, and angiosarcoma are most frequently seen. In children, infantile hemangioendothelioma is seen before 6 months of age, while the peak incidences of hepatoblastoma and mesenchymal hamartoma are similar at 18 months. In older children and adolescents, HCC and UES may be seen. Regarding sex, benign primary hepatic tumors are generally more frequent in women, while malignant primary hepatic tumors are more frequent in men. Overall, metastatic disease is much more common than primary liver neoplasms in adult as well as in pediatric age groups, except in cirrhotic patients, in whom HCC is more common.[161]

Other important clinical information includes the long-term use of steroids or oral contraceptives. Neoplasms related to such use include HCA and to a lesser degree FNH, NRH, hemangioma, and HCC.[39] With multiple hepatic masses, it should be remembered that metastases, although common, are not the only cause of multiple hepatic lesions. Abscesses, cysts, multifocal or diffuse HCC, I-CAC, angiosarcoma, nodular regenerative hyperplasia, and hemangioma may all present as multiple liver lesions.

The major goal in the evaluation of a suspected hepatic neoplasm is determining whether it is a surgical or nonsurgical lesion. The two most common nonsurgical primary hepatic neoplasms in adults are hemangioma and FNH. All other primary hepatic neoplasms are surgical lesions if resectable. In children, hepatoblastoma, UES, HCC, and mesenchymal hamartoma are considered surgical lesions. Infantile hemangioendothelioma need not be resected if the patient can survive with supportive care or embolization until the tumor spontaneously regresses.

REFERENCES

1. Ackerman NB, Lin WM, Conde ES, et al: The blood supply of experimental liver metastases: I. Distribution of hepatic artery and portal vein blood to "small" and "large" tumors. *Surgery* 66:1067, 1969.
2. Acunas B, Rozanes I, Acunas G, et al: Hydatid cyst of the liver identification of detached cyst lining on CT scans obtained after cyst puncture. *AJR* 156:751-752, 1991.
3. Acunas B, Rozanes I, Celik L, et al: Purely cystic hydatid disease of the liver: treatment with percutaneous aspiration and injection of hypertonic saline. *Radiology* 182:541-543, 1992.
4. Agildere AM, Haliloglu M, Akhan O: Biliary cystadenoma and cystadenocarcinoma. *AJR* 156:1113, 1991.
5. Allard JC, Kuligowska E: Percutaneous treatment of an intrahepatic abscess caused by a penetrating duodenal ulcer. *J Clin Gastroenterol* 95:603-606, 1987.
6. Altmeir WA, Schowenger DT, Whiteley DH: Abscess of the liver: surgical considerations. *Arch Surg* 101:258-267, 1982.
7. Araki T, Hayakawa K, Okada J, et al: Hepatic schistosomiasis japonica identified by CT. *Radiology* 157:757-760, 1985.
8. Balfe DM: Hepatic metastases from colorectal cancer: radiologic streategies for improved selection. *Radiology* 185:18-19, 1992.
9. Barnes PA, Thomas JL, Bernardino ME: Pitfalls in the diagnosis of hepatic cysts by computed tomography. *Radiology* 141:129-133, 1981.
10. Baron RL, Freeny PC, Moss AA: The liver. In Moss AA, Gamau G, Genant HK, editors: *Computed tomography of the whole body*, ed 2, Philadelphia, 1992, WB Saunders, pp 735-822.
11. Bean WJ, Rodan BA: Hepatic cysts: treatment with alcohol. *AJR* 144:237-241, 1985.
12. Behans KE, van Heerden JA: Surgical management of hepatic hydatid disease. *Mayo Clin Proc* 66:1193-1197, 1971.
13. Berland LL: Additional comment: dynamic hepatic CT. *Radiology* 181:22-23, 1991.
14. Berland L, Lee JKT, Stanley RJ: Liver and biliary tract, in Lee JKT, Sagel SS, Stanley RJ, editors: *Computed body tomography with MRI correlation*, ed 2, New York, 1989, Raven Press, pp 593-660.
15. Berlow ME, Spirt BA, Weil L: CT follow-up of hepatic and splenic fungal microabscesses. *J Comput Assist Tomogr* 8:42-45, 1984.
16. Berman MA, Burnham JA, Sheahan DG: Fibrolamellar carcinoma of the liver: an immunohistochemical study of nineteen cases and a review of the literature. *Hum Pathol* 19:784-794, 1988.
17. Bernardino ME, Ervin BC, Steinberg HV, et al: Delayed hepatic CT scanning: increased confidence and improved detection of hepatic metastases. *Radiology* 159:71-74, 1986.
18. Bernardino ME, et al: Computed tomography of calcified liver metastases. *J Comput Assist Tomogr* 3:32-35, 1979.
19. Bertel CK, Van Heerden JA, Sheedy PF: Treatment of pyogenic hepatic abscesses. *Arch Surg* 121:554-558, 1986.
20. Biemer JJ: Hepatic manifestations of lymphoma. *Ann Clin Lab* 14:252-260, 1984.
21. Boechat MI, Kangarloo H, Ortega J, et al: Primary liver tumors in children: comparison of CT and MR imaging. *Radiology* 169:727-732, 1988.
22. Marti-Bonmati L, Menor F, Vizcaino J, et al: Lipoma of the liver: US, CT and MRI appearance. *Gastrointest Radiol* 14:155-157, 1989.
23. Marti-Bonmati L, Serrano FM: Complications of hepatic hydatid cysts: ultrasound, computed tomography, and magnetic resonance diagnosis. *Gastrointest Radiol* 15:119-125, 1990.
24. Bosniak MA, Ambos MA: Polycystic kidney disease. *Semin Roentgenol* 10:133-143, 1975.
25. Brandborg LL, Goldman IS: Bacterial and miscellaneous infections of the liver. In Zakim D, Boyer TD, editors: *Hepatology*. Philadelphia, 1990, WB Saunders, pp 1086-1098.
26. Braun P, Ducharme JC, Riopelle JL, et al: Hemangiomatosis of the liver in infants. *J Pediatr Surg* 10:121-126, 1975.
27. Bressler EL, Alpern MB, Glazer GM, et al: Hypervascular hepatic metastases: CT evaluation. *Radiology* 162:49-54, 1987.
28. Bret PM, Fond A, Bretagnolle M, et al: Percutaneous aspiration and drainage of hydatid cysts in the liver. *Radiology* 168:617-620, 1980.
29. Bruneton J-N, Falewee M-N, Francois E, et al: Liver, spleen, and vessels: preliminary clinical results of CT with perfluorooctylbromide. *Radiology* 170:179-183, 1989.
30. Bruneton JN, Schnider M: *Radiology of Lymphoma*, New York, 1986, Springer-Verlag.
31. Bydder GM: Magnetic resonance imaging of the liver. In Wilkins RA, Nunnerly HB, editors: *Imaging of the Liver, Pancreas, and Spleen*, Oxford, 1990, Blackwell Scientific Publications, pp 49-66.
32. Carr DH, Hadjis NS, Banks LM, et al: Computed tomography of hilar cholangiocarcinoma: a new sign. *AJR* 145:53-56, 1985.
33. Carrel TP, Matthews JB, Baer HU, Blumgart LH: Etiology, diagnosis and treatment of hepatic abscesses after biliary tract surgery. *Ann Chir* 44(9):746-751, 1990.
34. Castellino RA, Hoppe RT, Blank N, et al: Computed tomography, lymphography and staging laparotomy: correlations in initial staging of Hodgkin's disease. *AJR* 143:37-41, 1984.
35. Chen KT, Bocian JJ: Multiple hepatic adenomas. *Arch Pathol Lab Med* 107:274-275, 1983.
36. Cho J, Kim EE, Varma DGK, Wallace S: MR imaging of hepatosplenic candidiasis superimposed on hemochromatosis. *J Comput Assist Tomogr* 14:774-776, 1990.
37. Choi B, Lim JH, Han MC, et al: Biliary cystadenoma and cystadenocarcinoma: CT and sonographic findings. *Radiology* 171:57, 1989.

38. Choi BI, Han MC, Park JH, et al: Giant cavernous hemangioma of the liver: CT and MR imaging in 10 cases. *AJR* 152:1221-1226, 1989.

39. Christopherson WM, Mays ET, Barrows G: A clinicopathologic study of steroid-related tumors. *Am J Surg Pathol* 1:31-41, 1977.

40. Claudon M, Bessieres M, Regent D, et al: Alveolar echinococcosis of the liver: MR findings. *J Comput Assist Tomogr* 14:608-614, 1990.

41. Cohen JL, Martin FM, Rossi RL, et al: Liver abscess: the need for complete gastrointestinal evaluation. *Arch Surg* 124:561-564, 1989.

42. Conran RM, Stocker JT: Malignant fibrous histiocytoma of the liver—a case report. *Am J Gastroenterol* 80:813-815, 1985.

43. Cotran RS, Kumar V, Robbins SL: *Robbins Pathologic Basis of Disease,* ed 4, Philadelphia, 1989 WB Saunders, pp 421-422.

44. Cox IH, Foley WD: Right window for dynamic hepatic CT. *Radiology* 181:18-21, 1991.

45. Cox IH, Foley WD: Dynamic hepatic CT: Drs. Cox and Foley reply. *Radiology* 181:23-24, 1991.

46. Craig GR, Peters RL, Edmonson HA: Tumors of the liver and intrahepatic bile ducts. *Atlas of tumor pathology,* 2nd Series. Washington, DC: Armed Forces Institute of Pathology, 1989.

47. Craig JR, Peters RL, Edmondson JL: Fibrolamellar carcinoma of the liver. *Cancer* 46:372-379, 1980.

48. Dachman AH, Parker RL, Ros PR, et al: Hepatoblastoma: a radiologic-pathologic correlation in 50 cases. *Radiology* 164:15-19, 1987.

49. Dachman AH, Ros PR, Goodman ZD, et al: Nodular regenerative hyperplasia of the liver: clinical and radiologic observations. *AJR* 148:717-722, 1987.

50. Didier D, Weiler S, Rohmer P, et al: Hepatic alveolar echinococcosis: correlative US and CT study. *Radiology* 154:179-186, 1985.

51. De Cock KM, Reynolds TB: Amebic and pyogenic liver abscess, in Schiff L, Schiff ER, editors: *Diseases of the Liver,* ed 6, Philadelphia, 1987, JB Lippincott, pp 1235-1255.

52. Dehner LP, Ewing SL, Sumner HW: Infantile mesenchymal hamartoma of the liver: histologic and ultrastructural observations. *Arch Pathol Lab Med* 99:379-382, 1975.

53. Dehner LP: Hepatic tumors in the pediatric age group: a distinctive clinicopathologic spectrum. *Perspect Pediatr Pathol* 4:217-268, 1978.

54. Do H, Lambiase RE, Deyoe L, et al: Percutaneous drainage of hepatic abscesses: comparison of results in abscesses with and without intrahepatic biliary communication. *AJR* 157:1209-1212, 1991.

55. Ebara M, Ohto M, Wantanabe Y, et al: Diagnosis of small hepatocellular carcinoma: correlation of MR imaging and tumor histologic studies. *Radiology* 159:371-377, 1986.

56. Edmunson HA, Craig JR: Neoplasms of the liver. In Schiff L, Schiff ER, editors: *Diseases of the Liver,* ed 8, Philadelphia, 1987, JB Lippincott, pp 1109-1158.

57. Edmunson HA, Peters RL: Tumors of the liver: pathologic features. *Semin Roentgenol* 18:75-83, 1983.

58. Egglin TK, Rummeny E, Stark DD, et al: Hepatic tumors: quantitative tissue characterization with MR imaging. *Radiology* 176:107-110, 1990.

59. Elizondo G, Weissleder R, Stark DD, et al: Amebic liver abscess: diagnosis and treatment evaluation with MR imaging. *Radiology* 165:795-800, 1987.

60. Fan ZM, Yamashita Y, Harada M, et al: Intrahepatic cholangiocarcinoma: spin-echo and contrast-enhanced dynamic MR imaging. *AJR* 161:313-317, 1993.

61. Fatar S, Bassiony H, Satyanath S: CT of hepatic schistosomiasis mansoni. *AJR* 145:63-66, 1985.

62. Fernandez MDP, Murphy FB: Hepatic biopsies and fluid drainages. *Radiol Clin North Am* 29:1311-1328, 1991.

63. Ferrucci JT: MR imaging of the liver. *AJR* 147:1103-1116, 1986.

64. Ferrucci JT, Stark DD: Iron oxide-enhanced MR imaging of the liver and spleen: review of the first five years. *AJR* 155:943-950, 1990.

65. Filice C, Strosselli M, Brunetti E, et al: Percutaneous drainage of hydatid liver cysts. *Radiology* 184:579, 1992.

66. Alberti-Flor JJ, O'Hara MF, Weaver F, et al: Malignant fibrous histiocytoma of the liver. *Gastroenterology* 89:890-893, 1985.

67. Foley WD: Dynamic hepatic CT. *Radiology* 170:617-622, 1989.

68. Foley WD, Jochem RJ: Computed tomography: focal and diffuse disease. *Radiol Clin North Am* 29:1213-1233, 1991.

69. Francis IR, Agha FP, Thompson NW, et al: Fibrolamellar hepatocarcinoma: clinical, radiologic and pathologic features. *Gastrointest Radiol* 11:67-72, 1986.

70. Francis IR, Glazer GM, Amendola MA, et al: Hepatic abscesses in the immunocompromised patient: role of CT in detection, diagnosis, management, and follow-up. *Gastrointest Radiol* 2:257-262, 1986.

71. Freeny PC: Comparison of uniphasic versus biphasic bolus contrast material injections for dynamic hepatic CT. *Radiology* 181(P):95, 1991.

72. Freeny PC, Baron RL, Teefey SA: Hepatocellular carcinoma: reduced frequency of typical findings with dynamic contrast-enhanced CT in a non-Asian population. *Radiology* 182:143-148, 1992.

73. Freeny PC, Marks WM: Hepatic hemangioma: dynamic bolus CT. *AJR* 147:711-719, 1986.

74. Freeny PC, Marks WM: Patterns of contrast enhancement of benign and malignant hepatic neoplasms during bolus dynamic and delayed CT. *Radiology* 160:613-618, 1986.

75. Freeny PC, Marks WM: Hepatic perfusion abnormalities during CT angiography: detection and interpretation. *Radiology* 159:685, 1986.

76. Freeney PC, Marks WM: Computed tomographic arteriography of the liver. *Radiology* 148:193-197, 1983.

77. Fretz CJ, et al: Detection of hepatic metastases: comparison of contrast-enhanced CT, unenhanced MR imaging, and iron oxide-enhanced MR imaging. *AJR* 155:763-770, 1990.

78. Friedman AC, Fishman EK, Radecki PD, et al: Focal disease. In Friedman AC, editor: *Radiology of the liver, biliary tract, pancreas and spleen,* Baltimore, 1987, Williams & Wilkins, pp 151-264.

79. Friedman AC, Lichtenstein JE, Goodman Z, et al: Fibrolamellar hepatocellular carcinoma. *Radiology* 157:583-587, 1985.

80. Forman HP, Heiken JP, Brink JA, et al: Dynamic contrast-enhanced CT of the liver: comparison of uniphasic and biphasic bolus-injection protocols. *Radiology* 181(P):96, 1991.

81. Gabata T, Matsui O, Kadoya M, et al: MR imaging of hepatic adenoma. *AJR* 155:1009-1011, 1990.

82. Giacomantonio M, Ein SH, Mancer K, et al: Thirty years of experience with pediatric primary malignant liver tumors. *J Pediatr Surg* 19:523-526, 1984.

83. Giorgio A, Tarantino L, Francica G, et al: Unilocular hydatid liver cysts: treatment with US-guided, double percutaneous aspiration and alcohol injection. *Radiology* 184:705, 1992.

84. Goldberg MA, Saini S, Hahn PF, et al: Differentiation between hemangiomas and metastases of the liver with ultrafast MR imaging: preliminary results with T2 calculations. *AJR* 157:727-730, 1991.

85. Golding SJ, Fletcher EWL: The radiology of secondary malignant neoplasms of the liver. In Wilkins RA, Nunnerly HB, editors: *Imaging of the liver, pancreas and spleen.* Oxford, 1990, Blackwell Scientific Publications, pp 198-219.

86. Goldman JS, Brandborg LL: Parasitic diseases of the liver. In Zakim D, Boyer TD, editors: *Hepatology,* Philadelphia, 1990, WB Saunders, pp 1061-1065.

87. Goodman ZD: Benign tumors of the liver. In Okuda K, Ishak KG, editors: *Neoplasms of the liver,* Tokyo, 1987, Springer-Verlag, pp 105-125.

88. Goodman ZD, Ishak DG: Angiomyolipomas of the liver. *Am J Surg Pathol* 8:745-750, 1984.

89. Goodman ZD, et al: Kupffer cells in hepatocellular adenomas. *Am J Surg Pathol* 11:191-196, 1987.

90. Gordon SC, Watts JC, Vener RJ, et al: Focal hepatic candidiasis with perihepatic adhesions: laparoscopic and immunohistologic diagnosis. *Gastroenterology* 88:214-217, 1990.

91. Gowing NFC: Modes of death and post mortem studies. In Smithers D, editor: *Hodgkin disease.* Edinburgh, 1973 Churchill-Livingstone, pp 163-166.

92. Gupta RK: Amebic liver abscess: a report of 100 cases. *Int Surg* 69:261-264, 1984.

93. Haas JE, Muczynski KA, Krallo M, et al: Histopathology and prognosis in childhood hepatoblastoma and hepatocarcinoma. *Cancer* 64:1082-1095, 1989.

94. Hahn PF, Stark DD, Weissleder R, et al: Clinical application of superparamagnetic iron oxide to MR imaging of tissue perfusion in vascular liver tumors. *Radiology* 174:361-366, 1990.

95. Halvorsen RA, Korobkin M, Foster WL, et al: The variable CT appearance of hepatic abscesses. *AJR* 141:941-946, 1984.

96. Hamm B, Fischer E, Taupitz M: Differentiation of hepatic hemangiomas from metastases by dynamic contrast-enhanced MR imaging. *J Comput Assist Tomogr* 14:205-216, 1990.

97. Hamm B, et al: Focal liver lesions: MR imaging with Mn-DPDP—initial clinical results in 40 patients. *Radiology* 182:167-174, 1992.

98. Harmon BH, Berland LL, Lee JY: Effect of varying rates of low-osmolarity contrast media injection for hepatic CT: correlation with indocyanine green transit time. *Radiology* 184:379-382, 1992.

99. Heiken JP, Weyman PJ, Lee JKT, et al: Detection of focal hepatic masses: prospective evaluation with CT, delayed CT, CT during arterial portography, and MR imaging. *Radiology* 171:47-51, 1989.

100. Hoff FL, Aisen AM, Walden ME, Glazer GM: MR imaging in hydatid disease of the liver. *Gastrointest Radiol* 12:39-42, 1987.

101. Horowitz ME, Etcubanas E, Webber BL, et al: Hepatic differentiated (embryonal) sarcoma and rhabdomyosarcoma in children. Results of therapy. *Cancer* 59:396-402, 1987.

102. Ishak KG: Mesenchymal tumors of the liver. In Okuda K, Peter RL, editors: *Hepatocellular carcinoma,* New York, 1976, John Wiley & Sons, pp 228-587.

103. Ishak KG: Pathogenesis of liver diseases. In Farber E, Philips MJ, Kaufman N, editors: *International Academy of Pathology,* Monograph No. 28, Baltimore, 1987, Williams & Wilkins, pp 314-315.

104. Ishak KG, Glunz PR: Hepatoblastoma and hepatocarcinoma in infancy and childhood: report of 47 cases. *Cancer* 20:396-422, 1967.

105. Ishak KG, Rabin L: Benign tumors of the liver. *Med Clin North Am* 59:995-1013, 1975.

106. Ishak KG, Sesterhenn IA, Goodman MD, et al: Epithelioid hemangioendothelioma of the liver: a clinicopathologic and follow-up study of 32 cases. *Hum Pathol* 15:839-852, 1984.

107. Ishak KG, Willis GW, Cummins SD, et al: Biliary cystadenoma and cystadenocarcinoma: report of 14 cases and review of the literature. *Cancer* 39:322-338, 1977.

108. Itai Y, Araki T, Furui S, et al: Computed tomography of primary intrahepatic biliary malignancy. *Radiology* 147:485-490, 1983.

109. Itai Y, Ohnishi S, Ohtomo K, et al: Regenerating nodules of liver cirrhosis: MR imaging. *Radiology* 165:419-423, 1987.

110. Itai Y, Ohtomo K, Furui S, et al: Noninvasive diagnosis of small cavernous hemangioma of the liver: advantage of MRI. *AJR* 145:1195-1199, 1985.

111. Itoh K: Differentiation between small hepatic hemangiomas and metastases on MR images: importance of size-specific quantitative criteria. *AJR* 155:61-65, 1990.

112. Ito Y, Kojiro M, Nakashima T, et al: Pathomorphologic characteristics of 102 cases of Thorotrast-related hepatocellular carcinoma, cholangiocarcinoma, and hepatic angiosarcoma. *Cancer* 62:1153-1162, 1988.

113. Itoh K, Nishimura K, Togashi K, et al: Hepatocellular carcinoma: MR imaging. *Radiology* 164:21-25, 1987.

114. Jeffrey RB, Tolentino CS, Chang FC, et al: CT of small pyogenic hepatic abscesses: the cluster sign. *AJR* 151:487-489, 1988.

115. Johnson RD, Mueller PR, Ferrucci JT, et al: Percutaneous drainage of pyogenic liver abscesses. *AJR* 144:463-467, 1985.

116. Jones EC, Chezmar JL, Nelson RC, et al: The frequency and significance of small (≤15 mm) hepatic lesions detected by CT. *AJR* 158:535-539, 1992.

117. Juimo AG, Gervez F, Angwafo FF: Extraintestinal amebiasis. *Radiology* 182:181, 1992.

118. Kairaluoma M, Leinonen A, Stahlberg MM, et al: Percutaneous aspiration and alcohol sclerotherapy for symptomatic hepatic cysts. *Ann Surg* 210:208-215, 1989.

119. Kalovidouris A, Pissiotis C, Pontifex G, et al: CT characterization of multivesicular hydatid cysts. *J Comput Assist Tomogr* 8:839-845, 1984.

120. Kandel G, Marion NE: Pyogenic liver abscess: new concepts of an old disease. *Am J Gastroenterol* 79:65-71, 1984.

121. Kanematsu M, Imaeda T, Yamawaki Y, et al: Rupture of hepatocellular carcinoma: predictive value of CT findings. *AJR* 158:1247-1250, 1992.

122. Karhunen PJ: Benign hepatic tumors and tumor-like conditions in men. *J Clin Pathol* 39:183-188, 1986.

123. Kennedy SJ: Biliary, in Ros PR, Bidgood WD, editors: *Abdominal magnetic resonance imaging,* St. Louis, 1993, CV Mosby, pp 246-251.

124. Kerr DN, Harrison CV, Sherlock S, et al: Congenital hepatic fibrosis. *Q J Med* 30:91-133, 1961.

125. Keslar PJ, Buck JL, Selby DM: Infantile hemangioendothelioma of the liver revisited. *Radiographics* 13:657-670, 1993.

126. Khuroo MS, Zargar SA, Mahajan R: Echinococcus granulosus cysts in the liver: management with percutaneous drainage. *Radiology* 180:141-145, 1991.

127. Klatskin G: Adenocarcinoma of the hepatic duct at its bifurcation within the porta hepatis. *Am J Med* 38:241-256, 1965.

128. Knight R: Hepatic amebiasis. *Semin Liver Dis* 4:277-292, 1984.

129. Kojiro M, Nakashima T, Ito Y, et al: Thorium dioxide-related angiosarcoma of the liver: pathomorphic study of 29 autopsy cases. *Arch Pathol Lab Med* 109:853-857, 1985.

130. Korobkin MT, Stephens DH, Lee JKT, et al: Biliary cystadenoma and cystadenocarcinoma: CT and sonographic findings. *AJR* 153:507-511, 1989.

131. Kressel HY, Abbas YA: The liver and pancreas. In Higgins CB, Hricak H, Helms CA, editors: *Magnetic resonance imaging of the body,* ed 2, New York, 1992, Raven Press, pp 721-760.

132. Kunstlinger F, et al: Computed tomography of hepatocellular carcinoma. *AJR* 134:431-437, 1980.

133. LaBerge JM, Laing FC, Federle MP, et al: Hepatocellular carcinoma: assessment of resectability by computed tomography and ultrasound. *Radiology* 152:485-490, 1984.

134. Lambiase RE, Deyoe L, Cronan JJ, Dorfman GS: Percutaneous drainage of 335 consecutive abscesses: results of primary drainage with 1-year follow-up. *Radiology* 184:167, 1992.

135. Langer B, Gallinger S: Cystic disease of the liver. In Zuidema GD,

editor: *Shackelford's surgery of the alimentary tract,* ed 3, Philadelphia, 1991 WB Saunders, pp 428-442.

136. Langer JC, Rose DB, Keystone JS, et al: Diagnosis and management of hydatid disease of the liver. *Ann Surg* 199:412-417, 1984.

137. Lee MJ, Saini S, Compton CC: MR demonstration of edema adjacent to a liver metastasis: pathologic correlation. *AJR* 157:499-501, 1991.

138. Lee MJ, Saini S, Hamm B, et al: Focal nodular hyperplasia of the liver: MR findings in 35 proved cases. *AJR* 156:317-320, 1991.

139. Levick CB, Rubie J: Hemangioendothelioma of the liver simulating congenital heart disease in infants. *Arch Dis Child* 28:49-51, 1953.

140. Levine E, Cook LT, Grantham JJ: Liver cysts in autosomal-dominant polycystic kidney disease: clinical and computed tomographic study. *AJR* 145:229-233, 1985.

141. Levy DW, Rindsberg S, Friedman AC, et al: Thorotrast-induced hepatosplenic neoplasia: CT identification. *AJR* 146:997-1004, 1986.

142. Lewall DB, McCorkell SJ: Rupture of echinococcal cysts: diagnosis, classification and clinical implications. *AJR* 146:391-394, 1986.

143. Lim KO, Stark DD, Leese PT, et al: Hepatobiliary MR imaging: first human experience with Mn-DPDP. *Radiology* 178:79-82, 1991.

144. Litwin DEM, Taylor BR, Greig P, Langer B: Nonparasitic cysts of the liver: the case for conservative surgical management. *Ann Surg* 205:45-48, 1987.

145. Locker GY, Doroshow JH, Zwelling LA, et al: The clinical features of hepatic angiosarcoma: a report of four cases and a review of the English literature. *Medicine (Baltimore)* 58:48-64, 1979.

146. Lucaya J, Enriquez G, Amat L, et al: Computed tomography of infantile hepatic hemangioendothelioma. *AJR* 144:821-826, 1985.

147. Lui AF, Hirotza LF, Hirose FM: Multiple adenomas of the liver. *Cancer* 45:1001-1004, 1980.

148. Lupetin AR, Dash N: Intrahepatic rupture of hydatid cyst: MR findings. *AJR* 151:491-492, 1988.

149. Mahony B, Jeffrey RB, Federle MP: Spontaneous rupture of hepatic and splenic angiosarcoma demonstrated by CT. *AJR* 183:965-966, 1982.

150. Maki HS, Hubert BC, Sajjad SM, et al: Primary hepatic leiomyosarcoma. *Arch Surg* 122:1193-1196, 1987.

151. Marani SAD, Canossi GC, Nicoli FA, et al: Hydatid disease: MR imaging study. *Radiology* 175:701-706, 1990.

152. Mathieu D, Bruneton JN, Drouillard J, et al: Hepatic adenomas and focal nodular hyperplasia: dynamic CT study. *Radiology* 160:53-58, 1986.

153. Mathieu D, Grenier P, Larde D, et al: Portal vein involvement in hepatocellular carcinoma. Dynamic CT features. *Radiology* 152:127-132, 1984.

154. Mathieu D, Rahmouni A, Anglade M-C, et al: Focal nodular hyperplasia of the liver: assessment with contrast-enhanced turbo-FLASH MR imaging. *Radiology* 180:25-30, 1991.

155. Mathieu D, Vasile N, Fagniez P, et al: Dynamic CT features of hepatic abscesses. *Radiology* 154:749-752, 1985.

156. Matsui O, Kadoya M, Kameyama T, et al: Adenomatous hyperplastic nodules in the cirrhotic liver: differentiation from hepatocellular carcinoma with MRI. *Radiology* 173:123-126, 1989.

157. Matsui O, Kadoya M, Suzuki M, et al: Dynamic sequential computed tomography during arterial portography in the detection of hepatic neoplasms. *Radiology* 146:721-727, 1983.

158. Mattison GR, Glazer GM, Quint LE, et al: MR imaging of hepatic focal nodular hyperplasia: characterization and distinction from primary malignant hepatic tumors. *AJR* 148:711-715, 1987.

159. Mattrey RF: Potential role of perfluorooctylbromide in the detection and characterization of liver lesions with CT. *Radiology* 170:18-20, 1989.

160. McLean RH, Moller JH, Warwick WJ: Multinodular hemangiomatosis of the liver in infancy. *Pediatrics* 49:563-573, 1972.

161. Melato M, Laurino L, Mueli E, et al: Relationship between cirrhosis, liver cancer, and hepatic metastases: an autopsy study. *Cancer* 64:455-459, 1989.

162. Miedema BW, Dineen P: The diagnosis and treatment of pyogenic liver abscesses. *Ann Surg* 200:328-335, 1984.

163. Mitchell DG, Rubin R, Siegelman ES, et al: Hepatocellular carcinoma within sideritic regenerative nodules: appearance as a nodule within a nodule on MR images. *Radiology* 178:101-103, 1991.

164. Miller DL, Simmons JT, Chang R, et al: Hepatic metastasis detection: comparison of three CT contrast enhancement methods. *Radiology* 165:785-790, 1987.

165. Miller DL, Vermess M, Doppman JL, et al: CT of the liver and spleen with EOE-13: review of 225 examinations. *AJR* 143:235-243, 1984.

166. Miller WJ, Dodd GD III, Federle MP, et al: Epithelioid hemangioendothelioma of the liver: imaging findings with pathologic correlation. *AJR* 159:53-57, 1992.

167. Miller WJ, Federle MP, Campbell WL: Diagnosis and staging of hepatocellular carcinoma: comparison of CT and sonography in 36 liver transplantation patients. *AJR* 157:303-306, 1991.

168. Mones JM, Saldana MJ: Nodular regenerative hyperplasia of the liver in a 4-month-old infant. *Am J Dis Child* 138:79-81, 1984.

169. Monzawa S, Uchiyama G, Ohtomo K, Araki T: Schistosomiasis japonica of the liver: contrast-enhanced CT findings in 113 patients. *AJR* 161:323-327, 1993.

170. Mori W, Nagasako K: Cholangiocarcinoma and related lesions. In Okuda K, Peters RL, editors: *Hepatocellular carcinoma.* New York, 1976, John Wiley & Sons, pp 227-246.

171. Moss AA, Goldberg HJ, Stark DD, et al: Hepatic tumors: magnetic resonance and CT appearance. *Radiology* 150:141-147, 1984.

172. Mueller PR, Dawson SL, Ferrucci JT, et al: Hepatic echinococcal cyst: successful percutaneous drainage. *Radiology* 155:627-628, 1985.

173. Mueller PR, White EM, Glass-Royal M, et al: Infected abdominal tumors: percutaneous catheter drainage. *Radiology* 173:627-629, 1989.

174. Munoz M, Bosch Y: Epidemiology of hepatocellular carcinoma. In Okuda K, Ishak KG, editors: *Neoplasms of the liver.* Tokyo, 1987, Springer-Verlag, pp 3-19.

175. Munzer D: New perspectives in the diagnosis of echinococcus disease. *J Clin Gastroenterol* 13:415-423, 1991.

176. Murphy BJ, Castillas J, Ros PR, et al: The CT appearance of cystic masses of the liver. *Radiographics* 9:307-322, 1989.

177. Nakanuma Y, Ohta G, Sasaki K: Nodular regenerative hyperplasia of the liver associated with polyarteritis nodosa. *Arch Pathol Lab Med* 108:133-135, 1984.

178. Nakashima T, Okuda K, Kojiro M, et al: Pathology of HCC in Japan: 232 consecutive cases autopsied in ten years. *Cancer* 51:863-877, 1983.

179. Nelson RC, Chezmar JL, Sugarbaker PH, et al: Preoperative localization of focal liver lesions to specific liver segments: utility of CT during arterial portography. *Radiology* 176:89-94, 1990.

180. Nelson RC, Chezmar JL, Sugarbaker PH, et al: Hepatic tumors: comparison of CT during arterial portography, delayed CT, and MR imaging for preoperative evaluation. *Radiology* 172:27-34, 1989.

181. Nelson RC, Moyers JH, Chezmar JL, et al: Hepatic sequential CT: section enhancement profiles with a bolus of ionic and nonionic contrast agents. *Radiology* 178:499-502, 1991.

182. Noguchi S, Yamamoto R, Tatsuta M, et al: Cell features and patterns in fine-needle aspirates of hepatocellular carcinoma. *Cancer* 58:321-328, 1986.

183. Nokes SR, Baker ME, Spritzer CE, et al: Hepatic adenoma: MR appearance mimicking focal nodular hyperplasia. *J Comput Assist Tomogr* 12:885-887, 1988.

184. Nompleggi DJ, Farraye FA, Singer A, et al: Hepatic schistosomiasis: report of two cases and literature review. *Am J Gastroenterol* 86:1658-1664, 1991.

185. Ohtomo K, Itai Y, Fururi S, et al: MR imaging of portal vein thrombus in hepatocellular carcinoma. *J Comput Assist Tomogr* 9:328-329, 1985.

186. Ohtomo K, Itai Y, Yoshida H, et al: Regenerating nodules of liver cirrhosis: MR imaging with pathologic correlation. *AJR* 154:505-507, 1990.

187. Ohtomo K, Itai Y, Yoshikawa K, et al: Hepatic tumors: dynamic MR imaging. *Radiology* 163:27-31, 1987.

188. O'Neil J, Ros PR: Knowing hepatic pathology aids MRI of liver tumors. *Diagn Imaging* 11(12):58-65, 1989.

189. Oudkerk M, van Ooijen B, Mali SPM, et al: Liver metastases from colorectal carcinoma: detection with continuous CT angiography. *Radiology* 185:157-161, 1992.

190. Outwater E, Tomaszewski JE, Daly JM, et al: Hepatic colorectal metastases: correlation of MR imaging and pathologic appearance. *Radiology* 180:327-332, 1991.

191. Palacios E, Shannon M, Solomon C, et al: Biliary cystadenoma: ultrasound, CT and MRI. *Gastrointest Radiol* 15:313-316, 1990.

192. Paling MR, Abbitt PL, Mugler JP, et al: Liver metastases: optimization of MR imaging pulse sequences at 1.0 T. *Radiology* 167:695-699, 1988.

193. Pandolfo I, Blandino G, Scribano E, et al: CT findings in hepatic involvement by echinococcus granulosus. *J Comput Assist Tomogr* 8:839-845, 1984.

194. Pardes JG, Bryan PJ, Gauderer MWL: Spontaneous regression of infantile hemangioendotheliomatosis of the liver. *J Ultrasound Med* 1:349-353, 1982.

195. Paushter DM, Zeman RK, Schiebler MJ, et al: CT evaluation of suspected hepatic metastases: comparison of techniques for IV contrast enhancement. *AJR* 152:267-271, 1989.

196. Peterson MS, Baron RL, Dood III GD, et al: Hepatic parenchymal perfusion defects associated with CTAP: imaging-pathologic correlation. *Radiology* 185:149-155, 1992.

197. Pitt HA: Surgical management of hepatic abscesses. *World J Surg* 14:498-504, 1990.

198. Pitt HA: Liver abscess. In Zuidema GD, editor: *Shackelford's surgery of the alimentary tract*, ed 3, Philadelphia, 1991, WB Saunders, pp 443-465.

199. Radin DR, Craig JR, Colletti PM: Hepatic epithelioid hemangioendothelioma. *Radiology* 169:145-148, 1988.

200. Radin DR, Ralls PW, Colletti PM, et al: CT of amebic liver abscess. *AJR* 150:1297-1301, 1988.

201. Ralls PW, Barnes PF, Johnson MB, et al: Medical treatment of hepatic amebic abscess: rare need for percutaneous drainage. *Radiology* 165:805-807, 1987.

202. Ralls PW, Henley DS, Colletti PM, et al: Amebic liver abscess: MR imaging. *Radiology* 165:801-804, 1987.

203. Reed SL: Amebiasis: an update. *Clin Infect Dis* 14:385-393, 1992.

204. Reinig JW: Differentiation of hepatic lesions with MR imaging: the last word. *Radiology* 179:601-602, 1991.

205. Reinig JW, Dwyer AJ, Miller DL, et al: Liver metastasis detection: comparative sensitivities of MR imaging and CT scanning. *Radiology* 163:43-47, 1987.

206. Roberts JL, Fishman EK, Hartman DS, et al: Lipomatous tumors of the liver: evaluation with CT and US. *Radiology* 158:613-617, 1986.

207. Rolfes DB: Fibrolamellar carcinoma of the liver. In Ishak KG, Okuda K, editors: *Neoplasms of the liver*, Tokyo, 1987, Springer-Verlag, pp 137-142.

208. Rooks JB, Ory HW, Ishak KG, et al: Epidemiology of hepatocellular adenoma: the role of contraceptive steroid use. *JAMA* 242:644-648, 1979.

209. Ros PR: Malignant liver tumors. In Ros PR, Bidgood WD, editors: *Abdominal magnetic resonance imaging*. St. Louis, 1993, CV Mosby, pp 208-218.

210. Ros PR: Benign tumors and tumor-like conditions. In Ros PR, Bidgood WD, editors: *Abdominal magnetic resonance imaging*, St. Louis, 1993 CV Mosby, pp 195-208.

211. Ros PR: Computed tomography-pathologic correlations in hepatic tumors. In Ferrucci JT, Mathieu DG, editors: *Advances in hepatobiliary radiology*, St. Louis, 1990, CV Mosby, pp 75-108.

212. Ros PR, Buck JL, Goodman ZD, et al: Intrahepatic cholangiocarcinoma: radiologic-pathologic correlation. *Radiology* 167:689-693, 1988.

213. Ros PR, Goodman ZD, Ishak KG, et al: Mesenchymal hamartoma of the liver: radiologic-pathologic correlation. *Radiology* 158:619-624, 1986.

214. Ros PR, Lubbers PR, Olmsted WW, et al: Hemangioma of the liver: magnetic resonance-gross morphologic correlation. *AJR* 149:1167-1170, 1987.

215. Ros PR, Murphy BJ, Buck JL, et al: Encapsulated hepatocellular carcinoma: radiologic findings and pathologic correlation. *Gastrointest Radiol* 15:233-237, 1990.

216. Ros PR, Olmsted WW, Dachman AH, et al: Undifferentiated (embryonal) sarcoma of the liver: radiologic-pathologic correlation. *Radiology* 160:141-145, 1986.

217. Ros PR, Rasmussen JF, Li KCP: Radiology of malignant and benign liver tumors. *Curr Probl Diagn Radiol* 18:95-155, 1989.

218. Rozanes I, Acunas B, Celik L, et al: CT in lobar atrophy of the liver caused by alveolar echinococcus. *J Comput Assist Tomogr* 16:216-218, 1992.

219. Rummeny E, Weissleder R, Stark DD, et al: Primary liver tumors: diagnosis by MR imaging. *AJR* 152:63-72, 1989.

220. Ryan J, Straus DJ, Lange C: Primary lymphoma of the liver. *Cancer* 61:370-375, 1988.

221. Sanfelippo PM, Beahrs OH, Weiland LK: Cystic diseases of the liver. *Ann Surg* 179:922-925, 1974.

222. Saraswat VA, Agarwal DK, Baijal SS, et al: Percutaneous catheter drainage of amebic liver abscess. *Clin Radiol* 45:187, 1992.

223. Saremi F: Percutaneous drainage of hydatid cysts: use of a new cutting device to avoid leakage. *AJR* 158:83-85, 1992.

224. Scatarige JC, Kenny JM, Fishman EK, et al: CT of giant cavernous hemangioma. *AJR* 149:83-85, 1987.

225. Scatarige JC, et al: Computed tomography of calcified liver masses. *J Comput Assist Tomogr* 7:83-89, 1983.

226. Scherer U, Weinzerl M, Sturm R, et al: Computed tomography of hydatid disease of the liver: a report on 13 cases. *J Comput Assist Tomogr* 2:612-617, 1978.

227. Schmiedl U, Paajanen H, Arakawa M, et al: MR imaging of liver abscesses: application of Gd-DTPA. *Magn Reson Imaging* 6:9-16, 1988.

228. Sherlock S: *Diseases of the liver and biliary system*, Oxford, 1981, Blackwell Scientific Publications, pp 431-435.

229. Shirkhoda A: CT findings in hepatosplenic and renal candidiasis. *J Comput Assist Tomogr* 11:795-798, 1987.

230. Shirkhoda A, Lopez-Berestein G, Holbert JM, et al: Hepatosplenic fungal infection: CT and pathologic evaluation after treatment with liposomal amphotericin B. *Radiology* 159:349-353, 1986.

231. Shirkhoda A, Ros PR, Farah J, et al: Lymphoma of the solid abdominal viscera. *Radiol Clin North Am* 28:785-799, 1990.

232. Silverman PM, Ram PC, Korobkin M: CT appearance of induced angiosarcoma of the liver. *J Comput Assist Tomogr* 4:655-658, 1983.

233. Stain SC, Yellin AE, Donovan AJ, et al: Pyogenic liver abscess. *Arch Surg* 126:991-996, 1991.

234. Stanley P, Hall TR, Woolley MM, et al: Mesenchymal hamartomas of the liver in childhood: sonographic and CT findings. *AJR* 147:1035-1039, 1986.

235. Stark DD, Felder RC, Wittenberg J, et al: Magnetic resonance imaging of cavernous hemangioma of the liver: tissue-specific characterization. *AJR* 145:213-222, 1985.

236. Stark DD, Weissleder R, Elizondo G, et al: Superparamagnetic iron oxide: clinical application as a contrast agent for MR imaging of the liver. *Radiology* 168:297-301, 1988.

237. Stark DD, Wittenberg J, Butch RJ, et al: Hepatic metastases: randomized, controlled comparison of detection with MR imaging and CT. *Radiology* 165:399-406, 1987.

238. Stark DD, Wittenberg J, Edelman RR, et al: Detection of hepatic metastases: analysis of pulse sequence performance in MR imaging. *Radiology* 159:365-370, 1986.

239. Steiner PE: Nodular regenerative hyperplasia of the liver. *Am J Pathol* 49:943-953, 1959.

240. Stephens DHL: The liver. In Haaga JR, Alfidi RJ, editors: *Computed tomography of the whole body*, St. Louis, 1988, CV Mosby, pp 792-853.

241. Stocker JT, Ishak KG: Undifferentiated (embryonal) sarcoma of the liver: report of 31 cases. *Cancer* 42:336-348, 1978.

242. Stocker JT, Ishak KG: Mesenchymal hamartoma of the liver: report of 30 cases and review of the literature. *Pediatr Pathol* 1:245-267, 1983.

243. Stromeyer FW, Ishak KG: Nodular transformation (nodular "regenerative" hyperplasia) of the liver: a clinicopathological study of 30 cases. *Hum Pathol* 12:60-71, 1981.

244. Subramanyan BR, Balthazar EJ, Hilton S, et al: Hepatocellular carcinoma with venous invasion: sonographic-angiographic correlation. *Radiology* 150:793-796, 1984.

245. Sutton CA, Eller JL: Mesenchymal hamartoma of the liver. *Cancer* 22:29-34, 1968.

246. Takayasu K, Moriyama N, Muramatsu Y, et al: The diagnosis of small hepatocellular carcinomas: efficacy of various imaging procedures in 100 patients. *AJR* 155:49-54, 1990.

247. Teefey SA, et al: Computed tomography and ultrasonography of hepatoma. *Clin Radiol* 37:339-345, 1986.

248. Thaler M, Pastakia B, Shawker TH, et al: Hepatic candidiasis in cancer patients: the evolving picture of the syndrome. *Ann Intern Med* 108:88-100, 1988.

249. Tham R, et al: Focal nodular hyperplasia of the liver: features on Gd-DTPA-enhanced MR. *AJR* 153:884-885, 1989.

250. Thoeni RF: Clinical applications of magnetic resonance imaging of the liver. *Invest Radiol* 26:266-273, 1991.

251. Thompson WM, Chisholm DP, Tank R: Plain film roentgenographic findings in alveolar hydatid disease—*Echinococcus multilocularis*. *AJR* 116:345-358, 1972.

252. Thorsen MK, Quiroz F, Lawson TL, et al: Primary biliary carcinoma: CT evaluation. *Radiology* 142:479-483, 1984.

253. Titelbaum DS, Burke DR, Meranze SG, et al: Fibrolamellar hepatocellular carcinoma: pitfalls in nonoperative diagnosis. *Radiology* 167:25-30, 1988.

254. Titelbaum DS, Hatabu H, Schiebler ML, et al: Fibrolamellar hepatocellular carcinoma: MR appearance. *J Comput Assist Tomogr* 12:588-591, 1988.

255. Van Allan RJ, Katz MD, Johnson MB, et al: Uncomplicated amebic liver abscess: prospective evaluation of percutaneous therapeutic aspiration. *Radiology* 183:827, 1992.

256. Van Beers B, Roche A, Mathieu D, et al: Epithelioid hemangioendothelioma of the liver: MR and CT findings. *J Comput Assist Tomogr* 16:420-424, 1992.

257. VanSonnenberg E, Mueller PR, Schiffman HR, et al: Intrahepatic amebic abscesses: indications for and results of percutaneous catheter drainage. *Radiology* 156:631-635, 1985.

258. Vilgrain V, Flejou J-F, Arrivé L, et al: Focal nodular hyperplasia of the liver: MR imaging and pathologic correlation in 37 patients. *Radiology* 184:699-703, 1992.

259. von Sinner W, te Starke L, Clark D, Sharif H: MR imaging in hydatid disease. *AJR* 157:741-745, 1991.

260. Walkey MM: Dynamic hepatic CT: Dr. Walkey replies. *Radiology* 181:22-23, 1991.

261. Walkey MM: Dynamic hepatic CT: how many years will it take 'til we learn? *Radiology* 181:17-18, 1991.

262. Wall SD, Fisher MR, Amparo EG, et al: Magnetic resonance imaging in the evaluation of abscesses. *AJR* 144:1217-1221, 1985.

263. Wanless IR, Mawdsley C, Adams R: Pathogenesis of focal nodular hyperplasia. *Hepatology* 5:1194-1200, 1985.

264. Wanless IR, Solt LC, Kortan P, et al: Nodular regenerative hyperplasia of the liver associated with macroglubulinemia. *Am J Med* 170:1203-1209, 1981.

265. Weinberg AG, Finegold MJ: Primary malignant tumors of childhood. *Hum Pathol* 14:512-537, 1983.

266. Weiss L, Gilbert HA: *Liver metastases*, Boston, 1992 GK Hall.

267. Weissleder R, Saini S, Stark DD, et al: Pyogenic liver abscess: contrast-enhanced MR imaging in rats. *AJR* 150:115-120, 1988.

268. Weissleder R, Stark DD: MRI of the liver. In Silverman PM, Zeman RK, editors: *CT and MRI of the liver and biliary system*, New York, 1990, Churchill-Livingstone, pp 39-62.

269. Weissleder R, Stark DD, Elizondo G: MRI of hepatic lymphoma. *Magn Reson Imaging* 6:675-681, 1988.

270. Welch TJ, Sheedy PF, Johnson CM, et al: Radiographic characteristics of benign liver tumors: focal nodular hyperplasia and hepatic adenoma. *Radiographics* 5:673-682, 1985.

271. Wheeler DA, Edmondson HA: Cystadenoma with mesenchymal stroma (CMS) in the liver and bile ducts: a clinico-pathologic study of 17 cases, 4 with malignant change. *Cancer* 56:1434-1445, 1985.

272. Wilcox DM, Weinreb JC, Lesh P: MR imaging of a hemorrhagic hepatic cyst in a patient with polycystic liver disease. *J Comput Assist Tomogr* 9:183-185, 1985.

273. Wilson MA: Metastatic disease of the liver. In Wilson MA, Ruzicka FF, editors: *Modern imaging of the liver*. New York, 1989, Marcel Dekker, pp 631-659.

274. Wittenberg J: MRI of hepatic metastatic disease. In Ferrucci JT, Stark DD, editors: *Liver imaging: current trends and new techniques*, Boston, 1990, Andover Medical Publishers, pp 153-161.

275. Wittenberg J, Stark DD, Forman BH, et al: Differentiation of hepatic metastases from hepatic hemangiomas and cysts by using MR imaging. *AJR* 151:79-84, 1988.

276. Wojtasek DA, Teixidor HS: Echinococcal hepatic disease: magnetic resonance appearance. *Gastrointest Radiol* 14:158-160, 1989.

277. Wooten WB, Bernardino ME, Goldstein HM: Computed tomography of necrotic hepatic metastases. *AJR* 131:839-842, 1978.

278. Yoshida H, Itai Y, Ohtomo K, et al: Small hepatocellular carcinoma and cavernous hemangioma: differentiation with dynamic FLASH MR imaging with Gd-DTPA. *Radiology* 171:339-342, 1989.

279. Yoshikawa J, Matsui O, Takashima T, et al: Fatty metamorphosis in hepatocellular carcinoma: radiologic features in 10 cases. *AJR* 151:717-720, 1988.

280. Zornoza J, Ginaldi S: Computed tomography in hepatic lymphoma. *Radiology* 138:405-410, 1981.

30

Liver: Normal Anatomy, Imaging Techniques, and Diffuse Diseases

RICHARD L. BARON

NORMAL ANATOMY: CT/MRI APPEARANCES

The liver is the largest abdominal organ and lies predominantly in the right upper quadrant, extending into the epigastrium and occasionally into the left upper quadrant. Most surfaces of the liver are covered by peritoneal reflections, with the exceptions of the fossa for the inferior vena cava, the fossa for the gallbladder, and the bare area of the liver, posteriorly where the liver comes in direct contact with the diaphragm (Fig. 30-16). The superior aspect of the liver as it abuts the diaphragm and ribs is generally smooth with a rounded margin, while inferiorly the visceral surface of the liver with its convex margin has an irregular and changing shape as it accommodates the various subhepatic organs. Cross-sectional computed tomography (CT) and magnetic resonance (MR) images display in detail the adjacent border-forming organs (Figs. 30-1, 30-2). Anteriorly lies the anterior slips of the diaphragm and the anterior abdominal wall, although occasionally colon can extend anterior to the liver. Posteriorly lies the diaphragm, and more posterior, inferior, and medially, the right kidney and the right adrenal gland. Medially lies the stomach. Inferiorly at different levels are the gallbladder, duodenum, and colon. The liver comes in close contact with the inferior vena cava, posteriorly at inferior levels and surrounding the inferior vena cava at more superior levels.

The vascular supply to the liver enters through the porta hepatis, a transverse fissure at the hilus of the liver. Contained within the layers of the hepatoduodenal ligament[138] are the portal vein, hepatic artery, and the major bile ducts. The hepatic artery delivers 20% to 25% of the blood flow to the liver, and the portal vein 75% to 80%. In the porta hepatis, the portal vein and hepatic artery

bifurcate to provide trunks to the left and right lobes of the liver. Similarly, bile ducts from the right and left lobes converge at the hilus to form the common hepatic duct. The relationships of these vessels in the porta hepatis is constant, with the larger portal vein lying in the posterior aspect, the common hepatic duct seen anterolateral to the portal vein, and the hepatic artery anteromedially.

The hepatic anatomic nomenclature is based on the distribution of blood vessels and bile ducts within the liver. As the branches of the portal vein, hepatic artery, and bile ducts course together as a portal triad, they serve specific lobes and segments. Similarly, hepatic veins drain in an organized fashion from specific segments and lobes to the inferior vena cava. The portal triad (portal veins, hepatic artery, and bile ducts) course within the segments of the liver, while the venous drainage (hepatic veins) course between segments and lobes and form the marginal anatomy of the liver segments, along with other fissures and ligaments.

The liver structure is based on the lobar anatomy of a large right and smaller left lobe as well as an anatomically distinct caudate lobe. The caudate lobe abuts the inferior aspect of the right lobe and is separated from the left lobe by the fissure of the ligamentum venosum. Superiorly, the hepatic veins demarcate the anatomic landmarks for the lobes and segments of the liver. The middle hepatic vein delineates the separation between the right and left lobes. The right lobe is comprised of an anterior and posterior segment, and the right hepatic vein superiorly depicts the boundary between these two segments. The left lobe is comprised of a medial and lateral segment, and superiorly the left hepatic vein depicts the boundary between these two segments.

Inferiorly, the landmarks for the liver segments are

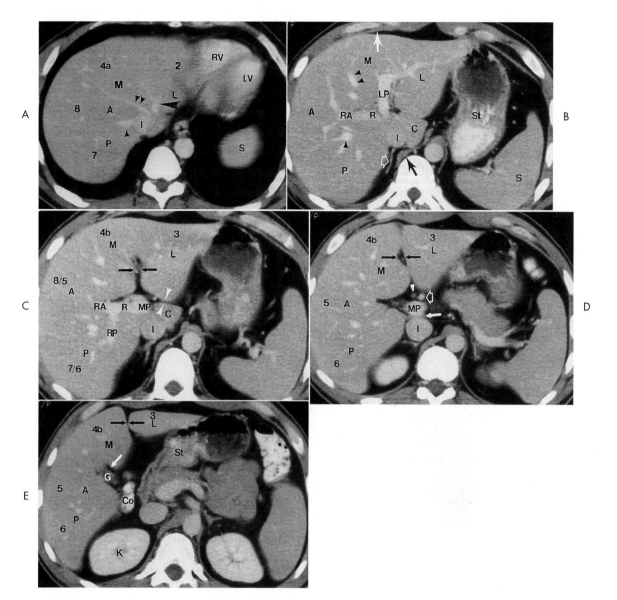

Fig. 30-1. Normal anatomy of the liver and adjacent organs. **A,** Contrast-enhanced CT scan superiorly shows the liver to the right of midline. The heart with contrast within the right ventricle *(RV)* and left ventricle *(LV)* are seen above the diaphragm and in the left side of the chest. The superior aspect of the spleen *(S)* can be seen posteriorly in the left abdomen. The hepatic venous branches can be well identified, with the right hepatic vein *(single small arrowhead)* coursing between the posterior segment *(P)* and the anterior segment *(A)* of the right lobe. The middle hepatic vein *(double arrowheads)* courses between the anterior segment *(A)* of the right lobe and medial segment *(M)* of the left lobe. The left hepatic vein *(large arrowhead)* courses between the medial segment *(M)* and the lateral segment *(L)* of the left lobe. The Bismuth classification at this level for segments 2, 4, 7, and 8 are labeled, representing the superior aspect of each of the traditional segments. The inferior vena cava *(I)* is entering its intrahepatic portion. **B,** Scan inferiorly is at the level of the right *(R)* and left *(LP)* portal veins. The continuation of the right portal vein at this level is the anterior branch *(RA)* of the right portal vein. According to the Bismuth classification, this level is the cranio-caudal demarcation separating the superior (segments 2, 4a, 7, 8) and inferior (segments 3, 4b, 5, 6) segments. Under that schema, the caudate lobe *(C)* is called segment 1. The right hepatic vein *(single arrowhead)* and the left hepatic vein *(double arrowhead)* course between the major segments separating the anterior *(A)* and posterior *(P)* segments of the right lobe and the anterior segment and the medial segment *(M)* of the left lobe. The demarcation between the medial segment and lateral *(L)* segment of the left lobe is the intersegmental fissure, which at this level contains the left portal vein *(LP)*. Predominately the portal venous branches course within the segments, and the hepatic venous branches between the segments. The adjacent organs at this level can be easily identified with the stomach *(St)* to the left, the right adrenal gland *(open arrow)* posteriorly and to the left, and the diaphragm seen anteriorly *(white arrow)* and posteriorly *(black arrow)*. S = spleen; I = inferior vena cava.

*Legend for **C** to **E** on p. 947.*

also well defined. The left intersegmental fissure contains fat, the ligamentum teres, and portions of the left portal vein; it extends sagitally through the left lobe of the liver along its mid and inferior portions. This divides the medial and lateral segments of the left lobe. The interlobar fissure is depicted as a plane extending from the recess of the gallbladder through the fossa of the inferior vena cava. Occasionally this will extend superior to the gallbladder as a fat-filled cleft, but most often does not, making delineation on CT or MRI an approximation at the levels between the inferior and superior portions of the liver. There is not a well-defined right intersegmental fissure making separation of the exact borders between the

---

Fig. 30-1, cont'd. C, Scan 1 cm below that of *(B)* shows the main portal vein *(MP)* giving rise to the right portal vein *(R),* which in turn bifurcates into the anterior *(RA)* and posterior *(RP)* branches. The left intersegmental fissure (or fissure for the ligamentum teres) *(arrows)* with the obliterated remnants of the round ligament centrally is seen separating the lateral *(L)* and medial *(M)* segments of the left lobe of the liver. Lying inferior to the level of the transverse scissura containing the left portal vein, the Bismuth classification of these segments represents segments 3 and 4b, respectively. The right lobe segments are at the junction between the superior and inferior subsegments of the anterior *(A)* segment (8, 5) and the posterior *(P)* segment (7, 6). Separating the lateral segment and the caudate lobe is the fissure for the ligamentum venosum *(white arrowheads).* **D,** Scan further inferiorly to *(C)* shows the main portal vein *(MP)* in the porta hepatis. Anterior and medial to the portal vein lies the hepatic artery *(open arrow)* and anterior and lateral lies the common bile duct *(arrowhead).* It is not possible to differentiate the hepatic venous branches from the portal venous branches at this level, and thus the landmarks dividing the segments are difficult to locate with precision. The left intersegmental fissure *(black arrows)* remains an accurate landmark separating the lateral *(L)* segment from the medial *(M)* segment, but the approximations of the right anterior *(A)* and right posterior *(P)* segments are less exact. Lying below the transverse scissura, the Bismuth classification segments are noted as 3, 4b, 5, and 6, appropriately. A thin soft tissue structure can be seen between the main portal vein and the inferior vena cava *(I)* representing the papillary process *(white arrow)* of the caudate lobe. When prominent, this can simulate adenopathy. **E,** Scan further inferiorly to *(D)* shows the superior aspect of the gallbladder *(G)* and the invagination of the gallbladder fossa *(white arrow)* into the liver separating the medial *(M)* (segment 4b) and anterior *(A)* (segment 5) segments of the liver. One can only approximate the demarcation between the anterior segment and posterior *(P)* segment (segment 6). The inferior extension of the left intersegmental fissure *(black arrows)* can be seen separating the lateral *(L)* segment (segment 3) from the medial segment. Organs bordering the liver are the stomach *(St),* the colon *(Co)* filled with contrast, and the right kidney *(K).*

anterior and posterior segments of the right lobe in the mid and inferior portions of the liver an approximation. This border is approximated by a plane bisecting the liver parenchyma between the anterior and posterior branches of the right portal vein, continuing superiorly to the right hepatic vein.

Intrahepatic vascular structures are easily seen on CT and MRI (Figs. 30-1, 30-2). On non–contrast-enhanced CT the vessels appear as slightly hypodense compared with normal surrounding liver parenchyma. If the liver has fatty infiltration, the vessels may be obscured and appear with the same attenuation as the liver parenchyma. Conversely, if the liver is of abnormally high attenuation (as in hemosiderosis) or the blood is of abnormally lower attenuation (as in notable anemia), the vessels may be significantly less dense than the liver parenchyma. Following a rapid infusion of intravenous contrast material, the vessels can be seen as enhancing structures greater than the attenuation of liver. With spin-echo MRI, generally vessels are delineated as areas of signal void, although there may be a central increase in signal in the vessel lumen seen normally as a result of entry slice phenomena, even echo rephasing or slow flow[141] (Fig. 30-3). When spatial saturation and gradient moment nulling techniques are used, vessels with blood flowing in the plane of section will be of increased signal intensity. With gradient echo imaging and appropriate technical factors, the vessels can be demonstrated as homogeneous high-signal intensity, an excellent approach to determine the vascular anatomy and to document patency of a vessel (Figs. 30-3, 30-4).

The largest vessel supplying the liver is the portal vein. The main portal vein is formed by the confluence of the superior mesenteric vein and the splenic vein, usually seen on axial images at CT and MRI. The course of the vein is seen in its cross section on axial images as it passes from its retropancreatic location, through the hepatoduodenal ligament, and into the porta hepatis. Reconstruction CT images or oblique coronal MRI can demonstrate the entire length of the main portal vein. In the porta hepatis the vein bifucates into the right and left portal veins. The left portal vein initially extends anteriorly and leftward over the anterior surface of the caudate lobe, supplying small branches to the caudate lobe. The left portal vein then extends into the left intersegmental fissure, coursing cranially and anteriorly as the umbilical segment, providing branches to the medial and lateral segments of the left hepatic lobe. The right portal vein flows superiorly and rightward from the main portal vein, also providing small branches to the caudate lobe. The vein bifurcates within the substance of the right lobe, providing an anterior branch and a posterior branch, which, unlike the hepatic venous blood supply, course in the central portions of the anterior and posterior segments of the right lobe.

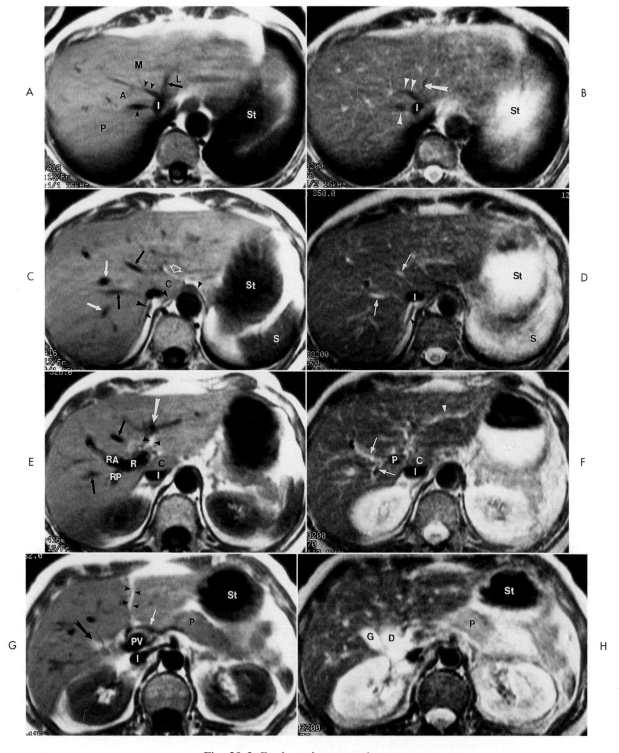

Fig. 30-2. For legend see opposite page.

Also coursing in the hepatoduodenal ligament with the portal vein is the hepatic artery. The proper hepatic artery usually arises from the celiac artery; after giving rise to the gastroduodenal artery, it becomes the common hepatic artery. This can be seen on MRI and CT in the axial plane anterolateral to the portal vein and medial to the bile duct in the porta hepatis. While this anatomy is seen most commonly, variants occur frequently, the most common being replacement of the right hepatic artery from the superior mesenteric artery, which can be demonstrated on axial CT or MRI (Fig. 30-4). Usually only the large hepatic artery branches are seen on CT and MRI. The smaller intrahepatic branches can only occasionally be seen as small enhancing structures in cross section, adjacent to the portal venous radicals and biliary ducts. These three channels together comprise the portal triad; as previously mentioned, they course within the functional segments of the liver.

The systemic hepatic veins, however, course between the lobes and segments (Fig. 30-1). The three major hepatic venous trunks—the right, middle, and left hepatic veins—are usually well displayed on axial CT and MRI images as they approach the inferior vena cava at the posterior superior aspect of the liver. The smaller and more proximal branches arise more inferiorly and course in a craniocaudal direction; they are thus seen in cross section only and are difficult to define as hepatic veins. Occasionally if one scans too early following contrast administration, these smaller veins in cross section can simulate a round, space-occupying lesion, such as a neoplasm (Fig. 30-5). By appreciating that these structures are actually a linear channel that connect on serial images to the hepatic veins, one can avoid the mistaken diagnosis of tumor for these normal structures.

Because of new surgical techniques allowing for subsegmentectomy, Bismuth et al proposed a more detailed classification of liver segmental anatomy lending itself well to axial imaging and surgical relevancy.[13,23,39]

Fig. 30-2. Normal anatomy of the liver and adjacent organs: MRI. **A,** T1-weighted spin echo MR image superiorly demonstrates the hepatic veins (right = *arrowhead;* middle = *double arrowheads;* left = *arrow*) as they join the inferior vena cava *(I).* The hepatic veins course between the major liver segments and delineate major landmarks separating the posterior *(P),* anterior *(A),* medial *(M)* and lateral *(L)* segments of the liver. Appearing as a signal void, they are easily identified. *St =* stomach. **B,** T2-weighted spin-echo MR image at approximately the same level as above, shows the hepatic veins (right = *arrowhead;* middle = *double arrowhead;* left = *arrow*) as they join the inferior vena cava *(I).* These vessels appear as a signal void and are easily identified. The liver parenchyma is of lower signal intensity on T2-weighted images than on T1-weighted images. Other small portal venous branches are seen as high-signal intensity structures scattered throughout the otherwise homogeneous-appearing parenchyma. The vessels are of increased signal intensity because of the spatial saturation and gradient moment nulling (flow compensation) techniques used. **C,** T1-weighted spin echo image slightly inferiorly shows the right and middle hepatic veins *(black arrows)* and right portal vein branches *(white arrows).* The fissure for the ligamentum venosum *(open arrow)* can be seen separating the caudate lobe *(C)* and lateral segment of the left lobe. The border forming organs identified include the diaphragm *(small arrowheads),* stomach *(St)* and right adrenal gland *(large arrowhead).* S = spleen. **D,** T2-weighted spin-echo image at the same level as *C* shows the liver parenchyma to be of homogeneous lower signal intensity other than the high signal intensity vessels. The vessels are not as well defined using the spatial saturation and gradient moment nulling techniques necessary to reduce phase-directed flow artifacts. Vessels flowing perpendicular to the plane of the image still retain a signal void appearance *(I* = inferior vena cava). The spleen *(S)* is of high signal intensity, with a greater liver-spleen signal intensity difference than on the T1-weighted image. *Arrows* = hepatic veins. *Arrowhead* = right adrenal gland. **E,** T1-weighted spin-echo image inferior to the above images shows the right portal vein *(R)* bifurcating into the right anterior *(RA)* and right posterior *(RP)* branches. These portal branches course within the respective lobar segments, while the hepatic veins *(black arrows)* course between the segments (see Fig. 1). Anteriorly, the left portal vein *(white arrow)* is present in the left intersegmental fissure *(arrowheads).* The fissures are of high signal intensity because of the presence of fat; they clearly separate the lateral segment from the medial segment of the left lobe. The fissure for the ligamentum venosum separates the lateral segment from the caudate lobe *(C).* **F,** T2-weighted sequence at the same level as *E* again shows the lower signal intensity of the liver parenchyma. While portions of the right portal vein are seen as a signal void *(P),* most of the branches of the right *(arrows)* and left *(arrows)* portal vein are predominately of high signal intensity as described above. C = caudate lobe, I = inferior vena cava. **G,** T1-weighted image lower than the above slices shows the full extent of the left intersegmental fissure *(arrowheads)* separating the lateral and medial segments of the liver. At this level, the superior aspect of the gallbladder fossa can be seen *(black arrow),* with the axis of the arrow delineating the margins of the right and left lobes. I = inferior vena cava, *PV* = main portal vein, *P* = pancreas, *St* = stomach, *white arrow* = hepatic artery. **H,** T2-weighted image at approximately the same level as *G.* The intersegmental fissure cannot be identified in the left lobe. The gallbladder *(G)* is of high signal intensity, and demarcates the separation between the right and left lobes. At this level it is difficult to delineate the landmarks separating the anterior and posterior segments of the right lobe. *D* = duodenum, *P* = pancreas, *St* = stomach.

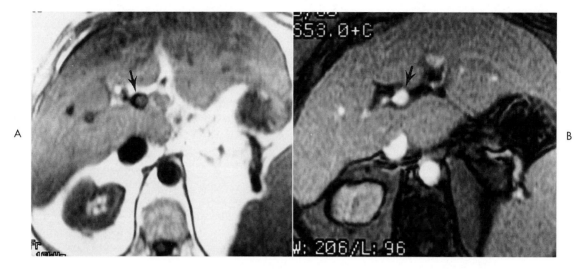

Fig. 30-3. Pseudothrombus at MR imaging in normal portal vein. **A,** T1-weighted spin-echo image in patients with cirrhosis shows only a peripheral rim of signal void in the portal vein *(arrow)*, with increased signal intensity centrally simulating a thrombust. The key to the proper diagnosis is that the increased signal is restricted to the central lumen and does not extend to the periphery. Note the hypertrophy of the lateral segment of the left lobe and atrophy of the right lobe of the liver, typical of cirrhosis. **B,** Contrast-enhanced gradient-echo MR image at the same level as *A* shows increased signal intensity throughout the entire lumen of the portal vein *(arrow)* confirming its patency. The gradient-echo technique demonstrates the vessels with a high signal intensity.

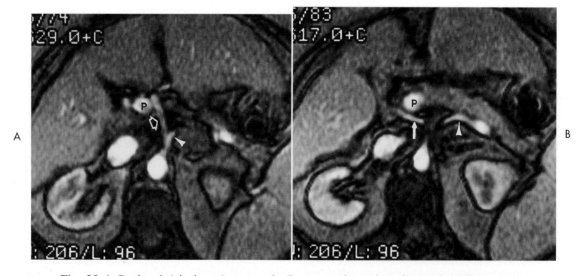

Fig. 30-4. Replaced right hepatic artery. **A,** Contrast-enhanced gradient-echo MR image at the level of the celiac axis shows the origins of the proper hepatic artery *(open arrow)* coursing medial and anterior to the portal vein *(P)*, and the splenic artery *(arrowhead)* heading to the left. **B,** Level just inferior to *A* shows the replaced right hepatic artery *(solid arrow)* after arising from the proper hepatic artery, coursing posterior to the portal vein *(P)*. *Arrowhead =* splenic artery.

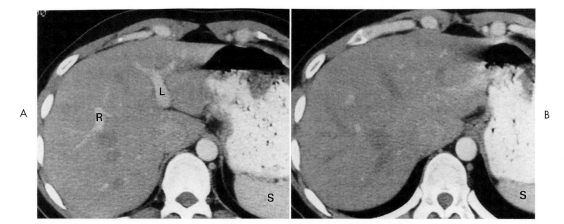

Fig. 30-5. Early scanning with unopacified hepatic veins simulating tumor. **A,** Contrast-enhanced CT shows enhancement of the right *(R)* and left *(L)* portal veins. Multiple rounded lesions seen as less dense than the enhanced liver parenchyma represent the hepatic veins. *S =* spleen. **B,** Enhanced CT image at level slightly higher than *(A)* shows the veins as they continue towards the inferior vena cava. At this level one can appreciate the branching structure and course of the lucencies, and make the proper diagnosis of normal veins. When imaged early following contrast enhancement, the veins may not be opacified, simulating neoplasm. Another clue to the early time frame of enhancement is that the liver is not as enhanced as the spleen *(S)*.

Using the same vertical landmarks separating the traditional segments, this anatomic classification scheme uses the planes of the right and left portal branches, the so-called transverse scissura, to divide each segment into superior and inferior subsegments (see Fig. 30-1). Table 30-1 lists and compares the nomenclature using this more detailed anatomic delineation with the traditional anatomy of the liver proposed by Goldsmith and Woodburne.[42]

While the morphology of the liver is fairly uniform and constant, variations do occur. The lateral segment of the liver may extend as a thin extension across the midline, even as far as lateral to the spleen. Alternatively, it can be very short and not even reach the midline. Rarely, congenital absence of the left or right lobes of the liver can be found, usually with associated hypertrophy of the remaining lobe.[7,110] Similarly, following resection of a liver lobe, there usually is extensive hypertrophy of the remaining lobe that at times can make it difficult to appreciate the morhologic or vascular anatomy, which becomes distorted. When the caudate lobe is prominent, and even with a normal caudate lobe, the inferior caudate extension, termed the *papillary process,* can simulate a mass in the portocaval region.[3] The correct diagnosis can be determined by recognizing the continuity of this process with the caudate lobe on contiguous axial sections (Fig. 30-1, *D*). Finally, slips of the diaphragm may compress the peripheral liver paren-

Table 30-1. Comparison of liver segmental nomenclature

Goldsmith classification	Bismuth classification
Caudate lobe	Segment 1
Left lateral segment	
superior subsegment	Segment 2
inferior subsegment	Segment 3
Left medial segment	
superior subsegment	Segment 4a
inferior subsegment	Segment 4b
Right anterior segment	
inferior subsegment	Segment 5
superior subsegment	Segment 8
Right posterior segment	
inferior subsegment	Segment 6
superior subsegment	Segment 7

The Bismuth classification numbers the eight segments based on a clockwise orientation from a frontal projection.

chyma and be visualized along the peripheral contour of the liver.[4] This may simulate a peripheral mass lesion; however, an awareness of the presence of this abnormality over serial sections often in contiguity with extrahepatic diaphragmatic slips, its usual wedge-shaped configuration, and the detection of low attenuation surrounding the wedge-shaped lesion representing fat between the diaphragm tendon and the liver almost always allows one to recognize these normal structures.

Hepatic parenchyma

The liver exhibits a wide range of CT attenuation measurements, between 38 and 80 Hounsfield units on non–contrast-enhanced images.[108,115] However, within any individual patient, the range is narrow with the liver appearing homogeneous and approximately 8 HU greater in attenuation than a normal spleen. The wide range of attenuation values for the normal liver relates to the complex components of the liver, including fat (lowering the attenuation) and glycogen (raising the attenuation). The slightly higher attenuation of the liver compared with other soft-tissue organs apparently relates to its glycogen content.[27] Glycogen content can vary greatly depending on the fasting state of the patient and other metabolic aspects and can affect the attenuation of the liver. Coursing through the liver parenchyma are the portal and hepatic venous branches extending to the peripheral regions of the liver. With newer quality scanners and increased low-contrast resolution, often normal intrahepatic bile ducts can be seen as thin (<2 mm) focal low-attenuation structures adjacent to portal venous branches.[67] These should never be long confluent segments, which is associated with biliary dilatation.

At MRI, the liver parenchyma also appears homogeneous (Fig. 30-2). With a T1 and T2 between that of fat and that of muscle, it demonstrates moderate signal intensity on T1-weighted images, similar to the pancreas but brighter than the spleen or kidneys. On T2-weighted images the liver has a lower signal intensity appearance, similar to that of muscle and less than that of the kidneys and spleen. Liver neoplasms typically have prolonged T1 and T2 relaxation times, which are similar to that of the spleen. Therefore liver-spleen contrast differences can be used to assess whether specific pulse sequences will be appropriate for liver tumor detection.[131] Intrahepatic biliary radicles are not typically identified on MR images.

CT/MR EXAMINATION TECHNIQUES
Noncontrast CT

Noncontrast CT can be used either as an adjunct before contrast-enhanced CT or as the sole CT technique. Usually the latter is performed if the patient has a known allergy to iodinated contrast agents, if he or she is in renal failure, or if the liver is not the suspected organ to be evaluated, such as in a postoperative abscess search. If liver lesions have a difference in attenuation between the lesion and the liver because of necrosis or less glycogen content, there may be enough inherent contrast difference between the liver parenchyma and the lesion to allow for its detection. While detection of liver neoplasms is generally best performed with dynamic, contrast-enhanced techniques, there are several situations in which noncontrast CT may be of benefit. High-attenuation lesions, such as calcified metastases from a mucinous adenocarcinoma, can be obscured by the enhanced liver parenchyma. Vascular tumors may rapidly accumulate contrast and become isodense with liver parenchyma; they may thus be more conspicuous on noncontrast images. Prior reports have shown that up to 39% of hypervascular metastases in patients with pancreatic islet cell carcinoma, renal cell carcinoma, pheochromocytoma, and breast and carcinoid metastases will be seen only on noncontrast CT and appear isodense with liver parenchyma following dynamic intravenous contrast administration.[15,26] In my experience I would add melanoma, cholangiocarcinoma, and hepatocellular carcinoma to that list. In addition, noncontrast CT demonstrates these tumors with a similar appearance between scans, allowing for assessment of tumoral growth or shrinkage and necrosis. Contrast-enhanced CT with vascular tumors may mistakenly give the appearance of larger or smaller tumors on sequential imaging as a result of varying aspects of the tumor becoming isodense with liver parenchyma.

Dynamic contrast-enhanced CT

In order to maximize liver-to-lesion contrast, intravenous iodinated contrast has become the standard imaging technique to evaluate the liver for potential neoplastic involvement. Numerous studies have shown that the sensitivity of contrast-enhanced techniques have a higher sensitivity than do noncontrast techniques by approximately 15%[8,35,117] when evaluating all patients referred for evaluation. By rapidly administering large volumes of contrast (generally 150 ml of a 60% iodinated agent) and scanning rapidly, one enhances the liver while the hypovascular neoplasms remain hypodense. This is accentuated by the fact that the portal vein supplies 75% to 80% of blood flow to the liver, providing the dominant enhancement effect on the liver. Yet tumors receive virtually all of their blood supply from the hepatic artery.[76] Soon after a rapid infusion of contrast, the liver parenchyma will receive a faster bolus of iodine if scans are obtained before equilibrium of contrast into the extravascular space occurs and before recirculation of hepatic artery delivery of iodine results in the tumors increasing their attenuation and lessening liver-lesion differences. Typically, determination of when to scan the liver following a rapid infusion depends on how long it will take the scanner to complete scanning the liver. With older equipment requiring 2 to 3 minutes to image the liver, one attempted to complete the scanning before the equilibrium phase was reached; thus scanning began at 40 seconds, before achieving optimal enhancement of the liver. With helical scanners capable of scanning the entire liver in 20 to 30 seconds, one can delay scanning until 70 to 80 seconds when greater enhancement of the liver occurs, and still complete the liver acquisition by 100 seconds, before equilibrium. When one anticipates imaging a hypervascular mass, consideration should be made to begin imaging the liver earlier to allow for visualization of an enhancing mass before the liver parenchyma has also enhanced. Because hypervascular neoplasms are less common, most CT techniques are optimized for detecting the hypovascular masses that typify the vast majority of neoplasms. A power injector is strongly recommended to provide a precise and sustained contrast enhancement, and to thus improve enhancement of the liver parenchyma.[34,123]

Delayed high dose contrast CT (delayed CT)

This technique is based on the ability of the liver to excrete a small percentage of the iodinated contrast into the biliary tract on a delayed basis. When administering a high dose (usually 60 gm iodine) of contrast material and waiting 4 to 6 hours, there will be extremely low levels of iodine within the circulating blood; yet retention of iodine within the hepatocytes will increase the attenuation of the liver parenchyma approximately 20

HU.[107] This increase in the background liver attenuation affords increased liver-lesion attenuation differences, as tumors, cysts, and hemangiomas will not retain iodine (Fig. 30-6). Because small vessels will also appear hypodense and can simulate a neoplasm, this technique cannot be used as a screening technique. It is used in conjunction with other contrast-enhanced CT techniques as an adjunct when increased sensitivity for tumor detection is required, or to clarify questionable lesions seen with other contrast techniques.[10,79]

Angiographic-assisted CT

Although this is the most sensitive CT technique for detecting liver neoplasms,[48,94] it is the most invasive. An angiographic catheter is placed in either the hepatic artery (CT-angiography) or the superior mesenteric artery or splenic artery (CT-portography). The patient is brought to the CT scanner where contrast is administered through the angiographic catheter. Even hypovascular tumors usually have peripheral vasculature that results in a hyperdense periphery at CT-angiography, and more vascular tumors will appear as a homogeneously enhancing focus (Fig. 30-7). CT-angiography is often limited by the variant arterial anatomy, which makes delivery of contrast medium to the entire liver difficult. CT-

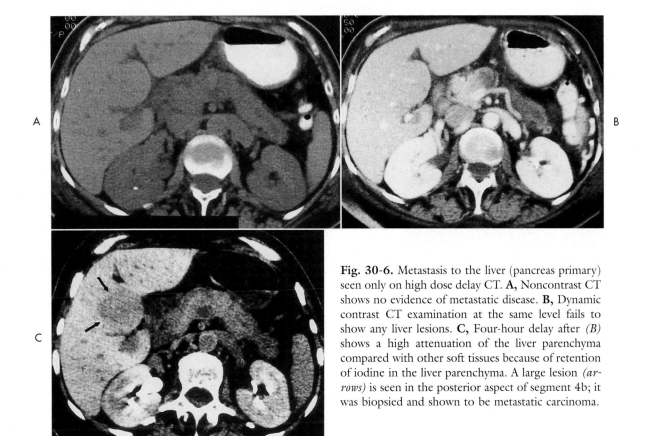

Fig. 30-6. Metastasis to the liver (pancreas primary) seen only on high dose delay CT. **A,** Noncontrast CT shows no evidence of metastatic disease. **B,** Dynamic contrast CT examination at the same level fails to show any liver lesions. **C,** Four-hour delay after *(B)* shows a high attenuation of the liver parenchyma compared with other soft tissues because of retention of iodine in the liver parenchyma. A large lesion *(arrows)* is seen in the posterior aspect of segment 4b; it was biopsied and shown to be metastatic carcinoma.

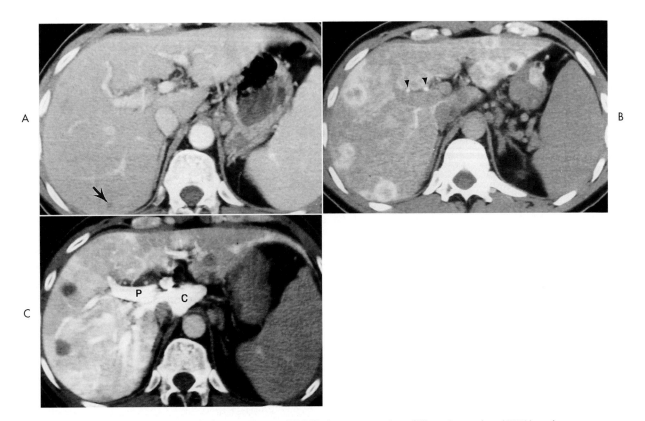

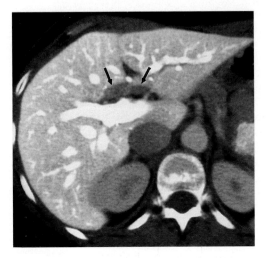

Fig. 30-7. Hepatocellular carcinoma *(HCC)* demonstrated at CT-angiography *(CTA)* and CT-portography *(CT-P)*. **A,** Contrast-enhanced CT visualizes one small focus *(arrow)* of HCC. **B,** CT-A at the same level as *A* shows numerous foci of HCC as lesions with peripheral enhancement. Note the intense enhancement of the hepatic artery *(arrowheads)*, while the other vessels are unenhanced. Because of the vast majority of blood flow to the liver coming from the portal vein, the liver parenchyma does not enhance to a great degree at CT-A. **C,** CT-P at the same level as *B* shows the significant enhancement of the portal vein *(P)*, resulting in significant enhancement of the liver parenchyma. Neoplasms that do not receive portal venous blood supply appear as unenhanced lesions. In this case, the CT-A shows more lesions than does the CT-P because of the length of time required in this case to cover the entire liver, with resultant arterial recirculation enhancing some lesions. The caudate lobe *(C)* is significantly enhanced as a result of portal flow patterns in this patient. Flow-induced heterogeneity in the liver parenchyma can make CT-P difficult to evaluate at times.

Fig. 30-8. Normal appearance of the liver at CT-portography. Note the significant enhancement of the portal venous branches throughout the liver as well as the marked enhancement of the liver parenchyma compared with the attenuation of the adjacent muscles. In the posterior aspect of the medial and lateral segments of the left lobe is a pseudolesion *(arrows)* frequently encountered at CT-portography. It is felt to be because of this region of the liver receiving a higher percentage of arterial blood supply or portal venous collateral flow. The location and flat nature of the lesion is the key to the correct diagnosis.

portography works on the principle that normal liver parenchyma receives the bulk of its blood supply from the portal venous system, and thus will significantly enhance with a large bolus of contrast medium administered through the portal circulation (Fig. 30-8). Hepatic tumors, however, typically do not receive any portal blood supply and are fed by the hepatic arterial circulation. If one administers contrast rapidly and scans rapidly before significant recirculation can bring large amounts of contrast medium to the hepatic arterial circulation, liver-lesion differences in attenuation will be maximized. CT-portography is felt to be more sensitive in detecting liver lesions, with the background liver parenchyma greatly enhanced via the portal circulation; neoplasms, not receiving portal circulation, appear as hypodense foci. Unfortunately, many lesions other than neoplasms also do not have a portal blood supply. These include cysts, hemangiomas, fibrous scars, and other benign lesions; they can appear as hypodense lesions as well. Thus any lesion seen at portography should be biopsied for confirmation before assumptions are made that such lesions are neoplastic. The exception in my practice is that if I see numerous rounded lesions throughout the liver, I conclude that neoplasm is virtually always the underlying diagnosis. Small, peripheral wedge-shaped lesions, reaching a fine point rather than a rounded apex and often of only slightly lower attenuation than surrounding liver parenchyma are virtually always benign perfusion defects.[106] The posterior aspect of the medial segment of the liver abutting the porta hepatis is another area where one normally can see hypodense foci.[32,106] These lesions each appear as a flat hypodense lesion (Fig. 30-8) rather than as a rounded lesion typical of neoplasia. These latter lesions presumably represent either foci supplied by collateral, unopacified veins or foci with a more prominent hepatic artery perfusion.[106]

Noncontrast MR imaging

While MRI offers the opportunity for multiplanar imaging that can be of help in selective instances, in the majority of cases, axial imaging of the liver provides the anatomic relationships and ability to detect neoplastic lesions. Unlike CT, a variety of noncontrast techniques are possible, each with different imaging characteristics of liver parenchyma and associated structures. The specifics of different MRI techniques are found elsewhere in this book, but the relative roles of the different techniques can be summarized as follows. T1-weighted spin-echo images are always obtained in evaluating the liver, providing the best anatomic detail using a repetition time of <300 ms and an echo delay time <20 ms. T1-weighted images are also important to characterize abnormal regions of the liver. Some authors have found that at midfield strengths, T1-weighted images had the highest sensitivity for detecting neoplasm with the highest signal-to-noise and contrast-to-noise ratios.[113,131] Others, however, found that T1-weighted inversion recovery images and T2-weighted spin-echo images had higher sensitivities at midfield strengths.[132] At field strengths of 1 to 1.5 T, it has been found that as a result of reduced T1 differences between normal liver and liver tumors, T2-weighted spin-echo sequences have the highest sensitivity for detecting neoplasms.[37,113,132] Conversely, some authors have found, even at high field, equal sensitivity in detecting tumors with T1- or T2-weighted sequences.[118] In practical terms, studies should be done with both T1- and T2-weighted sequences to allow for highest sensitivity and characterization capabilities as well as anatomic depiction. The use of T2-weighted sequences, particularly with a long echo delay time of >120 ms, is felt to optimize characterization of many liver lesions, particularly cysts and hemangiomas.

Gradient-echo techniques permit acquisition of either a single breathhold image or a rapid multislice technique that can be obtained within a breathhold with scan times down to 1 sec/image. These are the optimal imaging techniques when using extravascular contrast agents such as gadolinium complexes, which require rapid imaging in a similar fashion to iodinated CT contrast agents. In addition, because of their ability to demonstrate flowing blood with increased signal intensity, they are useful techniques to document vascular anatomy and patency.

Fat suppression techniques have been found helpful in maximizing liver-lesion conspicuity. These techniques include inversion recovery techniques with a short inversion time,[102,124] as well as T2-weighted spin-echo images with fat suppression.[121]

Contrast MR imaging

Gd-DTPA is a paramagnetic contrast agent that reduces T1 and T2 relaxation times, producing signal enhancement because of T1 shortening. Similar to iodinated contrast agents used for CT, Gd-DTPA rapidly distributes into the extravascular space. Thus, using fast scan techniques (gradient-echo or fast T1-weighted spin-echo sequences), scans obtained immediately after contrast administration may show liver lesions as hypointense to the enhanced surrounding liver parenchyma, with an improvement in lesion/liver signal intensity differences. Vascular lesions may appear as hyperintense to the liver parenchyma if imaged early before maximal liver enhancement. As with CT, delayed imaging several minutes after injection (as with conventional T1-weighted spin-echo imaging) represents the least effective time to image neoplasms because they will be isointense with parenchyma in many instances. Dynamic imaging with gradient-echo imaging or fast spin-echo techniques are necessary to achieve visualization of the majority of liver neoplasms.

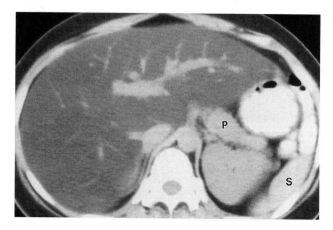

Fig. 30-9. Diffuse fatty infiltration of the liver. Non–contrast-enhanced CT shows the liver parenchyma to be of diffusely low attenuation, less than that of spleen (S), pancreas (P), and other soft-tissue attenuation organs. The vessels appear of a higher attenuation than the liver parenchyma, simulating a contrast-enhanced image.

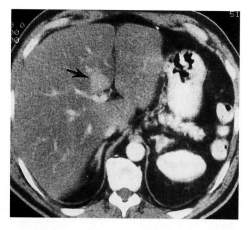

Fig. 30-10. Diffuse fatty infiltration of the liver with focal sparing simulating a neoplastic lesion. Contrast-enhanced CT shows a diffuse low-attenuation appearance of the liver as a result of fatty infiltration. In the posterior medial segment, a rounded foci of higher attenuation (arrow) is seen which represented a foci of unaffected, normal liver parenchyma.

Organ-specific contrast agents are under investigation, including ferrite particles[33] and Mn-DPDP,[30,44] which may improve lesion detection. Iron particles (taken up by the reticuloendothelial system) significantly decrease the signal intensity of the liver, and the lesions are thus seen as foci of higher signal intensity. Mn-DPDP (taken up by hepatocytes) increases the signal intensity of liver parenchyma with lesions appearing of lower signal intensity. Preliminary studies have found these agents helpful; however, they are not yet commercially available, and further testing of their utility will be necessary to determine their value in detecting and characterizing liver lesions.

DIFFUSE DISEASES OF THE LIVER
Fatty infiltration

Excessive deposition of triglycerides within hepatocytes occurs in association with a variety of disorders. Fatty infiltration is a nonspecific response to certain metabolic insults, and although indicative of significant hepatic abnormality, it is a reversible process. The disorders most often associated with this process include alcohol abuse, obesity, malnutrition, chemotherapy, hyperalimentation, diabetes, steroid administration, Cushing's syndrome and radiation hepatitis.[63]

Fatty infiltration of the liver results in a lowering of the attenuation of the liver parenchyma, seen on CT. This is best appreciated on noncontrast CT, in which the liver should have an attenuation greater than the spleen by approximately 8 HU. With fatty infiltration, the attenuation of liver parenchyma falls below that of the spleen. When the infiltration is severe, the normal hepatic vasculature will appear of higher attenuation than normal liver, simulating a contrast-enhanced image (Fig.

30-9). Although fatty infiltration can be depicted on contrast-enhanced images with liver parenchyma seen as lower attenuation than that of the spleen, contrasted images are less reliable and less specific for detecting fatty infiltration. The spleen can normally enhance to degrees greater than can the liver, particularly early during bolus injections, and can falsely lead one to the suggestion of fatty infiltration. Following contrast administration, significant fatty infiltration can be suggested if the liver parenchyma is less than that of muscle.

It is important when one encounters diffuse fatty infiltration on CT to realize that this can obscure the detection of liver lesions such as neoplasms or abscess by bringing the background liver attenuation down to the same level as the otherwise hypodense lesion.[66] Similarly, it can obscure the visualization of abnormal intrahepatic bile ducts.[109] Another problem is that residual foci of normal, unaffected liver parenchyma can be present, most often in the periphery of the liver or abutting the porta hepatis and gallbladder fossa. These foci may be confused with a neoplastic lesion unless one is aware of this process[66] (Fig. 30-10). At times, heterogeneous zones of normal liver and fatty infiltration can result in a bizarre appearance to the liver parenchyma, particularly at contrast-enhanced CT, which can also simulate neoplasia (Fig. 30-11).

Fatty infiltration itself can affect the liver in a focal distribution. When focal, it appears as hypodense to the remaining liver. It commonly has a lobar or segmental distribution, often with a straight line margin that provides a clue to the diagnosis (Figs. 30-11, 30-12). These large irregular-shaped lesions typically extend to the capsule of the liver, usually without associated bulging of the contour to suggest an underlying mass. In ad-

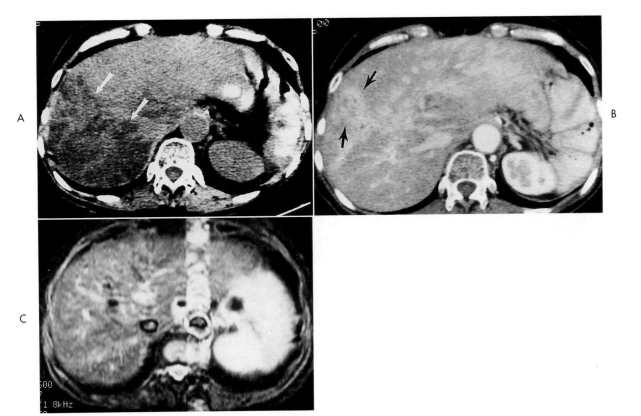

Fig. 30-11. Fatty infiltration of the liver. **A,** Non–contrast-enhanced CT shows focal fatty infiltration in the right lobe of the liver with a typical straight line margin to the affected area *(arrows)*. The fatty infiltration results in the affected portions of the liver appearing of lower attenuation. **B,** Contrast-enhanced CT at the same level as *A* shows much of the liver parenchyma to have a lower attenuation than expected because of the fatty infiltration. In the anterior right lobe of the liver is a foci of mixed attenuation enhancement because of residual foci of unaffected liver, simulating neoplasia *(arrows)*. **C,** STIR MR imaging at the same level as *(B)* resulting in fat suppression demonstrates a homogeneous appearance to the liver without any mass evident.

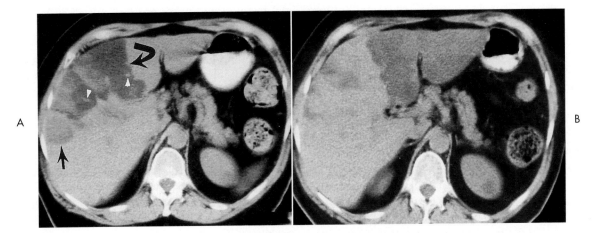

Fig. 30-12. Focal fatty infiltration of the liver. **A,** Non–contrast-enhanced CT shows the anterior segment of the right lobe to be involved with fatty deposition. The key to the diagnosis lies in the straight line margin of the lesion *(curved arrow)* and the lack of displacement of vessels *(arrowheads)*. While portions of the lesion are of extremely low attenuation and measured −45 HU, other portions with lesser fat measured 20 HU *(straight arrow)*, and could simulate a neoplasm. **B,** Non–contrast-enhanced CT at the same level as *A*, 2 months later shows the rapid changes that can occur with focal fatty infiltration. Most of the prior involved areas appear normal, and new areas of involvement are seen in the medial and lateral segments.

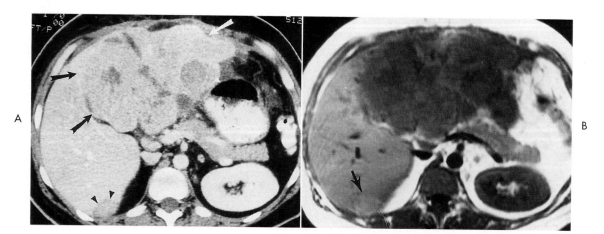

Fig. 30-13. Hepatocellular carcinoma and focal fat affecting the liver. **A,** Contrast-enhanced CT shows a large hepatocellular carcinoma *(arrows)* in the left lobe of the liver with a heterogeneous appearance. The lesion in the posterior right lobe *(arrowheads)*, the only lesion in the right lobe, has a similar appearance to the tumor and if malignant, would alter treatment away from a surgical resection. **B,** T1-weighted MR image at the same level as *A* showed the two lesions to have very different imaging characteristics. The tumor was hypointense, while the right lobe lesion was hyperintense *(arrow)*. Biopsy confirmed that the right lobe lesion was focal fat. While spin-echo imaging is insensitive to detecting fat in the liver, when seen it has a high signal intensity on T1- and T2-weighted sequences.

dition, vessels coursing through the area of abnormality are not displaced (Fig. 30-12), as it usually the case with neoplasms. Caution must be used in patients at high risk for hepatocellular carcinoma, however, because these lesions can contain macroscopic fat and can infiltrate (but not displace) vessels. When focal fatty infiltration is seen in a nodular presentation, the differentiation from neoplasm can be difficult on CT.[144] Absolute CT attenuation values are not reliable because often the infiltration does not cause the focus in the liver to measure in the range of fat, but merely lower than normal liver parenchyma (Figs. 30-12, 30-13). The medial segment of the liver anteriorly, adjacent to the falciform ligament and the fissure for the ligamentum teres has been found to be a common location for such nodular infiltration (Fig. 30-14), and knowledge of the location can help in suggesting the proper diagnosis. Often the diagnosis of focal fat can be made by changes appearing or clearing rapidly on follow-up imaging (Fig. 30-12). Occasionally a biopsy is necessary, either to make the diagnosis or because fatty infiltration was not considered before the biopsy. In the absence of hemochromatosis, dual-energy CT techniques can differentiate focal fatty infiltration from other lesions by showing a greater than 10 HU change in attenuation from 80 to 140 kVp.[111] When suspected, MR imaging can be helpful by demonstrating characteristics of fat within focal lesions (as bright on T1- and T2-weighted imaging, and suppressing with STIR imaging or other fat-suppression techniques). Again, caution must be used when dealing with patients at risk for hepatocellular carcinoma because well-differentiated lesions

can appear hyperintense on T1-weighted images and because these lesions can contain macroscopic fat with appropriate signal intensities for fat.

Spin-echo MR imaging is generally insensitive to fatty infiltration,[66,139] although when severe it will appear hyperintense on T1- and T2-weighted imaging (Fig. 30-15). In contrast, proton chemical-shift imaging techniques (or phase-contrast imaging) can differentiate signal from fat and water protons and allow for the accurate detection of the presence of fat.[47] By subtracting the intensity of fat signal from that of the water signal on the opposed-phase images, the fatty regions will appear as areas of significantly diminished signal intensity.[22] This is in notable contrast to neoplastic lesions, which appear of high signal intensity. These sequences, while extremely sensitive for detecting and differentiating fat from other lesions, are not commercially available on many MR scanners.

Other MR techniques for confirmation of suspected focal fat seen at CT or ultrasound have used fat-suppression MR sequences. Inversion recovery with a short inversion time (STIR) sequences have been shown to be sensitive in suppressing the signal from fat.[102,124] On these sequences, the presence of fat is confirmed indirectly by demonstrating no focal abnormality in the region of fat, in contrast to neoplastic lesions, which would be expected to show increased signal intensity (Fig. 30-11). Software with fat-suppression techniques applicable to spin-echo or gradient-echo imaging are now also commercially available. In my experience, however, these are less sensitive to documenting moderate fat accumulation.

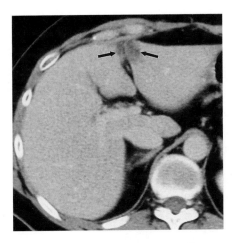

Fig. 30-14. Contrast CT shows focal fatty infiltration *(arrows)* adjacent to the fissure for the ligamentum teres. This is a common location for focal fatty infiltration, and simulates a focal neoplastic lesion. An awareness of the propensity for fat to accumulate here aids in avoiding a mistaken diagnosis.

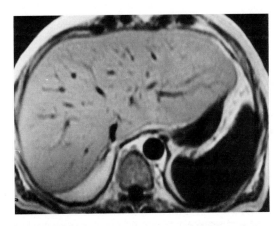

Fig. 30-15. Diffuse fatty infiltration at 1.5T MR imaging. While spin-echo imaging is generally insensitive to fat deposition, when excessive it will result in increased signal intensity to the affected liver. In this case, on T1-weighted imaging the liver is diffusely increased in signal intensity, compared with the spleen.

Occasionally water-suppression techniques will be helpful in suppressing most signal from the liver except in the regions of fatty infiltration. The morphologic appearances of the abnormal signal areas due to fat share similar appearances with CT: often there is a straight line margin and a segmental or lobar distribution, as well as a lack of associated displacement of vessels. Neoplastic lesions containing fat are not homogeneously composed of fat, and thus their MR images will show areas within the tumor corresponding to typical tumor signal intensity—low on T1-weighted images and high on T2-weighted images. On fat-suppressed images, the foci of the tumor containing fat will suppress, but the remainder of the lesion will typically be of high signal intensity.

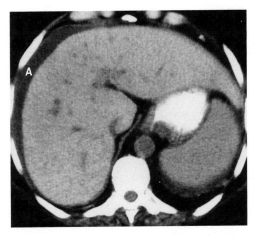

Fig. 30-16. Hemochromatosis. Noncontrast CT shows the liver to be of diffusely increased attenuation compared with the spleen and other soft tissues. The unenhanced vessels within the liver appear more prominent than normal. Ascites *(A)* is seen around the liver laterally, but it does not accumulate posteriorly in the region of the "bare area" where the liver is not covered by the peritoneum. The inability of ascites to accumulate in the most dependent portion of the abdomen here can be of help in differentiating pleural fluid collections from ascites in complex cases.

Hemochromatosis

Hemochromatosis is a disorder of excessive total body iron stores. Primary hemochromatosis (idiopathic) is an inherited disorder with increased intestinal absorption of iron, leading to abnormal iron accumulation within hepatic parenchyma (within hepatocytes), pancreas, heart, spleen, lymph nodes, kidney, endocrine glands, and skin.[56] With persistent hemochromatosis affecting the liver, there is associated development of cirrhosis and an increased incidence of hepatocellular carcinoma. Secondary hemochromatosis is not inherited and represents organ damage from iron overload because of an associated condition such as hemolytic anemias and multiple blood transfusions. In these situations, the iron accumulation is within the reticuloendothelial system and not the hepatocytes.[125]

Because of iron's high atomic number, excessive iron stores within the liver results in an increased attenuation of liver parenchyma on CT. Almost always this is a diffuse and homogeneous process (Fig. 30-16), although in rare instances it can be focal in its presentation.[92] The increased liver attenuation displays the liver as significantly higher attenuation than associated soft-tissue organs and muscles on noncontrast images. The blood vessels coursing through the liver are particularly lower in attenuation and stand out in sharp detail. The appearance by itself is not diagnostic and is similar to that seen in other disorders causing increased liver attenuation such as amiodarone toxicity and glycogen storage disease.

Some patients with proven hemochromatosis affecting the liver have attenuation values within the range of normal due to either lesser iron accumulations or associated fatty infiltration offsetting the effect of iron. Conversely, CT images showing elevated attenuation of liver parenchyma in patients at high risk for hemochromatosis are virtually diagnostic for the disorder.

A close correlation exists between the attenuation of liver parenchyma at CT and iron content of liver. However, the effect of glycogen, which also raises the attenuation of liver, must be differentiated for accurate estimation of hepatic iron content. Dual-energy CT (80 and 120 kVp) has been proposed as a means of differentiating between the glycogen and iron effect and more accurately correlate CT attenuation values with iron content.[40] Iron responds differently to energies of different kilovoltage, while attenuation values of glycogen remain stable at different kilovoltage levels.

When changes of cirrhosis occur in these patients, the CT images will show the secondary changes associated with that disorder. When hepatocellular carcinoma or metastases are present in these patients, they are usually best demonstrated on the noncontrast images because of the inherent contrast between the high-attenuation liver and lower-attenuation neoplastic lesion. In fact, contrast administration may occasionally obscure neoplastic lesions by affording an increased attenuation to the tumor relative to the liver.

Iron deposition with associated hemosiderin results in a shortening predominantly of T2 relaxation times, and to a lesser extent T1 relaxation times.[14,130] This results in a notable decrease in liver signal intensity homogenously throughout the liver, affecting the T2-weighted images to a greater degree (Fig. 30-17). This notable decrease in signal intensity affords excellent contrast for detecting neoplasms that are of increased signal intensity on T2-weighted images. Primary hemochromatosis tends to involve solely the liver and does not result in a decreased intensity of the spleen, while the reticuloendothelial iron accumulation seen in secondary hemochromatosis affects both the liver and spleen.

Early studies reported that while MR was more sensitive than CT to low quantities of iron, MR could not quantitate iron content, particularly at low levels.[16,18] A more recent report[43] using different techniques with a shorter echo time (TE = 13.4 msec) suggested that accurate quantification of iron is possible and was more accurate than CT in 10 severely iron-overloaded patients.

Glycogen storage disease

Glycogen storage diseases are genetic disorders of carbohydrate metabolism. Categorized into six groups, they all result in excessive storage of glycogen, with the liver involved in types I, II, III, IV, and VI.[80] Patients often present in infancy with hepatomegaly. The liver on noncontrast CT may demonstrate diffuse high-attenuation parenchyma (Fig. 30-18), normal attenuation, or lower-than-normal attenuation.[24,116] An increased liver attenuation is due to the large amount of glycogen, with a high physical density. The low-attenuation changes seen in some patients are due to areas of fatty infiltration that often are present with glycogen storage disease.[12,24] When the fatty infiltration is focal, it can be difficult to differentiate from tumor. Since patients with Type I glycogen storage disease are at an increased risk for hepatocellular adenoma and carcinoma,

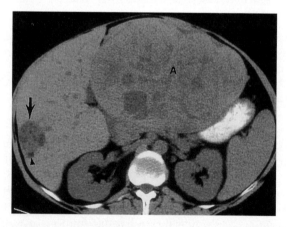

Fig. 30-18. Glycogen storage disease with multiple hepatocellular adenomas. Non–contrast-enhanced CT shows the liver to be of diffusely increased attenuation compared with the spleen and other soft-tissue attenuation organs. A large adenoma *(A)* protruding off the lateral segment of the liver, and a smaller adenoma *(arrow)* in the right lobe are present. The latter contains foci of extremely low attenuation *(arrowhead)*, indicative of fat accumulation occasionally seen in adenomas.

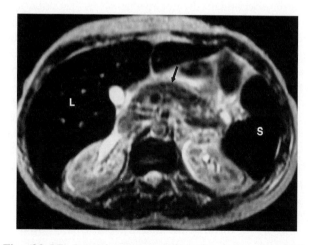

Fig. 30-17. Iron deposition in the liver and spleen. T2-weighted image shows the liver *(L)* and spleen *(S)* to be of extremely low signal intensity compared with other organs such as the pancreas *(arrow)*.

this can be an important distinction. Patients may have a liver within normal attenuation range because of off-setting factors of glycogen and fat storage. Other abnormalities that may seen on CT in these disorders include renomegaly with increased cortical density (Type I), splenomegaly (Types I, II, and VI), renal calculi (Type I), and liver cell adenoma or hepatocellular carcinoma (Type I).[12]

Thorotrast deposition

Thorotrast (thorium dioxide in a colloidal solution) was used as an angiographic contrast agent until the 1960s. The biologic half-life of thorotrast is 400 years; the agent accumulates in the reticuloendothelial system in the liver, spleen, bone marrow, and lymphatics emitting alpha radiation. Complications of the prolonged retention of this agent include fibrosis and the development of neoplasms. In the liver, the most common neoplasms found in thorotrast patients are angiosarcoma, hepatocellular carcinoma, and cholangiocarcinoma.

The hallmark of thorotrast within the liver is the significantly increased attenuation of the liver (Fig. 30-19). The thorotrast accumulates diffusely within the liver, but often may be patchy in its retention pattern.[64,127] The high-attenuation areas often have a reticulated appearance felt to be due to lymphatic migration of thorotrast.[64] Associated morphologic changes of cirrhosis may also be seen. When tumors interrupt the homogeneous pattern of increased attenuation, they are easily visible. In contrast, when a patchy accumulation of thorotrast is present, this can make detection of underlying neopasia difficult.

Thorotrast deposition can be differentiated from other causes of high-attenuation liver parenchyma because of the associated changes in the spleen and lymph nodes[127] (Fig. 30-19). The spleen is usually small and homogeneously of extremely high attenuation. The lymph nodes also appear of homogeneously high attenuation.

Other deposition diseases

Minerals with a high atomic number accumulating in the liver may result in abnormally high CT attenuation of liver parenchyma. Amiodarone, an iodinated drug used to treat cardiac arrythmias can result in elevated liver attenuation[41,70] in a homogeneous fashion. Colloidal gold used in the treatment of arthritis and cisplatin therapy have been reported to increase liver attenuation.[2,20] Patients with excessive copper accumulation in Wilson's disease do not typically demonstrate increased liver parenchymal attenuation,[21] most likely because of the minimal amounts of copper present as well as accompanying fatty infiltration, which lowers liver attenuation. Wilson's disease often is associated with cirrhosis, and therefore the morphologic changes of cirrhosis may also be seen in these patients. Cirrhosis may also demonstrate increased attenuation of liver parenchyma within regenerating nodules containing iron, discussed in the section on cirrhosis.

Radiation changes in the liver

Radiation therapy can induce hepatocellular damage in a geographic distribution corresponding to the radiation ports. Acute radiation changes in the liver usually occurs 2 to 6 weeks after therapy and generally requires greater than 3500 rad (35 Gy) delivered to the liver.[51] Histologically, radiation injury is associated with vascular congestion and fat deposition.[112] These changes are reflected on CT as areas of focal hypodense parenchyma, often with straight line margins corresponding to the radiation port (Fig. 30-20). These changes clear after several months with a return either to normal or with atrophy of the affected liver.[54,135]

MR findings in such patients also show signal abnormalities with a similar distribution to the radiation port; the imaging findings are what one would expect from the associated edema and vascular congestion. The affected regions demonstrate decreased intensity compared with unaffected liver on T1-weighted images and increased signal intensity on T2-weighted images.[135]

VASCULAR DISEASES
Passive hepatic congestion

The syndrome of passive hepatic congestion results from elevated right heart pressures transmitted as elevated hepatic venous pressure. Most often this is

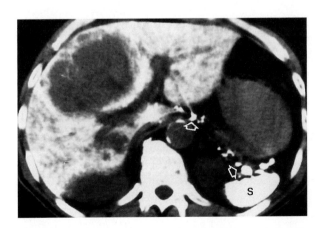

Fig. 30-19. Thorotrast deposition in the liver with associated angiosarcoma. Noncontrast CT shows a diffusely increased attenuation of the liver parenchyma from the thorotrast. The large mass seen as soft-tissue attenuation in the medial segment was found to be an angiosarcoma, associated with thorotrast deposition. Note also the extremely dense spleen *(S)* and lymph nodes *(open arrows)* typical of thorotrast deposition.

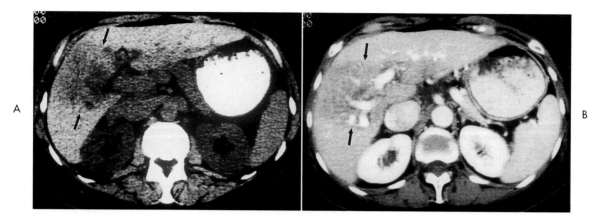

Fig. 30-20. Radiation changes to the liver. **A, B,** Noncontrast *(A)* and contrast-enhanced *(B)* CT shows a sharply demarcated zone of low attenuation *(arrows)* conforming to the radiation port.

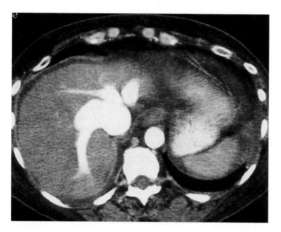

Fig. 30-21. Passive hepatic congestion in a patient with tricuspid valve regurgitation. In severe congestion, significant dilatation of the inferior vena cava and hepatic veins is seen on CT, as in this case. In addition, note that the contrast in these venous structures is equal in intensity to that of the aorta, indicating that this is not venous blood but blood refluxed from the right atrium and down into the hepatic veins.

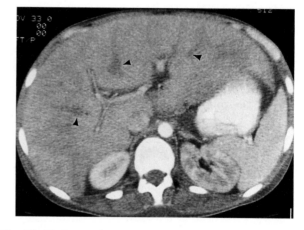

Fig. 30-22. Passive hepatic congestion in a patient with severe congestive heart failure. Contrast-enhanced CT shows a mottled appearance to the liver parenchyma with delayed filling of the hepatic veins *(arrowheads)*. Note also the periportal low attenuation often seen in hepatic congestion.

found in congestive heart failure or constrictive pericarditis and can lead to clinical and pathologic abnormalities.[140] Centrilobular congestion predominates, leading to hepatomegaly and dysfunction.

Morphologic changes seen on CT include enlargement of the inferior vena cava and hepatic veins, particularly prominent with tricuspid regurgitation where right ventricular pressure is forcing blood flow in a retrograde fashion to the inferior vena cava and hepatic veins (Fig. 30-21). On noncontrast CT, these are the only findings usually seen and no parenchymal abnormalities are present. Following intravenous contrast ad-

ministration, the liver enhances in a heterogeneous, patchy pattern during the dynamic phase (Fig. 30-22), with the liver becoming homogeneous with delayed imaging.[49,89] With intravascular fluid overload or in passive hepatic congestion, periportal low-attenuation edema can be seen tracking around peripheral portal vessels.[58]

Even without the presence of the clinical syndrome or pathologic evidence of passive hepatic congestion, these enhancement findings and morphologic changes can be seen in the presence of elevated right-heart pressures. In such situations, the liver appearance should not be mistaken for a diffuse infiltrative disorder or other vascular disorder, such as Budd-Chiari disorder.

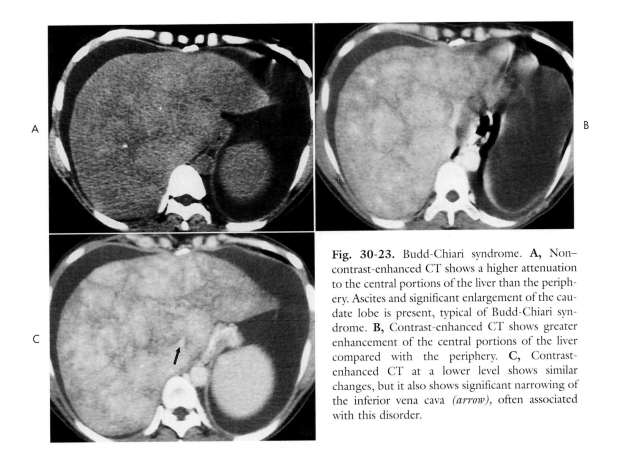

Fig. 30-23. Budd-Chiari syndrome. **A,** Non–contrast-enhanced CT shows a higher attenuation to the central portions of the liver than the periphery. Ascites and significant enlargement of the caudate lobe is present, typical of Budd-Chiari syndrome. **B,** Contrast-enhanced CT shows greater enhancement of the central portions of the liver compared with the periphery. **C,** Contrast-enhanced CT at a lower level shows similar changes, but it also shows significant narrowing of the inferior vena cava *(arrow)*, often associated with this disorder.

Budd-Chiari syndrome

Budd-Chiari syndrome is a rare clinical entity resulting from obstruction of hepatic venous outflow. The level of occlusion may be at the level of the intrahepatic venules, the hepatic veins, or the inferior vena cava. The venous obstruction may be idiopathic in origin or associated with underlying diseases including hypercoagulable states, oral contraceptive use, pregnancy, obstructing tumors (renal, liver, right atrial, inferior vena cava leiomyosarcoma, or adrenal), and membranous webs in the inferior vena cava.[69,128] Clinically, patients present with hepatomegaly and liver dysfunction leading to portal hypertension and liver failure.[128]

In imaging these patients, hepatomegaly and ascites is virtually always present. Significant enlargement of the caudate lobe, out of proportion to the remainder of the liver, is frequently present. On CT, regional differences in attenuation of the liver parenchyma characterize this disorder[74,137] (Fig. 30-23). On noncontrasted images, the periphery of the liver is typically of lower attenuation than the central portions and the caudate lobe. Scanning early during intravenous contrast administration shows patchy enhancement, usually greatest centrally, with less enhancement in the periphery. A reversal of this pattern can be seen on slightly later images, with delayed increased enhancement seen in the periphery; however, in many cases only the peripheral spread of the increased central enhancement toward the periphery may be seen. On delayed or equilibrium-phase imaging, the liver will appear homogeneously enhanced without regional differences seen. Associated vascular abnormalities are often noted. The hepatic veins are usually not visualized, and the intrahepatic portion of the inferior vena cava may be narrowed significantly (Fig. 30-23), often with collateral azygos or other veins seen.[5] The separate venous drainage for the caudate lobe often preserves the function of the caudate lobe and is felt to be an underlying reason for its notable hypertrophy. Similarly, central regions of the right and left lobes may also be spared because of collateral flow into the caudate lobe venous system and may explain why central portions of those lobes have attenuation and contrast characteristics similar to the caudate lobe.[136] Less often, chronic thrombus may be seen within the veins as low-attenuation defects within the contrast enhanced lumen, sometimes with peripheral enhancement.[74,137]

Rarely, patients are imaged on CT during the acute phase of hepatic venous obstruction. In these in-

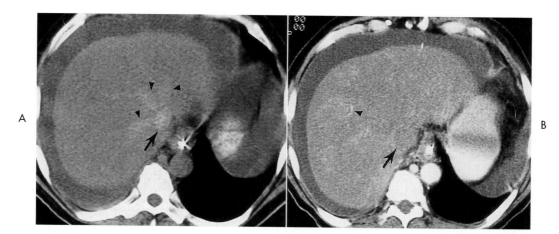

Fig. 30-24. Acute Budd-Chiari syndrome. **A,** Non–contrast-enhanced CT shows thrombus within the inferior vena cava *(arrow)* and hepatic veins *(arrowheads)* as high attenuation structures relative to the liver. **B,** Contrast-enhanced CT shows patchy enhancement throughout the liver parenchyma without visualization of the hepatic veins or enhancement within the inferior vena cava *(arrow)*. Curvilinear enhanced vessels *(arrowhead)* can be seen representing collateral venous flow.

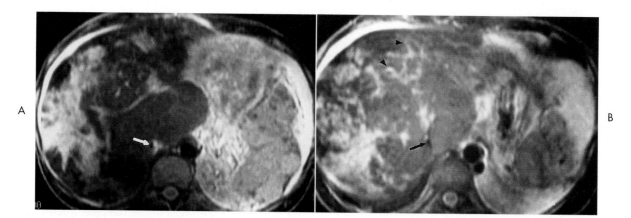

Fig. 30-25. MR appearance in the Budd-Chiari syndrome. **A,** T2-weighted image shows significant caudate enlargement, typical of Budd-Chiari patients. In the periphery of the liver, diffuse irregular increase in intensity is seen as a result of congestion and necrosis. Note the slit-like appearance of the inferior vena cava *(arrow)*. **B,** At another level, similar parenchymal changes are seen in the periphery. In addition, curvilinear, tortuous collateral vessels are identified *(arrowheads)*. The inferior vena cava *(arrow)* is again seen as extremely narrowed.

stances, thrombus may be seen in the hepatic veins or inferior vena cava as high-attenuation foci on non–contrast-enhanced images (Fig. 30-24), and as nonenhancing defects in the lumen following contrast administration.[88]

MR images also show the morphologic changes as seen on CT as well as the associated absence of visualization of the hepatic veins and/or significant narrowing of the intrahepatic inferior vena cava.[129] With its ex-

cellent vascular depiction, both spin-echo and gradient-echo imaging is sensitive in the detection of tumor thrombus within the inferior vena cava, right atrium, and hepatic veins. Intrahepatic collaterals can be demonstrated within the liver parenchyma as curvilinear areas of signal void on spin-echo images,[129] or high intensity structures on gradient-echo images or spin-echo images when spatial saturation and gradient moment nulling techniques are used (Fig. 30-25). Similar to CT, regional

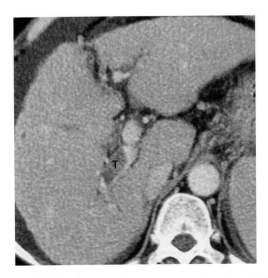

Fig. 30-26. Benign portal venous thrombus in cirrhosis. Contrast-enhanced CT shows the thrombus *(T)* as a foci of nonenhancement within the right portal vein. The contrast does course around the periphery of the vein, creating a "train-track" appearance of contrast. Evidence of cirrhosis is present with patent paraumbilical collateral veins, nodular liver contour, and ascites.

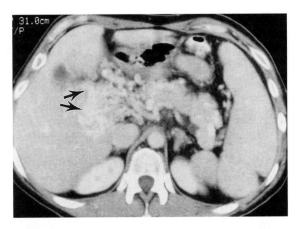

Fig. 30-27. Chronic portal venous thrombosis with collateral vessels. Contrast-enhanced CT shows numerous small vessels replacing the single large main portal vein. These reconstitute the distal right and left portal veins *(arrows)*.

differences in signal intensity may be seen throughout the liver parenchyma, presumably representing differences in hepatic vascular congestion and central lobular necrosis.[85] This can result in decreased signal intensity in the liver periphery on T1-weighted images and increased signal on the T2-weighted images (Fig. 30-25).

Portal venous thrombosis

Thrombosis of the portal vein can be caused by a variety of disorders, most commonly neoplasm (extrinsic compression or direct invasion), cirrhosis (presumably because of slow flow and congestion), infection, trauma, hypercoagulable states, inflammatory changes from pancreatitis, and hepatic venous obstruction.[72,73] When the thrombus is small and nonocclusive, it can be seen on CT as a filling defect to the contrast-enhanced lumen. When larger with total venous occlusion, the vein typically will not show expected contrast enhancement, although contrast may track around the peripheral portion of the vessels creating a "train track" appearance of enhancement[6] (Fig. 30-26). The vessel may have a prominent vaso vasorum, which may also enhance the periphery of the vessel dramatically.[73] On non–contrast-enhanced images, the thrombus is usually not visualized as different from the attenuation of flowing blood, although rarely in the acute phase it may be of higher attenuation.[73] Chronic thrombosis usually results in the development of numerous adjacent portal venous collat-

erals, or eventual recanalization of the thrombosis.[73,114] With the atrophy of the main portal vein from chronic thrombosis and inflammation, the former lumen often is obliterated, and these small vessels or channels may be the only visualized structures in the expected distribution of the portal vein (Fig. 30-27).

There may be secondary effects on the liver parenchyma resulting from portal venous occlusion. When the occlusion only affects one portion of the liver, there will be a segmental or focal decrease in enhancement to the regions supplied by the occluded portal venous branches. Similarly, on CT-portography, occluded branches of the portal vein may prevent contrast from reaching affected segments of the liver and may simulate tumor replacing liver parenchyma. A key to this effect is a straight line margin of the unenhanced areas, representing the margin of portal venous distribution affected (using caution because a small central tumor can also occlude peripheral portal venous branches and result in an unenhanced zone with a straight line margin).[134]

MRI can accurately evaluate flow and determine patency within the portal venous system.[29,65,133,143,145] Spin-echo imaging usually shows flowing vessels with a signal void lumen, while a thrombosed vessel will demonstrate increased intraluminal signal intensity, although one must be sure to exclude such artifacts as entry slice phenomena and even-echo rephasing as well as central intraluminal signal from slow flow.[141] Intraluminal thrombus is usually isointense with liver on T1-weighted sequences and hyperintense on T2-weighted sequences with a similar distribution on all sequences imaged and extending to the periphery of the vessel,[65] in contrast to the artifacts mentioned previously. Fresh thrombi may show a high signal intensity on T1-weighted images.[145]

Gradient-echo imaging[126] provides sharp delineation of vascular structures and should be used to document the extent of portal venous thrombosis and clarify confusing spin-echo images.

Quantitative measurements of portal venous blood flow are possible with MR[29,133] and have similar accuracy as Doppler ultrasound.

Liver infarction

Liver infarction is rare, in large part because of the dual blood supply provided by the hepatic arteries and

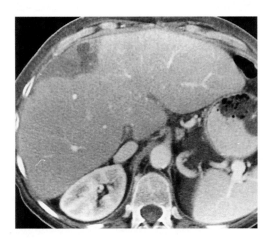

Fig. 30-28. Hepatic infarct following liver transplantation. Contrast-enhanced CT shows the area of infarction as a peripheral wedge-shaped area of low attenuation compared with the normal liver parenchyma.

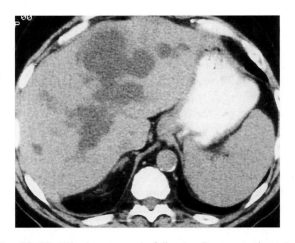

Fig. 30-29. Bile-duct necrosis following liver transplantation in patient with hepatic artery thrombosis. Noncontrast CT shows irregular low-attenuation areas radiating from the porta hepatis in the same distribution as the bile ducts. The ducts, however, are significantly enlarged because of the bile duct wall necrosis. Some of the areas show large round collections, which if seen in an area of focal infarction results in the formation of "bile duct cysts."

portal veins, as well as the extensive collateral system provided for these systems between segments and lobes. Hepatic arterial occlusion is most often seen following surgical procedures on the hepatic artery (particularly following transplantation), but can also be seen as a result of atherosclerosis, embolism, thrombosis, vasculitis, and severe hypotension. It also can be seen in preeclamptic or postpartum patients as part of the HELLP syndrome (hemolytic anemia, elevated liver enzymes, low platelets).[60]

When seen on CT, infarcts often have a peripheral, wedge-shaped distribution of lower attenuation than normal liver on postcontrast images[1] (Fig. 30-28). Necrosis can occur and result in air collections centrally without the presence of infection.[1] Chronic loss of blood supply can result in atrophy of the involved liver segment. The bile duct walls receive their blood supply solely from the hepatic artery and thus are more susceptible to injury from hepatic artery occlusion. In such cases, bile duct necrosis can occur, with associated inflammation of the surrounding hepatic parenchyma (Fig. 30-29). This leads to cystic areas that have been shown to be caused by bile duct cyst formation secondary to necrosis of the duct epithelium and bile extravasation.[25,105] This process, with the associated adjacent parenchymal inflammation, may explain why some authors have found liver infarcts to appear on CT as round and central in location.[62]

Little has been written on MR findings in hepatic infarction. When seen, it has been reported as areas of low signal intensity on T1-weighted images and high signal intensity on T2-weighted images.[60]

HEPATITIS

The liver appears normal at CT in most cases of hepatitis, although if severe and fulminant, edema may

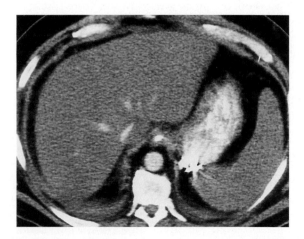

Fig. 30-30. Severe, fulminant hepatitis. Contrast-enhanced CT shows a diffuse low-attenuation liver as a result of the significant edema. Narrowing of the inferior vena cava and hepatic veins from the adjacent edema is also noted.

be present, diffusely lowering the parenchymal attenuation and making visualization of internal vascular structures difficult compression (Fig. 30-30). With acute viral hepatitis, a periportal low-attenuation ring has been attributed at CT to the histopathologic correlate of lymphocytic portal infiltration and edema.[53] Similarly, periportal high signal intensity can be seen cuffing around portal vessels on T2-weighted MR images in this condition.[53,77] Rarely, viral herpes hepatitis may show diffuse, patchy, and irregular liver parenchymal enhancement.

When hepatocyte necrosis is notable and regeneration occurs with associated inflammation, CT may show focal areas of decreased attenuation on noncontrast scans that enhance significantly following intravenous contrast administration.[52]

CIRRHOSIS

Cirrhosis can result from a variety of causes and results in morphologic changes seen at CT and MR. The pathologic process of cirrhosis represents irreversible hepatic fibrosis bridging between portal tracts. Conditions leading to cirrhosis include alcohol abuse, viral infections, hemochromatosis, chronic hepatitis, chemical/drug toxicity, chronic biliary obstruction and infections, and other rare entities. When the inciting cause is unknown, the process is referred to as cryptogenic cirrhosis. In general, cirrhosis represents the end process of chronic insults to liver, passing through phases of steatosis, inflammation, edema, and finally fibrosis. The fibrous deposition with nodular regeneration of liver parenchyma results in distortion of the normally smooth liver architecture and often results in a grossly nodular appearance to the liver, also seen at CT and MR. Pathologi-

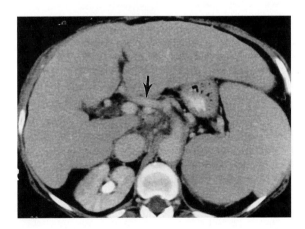

Fig. 30-31. Morphologic changes of cirrhosis. Contrast-enhanced CT scan shows an atrophic right lobe of the liver, with hypertrophied medial and lateral segments of the liver. The fissures (transverse fissure and fissure for the ligamentum teres) are widened. Note also the hypertrophied hepatic artery *(arrow)*, often seen in cirrhosis. Splenomegaly is present as evidence of portal hypertension.

cally these regenerating nodules may be uniformly small (<3 mm termed *micronodular cirrhosis*), larger (>3 mm, termed *macronodular cirrhosis*), or mixed. When the nodularity is micronodular, often CT or MRI may not demonstrate the underlying nodular architecture.

Computed tomography

CT demonstrates characteristic morphologic appearances to the liver, as are also seen on ultrasound and MRI. These typically reflect a nodular appearance to the contour of the liver, often with atrophy of the right lobe, and hypertrophy of the caudate lobe and lateral segment of the left lobe (Fig. 30-31). This results in alteration of relative sizes of the liver lobes from normal patients. The ratio of the transverse caudate lobe width (as measured from the medial aspect of the caudate lobe to the lateral aspect of the main portal vein) to the width of the transverse right hepatic lobe width (as measured from the lateral aspect of the main portal vein to the lateral margin of the right lobe) is increased in cirrhotic patients. In the study by Harbin et al,[46] no normal liver had a ratio greater than 0.55, and only one cirrhotic liver had a ratio less than 0.6. While the atrophic process affects the right lobe to the greatest degree, there usually is diffuse atrophy throughout the liver with subsequent regeneration giving the appearance of hypertrophy of the lateral segment, which in many instances is only relative enlargement to the smaller right lobe. Thus, the fibrotic process in most cases causes global shrinkage, with resulting enlargement of the fissures (left intersegmental fissure, fissure for the ligamentum venosum, and the gallbladder fossa).

Usually the fibrosis present in cirrhosis is a diffuse, lacy process, interweaving around regenerating nodules. Most regenerating nodules are not identified on CT other than by appreciating a nodular contour to the surface of the liver. A small percentage of nodules are of higher attenuation than the surrounding parenchyma on noncontrast CT; they can be seen as distinct foci, sometimes accentuated by surrounding fibrous septa (Fig. 30-32).

Massive, confluent fibrosis replacing even the cirrhotic, regenerating parenchyma that can simulate tumor[96] can be seen. This can appear as hypodense to remaining liver parenchyma on noncontrast CT and often becomes either isodense or slightly hypodense following contrast administration (Fig. 30-33). In a small number of cases these areas can show bizarre contrast enhancement as well, further confusing these lesions with neoplasm. Several characteristic morphologic changes occur with this process; this often allows for accurate diagnosis. One important feature is focal retraction of the liver capsule over the areas of fibrosis, which in contrast to untreated neoplasms would most often be expected to bulge the liver contour. Other findings include a charac-

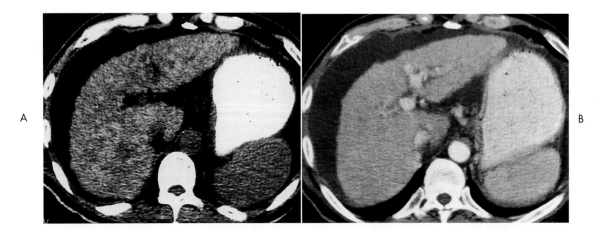

Fig. 30-32. Cirrhosis with regenerating nodules seen at CT. **A,** Noncontrast CT demonstrates numerous regenerating nodules as small, rounded foci of higher attenuation than surrounding fibrosis and lesser-affected parenchyma. High attenuation of regenerating nodules may be due to increased iron or glycogen content. **B,** The liver parenchyma, regenerating nodules, and fibrosis all enhance to the same degree, hiding the internal architecture so well demonstrated on noncontrast CT. The only visualized nodules are those on the periphery, isodense with liver, but protruding from the liver surface, creating a nodular liver contour, so typical of cirrhosis.

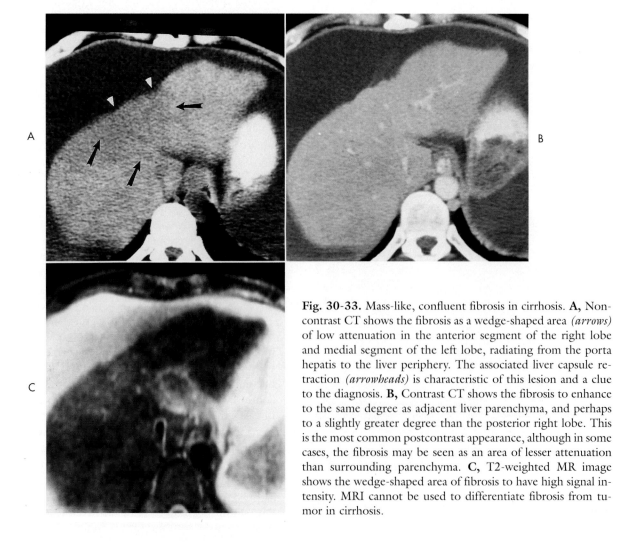

Fig. 30-33. Mass-like, confluent fibrosis in cirrhosis. **A,** Noncontrast CT shows the fibrosis as a wedge-shaped area *(arrows)* of low attenuation in the anterior segment of the right lobe and medial segment of the left lobe, radiating from the porta hepatis to the liver periphery. The associated liver capsule retraction *(arrowheads)* is characteristic of this lesion and a clue to the diagnosis. **B,** Contrast CT shows the fibrosis to enhance to the same degree as adjacent liver parenchyma, and perhaps to a slightly greater degree than the posterior right lobe. This is the most common postcontrast appearance, although in some cases, the fibrosis may be seen as an area of lesser attenuation than surrounding parenchyma. **C,** T2-weighted MR image shows the wedge-shaped area of fibrosis to have high signal intensity. MRI cannot be used to differentiate fibrosis from tumor in cirrhosis.

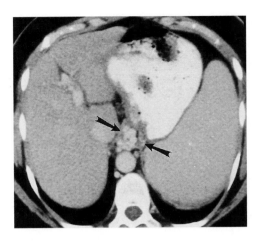

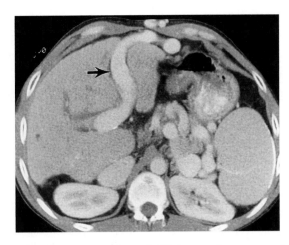

Fig. 30-34. Esophageal varices. Contrast-enhanced CT shows numerous large collaterals *(arrows)* in the wall of the esophagus and the paraesophageal region.

Fig. 30-35. Contrast-enhanced CT shows a large paraumbilical collateral vein *(arrow)* coursing from the left portal vein and exiting the liver via the fissure for the ligamentum teres.

teristic location (anterior segment of the right lobe and medial segment of the left lobe) and wedge shape radiating from the porta hepatis.

Associated processes with cirrhosis that can also be seen on CT include ascites and evidence of portal hypertension. Splenomegaly is the most common finding of portal hypertension, and varices are also often found. The spectrum of portal venous collaterals through varices is wide; this can be seen on CT as enhancing tortuous vessels in the paraesophageal and gastric cardia region (Fig. 30-34), the porta hepatis, in the peritoneal cavity, retroperitoneum, and through the liver via paraumbilical collaterals (Figs. 30-26, 30-35). The latter can be seen arising from the left portal vein and coursing toward the umbilicus from the anterior surface of the liver. Occasionally these collaterals can course thorugh the liver parenchyma and can simulate mass lesions if only noncontrast images are obtained, although usually a tortuous appearance can be seen. Occasionally the portal vein is obliterated from longstanding prior thrombosis, with only tortuous collateral vessels seen in the porta hepatis. This process has been termed *cavernous transformation* of the portal vein, but in most instances it does not represent recanalization but rather numerous adjacent collateral vessels (Fig. 30-27).

Adenopathy can be seen in the porta hepatis and peripancreatic regions in some cases of cirrhosis. These nodes are occasionally large and bulky and at first can be a cause of concern for possible neoplastic involvement. This process is most prominent in primary biliary cirrhosis[101] (Fig. 30-36), but it can be seen in lesser degrees with any type of cirrhosis.

The detection of hepatocellular carcinoma can be difficult in severe cirrhosis. The bizarre morphology of

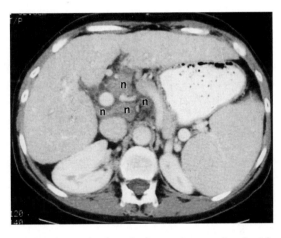

Fig. 30-36. Extensive lymphadenopathy associated with primary biliary cirrhosis. Contrast-enhanced CT shows bulky lymph nodes *(n)* in the porta hepatis and portocaval space.

large regenerating nodules can simulate neoplasm, and conversely, the nodular architecture can make detection of small tumor nodules difficult. The incidence of hepatocellular carcinoma in severe cirrhosis is high and ranges from 3% to 11%;[19,81,99] it is therefore important to search for these lesions on all imaging studies. Their detection is compounded by the close similarity of well-differentiated tumors with regenerating nodules on CT. Because of the poor portal venous flow, contrast-enhanced CT in the portal venous phase may be suboptimal in many cases for achieving adequate differences between liver parenchyma and tumor for detection. As the hepatic artery can hypertrophy with a twofold or threefold increase in arterial flow, this further decreases the chances of detecting small tumors. In my experience,

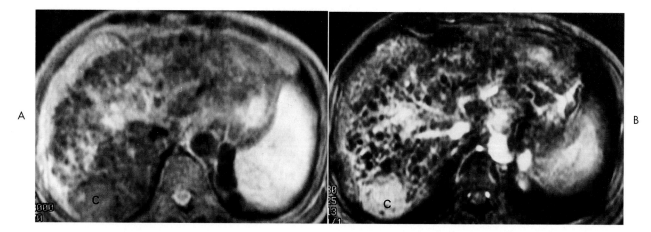

Fig. 30-37. Regenerating nodules of cirrhosis seen on MR imaging. **A,** T2-weighted image shows the nodules as small diffuse foci of very low intensity. Posteriorly in the liver is a hepatocellular carcinoma *(C)*, nearly isointense with the liver. **B,** Gradient-echo imaging shows the areas of nodular regeneration as larger and more prominent low signal intensity because of their iron content. The carcinoma *(C)* is more prominent as it breaks up the pattern of extremely nodular, low signal intensity.

imaging during the arterial phase, which is capable with helical scanners, may increase detection of small tumor nodules seen as enhancing foci. Similarly, because of the lack of portal blood flow to the liver, CT-portography is often a failure in cirrhotic patients and should in most cases be avoided.[100] The presence or absence of varices or severe parenchymal distortion is not a good predictor of whether a portogram can be successful in these patients.[100]

Magnetic resonance imaging

MR imaging demonstrates the morphologic liver changes of cirrhosis as described on CT. The nodular liver contour, prominent caudate lobe and lateral segment of the left lobe (Fig. 30-3), widening of the hepatic fissures, and ascites are well demonstrated. MR is able to delineate well the collateral variceal vessels as signal void tubular structures on spin-echo sequences or as high-intensity signal on gradient-echo sequences.[97] These techniques can be used to evaluate the patency of portosystemic shunts.[11]

While MR imaging is more sensitive than CT in detecting the underlying regenerating nodules typical of cirrhosis,[90] it still fails to visualize many patients with regenerating nodules. When regenerating nodules are visualized on MR images, they are most often seen as small, focal areas of significantly low signal intensity. If iron is contained in the nodules, these are best seen on gradient-echo images, and to a lesser degree on long TR spin-echo images (Fig. 30-37). The gradient-echo techniques are more sensitive to the magnetic susceptibility

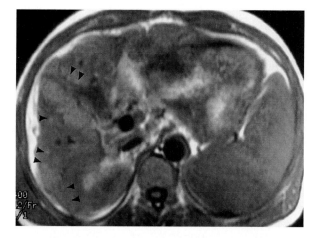

Fig. 30-38. Cirrhosis with high intensity regenerating nodules. T1-weighted MR imaging shows a cirrhotic morphology to the liver with splenomegaly. Multiple small foci of high attenuation *(arrowheads)* are seen scattered throughout the liver. At pathology only small regenerating nodules were found.

of paramagnetic hemosiderin deposits and thus nodules appear larger on these sequences when iron is present.[142] When iron is not present, they are seen less well and only on the long TR spin-echo images.[90,98] In a smaller percentage of patients, regenerating nodules are seen as hyperintense on T1-weighted images and isointense on T2-weighted images[59] (Fig. 30-38). Though the causes are uncertain, hyperintensity on T1-weighted images may reflect shortening of T1 because of increased glycogen

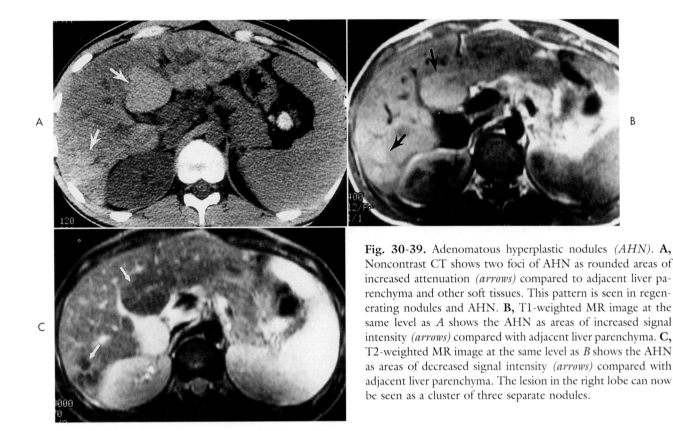

Fig. 30-39. Adenomatous hyperplastic nodules *(AHN)*. **A,** Noncontrast CT shows two foci of AHN as rounded areas of increased attenuation *(arrows)* compared to adjacent liver parenchyma and other soft tissues. This pattern is seen in regenerating nodules and AHN. **B,** T1-weighted MR image at the same level as *A* shows the AHN as areas of increased signal intensity *(arrows)* compared with adjacent liver parenchyma. **C,** T2-weighted MR image at the same level as *B* shows the AHN as areas of decreased signal intensity *(arrows)* compared with adjacent liver parenchyma. The lesion in the right lobe can now be seen as a cluster of three separate nodules.

stores, increased copper content, or fatty accumulation.[28]

The pathologic spectrum of regenerating nodules is larger, including size range and evolution from cellular atypia to dysplasia and frank malignancy. Recently, differentiation of adenomatous hyperplastic nodules (AHN) as distinct from other regenerating nodules has been defined pathologically.[38,95] These dominant nodules have an increased incidence of dysplasia and frank malignancy.[91] Lencioni et al[61] reported that of 11 such lesions followed in 9 patients, 7 evolved into hepatocellular carcinoma in a mean follow-up time of 11 months. Because of this high incidence of malignant degeneration, these authors recommend treating AHN with percutaneous alcohol ablation. AHN has a characteristic appearance on MR with a high signal intensity appearance on T1-weighted sequences and low signal intensity on T2-weighted images[75] (Fig. 30-39). When these lesions develop carcinomatous changes, foci of high intensity on T2-weighted images within the low signal intensity nodule may give a "nodule-within-a-nodule" appearance[84] and be a clue to early development of carcinoma.

DIFFUSE NONVIRAL INFECTIONS

Diffuse nonviral infections occur almost exclusively in immunocompromised patients. The most com-

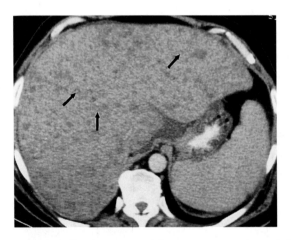

Fig. 30-40. Diffuse hepatic candidiasis. Contrast-enhanced CT shows numerous small lesions hypodense to the surrounding parenchyma as a result of multiple foci of infection with candidiasis. Notice that many of the lesions have a central foci of soft-tissue attenuation (some noted with *arrows*).

mon agents are fungal, most often *Candida* and less commonly *Aspergillus* and *Cryptococcus*. These lesions appear on noncontrast and contrast-enhanced CT as small (<1 cm) hypodense lesions (Fig. 30-40) scattered throughout the liver and often the spleen.[9,122] Small central opacities can be seen within the lesions thought to represent hyphae.[103] Faint peripheral contrast enhancement can occasionally be seen around the lesions. While these lesions may be seen regressing on CT with successful therapy,[9,122] the persistence of the lesions does not imply lack of adequate treatment. Because of focal areas of necrosis, granuloma formation, or fibrosis, lesions can persist without persisting infection.[122] These lesions can be well demonstrated on MR imaging as low signal intensity small lesions on T1-weighted sequences and high signal intensity on T2-weighted sequences, and without contrast enhancement when using Gd-DTPA.[120] Semelka et al reported that MR was more sensitive than CT in detecting liver and splenic involvement with candidiasis.[120]

Other infections including *mycobacterium avium intracellular* (Fig. 30-41) and unusual bacterial sepsis can occasionally also cause diffuse, small low-attenuation lesions throughout the liver in the immunocompromised host. These have a similar appearance on CT as diffuse fungal infections. Because of this similarity, CT cannot be used to predict the infecting organism.

GRANULOMATOUS DISEASES

Sarcoidosis can involve the liver with noncaseating granulomas seen pathologically in liver biopsy specimens.[71] Usually these lesions are less than 2 mm in size and are not appreciated on CT or MR as discrete lesions, although hepatomegaly may be seen. When the lesions are larger, CT may demonstrate multiple, diffuse low-attenuation areas throughout the liver parenchyma[93]

(Fig. 30-42). This can simulate diffuse infections as described above.

TRAUMA

Probably in no other area has CT had a greater effect on patient management than in cases of the traumatized patient. CT provides unique information concerning the presence or absence as well as the extent of abdominal trauma and has been shown to be an excellent screening tool in the hemodynamically stable patient.[45,78,83,86] It is important to remember that in evaluating the trauma patient, one is not looking at isolated organs but rather is searching the entire abdomen for potential injury to numerous organs as well as for distant evidence of bleeding from organs into the peritoneum. Such trauma can be seen as the result of direct penetrating injuries (knife wounds, surgical complications) or from blunt, nonpenetrating injuries such as motor vehicle accidents and falls.

Liver traumatic lesions can be classified as contusions, lacerations, hematomas (subcapsular and intraparenchymal), and fractures. Injuries can be graded based on the extent and location of these abnormalities (particularly important is documenting injuries in close approximation to the major hepatic veins and inferior vena cava).[87] The necessity for surgery does not depend on the severity of findings as depicted by CT; it relates rather to the hemodynamic status of the patient. Thus, any useful clinical grading system for trauma must take into consideration the anatomic depiction afforded by CT and the clinical effects of these changes. As an example, none of the most severely affected liver-injury patients (as depicted by CT in a series by Mirvis et al) who were hemodynamically stable required surgical intervention.[83]

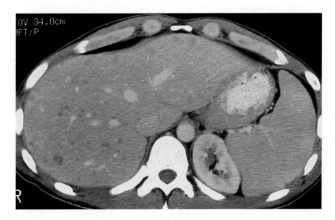

Fig. 30-41. *Mycobacterium avium intracellulare* in the liver in a patient with AIDS. Contrast-enhanced CT shows numerous small low-attenuation lesions scattered randomly throughout the liver. Note that some of these lesions have central foci of increased attenuation simulating findings often found in fungal infections (see Fig. 30-39).

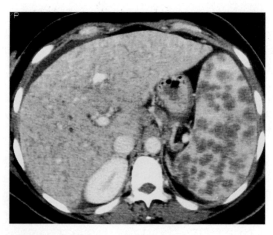

Fig. 30-42. Hepatosplenic sarcoidosis. Contrast-enhanced CT shows numerous small hypodense lesions scattered throughout the liver. Note the larger granulomatous lesions in the spleen.

However, it has also been shown to be important to serially monitor patients with clinical and CT evaluations when conservatively treating patients with liver injury.[36,83]

Most centers perform contrast-enhanced imaging to maximize detection of hepatic traumatic lesions.[31,55,82] While this detects most abnormalities, non–contrast-enhanced imaging can be of benefit to detect subtle hematomas that can be obscured by the enhancement of liver or splenic parenchyma.[57] Whether one performs contrast-enhanced imaging as a sole method or adds several non–contrast-enhanced images is a matter of personal preference and comfort.

Hepatic contusions without frank disruption of the liver parenchyma or associated hematoma are rare.[55] As compared with the normal liver parenchyma, they appear as ill-defined areas of decreased attenuation on contrast-enhanced scans, without fluid collections or hematoma. Presumably, this represents areas of edema or microscopic hemorrhage, but without gross bleeding.[82] These lesions typically heal rapidly without complications.

Lacerations of the liver appear as linear low-attenuation abnormalities, which can be isolated (Fig. 30-43) or appear clustered in a branching or parallel configuration (Fig. 30-44).[55,83] Typically, liver lacerations parallel the intrahepatic vasculature. On contrast-enhanced images, these lesions appear less dense than the normal enhanced parenchyma, although an acute blood clot can be of higher attenuation. On non–contrast-enhanced imaging, these lesions can be isodense, hypodense, or hyperdense to parenchyma, depending on the composition of the fluid within the laceration. It is important to document whether these lesions are superficial, perihilar, or deep (extending to the first or second order of major portal venous branches), because the perihilar and deep lesions have a higher incidence of complications.[55,87] The evolution of these lesions on CT is typically to show sharper demarcation of the margins over the first week, and then the lesions typically show indistinct margins and decrease in size over time.[36]

Hematomas from liver injury can present in a sub-

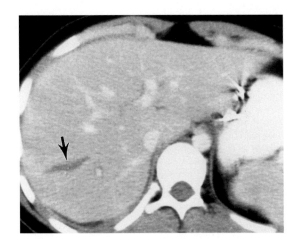

Fig. 30-43. Hepatic laceration. Contrast-enhanced CT shows the laceration *(arrow)* as a narrow linear focus of lower attenuation than the enhanced parenchyma.

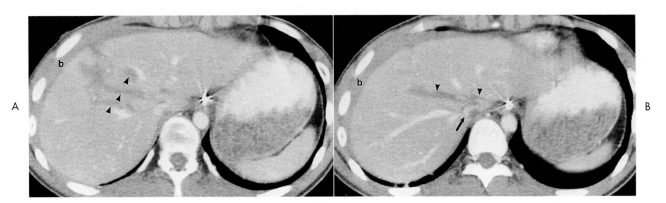

Fig. 30-44. Hepatic laceration. **A,** Contrast-enhanced CT shows parallel liver lacerations *(arrowheads)* that course adjacent to and in the same plane as the major hepatic vasculature. Peritoneal blood can be seen as a relatively high attenuation fluid collection adjacent to the liver laterally *(B)*. Because there is no peritoneal space covering the "bare area" of the liver posteriorly, no blood can be seen posterior to the liver. **B,** Scan slightly cephalad to *A* shows that the laceration *(arrowheads)* abuts the inferior vena cava at the confluence of the hepatic veins. A small hematoma can be seen posterior to the inferior vena cava. Relationships of lacerations to major vessels should be ascertained when evaluating liver trauma. *b* = blood in the perihepatic peritoneal space.

capsular or intraparenchymal location. Subcapsular hematomas typically appear lenticular in shape and with a sharp margin with the liver parenchyma. The attenuation of the fluid collection will appear either hypodense, isodense or hyperdense to the normal liver parenchyma on unenhanced imaging, and with contrast appears hypodense. However, the hypodense hematoma does not measure within the expected range of water attenuation, but usually higher. Over time, the attenuation of the hematoma will decrease to close to water attenuation.[119]

Intraparenchymal hematomas are typically round or oval, with central high-attenuation collections as a result of clotted blood. As the clot lyses, the attenuation of the hematoma will decrease and the collection will decrease in size; however, initially, perhaps because of osmotic effects, the collection may increase slightly in size.[82]

Hepatic fracture represents a laceration that extends through an entire region of the liver from one surface to the opposite surface. This fragmentation of the liver may result in lack of enhancement of the distal portion of the liver if the vascular blood supply is disrupted. These types of lesions are rarely seen at CT because of the instability of the patient who most often is handled immediately with surgical intervention partly because of the severity of this type of lesion and partly because of the high incidence of other associated injuries.[55]

Low-attenuation collections surrounding portal venous branches have been described in patients with liver injury and attributed to blood tracking along portal venous radicals.[68] Furthermore, similar findings can be seen in liver trauma due to lymphedema from obstruction of lymphatics.[58,104] In the pediatric population, this has been found to correlate with greater severity of trauma,[104] although because of the lack of specificity of this finding, caution is recommended in relying on this finding as a sole indicator of traumatic injury to the liver.

Lesions abutting the major hepatic veins, often at their confluence at the inferior vena cava, deserve special attention and discussion (Fig. 30-43). These are difficult lesions to approach surgically, and preference at my institution in such cases is often to attempt to handle these cases nonsurgically for fear of disrupting the major vascular system during surgery.

REFERENCES

1. Adler DD, et al: Computed tomography of liver infarction. *AJR* 142:315-318, 1984.
2. Aihara T, et al: Increased CT density of the liver due to cis-diaminedichloro platinum (II). *Pediatr Radiol* 17:75-76, 1987.
3. Auh YH, et al: CT of the papillary process of the caudate lobe of the liver. *AJR* 142:535-538, 1984.
4. Auh YH, et al: Accessory fissures of the liver: CT and sonographic appearance. *AJR* 143:565-572, 1984.
5. Baert AL, et al: Early diagnosis of Budd-Chiari syndrome by computed tomography and ultrasonography: report of five cases. *Gastroenterology* 84:587-595, 1983.
6. Baron RL, et al: The Liver. In Moss AA, Gamsu G, Genant HK, editors: *Computed tomography of the body with magnetic resonance imaging.* Philadelphia, 1992, WB Saunders Co.
7. Belton RL, et al: Congenital absence of the left lobe of the liver: a radiologic diagnosis. *Radiology* 147:184, 1983.
8. Berland LL, et al: Comparison of pre- and post-contrast CT in hepatic masses. *AJR* 138:853-858, 1982.
9. Berlow ME, et al: CT follow-up of hepatic and splenic fungal microabscesses. *J Comput Assist Tomogr* 8:42-45, 1984.
10. Bernardino ME, et al: Delayed hepatic CT scanning: increased confidence and improved detection of hepatic metastases. *Radiology* 159:71-74, 1986.
11. Bernardino ME, et al: Shunts for portal hypertension: MR and angiography for determination of patency. *Radiology* 158:57-61, 1986.
12. Biondetti PR, et al: Computed tomography of the liver in Von Gierke's disease. *J Comput Assist Tomogr* 4:685-686, 1980.
13. Bismuth H, et al: Major and minor segmentectomies "reglees" in liver surgery. *World J Surg* 6:10-24, 1982.
14. Brasch RC, et al: MRI of transfusional hemosiderosis complicating thalassemia major. *Radiology* 150:767-771, 1984.
15. Bressler EL, et al: Hypervascular hepatic metastases: CT evaluation. *Radiology* 162:49-51, 1987.
16. Brown DW, et al: Nuclear magnetic resonance study of iron overload in liver tissue. *Magnetic Resonance Imaging* 3:275-282, 1985.
17. Chapman RWG, et al: Computed tomography for determining liver iron content in primary hemochromatosis. *Br Med J* 280:440-442, 1980.
18. Chezmar JL, et al: Hepatic iron overload: diagnosis and quantification by noninvasive imaging. *Gastrointest Radiol* 15:27-31, 1990.
19. Colombo M, et al: Hepatocellular carcinoma in Italian patients with cirrhosis. *N Engl J Med* 325:675-680, 1991.
20. DeMaria M, et al: Gold storage in the liver: appearance on CT scans. *Radiology* 159:355-356, 1986.
21. Dixon AK, et al: Computed tomography of the liver in Wilson disease. *J Comput Assist Tomogr* 8:46-49, 1984.
22. Dixon WT: Simple proton spectroscopic imaging. *Radiology* 153:189-194, 1984.
23. Dodd GD III: An American's guide to couinaud's numbering system. *AJR* 161:574-575, 1993.
24. Doppman JL, et al: Computed tomography of the liver and kidneys in glycogen storage disease. *J Comput Assist Tomogr* 6:67-71, 1982.
25. Doppman JL, et al: Bile duct cysts secondary to liver infarction. *Radiology* 130:1-5, 1979.
26. DuBrow RA, et al: Detection of hepatic metastases in breast cancer: the role of nonenhanced and enhanced CT scanning. *J Comput Assist Tomogr* 14:366-369, 1990.
27. Dwyer A, et al: Influence of glycogen on liver density: computed tomography from a metabolic perspective. *J Comput Assist Tomogr* 7:70-73, 1983.
28. Ebara M, et al: MR imaging of small hepatocellular carcinoma: effect of intratumoral copper content on signal intensity. *Radiology* 180:617-621, 1991.
29. Edelman RR, et al: MR angiography and dynamic flow evaluation of the portal venous system. *AJR* 153:755-760, 1989.
30. Elizondo G, et al: Preclinical evaluation of MnDPDP: new paramagnetic hepatobiliary contrast agent for MR imaging. *Radiology* 178:73-78, 1991.
31. Federle MP: CT of upper abdominal trauma. *Semin Roentgenol* 19:269-280, 1984.

32. Fernandez MP, et al: Hepatic pseudolesions: appearance of focal low attenuation in the medial segment of the left lobe at CT-arterial portography. *Radiology* 181:809-811, 1991.

33. Ferrucci JT, et al: Iron oxide-enhanced MR imaging of the liver and spleen: review of the first 5 years. *AJR* 155:943-950, 1990.

34. Foley WD: Dynamic hepatic CT. *Radiology* 170:617-622, 1989.

35. Foley WD, et al: Contrast enhancement technique for dynamic hepatic computed tomographic scanning. *Radiology* 147:797-803, 1983.

36. Foley WD, et al: Treatment of blunt hepatic injuries: role of CT. *Radiology* 164:635-638, 1987.

37. Foley WD, et al: Contrast optimization for the detection of focal hepatic lesions by MR imaging at 1.5T. *AJR* 149:1155-1160, 1987.

38. Furuya K, et al: Macroregenerative nodule of the liver: a clinicopathologic study of 345 autopsy cases of chronic liver disease. *Cancer* 61:99-105, 1988.

39. Gazelle GS, et al: Hepatic neoplasms: surgically relevant segmental anatomy and imaging techniques. *AJR* 158:1015-1018, 1992.

40. Goldberg HI, et al: Noninvasive quantitation of liver iron in dogs with hemochromatosis using dual energy CT scanning. *Invest Radiol* 17:375-380, 1982.

41. Goldman IS, et al: Increased hepatic density and phospholipidosis due to amiodarone. *AJR* 144:541-546, 1985.

42. Goldsmith MA, et al: Surgical anatomy pertaining to liver resection. *Surg Gynecol Obstet* 141:429-437, 1957.

43. Gomori HM, et al: Hepatic iron overload: quantitative MR imaging. *Radiology* 179:367-369, 1991.

44. Hamm B, et al: Focal liver lesions: MR imaging with Mn-DPDP—initial clinical results in 40 patients. *Radiology* 182:167-174, 1992.

45. Haney PJ, et al: Liver injury and complications in the postoperative trauma patient: CT evaluation. *AJR* 139:271-275, 1982.

46. Harbin WP, et al: Diagnosis of cirrhosis based on regional changes in hepatic morphology. *Radiology* 135:273-283, 1980.

47. Heiken JP, et al: Fatty infiltration of the liver: evaluation by proton spectroscopic imaging. *Radiology* 157:707-710, 1985.

48. Heiken JP, et al: Detection of focal hepatic masses: prospective evaluation with CT, delayed CT, CT during arterial portography, and MR imaging. *Radiology* 171:47-51, 1989.

49. Holley HC, et al: Inhomogeneous enhancement of liver parenchyma secondary to passive congestion: contrast-enhanced CT. *Radiology* 170:795-800, 1989.

50. Howard HM, et al: Diagnostic efficacy of hepatic computed tomography in the detection of body iron overload. *Gastroenterology* 84:209-215, 1983.

51. Ingold J, et al: Radiation hepatitis. *AJR* 93:200-208, 1965.

52. Itai Y, et al: CT and MR imaging of postnecrotic liver scars. *J Comput Assist Tomogr* 12:971-975, 1988.

53. Itoh H, et al: Periportal high intensity on T2-weighted MR images in acute viral hepatitis. *J Comput Assist Tomogr* 16:564-567, 1992.

54. Jeffrey RB, et al: CT of radiation-induced hepatic injury. *AJR* 135:445-448, 1980.

55. Jeffrey RB, et al: Imaging of blunt hepatic trauma. *Radiol Clin North Am* 29:1299-1310, 1991.

56. Jensen PS: Hemochromatosis: a disease often silent but not invisible. *AJR* 126:343-351, 1976.

57. Kelly J, et al: The value of non-contrast-enhanced CT in blunt abdominal trauma. *AJR* 152:41-46, 1989.

58. Koslin DB, et al: Hepatic perivascular lymphedema: CT appearance. *AJR* 150:111-113, 1988.

59. Koslow SA, et al: Hyperintense cirrhotic nodules on MRI. *Gastrointest Radiol* 16:339-341, 1991.

60. Kronthal AJ, et al: Hepatic infarction in preeclampsia. *Radiology* 177:726-728, 1990.

61. Lencioni R, et al: Management of adenomatous hyperlastic nodules in the cirrhotic liver: US follow-up or percutaneous alcohol ablation. *Abdom Imaging* 18:50-55, 1993.

62. Lev-Toaff AS, et al: Hepatic infarcts: new observations by CT and sonography. *AJR* 149:87-90, 1987.

63. Levy CM: Fatty liver: a study of 270 patients with biopsy proven fatty liver and a review of the literature. *Medicine* 41:249-276, 1962.

64. Levy DW, et al: Thorotrast-induced hepatosplenic neoplasia: CT identification. *AJR* 146:977-1004, 1986.

65. Levy HM, et al: MR imaging of portal vein thrombosis. *AJR* 151:283-286, 1988.

66. Lewis E, et al: The fatty liver: pitfalls in the CT and angiographic evaluation of metastatic disease. *J Comput Assist Tomogr* 7:235-241, 1983.

67. Liddell RM, et al: CT depiction of intrahepatic bile ducts. *Radiology* 176:633-635, 1990.

68. Macrander SJ, et al: Periportal tracking in hepatic trauma: CT features. *J Comput Assist Tomogr* 13:952-957, 1989.

69. Maddrey WC: Hepatic vein thrombosis (Budd-Chiari syndrome). *Hepatology* 4:445-465, 1984.

70. Markos J, et al: Value of hepatic computerized tomographic scanning during amiodarone therapy. *Am J Cardiol* 56:89-92, 1985.

71. Mather G, et al: Liver biopsy in sarcoidosis. *Q J Med* 24:331-350, 1955.

72. Mathieu D, et al: Portal vein involvement in hepatocellular carcinoma: dynamic CT features. *Radiology* 152:127-132, 1984.

73. Mathieu D, et al: Portal thrombosis: dynamic CT features and course. *Radiology* 154:737-741, 1985.

74. Mathieu D, et al: Budd-Chiari syndrome: dynamic CT. *Radiology* 165:409-413, 1987.

75. Matsui O, et al: Adenomatous hyperplastic nodules in the cirrhotic liver: differentiation from hepatocellular carcinoma with MR imaging. *Radiology* 173:123-126, 1989.

76. Matsui O, et al: Benign and malignant nodules in cirrhotic livers: distinction based on blood supply. *Radiology* 178:493-497, 1991.

77. Matsui O, et al: Intrahepatic periportal abnormal intensity on MR imaging: an indication of various hepatobiliary diseases. *Radiology* 171:335-338, 1989.

78. Meyer AA, et al: Selective nonoperative management of blunt liver injury using computed tomography. *Arch Surg* 120:550-554, 1985.

79. Miller DL, et al: Hepatic metastasis detection: comparison of three CT contrast enhancement methods. *Radiology* 165:785-790, 1987.

80. Miller JH, et al: Radiography of glycogen storage diseases. *AJR* 132:379-387, 1979.

81. Miller WJ, et al: CT sensitivity and specificity in detecting malignancy in cirrhotic patients with pathologic correlation. *Radiology* 181(P):95, 1991.

82. Mirvis SE, et al: Computed tomography in hepatobiliary trauma. In Ferrucci, JT, Mathieu, DG, editors: *Advances in hepatobiliary radiology,* St. Louis, 1990, Mosby–Year Book, Inc.

83. Mirvis SE, et al: Blunt hepatic trauma in adults: CT-based classification and correlation with prognosis and treatment. *Radiology* 171:27-32, 1989.

84. Mitchell DG, et al: Hepatocellular carcinoma within siderotic regenerative nodules: appearance as a nodule within a nodule on MR images. *Radiology* 178:101-103, 1991.

85. Mitchell DG, Stark DD: *Hepatobiliary MRI,* St. Louis, 1992, Mosby–Year Book, Inc.

86. Moon KL, et al: Computed tomography in hepatic trauma. *AJR* 141:309-314, 1983.

87. Moore EE, et al: Organ injury scaling spleen, liver, and kidney. *J Trauma* 29:1664-1665, 1989.

88. Mori H, et al: Acute thrombosis of the inferior vena cava and hepatic veins in patients with Budd-Chiari syndrome: CT demonstration. *AJR* 153:987-991, 1989.

89. Moulton JS, et al: Passive hepatic congestion in heart failure: CT abnormalities. *AJR* 151:939-942, 1988.

90. Murakami T, et al: CT and MRI of siderotic regenerating nodules in hepatic cirrhosis. *J Comput Assist Tomogr* 16:578-582, 1992.

91. Muramatsu Y, et al: Early hepatocellular carcinoma: MR imaging. *Radiology* 181:209-213, 1991.

92. Murphy FB, et al: MR imaging of focal hemochromatosis. *J Comput Assist Tomogr* 10:1044-1046, 1986.

93. Nakata K, et al: Computed tomography of liver sarcoidosis. *J Comput Assist Tomgr* 13:707-708, 1989.

94. Nelson RC, et al: Hepatic tumors: comparison of CT during arterial portography, delayed CT, and MR imaging for preoperative evaluation. *Radiology* 172:27-34, 1989.

95. Ohta G, et al: Comparative study of three nodular lesions in cirrhosis: adenomatoid hyperplasia, adenomatoid hyperplasia with intermediate lesion and small hepatocellular carcinoma. In Okuda, K, Ishak, KG, editors: *Neoplasms of the liver,* Tokyo, 1987, Springer.

96. Ohtomo K, et al: Confluent hepatic fibrosis in advanced cirrhosis: appearance at CT. *Radiology* 188:31-35, 1993.

97. Ohtomo K, et al: Portosystemic collaterals on MR imaging. *J Comput Assist Tomogr* 10:751-755, 1986.

98. Ohtomo K, et al: Regenerating nodules of liver cirrhosis: MR imaging with pathologic correlation. *AJR* 154:505-507, 1990.

99. Oka H, et al: Prospective study of early detection of hepatocellular carcinoma in patients with cirrhosis. *Hepatology* 12:680-687, 1990.

100. Oliver JC, et al: Efficacy of CT portography in the evaluation of cirrhotic patients for hepatocellular carcinoma. *Radiology* 181(P):167-168, 1991.

101. Outwater E, et al: Lymphadenopathy in primary biliary cirrhosis: CT observations. *Radiology* 171:731-733, 1989.

102. Paling MR, et al: Liver metastases: optimization of MR imaging pulse sequences at 1.0 T. *Radiology* 167:695-699, 1988.

103. Pastakia B, et al: Hepatosplenic candidiasis: wheels within wheels. *Radiology* 166:417-421, 1988.

104. Patrick LE, et al: Pediatric blunt abdominal trauma: periportal tracking at CT. *Radiology* 183:689-691, 1992.

105. Peterson IM, et al: Focal hepatic infarction with bile lake formation. *AJR* 142:1155-1156, 1984.

106. Peterson MS, et al: Hepatic parenchymal perfusion defects detected with CTAP: imaging-pathologic correlation. *Radiology* 185:149-155, 1992.

107. Phillips VM, et al: Delayed iodine scanning of the liver: promising CT technique. *J Comput Assist Tomogr* 9:415-416, 1985.

108. Piekarski J, et al: Difference between liver and spleen CT numbers in the normal adult: its usefulness in predicting the presence of diffuse liver disease. *Radiology* 137:727-729, 1980.

109. Quint LE, et al: CT evaluation of the bile ducts in patients with fatty liver. *Radiology* 153:755-756, 1984.

110. Radin DR, et al: Agenesis of the right lobe of the liver. *Radiology* 164:639-642, 1987.

111. Raptopoulos V, et al: Value of dual-energy CT in differentiating focal fatty infiltration of the liver from low-density masses *AJR* 157:721-725, 1991.

112. Reed GB, et al: The human liver after radiation injury. *Am J Pathol* 45:597-611, 1965.

113. Reinig JW, et al: Liver metastases: detection with MR imaging at 0.5 and 1.5T. *Radiology* 170:149-153, 1989.

114. Reinig JW, et al: Hemodynamics of portal blood flow shown by CT portography. *Radiology* 154:473-476, 1985.

115. Ritchings RJT, et al: An analysis of the spatial distribution of attenuation values in computed tomographic scans of liver and spleen. *J Comput Assist Tomogr* 3:36-39, 1979.

116. Royal SA, et al: Detection and estimation of iron, glycogen and fat in liver of children with hepatomegaly using computed tomography (CT). *Pediatr Res* 13:408, 1979.

117. Sager EM, et al: Increased detectability of liver metastases by the use of contrast enhancement in computed tomography. *Acta Radiol* 26:369-374, 1985.

118. Saini S, et al: MR imaging of liver metastases at 1.5T: similar contrast discrimination with T1- and T2-weighted pulse sequences. *Radiology* 181:449-453, 1991.

119. Savolaine ER, et al: Evolution of CT findings in hepatic hematoma. *J Comput Assist Tomogr* 9:1090-1096, 1985.

120. Semelka RC, et al: Detection of acute and treated lesions of hepatosplenic candidiasis: comparison of dynamic contrast-enhanced CT and MR imaging. *JMRI* 2:341-345, 1992.

121. Semelka RC, et al: Focal liver disease: comparison of dynamic contrast-enhanced CT and T2-weighted fat-suppressed, FLASH, and dynamic gadolinium-enhanced MR imaging at 1.5T. *Radiology* 184:687-694, 1992.

122. Shirkhoda A, et al: Hepatosplenic fungal infection: CT and pathologic evaluation after treatment with liposomal amphotericin B. *Radiology* 159:349-353, 1986.

123. Shuman WP, et al: Use of a power injector during dynamic computed tomography. *J Comput Assist Tomogr* 10:1000-1002, 1986.

124. Shuman WP, et al: Comparison of STIR and spin-echo MR imaging at 1.5T in 90 lesions of the chest, liver, and pelvis. *AJR* 152:853-859, 1989.

125. Siegelman ES, et al: Parenchymal versus reticuloendothelial iron overload in the liver: distinction with MR imaging. *Radiology* 179:361-366, 1991.

126. Silverman PM, et al: MR imaging of the portal venous system: value of gradient-echo imaging as an adjunct to spin-echo imaging. *AJR* 157:297-302, 1991.

127. Silverman PM, et al: CT appearance of abdominal Thorotrast deposition and Thorotrast-induced angiosarcoma of the liver. *J Comput Assist Tomogr* 7:655-658, 1983.

128. Stanley P: Budd-Chiari syndrome. *Radiology* 170:625-627, 1989.

129. Stark DD, et al: MRI of the Budd-Chiari syndrome. *AJR* 146:1141-1148, 1986.

130. Stark DD, et al: MRI and spectroscopy of hepatic iron overload. *Radiology* 154:137-142, 1985.

131. Stark DD, et al: Detection of hepatic metastases: analysis of pulse sequence performance in MR imaging. *Radiology* 159:365-370, 1986.

132. Steinberg HV, et al: Focal hepatic lesions: comparative MR imaging at 0.5 and 1.5 T, *Radiology* 174:153-156, 1990.

133. Tamada T, et al: Portal blood flow: measurement with MR imaging. *Radiology* 173:639-644, 1989.

134. Tyrrel RT, et al: Straight line sign: appearance and significance during CT portography. *Radiology* 173:635-637, 1989.

135. Unger EC, et al: CT and MR imaging of radiation hepatitis. *J Comput Assist Tomogr* 11:264-268, 1987.

136. Van Beers B, et al: Hepatic heterogeneity on CT in Budd-Chiari syndrome: correlation with regional disturbances in portal flow. *Gastrointest Radiol* 13:61-66, 1988.

137. Vogelzang RL, et al: Budd-Chiari syndrome: CT observations. *Radiology* 163:329, 1987.

138. Weinstein JB, et al: High resolution CT of the porta hepatis and hepatoduodenal ligament. *RadioGraphics* 6:55-74, 1986.

139. Wenker JC, et al: Focal fatty infiltration of the liver: demonstration by magnetic resonance imaging. *AJR* 143:573-574, 1984.

140. White TJ, et al: The liver in congestive heart failure. *Am Heart J* 49:250-257, 1955.

141. Williams DK, et al: Portal hypertension evaluated by MR imaging. *Radiology* 157:703-706, 1985.

142. Winkler ML, et al: Hepatic neoplasia: breath-holding MR imaging. *Radiology* 170:801-806, 1989.

143. Winn JP, et al: Liver transplantation: MR angiography with surgical validation. *Radiology* 179:265-269, 1991.

144. Yates CK, et al: Focal fatty infiltration of the liver simulating metastatic disease. *Radiology* 159:83-84, 1986.

145. Zirinsky K, et al: MR imaging of portal venous thrombosis: correlation with CT and sonography. *AJR* 150:283-288, 1988.

31

The Gallbladder and Biliary Tract

THOMAS E. HERBENER

THE GALLBLADDER

The gallbladder is a blind pear-shaped pouch lying along the undersurface of the liver. The gallbladder fossa is located in the plane of the interlobar fissure, which lies between the right and left hepatic lobes (Fig. 31-1). It is approximated by a plane passing longitudinally through the middle hepatic vein and the inferior vena cava. Knowledge of the normal gallbladder location aids in differentiating the gallbladder from other structures and in determining whether the gallbladder location is normal or ectopic.

Normal anatomy

On axial CT images, the gallbladder is a rounded structure with a maximum diameter of less than 4 to 5 cm and an average volume of 30 to 50 cc in the distended state (Fig. 31-1).[94] On consecutive axial images, the diameter of the gallbladder usually increases from the more cephalad and medially located neck to the more caudal and typically more laterally located fundus. The neck of the gallbladder may not be readily obvious except on thin section axial images focused on the porta hepatis (Fig. 31-90). If contracted, the gallbladder is a smaller tubular structure with a readily discernible wall (Fig. 31-2). Visualization of the gallbladder wall depends on the degree of gallbladder distention, clarity of visualization of the gallbladder, or the presence of abnormality. Several values for normal gallbladder wall thickness have been published; these range from 1 to 3.5 mm.[198,201,202,217,230] In a series by Whitehouse et al,[231] 95% of normal patients had a gallbladder wall thickness of less than 2.8 mm. As with ultrasound, 3 mm is therefore a reasonable upper limit of normal. The accuracy of the wall thickness measurement will depend on technical factors such as small pixel size, thin slice collimation, field of view, and appropriate window width and level. In addition, contrast administration may aid in de-fining the wall. There can be enhancement in the gallbladder wall normally after intravenous contrast administration, especially if given in bolus form with dynamic scanning.[206,230] A 20-HU increase in gallbladder-wall density has been shown in normal gallbladder walls after contrast administration.[115,230] Enhancement may persist normally in the gallbladder wall up to 2 hours after angiographic studies if more than 37 g of iodine were administered.[206]

The density of the gallbladder lumen is usually that of water (0 to 20 HU).[94] After intravascular contrast administration, an increase in density of the gallbladder lumen can be seen normally on CT. This is due to normal hepatic excretion of a small fraction of the contrast into the biliary tree. This amount is usually too small to be seen on plain film but can be seen on CT because of the superior contrast sensitivity.[206,222] In the setting of abnormal renal function, hepatobiliary excretion of contrast may be pronounced with increased density of the gallbladder lumen on CT and plain films.[197,206] Certainly, oral cholecystographic agents will increase the density of bile and have been used to perform CT cholangiography.[85,86]

Abnormal density of bile in the gallbladder lumen can be seen in various pathologic conditions by CT. Hemobilia can increase the density of bile toward that of blood (50 to 60 HU) as in hepatobiliary trauma or hemorrhage from a neoplasm or vascular abnormality (Fig. 31-3).[125] Multiple tiny stones may appear simply as increased bile density in the gallbladder lumen if the stones are too small to be individually resolved (Fig. 31-4). However, the most common cause of increased bile density in the gallbladder lumen is due to cystic duct obstruction secondary to an impacted stone or neoplasm. In acute and chronic cholecystitis, the density of the gallbladder lumen may be increased because of inflammatory debris (Fig. 31-5).[221,222] More commonly, how-

978

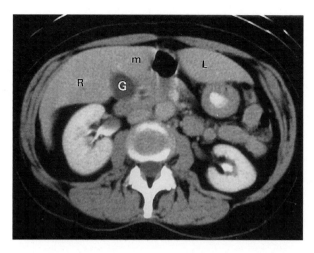

Fig. 31-1. Normal gallbladder fossa. Gallbladder *(G);* right hepatic lobe *(R);* medial segment *(M);* and lateral segment *(L)* of left hepatic lobe.

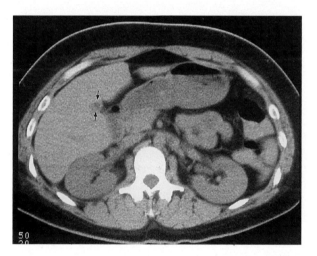

Fig. 31-2. Small contracted gallbladder *(arrows)* with visible wall.

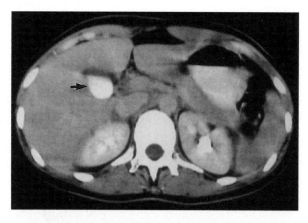

Fig. 31-3. Hemobilia with hyperdense blood in gallbladder *(arrow)* from liver laceration.

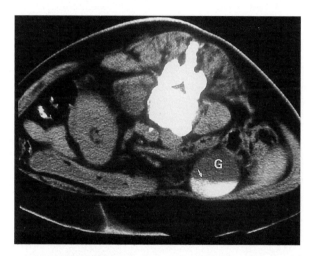

Fig. 31-4. Prone CT scan of multiple tiny layering gallstones *(arrow)* in the gallbladder *(G).*

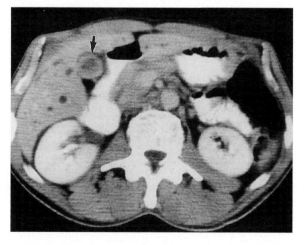

Fig. 31-5. Chronic cholecystitis with contracted gallbladder *(arrow)* with thickened wall and internal debris with increased density of bile.

ever, milk of calcium bile, which is a suspension of calcium carbonate and calcium bilirubinate, will form with cystic duct obstruction (Figs. 31-6 and 31-7; see also Fig. 31-43). This calcium salt suspension may form from a change in bile alkalinity as a result of cystic duct obstruction and inflammation or may result from secretion of calcium by the injured gallbladder mucosa. It also has been described in the setting of ischemic injury to the gallbladder following transcatheter embolization of the cystic artery.[37,222] Milk of calcium bile may completely fill the gallbladder or produce a fluid-fluid level with the denser calcium salt suspension layering dependently. Blood is usually less dense (less than 90 HU) than milk of calcium bile, which may have a density as high as 1000 HU (Figs. 31-3; see also Figs. 31-22 and 31-99).[102]

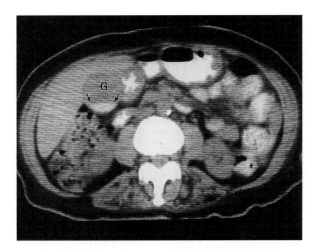

Fig. 31-6. Gallbladder *(G)* with milk of calcium bile *(arrows)*.

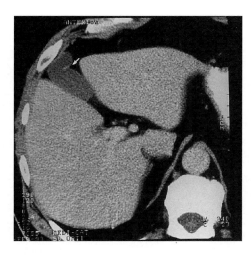

Fig. 31-8. Phrygian cap with small luminal septation *(arrow)*.

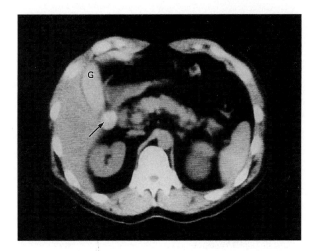

Fig. 31-7. Milk of calcium bile. The intraluminal contents of the gallbladder *(G)* are hyperdense rather than the normal water-density bile. There is also an obstructing calcified gallstone *(arrow)* in the gallbladder neck. Bile stasis, often secondary to cystic duct obstruction, is the cause of milk of calcium bile. (Courtesy of Dr. Avram Pearlstein, Mount Sinai Hospital, Cleveland, Ohio)

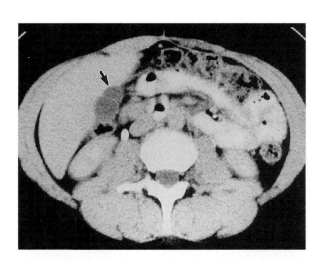

Fig. 31-9. A septation in the gallbladder may give appearance of a pericholecystic fluid collection *(arrow)*.

Congenital variants

Most anomalies of the gallbladder occur as a result of alterations in budding from the primitive foregut or recanalization of the originally solid gallbladder anlage.[191] Abnormalities in gallbladder form, number, and location occur. Abnomalies in number, such as agenesis or duplication, have been described and are rare.[140]

The most common anomalies are those of form, particularly septations of the gallbladder lumen. The most common anomaly of the entire biliary tree is a septation in the distal fundus, which gives the configuration

called a phrygian cap (Fig. 31-8). Septations may occur elsewhere in the gallbladder but are less common and may be multiple. Septations may predispose to bile stasis and stone formation.[140] In addition, septations in the gallbladder may cause an appearance that mimics pericholecystic fluid collections (Fig. 31-9).

Anomalies of gallbladder position are rare. The most common ectopic locations are under the left lobe, intrahepatic, transverse, and retroplaced.[140,154] The intrahepatic gallbladder is typically subcapsular in location along the anteroinferior aspect of the right hepatic lobe and may be surrounded by fat (Figs. 31-10, 31-11).[23] With hypoplasia, aplasia, atrophy, or hypertrophy of one of the hepatic lobes, the gallbladder may be displaced or rotated abnormally to one side.[140] With cirrhosis and associated atrophy of the right hepatic lobe, the gallblad-

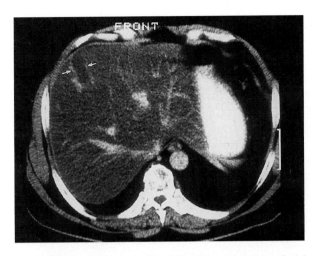

Fig. 31-10. Intrahepatic gallbladder *(arrows)* surrounded by liver parenchyma infiltrated with fat.

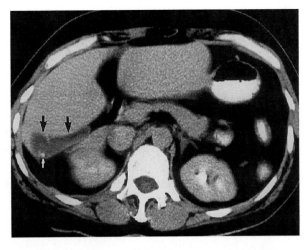

Fig. 31-12. Retroplaced gallbladder *(black arrows)* secondary to hypoplasia of the right hepatic lobe. Note small gallstone *(white arrow).*

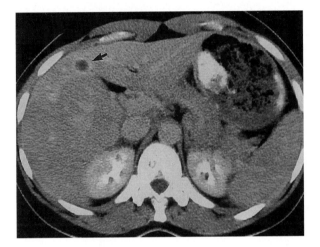

Fig. 31-11. Intrahepatic gallbladder *(arrow)* surrounded by liver parenchyma.

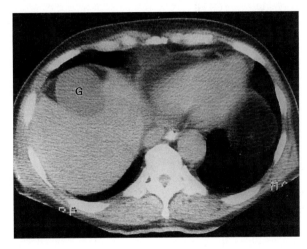

Fig. 31-13. Suprahepatic gallbladder *(G)* just below hemidiaphragm.

der may be retroplaced and be posterior to the liver (Fig. 31-12).[157] A suprahepatic gallbladder was described with hypoplasia of the right hepatic lobe and eventration of the diaphragm (Fig. 31-13).[66] Patients with situs inversus will have a gallbladder in the left upper quadrant, and those with polysplenia syndrome may have a spectrum of hepatobiliary anomalies including a centrally located gallbladder.[74]

Approximately 10% of gallbladders are completely surrounded by peritoneum and may have a long mesentary that allows the gallbladder to lie in abnormal locations such as the pelvis (Fig. 31-14). These are the so called "floating" gallbladders. These gallbladders may be prone to torsion or volvulus.[191] In one reported case,

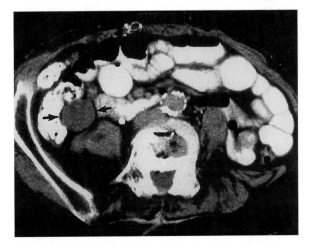

Fig. 31-14. A gallbladder *(arrows)* located in the pelvis because of a long mesentery.

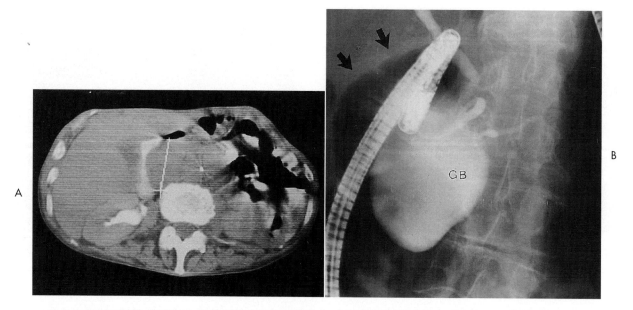

Fig. 31-15. A, The ectopic, floating gallbladder appears as a mass in the region of the head of the pancreas. Associated indentation of the medial wall of the contrast-filled duodenum is seen. **B,** Endoscopic retrograde cholangiopancreatography (ERCP) reveals normal pancreatic and common bile ducts. The normal, contrast-filled gallbladder *(GB)* is located medial to the air-filled C loop of the duodenum *(arrows).* (From Morse J, et al: *Gastrointest Radiol* 10:111-113, 1985.)

such a gallbladder presented as a mass in the region of the head of the pancreas (Fig. 31-15).[154]

Patients with disease in an ectopic gallbladder may present diagnostic challenges because their symptoms may be atypical particularly as to the location of the pain (Fig. 31-12). The key to the diagnosis on CT is absence of the gallbladder in its typical location in the gallbladder fossa. Identifying the abnormally located gallbladder is imperative to ensure the appropriate surgical approach if needed.

Cholecystitis

The findings on CT of cholecystitis are individually nonspecific. Gallbladder wall thickening, gallbladder distension, gallbladder wall enhancement, gallstones, and pericholecystic fluid can be seen in both acute and chronic cholecystitis but also in other conditions such as gallbladder carcinoma. The overall specificity of CT depends on both the constellation of radiographic findings and the appropriate clinical setting. Since the clinical presentation of patients with cholecystitis is often unclear, CT may be the first exam performed. Knowledge of the characteristics of cholecystitis on CT will be helpful for appropriate diagnosis.

Acute cholecystitis. The most common finding on CT of acute cholecystitis is thickening of the gallbladder wall, often nodular in contour (Fig. 31-16).[117,216]

Thickening of the wall alone is not specific for acute cholecystitis and can be seen in a contracted gallbladder, cirrhosis, hepatitis, ascites, pancreatitis, congestive heart failure, renal failure, hypoalbuminemia, adenomyomatosis, portal hypertension, multiple myeloma and gallbladder carcinoma (Fig. 31-17; see also Figs. 31-45, 31-47, and 31-49).[34,116,129,160,170] The wall thickness in acute cholecystitis is 3 to 5 mm or more and is due to mural inflammation and edema. Subserosal edema may present as a hypodense rim surrounding inner, more dense layers of the wall (Figs. 31-18; see also Fig. 31-21).[160] On CT, differentiation of this subserosal edema from pericholecystic fluid may be difficult. Pericholecystic fluid, however, tends to be more focal, and mural edema is more circumferential (Fig. 31-18). With mural edema, an inner enhancing layer of mucosa and an outer enhancing layer of serosa will "sandwich" the hypodense layer of mural edema.[84] Pericholecystic fluid will not be surrounded by an enhancing serosa. In addition, enhancing blood vessels may be seen passing through the mural edema but not through the pericholecystic fluid.[84]

Distension of the gallbladder to greater than 5 cm in diameter can be seen in acute cholecystitis. This, however, is also a nonspecific finding if it is the only abnormality. Diabetes, toxic hepatitis, and distension secondary to neoplastic obstruction of the common bile duct can produce enlarged gallbladders.[94,115] In these set-

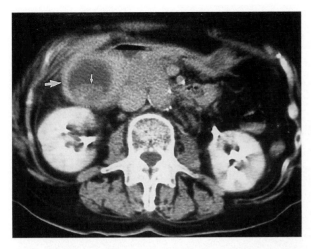

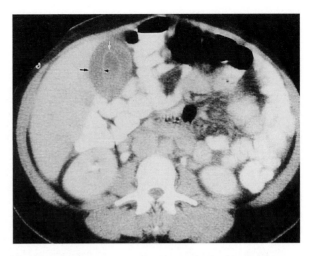

Fig. 31-16. Acute cholecystitis with thickened gallbladder wall *(large arrow)* with debris in the gallbladder lumen *(small arrow)*.

Fig. 31-17. Thickened gallbladder wall *(between black arrows)* due to hepatitis. Note enhancing mucosa along inner wall *(white arrow)*.

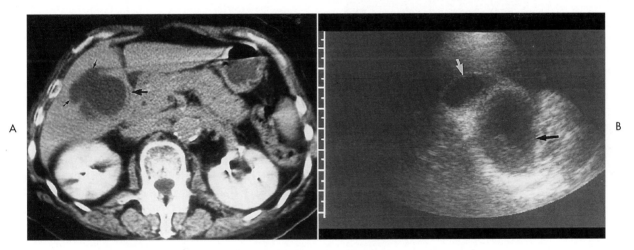

Fig. 31-18. A, Gangrenous cholecystitis with pericholecystic fluid *(small arrows)* and "halo" of subserosal edema *(large arrow).* **B,** Ultrasound of same patient with gangrenous cholecystitis with pericholecystic fluid *(white arrow)* adjacent to gallbladder containing debris *(black arrow).*

tings, however, the gallbladder wall is usually not thickened. Distension and wall thickening together are more specific for cholecystitis.

Poor definition of the gallbladder wall and inflammatory changes in the pericholecystic fat are important findings of cholecystitis on CT. The strand-like water and soft-tissue densities in the pericholecystic fat represent edema and inflammation (Figs. 31-19, 31-20). Transmural inflammation with edema in the tissues around the gallbladder wall will cause loss of sharpness of the wall, and the fatty interface between the gallbladder and ad-

jacent liver parenchcyma will be obscured. One report suggests that these pericholecystic changes are one of the most reliable signs of acute cholecystitis on CT.[216]

Gallstones alone are not themselves a reliable sign of the presence of acute cholecystitis since they may be seen with or without inflammation of the gallbladder. In addition, CT is not as sensitive as ultrasound for detecting gallstones (see Fig. 31-41). Pure cholesterol stones may not be visualized on CT due to the similar density with adjacent bile. Finally, acalculous cholecystitis may demonstrate similar CT findings as acute calculous cho-

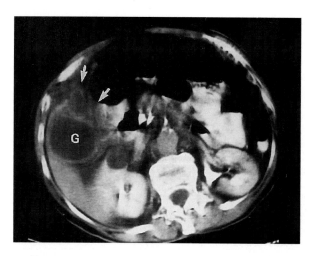

Fig. 31-19. Acute cholecystitis with pericholecystic inflammatory changes *(arrows)* and distended gallbladder *(G)*.

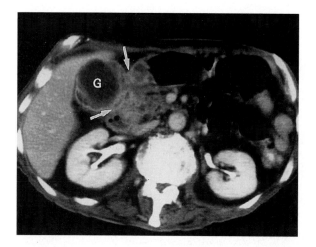

Fig. 31-20. Acute cholecystitis *(G)* with pericholecystitic inflammation *(arrows)* extending into adjacent bowel.

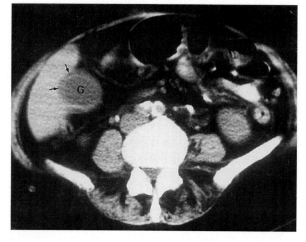

Fig. 31-21. Acalculous cholecystitis *(G)* with no visible gallstones and thin rim of wall edema *(arrows)*.

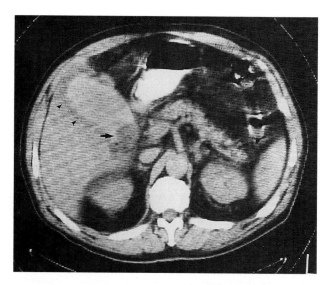

Fig. 31-22. Hemorrhagic cholecystitis. The gallbladder wall is thickened *(arrowheads)*, and its intraluminal contents are abnormally increased in density, representing blood mixed with bile. The rounded area of decreased density within the neck of the gallbladder *(arrow)* is a calculus. (From Jenkins M, et al: *AJR* 140:1197-1198, © by American Roentgen Ray Society, 1983.)

lecystitis such as wall thickening, pericholecystic fluid, and pericholecystic inflammation but without demonstrable gallstones (Fig. 31-21).[145,223]

Complicated cholecystitis. CT is helpful in diagnosing complications of acute cholecystitis since it demonstrates the pericholecystic abnormalities better than ultrasound.[223] Progression to complicated cholecystitis such as empyema, gangrene, and perforation occurs in 25% to 30% of cases of acute cholecystitis.[127,216] As transmural inflammation progresses, ischemia and necrosis may develop and lead to perforation. A focal pericholecystic fluid collection in the setting of gallstones, wall thickening, and pericholecystic edema should suggest acute gangrenous cholecystitis (Fig. 31-18).[216,223] Phlegmon or a complex abscess adjacent to the gallbladder may have a density higher than bile in the gallbladder lumen. In addition, with perforation, gallstones may be detected outside the gallbladder lumen. These stones may erode into adjacent structures such as the duodenum, colon, and biliary tree, causing fistulae. If there is communication into bowel, air may be seen in the gallbladder and biliary tree. Gallstone ileus can occur when a stone erodes into the small bowel with subsequent small bowel obstruction (Fig. 31-25).

Empyema of the gallbladder may not appear differently on CT than uncomplicated acute cholecystitis because pus in the gallbladder lumen may have normal water density. Increased luminal density, however, may

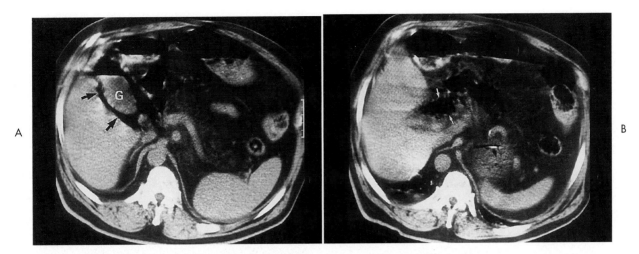

Fig. 31-23. **A,** Emphysematous cholecystitis with gas in the gallbladder wall *(arrows)* surrounding the gallbladder lumen *(G)*. **B,** Emphysematous cholecystitis with gas extending into porta hepatis *(arrows)*.

be seen as a result of the inflammatory debris. A case of hemorrhagic cholecystitis has been reported with hyperdense fluid in the gallbladder lumen, as a result of hemorrhage (Fig. 31-22).[115] Although milk of calcium bile and contrast can increase the density of bile in the gallbladder, empyema and hemorrhagic cholecystitis should be another consideration.

Emphysematous cholecystitis. The only single specific sign for acute cholecystitis on CT is gas in the wall or lumen of the gallbladder as seen in emphysematous cholecystitis.[5,139] The gas develops in acute cholecystitis with bacterial infection secondary to gas-producing organisms such as *E. coli, Enterobacter aerogenes,* and *Clostridium.* The gas may appear as bubbles in the gallbladder lumen, or it may lie within the gallbladder wall, giving a gas density rim to the gallbladder that is pathognomonic (Figs. 31-23 & 31-24). CT is an excellent technique to diagnose emphysematous cholecystitis because it detects and localizes gas easily as a result of its superior contrast and spatial resolution. No intravenous or oral contrast is required and, unlike on plain film or ultrasound, bowel gas is usually readily differentiated.

Gallstone ileus. Gallstone ileus is an uncommon complication of chronic cholecystitis in which a gallstone erodes through the gallbladder wall and into adjacent bowel, causing subsequent bowel obstruction. The duodenum is the most common site of erosion, with the stone migrating distally in the bowel lumen and causing distal small bowel obstruction (Fig. 31-25).

Patients with gallstone ileus often present with nonspecific abdominal pain. Biliary symptoms are often absent. The preoperative diagnosis is difficult to make. The plain film findings have been described and include

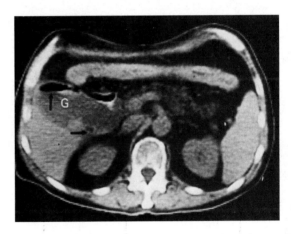

Fig. 31-24. This scan is of a patient with *Clostridium* infection of the gallbladder *(G)*, producing gas *(arrows)* within the gallbladder lumen.

the triad of small bowel obstruction, pneumobilia, and an ectopic gallstone. However, not all gallstones are radiopaque on plain film, and pneumobilia may not be present. Therefore, plain film diagnosis may be difficult and is seen in only 30% to 35% to cases.[88]

The findings on CT have been described and include dilated loops of small bowel, pneumobilia with air in the bile ducts and gallbladder, and a stone within the bowel lumen—usually distal small bowel.[88]

Mirizzi syndrome. Mirizzi syndrome is the condition of biliary obstruction of the common hepatic duct at the level of the gallbladder neck caused by inflammation associated with an impacted gallstone in the gallbladder neck or cystic duct. It is typically a complication of chronic cholecystitis. Congenital anomalies of the ex-

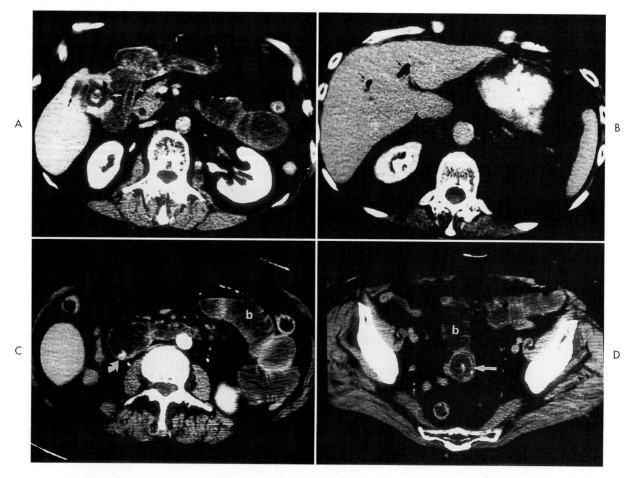

Fig. 31-25. Gallstone ileus. **A,** A stone *(S)* is seen in the gallbladder with a visible fistula between the gallbladder and the adjacent duodenum (*white arrow* shows defect in medial gallbladder wall). *Black arrow* shows pericholecystic fluid. **B,** Pneumobilia *(black arrows).* **C,** Stone in second portion of dilated duodenum *(arrow).* Note dilated small bowel *(b)* due to distal obstruction. **D,** Stone in distal small bowel lumen *(arrow)* causing obstruction with dilated small bowel *(b)* proximally.

trahepatic bile ducts may predispose patients to this condition.[20] Because of the inflammation, fibrosis, and distortion of structures at the level of obstruction, both preoperative and intraoperative diagnoses are difficult.

These patients typically present with symptoms suggestive of gallbladder disease and jaundice. US and CT are often the initial exams performed to evaluate such a clinical presentation. On CT, dilated bile ducts may be seen with the CHD dilated to the level of the gallbladder neck or cystic duct (Fig. 31-26).[20,22] Often a stone may be seen in the neck or cystic duct at this level. The CHD diameter abruptly decreases below the level of the stone. Nonspecific signs of cholecystitis may be present.

The stone in the neck of the gallbladder or cystic duct may obstruct the CHD as a result of extrinsic compression. However, the stone may erode into the CHD by pressure necrosis, or it may erode into the surrounding tissues of the hepatoduodenal ligament and be detected outside the bile duct. A cholecystobiliary fistula may occur but will be difficult to directly visualize on CT.[20] Cholangiography (ERCP, PTC) is the gold standard to evaluate for a fistula.

Mirizzi syndrome may mimic a malignancy especially if the stone in the neck of the gallbladder or cystic duct is not visualized. Abrupt change in caliber of the CHD can be seen in malignancy such as cholangiocarcinoma. PTC or ERCP may demonstrate a stricture in the CHD that also may mimic malignancy. Carcinoma of the cystic duct has been described as mimicking Mirizzi syndrome because of associated CHD obstruction.[175] However, CT, especially high-resolution CT, will show no evidence of mass or lymphadenopathy in the setting of Mirizzi syndrome as expected with malignancy; this is an extremely important observation.[22]

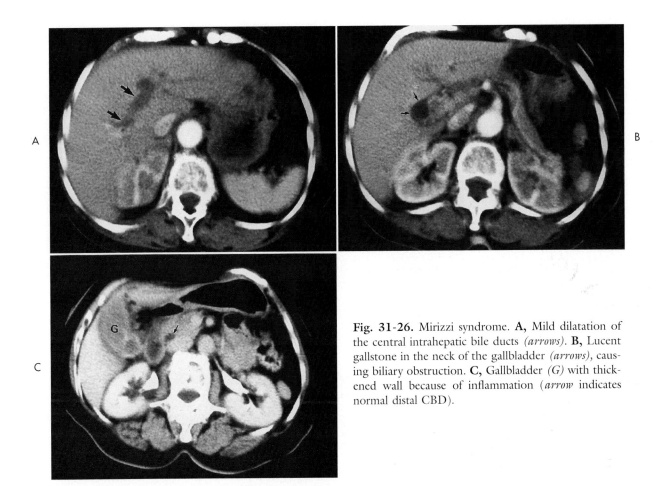

Fig. 31-26. Mirizzi syndrome. **A,** Mild dilatation of the central intrahepatic bile ducts *(arrows).* **B,** Lucent gallstone in the neck of the gallbladder *(arrows),* causing biliary obstruction. **C,** Gallbladder *(G)* with thickened wall because of inflammation *(arrow* indicates normal distal CBD).

Chronic cholecystitis. Chronic cholecystitis may have similar findings as acute cholecystitis, such as wall thickening, stones, and wall enhancement (Figs. 31-27, 31-28). The gallbladder, however, often is contracted around the gallstones rather than distended. A "porcelain" gallbladder is an uncommon manifestation of chronic cholecystitis where calcium is deposited in the gallbladder wall. The calcium may be found in coarse plaques in the muscularis or as diffuse punctate foci in the mucosa (Fig. 31-29). Although plain film and ultrasound may demonstrate a porcelain gallbladder, CT is better at detecting and localizing the calcium to the wall of the gallbladder.[118] In addition, because of the association of porcelain gallbladder and gallbladder carcinoma, the CT examination should be carefully viewed for any sign of carcinoma (Fig. 31-45).[75,102,169] Porcelain gallbladders may in fact be removed prophylactically because of the association with carcinoma. Occasionally, the calcified rim of a large gallstone may mimic calcification in the wall of the gallbladder.

Xanthogranulomatous cholecystitis. Xanthogranulomatous cholecystitis is a rare condition associated with chronic recurrent inflammation of the gallbladder due to gallstones. It is a benign process but may mimic gallbladder malignancy with its slow insidious onset and its appearance on imaging studies. Preoperative diagnosis is rare.[55,61]

Pathologically, this process consists of a mixed inflammatory infiltrate in the gallbladder wall with foamy histiocytes, foreign body giant cells, and diffuse fibrotic reaction. This is a similar xanthogranulomatous reaction as elsewhere in the body. Grossly, diffuse nodules may appear in the gallbladder wall, a large "tumor" mass may form, or an ill-defined infiltrative process may occur.[55]

On CT, irregular thickening of the gallbladder wall is the most common abnormality in addition to gallstones. However, a mass may be present in the gallbladder fossa.[51] The appearance may be impossible to separate from that of gallbladder carcinoma on both US and CT. However, no evidence of metastases or biliary dilatation will be seen with xanthogranulomatous cholecystitis.[55,61]

Hyperplastic cholecystoses. The hyperplastic cholecystoses are noninflammatory conditions of the gallbladder that consist of benign proliferation of normal tissue of the gallbladder and include cholesterolosis

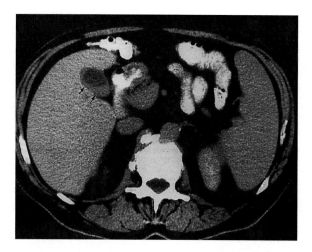

Fig. 31-27. Chronic cholecystitis with thickened gallbladder wall *(arrows)*.

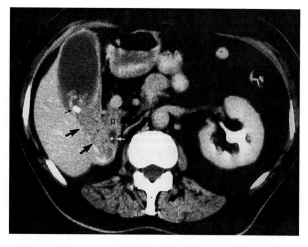

Fig. 31-28. Chronic cholecystitis with thickened gallbladder wall *(large black arrows)*, gallstones *(small black arrow)*, and distal CBD stone *(small white arrow)* in the head of the pancreas *(P)*.

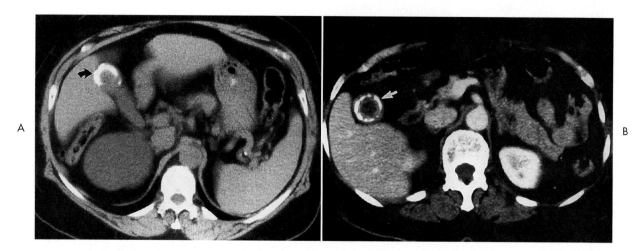

Fig. 31-29. Porcelain gallbladder. **A,** Focal course calcified plaque in fundus *(arrow)*. **B,** Diffuse calcific plaques throughout gallbladder wall.

and adenomyomatosis. Cholesterolosis consists of multiple focal deposits of cholesterol-laden macrophages in the lamina propria of the gallbladder wall and formation of cholesterol polyps. These are very small, however, and not typically seen on CT but better appreciated on ultrasound.

The CT findings in adenomyomatosis have been described. This condition consists of thickening of the muscular wall of the gallbladder with proliferation of mucosal epithelium and outpouching of the mucosa into or through the wall, forming intramural diverticula. CT demonstrates the gallbladder wall thickening, which may

be focal and may show the intramural diverticular especially if an oral cholecystographic agent is administered or if small stones are within the diverticula (Figs. 31-30 and 31-31).[27,47,109,147] Fatty proliferation in the subserosal portion of the gallbladder has been reported.[147] Thickening of the gallbladder wall may be the only finding on CT, and exclusion of other processes such as cholecytitis or gallbladder carcinoma may be difficult (Fig. 31-53).[109]

Postcholecystectomy. After cholecystectomy via laparotomy (open cholecystectomy), CT can be used to evaluate patients with persistent fever, abdominal pain,

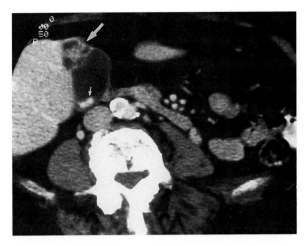

Fig. 31-30. Focal adenomyomatosis *(large arrow)* in fundus of gallbladder with small gallstones in the lumen *(small arrow).*

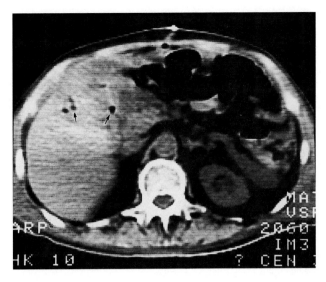

Fig. 31-32. After cholecystectomy, abnormal soft tissue density, with a few small collections of gas *(arrows),* is present in the region of the gallbladder fossa. On aspiration, this proved to be an infected hematoma.

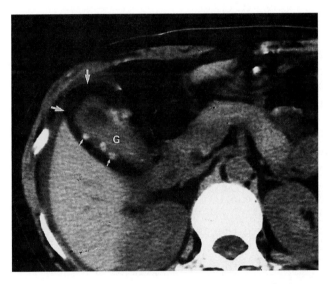

Fig. 31-31. Adenomyomatosis with proliferation of subserosal fat *(large arrows),* intramural diverticula containing stones *(small arrows),* and soft-tissue mass *(G)* in gallbladder lumen. (From Miyake H, et al: *Gastrointest Radiol* 17:21-23, 1992.)

or abnormal liver function tests. Biliary scintigraphy (DISIDA) and cholangiography will often be the first line examinations to evaluate for bile leak or duct injury.[76] However, CT may be used to evaluate for abscess, hematoma, or an unexpected postoperative complication. Subhepatic fluid collections have been shown by ultrasound in 20% of postcholecystectomy patients.[137] In addition, 44% of such patients have been shown in one series to have bile leaks on DISIDA scans, with the majority being clinically insignificant.[226] CT can identify these collections but unfortunately often cannot differentiate

a postoperative seroma, abscess, hematoma, or biloma, unless percutaneous aspiration is performed (Fig. 31-32).

Laparoscopic cholecystectomy is rapidly becoming a popular treatment for gallbladder disease. Typical postoperative changes on CT have been described and include pneumoperitoneum, subcutaneous emphysema, subhepatic fluid collections, ascites, and gallbladder fossa edema.[137] Small fluid collections in the gallbladder fossa immediately in the postoperative period are common and probably represent small bile leaks because of disruption of ducts of Luschka, which are accessory ducts draining directly from liver parenchyma into the gallbladder (Fig. 31-33).[226] Significant bile leakage is one of the more common postoperative complications and occurs as a result of injury to the extrahepatic bile ducts, leak from the cystic duct remnant, or leak from transection of large unrecognized accessory bile ducts. A DISIDA scan will be the most useful exam in demonstrating the bile leak, and ERCP can define the exact site of leakage. CT will demonstrate a fluid collection in the porta hepatis, subhepatic fluid, or diffuse ascites. Endoscopic management of such leaks has been shown to be nearly 95% successful.[226] If the DISIDA and ERCP are not helpful, CT may be used to examine the patient for other postoperative complications such as abscess or hematoma. Ligation of aberrant bile ducts or unrecognized accessory bile ducts may be demonstrated on CT and has been reported as focally dilated subsegmental intrahepatic bile ducts typi-

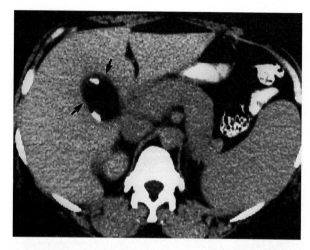

Fig. 31-33. Abscess *(arrows)* in the gallbladder fossa following laparoscopic cholecystectomy.

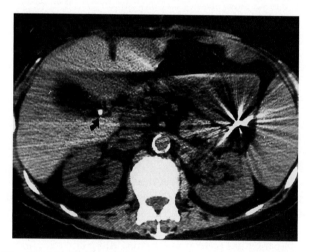

Fig. 31-34. Retained stone within cystic duct remnant *(arrow)*.

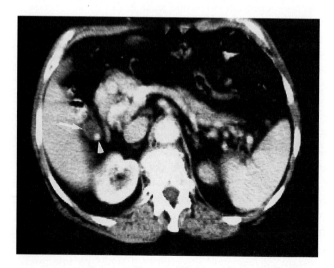

Fig. 31-35. Dilated cystic duct remnant *(large arrow)* containing dense stone *(arrow head)*.

cally in the posterior portion of the right lobe of the liver.[46]

Cystic duct remnant. Following cholecystectomy, a small remnant of the cystic duct remains in place. Rarely, patients may develop symptoms because of the residual cystic duct that mimic symptoms of cholecystitis or cholelithiasis (Fig. 31-34).[83] The remnant itself can enlarge over time and may function as a gallbladder developing similar diseases such as gallstones and even carcinoma (Fig. 31-35).[186]

Gallstones

The appearance of gallstones on CT depends on the complex relationship of several factors. The major determinant of appearance is the composition of the stone. Gallstones may be composed of, in general, three components: bile pigments, cholesterol, and calcium. Pure cholesterol or pure bile pigment stones are rare. Pure cholesterol stones will have a low density compared to bile (−100 HU in vitro).[72] Most stones, however, are a mixture of calcium, bile pigment, and cholesterol. The density of the mixed stone will vary, depending on the amount of each component present. There is some controversy in the literature as to whether calcium or cholesterol play the predominant role in determining stone density on CT.[14,17,18,28,31,236] In general, calcium content is responsible for increasing the density of the stone. Up to 60% of gallstones demonstrate calcium on CT scan in vivo and are dense.[11,31] Other mixed composition stones with less calcium may have a density equal to bile and may be difficult to visualize on CT (Figs. 31-36 to 31-43).[11,13,21,72]

The pattern in which the components of the stone are distributed will affect the appearance of the stone. Calcium bilirubinate stones are often homogeneously dense (Fig. 31-36). Mixed composition stones may have several patterns, depending on the distribution of cal-

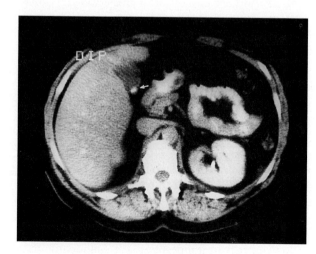

Fig. 31-36. Tiny dense gallstone *(arrow)*.

cium. They may have a dense rim of calcium peripherally with a low density cholesterol center (Figs. 31-37, 31-38). They may also have a laminated appearance with alternating layers of calcification. Also, these stones may have punctate foci of increased density scattered throughout.

Stones may also have clefts centrally in their matrix that contain gas (Figs. 31-37, 31-39). Gas in these clefts appears as low-density fissures in various patterns giving the so-called Mercedes-Benz sign, crow's feet sign, or seagull sign. Gas probably forms after shrinkage of the stone matrix.[72] The gas consists mostly of nitrogen. The significance of the gas clefts is little if any, except that it may contribute to gallstones floating and it may aid in detecting stones on CT that are otherwise isodense with bile (Fig. 31-40).

The ability of CT to detect gallstones depends on several factors including stone composition, size, number, shape, bile density, and scanning technique. There have been numerous reports of varying degrees of sensitivity of CT for detecting stones ranging from 78% to 83%.* Uchida[220] reported a 100% sensitivity for calcified stones. Havrilla reported a 78% sensitivity prospectively with a 94% sensitivity retrospectively.[94] The stone composition greatly affects the detection rate. Calcified stones that are hyperdense will be seen more readily than will composite stones, which are isodense to bile (Fig. 31-41). In addition, the presence of matrix gas will increase detection rate (Fig. 31-40). The size of stones will

*References 11, 13, 28, 31, 94, 102, 220.

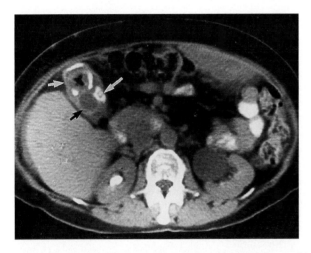

Fig. 31-37. Gallbladder containing rim calcified stone with central gas *(short white arrow)* and relatively lucent stone *(black arrow),* with coarse calcified plaque *(long white arrow)* in gallbladder wall (porcelain gallbladder).

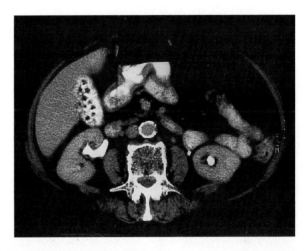

Fig. 31-39. Multiple small lucent stones floating in gallbladder presenting as negative filling defects due to contrast in gallbladder following ERCP.

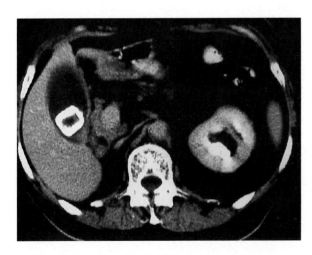

Fig. 31-38. Densely calcified, laminated gallstone.

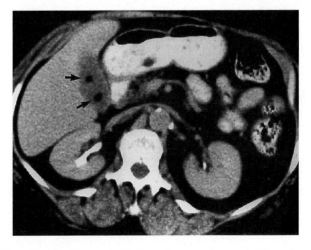

Fig. 31-40. Gas centrally in gallstones *(arrows).* These isodense stones would not be visible without the gas.

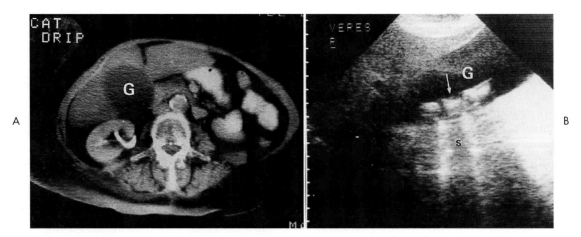

Fig. 31-41. A, The gallbladder *(G)* is distended, but no filling defects are perceptible on this CT scan. **B,** Sagittal ultrasound scan through the gallbladder *(G)* demonstrates large, echogenic structures *(arrow)* within the gallbladder lumen, with associated acoustic shadowing *(s)* diagnostic of gallstones.

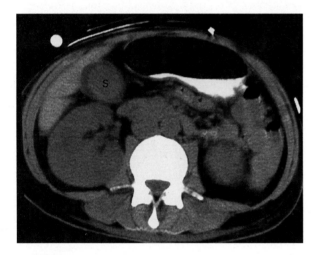

Fig. 31-42. Large nearly isodense stone *(S)* that almost fills the gallbladder lumen.

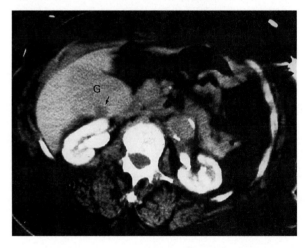

Fig. 31-43. Low-density gallstone *(arrow)* presents as negative filling defect because of high density bile in gallbladder *(G)*.

also affect detection rate, with small stones being missed because of partial voluming. Large stones that completely fill the lumen may not be detected if they are isodense with bile (Fig. 31-42). In addition, if there are multiple tiny stones, they may layer and mimic milk of calcium bile (Fig. 31-4). The density of bile may also affect stone detection. If the bile density is increased, lower density stones will appear as negative filling defects while higher density stones may be obscured (Fig. 31-43). Oral cholangiographic agents have been used to increase the density of bile to improve CT detection rates of gallstones. Finally, the technique of the CT examination will determine detection rates of stones. High-resolution CT

that is targeted to the gallbladder with thin collimation is recommended.[14]

In recent years, a large volume of literature has considered the use of CT in selecting patients for nonsurgical therapy of gallstones. The nonsurgical options include extracorporeal shock-wave lithotripsy (ESWL), direct-contact dissolution with methyl tert-butyl ether (MTBE) and oral agents (cheno- and ursodeoxycholic acid). In the past, plain film was used to detect gallstones containing calcium, which precluded nonsurgical therapy. The problem is that 14% of patients with lucent stones based on plain films have pigment stones that are not candidates for dissolution. In addition, 33%

of dense stones on plain film are cholesterol stones and would be candidates for nonsurgical therapy.[14] Therefore, CT has been proposed as a more accurate method to evaluate which stones would be ideal for the nonsurgical therapies.

Studies have shown correlation between the CT attenuation of gallstones and the cholesterol and calcium content of the stone, and both in vitro and in vivo studies have demonstrated this finding.[8,14,28,111,237] Although there have been disagreements over whether it is the calcium or the cholesterol content which most determines the CT attenuation number, the basic finding is that the homogeneously dense stone with high attenuation numbers contains high levels of calcium and is a poor candidate for nonsurgical therapy. The less dense the stone, with lower attenuation values, the better the success with nonsurgical therapy. Unfortunately, the issue is not this straightforward. Concerning the success of dissolution, Baron et al reported that the pattern of calcium within the stone may play a more important role than does simply the amount of calcium.[18] For example, densely calcified stones do poorly with MTBE dissolution. However, if the calcium is arranged in lamina or a peripheral rim, the stone dissolves well. Those that dissolve best are isodense or hypodense with bile and contain a high amount of cholesterol. In addition, stones with a central nidus of calcium or peripheral rim of calcium have been shown to fragment with ESWL; these have now been approved for such therapy.[31] Therefore, success at nonsurgical treatment may not simply depend on the attenuation number of the stone but on multiple factors such as the pattern of calcification in the stone. CT may therefore be important in evaluating which patients will have the greatest success with the nonsurgical therapies; however, large-scale clinical trials will have to be performed.

Gallbladder neoplasms

Gallbladder carcinoma is the most common malignant tumor of the gallbladder. Adenocarcinoma is the most common histologic type, in 90% of cases. Squamous carcinomas, mixed-type carcinomas, and sarcomas have been described in the gallbladder (Fig. 31-44).

Many benign neoplasms of the gallbladder have been reported such as a fibroma, lipoma, myxoma, granular cell tumor, leiomyoma, hemangioma, and neurofibroma.[101,153] The most common benign tumor of the gallbladder is the adenoma, which appears on CT as a small mass along the gallbladder wall.

Gallbladder carcinoma is the most common malignancy of the biliary tree and is the fifth most common gastrointestinal malignancy. Its peak occurrence is in the sixth decade or older, and there is a female predilection of 3-4:1 (F:M).[141,198] The female predominance may be related to underlying inflammatory disease, and gall-

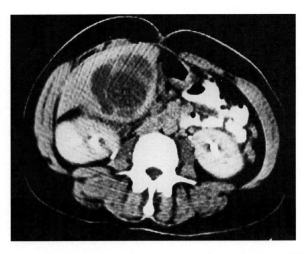

Fig. 31-44. Squamous cell carcinoma of the gallbladder *(M)*.

stones are detected in 65% to 95% of gallbladder carcinoma cases.[141,198] With new therapeutic methods for treating gallstones, such as lithotripsy or stone dissolution, that spare the gallbladder and leave it in place, surveillance of the gallbladder is recommended because of the increased risk of carcinoma.[199] Calcification in the gallbladder wall (porcelain gallbladder) is associated with gallbladder carcinoma in 11% to 33% of cases (Fig. 31-45).[75,102,169] In addition, an increased risk of gallbladder carcinoma has been reported in patients with choledochal cysts.[238]

The clinical presentation of gallbladder carcinoma is often nonspecific and mimics other right upper quadrant diseases such as cholecystitis. Symptoms of jaundice and weight loss may not appear until the carcinoma has spread. Local extension of tumor is seen in 75% to 85% of patients at the time of presentation.[141] Therefore a large portion of patients are unresectable at presentation, and prognosis is poor with a 5-year survival rate of less than 12% even if the carcinoma is incidentally detected.[141] An estimated 1% of gallbladder carcinoma is detected incidentally at the time of cholecystectomy.[228]

The appearance on CT scan is also nonspecific and often mimics benign disease. The typical findings of gallbladder carcinoma include three patterns: a mass replacing the gallbladder fossa, an intraluminal mass, and gallbladder-wall thickening. The mass replacing the gallbladder fossa is the most common appearance in several series (Figs. 31-44 to 31-46 and 31-50 to 31-52).[103,107,228,236] Such a mass may contain gallstones within it and demonstrate central necrosis when large. A normal gallbladder cannot be detected (Fig. 31-46). This form typically has invaded adjacent structures at the time of presentation. The thickened gallbladder-wall type is less common but is very difficult to differentiate from

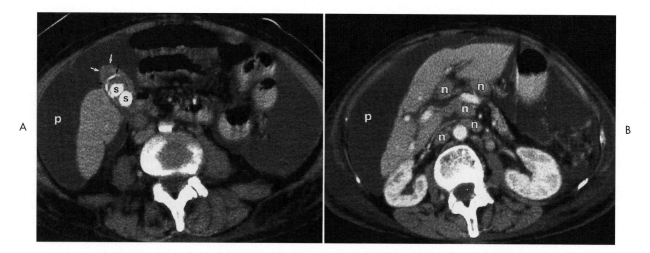

Fig. 31-45. Gallbladder carcinoma arising from a porcelain gallbladder. **A,** Gallbladder containing dense stones *(s)* and calcified mural plaque *(black arrows)* with focal carcinoma in the wall *(white arrows)*. P, ascites. **B,** Diffuse metastatic lymphadenopathy *(n)* and ascites *(p)* with peritoneal metastases.

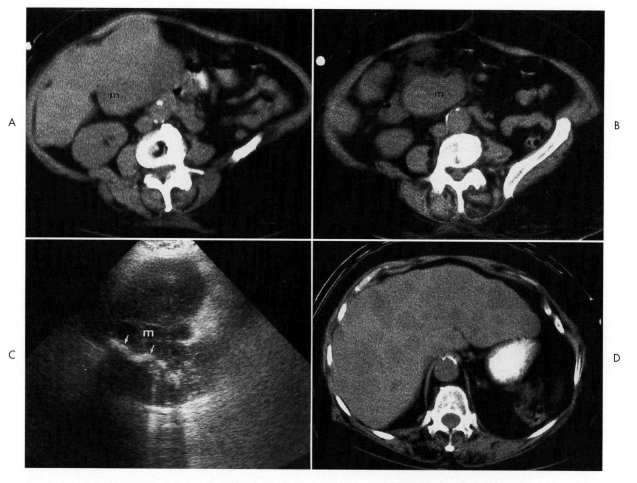

Fig. 31-46. Gallbladder carcinoma. **A,** Ill-defined mass *(m)* in the gallbladder fossa. **B,** Several centimeters caudal to level of *A* with mass *(M)* extending from gallbladder fossa. **C,** Ultrasound of mass in gallbladder fossa shows stones *(arrows)* within hypoechoic mass *(M)*. **D,** Multiple metastases to liver.

benign cholecystitis (Fig. 31-47). The wall is usually 4 to 13 mm or greater in thickness, often asymmetrically thickened, and often nodular.[103] The intraluminal mass type is less common and presents as a polypoid mass in the gallbladder lumen (Fig. 31-48). Lesions less than 10 mm in diameter are difficult to detect on CT.[102] Such lesions are difficult to differentiate from benign polyps or low-density adherent stones.

Associated findings on CT typically involve the spread of the tumor and aid in diagnosis. Gallbladder carcinoma most commonly spreads via direct invasion into adjacent structures such as liver, porta hepatic structures, colon, duodenum, and pancreas. The liver is the most common site of invasion in 34% to 89% of patients, de-

pending on the series, at the time of presentation.[198] When the tumor invades the liver, the medial segment of the left lobe and the anterior segment of the right lobe are the most common targets (Figs. 31-49 and 31-50). The area of invasion is usually hypodense relative to surrounding liver parenchycyma on enhanced CT scan. Direct invasion of the liver versus simple contact of the tumor with the liver surface may be difficult to differentiate on CT. An irregular boundary with normal liver parenchyma suggests invasion (Fig. 31-51).

Gallbladder carcinoma can metastasize to local nodes or distantly, primarily to the liver. Lymph nodes in the porta hepatis, peripancreatic region, and celiac axis may be involved. Engels reported that the foramen of Winslow lymph node and the superior pancreaticoduodenal node are the most frequent sites of nodal metastases (Figs. 31-45 and 31-47).[64] Nodal masses may cause biliary obstruction and mimic a primary pancreatic tumor.[228] Distant metastases to the liver appear as hypodense lesions relative to adjacent liver parenchyma on enhanced CT scans (Fig. 32-47). Hepatic metastases are less common, however, than direct invasion.[102] Peritoneal carcinomatosis may occur (Figs. 31-45 and 31-50).

Biliary obstruction is reported in 50% of cases of gallbladder carcinoma (Fig. 31-49).[141] This may be due to direct invasion into the porta hepatis, obstructing lymphadenopathy, or intraductal spread of tumor. Intraductal spread of tumor was reported in only 4% of cases by Weiner et al but is difficult to differentiate from cholangiocarcinoma (Fig. 31-52).[228]

The differential diagnosis of gallbladder carcinoma on CT scan may be difficult. Gallbladder carcinoma often mimics cholecystitis (acute, chronic, and xanthogranulomatous) radiographically and clinically.

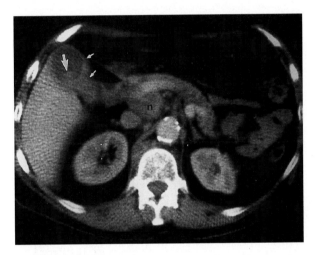

Fig. 31-47. Gallbladder carcinoma *(small arrows)* presenting as thickening of the gallbladder wall with a gallstone *(large arrow)* and metastasis to lymph nodes *(N).*

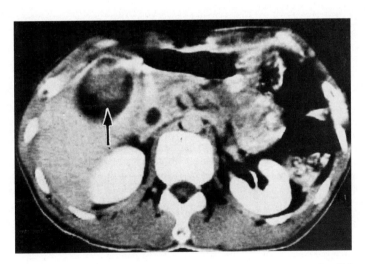

Fig. 31-48. Intraluminal type of gallbladder neoplasm. (From Itani Y: *Radiology* 137:715, 1980.)

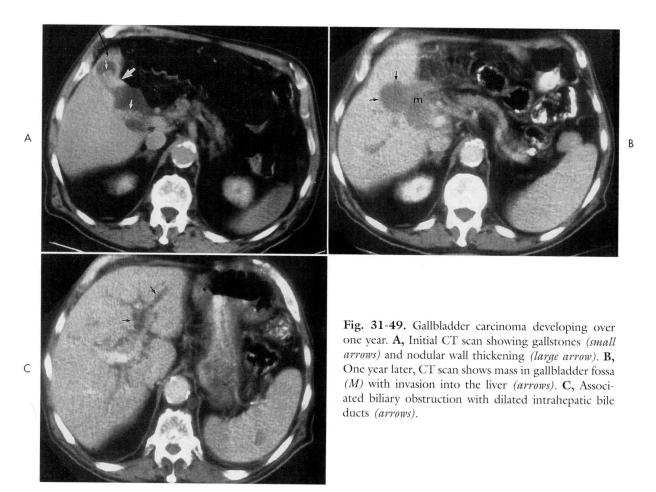

Fig. 31-49. Gallbladder carcinoma developing over one year. **A,** Initial CT scan showing gallstones *(small arrows)* and nodular wall thickening *(large arrow).* **B,** One year later, CT scan shows mass in gallbladder fossa *(M)* with invasion into the liver *(arrows).* **C,** Associated biliary obstruction with dilated intrahepatic bile ducts *(arrows).*

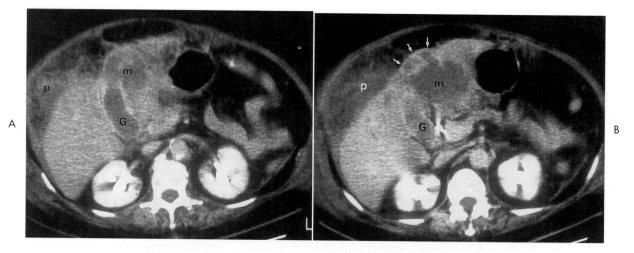

Fig. 31-50. **A,** Gallbladder carcinoma extending from gallbladder *(G)* into medial segment of left lobe of the liver *(M)* with peritoneal carcinomatosis *(P).* **B,** Gallbladder carcinoma bulging anterior surface of medial segment of left lobe *(arrows).*

Findings common to both on CT scan include gallbladder wall thickening, gallstones, mass in the gallbladder fossa, edema in pericholecystic fat, and thickening of the hepatoduodenal ligament. A hypodense "halo" in the thickened gallbladder wall has been described as a helpful sign on CT of cholecystitis rather than carcinoma (Fig. 31-18).[198] The halo represents mural edema. Direct invasion into the liver suggests carcinoma; however, in rare cases abscess formation may occur in liver parenchyma adjacent to gangrenous cholecystitis. Smathers et al reported signs on CT that were helpful to differentiate gallbladder carcinoma from complicated cholecystitis

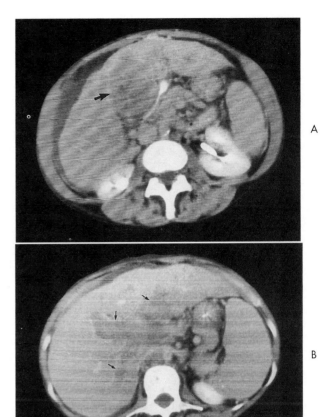

Fig. 31-52. Gallbladder carcinoma. A, Mass in gallbladder fossa *(arrow)*. B, Intraductal spread of tumor throughout the biliary tree *(arrows)*.

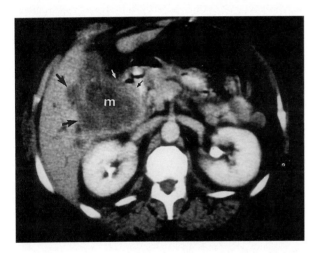

Fig. 31-51. Gallbladder carcinoma presenting as mass in the gallbladder fossa *(M)* with invasion into adjacent liver *(large arrows)* and duodenum *(small arrows)*.

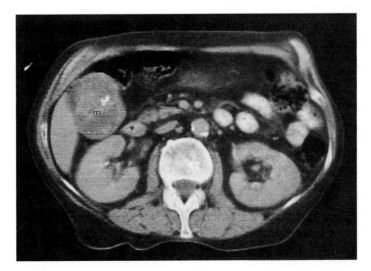

Fig. 31-53. Adenomyomatosis presenting as mass in the gallbladder fossa *(M)* and mimicking gallbladder carcinoma. (From Gerard PS, et al: *J Comput Assist Tomogr* 14(3):490-491, 1990.)

including: a mass less than half the size of the gallbladder, direct invasion of the liver with focal bulge of the anterior contour of the liver, biliary obstruction at the level of the porta hepatis, and lymphadenopathy.[198]

Primary malignant tumors of the liver may extend into the gallbladder fossa and mimic gallbladder carcinoma. Visualizing a normal gallbladder on CT scan, even if displaced by tumor, suggests a hepatic primary rather than gallbladder primary. Occasionally, the scirrhous type of gallbladder carcinoma may present as a contracted gallbladder with a thickened wall, mimicking a cholangiocarcinoma (Fig. 31-53).[141]

The diagnostic accuracy of CT scan with gallbladder carcinoma has been reported in several series. Itai reported successful detection of 27 of 30 cases of gallbladder carcinoma on CT scan for an accuracy of 90%.[102] Ryu et al reported detection of 31 of 37 cases (89%).[102] In addition, CT and ultrasound were compared by Weiner et al and of 22 cases, ultrasound detected seven of 11 cases, and CT detected 10 of 11 cases.[228] The conclusion was that CT and ultrasound were complementary.

Metastases

Metastases to the gallbladder are rare and often detected incidentally at autopsy. The most common primary malignancies with metastases reported to the gallbladder are pancreatic, gastric, renal cell, ovarian, and melanoma.[26,33,141] Typically metastases are focal, nodular thickenings of the gallbladder wall and are often serosal in location. Such a finding in a patient with a known primary malignancy should raise suspicion for gallbladder metastasis.

THE BILIARY TRACT

Normal anatomy

Normal intrahepatic bile ducts can be visualized in the liver parenchyma, especially on the newer-generation high-resolution CT scanners (Fig. 31-54). In 40% of their patients, Liddell et al reported seeing normal intrahepatic bile ducts as linear water-density structures accompanying the portal vein branches peripherally in the liver parenchyma.[130] The normal intrahepatic bile ducts measure less than 3 mm, are few in number, and are randomly scattered throughout the liver. Such random scattering is a key observation, since visualization of intrahepatic bile ducts confluent with the hilum should raise suspicion of obstruction (Fig. 31-55). In addition, certain pathologic conditions may be difficult to differentiate from visualization of normal intrahepatic bile ducts. For example, sclerosing cholangitis and biliary obstruction in cirrhosis may present with a few, scattered, and small visible intrahepatic bile ducts (Fig. 31-68, A). The clinical setting will aid in differentiating these conditions. Finally, normal intrahepatic ducts are

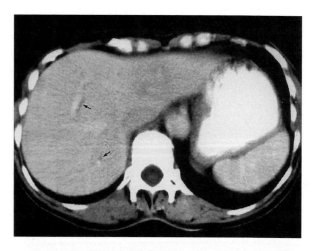

Fig. 31-54. Normal intrahepatic bile ducts *(arrows)*.

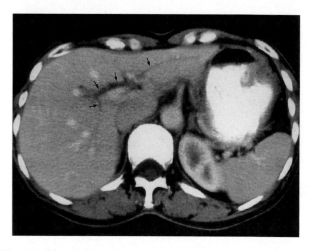

Fig. 31-55. Mild intrahepatic biliary dilatation *(arrows)*. Note the confluence of the ducts into the hilum.

linear structures seen along one side of the portal vein. In contrast, periportal lymphedema will appear as low density accompanying the portal vein branches but will completely surround the portal vein and usually will be confluent with the hilum (Fig. 31-56).[124,227]

The normal intrahepatic ducts may lie on any side of the accompanying portal vein. As they course toward the hilum, the intrahepatic bile ducts from each lobe unite to form the right and left hepatic ducts, which have a constant location just anterior to the main portal vein bifurcation (Fig. 31-57, A). The right and left hepatic ducts unite in the hilum to form the common hepatic duct (CHD). The CHD is usually imaged as a round or elliptical structure sitting anterior and often slightly lateral to the main portal vein (Fig. 31-57, B). On consecutive axial images, the CHD usually courses along a 40 to

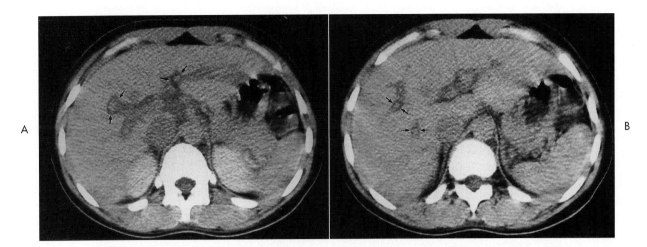

Fig. 31-56. Periportal edema. **A,** Edema around hilar portal vein branches *(arrows).* **B,** Edema forms lucent "collar" around portal vein branches *(arrow).* Note how low density completely surrounds the vein.

45° oblique plane with reference to the midline sagittal plane (Fig. 31-57, *C & D*).[165,166] It may, however, lie transversely; previously this was considered a sign of obstruction and is now known to be an anatomic variant.[85,110] The CHD lies to the right and lateral to the proper hepatic artery. The right hepatic artery typically branches off the proper hepatic artery and passes between the CHD and main portal vein in 75% to 85% of patients.[229] Contrast enhancement often aids in differentiating the water-density CHD from the enhanced hepatic artery and portal vein.

The common bile duct (CBD) forms when the cystic duct joins with the CHD. This union can occur at varying levels from high in the porta hepatis to near the ampulla of Vater. The confluence is rarely imaged on CT (Fig. 31-77, *B*). The CBD enters the pancreas and typically lies along the posterior and lateral aspect of the pancreatic head. It can be used as a landmark to indicate the lateral border of the pancreatic head (Fig. 31-57, *E*).

The extrahepatic bile ducts (CHD and CBD) are readily visualized if the anatomy is recognized and the study tailored appropriately. Schulte et al demonstrated the CHD in 66% of their patients and CBD in 82%.[193] The CHD usually measures 3 to 6 mm in short axis diameter, and the CBD usually measures up to 8 mm.[13] The diameter should be measured in short axis since the duct often courses obliquely through the axial image making the long axis diameter inaccurate.[71] In some patients, the CBD may be larger than 8 mm, and in postcholecystectomy patients it may measure up to 10 mm without obstruction.[13,48] The wall of the CHD and CBD can normally be visualized and measures less than 1.5 mm.[193] The wall may also enhance normally and be brighter than the adjacent pancreas (Fig. 31-81, *B*).

The CT examination should be tailored to examine the extrahepatic bile ducts. Narrow collimation of 4 to 5 mm at 5 to 10-mm intervals with bolus intravenous contrast enhancement injected at 1 to 2 cc/sec can be used. In addition, a small field of view should be used with the image targeted to the porta hepatis and pancreatic head (Fig. 31-57). Oral cholangiographic agents have been used to demonstrate the biliary tree on CT scan;[85,86] however, these are probably not needed with the new higher-resolution scanners.

Congenital biliary anomalies

Biliary atresia. In extrahepatic biliary atresia, ultrasound and a DISIDA scan are typically the imaging studies performed initially to evaluate the biliary tree. Extrahepatic biliary atresia, however, is associated with other anomalies in 10% to 23% of patients.[74] Such anomalies include polysplenia, bilateral bilobed lungs, azygous continuation of the IVC, intestinal malrotation, and situs inversus.[54] CT can be used to demonstrate these associated anomalies. In addition, CT can be used to assess patients who, after corrective surgery, develop cholangitis, bile duct dilatation, bilomas, or intrahepatic calculi (Fig. 31-94).[54] CT can also evaluate the development of cirrhosis, varices, splenomegaly, and ascites and play an important role in pre-liver transplant evaluation in such patients.

Choledochal cyst. Congenital dilatation of the biliary tract the so-called choledochal cyst may occur and has been classified based on the spectrum of morphologic changes in the bile ducts.[32] The most common classification scheme of Alonso-Lej includes: Type I, which is dilatation of the CBD; Type II, which is a diverticulum of the CBD; and Type III, which is the rare chole-

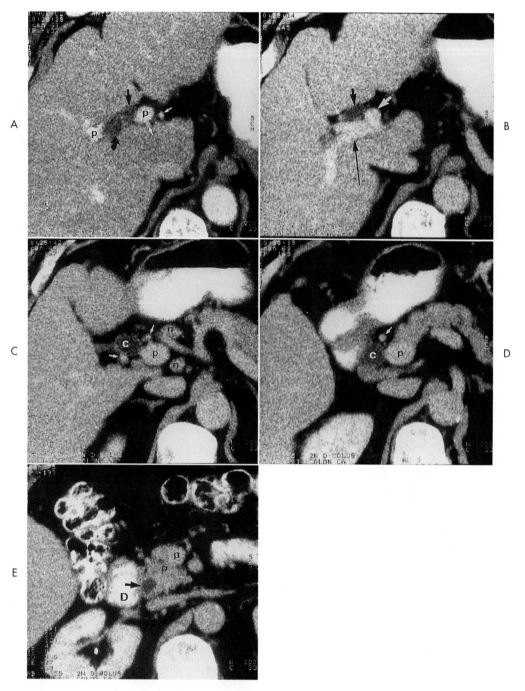

Fig. 31-57. Normal anatomy of extrahepatic bile duct. Exam is high-resolution study with 4-mm–thick images, with bolus IV contrast and targeted field of view. **A,** First level at the confluence of the right hepatic duct *(curved black arrow)* with the left hepatic duct *(straight black arrow)*. Portal vein branches *(p)* and hepatic artery branches *(white arrows)*. **B,** Level 8 mm caudal to *A*. CHD *(short black arrow)* has formed and lies anterior to bifurcation of portal vein into right *(long black arrow)* and left *(large white arrow)* branches. Hepatic artery branch *(small white arrow)*. **C,** Level 12 mm caudal to *B*. Common duct *(C)* lies anterolateral to main portal vein *(p)*. Branches of hepatic artery *(small white arrows)*; small lymph nodes *(n)*. **D,** Level 12 mm caudal to *C*. Common duct *(c)* is lateral to main portal vein *(p)* and posterolateral to the hepatic artery *(small white arrow)*. **E,** Level 24 mm caudal to *D* at the level of the pancreatic head. Distal common duct *(black arrow)* lies in posterolateral aspect of pancreatic head *(P)*. The descending duodenum *(D)* is filled with contrast just lateral to the pancreatic head. Superior mesenteric vein *(p)*.

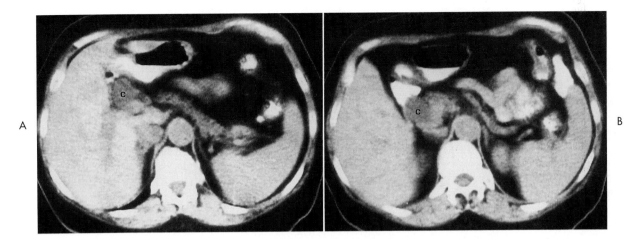

Fig. 31-58. Choledochal cyst. **A,** Choledochal cyst with dilatation of the extrahepatic common bile duct *(c).* **B,** CBD dilated *(c)* down to the pancreatic head. No intrahepatic biliary dilatation.

dochocele. Type I has been subdivided into cystic dilatation of the entire CBD and CHD, a small cyst of the distal CBD, or diffuse fusiform dilatation of the CBD. Todani et al added to this classification Type IV-A representing multiple cysts of the IHBD and EHBD; Type IV-B representing multiple cysts of the EHBD; and Type V representing multiple cysts of the IHBD, or Caroli disease.[190,219] Placing a patient into a specific category is not as important to the patient's management as is describing the extent of involvement of the IHBD and EHBD.

The choledochal cyst is not truly a cyst of the biliary tract but rather some variation of duct dilatation. The etiology of this condition is not clear but may be multifactorial. Landing proposed that biliary atresia, neonatal hepatitis, and choledochal cyst are part of the same spectrum of disease.[62] In addition, biliary atresia may be coexistent with choledochal cyst.[213] An anomalous union of the distal CBD and pancreatic duct has been reported in patients with a choledochal cyst; this may lead to pancreatic enzyme reflux into the CBD causing dilatation. This anomalous union is seen in 10% to 58% of such patients.[190] The choledochocele may have a different cause and may form as a result of obstruction at the ampulla with formation of a diverticulum of the sphincter, or it may represent a distal choledochal cyst that prolapses into the duodenum.

On CT, choledochal cyst can have varying appearances depending on the extent of ductal involvement and the degree of dilatation. There may only be mild EHBD dilatation (Fig. 31-58) or a large water-density mass in the porta hepatis or adjacent to the head of the pancreas (Fig. 31-59). Reportedly, 60% of patients with choledochal cyst will have associated congenital IHBD dilata-

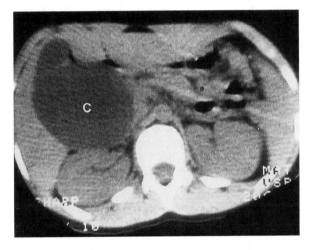

Fig. 31-59. Large choledochal cyst *(c).*

tion. This is usually limited to the central IHBD.[6,233] Congenitally dilated IHBD often have a lobulated cystic appearance with an abrupt transition zone at the junction with the normal ducts. Acquired biliary dilatation usually does not have the lobulated cystic appearance, and the dilated ducts usually taper gradually toward the periphery of the liver. With congenitally dilated ducts, the gallbladder is often normal. Direct communication of the cystic duct to the dilated EHBD will aid in making the diagnosis of choledochal cyst, but this connection is often difficult to visualize on CT. Direct communication of nondilated ducts with the dilated portion is important to visualize and can be seen on CT unless the choledochal cyst is large. The differential diagnosis of choledochal cysts will include gastrointestinal tract duplication cysts, mesenteric cysts, hepatic cysts, pseudo-cysts, ovarian cyst, and a renal cyst.

Ultrasound and CT can make the diagnosis if direct communication with the biliary tree and the choledochal cyst is demonstrated. Often this cannot be accomplished, and a DISIDA scan is required. CT cholangiography can be diagnostic and has been described revealing a contrast-fluid level within the choledochal cyst.[233]

The choledochocele is typically seen as a round fluid-density structure in or medial to the pancreatic head or may lie completely within the lumen of the duodenum (Fig. 31-60). If oral contrast has been given, the lesion may be circumscribed by the contrast. The IHBD and EHBD are often not dilated. Differential diagnostic considerations would include an intraluminal duodenal diverticulum, small pseudocyst, duodenal duplication cyst, or small cystic neoplasm of the pancreas. CT cholangiography with administration of an oral cholangiographic agent may make the diagnosis.[13,50]

Most patients with choledochal cyst present with jaundice; therefore, imaging usually with CT or US is performed. Only about 25% of patients present with the classic triad of pain, jaundice, and a right upper quadrant mass. Surgical correction is usually required and involves excision with a biliary-enteric anastomosis.

Complications of the choledochal cyst usually involve bile stasis with stone formation and infection, pancreatitis, biliary cirrhosis, and portal hypertension. There is however a reported increased incidence (4% to 28%) of malignancy involving the hepatobiliary system.[6,13,82,190,238] The increased risk of malignancy is most likely due to chronic mucosal irritation, but it is not limited only to the choledochal cyst. Malignancy can

develop anywhere in the biliary tree in such patients.[238] Cholangiocarcinoma arising in the choledochal cyst will appear as a soft-tissue density mass or irregular thickening of the cyst wall (Fig. 31-96). Tumor arising in a choledochal cyst that was bypassed but not excised has been reported.[213] Gallbladder carcinoma has been reported in patients with a choledochal cyst and will appear as described previously in this chapter.

Caroli disease. Caroli disease is also called communicating cavernous ectasis of the biliary tract. This is a rare disease that is part of the spectrum of congenital anomalies affecting the biliary tree and the kidney. The uncommon pure form of this entity involves congenital saccular dilatation of only the IHBD. The second more common or "classical" form consists of the saccular bile duct dilatation with associated congenital hepatic fibrosis and portal hypertension.[45,189] In addition, there may be associated congenital dilatation of the EHBD, suggesting that Caroli disease is part of the spectrum of choledochal cyst. Two thirds of such patients have been reported to have extrahepatic biliary abnormalities.[190] In addition, there is a high association with renal tubular ectasis and other renal cystic disease that may be part of the same underlying disorder.

On CT, the saccular cystic dilatation of the IHBD may mimic multiple hepatic cysts. Several signs, however, aid in differentiating Caroli disease. Most importantly, the cystic areas often can be shown to communicate directly with the bile ducts.[13] The distribution of cystic dilatation is often segmental. Finally, the "central dot sign" has been suggested as a pathognomonic sign of Caroli disease (Fig. 31-61).[45] This sign consists of cystic dilatation of the IHBD with a small focus or "dot" of in-

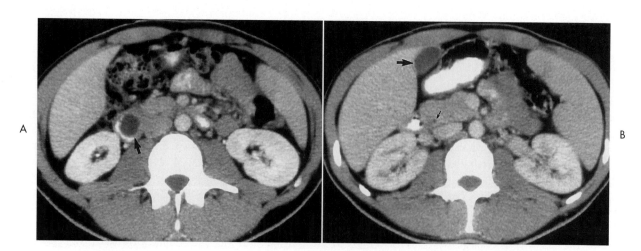

Fig. 31-60. A, Choledochocele *(arrow)* appears as fluid density mass pushing laterally into barium-filled duodenum. **B,** Note common bile duct *(small arrow)* proximal to the choledochocele is not dilated, nor is gallbladder distended *(large arrow).*

creased density lying apparently within the lumen of the duct. This "dot" represents the portal radicle which has become engulfed by the dilating adjacent bile duct. The vessel is not truly in the lumen but is surrounded by the duct. The "dot" will enhance with intravenous contrast. One case report documented a case of the "central dot sign" being seen with large hepatic cysts that occurred centrally in the liver and most likely represented retention cysts in periductal glands.[97]

Complications of Caroli disease will include problems with bile stasis such as stone formation and cholangitis. In addition, pancreatitis, abscess formation, hepatic

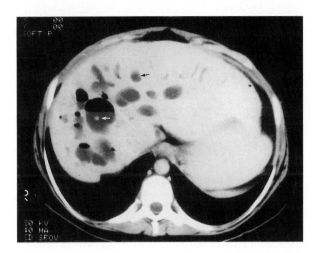

Fig. 31-61. Caroli disease with cystic dilatation of the intrahepatic bile ducts. *Arrows* show "central dot sign." Air in ducts due to previous intervention. (Courtesy RL Baron, M.D., Pittsburgh, Pa.)

amyloidosis, and biliary malignancy have been associated with Caroli disease.[98,131] CT can document the extent of the disease and the presence of intrahepatic calculi, abscess formation, etc. With congenital hepatic fibrosis, CT can document the presence of splenomegaly and varices. Finally, because of the association with renal cystic disease, the kidneys should be carefully evaluated for the presence of obvious cysts or calculi.

Cholangitis

Suppurative cholangitis. Acute cholangitis is typically found in patients with obstruction or stone disease. Gram-negative organisms, such as *E. coli,* are often responsible. The disease can become quite severe and life-threatening, requiring immediate relief of the obstruction as well as antibiotic therapy.

On CT, dilatation of the IHBD and EHBD may be present unless early obstruction or partial obstruction is present.[13] There may be increased density of the bile within the ducts because of purulent material (Fig. 31-62). The bile duct wall may be thickened concentrically and diffusely with prominent contrast enhancement (Fig. 31-62).[193] High-resolution CT will best demonstrate this finding. Finally, gas-forming organisms can cause pneumobilia, which can be seen on CT especially in the nondependent portion of the biliary tract, typically in the left lobe.

CT can also be used to assess for complications of suppurative cholangitis, such as abscesses, which will appear as hypodense or fluid density areas adjacent to the bile ducts. Areas of liver parenchyma enhancement around the bile ducts may represent focal pyogenic hepatitis (Fig. 31-66).[39]

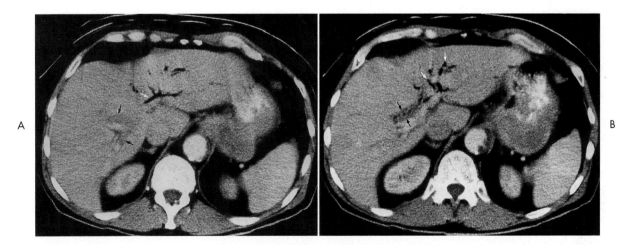

Fig. 31-62. A, Suppurative cholangitis with dilated intrahepatic ducts *(black arrows)* filled with dense inflammatory debris. Pneumobilia *(white arrow)* secondary to previous biliary enteric anastomosis. **B,** Suppurative cholangitis. Note thickened wall of the hepatic ducts *(black arrows)* and pneumobilia *(white arrows).*

AIDS cholangitis. Several abnormalities in the biliary tract have been described in patients with AIDS. Although difficult to directly prove, the major cause of these biliary abnormalities is opportunistic infection with the typical agents being *Cryptosporidium*, cytomegalovirus, *Mycobacterium avium intracellular, Candida albicans,* and *Klebsiella pneumoniae*.[38,182]

One of the most common biliary abnormalities is diffuse gallbladder-wall thickening. This may be due to edema in the gallbladder wall and can rapidly change over time. The exact cause of the wall edema is not clear but may be due to lymphatic obstruction as has been shown in patients with adenopathy secondary to Kaposi's sarcoma or lymphoma.[182] The gallbladder-wall thickening may also be due to inflammation associated with acalculous cholecystitis. Both *Cryptosporidium* and cytomegalovirus has been implicated in causing acalculous cholecystitis in AIDS patients.[214,215] The diagnosis may be difficult with imaging studies. However, if there is pericholecystic fluid or inflammatory changes on CT or US, acalculous cholecystitis should be suspected in the appropriate clinical setting over noninflammatory gallbladder-wall edema.

Bile duct abnormalities in patients with AIDS can be arranged into two patterns. The first pattern involves narrowing only of the distal CBD; this may be due to acute papillitis or stricture and may mimic papillary stenosis.[57,214,215] The remainder of the biliary tract in those cases may be dilated but otherwise normal. Acute inflammation or an inflammatory stricture of the distal CBD/ampulla have been attributed to infection by *Cryptosporidium* and CMV, both of which have been isolated on ampullary biopsies.[57]

The second pattern of bile duct abnormalities mimics sclerosing cholangitis (PSC) with multiple strictures occurring throughout the biliary tree with or without distal CBD/ampullary strictures (Fig. 31-63). Focal dilatation of the ducts and pruning of the intrahepatic ducts can occur as in PSC.[57] Thickening of the duct wall can be appreciated on CT or US. The cause of these strictures has been linked to *Cryptospordium* and CMV.

AIDS patients with such biliary infections usually present with recurrent nonspecific abdominal pain, nausea, vomiting, fever, diarrhea, and cholestasis. US and CT can be performed to evaluate the biliary tract and rule out other abnormalities such as stone disease. The biliary abnormalities in AIDS patients may rapidly progress; therefore, US and CT can be used for follow-up examinations.[215] ERCP is helpful in evaluating these patients by allowing for simultaneous ductal evaluation, biopsy, and papillotomy if required.

Parasitic cholangitis. Parasitic infection of the biliary tract is rare in the United States. It is seen, however, in areas where there are large populations of immi-

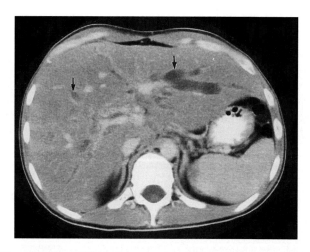

Fig. 31-63. AIDS cholangitis with dilated intrahepatic ducts (*arrows*). Note asymmetry of dilatation with greater dilatation of the left ducts. (From Dolmatch BL, et al: *Radiology* 163:313-316, 1987.)

grants particularly from Southeast Asia. *Clonorchis sinensis* and *Ascaris lumbricoides* are the two major biliary tract parasites.

Ascariasis can involve the biliary tract when the worms migrate through the ampulla. This may produce biliary colic, pyogenic cholangitis, and acalculous cholecystitis.[176] Stones may form around the worms or ova, and ductal stricture formation may occur as a result of inflammatory reaction. Liver abscesses may develop secondary to infected and obstructed bile ducts. On CT, signs of cholangitis may be visualized with biliary dilatation, increased density of bile, pneumobilia, and parenchymal abscesses.[176]

Clonorchiasis typically appears on CT scan as biliary dilatation. The degree of biliary dilatation will vary but is usually mild and involves only the intrahepatic bile ducts (Fig. 31-64). The extrahepatic bile ducts are characteristically not dilated. Dilatation of the intrahepatic ducts is due to obstruction by the parasites or associated inflammatory debris. Thickening of the bile duct walls and the parasites themselves are usually not seen on CT but may be appreciated on US.[43] CT may, however, demonstrate complications of the infection such as calculi, suppurative cholangitis, abscesses, or cholangiohepatitis. There is an increased incidence of cholangiocarcinoma associated with chronic *Clonorchis* infection. If prominent biliary dilatation is seen, an underlying biliary neoplasm should be suspected since significant biliary dilatation is not common with *Clonorchis* infection alone.[41,43] Finally, CT may demonstrate an intrahepatic mass due to cholangiocarcinoma (Fig. 31-64).

Recurrent pyogenic cholangitis. Recurrent pyogenic cholangitis (RPC) or oriental cholangiohepatitis is

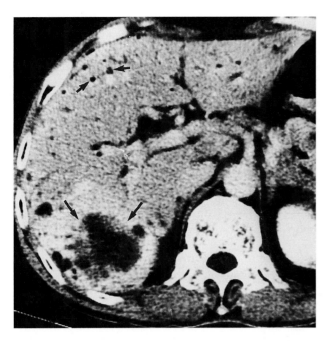

Fig. 31-64. Clinorchis infection with dilated intrahepatic bile ducts *(short arrows)* and an intrahepatic cholangiocarcinoma *(long arrows).* (From Choi BI: *AJR* 152:281-284, 1989.)

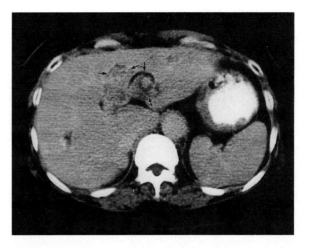

Fig. 31-65. Recurrent pyogenic cholangitis with significantly dilated intrahepatic bile ducts containing debris and stones *(between arrows).*

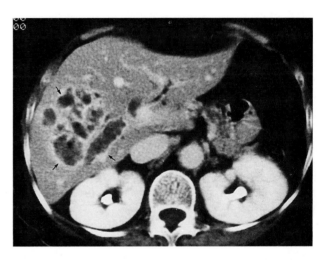

Fig. 31-66. Acute exacerbation of recurrent pyogenic cholangitis with dilated right intrahepatic bile ducts and periductal enhancement *(arrows).* (From Chan F, et al: *Radiology* 170, 165-169, 1989.)

a common disease in Asia and is being seen more in Western countries because of immigration. It is reported to be a very common cause of an acute abdomen requiring surgery in Southeast Asia.[113] The disease involves recurrent episodes of infectious cholangitis that eventually leads to bile duct strictures, ductal obstruction, and biliary calculi. Clinically, the patients present with episodic abdominal pain, sepsis, and jaundice.

The findings on CT reflect the pathologic changes. There is usually significant intrahepatic and extrahepatic biliary dilatation. "Pruning" of the intrahepatic ducts can occur where there is notable dilatation of the duct, blunting of the peripheral end of the duct, and nonvisualization of the secondary duct branches. Debris and calculi are often seen within the ducts (Fig. 31-65). The stones are usually bile pigment stones with varying degrees of calcium content. Depending on the calcium content, the stones may vary from isodense to hyperdense with bile.[13,68] CT demonstrates the stones better than can ultrasound, because often these stones are the consistency of paste and do not shadow on ultrasound.[68,113,180] In addition, pneumobilia is often present, which limits ability to visualize the ducts optimally with ultrasound.

The intrahepatic bile ducts in the left lobe of the liver are usually the most common site of involvement and often the most severely involved.[39] There may be diffuse areas of involvement in the liver with varying de-

grees of severity. However, solitary segmental involvement may occur. CT can demonstrate the areas of involvement quite well; this is important for surgical treatment planning.

Periductal and duct-wall enhancement can be seen on contrasted CT scans. This suggests acute inflammation (Fig. 31-66).[39] In addition, periductal hepatic abscesses can be detected as a complication of acute episodes. Chronically, the disease can lead to lobar atrophy, cirrhosis, and portal hypertension.

The extrahepatic bile duct is often significantly dilated up to as much as 3 to 4 cm in diameter. The grossly

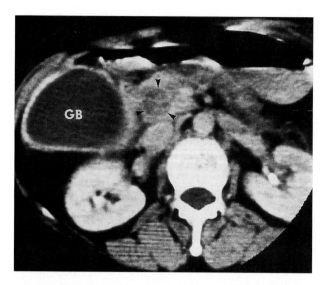

Fig. 31-67. Arrowheads show dilated common duct in the pancreatic head, filled with a calculus of higher attenuation than bile in the gallbladder *(GB)*. (From Choi BI: *AJR* 152:281-284, 1989.)

distended common duct may be full of stones and debris, producing a cast of the duct (Fig. 31-67). This finding is very suggestive of RPC.[113] On high-resolution CT, the wall of the common duct may be seen to be eccentrically and diffusely thickened.[193] Differential diagnosis of RPC includes primary sclerosing cholangitis (PSC). However, the ducts are usually not as dilated in PSC and intrahepatic calculi are more common in RPC. Caroli disease may be difficult to differentiate from RPC, but the extrahepatic bile duct is usually not as dilated in Caroli disease.

CT is probably the best examination for evaluating patients with RPC. Since the biliary tree in these patients is colonized with bacteria and parasites, biliary sepsis can occur from an invasive procedure such as ERCP and PTC. CT, however, will noninvasively demonstrate the distribution, extent, and severity of ductal and hepatic parenchymal involvement.

Sclerosing cholangitis. Sclerosing cholangitis is a rare disease of the biliary tract that may be primary (PSC), in which case it is idiopathic or associated with several diseases such as ulcerative colitis, Crohn's disease, retroperitoneal fibrosis, and Reidel's stroma. It has been described in association with histiocytosis X, angioimmunoblastic lymphadenopathy, and AIDS.[162] Secondary sclerosing cholangitis can occur as a result of stone disease, previous biliary surgery, or recurrent infection, and these conditions must be excluded to diagnose primary sclerosing cholangitis. The clinical course is insidious and manifested by intermittent jaundice. Cirrhosis may result because of chronic cholestasis.

The pathology of sclerosing cholangitis is characterized by ductal and periductal fibrosis causing focal strictures with alternating areas of ductal dilatation. This pattern produces the "beaded" appearance of the ducts on cholangiography. Classically, both the intrahepatic and extrahepatic bile ducts are involved. However, cases have been reported of only the extrahepatic bile ducts being involved.[4]

The classically described findings of sclerosing cholangitis on CT reflect the cholangiographic and pathologic findings.[4,178,211,212] Randomly scattered, focal areas of bile duct dilatation are seen. The focally dilated ducts do not directly communicate, nor are they confluent with the hilum (Fig. 31-68, *A*). There often is a segmental distribution to the involved ducts. The dilated ducts may demonstrate a beaded appearance reflecting alternating areas of strictures and dilatation. Pruning of the ducts may be seen where there is dilatation of the segmental ducts without dilatation of their secondary branches (Fig. 31-68, *B*). Teefey et al[212] reported a series of 100 patients in which pruning and beading of the IHBD was not specific for PSC but was also seen in infectious and malignant processes. Skip dilatations or areas of alternating stricture and duct dilatation were considered the strongest sign for PSC, especially in the absence of a mass or evidence of recurrent pyogenic cholangitis.

In PSC, the extrahepatic bile duct is often not dilated but may have a serpentine course. With high-resolution CT of the extrahepatic duct, subtle changes in the wall of the duct may be appreciated. Teefey et al[211] described such findings in the extrahepatic duct, including wall thickening with enhancement, mural nodules, and focal ductal stenosis (Fig. 31-68, *E*).

The differential diagnosis of sclerosing cholangitis includes recurrent infectious cholangitis, diffuse sclerosing cholangiocarcinoma, early Caroli disease, ductal sclerosis following transcatheter arterial chemotherapy administration, and posttraumatic stricture.[25,168] The clinical setting may allow differentiation of several of these entities, but the CT appearances are often similar. Diffuse sclerosing cholangiocarcinoma is difficult to differentiate and often requires a biopsy for the diagnosis. Brush biopsies of the ducts may not be helpful, because of the large component of fibrosis found in both PSC and sclerosing cholangiocarcinoma. There is an increased incidence of cholangiocarcinoma in sclerosing cholangitis, and sclerosing cholangitis is considered to be a premalignant condition.[159] In a series of patients receiving liver transplants for primary sclerosing cholangitis, 10% of the patients were found to have cholangiocarcinoma in their native livers.[96] Some of these cases were not discovered until later when the hepatectomy specimens were histologically examined. In sclerosing cholangitis,

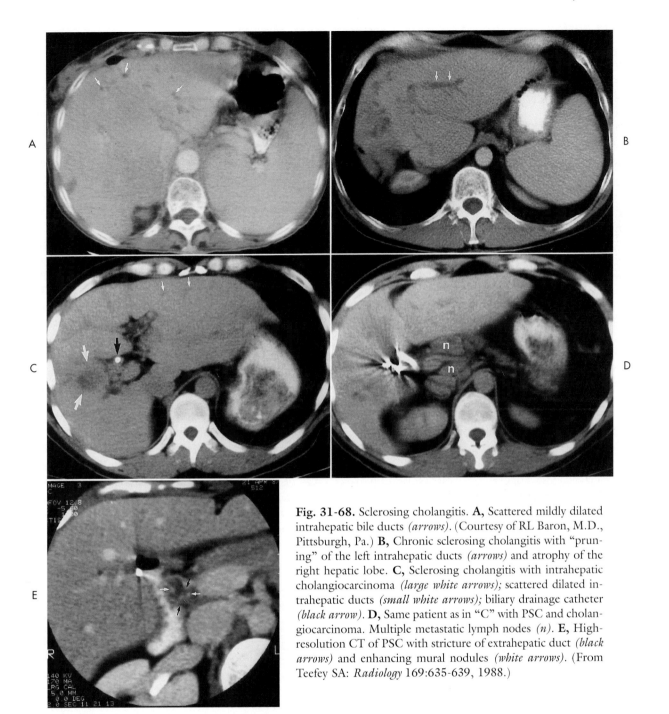

Fig. 31-68. Sclerosing cholangitis. **A,** Scattered mildly dilated intrahepatic bile ducts *(arrows).* (Courtesy of RL Baron, M.D., Pittsburgh, Pa.) **B,** Chronic sclerosing cholangitis with "pruning" of the left intrahepatic ducts *(arrows)* and atrophy of the right hepatic lobe. **C,** Sclerosing cholangitis with intrahepatic cholangiocarcinoma *(large white arrows);* scattered dilated intrahepatic ducts *(small white arrows);* biliary drainage catheter *(black arrow).* **D,** Same patient as in "C" with PSC and cholangiocarcinoma. Multiple metastatic lymph nodes *(n).* **E,** High-resolution CT of PSC with stricture of extrahepatic duct *(black arrows)* and enhancing mural nodules *(white arrows).* (From Teefey SA: *Radiology* 169:635-639, 1988.)

ductal dilatation is often not dramatic; this is due to periductal fibrosis. However, if prominent duct dilatation, particularly segmental dilatation, is seen in a patient with known sclerosing cholangitis, or if ductal dilatation rapidly progresses, cholangiocarcinoma should be suspected (Fig. 31-68, *C*).[181] Lymphadenopathy in the upper abdomen has been reported in PSC without cholangiocarcinoma.[162] Such enlarged nodes often occur in the gastrohepatic ligament and in the pancreaticoduodenal

chain. Lymphadenopathy in the porta hepatis has been reported as a sign suggesting a malignant, rather than benign, biliary process (Fig. 31-68, *D*).[181] However, in PSC the mere presence of lymphadenopathy is not as useful. Therefore, biopsy of the lymph nodes may be required.

PTC and ERCP have been the gold standards for demonstrating sclerosing cholangitis. However, cholangiographically, ducts peripheral to tight strictures may not be filled adequately, and CT may show these areas better. In addition, given the possibility of underlying cholangiocarcinoma, CT can evaluate for an extraductal mass or lymphadenopathy better than can cholangiography.

Biliary obstruction

CT is often the initial examination performed in patients with clinical presentation of jaundice, or CT may be performed as a correlative examination after ultrasound. The main goals of the CT examination are to determine the presence of obstruction, determine the level and extent of obstruction, and determine the cause. The overall accuracy of CT for diagnosing biliary obstruction has been reported at 85% to 97%.[15,128,151,218] The hallmark of biliary obstruction on CT is biliary dilatation (Figs. 31-72 to 31-77, 31-79). Such intrahepatic dilatation appears as confluent linear structures of water density that course with the portal vein branches and gradually increase in size as they course toward the hilum. As mentioned previously, normal intrahepatic ducts may occasionally be visualized, but these are few in number, scattered, and not confluent (Figs. 31-54, 31-55). The dilated extrahepatic bile duct measures greater than 8 to 10 mm in short axis measurement. With intravenous enhancement, dilated bile ducts can more easily be differentiated from enhancing vascular structures.

False negatives for biliary obstruction being diagnosed by CT do exist. For example, biliary dilatation may not be present in early obstruction. Animal studies have demonstrated that 4 days may be required before dilatation occurs following duct obstruction.[13] In addition, obstruction may be present in certain cases without dilatation, as can happen in cirrhosis and in liver transplants.[13,126,240] In such cases, cholangiography is required to make the diagnosis. In partial or intermittent obstruction, ductal dilatation may not be present. Choledocholithiasis has been reported to cause partial and intermittent obstruction without dilatation. A number of series have reported the lack of sensitivity of CT to detect obstruction in cases of distal common duct stones because of the lack of dilatation (Fig. 31-69).[13,52,80,81,163] Finally, ductal dilatation, particularly intrahepatic, may be difficult to detect in the setting of diffuse fatty infiltration of the liver because of less contrast between the water density ducts and the fatty liver (Fig. 31-70).[173]

In CT, false positives for biliary dilatation, hence obstruction, do exist. Morehouse reported a case of metastatic pancreatic carcinoma extending along the portal vein branches mimicking biliary dilatation.[151] In addition, this author has seen a case of a neurofibroma in the portahepatis with extension along the portal vein branches mimicking biliary dilatation on US, CT, and MRI (Fig. 31-71). Periductal tumor will often enhance and thereby be differentiated from dilated bile ducts. Periportal lymphedema and ascites tracking along the hepatoduodenal ligament may also mimic ductal dilatation (Fig. 31-56). Finally, thrombosis of the portal vein can mimic dilated bile ducts.[151]

In early obstruction and in some cases of prolonged obstruction, only extrahepatic biliary dilatation may be seen.[16,193,196] This has been described with common bile duct stones. In postcholecystectomy patients, the extrahepatic duct is considered normal in size up to 10 mm in short axis diameter.[13,48,155,193] If there is any question of obstruction in such patients, a fatty meal challenge or intravenous cholecystokinin may be given

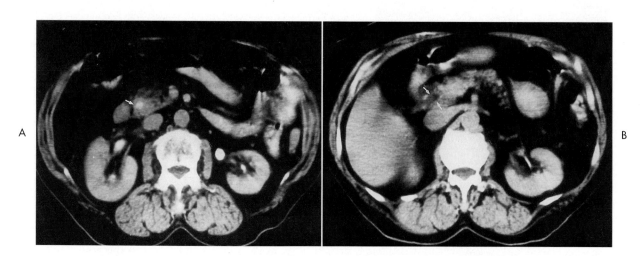

Fig. 31-69. Distal CBD stone without biliary dilatation. **A,** Dense stone in distal CBD *(arrow)*. **B,** Nondilated CBD *(arrows)* just above level of stone.

with measurement of the extrahepatic duct prior to and 10 to 15 minutes after administration. A normal response is seen if the duct remains stable or decreases in diameter. If there is an increase in the size of the duct or onset of pain, the response is abnormal.[13] Further evaluation of the duct with ERCP will be necessary.

Level and extent of obstruction. Depending on the series, the accuracy of CT for determining the level of obstruction has been reported to be 80% to 97%.[15,81,165,166] The dilated bile ducts can be traced on the same image or consecutive images to the transition point at which the caliber of the duct decreases or the duct disappears. This transition point is best demonstrated with thin collimation axial images along the course of the biliary tree. Associated findings may aid in determining the level. Gallbladder dilatation can be seen with distal duct obstruction, but it is not a sensitive indicator and may be seen only in 50% of cases.[16] Pancreatic duct dilatation points to an obstructing lesion in the distal common duct or even the ampulla (Fig. 31-77).

The extent of the biliary tree that is obstructed can be determined by CT and can aid in therapy plan-

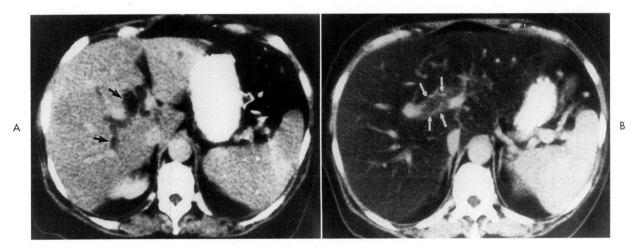

Fig. 31-70. Biliary dilatation in a fatty liver. **A,** Postcontrast CT shows mild fatty infiltration of the liver with biliary dilatation *(arrows).* **B,** Five months after *(A),* dilated bile ducts *(arrows)* are indistinguishable from the hypodense fatty liver on this postcontrast scan. (From Quint LE: *Radiology* 153:755-756, 1984.)

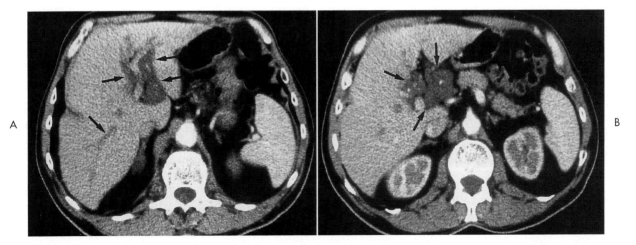

Fig. 31-71. Peribiliary neurofibroma. **A,** Hypodense structures *(arrows)* mimicking dilated bile ducts are actually a neurofibroma branching along the biliary tract and portal structures. No dilated ducts were seen on ERCP. **B,** Hypodense neurofibroma *(arrows)* in the porta hepatis mimics dilated bile ducts.

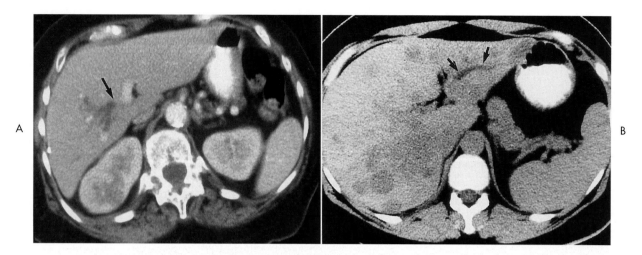

Fig. 31-72. Focal intrahepatic dilatation. **A,** Isolated intrahepatic biliary dilatation in the posterior segment of the right hepatic lobe because of focal stricture *(arrow)* secondary to stone disease and cholangitis. **B,** Focal intrahepatic biliary dilatation *(arrows)* due to breast carcinoma metastases.

ning. For example, intrahepatic biliary obstruction proximal to the right or left hepatic duct is rarely amenable to surgical correction. Such obstruction is usually treated with percutaneous transhepatic catheter drainage. CT can demonstrate which dilated segmental ducts communicate and whether more than one catheter is required.[181] If the ducts in more than three segments are obstructed and do not communicate, these cases are poor candidates for surgery and catheter drainage. More distal extrahepatic bile duct obstruction is usually more amenable to surgical correction and percutaneous or endoscopic intervention.

Cause of obstruction. The reported accuracy of CT for determining the cause of biliary obstruction ranges from 63% to 94%.[15,80,81,165,166] The wide range of accuracies is most likely due to different generations of CT scanners, different scanning techniques, and different types of pathology in each series. High-resolution scanning of the bile ducts with small field of view and thin collimation is the optimum technique (Figs. 31-77, 31-90). However, even with optimum technique, certain pathologic conditions such as cholesterol stones in the common duct are difficult to detect (see section on choledocholithiasis).

Differential diagnostic categories can be formulated based on the level at which obstruction occurs. Intrahepatic ductal obstruction can be due to strictures secondary to sclerosing cholangitis, infection, or neoplasm such as cholangiocarcinoma (Fig. 31-72, *A*). Rarely, metastases may cause intrahepatic ductal obstruction (Fig. 31-72, *B*). Christensen reported focal dilatation of intrahepatic bile ducts limited to a subsegment in the poste-

rior segment of the right hepatic lobe as a result of inadvertent ligation of an aberrant right hepatic duct during cholecystectomy.[46] At the hilum, obstruction is commonly a result of tumor such as cholangiocarcinoma or a hepatic neoplasm extending into the hilum (Figs. 31-86 to 31-88). In the suprapancreatic portion of the extrahepatic duct, strictures can be due to benign disease such as sclerosing cholangitis, infectious cholangitis, surgery, or trauma. However, malignant strictures due to cholangiocarcinoma or secondary involvement by tumor of the gallbladder, pancreas, liver, or duodenum may occur (Figs. 31-73; see also Figs. 31-89 and 31-90). In addition, adenopathy secondary to inflammatory conditions or malignancy may obstruct the suprapancreatic duct (Fig. 31-74). Finally, obstruction of the distal common duct can be a result of benign inflammatory strictures due to cholangitis or pancreatitis, common duct stones, adenopathy, or tumor (pancreatic carcinoma or ampullary carcinoma) (Figs. 31-75 to 31-78).

Once the level of obstruction is determined and various etiologies care considered, CT can be used to narrow the possibilities. A clue to the cause of obstruction is the manner in which the duct terminates at the site of obstruction (Fig. 31-79). Different pathology may have different appearances at the level of obstruction. Gradual tapering of the bile duct over a distance of 1 cm or greater is typically due to benign disease such as an inflammatory stricture (Fig. 31-75). However, abrupt termination of the dilated bile duct over less than 5 mm is highly suggestive of malignancy, especially if seen in the suprapancreatic portion of the duct or near the ampulla (Figs. 31-76, 31-90). In a series by Reiman et al,

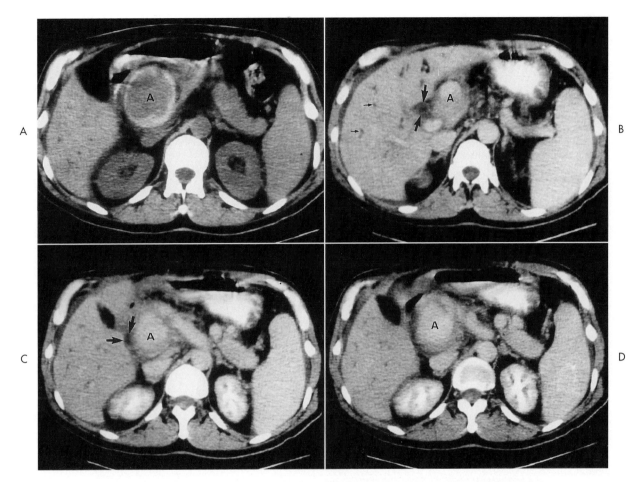

Fig. 31-73. Obstruction of suprapancreatic portion of common duct by aneurysm of gastroduodenal artery. **A,** Precontrast scan of HIV+ patient showing dense gastroduodenal artery aneurysm *(A)*. **B,** Postcontrast scan at level of CHD *(large arrows)* with mild intrahepatic biliary duct dilatation *(small arrows)* and enhancing aneurysm *(A)*. **C,** Level caudal to "B." Shows compression of common duct *(arrows)* by aneurysm *(A)*. **D,** Level caudal to "C" shows aneurysm *(A)*, which has occluded the common duct.

abrupt termination of the suprapancreatic common duct was seen in all cases of malignancy but also in 50% of benign causes of obstruction.[181] Benign strictures occasionally may cause abrupt termination of the duct.[13] In addition, obstructing cholesterol stones in the common duct may cause abrupt termination of the duct and escape visualization because of its density being similar to bile (Fig. 31-80, 31-81). However, if a soft-tissue mass or lymphadenopathy is seen with the abrupt ductal termination, then malignancy should be suspected (Fig. 31-90).[80,81,181] CT is much better than colangiography for demonstrating mass outside the duct or periductal lymphadenopathy.

Schulte et al described the appearance of the bile duct at or proximal to the level of obstruction as being helpful in determining the cause of obstruction.[193] High-resolution CT with thin collimation of images is

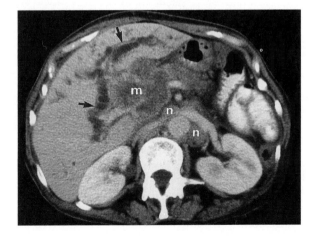

Fig. 31-74. Obstruction of suprapancreatic portion of common duct by metastatic nodal mass *(m)* from lung carcinoma. Dilated intrahepatic ducts *(arrows)*, lymphadenopathy *(n)*.

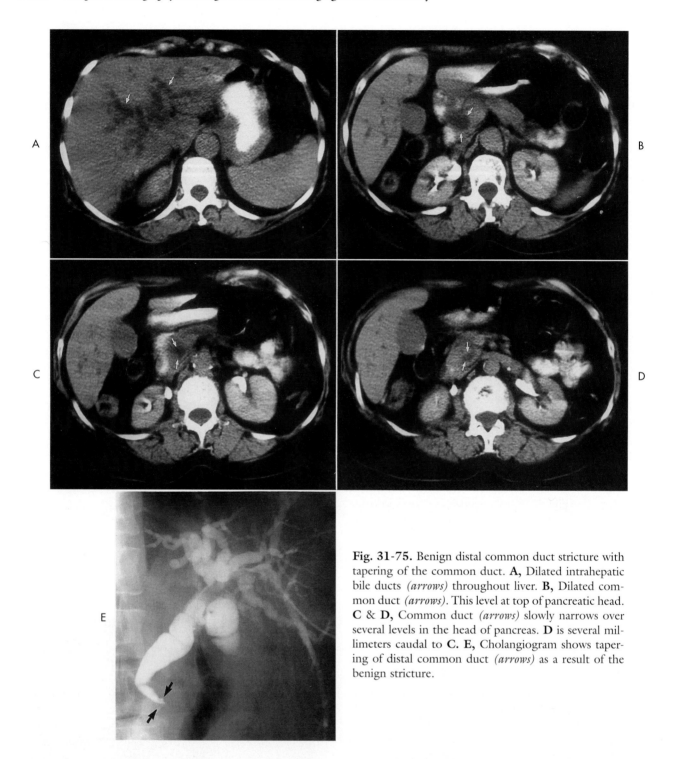

Fig. 31-75. Benign distal common duct stricture with tapering of the common duct. **A,** Dilated intrahepatic bile ducts *(arrows)* throughout liver. **B,** Dilated common duct *(arrows)*. This level at top of pancreatic head. **C & D,** Common duct *(arrows)* slowly narrows over several levels in the head of pancreas. **D** is several millimeters caudal to **C. E,** Cholangiogram shows tapering of distal common duct *(arrows)* as a result of the benign stricture.

optimum for this evaluation. Thickening of the duct wall (greater than 1.5 mm) can be observed and classified as concentric or eccentric, and focal or diffuse.[193] Focal concentric thickening in the distal common duct was nonspecific and attributed to stones, pancreatitis, or pancreatic carcinoma (Fig. 21-81, *B*). Diffuse concentric wall thickening was relatively specific and seen in infectious cholangitis (Fig. 31-62, *B*). Focal concentric

or eccentric thickening elsewhere in the common duct may be seen in primary sclerosing cholangitis, but this pattern may also be seen in cholangiocarcinoma, especially with pronounced wall thickening (Figs. 31-68, *E,* 31-90).

Choledocholithiasis. The diagnosis of common duct stones can be difficult to make on noninvasive imaging. Ultrasound is often the first line study requested

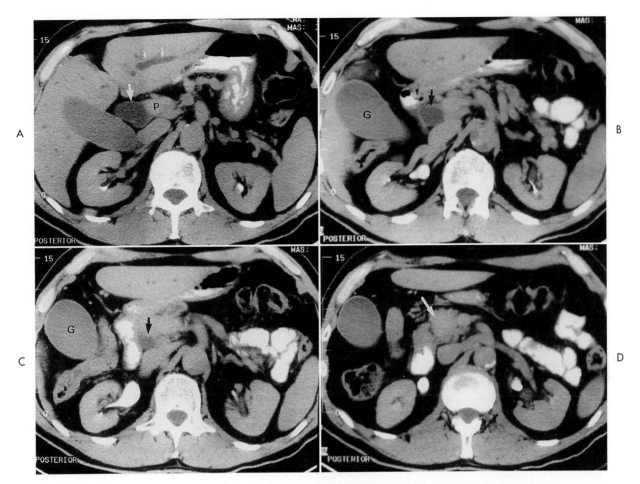

Fig. 31-76. Distal biliary obstruction secondary to pancreatic carcinoma. **A,** Dilated common duct *(large arrow)* next to portal vein *(p)* with dilated intrahepatic ducts *(small arrows)*. **B,** Dilated common duct *(arrow)* at level 8 mm caudal to *A*. Note dilated gallbladder *(G)*. **C,** Dilated common duct *(arrow)* in head of pancreas. Note irregularity in ventral wall of dilated duct *(at arrow tip)* secondary to pancreatic carcinoma. Dilated gallbladder *(G)*. **D,** Level just caudal to *C*. Shows abrupt termination of common duct with mass *(arrow)*, which is the pancreatic carcinoma.

to evaluate the patient with biliary colic or jaundice. Its reported sensitivity ranges up to 80% to 82%, but many series suggest lower sensitivity.[163] These studies are limited by the patient's body habitus, bowel gas, and experience of the operator. CT on the other hand is not limited by bowel gas or the patient's body habitus. The reported sensitivities of CT for choledocholethiasis vary but range up to 90%.[12,13,15,114,166] The sensitivity of CT greatly depends on the type of stone in the duct and the technique of the examination. Though invasive, ERCP remains the gold standard technique for diagnosing common duct stones.

Strict attention to the technique of the CT examination will improve the ability to detect common duct stones. High-resolution CT should be performed with a small field of view targeted to the right upper quadrant with specific attention to the distal common duct. Thin collimation of axial images (3 to 5 mm thick) should be used with contiguous spacing at 3- to 5-mm intervals. Baron suggests that overlapping images are helpful in the distal common duct.[12] Intravenous contrast is helpful in defining structures in the porta hepatis. Contrast enhancement will aid in detecting subtle intrahepatic biliary dilatation and will also increase the visibility of the distal common duct contrasted with the pancreatic head. Oral contrast may confuse the picture since dense contrast in the duodenum may obscure or mimic a calcified stone near the ampulla (Fig. 31-82). Therefore, studies should be performed without oral contrast. In addition, glucagon administered intravenously or intramuscularly

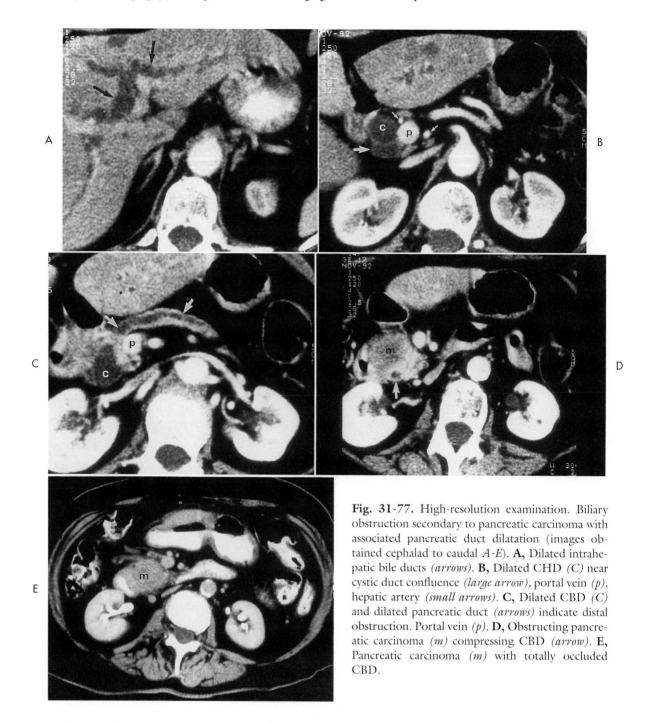

Fig. 31-77. High-resolution examination. Biliary obstruction secondary to pancreatic carcinoma with associated pancreatic duct dilatation (images obtained cephalad to caudal *A-E*). **A,** Dilated intrahepatic bile ducts *(arrows)*. **B,** Dilated CHD *(C)* near cystic duct confluence *(large arrow)*, portal vein *(p)*, hepatic artery *(small arrows)*. **C,** Dilated CBD *(C)* and dilated pancreatic duct *(arrows)* indicate distal obstruction. Portal vein *(p)*. **D,** Obstructing pancreatic carcinoma *(m)* compressing CBD *(arrow)*. **E,** Pancreatic carcinoma *(m)* with totally occluded CBD.

will decrease artifact from bowel peristalsis. Finally, these examinations should be closely monitored so that they may be tailored to the individual patient.

Even given optimum scan technique, common duct stones may elude detection because of the stone composition. Some stones are isodense with bile and may not be detected within the dilated common duct (Figs. 31-1 31-80). Mixed composition stones may have densities similar to soft tissue and may be difficult to detect

when surrounded by pancreatic tissue. Calcium bilirubinate stones are the easiest to detect and appear as radiopaque calcified filling defects in the duct (Figs. 31-78, 31-81). However, calcium bilirubinate stones are the minority of stones (15% to 20%) with pure cholesterol and mixed composition stones being the most common (80% to 85%). Secondary signs of common duct stones must be employed to detect these noncalcified stones.

The primary sign of a stone in the common duct

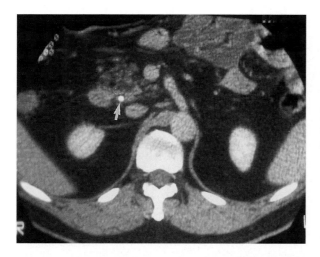

Fig. 31-78. Homogeneously dense stone *(arrow)* in distal CBD on high-resolution axial image at level of uncinate process of pancreas.

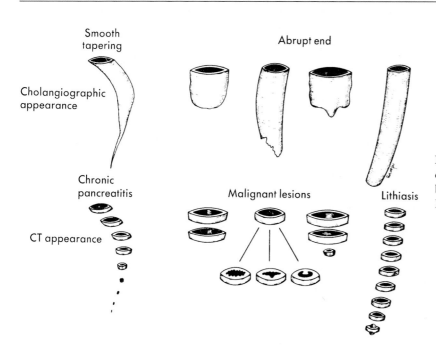

Fig. 31-79. Diagrammatic representation of cholangiographic and CT appearance of the bile duct in the most common lesions. (From Pedrosa, CS: *Radiology* 139:636, 1981.)

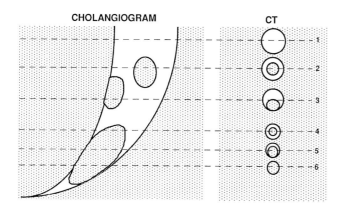

Fig. 31-80. Appearance of distal CBD seen on cholangiogram *(left)* and CT *(right). 1,* CT shows rounded CBD with only water density bile. *2,* Target sign shows central, the stone, surrounded by water density bile "halo" (see *4*). *3,* Crescent sign shows rim of water density bile anterior to dependent stone (see *5*). *4,* Target sign can be seen when the image cuts through only one end of the stone. *5,* Crescent sign can be seen when the stone does not fill the duct. *6,* If stone is soft-tissue density, no duct may be seen at this level mimicking abrupt termination of the duct as if due to carcinoma. (From Baron RL: *Radiol Clin North Am* 29(6):1235-1250, 1991.)

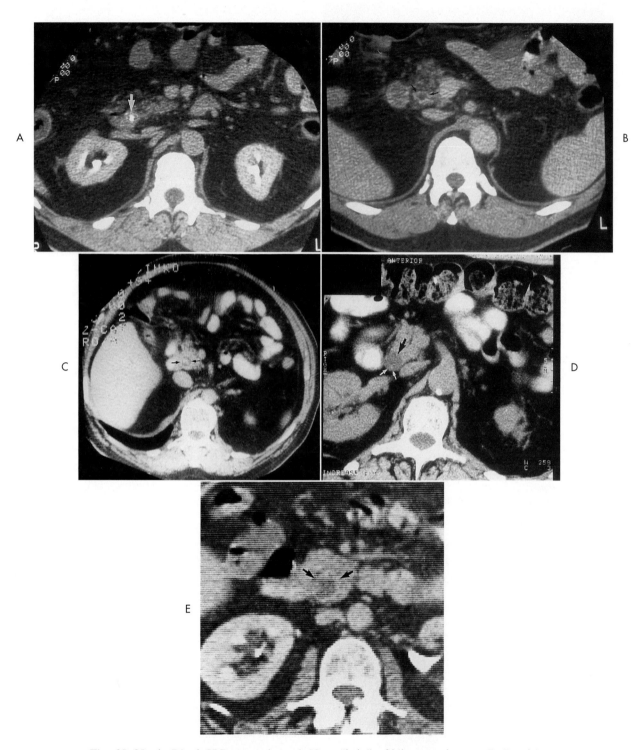

Fig. 31-81. A, Distal CBD stone *(arrow)*. Note "halo" of bile around stone. **B,** Level just cephalic to *A*. Normal size CBD *(arrows)*. Note enhancement in the wall of the CBD relative to surrounding pancreas. **C,** Distal CBD stone *(arrows)* of density similar to soft tissue. Note surrounding hypodense "halo" of bile. **D,** Subtle stone *(white arrows)* in the distal CBD *(black arrow)*. Stones proved on US and ERCP. **E,** Cholesterol calculus in distal CBD with low-density matrix, increased density rim along margin of stone *(arrows)*.

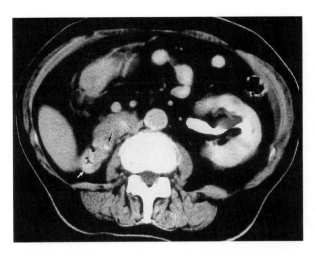

Fig. 31-82. Barium in duodenum *(black arrow)* mimics stones in distal common duct. *White arrow* shows barium and gas in descending duodenum.

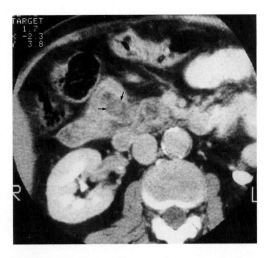

Fig. 31-83. Protrusion of pancreatic carcinoma into distal common duct *(arrows)* mimics soft-tissue density stone. (From Baron RL: *Radiol Clin North Am* 29(2):1235-1250, 1991.)

is a radiopaque filling defect in the lumen (Figs. 31-78, 31-81). This sign may be detected even if the duct is not dilated (Fig. 31-69). Common duct stones may not have associated biliary dilatation in 24% to 36% of cases even with obstruction.[13,52] Another sign, the target sign, consists of higher central density (the stone), surrounded by a water-density "halo" of bile, which is surrounded by the duct wall (Fig. 31-81). If the stone lies in the dependent portion of the duct, the surrounding bile will form a crescent of lower density anteriorly. Rarely, a papillary tumor may project into the lumen of the duct, giving a target sign and mimicking a stone (Fig. 31-83).

Secondary signs of duct stones include abrupt termination of the common duct without an associated mass. This sign, however, is not specific for stones and can be seen with obstructing malignancies, particularly pancreatic carcinoma. A second sign is a thin rim of increased density around a central portion of lower density (Fig. 31-81, *E*). The whole complex is thought to represent an impacted stone with the high-density rim representing a peripheral calcified layer in the stone. The density of the central portion will be hypodense or isodense with bile if the stone is composed of cholesterol, and soft-tissue density if of mixed composition. It has been reported, however, that the thin dense rim represents the wall of the common duct and not part of the stone.[13] There may be inflammation in the wall of the duct at the level of an impacted stone, which on high-resolution CT will show prominent contrast enhancement and concentric thickening.[193] A final secondary sign of a common duct stone is subtle soft tissue densities in the lumen of the duct; this may represent areas of different composition within the stone matrix (Fig. 31-

81, *D*). Unfortunately, none of these secondary signs are specific for choledocholithiasis. Intraluminal neoplasm may demonstrate any of these signs. If there is an irregular termination to the dilated duct, visible mass, or lymphadenopathy, then neoplasm rather than a stone should be suspected. For calcified distal common duct stones, there are several false positives. Barium in the duodenum adjacent to the ampulla may mimic a common duct stone especially if the barium is within a duodenal diverticulum (Fig. 31-82). Barium may reflux into the distal duct if there is a sphincterotomy or incompetent sphincter. In addition, a pancreatic duct stone or calcification in the pancreatic parenchyma may mimic a common duct stone. With high-resolution CT, most of these entities can be differentiated.

Intrahepatic calculi. Intrahepatic biliary calculi are rare in Western countries. They typically occur in the setting of an underlying biliary abnormality such as congenital duct dilatation, strictures, cholangitis, or previous biliary surgery.[141] They do occur in patients with biliary atresia status-post portoenterostomy and in cystic fibrosis.[65] The density of the stones on CT depends on the amount of calcium within the stone. CT, however, demonstrates the location of intrahepatic stones well and, unlike US, is not inhibited by pneumobilia in visualizing these stones. (See section on recurrent pyogenic cholangitis).

Neoplasms of the biliary tree

Bile duct carcinoma or cholangiocarcinoma (CCA) is a rare malignancy comprising 0.5% to 1.0% of all malignancies.[158] Of the hepatobiliary tumors, it is much less common than other hepatobiliary tumors. It is much less common than hepatocellular or gallbladder

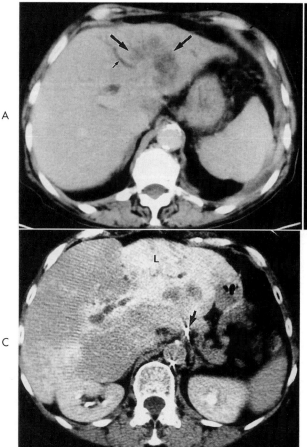

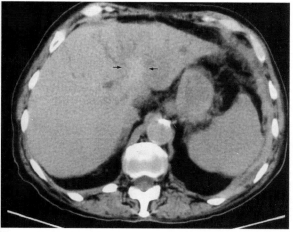

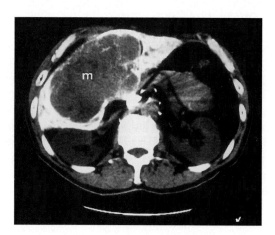

Fig. 31-84. Intrahepatic cholangiocarcinoma diagnosed in a patient with a malignant left pleural effusion. **A,** Hypodense mass relative to enhancing liver parenchyma with ill-defined margins *(large arrows)* and focal intrahepatic bile duct dilatation *(small arrow)*. **B,** Delayed image approximately 15 minutes after initial contrast bolus shows persistent enhancement in the mass *(arrows)*. **C,** Pronounced enhancement in the left hepatic lobe *(L)* during catheter injection of contrast directly into the celiac artery *(arrow)* in patient with cholangiocarcinoma in left hepatic lobe. The abnormal enhancement pattern is due to vascular invasion by the tumor.

Fig. 31-85. Mass *(M)* arising in liver with pathology revealing a mixed tumor containing cholangiocarcinoma and hepatoma. Note the density of the liver is increased because of previous thoratrast administration.

carcinomas. The vast majority of bile duct malignancies are adenocarcinomas, but squamous carcinoma, carcinoid, leiomyosarcoma, and rhabdomyosarcoma of the bile ducts have been reported.[73,141,218,224] The peak age

of onset for adenocarcinoma is usually in the sixth to seventh decade, though patients with predisposing inflammatory bowel disease or primary sclerosing cholangitis may present earlier.[134] There is a slight male predominance (1.5:1.0), but this is not as great as with hepatocellular carcinoma.

The clinical presentation depends on where in the biliary tree the tumor arises. If the tumor arises intrahepatic, it usually presents late with abdominal pain. However, if the tumor arises in the hilum or the extrahepatic bile duct, presentation is usually earlier with painless jaundice.

There are a number of predisposing conditions for CCA, including inflammatory bowel disease (ulcerative colitis and Crohn's disease), sclerosing cholangitis, *Clonorchis sinensis* infestation, biliary-enteric anastomosis, biliary tract stones and gallstones, thoratrast exposure, choledochal cyst, Caroli's disease, congenital hepatic fibrosis, and pancreatico-choledochal junction anomalies.* A case of CCA arising in a patient with cystic fibrosis has been reported.[1] Chronic inflammation of

*References 41, 43, 62, 133, 141, 224.

the bile ducts seems to be a common element leading to CCA. Sclerosing cholangitis with chronic biliary inflammation and fibrosis is most likely the underlying cause of an increased risk of CCA in patients with ulcerative colitis and Crohn's disease. Chronic inflammation is also probably the underlying cause of predisposition to CCA with chronic *Clonorchis* (liver fluke) infestation, stone disease, choledochal cyst, and biliary-enteric anastomoses.[41,43,95,149]

If CCA arises peripherally in the liver parenchyma from small intrahepatic bile ducts, it usually presents as a well-defined mass (Figs. 31-84, 31-85; see also Fig. 31-91). Rarely, a diffusely infiltrating or sclerosing type can occur.[159] The mass is usually heterogeneous but hypodense relative to the liver on unenhanced scans. High-attenuation areas in the mass may be seen because of the presence of mucinous material.[45] These tumors can produce mucin, which may accumulate in adjacent bile ducts and, if dense, may mimic stones. Low-attenuation areas in the mass may be due to mucin or necrosis.[105] With intravenous contrast, heterogeneous enhancement is seen, often peripherally. The differential diagnostic considerations of such as mass would include hepatocellular carcinoma, biliary cystadenoma or cystadenocarcinoma, and metastases. Hepatocellular carcinoma is much more common than CCA and typically arises in cirrhotic livers. The serum alpha-fetoprotein is usually not elevated in CCA, but the bilirubin may be higher than typically seen with hepatocellular carcinoma.[141] In addition, if intrahepatic biliary dilatation is associated with the mass, then CCA should be suspected over hepatocellular carcinoma. Biliary cystadenoma and cystadenocarcinoma may mimic this form of CCA, but they are usually more cystic than is CCA. Finally, metastases may have a similar appearance to this form of CCA and are far more common (Fig. 31-86). Percutaneous needle biopsy is usually the only definite way to differentiate these lesions.

CCA arising from the extrahepatic bile ducts is the most common form of this tumor. Grossly, the extrahepatic type of tumor is typically sclerosing and infiltrative, though it may be exophytic with an associated mass or polypoid with an intraluminal mass. The most common extrahepatic site is the confluence of the right and left hepatic ducts with the CHD. Such hilar CCA comprise up to 85% of extrahepatic CCA, depending on the series.[12,13,224] A distinct pathologic variant of CCA found at the hilum is the so-called Klatskin tumor, which spreads along the ducts with extensive fibrosis.[62] These infiltrating tumors are often difficult to visualize directly on CT scans since there may only be focal thickening of the duct wall and little associated mass (Fig. 31-87).[36,44] A reported sensitivity of CT for such a hilar CCA has been reported in the range of only 40%.[44,234] The typi-

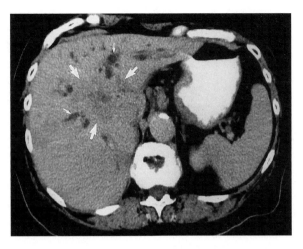

Fig. 31-86. Ill-defined mass in hilum of liver *(large white arrows)* causing biliary dilatation *(small white arrows)*. The mass proved to be metastatic adenocarcinoma but mimicked cholangiocarcinoma.

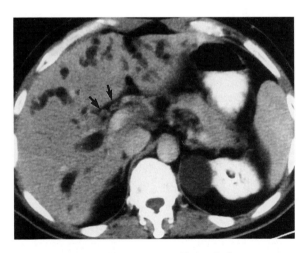

Fig. 31-87. Subtle infiltrative type of hilar cholangiocarcinoma presents with only mild thickening of the walls of the right and left hepatic ducts *(arrows)*. Note dilated intrahepatic ducts.

cal finding on CT is dilatation of the intrahepatic bile ducts in both the right and left lobes with nonunion of the dilated ducts at the hilum. Occasionally a mass may be detected at the hilum, and it is typically hypodense relative to adjacent liver parenchycyma on enhanced scans (Fig. 31-88). Yamashita, however, reported hypervascular densely enhancing exophytic-type mass as one appearance of hilar CCA.[234] The density of the hypodense masses may increase relative to liver parenchyma on delayed scans (8 to 15 min postinjection) (Fig. 31-84).[208]

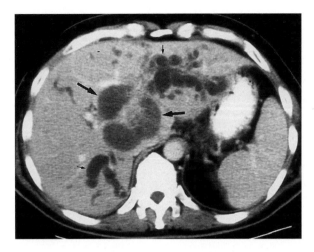

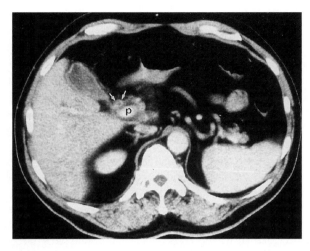

Fig. 31-88. Hilar cholangiocarcinoma *(large arrows)* presenting as a hypodense mass expanding out into the hepatic parenchyma. Because of the location of the tumor, intrahepatic biliary dilatation in both lobes of the liver occurs *(small arrows)*.

Fig. 31-89. Infiltrative type of cholangiocarcinoma causing wall thickening of the common hepatic duct *(white arrows)*; portal vein *(p)*.

CCA can arise elsewhere in the remainder of the extrahepatic bile ducts. Typically these tumors are of the infiltrating type, with little detectable mass (Fig. 31-89). Biliary dilatation down to the level of the tumor will be present, and the appearance may mimic a benign stricture or obstruction secondary to a cholesterol stone. Thin-section CT scanning targeted to this area, however, may reveal wall thickening or a small intraluminal mass consistent with tumor (Fig. 31-90).[13,193] CCA should be suspected if there is an abrupt end to the biliary dilatation without a visible mass, especially if it occurs between the hilum and the pancreatic head.[13]

Hilar CCA tends more to present early because of earlier biliary obstruction than does the peripheral intrahepatic form of CCA. However, Torsen et al reported that 57% of their patients with hilar CCA were nonresectable at presentation because of local liver invasion.[218] Resectability depends on location of the tumor and local or distant metastasis. If there is extensive ductal involvement, liver or vascular invasion, or nodal involvement, resection is difficult. Generally, distal duct tumors tend to be more resectable than are proximal tumors. Proximal tumors invade locally with nodal metastases earlier than do distal tumors. Common sites for nodal metastases involve primarily the foramen of Winslow node, superior pancreaticoduodenal nodes, and posterior pancreaticoduodenal nodes (Fig. 31-68,D). Distant metastases to liver, lung, and bones may occur but late in the disease. Portal vein invasion occurs less frequently with CCA than with hepatocellular carcinoma grossly

(Fig. 31-91). However, microscopically, portal vein invasion is common (89% to 90%).[235] Enhancement of liver parenchyma peripheral to a CCA may be altered as a result of portal vein invasion. Increased enhancement of the liver parenchyma distal to the tumor on bolus-enhanced CT and decreased enhancement of the same area on CT arterioportography has been described in the setting of portal vein invasion (Fig. 31-84, C).[107,235] The same area may appear hyperintense on T2-weighted MRI imaging.[107]

Lobar atrophy has been described with CCA, particularly hilar CCA (Fig. 31-92). The exact mechanism of lobar atrophy is not clear. One of the major causes is biliary obstruction, which secondarily leads to diversion of portal vein flow with resultant atrophy of the affected hepatic parenchyma.[36,207] Some have argued that lobar atrophy is a sign of nonresectability because it implies portal vein invasion.[36,224] However, others have demonstrated lobar atrophy with only biliary obstruction without venous involvement, and therefore these patients are still resectable.[181] Lobar atrophy was once used as a sign of the presence of malignancy but also has been reported in benign biliary disease.

The staging of CCA is best performed by US, CT, and cholangiography (PTC and ERCP) (Figs. 31-93 to 31-96). The overall accuracy of US, CT, and cholangiography at staging CCA is reported at 70% to 90%.[81,158] Cholangiography demonstrates the extent of bile duct involvement better than do US and CT especially for infiltrative tumors, and it provides a route for biopsy. MRI

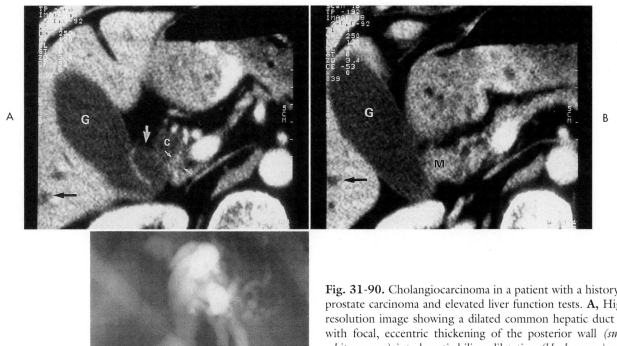

Fig. 31-90. Cholangiocarcinoma in a patient with a history of prostate carcinoma and elevated liver function tests. **A,** High-resolution image showing a dilated common hepatic duct *(c)* with focal, eccentric thickening of the posterior wall *(small white arrows);* intrahepatic biliary dilatation *(black arrow);* gallbladder *(g);* neck of the gallbladder and cystic duct *(large white arrow).* **B,** Image 6 mm caudal to *A* shows abrupt termination of the common duct with a small mass *(M)* at the level of termination; *(G)* gallbladder; intrahepatic biliary dilatation *(black arrow).* **C,** ERCP showing dilatation of the intrahepatic bile ducts and the extrahepatic duct down to the level of a tight stricture *(white arrows),* which correlates with the level of the mass in image "B."

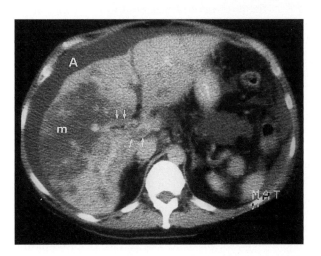

Fig. 31-91. Multiple intrahepatic foci of cholangiocarcinoma *(m)* presenting as hypodense masses. Note thrombus in the main and right branch of the portal vein *(arrows);* ascites *(A).*

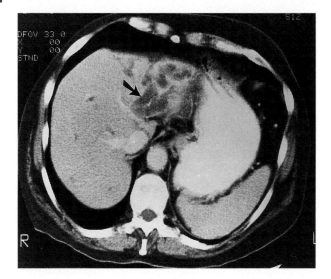

Fig. 31-92. Biliary dilatation *(arrow)* and atrophy of the left hepatic lobe as a result of cholangiocarcinoma. (From Vasquez J, et al: *AJR* 144:542-548, 1985.)

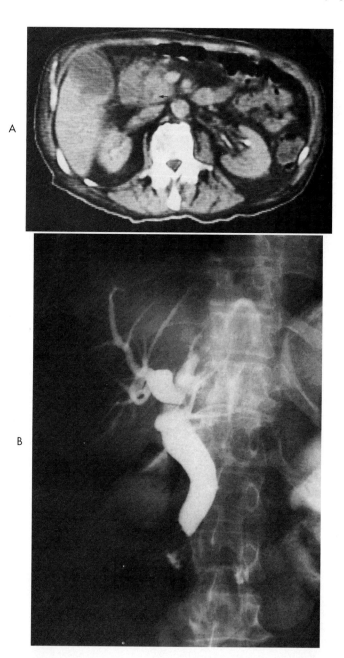

Fig. 31-93. **A,** This scan shows a calcification *(arrow)* below the level of a dilated bile duct that was believed to be a calculus. Gallstones were present on another scan. **B,** The transhepatic cholangiogram shows a dilated common bile duct with narrowing distally, which is diagnostic of a malignancy.

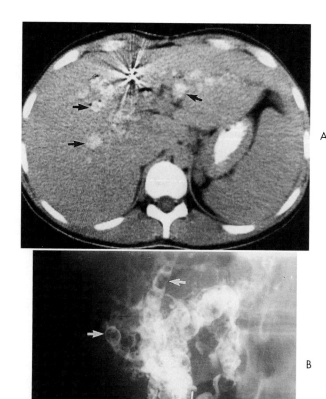

Fig. 31-94. Patient with biliary atresia, cirrhosis, and portoenterostomy. **A,** Multiple intrahepatic calculi *(arrows)*. **B,** Cholangiogram revealing multiple filling defects consistent with stones *(arrows)*.

is gaining in its use forstaging because of its sensitivity for vascular invasion and invasion into the hepatoduodenal ligament. Itoh compared US, CT, and MRI for staging hilar or proximal bile duct carcinoma and concluded that CT was the best overall examination for tumor depiction but that MRI was more useful for evaluating portal vein invasion.[108] Nesbit et al reported a 78% accuracy by CT for deter-mining unresectability of CCA but only a 44% accuracy in suggesting resectability. False negatives were due to metastases to lymph nodes and liver or portal vein invasion detected at surgery that were not detected by CT examination. Normal-sized positive lymph nodes and small hepatic metastases (<1 to 2 cm) may not be detected on CT.[89] Tailoring of the CT examination with thin collimation axial images, bolus administration of intravenous contrast, and a targeted small field of view will improve the ability to stage CCA.

Biliary cystadenoma and cystadenocarcinoma. The biliary cystadenoma and cystadenocarcinoma are rare neoplasms of the biliary tree. They typically arise from intrahepatic bile ducts but in rare cases are found in extrahepatic ducts. The vast majority arise in women and in patients over 30 years of age. These lesions are usually large, well-defined, solitary masses that are multiloculated and hypodense relative to liver (Fig. 31-97).

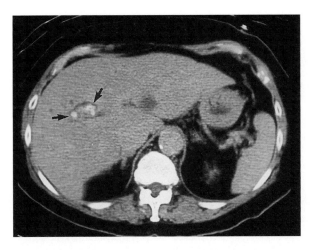

Fig. 31-95. Intrahepatic biliary calculi *(arrows)* in patient with repeated episodes of cholangitis.

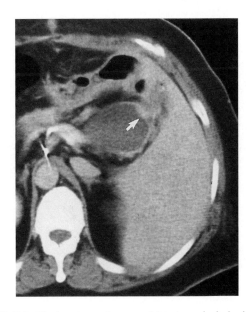

Fig. 31-96. Cholangiocarcinoma arising in a choledochal cyst. The tumor presents as a focal thickening in the cyst wall *(arrow)*. (From Baron RL: *Radiol Clin North Am* 29(6):1235-1250, 1991.)

Rarely, they may be multifocal.[42] There have been case reports of unilocular lesions, but most have multiple septations. The septations in the benign cystadenoma are usually thin, whereas those seen in the cystadenocarcinoma are often thicker with nodularity or papillary projections. These septations typically enhance on CT. Often, these lesions contain mucin and are low in density. However, the cystic spaces may vary in density because of the presence of serous fluid, pus, or high amounts of cholesterol.[78] They may communicate with the intrahepatic bile ducts and secrete mucinous material into the ducts. Calcifications may be present in the septations;

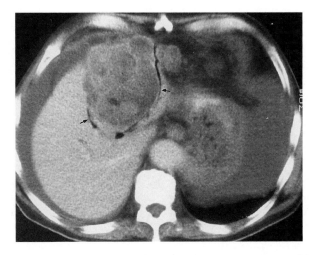

Fig. 31-97. Papillary cystadenocarcinoma appears as a multiseptated mass with areas of high and low density. Pneumobilia around mass *(arrows)* is secondary to recent biliary intervention.

when coarse and associated with nodular projections, they are more suggestive of cystadenocarcinoma.[123]

The differential diagnosis of these lesions would include a complex benign cyst, abscess, hematoma, Echinoccocal cyst, mesenchymal hamartoma, undifferentiated embryonal sarcoma, and cystic metastases. Diagnosis has been performed with percutaneous biopsy.[40,100] Resection of these lesions is usually complete and leads to cure.

Other neoplasms of the biliary tract. Other benign neoplasms of the bile ducts are very rare. Papillomas, bile duct hamaratomas, neurofibromas, and granular cell tumors have been reported (Fig. 31-71).[62,63,141] These lesions may appear as intraluminal filling defects or may simply occur with ductal obstruction. Cholangiography is typically most helpful at evaluating such lesions.

Lymphoma in the bile ducts has been described.[210] Typically, lymphomatous involvement of the biliary tract involves extrinsic compression by hepatoduodenal ligament and pancreaticoduodenal lymph nodes. Direct infiltration of the bile duct wall can occur, and it may cause biliary obstruction with a smooth stricture. Only bile-duct wall thickening may be seen without apparent mass on CT scan (Fig. 31-98).

Trauma to the biliary tree

Trauma to the gallbladder and biliary tree is uncommon and is almost always associated with hepatic injury.[77,200] Because of the location of the gallbladder, it is protected from injury to some degree by ribs and the liver. With blunt trauma however, perforation, avulsion, or contusion of the gallbladder can occur in rare cases.

Perforation or laceration of the gallbladder is the

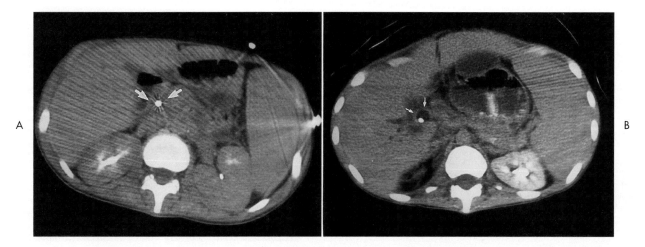

Fig. 31-98. Lymphoma involving wall of distal CBD. **A,** Pretreatment examination shows thickened tissue *(arrows)* around biliary stent. **B,** Posttreatment examination shows residual thickening of CBD wall *(arrows)*.

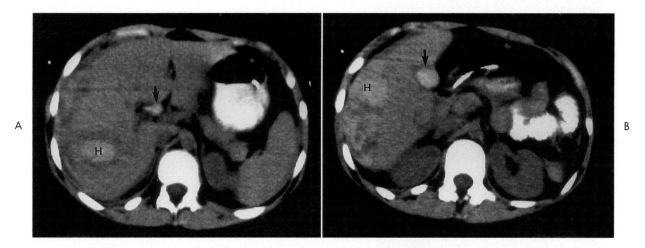

Fig. 31-99. Hemobilia secondary to liver trauma. **A,** Hyperdense blood in central bile ducts *(arrow)*. Liver hematoma *(H)*. **B,** Hyperdense blood in gallbladder *(arrow);* liver hematoma *(H)*.

most common type of injury and can result in bile leakage. Unfortunately, such leakage may not be detected for days to weeks.[10,53] On CT, ascites or a localized fluid collection around the gallbladder may be seen. The diagnosis can be made more accurately with aspiration of the fluid or a DISIDA scan.

A contusion of the gallbladder may simply appear as gallbladder wall thickening on CT, a nonspecific finding. Avulsion of the gallbladder is usually associated with bile ascites or hemoperitoneum on CT.[112] Both conditions are difficult radiologic diagnoses.

Trauma to the bile ducts is usually associated with an hepatic injury. Bilomas may occur, particularly with perihilar hepatic injuries.[144] Such bilomas may develop slowly over several days to weeks and may be asymptomatic. On CT, these bilomas will be focal collections of water density and may mimic abscesses or old hematomas. The diagnosis, however, can be made with DISIDA scans, aspiration, or cholangiography.

Hemobilia is a rare occurrence with hepatobiliary trauma but can result in increased density in the gallbladder or biliary tree on CT scan (Fig. 31-99). The differential diagnostic considerations for hemobilia include vicarious excretion of intravascular contrast, milk of calcium bile, or multiple small stones (Figs. 31-3, 31-4, 31-6, 31-7, 31-22).

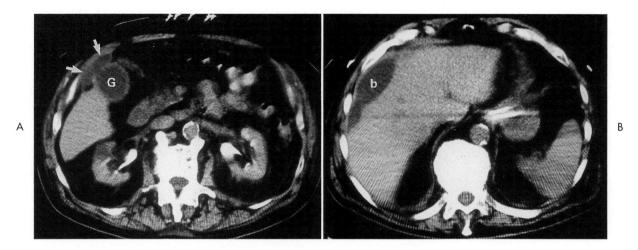

Fig. 31-100. Biloma secondary to gallbladder perforation. **A,** Gallbladder *(G)* with adjacent biloma *(arrows)*. **B,** Biloma *(b)* tracking superiorly along the right side of the liver.

Bilomas

Bilomas are focal collections of bile that may occur in a variety of locations such as intrahepatic, subcapsular, in the porta hepatis, and subhepatic (Fig. 31-100). Typically, they appear on CT as near-water–density collections, though if infected or associated with hemorrhage, the density may be higher. Most bilomas occur following surgery such as cholecystectomy or liver transplantation. However, they can occur as a result of trauma particularly with blunt trauma to the gallbladder or with a penetrating laceration of the liver.[76,144] They may also occur iatrogenically following a liver biopsy. Bilomas may rarely occur following gallbladder perforation due to severe acute cholecystitis; however, most pericholecystic fluid collections associated with acute cholecystitis are abscesses. Rare reports of spontaneous performation of the CBD described bile leakage with biloma formation occurring spontaneously, particularly in children. The cause is not known but may be related to occult distal biliary obstruction or congenital weakness in the duct wall near the cystic duct and CBD junction.[91]

CT cannot definitively diagnose a biloma, because they appear like other fluid collections. DISIDA scans or cholangiography better define leaks and bilomas. However, CT can be used to percutaneously aspirate or drain such collections.

Biliary complications in liver transplants

Biliary complications following liver transplantation are the second most common cause of hepatic dysfunction following rejection, and may occur in up to 20% of patients.[161,240,241,242] Biliary obstruction and bile leak are the two major categories of posttransplant biliary complications. Although cholangiography is the gold standard method for evaluating biliary complications, the clinical presentation of such problems is often nonspecific, and CT scans are initially obtained as general surveys of the abdomen. Therefore, recognition of the CT appearance of these biliary complications can aid in directing the work-up and therapy.

Bile leaks typically occur at the duct anastomosis. The preferred type of anastomosis is the duct-duct or choledochocholedochostomy, which preserves the recipient ampulla of Vater. If the recipient duct is diseased, as for example in recurrent cholangitis, then a biliary-enteric anastomosis or choledochojejunostomy is performed. In the latter case, a Roux loop of bowel is brought up into the porta hepatis and connected to the donor CBD. The Roux loop itself may be fluid-filled and mimic a fluid collection such as a biloma in the port hepatis.[87] Bile leaks will appear as focal fluid collections in the porta hepatis, or if nonfocal may appear as ascites. Unfortunately, CT cannot differentiate bile from other fluid such as lymph, blood, or pus. A DISIDA scan or cholangiogram will be required to more definitively diagnose a bile leak. CT, however, can be used to percutaneously aspirate or drain such collections.

Bile leaks with associated bilomas can occur away from the anastomosis and should be recognized as a sign of a hepatic arterial complication, particularly thrombosis.[239] In liver allografts, the biliary tree is highly dependent on the hepatic artery for its blood supply. Hepatic arterial occlusion results in bile duct necrosis with bile leak and biloma formation. Bilomas in the liver appear as focal fluid collections along the biliary tree (Fig. 31-101). They may or may not become infected. Hepatic infarcts may also be seen presenting as hypodense areas of liver parenchyma.

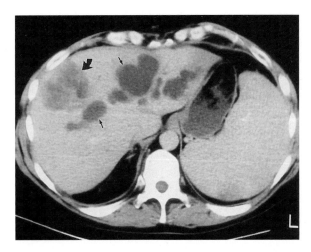

Fig. 31-101. Liver transplant with hepatic arterial occlusion and resultant hepatic infarct *(large arrow)* and bile duct necrosis with formation of bilomas *(small arrows)*.

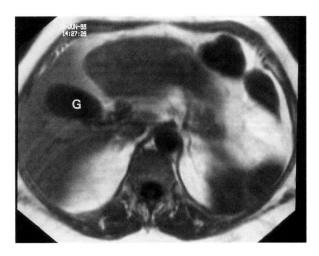

Fig. 31-102. Normal appearance of gallbladder on short TR (T1-weighted) image. Note hypointense signal of gallbladder *(G)*. TR, 700; TE, 10.

Biliary obstruction can occur because of strictures, occluded or trapped internal stent, T-tube dysfunction, common duct redundancy, stones, or mucocele of the cystic duct.[161] A stricture at the biliary anastomosis is the most common cause of obstruction. Cholangiography is the best method for evaluating posttransplant biliary obstruction and can provide subsequent therapy via stenting or balloon dilatation. The hallmark of biliary obstruction on CT or US is duct dilatation. However, in liver allografts, dilatation may not be present at the time that biliary obstruction is clinically suspected, and biliary obstruction may not be diagnosed by CT or US.[240] Cholangiography would be required in such cases. Obstructing stones or sludge may be recognized on CT as increased density in the bile ducts. In addition, a mucocele of the cystic duct remnant has been reported as a small round collection in the porta hepatitis on CT.[242] On cholangiography, it can be seen to compress the extrahepatic bile duct and cause obstruction. The differential diagnosis of such a small collection should include a seroma, abscess, pseudoaneurysm of the hepatic artery, hematoma, biloma, or Roux limb of the biliary-enteric anastomosis.

Diffuse dilatation of the extrahepatic bile duct after liver transplantation has been reported and may be seen with or without obstruction. This generalized dilatation of only the extrahepatic duct can occur gradually and may be due to sphincter of Oddi dysfunction or denervation and devascularization of the duct during surgery.[35,143,161,241] Clinically the patient may present with signs of biliary obstruction, or the dilatation may simply occur with no apparent obstruction to bile flow. If the degree of dilatation is significant, some element of obstruction should be suspected and further investigation

with a DISIDA scan or cholangiography should be performed.

MRI of the biliary tract

Only a brief overview of MRI of the biliary tract will be provided here because currently it is not one of the primary imaging modalities of the biliary tract. Cholangiography, US, and CT are more useful in evaluating the biliary tract. However, familiarity with the MR appearance of the biliary tract and biliary diseases is essential when interpreting MRI examinations of the upper abdomen.

Bile has varying signal on MRI, depending on the fasting state of the individual, the pulse sequence used, and the presence of pathology.[56,99,119,120] In a fasting individual, bile is concentrated with little water content and increased concentrations of bile acids, cholesterol, and phospholipids. The T1 value of concentrated bile is shortened and on short TR/TE images (T1-weighted images) it can appear hyperintense compared with other body fluids such as CSF.[99,119] On long TR/TE images (T2-weighted images), concentrated bile will still have high signal comparable to CSF. In the nonfasting individual with rapid release of bile, concentration does not occur and the water content remains relatively high. Such bile behaves similar to other fluid such as CSF with hypointensity on T1-weighted images and hyperintensity on T2-weighted images (Fig. 31-102). Layering of various concentrations of bile can occur in the gallbladder. Because of a higher specific gravity, the more concentrated bile will layer dependently (Fig. 31-103).

Lack of concentrating ability of the gallbladder in fasting patients has been reported with acute cholecystitis.[138] Such patients demonstrate low signal intensity bile

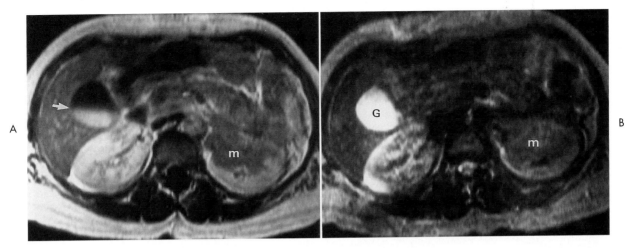

Fig. 31-103. Layering bile in gallbladder. Note patient also has left renal neoplasm *(m)*. **A,** T1-weighted image showing concentrated bile (hyperintense) layering dependently beneath the less concentrated bile (hypointense) in the gallbladder *(white arrow)*. TR, 700; TE, 10. **B,** T2-weighted image showing all bile in gallbladder *(G)* turned hyperintense. TR, 2000; TE, 80.

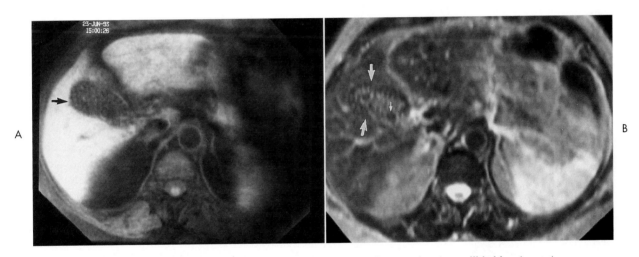

Fig. 31-104. Gallstones. **A,** Fat-suppression T1-weighted image showing gallbladder *(arrow)* with multiple tiny stones presenting as signal voids. **B,** T2-weighted image of same patient. Gallbladder *(large arrows)*; gallstones *(small arrow)*.

on T1-weighted images rather than the high signal of concentrated bile. This finding in a fasting patient is suggestive of a concentrating problem in the gallbladder, as can be seen in acute cholecystitis. Unfortunately it is not a consistent finding in all cases of acute cholecystitis.[120,138,230] In chronic cholecystitis, the concentrating function of the gallbladder is typically preserved so that the signal of bile is as expected in fasting and nonfasting patients.[120] Therefore, the signal characteristics of the gallbladder bile alone are not diagnostic for cholecystitis on MRI but must be used in conjunction with other signs such as gallbladder wall thickening, gallstones, and pericholecystic fluid.

Gallstones typically have no signal on MRI because of their solid nature, with little free water, rather than their chemical composition (Figs. 31-104, 31-105).[18,150] There may, however, be retraction clefts centrally in the stone that contain fluid and appear hyperintense on T2-weighted images.[90] An atypical appearance of gallstones on MRI was reported where the stones demonstrated high signal on T1-weighted images because of high fatty acid content.[148]

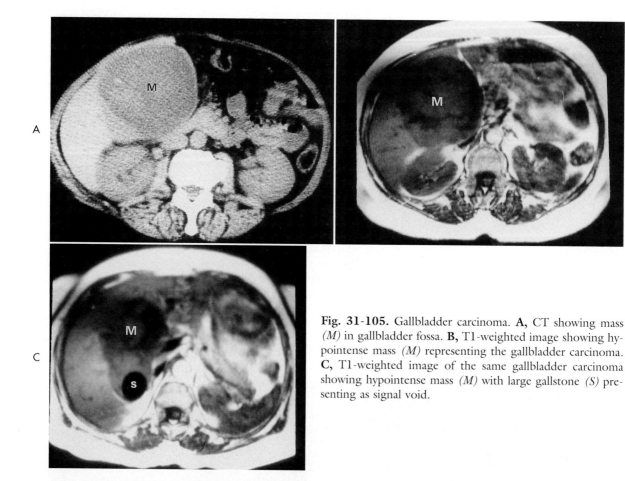

Fig. 31-105. Gallbladder carcinoma. **A,** CT showing mass *(M)* in gallbladder fossa. **B,** T1-weighted image showing hypointense mass *(M)* representing the gallbladder carcinoma. **C,** T1-weighted image of the same gallbladder carcinoma showing hypointense mass *(M)* with large gallstone *(S)* presenting as signal void.

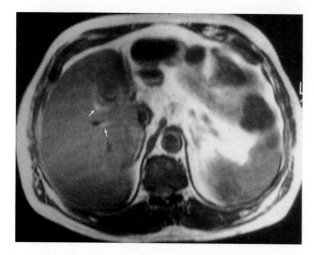

Fig. 31-106. T1-weighted image of subtle intrahepatic biliary dilatation *(arrows)*. The dilated ducts are hyperintense because of the concentration of the bile. Adjacent vessels have relatively low signal. TR, 500; TE, 20.

Carcinoma of the gallbladder has been described as a mass in the gallbladder fossa with hypointensity on T1-weighted images and hyperintensity on T2-weighted images relative to liver.[185,188,232] Low signal gallstones

may be seen within the gallbladder or engulfed within the mass. MRI is helpful in evaluating spread of tumor into the liver with hyperintensity of the tumor relative to liver parenchyma on T2-weighted images. In addition, MRI is reported to be more accurate than CT or US for invasion of the hepatoduodenal ligament or spread to pancreaticoduodenal lymph nodes.[188] MRI performs as well as CT for direct spread to the liver and for hepatic metastases. The ability of MRI to detect small gallbladder tumors is not yet evident.

Visualization of the intrahepatic bile ducts on MRI depends on the size of the ducts, concentration of the bile, pulse sequences used, motion artifact, and periportal high signal. Rapid pulse sequences, as in single-breath hold techniques, reduce respiratory and motion artifact and aid in evaluating the intrahepatic bile ducts, which are normally not visible. In our experience, T1- and T2-weighted sequences with fat-suppression techniques are required for visualizing the intrahepatic bile ducts especially if they are only mildly dilated. Detecting mildly dilated intrahepatic bile ducts may still be difficult even with optimum imaging because the signal characteristics of bile will vary, depending on its concentration (Fig. 31-106). Signal contrast between the bile ducts and the liver therefore may be low, depending on

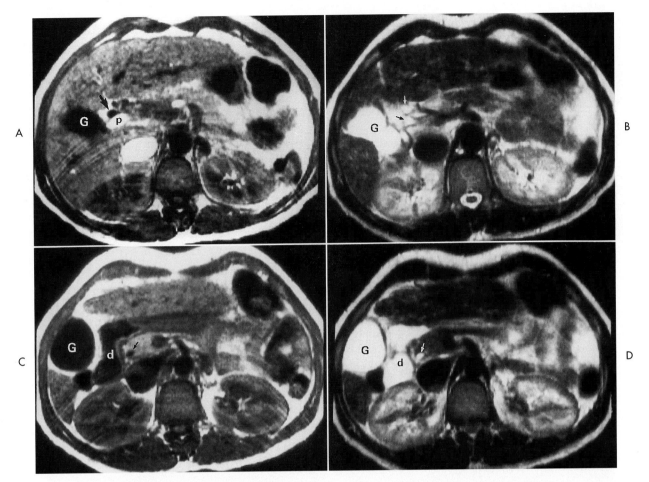

Fig. 31-107. Normal extrahepatic bile duct. **A,** Common hepatic duct *(arrow)* is hypointense on the T1-weighted image. Gallbladder *(G)*; portal vein *(p)*. TR, 578; TE, 15. **B,** T2-weighted image at level comparable to "A." CHD *(white arrow)* is now hyperintense. Gallbladder *(G)*; portal vein (black arrow) TR, 1995; TE, 90. **C,** T1-weighted image of distal CBD *(arrow)* in pancreatic head. Gallbladder *(g)*; duodenum *(d)*. TR, 578; TE, 15. **D,** T2-weighted image at comparable level to "C." Note distal CBD *(arrow)* now turns hyperintense. Gallbladder *(G)*; duodenum *(d)*. TR, 1995; TE, 90.

the bile concentration. CT and US are more sensitive for mild intrahepatic bile duct dilatation than is MRI.[58,90]

The extrahepatic bile duct can be visualized with varying normal diameters being reported (Fig. 31-107). The upper limit of normal size of the extrahepatic bile duct on T1-weighted images is 10 mm and on T2-weighted images is 11.8 mm.[205] The distal CBD appears as a relatively hypointense round structure in the posterolateral portion of the pancreatic head on T1-weighted images and is relatively hyperintense on T2-weighted images.

The characteristics of several types of bile duct pathology on MRI have been described. The appearance of a choledochal cyst has been reported as a mass near the porta hepatis with a long T1 and T2 with associated biliary dilatation.[3,24] Cholangiocarcinoma (CCA) has

two basic appearances on MRI. Peripheral CCA often appears as a focal well-defined mass with homogeneous relatively high signal as compared with the liver on T2-weighted images. There may be a central scar and satellite nodules.[67,92] The detection rate of such tumors has been reported to be 78% to 100%.[209] This appearance, however, is not diagnostic for CCA, and other liver lesions such as hepatomas may have a similar appearance.[67,187] The second type of CCA is the more infiltrative and scirrhous type that may have relatively low signal on all sequences because of high fibrous tissue content.[59] Biliary dilatation that abruptly terminates is an important sign for malignancy as on CT, US, and cholangiography. MRI is not as sensitive as CT for showing subtle duct-wall thickening associated with CCA because of the lower spatial resolution and more artifacts. MRI,

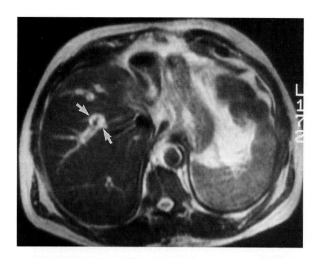

Fig. 31-108. Periportal high signal intensity *(arrows)* seen around low signal vessel centrally, in patient with liver disease. TR, 2000; TE, 80.

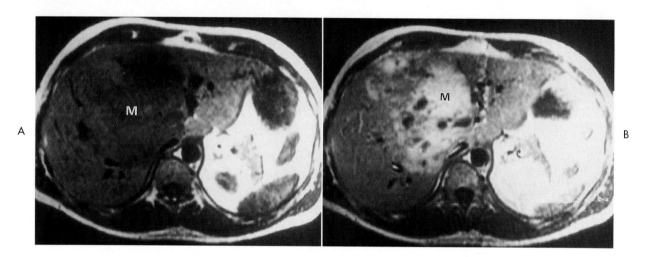

Fig. 31-109. Gallbladder carcinoma invading liver. **A,** Invasion into liver appears as hypointense mass *(M)* on T1-weighted image. TR, 500; TE, 15. **B,** Tumor invasion into liver *(M)* becomes hyperintense on T2-weighted image. TR, 2357; TE, 80.

however, can demonstrate the hepatic lobar or segmentaltumor location and detect intrahepatic metastases well. In addition, MRI may be quite useful at determining resectability.[108,195] It can demonstrate vascular invasion by showing loss of normal vascular flow void, tumor enhancement within the vessel, or abnormal signal in the liver parenchymal affected by the vascular invasion or occlusion.[107]

Abnormal signal can be seen surrounding intrahepatic vascular structures and has been described by Matsui as periportal abnormal intensity.[136] PAI is a nonspecific finding seen in diseases affecting the biliary tract such as cholangitis, CCA, obstructive jaundice of any cause, and lymphedema secondary to malignant portal lymph nodes. Matsui reported that PAI was not seen in cases of choledocholithiasis, pancreatic disease, or nonobstructive biliary dilatation.[136] However, similar abnormal signal can be found in a variety of conditions including trauma, CHF, and in rejection in liver allografts, and

it has been described on CT as periportal lymphedema.[7,121,124,135,227] Matsui reported that the PAI represents edema, ductal proliferation, dilated lymphatics, and inflammatory infiltrates in periportal tissues.[136] Typically, the PAI is low signal on T1-weighted images and relatively high signal on T2-weighted images. It differs from biliary dilatation in that PAI completely surrounds the portal vein, whereas dilated bile ducts are found on only one side of the vessel (Fig. 31-108).

Recently literature has been published concerning three-dimensional MR cholangiography. The technique employs two- and three-dimensional fast scanning sequences with multiplanar reconstruction so that the biliary tree can be visualized in three-dimensional projections (Figs. 31-109, 31-110).[152] Such techniques will provide similar information as direct cholangiography, without the risks of an invasive procedure such as ERCP or PTC.

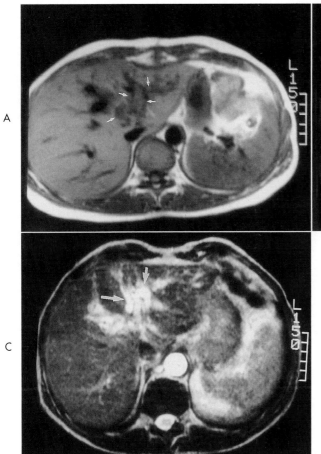

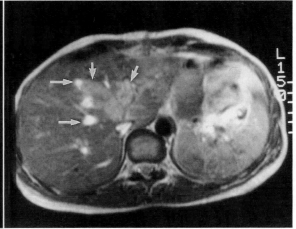

Fig. 31-110. Biliary obstruction. **A,** T1-weighted image showing dilated intrahepatic bile ducts *(arrows)* of intermediate intensity; vessels have black signal void. TR, 500; TE, 20. **B,** Spin density T2-weighted image showing ducts *(short arrows)* to have slightly higher signal than adjacent liver but lower signal than vessels *(long arrows)*. TR, 2857; TE, 30. **C,** T2-weighted image showing dilated ducts to be hyperintense *(short arrow)* as are the vessels *(long arrow)*. TR, 2571; TE, 80.

REFERENCES

1. Abdul-Karim FW, et al: Carcinoma of the extrahepatic biliary system in an adult with cystic fibrosis, *Gastroenterology* 82:758-762, 1982.
2. Alagille D: Extrahepatic biliary atresia. *Hepatology* 4:75, 1984.
3. Alexander MC, Haaga JR: MR imaging of the choledochal cyst. *J Comput Assist Tomogr* 9(2):357, 1985.
4. Ament AE, et al: Primary sclerosing cholangitis: CT findings. *J Comput Assist Tomogr* 7:795-800, 1983.
5. Andreu J, et al: Computed tomography as the method of choice in the diagnosis of emphysematous cholecystitis. *Gastrointest Radiol* 12:315-318, 1987.
6. Araki T, Itani Y, Tasaka A: CT of choledochal cyst. *AJR* 135:729-734, 1980.
7. Aspestrande F, et al: Increased lymphatic flow from the liver in different intra- and extrahepatic disease demonstrated by CT. *J Comput Assist Tomogr* 15(4):550-554, 1991.
8. Auteri AG, Malet PF: Radiographic imaging to predict gallstone dissolution: more than meets the eye. *Gastroenterology* 98(6):1715-1716, 1990.
9. Baker ME, et al: Computed tomography of masses in periportal/hepatoduodenal ligament. *J Comput Assist Tomogr* 11:258-262, 1987.
10. Ball DS, et al: Avulsed gallbladder: CT appearance. *J Comput Assist Tomogr* 12:538, 1988.
11. Barakos JA, et al: Cholelithiasis: evaluation with CT. *Radiology* 162:415-418, 1987.
12. Baron RL: Common bile duct stones. Reassessment of criteria for CT diagnosis. *Radiology* 162:419-424, 1987.
13. Baron RL: Computed tomography of the biliary tree. *Radiologic Clin North Am* 29(6), 1235-1250, 1991.
14. Baron RL: Role of CT in characterizing gallstones: an unsettled issue. *Radiology* 178:635-636, 1991.
15. Baron RL, et al: A prospective comparison of the elevation of biliary obstruction using computed tomography and ultrasonography. *Radiology* 145:91-98, 1982.
16. Baron RL, et al: Computed tomographic features of biliary obstruction. *AJR* 140:1173, 1983.
17. Baron RL, et al: CT evaluation of gallstones in vitro: correlation with chemical analysis, *AJR* 151:1123-1128, 1988.
18. Baron RL, et al: In vitro dissolution of gallstones with MTBE: correlation with characteristics of CT and MR imaging. *Radiology* 173:117, 1989.
19. Barwick KW, Rosai J: Liver. In *Ackerman's surgical pathology,* ed 7, 1989, CV Mosby Co., St. Louis.
20. Becker CD, Hassler H, Terrier F: Preoperative diagnosis of the Mirizzi syndrome: limitations of sonography and computed tomography. *AJR* 143:591-596, 1984.
21. Becker CD, Vock P: Appearance of gas-containing gallstones on sonography and computed tomography. *Gastrointest Radiol* 9:323-328, 1984.
22. Berland LL, Lawson TL, Stanley RJ: CT appearance of Mirizzi syndrome. *J Comput Assist Tomogr* 8(1):165-166, 1984.

23. Blanton DE, Bream CA, Mandel SR: Gallbladder ectopia: a review of anomalies of position. *AJR* 121:396-400, 1974.

24. Boechant MI: Magnetic resonance imaging of abdominal and pelvic masses in children. *Top Magn Reson Imaging* 3(1):25-41, 1990.

25. Bofet JF, et al: Cholangitis complicating intraarterial chemotherapy in liver metastasis. *Radiology* 156:335-337, 1985.

26. Botting AL, et al: Metastatic hypernephroma masquerading as a polypoid tumor of the gallbladder and review of metastatic tumors of the gallbladder. *Mayo Clin Proc* 38:225-231, 1963.

27. Boukadoum M, et al: CT demonstration of adenomyomatosis of the gallbladder. *J Comput Assist Tomogr* 8(1):177-180, 1984.

28. Brakel K, et al: Predicting gallstone composition with CT: in vivo and in vitro analysis. *Radiology* 174:337-341, 1990.

29. Brandon JC, et al: Laparoscopic cholecystectomy: evolution, early results, and impact on nonsurgical gallstones therapies. *AJR* 157:235-239, 1991.

30. Brandt DJ, et al: Gallbladder disease in patients with primary sclerosing cholangitis. *AJR* 150:571-574, 1988.

31. Brink JA, Ferrucci JT: Use of CT for predicting gallstone composition: a dissenting view. *Radiology* 178:633-634, 1991.

32. Brodey PA, et al: Computed tomography of choledochocele. *J Comput Assist Tomogr* 8(1):162-164, 1984.

33. Bundy AL, et al: Ultrasonic diagnosis of metastatic melanoma of the gallbladder presenting as acute cholecystitis. *J Clin Ultrasound* 10:285-287, 1982.

34. Burrell MI, et al: The biliary tract: imaging for the 1990's. *AJR* 157:223-233, 1991.

35. Campbell WL, et al: Changes in extrahepatic bile duct caliber in liver transplant recipients without evidence of biliary obstruction. *AJR* 158:997-1000, 1992.

36. Carr DH, et al: Computed tomography of hilar cholangiocarcinoma a new sign. *AJR* 53-56, 1985.

37. Carrasco CH, et al: Chemical cholecystitis associated with hepatic artery infusion chemotherapy. *AJR* 141:703-706, 1983.

38. Cello JP, et al: Acquired immunodeficiency syndrome cholangiopathy: spectrum of disease. *Am J Med* 86:539-546, 1989.

39. Chan FL, et al: Evaluation of recurrent pyogenic cholangitis with CT: analysis of 50 patients. *Radiology* 170:165-169, 1989.

40. Cheung YK, et al: Biliary cystadenoma and cystadenocarcinoma: some unusual features. *Clin Radiol* 43:183-185, 1991.

41. Choi BI, et al: Peripheral cholangiocarcinoma and cholanorchiasis: CT findings. *Radiology* 169:149-153, 1988.

42. Choi BI, et al: Biliary cystadenoma and cystadenocaricnoma: CT and sonographic findings. *Radiology* 171:57-61, 1989.

43. Choi BI, et al: CT findings of clonorchiasis. *AJR* 152:281-284, 1989.

44. Choi BI, et al: Hilar cholangiocarcinoma: comparative study with sonography and CT. *Radiology* 172:689-692, 1989.

45. Choi BI, et al: Caroli disease: central dot sign in CT. *Radiology* 174:161-163, 1990.

46. Christansen RA, et al: Inadvertant ligation of the aberrant right hepatic duct at cholecystectomy: radiologic diagnosis and treatment. *Radiology* 183:549-553, 1992.

47. Clouston JE, Thorpe RJ: Case report-CT findings in adenomyomatosis of gallbladder. *Australas Radiol* 35:86-87, 1991.

48. Co CS, Shea WJ Jr, Goldberg HI: Evaluation of common bile duct diameter using high resolution computed tomography. *J Comput Assist Tomogr* 10(3):424-427, 1986.

49. Cooperberg PL, Gibney RG: Imaging of the gallbladder. *Radiology* 163:605, 1987.

50. Cory DA, Don S, West KW: CT cholangiography of a choledochocele. *Pediatr Radiol* 21:73-74, 1990.

51. Cossi AF, et al: Computed tomography of xanthogranulomatous cholecystitis. *Gastrointest Radiol* 12:154-155, 1987.

52. Cronan JJ, Mueller PR, Simeone JF: Prospective diagnosis of choledocholithiasis. *Radiology* 146:467, 1983.

53. Daneman A, Matzinger MA, Martin DJ: Post-traumatic hemorrhage into the gallbladder. *J Comput Tomogr* 7:59-61, 1983.

54. Day DL, et al: Post operative abdominal CT scanning in extrahepatic biliary atresia. *Pediatr Radiol* 19:379-382, 1982.

55. DeGaetano AM, et al: Xanthogranulomatous cholecystitis: echographic and CT patterns. *RAYS (Roma)* 10(2):63-67, 1985.

56. Demas BE, et al: Gallbladder bile: an experimental study in dogs using MR imaging and proton MR spectroscopy. *Radiology* 157:453, 1985.

57. Dolmatch BL, et al: AIDS-related cholangitis: radiographic findings in nine patients. *Radiology* 163:313-316, 1987.

58. Dooms GC, Fisher MR, Higgins CB: MR imaging of the dilated biliary tract. *Radiology* 158:337-342, 1986.

59. Dooms GC, et al: Cholangiocarcinoma: imaging by MR. *Radiology* 159:89-94, 1986.

60. Doppmann JL, et al: Segmental hyperlucent defects in the liver. *J Comput Assist Tomogr* 8:50-57, 1984.

61. Duber C, et al: Xanthogranulomatous cholecystitis mimicking carcinoma of the gallbladder: CT findings. *J Comput Assist Tomogr* 8(6):1195-1198, 1984.

62. Edmondson HA, Peters RL: Liver. In Kissane JM, editors: *Anderson's pathology*, St Louis, Mosby 1985, p 1194.

63. Eisenberg D, Hurwitz L, Yo AC: CT and sonography of multiple bile duct hamartomas simulating malignant liver disease (Case Report). *AJR* 147:279-280, 1986.

64. Engels JT, Balfe DM, le JKT: Biliary carcinoma: CT evaluation of extrahepatic spread. *Radiology* 172:35-40, 1989.

65. Enriquez G, et al: Intrahepatic biliary stones in children. *Pediatr Radiol* 22:283-286, 1992.

66. Faintuch J, Machado MCC, Raia AA: Suprahepatic gallbladder with hypoplasia of the right lobe of the liver. *Arch Surg* 115:658-659, 1980.

67. Fan ZM, et al: Intrahepatic cholangiocarcinoma: spin-echo and contrast-enhanced dynamic MR imaging, *AJR* 161:313-317, 1993.

68. Federle MP, et al: Recurrent pyogenic cholangitis in Asian immigrants. *Radiology* 143:151-156, 1982.

69. Ferrozzi F, et al: Gallbladder metastasis: CT appearance. *Rays* 13(2):23-25, 1988.

70. Ferrucci JT Jr, et al: The radiologic diagnosis of gallbladder disease: an imaging symposium. *Radiology* 141:49-56, 1981.

71. Foley WD, et al: Demonstration of the normal extrahepatic biliary tree with computed tomography. *J Comput Assist Tomogr* 4:48-52, 1980.

72. Fork FT, Nyman UIF, Sigurjonnson S: Recognition of gas in gallstones in routine computed tomograms of the abdomen. *J Comput Assist Tomogr* 7(5):805-809, 1983.

73. Friedburg H, et al: Sonographic and computed tomographic features of embryonal rhabdomyosarcoma of the biliary tract. *Pediatr Radiol* 14:436-438, 1984.

74. Gagner M, Munson JL, Scholz FJ: Hepatobiliary anomalies associated with polysplenia syndrome. *Gastrointest Radiol* 16:167-171, 1991.

75. Gale ME, Robbins AH: Computed tomography of the gallbladder: unusual disease. *J Comput Assist Tomogr* 9(3):439-443, 1985.

76. Gelman R, et al: The use of radionuclide imaging in the evaluation of suspected biliary damage during laparoscopic cholecystectomy. *Gastrointest Radiol* 16:201-204, 1991.

77. Gembala RB, et al: Sonographic diagnosis of traumatic gallbladder avulsion. *J Ultrasound Med* 5:399-301, 1993.

78. Genkins SM, et al: Biliary cystadenoma with mesenchymal stroma: CT and angiographic appearance. *J Comput Assist Tomogr* 12:527-529, 1988 (Case Report).

79. Gerard PS, Berman D, Zafarnloss S: CT and ultrasound of gallbladder adenomyomatosis mimicking carcinoma. *J Comput Assist Tomogr* 14(3):490-491, 1990.

80. Gibson RN: Suprapancreatic biliary obstruction: CT evaluation, *Radiology* 165:875-876, 1987 (Letter to the Editor).

81. Gibson RN, et al: Bile duct obstruction: radiologic evaluation of level, cause and tumor resectability. *Radiology* 160:43-50, 1986.

82. Ginaldi S: Cholangiocarcinomas arising in a choledochal cyst: diagnostic value of computed tomography and ultrasonography. *Gastrointest Radiol* 12:212, 1987.

83. Goldstein F: Cystic duct syndrome. In Bockus HL, editor: *Gastroenterology*, Philadelphia, 1976, WB Saunders Co.

84. Goldstein RB, et al: Computed tomography of the thick-walled gallbladder mimicking pericholecystic fluid. *J Comput Assist Tomogr* 10(1):55-56, 1986.

85. Greenberg M, Robin JM, Greenberg BM: Appearance of the gallbladder and biliary tree by CT cholangiography. *J Comp Assist Tomogr* 7:788-794, 1983.

86. Greenberg M, et al: Computed tomographic cholangiography. *Radiology* 144:363-368, 1982.

87. Greenler DP, Sumkin JH, Campbell WL: CT appearance of the Roux limb following choledochojejunostomy in liver transplantation, *Gastrointest Radiol* 16:41-44, 1991.

88. Grumbach K, Levine MS, Exler JA: Gallstone ileus diagnosed by computed tomography. *J Comput Assist Tomogr* 10(1):146-148, 1986.

89. Gulliver DJ, et al: Malignant biliary obstruction: efficacy of thin-section dynamic CT in determining resectability. *AJR* 159:503-507, 1992.

90. Gupta RK, et al: Magnetic resonance in obstructive jaundice. *Australas Radiol* 33:245-251, 1989.

91. Haller JO, et al: Spontaneous perforation of the common bile duct in children. *Radiology* 172:621-624, 1989.

92. Hamrick-Turner J, Abbitt PL, Ros PR: Intrahepatic cholangiocarcinoma: MR appearance. *AJR* 158:77-79, 1992.

93. Harshfield DL, et al: Obstructing villous adenoma and papillary adenomatosis of the bile duct. *AJR* 154:1217-1218, 1990.

94. Havrilla TR, et al: Computed tomography of the gallbladder. *AJR* 130:1059-1067, 1978.

95. Herba MJ, et al: Cholangiocarcinoma as a late complication of choledochoenteric anastomoses. *AJR* 147:513-515, 1986.

96. Herbener TE, et al: Recurrent cholangiocarcinoma of the biliary tree after liver transplantation. *Radiology* 1969:642-642, 1988.

97. Herman TE, Siegel MJ: Central dot sign on CT of liver cysts. *J Comput Assist Tomogr* 14(6):1019-1021, 1990.

98. Hopper KD: The role of computed tomography in the evaluation of Caroli disease. *Clin Imaging* 13:68-73, 1989.

99. Hricak H, et al: Nuclear magnetic imaging of the gallbladder. *Radiology* 147:481-484, 1983.

100. Iemoto Y, et al: Biliary cystadenocarcinoma diagnosed by liver biopsy performed under ultrasonographic guidance. *Gastroenterology* 84:399-403, 1983.

101. Iline B, et al: Solitary neurofibroma of the gallbladder: report of three cases and literature review. *Mt Sinai J Med* 52(6):473-477, 1985.

102. Itai Y: Computed tomographic evaluation of gallbladder disease. *CRC Crit Rev Diagn Imaging* 27(2):113-152, 1987.

103. Itai Y, et al: Computed tomography of gallbladder carcinoma. *Radiology* 137:713-718, 1980.

104. Itai Y, et al: Computed tomography and ultrasound in the diagnosis of intrahepatic calculi. *Radiology* 136:399-405, 1980.

105. Itai Y, et al: Computed tomography of primary intrahepatic biliary malignancy. *Radiology* 147:485-490, 1983.

106. Itai Y, et al: CT of hepatic masses: significance of prolonged and delayed enhancement. *AJR* 146:729-733, 1986.

107. Itai Y, et al: Segmental intensity differences in the liver on MR images: a sign of intrahepatic portal flow stoppage. *Radiology* 167:17-19, 1988.

108. Itoh K, et al: Staging of bile duct cancer: comparative study of US, CT, and MR imaging, presented at RSNA meeting 1992.

109. Izumi N, et al: Ultrasonography and computed tomography in adenomyomatosis of the gallbladder. *Acta Radiol Diagn* 26:689-692, 1985.

110. Jacobson JB, Brodey PA: The transverse common duct. *AJR* 136:91-96, 1981.

111. Janowitz P, et al: Computed tomography evaluation of radiolucent gallstones in vivo. *Gastrointest Radiol* 15:58-60, 1990.

112. Jeffrey RB Jr, et al: Computed tomography of blunt trauma to the gallbladder. *J Comput Assist Tomogr* 10(5):756-758, 1986.

113. Jeffrey, RB Jr: Diagnosis of intrahepatic calculi and choledocholithiasis.In Ferrucci JT, Mathieu DG, editors: *Advances in hepatobiliary radiology*, St. Louis, 1990, CV Mosby Co.

114. Jeffrey RB, et al: Computed tomography in choledocholithiasis. *AJR* 140:1179, 1983.

115. Jenkins M, Golding RH, Cooperberg PL: Sonography and computed tomography of hemorrhagic cholecystitis. *AJR* 140:1197-1198, 1983.

116. Juttner H, et al: Thickening of the gallbladder wall in acute hepatitis: ultrasound demonstration. *Radiology* 142:465, 1982.

117. Kane RA, Costella P, Duszlak E: Computed tomography in acute cholecystitis: new observations. *AJR* 141:697-701, 1983.

118. Kane RA, et al: Porcelain gallbladder: ultrasound and CT appearance, *Radiology* 152:137-141, 1984.

119. Kang YS, et al: Alternatives in MR relaxation of normal canine gallbladder bile during fasting. *Magn Reson Imaging* 4:399, 1986.

120. Kanzer GK, Weinreb JC: Magnetic resonance imaging of diseases of the liver and biliary system. *Radiol Clin North Am* 29(6):1259-1284, 1991.

121. Kaplan SB, Zajko AB, Koneru B: Hepatic bilomes due to hepatic artery thrombosis in liver transplant recipients: percutaneous drainage and clinical outcome. *Radiology* 174:1031-1035, 1990.

122. Kaplan SB, et al: Periportal low attenuation areas on CT: value as evidence of liver transplant rejection. *AJR* 152:285-287, 1988.

123. Korobkin M, et al: Biliary cystadenoma and cystadenocarcinoma: CT and sonographic findings. *AJR* 153:507-511, 1989.

124. Koslin DB, et al: Hepatic perivascular lymphedema: CT appearance. *AJR* 150:111-113, 1980.

125. Krudy AG, et al: Hemobilia: computed tomographic diagnosis. *Radiology* 148:785-789, 1983.

126. Laing FC et al: Biliary dilatation: defining the level and cause by real-time US. *Radiology* 160:36, 1986.

127. Lamki N, Raval B, St Ville E: Computed tomography of complicated cholecystitis. *J Comput Assist Tomogr* 10:319-324, 1985.

128. Levitt R, et al: Accuracy of computed tomography of the liver and biliary tract. *Radiology* 124:123-128, 1988.

129. Lewandowski BJ, Winsberg F: Gallbladder wall thickness distortion by ascites. *AJR* 137:519-521, 1981.

130. Liddell RM, et al: CT depiction of intrahepatic bile ducts. *Radiology* 176:633-635, 1990.

131. Lindsay KA, Hall JRW, Chapman AH: Radiology of excessive mucus production as a complication of congenital bile duct abnormalities. *Clin Radiol* 46:43-45, 1992.

132. Loflin TG, et al: Gallbladder bile in cholecystitis, in vitro MR evaluation. *Radiology* 157:457-459, 1985.

133. MacCarty RL, et al: Primary sclerosing cholangitis: findings on cholangiography and pancreatography. *Radiology* 149:39-44, 1983.

134. MacCarty RL, et al: Cholangiocarcinoma complicating primary sclerosing cholangitis: cholangiographic appearance. *Radiology* 156:43-46, 1985.

135. Marincek B, et al: CT appearance of impaired lymphatic drainage in liver transplants. *AJR* 147:519-523, 1986.

136. Matsui O, Kadoya M, Takashima T: Intrahepatic periportal abnormal intensity on MR images: an indication of various hepatobiliary diseases. *Radiology* 171:335-338, 1989.

137. McAllister JD, D'Altori RA, Synder A: CT findings after uncomplicated percutaneous laparoscopic cholecystectomy. *J Comput Assist Tomogr* 15(5):770-772, 1991.

138. McCarthy S, et al: Cholecystitis: detection with MR imaging. *Radiology* 158:333-336, 1986.

139. McMillin K: Computed tomography of emphysematous cholecystitis. *J Comput Assist Tomogr* 9(2)330-332, 1985.

140. Meilstrup JW, Hopper KD, Hieme GA: Imaging of gallbladder variants. *AJR* 152:1205-1208, 1991.

141. Menu Y, Lorphelin JM, Arrive L: Tumors of the gallbladder and bile ducts. In Ferrucci JT, Mathieu DG, editors: *Advances in hepatobiliary radiology*, St. Louis, 1990, CV Mosby Co.

142. Menu Y, et al: Sonographic and computed tomographic evaluation of intrahepatic calculi. *AJR* 145:579-583, 1985.

143. Miller WJ, et al: Obstructive dilatation of extrahepatic recipient and donor bile ducts complicating orthotopic liver transplantation: imaging and laboratory findings. *AJR* 157:959-964, 1991.

144. Mirvis SE, Whitley NO: Computed tomography in hepatobiliary trauma. In Ferrucci JT and Matthieu DG, editors: *Advances in hepatobiliary radiology*, St. Louis, 1990, CV Mosby Co.

145. Mirvis SE, et al: The diagnosis of acute acalculous cholecystitis: a comparison of sonography, scintigraphy, and CT. *AJR* 147:1171-1175, 1986.

146. Mitchell SE, Clark KA: A comparison of computed tomography and sonography in choledocholithiasis. *AJR* 142:729, 1984.

147. Miyake H, et al: Adenomyomatosis of the gallbladder with subserosal fatty proliferation: CT findings in two cases. *Gastrointest Radiol* 17:21-23, 1992.

148. Moeser PM, et al: Unusual presentation of cholelithiasis on T_1-weighted MR imaging. *J Comput Assist Tomogr* 12:150, 1988.

149. Montana MA, Rohromann CA: Cholangiocarcinoma in a choledochal cyst: preoperative diagnosis. *AJR* 147:516-517, 1986.

150. Moon KL Jr, et al: Nuclear magnetic resonance imaging characteristics of gallstones in vitro. *Radiology* 148:753-756, 1983.

151. Morehouse H, et al: Infiltrating periductal neoplasm mimicking biliary dilatation on computed tomography. *J Comput Assist Tomogr* 7(4):721-723, 1983.

152. Morimoto K, et al: Biliary obstruction: evaluation with three-dimensional MR cholangiography. *Radiology* 183:578-580, 1992.

153. Morizumi H, et al: Neurofibroma of the gallbladder seen as a papillary polyp. *Acta Pathol Jpn* 38(2):259-268, 1988.

154. Morse JMD, Lakshman S, Thomas E: Gallbladder ectopia simulating pancreatic mass on CT. *Gastrointest Radiol* 10:111-113, 1985.

155. Mueller PR, et al: Postcholecystectomy bile duct dilatation: myth or reality? *AJR* 136:355-358, 1981.

156. Muhletaler C, et al: Diagnosis of obstructive jaundice with non-dilated bile ducts. *AJR* 134:1149-1152, 1980.

157. Nardi PM, Yaghoobian J, Ruchman RB: CT demonstration of retrohepatic gallbladder in severe cirrhosis. *J Comput Assist Tomogr* 12(6):968-970, 1988.

158. Nesbit GM, et al: Cholangiocarcinoma: diagnosis and evaluation of resectability by CT and sonography as procedures complementary to cholangiography. *AJR* 151:933-938, 1988.

159. Nichols DA, et al: Cholangiographic evaluation of bile duct carcinoma. *AJR* 141:1291-1294, 1983.

160. Nymann U, et al: Intravenous computed tomographic cholangiography in acute cholecystitis. *Acta Radiol Diagn* 25:289-298, 1984.

161. Oliver JH, et al: Imaging the hepatic transplant. *Radiol Clin North Am* 29(6):1285-1298, 1991.

162. Outwater E, Kaplan MM, Bankoff MS: Lymphadenopathy in sclerosing cholangitis: pitfall in the diagnosis of malignant biliary obstruction. *Gastrointest Radiol* 17:157-160, 1992.

163. Pasanen P, et al: Ultrasonography, CT and ERCP in the diagnosis of choledochal stones. *Acta Radiologica* 33(1):53-55, 1992.

164. Pastakia B, Shawker TH, Horvath K: Biliary neoplasm simulating dilated bile ducts: Role of computed tomography and ultrasound. *J Ultrasound Med* 6:333, 1987.

165. Pedrosa CS, et al: Computed tomography in obstructive jaundice. Part I: The level of obstruction. *Radiology* 139:627-634, 1980.

166. Pedrosa CS, et al: Computed tomography in obstructive jaundice. Part II: The level of obstruction. *Radiology* 139:635-645, 1981.

167. Phillips G, et al: Ultrasound patterns of metastatic tumors in the gallbladder. *J Clin Ultrasound* 10:379-383, 1982.

168. Pien EH, et al: Iatrogenic sclerosing cholangitis following hepatic arterial chemotherapy infusion. *Radiology* 156:329-330, 1985.

169. Polk HC, Jr: Carcinoma and calcified gallbladder. *Gastroenterology* 50:582-585, 1966.

170. Pollack M, Shirkhoda A, Charnsangavej C: Computed tomography of choledochocele. *J Comput Assist Tomogr* 9(2):360-362, 1985.

171. Pombo F, Arrojo L, Soler R: Left hepatic atrophy in Mirizzi syndrome: CT appearance. *Eur J Radiol* 10(3):181-182, 1990.

172. Quinn SF, Fazzio F, Jones E: Torsion of the gallbladder: findings on CT and sonography and role of percutaneous cholecystostomy. *AJR* 148:881-882, 1987.

173. Quint LE, Glazer GM: CT evaluation of the bile ducts in patients with fatty liver. *Radiology* 153:755-756, 1984.

174. Radin DR, Cohen H, Halls JM: Acalculous inflammatory disease of the biliary tree in acquired immunodeficiency syndrome: CT demonstration. *J Comput Assist Tomogr* 11:775-778, 1987.

175. Radin DR, Parkrama C, Ralls PW: Carcinoma of the cystic duct. *Gastrointest Radiol* 15:49-52, 1990.

176. Radin DR, Vachon LA: CT findings in biliary and pancreatic ascariasis. *J Comput Assist Tomogr* 10(3):508-509, 1986.

177. Raghavendra BN: Ultrasound features of primary carcinoma of the gallbladder: report of five cases. *Gastrointest Radiol* 5:239-244, 1980.

178. Rahn NH, et al: CT appearance of sclerosing cholangitis. *AJR* 141:549-552, 1983.

179. Ralls PW, et al: Gallbladder wall thickening: patients without intrinsic gallbladder disease. *AJR* 137:65, 1981.

180. Ralls PW, et al: Sonography in recurrent oriental pyogenic cholangitis. *AJR* 136:1010-1012, 1981.

181. Reiman TH, Balfe DM, Weyman PJ: Suprapancreatic biliary obstruction: CT evaluation. *Radiology* 163:49-56, 1987.

182. Romano AJ, et al: Gallbladder and bile duct abnormalities in AIDS: sonographic findings in eight patients. *AJR* 150:123-127, 1988.

183. Ros PR, et al: Intrahepatic cholangiocarcinoma: radiologic-pathologic correlation. *Radiology* 167:689-693, 1988.

184. Rosai J: Gallbladder and extrahepatic bile ducts. In *Ackerman's surgical pathology*, ed. 7, 1989, CV Mosby Co., St. Louis.

185. Rossman MD, et al: MR imaging of gallbladder carcinoma. *AJR* 148:143-144, 1987.

186. Roth JL, Berk JE: Symptoms after cholecystectomy. In Bockus HL, editor: *Gastroenterology*, ed. 3, Philadelphia, 1976, WB Saunders Co.

187. Rummeny E, et al: Primary liver tumors: diagnosis by MR imaging. *AJR* 152:63, 1989.

188. Sagoh T, et al: Gallbladder carcinoma: evaluation with MR imaging. *Radiology* 174:131-136, 1990.

189. Sarno RC, Carter BL: Computed tomography in Caroli's disease. *Comput Radiol* 7(5):287-290, 1983.

190. Savader SJ, et al: Choledochal cysts: classification and cholangiographic appearance. *AJR* 156:327-331, 1991.

191. Schoenfield LJ: Gallstones and other biliary diseases. *Clin Symp CIBA*, 34(4), 1982.

192. Schoenefield LJ, Gallstones: an update. *Am J Gastroenterol* 84:999, 1987.

193. Schulte SJ, et al: CT of the extrahepatic bile ducts: wall thickness and contrast enhancement in normal and abnormal ducts. *AJR* 154:79-85, 1990.

194. Schulman A: Non-western patterns of biliary stones and the role of ascariasis. *Radiology* 162:425-430, 1987.

195. Semelka RC, et al: Bile duct disease: prospective comparison of ERCP, CT, and fat suppression MRI. *Gastrointest Radiol* 17:347-352, 1992.

196. Shanser JD, et al: Computed tomographic diagnosis of obstructive jaundice in the absence of intrahepatic ductal dilatation. *AJR* 131:389-392, 1978.

197. Shea TE, Pfister RC: Opacification of the gallbladder by urographic contrast media reflection of an alternate excretory pathway. *Am J Roentgenol Radium Ther Nucl Med* 107:763-768, 1969.

198. Smathers RL, Lee JKT, Heiken JP: Differentiation of complicated cholecystitis from gallbladder carcinoma by computed tomography. *AJR* 143:255-259, 1984.

199. So CB, Gibney RG, Swdamore CH: Carcinoma of the gallbladder: a risk associated with the gallbladder-preserving treatments for cholelithiasis, *Radiology* 174, 127-130, 1990.

200. Soderstrom CA, et al: Gallbladder injuries resulting from blunt abdominal trauma. *Ann Surg* 193:60-66, 1981.

201. Solomon A, Kreel L, Pinto D: Contrast computed tomography in the diagnosis of acute cholecystitis. *J Comput Assist Tomogr* 3:585-588, 1979.

202. Somer K, et al: Contrast enhanced computed tomography of the gallbladder in acute pancreatitis. *Gastrointest Radiol* 9:31-34, 1984.

203. Sons HV, Borchard F: Carcinoma of the extrahepatic bile ducts: a postmortem study of 65 cases and review of the literature. *J Surg Oncol* 34:6-12, 1987.

204. Sood GK, et al: Caroli disease: computed tomographic diagnosis. *Gastrointest Radiol* 16:243-244, 1991.

205. Spritzer C, et al: MR imaging of normal extrahepatic bile ducts. *J Comput Assist Tomogr* 11:248, 1987.

206. Strax R, et al: Gallbladder enhancement following angiography: a normal CT finding. *J Comput Assist Tomogr* 6:766-768, 1982.

207. Takayasu K, et al: Hepatic lobar atrophy following obstruction of the ipsilateral portal vein from hilar cholangiocarcinoma. *Radiology* 160:389-393, 1986.

208. Takayasu K, et al: CT of hilar cholangiocarcinoma: late contrast enhancement in six patients. *AJR* 154:1203-1206, 1990.

209. Tani K, et al: MR imaging of the peripheral cholangiocarcinoma. *J Comput Assist Tomogr* 15(6):975-978, 1991.

210. Tartar VM, Balfe DM: Lymphoma in the wall of the bile ducts: radiologic imaging. *Gastrointest Radiol* 15:53-57, 1990.

211. Teefey SA, et al: Sclerosing cholangitis: CT findings. *Radiology* 169:635-639, 1988.

212. Teefey SA, et al: Patterns of intrahepatic bile duct dilatation at CT: correlation with obstructive disease processes. *Radiology* 182:139-142, 1992.

213. Teele RL, Share JC: *Ultrasound of infants and children*, Philadelphia, 1991, WB Saunders Co.

214. Teixidor HS, Godwin TA, Ramirez EA: Cryptosporidiosis of the biliary tract in AIDS, *Radiology* 180:51-56, 1991.

215. Teixidor HS, et al: CMV infection of the alimentary canal: radiologic findings with pathologic correlation. *Radiology* 163:317-323, 1987.

216. Terrier F, et al: Computed tomography in complicated cholecystitis. *J Comput Assist Tomogr* 8:(1):58-62, 1984.

217. Thomas JL, Bernadino ME: Segmental biliary obstruction: its detection and significance. *J Comput Assist Tomogr* 4:155-158, 1980.

218. Thorsen MK, et al: Primary biliary caricinoma: CT evaluation, *Radiology* 152:479-483, 1984.

219. Todani T, et al: Congenital bile duct cysts: its classification, operative procedures, and review of 37 cases including cancer arising from a choledochal cyst. *Am J Surg* 1134:263-273, 1977.

220. Uchida H, et al: Computed tomography of gallstones. *Jpn Clin Exp Med* 62:2411, 1985.

221. Ueda J, Kobayashi Y, Nishida T: Computed tomography evaluation of high-density bile in the gallbladder. *Gastrointest Radiol* 15:22-26, 1990.

222. Ueda J, et al: High density bile in the gallbladder observed by computed tomography. *J Comput Assist Tomogr* 7(5):801-804, 1983.

223. Varma DGK, Faust JM: Computed tomography of gangrenous acute postoperative acalculous cholecystitis. *J Comput Assist Tomogr* 12:29-31, 1988.

224. Vazquez JL, et al: Atrophy of the left hepatic lobe caused by a cholangiocarcinoma. *AJR* 144:547-548, 1985.

225. Vujic I, et al: Computed tomographic demonstration of hemobilia. *J Comput Assist Tomogr* 7:219-222, 1983.

226. Walker AT, et al: Bile duct disruption and biloma after laparoscopic cholecystectomy: imaging evaluation. *AJR* 158:785-789, 1991.

227. Wechsler, RJ, et al: The periportal collar sign: a CT sign of liver transplant rejection. *Radiology* 165:57-60, 1987.

228. Weiner SN, et al: Sonography and computed tomography in the diagnosis of carcinoma of the gallbladder. *AJR* 142:735-739, 1984.

229. Weinstein JB, et al: High resolution CT of the porta hepatis and hepatoduodenal ligament. *Radiographics* 6:55-74, 1986.

230. Weissleder R, et al: Cholecystitis: diagnosis by MR imaging. *Magn Reson Imaging* 6:345, 1988.

231. Whitehouse RW, Martin DF: Contrast-enhanced computed tomography of the normal and abnormal gallbladder. *Br J Radiol* 59:1083-1085, 1986.

232. Wilbur AC, et al: High-field MRI of primary gallbladder carcinoma. *Gastrointest Radiol* 13:142-144, 1988.

233. Wolfe B: Contrast layering in a choledochal cyst: a new CT observation. *J Can Radiol Assoc* 39:51-53, 1988.

234. Yamashita Y, et al: Hilar cholangiocarcinoma: an evaluation of subtype with CT and angiography. *Acta Radiologica* 33(4):351-355, 1992.

235. Yamashita Y, et al: Parenchymal changes of the liver in cholangiocarcinoma: CT evaluation. *Gastrointest Radiol* 17:161-166, 1992.

236. Yeh H: Ultrasonography and computed tomography of carcinoma of the gallbladder. *J Comput Assist Tomogr* 133:167-173, 1979.

237. Yoneda M, et al: Measurement of calcium content of gallstones by computed tomography and the relationship between gallbladder function and calcification of gallstones. *Gastroenterol Jpn* 25(4):478-484, 1990.

238. Yoshida H, et al: Biliary malignancies occurring in choledochal cysts. *Radiology* 173:389, 1989.

239. Zajko AB, et al: Cholangiographic findings in hepatic artery occlusion after liver transplantation. *AJR* 149:485-489, 1987.

240. Zajko AB, et al: Percutaneous transhepatic cholangiography rather than ultrasound as a screening test for post-operative biliary complications in liver transplant patients. *Transplant Proc* 20:678-681, 1988.

241. Zajko AB, et al: Diagnostic and interventional radiology in liver transplantation. *Gastroenterol Clin North Am* 17(1):105-143, 1988.

242. Zajko AB, et al: Mucocele of the cystic duct remnant in eight liver transplant recipients: findings at cholangiography, CT and US. *Radiology* 177, 691-693, 1990.

243. Zeman RK, et al: The clinical and imaging spectrum of pancreaticoduodenal lymph node enlargement. *AJR* 144:1223-1227, 1988.

244. Zirinsky K, et al: The portacaval space: CT with MR correlation. *Radiology* 156:453-460, 1985.

32

The Pancreas

JOHN R. HAAGA

Before the advent of the modern cross-sectional imaging modalities of gray-scale ultrasonography and computed tomography (CT), the pancreas was truly one of the "hidden" organs within the abdomen. With CT, the exact anatomical characteristics of the pancreas and the peripancreatic region can be precisely and consistently visualized. Diagnosis and treatment of pancreatic disease are no longer restricted by the lack of anatomical detail but only by the inherent nature of the disease and the limitations of therapeutic regimens. This chapter discusses the normal anatomical appearance and relationships and pathological conditions of the pancreas as visualized by CT and magnetic resonance imaging (MRI).

CT ANATOMY

The pancreas is an exocrine and endocrine organ measuring approximately 15 cm in length and weighing 60 to 100 g. It is located in the anterior pararenal space of the retroperitoneum, just anterior to the perirenal (Gerota's) fascia and posterior to the parietal peritoneum (Fig. 32-1). Its gross anatomical relationships with the stomach, duodenum, colon, and spleen are fairly constant, but individual variations do occur. The uncinate portion of the pancreas (congenitally the ventral aspect of the pancreas) is in the inferior most portion of the head of the pancreas, just posterior to the superior mesenteric artery and vein (Fig. 32-2, A). The normal uncinate portion is triangular or wedge shaped with the narrow portion beneath the superior mesenteric artery and vein (Fig. 32-2, A). The head of the pancreas is medial and posterior to the bulb of the duodenum, bounded laterally by the second and inferiorly by the third portions of the duodenum (Fig. 32-2, B). The neck of the pancreas is anterior to the superior mesenteric artery and varies in thickness depending on the specific configuration (Fig. 32-2, C, 32-6). The tail and body of the pancreas lie immediately posterior to the fundus and antrum of the stomach (Fig. 32-2, C and D). The omental bursa, or lesser peritoneal sac, is a potential space between the stomach and the pancreas, which is never visualized unless it is filled with fluid. The entrance to this space, Winslow's foramen, is behind the free edge of the lesser omentum or the hepatoduodenal ligament, which contains the portal vein, common bile duct, and hepatic artery (Fig. 32-2, C). The tail of the pancreas is adjacent to the hilum of the spleen, just anterior to the left adrenal gland, upper pole of the left kidney, and medial portion of the spleen. The tail usually tapers gradually in constant plane, but occasionally it may be bulbous or angulated at the end. The tail may also be closely adherent to the left kidney or surrounded by the peritoneum in unusual cases.

Vascular anatomy in the peripancreatic region is also nearly constant and correlates well with vascular anatomy as demonstrated by angiography (Fig. 32-3, A, 32-4). The splenic vessels are intimately associated with the pancreas. The splenic artery lies along the cephalad border of the pancreas and may be relatively straight in young people (see Figs. 32-2, D and 32-5, B) or serpiginous in older patients (see Figs. 32-4, C, and 32-6, C). The splenic vein runs posterior from the hilum to the spleen along the posterior side of the pancreas and becomes confluent with the superior mesenteric vein to become the portal vein just anterior to the vena cava (see Figs. 32-4, B, and 32-6, B and C). The inferior mesenteric vein runs in the free edge of Treitz's ligament and joins the superior mesenteric and splenic veins at the fourth portion of the duodenum. At the uncinate portion of the pancreas, the superior mesenteric vein is to the right of the superior mesenteric artery, and both are anterior to the medial edge of the uncinate process (Figs. 32-4, A, 32-5, A, and 32-6, A). At the upper portion of the head of the pancreas, the superior mesenteric artery is posterior to the neck of the pancreas. A number of arteries, including the hepatic, gastroduodenal, and pancreaticoduodenal arteries, can be visualized when an adequate intravenous contrast agent is given appropriately by mechanical injection. Calcifications occur commonly in the splenic artery and others and should not be mistaken for pancreatic calcifications.

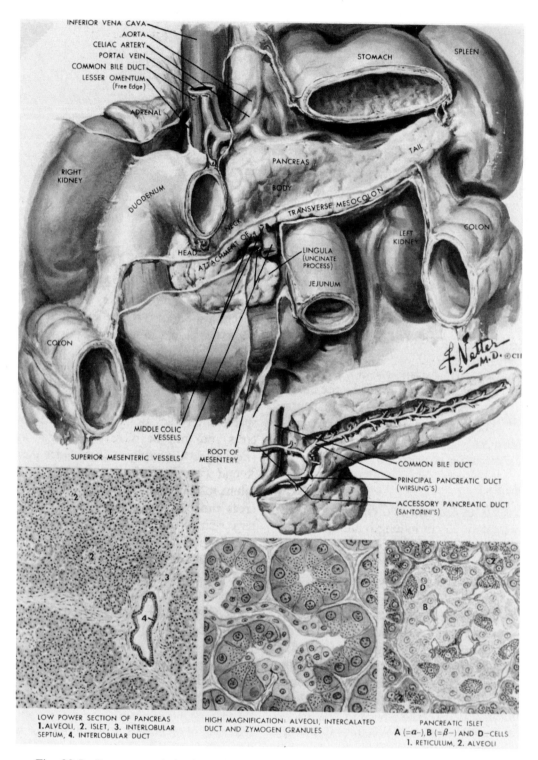

Fig. 32-1. Gross anatomical relationships of the pancreas. (From Netter F: *Atlas of human anatomy,* Summit, NJ, 1989, Ciba Geigy.)

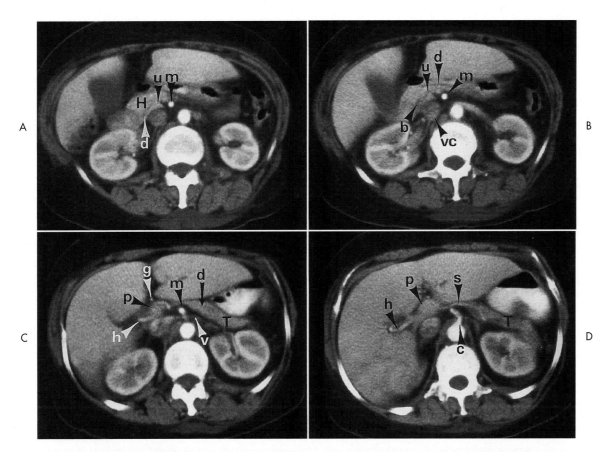

Fig. 32-2. Normal pancreas with appropriate intravenous contrast enhancement. **A,** The head portion *(H)* of the gland is seen adjacent to the superior mesenteric vein *(u)* and the superior mesenteric artery *(m).* The terminal portion of the minor duct *(d)* is seen adjacent to the ampulla. **B,** The normal pancreatic duct *(d)* is better visualized in the neck portion of the normal gland. The superior mesenteric artery *(m),* vena cava *(vc),* bile duct *(b),* and superior mesenteric vein *(u)* are noted. **C,** Normal enhancing body and tail *(T)* of the gland are seen. The superior mesenteric artery *(m),* gastroduodenal artery *(g),* hepatic artery *(h),* portal vein *(p),* and left renal vein *(v)* are visualized because of the contrast filling. The normal duct *(d)* can be seen in the middle of the normally enhancing gland but is faint because of the small size of the tapering duct. **D,** The tail *(T)* is located anterior to the kidney. The opacified celiac artery *(c),* splenic artery *(s),* portal vein *(p),* and hepatic artery *(h)* are seen.

The configuration of the pancreas may vary. There are several basic shapes; perhaps the most common is the gradually tapered pancreas in which the head is larger than either the body or tail (see Fig. 32-2, *A* and *C*). The narrowest portion is the neck, just anterior to the superior mesenteric artery. Another common variant is a dumbbell-shaped pancreas, which has a larger head and tail and a narrow neck immediately anterior to the superior mesenteric artery (see Fig. 32-6, *C*). The tail of the pancreas may vary in its appearance, with the end being bulbous, angled, or especially close to the left kidney (Fig. 32-7). In some patients, in whom the peritoneal spaces have developed abnormally in utero, the splenic flexure of the colon may actually be posterior to the pancreas and within the hilum of the spleen; in such cases, the pancreatic tail and the spleen are partially peritonealized.

One should be familiar with these various configurations because pathological processes may on occasion mimic them, and the only clue may be disproportion in the different portions of the gland. With the most common tapering configuration, there should be a gentle decrease in the size of the gland as one moves from the head to the tail. A pathological process may cause the head to be normal and the rest to be atrophied (see later sections). If a dumbbell-shaped gland is present, the size

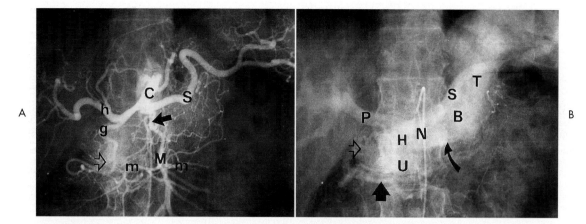

Fig. 32-3. A, Angiogram shows the major arterial vessels in the area of the pancreas. From the celiac artery *(C)* comes the splenic artery *(S)* and the common hepatic artery, which branches into the proper hepatic *(h)* and the gastroduodenal *(g)* arteries. The pancreatic magna *(arrow)* and the branches of the pancreaticoduodenal arteries *(open arrow)* are seen. Overflow from the injection into the celiac artery produces opacification of the superior mesenteric artery *(M)*, which supplies the middle colic branches *(m)* of the mesocolon and colon. **B,** Capillary and venous phase of the study shows the pancreas and veins. The major portion of the gland includes the uncinate process *(U)*, head *(H)*, neck *(N)*, body *(B)*, and tail *(T)*. The splenic *(S)* and the portal *(P)* veins are adjacent to the cephalad surface of the gland. Venous drainage of the gland includes the small pancreatic parenchymal veins *(curved arrow)*, network of inferior pancreaticoduodenal *(solid arrow)*, and superior pancreaticoduodenal veins *(open arrows)*.

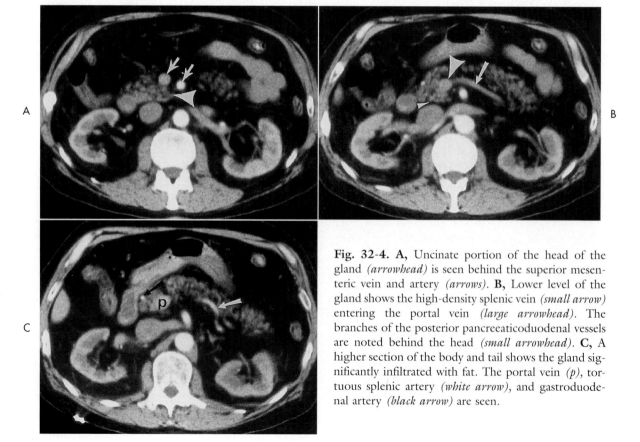

Fig. 32-4. A, Uncinate portion of the head of the gland *(arrowhead)* is seen behind the superior mesenteric vein and artery *(arrows)*. **B,** Lower level of the gland shows the high-density splenic vein *(small arrow)* entering the portal vein *(large arrowhead)*. The branches of the posterior pancreeaticoduodenal vessels are noted behind the head *(small arrowhead)*. **C,** A higher section of the body and tail shows the gland significantly infiltrated with fat. The portal vein *(p)*, tortuous splenic artery *(white arrow)*, and gastroduodenal artery *(black arrow)* are seen.

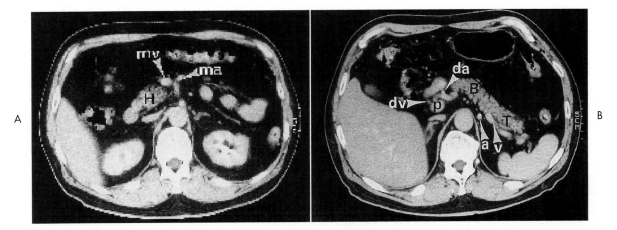

Fig. 32-5. A, In the region of the head *(H)*, the superior mesenteric vein *(mv)* and superior mesenteric artery *(ma)* are seen. **B,** The texture of the gland is varied with fat being interspersed among the margins of the gland. The pancreaticoduodenal artery *(da)*, pancreaticoduodenal vein *(dv)*, portal vein *(p)*, splenic artery *(a)*, and splenic vein *(v)* are noted around the body *(B)* and tail *(T)* of the gland. The splenic artery is almost always tortuous, so only circular cross-sectional portions are usually seen.

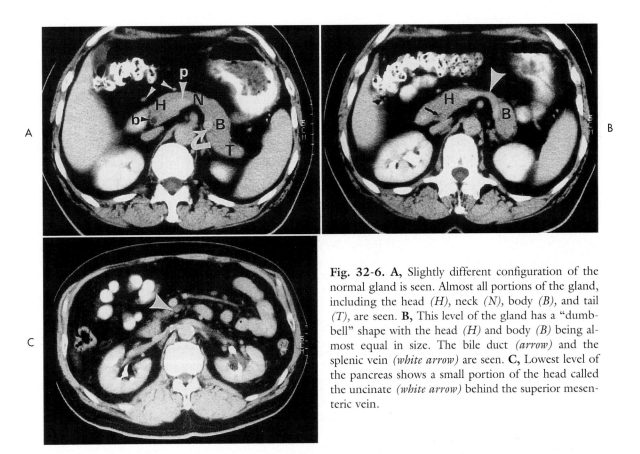

Fig. 32-6. A, Slightly different configuration of the normal gland is seen. Almost all portions of the gland, including the head *(H)*, neck *(N)*, body *(B)*, and tail *(T)*, are seen. **B,** This level of the gland has a "dumbbell" shape with the head *(H)* and body *(B)* being almost equal in size. The bile duct *(arrow)* and the splenic vein *(white arrow)* are seen. **C,** Lowest level of the pancreas shows a small portion of the head called the uncinate *(white arrow)* behind the superior mesenteric vein.

of both ends should be about equal. If the head or body is larger than the other, a pathological process should be considered.

The size of the normal pancreas may be measured several ways.[33,49] An average size or a range of sizes in the different regions of the pancreas can be used. The best anteroposterior measurements of the normal gland were made by Kreel and Sandin[128] as follows: head, 23

(+3) mm; neck, 19 (+2.5) mm; body, 20 (+3) mm; and tail, 15 (+2.5) mm. These measurements with CT differ from those with ultrasound because ultrasound is typically better for visualization of the splenic vein and artery, and so accordingly the ultrasound measurements tend to be smaller. The most accurate and noteworthy study of pancreatic size was performed by Muranaka and colleagues,[169] who studied the anteroposterior diameter of the head and body in various age groups (Fig. 32-8). He reconfirmed the observations by others that the size of the gland decreases with age, but the ratio of the head to the body remains almost constant.

Little attention has been given to the craniocaudad measurement of the gland until the description of pancreatic divisum, as described later. The first to measure the maximal craniocaudad dimension were Pochammer and associates.[188] They found that the mean length in women was 5.9 cm, with a range of 4.2 to 7.8 cm; the mean length in men was 6.2 cm, with a range of 4.8 to 7.6 cm. These measurements were made from older scanning devices, so the upper value limits are probably greater than they should be; more recent measurements have been made in conjunction with diagnosis of pancreatic divisum (see later section).

The main pancreatic duct—Wirsung's duct—runs the length of the pancreas and joins the common bile

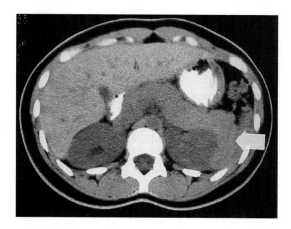

Fig. 32-7. Variation of the tail *(arrow)* may be slightly bulbous and almost wraps around the kidney.

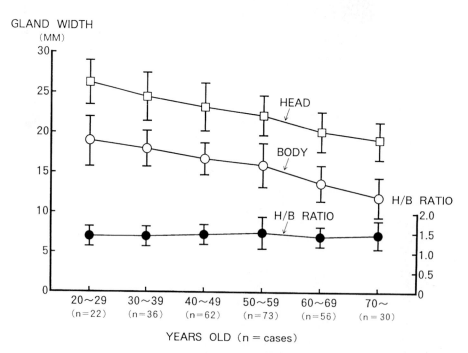

Fig. 32-8. Anteroposterior width of the pancreas and the head-to-body ratio (H/B ratio) in normal subjects. The head width was 22.4 ± 3.0 mm (mean ± SD). The body width was 15.8 ± 2.9 mm. The H/B ratio was 1.45 ± 0.03. (Data from Muranaka T, et al: Computed tomography and histologic appearance of pancreatic metastases from distant sources. *Acta Radiol* 30:615-619, 1989.)

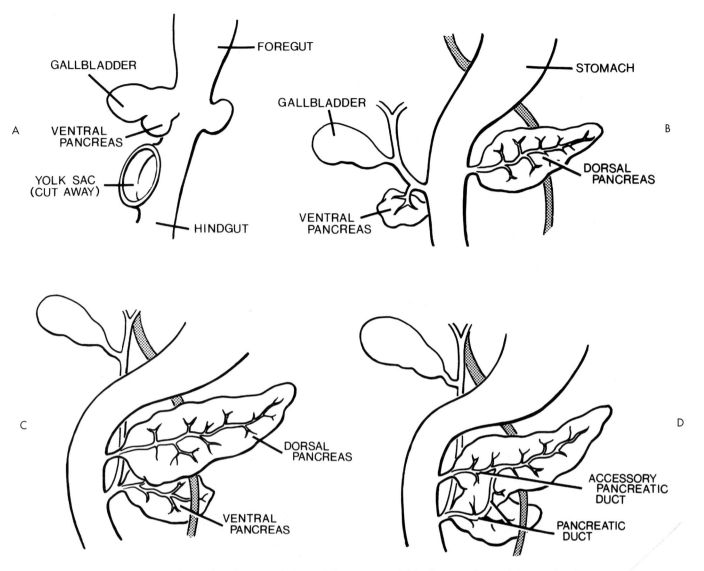

Fig. 32-9. A, Embryologic evolution of the pancreas. This diagram shows the ventral and dorsal bud of the pancreas forming off of the primitive gut. **B,** Dorsal and ventral pancreas evolves from the pancreatic buds. **C,** Without fusion of the dorsal and ventral pancreas, pancreatic divisum develops. **D,** Normal fusion of the gland should result in atrophy of the accessory duct to the duodenum with maintenance of main duct patency.

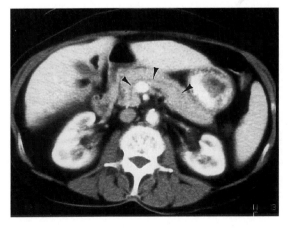

Fig. 32-10. Normal pancreactic duct seen within the normally enhanced gland. Note that because 8 mm sections were used, almost the entire length of the duct can be seen *(arrowheads).*

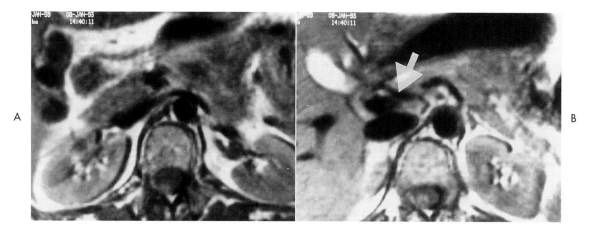

Fig. 32-11. A, MRI scan spin density, TR 2000/20, SE 2-90. Scan taken at the level of the head of the pancreas shows intermediate intensity pancreatic tissue. Superior mesenteric artery and vein are low signal. **B,** MRI scan spin density image at higher level. The neck (body) and tail of gland in front of the splenic vein can be seen. The hepatoduodenal ligament containing the portal vein, hepatic artery, and common duct *(arrow)* is low intensity.

duct at Vater's ampulla. The accessory pancreatic duct—Santorini's duct—is in the upper portion of the pancreas and is more horizontal than Wirsung's duct (Figs. 32-9 and 32-10). The common bile duct travels with the portal vein and hepatic artery in the edge of the lesser omentum or the hepatoduodenal ligament. The common bile duct appears as a low-density structure in the posterior portion of the head of the pancreas (see Figs. 32-2, *B* and 32-6, *B*). It and the normal pancreatic duct are seen during rapid injection of intravenous contrast material as described in the technique section. Although both of these are commonly visualized, their clear delineation is also variable.

The density or attenuation of the pancreas is normally the same as soft tissue, or somewhere between 30 and 50 HU, depending on whether contrast material has been administered. The normal pancreas increases in density after intravenous administration of urographic contrast material; the more rapid the administration (i.e., dynamic), the denser the enhancement.[127,151] If a bolus injection is administered, normal enhancement can be visualized during an arterial, capillary, and venous phase. This enhancement of the normal gland has become an important differential sign for excluding the presence of necrosis in pancreatitis (see later section on necrosing pancreatitis). The margin of the pancreas may be smooth (see Fig. 32-6, *C*) or somewhat irregular (see Fig. 32-4, *C*). In the normal gland, variable normal fat tissue may be present, either interspersed along the margin of the gland or within the glandular portions. The entire pancreas may be replaced by fat, and the patient may not have any clinical symptoms. Some pathological conditions, however, do produce infiltration of fat when atrophy of the gland occurs, such as cystic fibrosis.

The position of the pancreas may vary. In most patients, the head is more caudad than the tail, and the tail is located adjacent to the hilum of the spleen. In some patients, the head and tail may be more horizontal and below the spleen, and in others, the tip of the tail may be high. In postnephrectomy cases or with agenesis of the kidney, the appropriate portion of the gland moves posteriorly to fill in partially the space vacated by the kidney. One should not mistake the soft tissue density of the retropositioned pancreas for recurrent tumor.

Pancreatic vessels and lymphatic drainage

The vascular anatomy of the pancreas consists of arteries originating from the celiac and superior mesenteric arteries and veins that drain into the tributaries of the superior mesenteric and portal veins (see Figs. 32-2 and 32-3). The main arteries, consisting of the dorsal pancreatic, great pancreatic, transverse pancreatic, and pancreaticoduodenal branches, are almost always present, but the origin, size, and type of collateral supply may vary. The draining veins are also constant in that they parallel the arteries and they drain into the pancreaticoduodenal, superior mesenteric, splenic, or portal veins. Small circular structures representing these vessels may be seen in and around the pancreas, but specific identification may be difficult. When pathological occlusion of any of these vessels occurs, collateral vessels may open and become visible. A vein that has been reported to do this consistently is the posterior pancreaticoduodenal vein, as noted later.

The lymphatic drainage of the pancreas parallels the venous drainage. Small lymph nodes around vessels and in the various ligaments are commonly seen, but if nodes are 10 mm or larger, one should be suspicious of neoplasm.

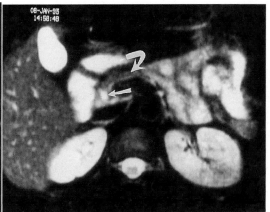

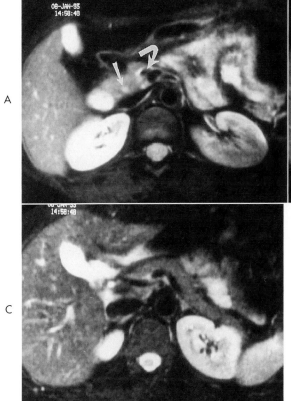

Fig. 32-12. A, MRI scan FSSE TR 2177/45 (with intermediate T2 signal). Intermediate signal glandular tissue is noted in the head. The common bile duct is high signal (arrow), and the superior mesenteric vessels are low signal (curved arrow). B, MRI scan same sequence, at level of the neck. Pancreatic duct (curved arrow) is seen in the neck, and the common bile duct (arrow) is seen in the head. C, MRI scan shows normal neck, body, and tail of the pancreas with intermediate intensity. The splenic vein, hepatic artery, and portal vein are seen as low signal.

NORMAL MRI OF THE PANCREAS

The appearance of the normal gland on MRI depends partially on the specific pulsing sequence used, but the overall configuration and intensity appearances are consistent. As one can note in Figs. 32-11 and 32-12, the gland, with its uniform texture and the adjacent blood vessels, is easily appreciated. The relationship of the splenic vessels, gastroduodenal vessels, common bile duct, and other structures is consistent. When there is less than optimal signal characteristics or motion artifacts, the best approach is to identify the location of the splenic vein and then extrapolate from that structure. Considering the many pulsing sequences that are now available, it is not possible to perform all pulsing sequences on all patients. The best two sequences that I have found are the standard spin-echo T1-weighted images, which give good anatomical detail with relatively high signal intensity. A variety of breathholding "flash" images are now available which minimize patient motion (see section on MRI Technique).

EMBRYOLOGY AND CONGENITAL VARIANTS

Although the embryology of many organs is well known to most physicians, knowledge of pancreatic development is less prevalent. In the early stages of the embryo, there is a dorsal and ventral pancreas, which are lo-
cated on opposite sides of the gut. When the rotation of the bowel occurs, the dorsal and ventral pancreas fuse into a single gland. The dorsal portion becomes the body and tail, and the ventral portion becomes the head and uncinate portion of the gland (see Figs. 32-9 and 32-10).

As one might anticipate, the outcome of these complex events is variable, and the final form of the gland has a wide spectrum of variation, including a prominence of the head in the approximate area of the fusion, agenesis of the dorsal or ventral portion, annular pancreas, pancreatic divisum, and left side of pancreas.[76] Furthermore, this embryologic information explains the wide variation in the ductal system.[152]

Ductal variations

Before the refinements of CT, discussion of ductal anatomy and variation was not relevant. With the current high-resolution systems and spiral scanning systems, one should be aware of possible variations because of the consistent visualization of the ductal systems during normal and pathological states. The main pancreatic duct in the dorsal pancreas combines with the ventral component to form the main duct, Wirsung's duct, which enters through the main papilla and ampulla of Vater. In most instances, the minor duct, Santorini's duct, becomes atretic. If the accessory Santorini's duct stays patent, it enters by means of the minor papilla.

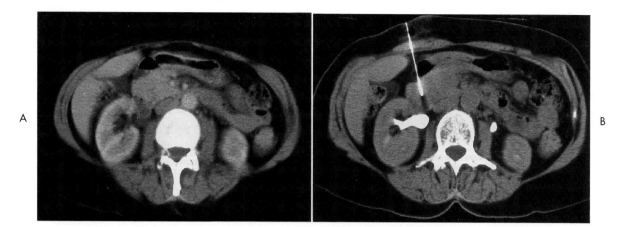

A B

Fig. 32-13. A, Unusually prominent head was suggested to be a neoplasm at another institution. Note the uniform pancreatogram with normal enhancement and density. **B,** At the insistence of the patient and clinical physician, a careful aspiration biopsy was performed. Normal cells were obtained.

Prominent fusion anomaly

One permutation of the variable anatomy is a prominent head of the pancreas at the junction point between the head and neck of the gland, close to the main portal vein (Fig. 32-13). The contour of the gland may be so prominent that there may be a concern about an early neoplasm. Fortunately, with experience one can learn to identify this normal variant by carefully noting the density resulting from intravenous contrast enhancement and the appearance of the uncinate portion of the gland. With contrast enhancement, the density of the normal head is increased in a comparable amount compared with the adjacent gland. Virtually all nonislet cell tumors are hypovascular and show a lower density than normal, whereas most islet cell tumors are hypervascular and show an increase in density. Notwithstanding this information, occasions may arise when the clinical suspicion is so high that percutaneous biopsy might be performed (see Chapter 46).

Pancreatic divisum

One of the most common anomalies is pancreatic divisum, the nonfusion of the dorsal and ventral ductal system. Frequency by autopsy studies is reported between 4% and 14%, whereas endoscopic retrograde cholangiopancreatography (ERCP) confirmation of this entity is stated to be between 1% and 7%. Normally during the 8 weeks of embryological life, fusion of the ductal bud occurs to form the adult system. When such fusion does not occur, two separate entry points through the major and minor papilla form, which are the exclusive ductal paths from the dorsal and ventral gland.

The mere presence of this problem is not in itself significant, but such patients are considered at risk for

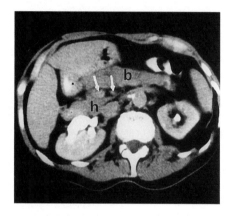

Fig. 32-14. Pancreatic divisum, which shows a fat cleft separating the head *(h)* from the body *(b)*. The superior mesenteric vessels *(arrows)* are noted within the cleft. This appearance was seen on all sections through the gland.

pancreatitis in the dorsal portion because of frequent narrowing of the duct at the papilla. Such pancreatitis is recurring unless corrective action is taken to eliminate the narrowing.

Diagnosis of this entity is best made by ERCP, but CT findings may suggest the correct diagnosis.[142,215,216] Two findings appear to be consistent among the various articles reporting on this topic: the increase in the cephalad caudad length and the occasional presence of a fat cleft separating the dorsal and ventral elements. Soulen and others[215,216] reported a size variation of the pancreas in a group of 12 patients with pancreatic divisum. They noted an increase in both the anteroposterior and the craniocaudad dimension; in the anteroposterior size, they noted a measurement of 3.2 cm compared with 2.7 cm for normals and in the craniocaudad size a

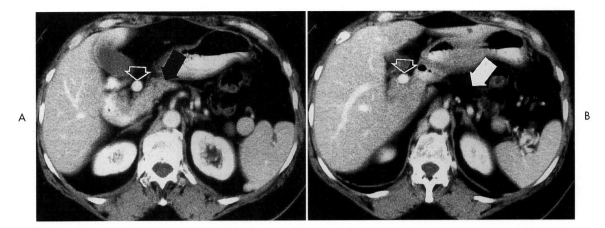

Fig. 32-15. A, Congenitally short pancreas or agenesis of dorsal gland. This level shows the head of the gland *(arrow)* behind the stomach. Note the preduodenal portal vein *(open arrow)*. **B,** A higher section through the gland shows absence of the gland in the body and tail *(white arrow)*. The preduodenal portal vein *(open arrow)* is again seen.

measurement of 5.4 cm in pancreatic divisum compared with 4.4 cm in the normal gland. Lindstrom and Ihse[142] found that the cephalad caudad length of the pancreatic head was 40% longer in patients with pancreatic divisum than in normal patients. They found that the anteroposterior dimensions and the total volume of the gland did not vary between the two groups. Zeman and colleagues[250] reported the occasional presence of the fat cleft separating the two segments (Fig. 32-14). An associated finding that is not specific is that the dorsal duct was visualized in a high percentage of cases, which incidentally was said to be normal; the ventral duct was infrequently seen.

With the occurrence of pancreatitis, secondary changes in the gland, such as focal enlargement, irregularity of the margins, and calcifications, can occur. These have been noted in the reports on pancreatic divisum and have been recognized as sequelae of the inflammation rather than primary findings of the problem. One author believed that the increased anteroposterior size noted by Soulen and others[215,216] might have been due to inflammation. Gold and coworkers[71] reported a case of pseudocyst associated with pancreatic divisum.

Annular pancreas

When rotation of the embryological analogues does not occur and fusion takes place, an annular pancreas results.[173] In such cases, the CT appearance suggests a mass in the head of the pancreas. Although most case reports have described these as false-positive cases for tumors, the prospective diagnosis should be possible with an adequate contrast enhancement, correlative studies, and clinical information.

Agenesis of the gland or short pancreas

Several case reports showing agenesis of the dorsal pancreas have been published under the topic of congenital short pancreas.[84,91] In these cases, the head of the pancreas is in a normal location, but the body and tail of the pancreas distal to the neck is absent (Fig. 32-15). With congenitally short pancreas, there is a high association with polysplenia and other gastrointestinal anomalies, such as partial situs inversus, common mesentery with or without malrotation, preduodenal portal vein, lobulation of the liver, agenesis of the gallbladder, biliary atresia, and absent omentum. The reported pancreatic anomalies associated with this include intraperitoneal location and annular shape. There has been a single case report of a carcinoma in such a case.

Ectopic pancreas

The most common sites for ectopic pancreatic tissue are the esophagus, stomach, duodenum, jejunum, and Meckel's diverticulum. Ectopic tissue can produce a mass in such areas if the primordial ductal system and acinar elements produce and retain excretions.

Other variants

In some other variants, the configuration of the gland varies or confusion arises because of embryological or pathological changes that occur in the adjacent structures (Figs. 32-16 and 32-17). Several problems occur that are associated with anomalous rotation of the bowel and formation of the peritoneum. The splenic flexure may reside between the tail of the pancreas and the spleen, with an associated abnormal contour and size (Fig. 32-18). When malrotation of the duodenum occurs, the third portion of the duodenum does not cross

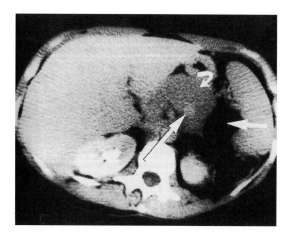

Fig. 32-16. Patients with fusion anomalies of the peritoneum can have the colon *(short arrow)* interposed between the spleen and pancreas. The gland *(curved arrow)* is anterior to the splenic vein *(long arrow)*. Note the normal enhancement of the portal vein *(long arrow)* and the normal parenchyma.

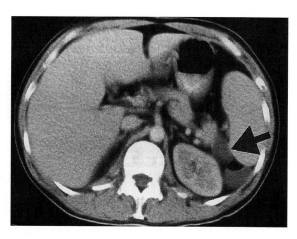

Fig. 32-18. Variant of normal related to incomplete rotation of bowel and fusion of the peritoneum. Note the splenic flexure of colon behind the spleen adjacent to the tail of the gland *(arrow)*.

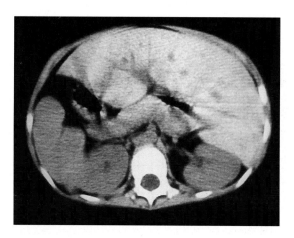

Fig. 32-17. Situs inversus with complete reversal of the abdominal anatomy.

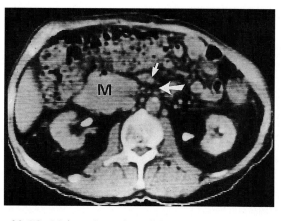

Fig. 32-19. Malrotation of small bowel produces a pseudomass *(M)* because of the unusual position of the duodenum. Note that the duodenum cannot be seen in the space *(large arrow)* behind the mesenteric vessel *(small arrow)*, where it should be crossing from right to left.

beneath the superior mesenteric artery and vein (Fig. 32-19). Other authors[174] have stated that a reversal of the position of the superior mesenteric vein and artery helps diagnose this entity (our cases did not show this finding). There has been a single case report[208] of a torsion of the tail of the pancreas, which probably occurred as a result of abnormal fusion of the peritoneum and retroperitoneum (Fig. 32-20).

Several unusual problems can produce the findings of a spurious mass.[171] In patients with severe scoliosis, the acute angulation of the body can distort the gland so its anteroposterior dimension may be increased because of "buckling." A spurious mass can also be pro-

duced by an enlarged caudate lobe of the liver (Fig. 32-21), accessory spleen (Fig. 32-22), fluid-filled diverticulum, or a benign lymph node enlargement.

CT AND MRI INDICATIONS

Considering the extensive experience and clinical track record of CT and the exciting new images available with MRI systems, it is worthwhile to define the current roles of these imaging systems for evaluation of the pancreas. It is quite apparent from the literature that remarkable strides are being made constantly with both MRI and CT, so any statement of current indications must be qualified with a caveat. One must continue to

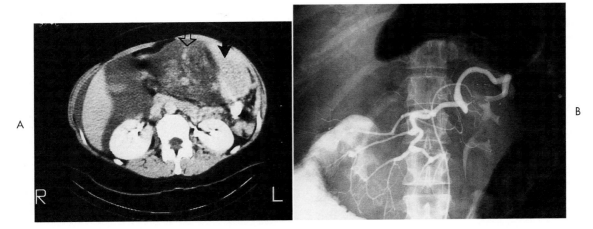

Fig. 32-20. A, Large mass in the midabdomen *(open arrow)* that is adjacent to the spleen *(arrow)*. The mass was the edematous tail of the pancreas from torsion of the gland. **B,** Angiogram shows a circular configuration of the splenic artery and a cutoff at the end. (From Sheflin J, Lee CM, Kretchmar KA: Torsion of wandering spleen and distal pancreas. *AJR* 142:100; copyright by American Roentgen Ray Society, 1984.)

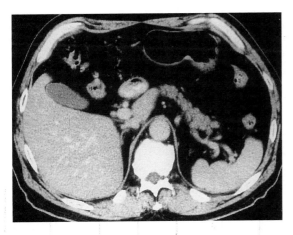

Fig. 32-21. This image shows the slightly higher density spurious "mass" in the head of the gland. This is the caudate lobe of the liver projecting down and effacing the normal gland.

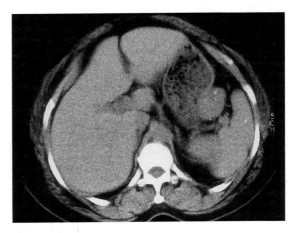

Fig. 32-22. Accessory spleen adjacent to stomach, simulating a pancreatic mass. There are small calcified granulomas in the spleen and the accessory spleen, which suggest the diagnosis.

read the literature because technology is producing remarkable progress in all aspects of imaging.

At the onset, it is important to note that CT and MRI have proved themselves equivalent in most areas of the abdomen and chest, whereas MRI is clearly superior for neurological and musculoskeletal areas. At the same time, there are certain body areas, such as the pancreas, for which MRI has not yet had significant impact. Although several authors have asserted that MRI is equivalent and perhaps slightly better than CT, most authors have not been so enthusiastic. Computerized ultrasound with gray scale combined Doppler and CT have remained the mainstay of pancreatic diagnosis. MRI, at

least in its current state of development, serves as a problem-solving tool. Ultrasound is the choice for screening or initial evaluation of the pancreas, CT is the gold standard for definitive evaluation of the pancreas, and MRI is as the problem-solving device.

GENERAL CT TECHNIQUE

The technique for examination of the pancreas is straightforward, but it may vary depending on some unusual circumstances, anatomy, and the information sought. Most commonly the patient is examined in the supine position and administered a large amount of intravenous contrast material.

Assuming that one has a modern high-speed scanner, the injection should be made through a moderate-sized needle with rapid injection rate. In most centers, a loading dose of 25 to 55 ml is given acutely and followed by an infusion rate of 1 to 1.5 ml/second to a maximal accumulated dose of 150 to 200 ml. The amount of contrast material given must be varied according to the patient's clinical and renal status. Using modern equipment with either cluster or spiral scanning, the pancreatic area is scanned during the course of several minutes. If one does not have the luxury of a high-speed scanner, the contrast material should be given with a 50-ml loading dose followed by a constant infusion during the entire time period of the scan; administration rates may need to be adjusted according to the scanning time. Appropriate amounts of intravenous contrast material are important to provide enhancement, which highlights and distinguishes tumors, vascular or avascular, and blood vessels, whether they are normal, neovascular, collaterals, or aneurysmal.[121]

In our laboratory, most examinations are performed with the following technical parameters. Because most of the studies are performed during the course of a general examination, the scan slices are typically contiguous 8 mm slices or spiral scans, over the entire upper abdomen. In special cases, if one is aware of pancreatic pathology and one wishes to optimize visualization of the pancreatic duct, thin section of 4 or 2 mm may be used. One should be aware of two shortcomings with these techniques, related to contrast material and radiation dosage. Because the thin sections require more time to cover the anatomy, the rate of contrast administration needs to be changed. Furthermore, because more x-ray output is required to make the images acceptable, the patient receives a higher radiation exposure.

It is also important to administer oral contrast material for opacification of the duodenum and the bowel. Although iodinated materials can be given, they are less palatable, and they stimulate peristalsis, which can produce a large number of artifacts. Dilute barium solutions are better accepted because of the pleasant taste, and they seldom produce artifacts. With slow scanning devices or with iodinated oral contrast material, one should be careful to distinguish the contrast from pancreatic calcification, so as not to miss or overcall calcifications.

On occasion even with modern scanners, portions of the pancreatic tail or head may be difficult to visualize if there is a paucity of fat in the retroperitoneum in front of the gland with the patient in a supine position. In such cases, examining the patient in the decubitus position after the ingestion of oral contrast material is helpful (Fig. 32-23). This particular technique is valuable because it eliminates three troublesome false-positive possibilities: (1) With contrast material gravitating into the antrum of the stomach and duodenum,[79,118,172] those structures can not be confused for masses in the head of the pancreas; (2) air in the fundus of the stomach eliminates the pseudomass that can be produced by the partial volume effect of the fluid-filled stomach fundus; and (3) the jejunum moves away from the body and tail of the pancreas, eliminating another pseudomass.

Scanning parameters

There are a number of scanning parameters that should be considered, which include the scanning matrix, slice thickness, field of view, reconstruction algorithms, and radiation dosage.

With advances in CT scanners and computers, the discussion of matrix size is no longer a germane factor.

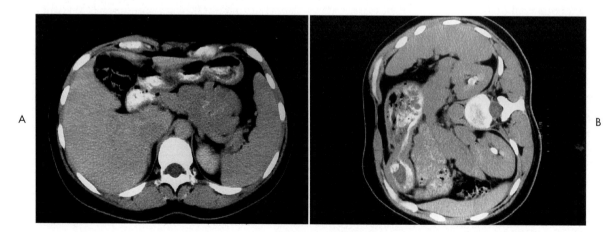

Fig. 32-23. A, Scan performed in the supine position shows a questionable mass in the body of the pancreas. **B,** Scan performed in the decubitus shows a normal body and tail of the gland.

All current scanning devices have available 512×512 pixel images, which provide excellent image quality. Even with these sophisticated scanners, one can improve the spatial resolution by using a smaller field of view, which uses all of the pixels for the smaller amount of anatomy. This provides more imaging pixels per distance of the anatomy and a larger image, which improves the perceived anatomical detail.

Another method of improving spatial resolution is to reduce the slice thickness. Considering that the configuration of the imaging pixel is a long, small rectangle (see Chapter 2), one can understand that if a structure being examined is less than the length of the pixel, it must be averaged within the overall pixel, thereby reducing its visibility. Stated differently from a clinical perspective, decreasing the slice thickness maximizes the visualization of small details that are less than 1 cm in the longitudinal axis. Therefore, if one wishes to identify the normal pancreatic duct reliably, a thinner slice thickness is helpful. If sagittal and coronal reconstructions are desired,[59] one must use thin sections to collect the information if suitable reconstructions are to be made; otherwise the images appear quite "coarse." There are several negative factors related to such thin sections, including increased scanning time and radiation dose to the patient. The increased scanning time is simply related to the fact that more slices must be taken to cover a given anatomical areas. The increased dosage results from the fact that if a thin section is taken without a corresponding increase in radiation photons, the resulting image is grainy and mottled; technical compensation is made by increasing the dose of the thin sections, thereby increasing the overall dosage (see Chapter 2).

Choice of reconstruction algorithms is actually simplified with the newer scanners because the equipment is so refined and resolution is so good that there are essentially no perceptible differences when the pancreas is being scanned (Fig. 32-24). In our example, normal, high, and super-high resolution algorithms were used on the Somatom Plus with little change in quality of the images. Although considerable progress has been made in many other technical areas related to CT, in my opinion, less progress has been made with radiation dose. Little progress has been made in regards to adjusting the radiation dosage appropriately for various sizes of patients. In our previous work, we had noted that diagnostically satisfactory scans were possible in small patients with a reduced dosage and that larger doses were necessary to obtain good quality scans in large patients. It would seem logical that commercial vendors would be more receptive to making devices that would permit adjustable doses either automatically (why not photo-timed

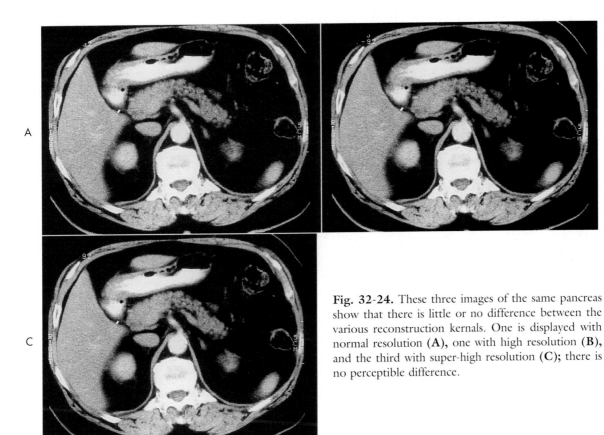

Fig. 32-24. These three images of the same pancreas show that there is little or no difference between the various reconstruction kernals. One is displayed with normal resolution (**A**), one with high resolution (**B**), and the third with super-high resolution (**C**); there is no perceptible difference.

CT scans?) or manually to minimize the dosage risk to small patients and to ensure good quality scans in large patients.

MRI TECHNIQUE

As for many other organ areas, MRI pulsing and scanning techniques for the pancreas vary significantly among the many groups who are reporting in the literature. Most scanning sequences have been spin-echo sequences with T1-weighted (approximately SE 250-400/14-20) and T2-weighted (approximately SE 2000/100) signals, but more recently breath-holding flash images have been reported (130/4.5. 80-degree flip angle). Although the earlier sequences are somewhat slow, the more recent sequences can acquire 14 images during a 19-second breath hold. Furthermore, paramagnetic contrast agents have come into common usage, and injection of gadolinum and oral contrast material is probably advisable for better delineation of the bowel and to show normal vascular enhancement of the pancreatic tissue and the vessels (similar to CT). Another sequence that I believe has considerable merit is the fat saturation spin echo.

The faster breath-hold types of imaging have been developed to reduce the acquisition time and thereby improve the quality of the images. These imaging methods have different commercial brand names, such as FLASH, GRASS, FISP, and FAST. These methods have improved the quality of the images so they may be more useful. Because development of these pulsing sequences is on-

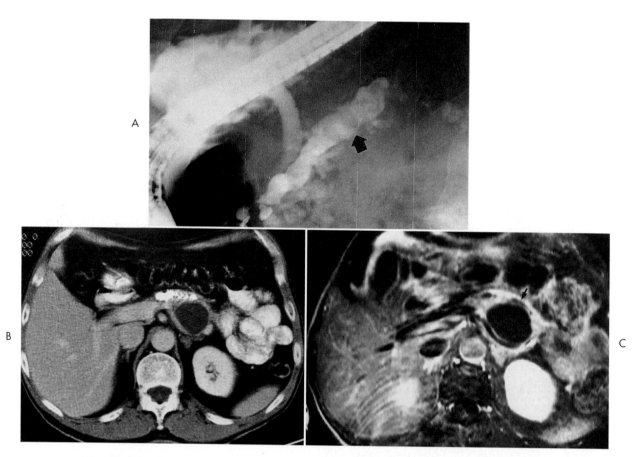

Fig. 32-25. Chronic pancreatitis with pseudocysts on **(A)** ERCP, **(B)** contrast-enhanced 5 mm CT, and **(C)** gadolinium-enhanced FSEE (500/15) images. A, ERCP shows dilatation of the pancreatic duct *(arrow)* with calcifications throughout the pancreas. No communication between the duct and pseudocyst is shown. B, CT image shows extensive calcification along the wall of the pancreatic duct and clearly shows the pseudocyst arising from the posterior aspect of the body of the pancreas. C, MRI clearly shows that the pancreatic duct *(arrow)* is anterior to the pseudocyst. Dilated duct and calcification could not be clearly distinguished. (From Semelka et al: RC, Pancreatic disease: prospective comparison of CT, ERCP, and 1.5-T MR imaging with dynamic gadolinium enhancement and fat suppression. *Radiology* 181:785, 1991.)

going and equipment dependent, consultation with the technical support groups of the major vendors is recommended.

PANCREATIC PATHOLOGY DETECTED BY MRI

Because MRI has had only a limited role in the evaluation of the pancreas, the use of MRI is explained in this small section at the beginning of the chapter. There is only limited data about MRI[203,206,213,225] and the various disease processes of the pancreas. Any attempt to interweave the MRI information with the CT information would seem somewhat artificial because the data about CT are so massive by comparison. Combining the MRI data in this short segment actually improves the comprehension of the advantages and disadvantages of MRI.

There are several obvious general advantages of MRI, which are also pertinent in the pancreas. MRI does not use ionizing radiation, and associated ill effects are eliminated.[206] The contrast resolution of soft tissue is remarkable and potentially can show subtle changes based on edema and relaxation times.

The disadvantages of MRI are several. First, the cost of MRI compared with CT is expensive because of the high technical cost. With the current trends of limiting health care cost, the cost issue must be critically examined. For those disease processes that can be equivalently diagnosed by CT, it is unlikely that MRI will become the primary diagnostic tool. From a more personal perspective, it is likely that if government agencies intend to limit the use of expensive technologies, the professional reimbursement will be more adversely affected by MRI. The second disadvantage of MRI is that for the pancreas, the image quality is not as consistent as with CT. Although it is true that under optimal circumstances, MRI images are equivalent to CT images, routine scans are not yet as consistently equal to CT images. Production of high-quality images is operator and equipment dependent. In many instances, substantial physician time is required to obtain optimal scans. Probably the most concrete example to validate this point is the continued development and publication of different pulsing sequences to address these issues.

Pancreatitis

Imaging of acute pancreatitis is possible with the newer sequences. Several authors, most recently Semelka

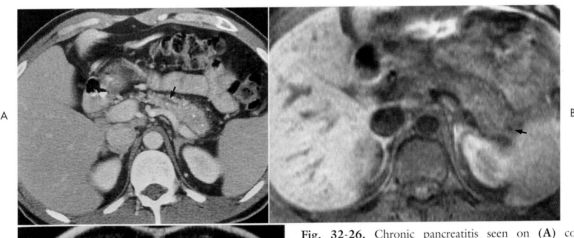
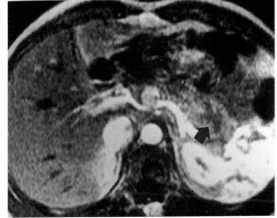

Fig. 32-26. Chronic pancreatitis seen on (A) contrast-enhanced 5 mm CT, (B) FSSE (500/15), and (C) immediate postcontrast FLASH (130/4.5) images obtained in a 32-year-old man. A, On the CT image, calcifications in the pancreas and mild dilatation of the pancreatic duct *(arrow)* are well demonstrated. B, On the FSSE image, the pancreas is of uniformly low SI, but the signal void calcifications are difficult to appreciate *(arrow)*. C, On the immediate postcontrast FLASH image, contrast enhancement is diminished, and the pancreas enhances inhomogeneously with an irregular region of low SI in the tail *(large arrow)*. Mild ductal dilatation can be appreciated *(small arrow)*. (From Semelka RC, et al: Pancreatic disease: prospective comparison of CT, ERCP, and 1.5-T MR imaging with dynamic gadolinium enhancement and fat suppression. *Radiology* 181:785, 1991.)

and colleagues,[206] have shown that the acute changes are quite consistently imaged with the new fast acquisition images.

The findings that can be noted include the overall morphology of the gland, the presence of edema, enlargement of the pancreatic duct, formation of fluid collections, and the presence of fibrotic tissue. Edema or fluid within the parenchyma shows a decrease in intensity with the T1-weighted images and increase in the intensity with the T2-weighted images. The evolution of the disease, with either an increase in fluid during exacerbation or a decrease in fluid during improvement, can be seen (Figs. 32-25 and 32-26). The dilatation of the pancreatic duct is seen as a tubular fluid density structure within the gland. The signal intensity varies from bright to dark depending on weighting of the signal (Fig. 32-25).

As the disease evolves, any pseudocyst is visualized as a fluid collection showing the appropriate signal intensity. T1-weighted images are dark (see Fig. 32-25, *A*), and T2-weighted images are bright.

As chronicity develops in the gland, fibrosis and calcification may occur. Fibrosis characteristically shows an absence of signal on both T1- and T2-weighted imaging. Calcifications may show a signal void on all signals if the calcium is quite mature or a normal signal depending on the amount of hydration of the calcium (see Fig. 32-25, *A* and *C*). All authors reporting note that the inability to detect and characterize calcium consistently is a definite disadvantage.

Cystic fibrosis

MRI has been used to evaluate cystic fibrosis by numerous authors. These authors have noted that because of the ability of MRI to visualize fat well, patterns of change resulting from atrophic changes were well seen. Tham and associates[232] reported on 15 cases and noted three appearances: complete replacement of the gland by fat resulting in a lobulated enlarged gland, small atrophic gland with partial fat replacement, and diffuse atrophy of the gland.

Pancreatic transplants

The ability of MRI to detect edema of the pancreas makes it well suited for evaluation of pancreatic transplants. The most notable article on this topic is by Yuh and colleagues.[248] In this report, the authors noted that configuration and density changes related to edema and rejection can be well evaluated by MRI. They noted that the progression and regression of rejection could be followed by the increase and decrease in the amount of fluid within the gland. Chronic rejection showed the progressive decrease in size as well as the decrease in signal associated with the development of fibrosis.

Another potential use of MRI is the prediction of rejection/infarction based on changes in enhancement produced by injection of gadopentetate dimeglumine-(Fig. 32-27). After injection of 0.1 mmol/kg, the authors obtained numerous gradient echo scans in the same anatomical location over the pancreas. They found that the normal gland in six cases increased enhancement by 98% during the first minute, whereas the rejecting gland increased enhancement at 1 minute by 42% six of six rejections) (see Fig. 32-10). They found that there was little or no change in the calculated T2 value. The abnormal scans preceded chemical evidence of rejection (urinary amylase levels) in four cases (four of six rejection cases). They concluded that T2 intensity was a poor indicator for rejection and favored the use of this new enhancement method.

PANCREATIC NONENDOCRINE TUMORS

Most tumors in the pancreas are adenocarcinoma, which produce characteristic configuration changes and occasional signal change. The two most significant reports on MRI of tumors are those by Steiner and associates[225] and Semelka and colleagues.[206] As with CT, these tumors produce contour alterations that exceed normal measurements or apparent discrepancy between various portions of the gland. On unenhanced scans, Steiner and associates reported that 61% (20 of 32) of the tumors had an intensity less than normal pancreas, whereas 40% (13 of 32) of the tumors had intensities greater than the normal gland. In a similar way that the avascular tumor produces a decreased density with intravenous urographic contrast material on CT, gadolinium-enhanced images can also show a difference in the intensity of such tumors when compared with the normal gland (Figs. 32-28, 32-29, and 32-30).

Although the point has not been emphasized, it is apparent that if problematic cases of staging for operability arise, MRI would be extremely well suited to evaluate the status of the peripancreatic vascular system. Encroachment of the portal or superior mesenteric vein would be quite easily detected by MRI.

MRI offers a viable alternative to CT if a specific case is problematic or contrast allergy is an issue. No authors have asserted that MRI is the preeminent study for tumor, but all including ourselves recognize the potential for the future.

Authors who have reported indicate that MRI offers no significant advantages over CT for evaluating the pancreas for neoplasia. Further progress is needed in refinement of signal-to-noise ratio, spatial resolution, motion suppression, and bowel opacification before MRI might become competitive with CT.

Cystic tumors

There is only one extensive report in the literature about the usefulness of MRI for the diagnosis and evaluation of cystic tumors of the neoplasm, by Minami

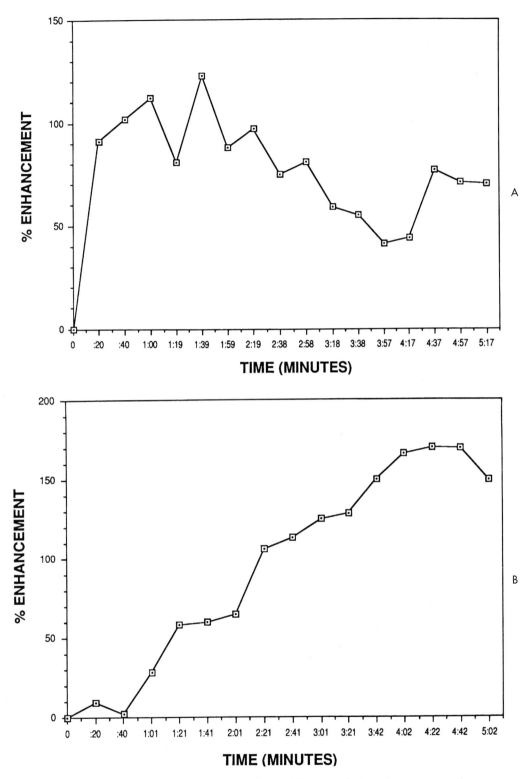

Fig. 32-27. A, Graph shows enhancement obtained for normally functioning pancreatic transplant. Enhancement during first minute after intravenous bolus of gadopentetate dimeglumine was 112%. **B,** Graph shows enhancement curve obtained for a pancreatic transplant undergoing early acute rejection. Maximal enhancement during first minute after intravenous bolus of gadopentetate dimeglumine was 28%. (From Fernandez et al: *AJR* 156:1171-1176, 1991.)

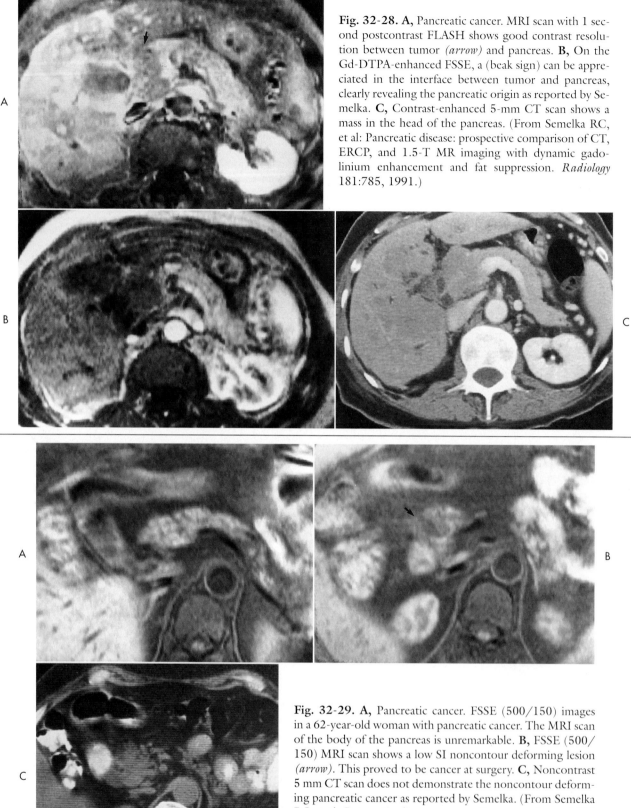

Fig. 32-28. A, Pancreatic cancer. MRI scan with 1 second postcontrast FLASH shows good contrast resolution between tumor *(arrow)* and pancreas. **B,** On the Gd-DTPA-enhanced FSSE, a (beak sign) can be appreciated in the interface between tumor and pancreas, clearly revealing the pancreatic origin as reported by Semelka. **C,** Contrast-enhanced 5-mm CT scan shows a mass in the head of the pancreas. (From Semelka RC, et al: Pancreatic disease: prospective comparison of CT, ERCP, and 1.5-T MR imaging with dynamic gadolinium enhancement and fat suppression. *Radiology* 181:785, 1991.)

Fig. 32-29. A, Pancreatic cancer. FSSE (500/150) images in a 62-year-old woman with pancreatic cancer. The MRI scan of the body of the pancreas is unremarkable. **B,** FSSE (500/150) MRI scan shows a low SI noncontour deforming lesion *(arrow)*. This proved to be cancer at surgery. **C,** Noncontrast 5 mm CT scan does not demonstrate the noncontour deforming pancreatic cancer as reported by Semelka. (From Semelka RC et al: Pancreatic disease: prospective comparison of CT, ERCP, and 1.5-T MR imaging with dynamic gadolinium enhancement and fat suppression. *Radiology* 181:785, 1991.)

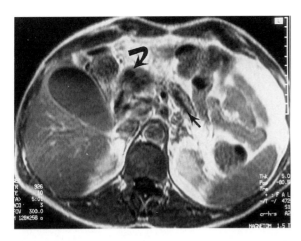

Fig. 32-30. Pancreatic cancer *(curved arrow)* noted in head of pancreas producing distal ductal dilatation *(arrow)* SE 926/10.

and associates.[65] In their report, they studied five microcystic adenomas and seven mucinous (macrocystic) neoplasms (not prospective nor blinded). Three cystadenomas and four cystadenocarcinomas were studied with both CT and MRI. The observations and conclusions of the authors were that MRI was equivalent or slightly better than CT for these tumors because MRI was better able to demonstrate the cystic content by virtue of the different signal on MRI (Fig. 32-31). The cystic material was low intensity on the T1-weighted images and high intensity on the T2-weighted images (Figs. 32-32 and 32-33). Attempts to characterize lesions as either microcystic and mucinous or benign from malignant (cystadenoma from cystadenocarcinoma) were not possible based on the MRI appearance alone. Variation in signal between different loculations is more common with mucinous tumors, but it can also occur with serous tumors.

The authors' conclusion was optimistic but cautious in stating that MRI was equivalent or slightly superior to CT by virtue of its sensitivity to difference in intensity of the different cavities and the better definition of the out contour of the masses. They also noted

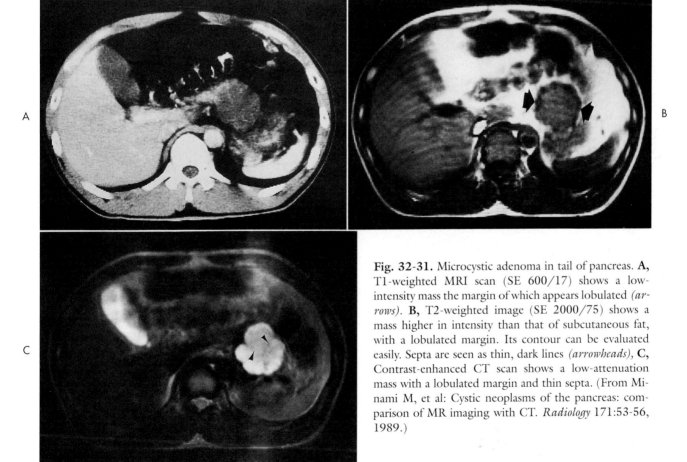

Fig. 32-31. Microcystic adenoma in tail of pancreas. **A,** T1-weighted MRI scan (SE 600/17) shows a low-intensity mass the margin of which appears lobulated *(arrows)*. **B,** T2-weighted image (SE 2000/75) shows a mass higher in intensity than that of subcutaneous fat, with a lobulated margin. Its contour can be evaluated easily. Septa are seen as thin, dark lines *(arrowheads)*, **C,** Contrast-enhanced CT scan shows a low-attenuation mass with a lobulated margin and thin septa. (From Minami M, et al: Cystic neoplasms of the pancreas: comparison of MR imaging with CT. *Radiology* 171:53-56, 1989.)

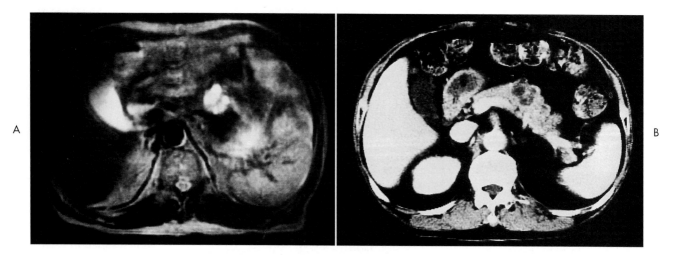

Fig. 32-32. Microcystic adenoma in the body of the pancreas. **A,** T2-weighted MRI scan (SE 2000/75) shows a hyperintense tumor that appears inhomogenous in intensity owing to the low intensity of a central scar. **B,** Enhanced CT scan shows a lobulated tumor with a calcified central stellate scar. (From Minami M, et al: Cystic neoplasms of the pancreas: comparison of MR imaging with CT. *Radiology* 171:53-56, 1989.)

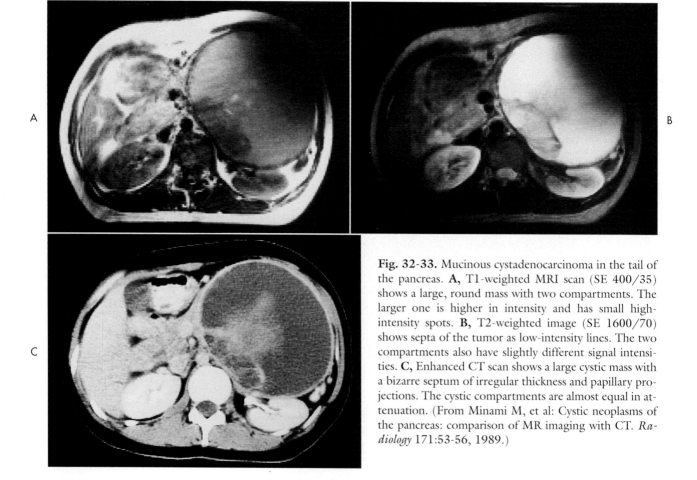

Fig. 32-33. Mucinous cystadenocarcinoma in the tail of the pancreas. **A,** T1-weighted MRI scan (SE 400/35) shows a large, round mass with two compartments. The larger one is higher in intensity and has small high-intensity spots. **B,** T2-weighted image (SE 1600/70) shows septa of the tumor as low-intensity lines. The two compartments also have slightly different signal intensities. **C,** Enhanced CT scan shows a large cystic mass with a bizarre septum of irregular thickness and papillary projections. The cystic compartments are almost equal in attenuation. (From Minami M, et al: Cystic neoplasms of the pancreas: comparison of MR imaging with CT. *Radiology* 171:53-56, 1989.)

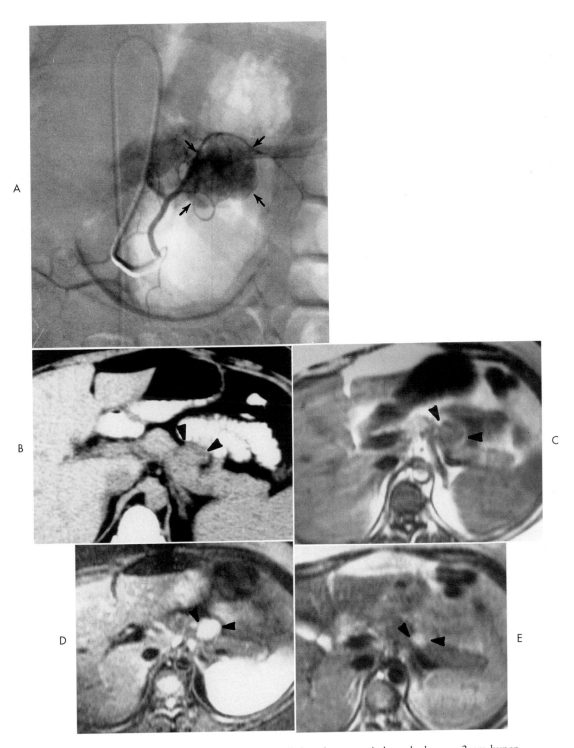

Fig. 32-34. A, Selective arteriogram of a small dorsal pancreatic branch shows a 3-cm hypervascular mass *(arrows)* in the body of the pancreas just to the left of the spine. **B,** CT scan shows the mass protruding from the anterior surface of the pancreas *(arrowheads)*. **C,** T1-weighted MRI scan shows the mass with an area of slightly decreased signal intensity compared with the pancreas *(arrowheads)*, but the mass is difficult to distinguish from the surrounding structures. **D,** On the T2-weighted image, the gastrinoma reveals increased signal intensity *(arrowheads)*. **E,** The tumor is far more apparent on the sequence with short inversion-recovery image (STIR) *(arrowheads)* as a focus of very high signal intensity. (From Frucht H, et al: Gastrinomas: comparison of MR imaging with CT, angiography, and US. *Radiology* 171:713-717, 1989.)

that further improvement would be important if better spatial resolution and differentiation between serous and mucinous material were to be achieved.

Endocrine tumors

A variety of endocrine tumors have been studied with MRI and reported in the literature. Although we have not accumulated a large number of such cases, we have observed the same advantages reported by others for MRI in evaluating these cases.

The signal intensity of endocrine tumors of the pancreas is much different than that for nonendocrine tumors. Such tumors show configuration changes as one might expect, but also the intensity of the tumor is higher on T2-weighted images than that of the normal pancreas or the typical pancreatic adenocarcinoma (Figs. 32-34 and 32-35).

One of the larger studies reported by Frucht and colleagues[67] evaluated the prospective usefulness of various imaging modalities, including CT, ultrasound, MRI, and angiography, for the detection of gastrinoma (outside of the liver). The results are rather surprising considering the theoretical advantage of MRI and CT. The authors used spin-echo imaging with T1 and T2 weighting as well as some short T1 inversion recovery imaging. Of the 22 cases of extrahepatic gastrinoma, 17 were within the pancreas and 3 were outside. MRI was successful in only 4 of the group, and CT was successful in detecting the lesion in only 9 of the group. The most effective imaging system used was angiography, which detected 16 lesions. The addition of MRI or CT did not improve the results because no additional lesions not seen on angiography were found. Tham and others[230-232] made similar observations, noting that MRI was superior to CT for detecting endocrine tumors, but angiography was still superior to both (Fig. 32-35).

Although these data seem somewhat disappointing at this time, several things should be considered. The cases evaluated by these authors were examined by early MRI devices. It is possible that newer devices capable of fast imaging, such as higher strength magnets or echo planar units, might produce better results for the primary detection. The development of contrast agents may also have a positive effect on the future diagnostic accuracy of MRI.

The second point that should be raised is that although MRI is not remarkably effective for the detection of lesions, it may be useful for the follow-up of metastatic disease. Surgical treatment of the metastatic disease is not effective in most cases, and chemotherapy is being used more consistently. Because MRI shows a significant signal difference between the tumor, increased T2 signal, and other tissues, one would expect better follow-up of therapeutic treatments (Figs. 32-36 and 32-37).

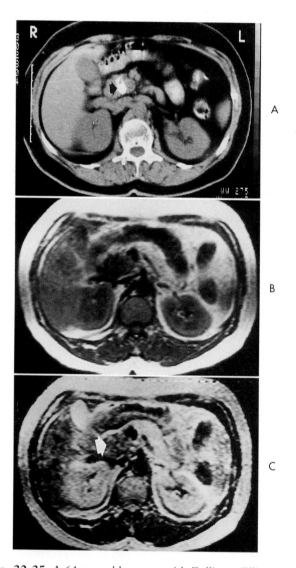

Fig. 32-35. A 64-year-old woman with Zollinger-Ellison syndrome for 5 years. The patient died 1 year after this examination from tumor progression. Autopsy demonstrates a gastrinoma in the pancreatic head and uncinate process. **A,** Nonenhanced CT scan shows gross calcifications in the uncinate process of the pancreas *(arrow).* **B,** T1-weighted (SE 650/30) MRI scan. Compared with the body and tail of the pancreas, the enlarged head and uncinate process have a low signal intensity. The lesion can be distinguished from the body and the tail of the pancreas. **C,** T2-weighted (SE 2000/50) MRI scan. The signal intensity of the pancreatic tumor remains low *(arrow)* compared with that of the normal body and tail of the pancreas. (From Tham RTOTA, et al: CT and MR imaging of advanced Zollinger-Ellison syndrome. J Comput Assist Tomogr 13:821-828, 1989.)

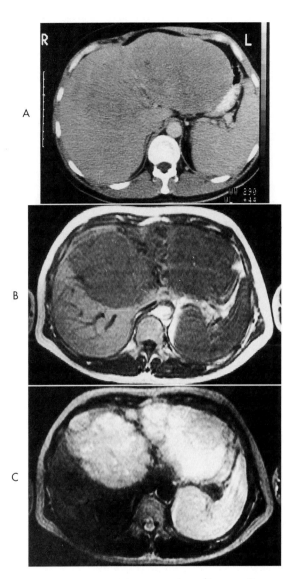

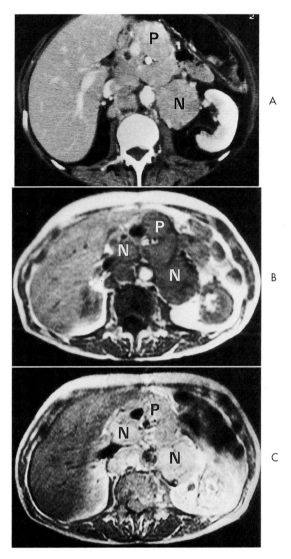

Fig. 32-36. A 37-year-old man with Zollinger-Ellison syndrome and multiple metastases in the liver. **A,** CT scan after intravenous contrast administration shows two large hypodense metastases in the left and right lobe of the liver. **B,** T1-weighted (SE 300/20) MRI scan taken at the same level shows the same hepatic metastases. Their signal is low compared with that of the normal liver parenchyma. **C,** T2-weighted (SE 2000/100) MRI scan. The hepatic metastases now produce a high signal compared with the normal liver parenchyma. The large metastases are composed of a cluster of five or six smaller lesions. (From Tham RTOTA, et al: CT and MR imaging of advanced Zollinger-Ellison syndrome. *J Comput Assist Tomogr* 13:821-828, 1989.)

Fig. 32-37. A 55-year-old woman with multiple endocrine neoplasia type I and Zollinger-Ellison syndrome for 18 years exhibits a tumor of the body of the pancreas with lymph node and bone metastases. **A,** CT scan after intravenous contrast administration demonstrates enlargement of the body of the pancreas *(P)* and lymph node metastases *(N)* that are isodense. **B,** T1-weighted (SE 300/20) MRI scan shows the pancreatic tumor *(P)* and the lymph node metastases *(N)* with a homogeneous low signal intensity compared with that of the normal liver parenchyma. The sharply delineated contours of the multiple lesions are readily visible. **C,** T2-weighted (SE 2000/50) MRI scan reveals the slightly inhomogeneous high signal intensity of the pancreatic tumor *(P)* and lymph node metastases *(N)*. (From Tham RTOTA, et al: CT and MR imaging of advanced Zollinger-Ellison syndrome. *J Comput Assist Tomogr* 13(5):821-828, 1989.)

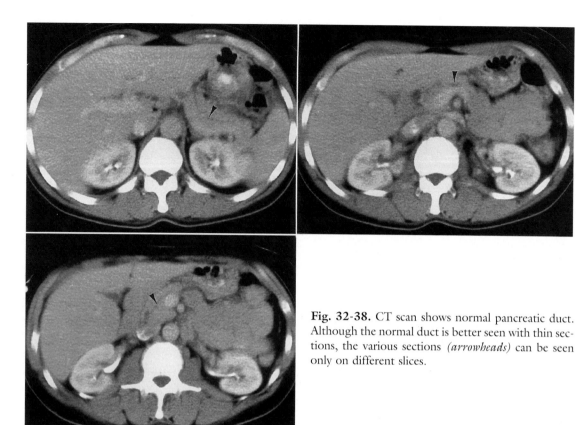

Fig. 32-38. CT scan shows normal pancreatic duct. Although the normal duct is better seen with thin sections, the various sections *(arrowheads)* can be seen only on different slices.

Pancreatic duct

The best technique to visualize the duct in both normal and abnormal situations requires the administration of urographic contrast material and selection of optimal scanning parameters.[58,86]

For best visualization, maximal enhancement of the parenchyma relative to the duct should be produced by a sustained intravenous injection of urographic contrast material by mechanical injector with simultaneous or immediately subsequent CT scanning of the pancreas (see Fig. 32-10). The recommendations of exact injection rates may vary from one institution to the next, but the dosage and rate suggested in the previous section on technique are adequate.

Occasionally the normal duct can be visualized with 8 mm thick scan slices. More consistent visualization of the duct can also be achieved by setting the scanning parameters to optimize contrast and spatial resolution. The best approach to do this is to optimize the spatial resolution in the XY as well as the longitudinal plane. Resolution in the XY plane is improved by using a small field of view to maximize the number of pixels within the anatomy being imaged and using thin scan slices of 2 to 4 mm. These thin sections are necessary to mini-

mize the partial volume effect in the longitudinal plane, considering that the diameter of the normal duct is 2 to 6 mm. The advantage of the thick slices is that the entire duct can be seen through the length of the gland, and most cases of pathological dilatation can be routinely imaged without the optimized scanning parameters. Thin slices are advantageous in that the anatomy is better defined, but in most cases the segments of the duct appear on different scans (Fig. 32-38).

Pancreatitis

Acute pancreatitis may produce dilatation of the duct, especially if there is superimposition of acute inflammation on a baseline of chronic changes or rarely an acute obstruction of the duct by a calculus (Fig. 32-39) or pseudocyst (Fig. 32-40).

Chronic inflammation produces fibrosis, which, depending on its anatomical location and extent of the fibrosis, may result in diffuse dilatation, diffuse stenosis, or segmental narrowing of the duct; the CT or MRI scan directly reflects these gross anatomical findings. In patients who have diffuse narrowing of the ductal system that is significantly attenuated, the CT scan is unlikely to show any positive findings.

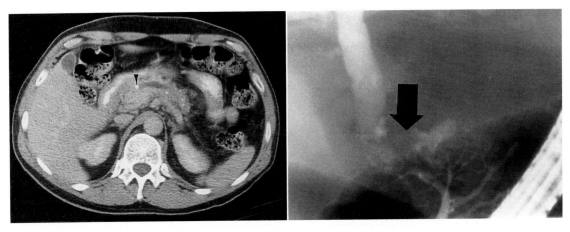

Fig. 32-39. Pancreatic duct enlargement can be caused acutely by a ductal calculus *(arrowhead)*.

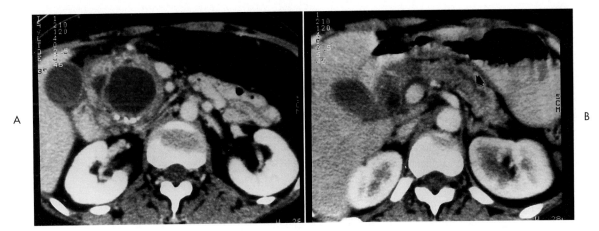

Fig. 32-40. A, Pseudocyst in the head is located in front of pancreatic calcifications. The mass effect is producing distal ductal dilatation. **B,** The midpart of the enlarged pancreatic duct appears smooth *(arrow)*.

When fibrosis occurs close to the head of the gland and is producing partial obstruction, moderate dilatation of the duct, which appears as a fluid-density tubular structure within the gland, occurs. When fibrosis occurs intermittently along the length of the duct, a string of ectatic areas is produced resulting in the appearance of sacculations on the duct on the CT scan (Fig. 32-40, *B*). On occasion, one portion of the duct is more isolated than the others, and a buildup of fluid in a localized area, which appears as a cystic mass on the scan, is produced. This cyst mass cannot be distinguished from a pseudocyst by imaging alone and is called a *retention cyst* (Figs. 32-41 and 32-42). It differs from a pseudocyst in that the wall is lined by epithelium of the duct; if the epithelium remains in place for a sufficient amount of time, the ductal lining may atrophy so ductal elements may not be detectable pathologically. Differentiation from pseudocysts may be difficult because pseudocysts may coexist with even causing ductal dilatation. The nature of a cystic abnormality can be best differentiated by ERCP. Dilatation of the secondary ductules produces clusters of cysts (Fig. 32-43), which are typically fluid density, but they may calcify if chronic disease persists.

Ductal calcification

The same type of calcium deposits that can occur in the parenchyma of the gland can also occur in the wall or the lumen of the duct (Figs. 32-43 and 32-44). The cause and pathophysiology of this process are not well understood. Their presence, however, should be detected at the earliest time so corrective measures, such as surgical ductal drainages, can be contemplated if clinically indicated. The spectrum of symptoms associated with a calculus in the duct is quite wide. Some patients are asymptomatic, some develop atrophy of the gland, and some may even develop life-threatening inflammation (Fig. 32-45) following ductal enterostomy.

Ductal gas

Air can appear in the duct, which may be a result of a fistula or other more benign conditions. Air can also occur after ERCP (see Fig. 32-46, *A*), as a result of papillotomy (Fig. 32-46, *B*), or in some patients simply as a result of a patulous sphincter of Oddi (Fig. 32-46, *D*). One could certainly hypothesize that cholangitis or another infectious process could spread gas to the duct, but I have not observed this nor seen it reported.

Ductal changes from neoplasm

Several authors have reported on this topic, including Berland and colleagues,[21] Freeny and others,[60-63] and Muranaka and associates.[169] There is a consensus among authors that high-quality, modern CT and MRI reliably demonstrate the appearance and status of the duct. Recognizing the changes produced by inflammation as noted previously, these authors point out that uniform, severe dilatation of the duct can be produced by either inflammation or neoplasm (Fig. 32-47). The frequency and reliability of differentiating inflammation from neoplasm has been variable among these authors.

Karasawa and coworkers[117] reported their experience with CT pancreatogram in patients with pancre-

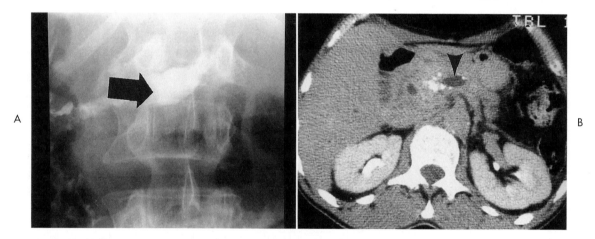

Fig. 32-41. A, Pancreatogram shows diffuse dilatation with a central ectasi *(arrow)*. B, CT scan shows central dilatation of the main pancreatic duct resulting in a small retention cyst.

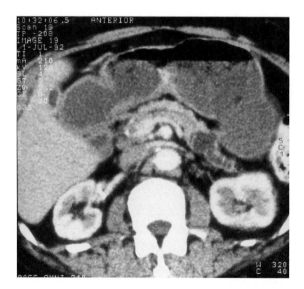

Fig. 32-42. CT scan shows mild dilatation of the central portion of the duct with saccular dilatation distally, resulting in a retention cyst.

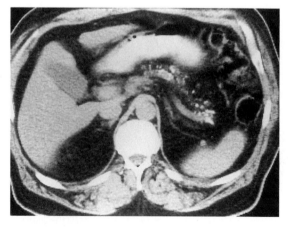

Fig. 32-43. Chronic inflammation has produced intense calcification in the pancreatic duct, atrophy of the gland, and calcifications of the secondary ductules of the gland.

atitis and carcinoma. They stated that ductal dilatation caused by these entities could be distinguished in a large number of cases. They reported that smooth or beaded dilatation was commonly associated with carcinoma; dilatation occurred in 56% of those patients with neoplasm. Ductal dilatation occurred in 58% of patients with pancreatitis, and irregular dilatation was seen in 73% of those patients. They found that patients with carcinoma tended

to have a larger duct, measuring on average 8.7 mm compared with 6.7 mm for patients with pancreatitis. They also noted that the ratio of the duct to the overall dimension of the gland was greater with carcinoma because of atrophy of the acinar elements associated with complete obstruction; if the ratio of duct to gland was greater than 0.5 mm, carcinoma was likely.

Freeny and others[60-63] reported that 108 of 159 patients (68%) had ductal dilatation. In 90 of 108 patients, the margins of the duct were smooth and parallel. In 18 of 108, they appeared beaded or irregular. Pancreatic parenchyma was atrophic in 82% of the patients with ductal dilatation.

Differentiating pathology by ductal changes

The information provided by these authors is helpful for an overall perspective of pancreatic duct assessment, but the most definitive work to date on this topic was by Muranaka and coworkers.[169] In their work, they noted that differentiation of benign and malignant disease in the specific case is still not always possible. The configuration and size of the duct depends on the degree and duration of obstruction. Muranaka reported that pancreatic duct dilatation is relatively uncommon in small tumors, but that dilatation of the duct and atrophy of the gland progresses with tumor growth. The increased ratio of duct to gland occurs with late tumor progression. Neoplasms and inflammatory processes can produce partial or complete and slow or quick obstruction of the duct. The guidelines proposed by earlier authors are beneficial; i.e., if the ratio of the diameter of

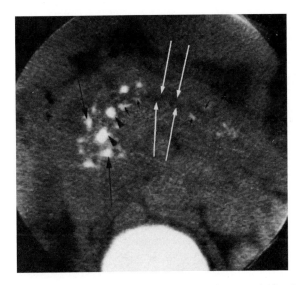

Fig. 32-44. High-resolution CT scan shows calcification *(small arrows)* in the wall of the dilated duct *(white arrows)*, in the parenchyma *(large arrows)*, and within the duct *(arrowheads)*.

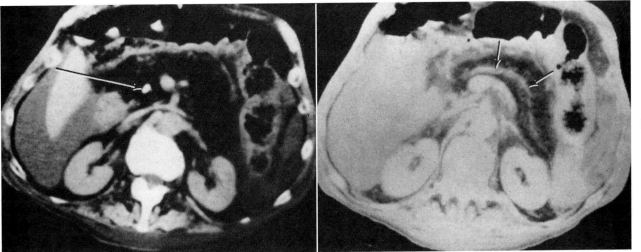

Fig. 32-45. A, A calculus in the ampulla *(arrow).* **B,** Obstruction of the pancreatic duct *(arrows)* resulting from calculus. The pancreas has autolyzed so only the fat remains within the parenchymal area. (From Patel S, et al: Fat replacement of the exocrine pancreas. *AJR* 135:843-845; copyright by American Roentgen Ray Society, 1980.)

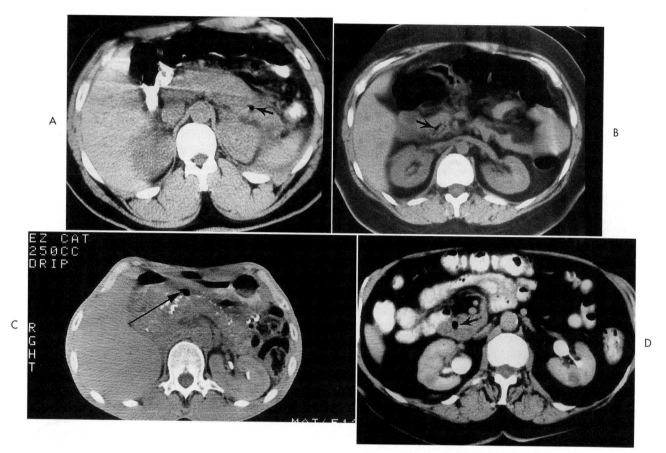

Fig. 32-46. **A,** Small bubbles of gas *(arrow)* can be introduced into the ductal system by pancreatograms. **B,** Following interventional procedures on the common or pancreatic duct, small air collections can be seen with the head of the gland *(arrow)*. **C,** Patient with calcifications has air *(arrow)* in the duct containing calculi. **D,** Air has refluxed from the bowel through an anastomosis through the duct.

the duct to the overall diameter of the parenchyma is 0.5 mm or greater, the chance of a neoplastic origin is more likely (Figs. 32-48, *A, B,* 32-49). The detailed analysis of these findings provided by Muranaka and coworkers is illuminating as a reference source (Table 32-1).

PANCREATITIS

Inflammation of the pancreas is produced by the release of proteolytic, lipolytic, and other enzymes; the acute process produces a serious clinical state that has numerous life-threatening complications. Chronic pancreatitis is associated with recurrent acute bouts and produces significant long-term morbidity.[6]

Causes of pancreatitis are numerous and include gallbladder disease, trauma,[149] alcohol ingestion, drug use, hypercalcemia, hyperlipidemia, vascular disease, infection, uremia, diabetic coma, heredity, and unknown causes. Regardless the initiating cause, once there has

been activation of the various enzymes, severe inflammation ensues. The spectrum of acute pancreatitis is broad, and it may produce a benign, self-limited episode or worsen into a self-perpetuating fulminant course.

The symptoms of pancreatitis include abdominal pain, nausea, and vomiting. Classic laboratory findings include elevated levels of serum amylase and lipase and depressed levels of serum calcium. Occasionally there are also elevations of the serum glucose and triglycerides.

Although the diagnosis of either acute or chronic pancreatitis usually is made clinically, imaging procedures at times may provide valuable information about the case, course, progression, prognosis, and complications of the disease.[4,245] The following sections discuss the different forms of pancreatitis and are intended to make the radiologist an integral part of the clinical team that cares for such patients.

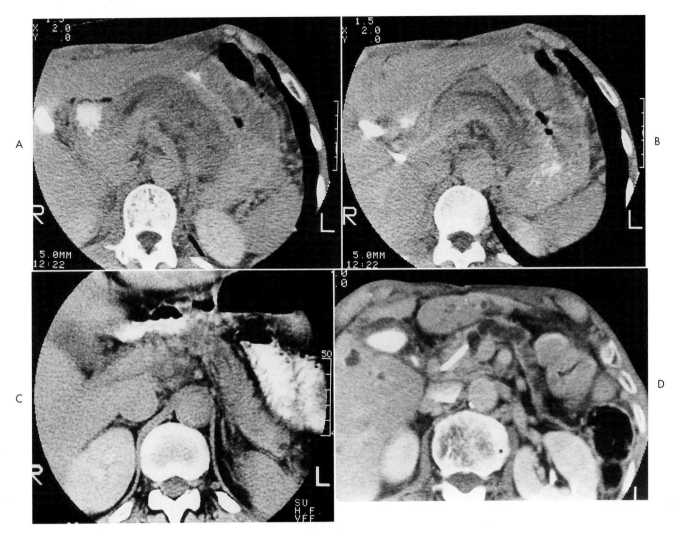

Fig. 32-47. Sequential changes in the pancreatic body on CT in patients with pancreatic head carcinoma. This patient was followed clinically because of poor respiratory function. Carcinoma was confirmed by postmortem examination. **A,** Initial CT scan shows marked enlargement of the pancreatic body. **B,** Two months later, the pancreatic body width is decreased, and a smooth, narrow pancreatic duct is seen continuously. **C,** Four months later, the pancreatic body became normal in size. **D,** Atrophy of the pancreatic body and marked dilatation of the pancreatic duct with a beaded contour are demonstrated 7 months later. (From Muranaka T, et al: *Acta Radiol* 31:483-488, 1990.)

Causative factors

The most valuable contribution that can be made by CT examination is the detection of the primary cause of the inflammatory process so remedial steps can be taken. The most important finding on a study of a patient with pancreatitis is the presence of biliary or gallbladder calculi. Calculi can be the cause of severe pancreatitis, and they are one of the few problems that can be easily remedied. The specific appearance of calculi is discussed in Chapter 31, but one should bear in mind that CT is not the modality of choice for biliary or gallbladder calculi. A CT scan may be negative in the presence of gallstones simply because there is minimal density between the stones and the surrounding bile. Ultrasound is the study of choice and should be performed in all patients with pancreatitis.

In cases of trauma, direct damage can be seen as well as significant trauma in the adjacent structures. In children with pancreatitis, the presence of calcification is usually indicative of familial pancreatitis. In most instances, the cause of pancreatitis is unknown, let alone detectable on CT or other imaging tests. The sensitivity of CT for detecting pancreatitis is exceptional, considering that even clinically asymptomatic pancreatitis caused

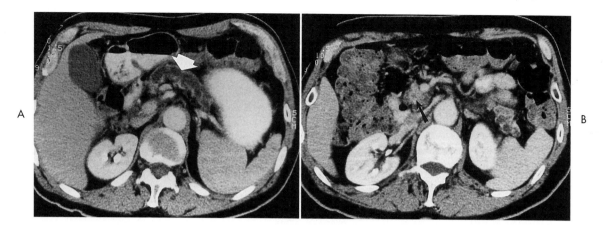

Fig. 32-48. A, CT scan of a patient with chronic pain, which shows severe dilatation of the pancreatic duct. The diameter of the duct is more than 0.5 the diameter of the gland. The duct is somewhat tortuous, which some authors suggest may be consistent with pancreatitis. **B,** A lower section on CT scan shows a small high-density mass *(arrow)* within the fat density gland.

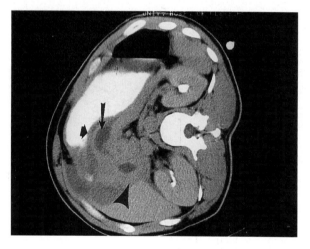

Fig. 32-49. CT scan of patient in the decubitus position. Asymmetrical enlargement of the pancreatic duct as a result of inflammation causes cystic dilatation or retention cysts *(long arrow)*. Note the thickening of the gastric wall *(small arrow)* and the diffuse enlargement of the head *(arrowhead)*.

by ERCP can be detected by CT, as noted by Thoeni and associates.[233]

Acute edematous pancreatitis

Acute pancreatitis is well suited for examination by CT because CT scanning is not impaired by gas, as is ultrasound. If there is an associated ileus or sentinal loop, it will not impede CT examination but may preclude an examination by ultrasound. The diagnostic signs of pancreatitis include alteration of the pancreatic density, duct dilatation (Fig. 32-49), morphological characteristics, contour, and peripancreatic edema and fluid collections.

Density alterations within the gland result from either fluid accumulation or necrosis. The most subtle finding is decreased density within the gland without alteration of the contour or peripancreatic anatomy (Fig. 32-50). Edematous pancreatitis can be differentiated from necrotizing pancreatitis by the injection of contrast material. Maier[148] studied this and found in operatively confirmed cases that edematous pancreatitis maintains uniform enhancement without alteration of density; necrotic areas devascularized do not enhance. In subtle

Table 32-1. Incidence of pancreatic duct visualization on CT scans in pancreatic head mass*

	Pancreatic carcinoma				Focal inflammatory mass No. (%)	Pseudocyst No. (%)
	T1 No. (%)	T2 No. (%)	T3 No. (%)	T4 No. (%)		
Pancreatic Duct	2 (18)	10 (71)	14 (70)	10 (91)	8 (80)	12 (100)

*Incidence of pancreatic duct visualization in carcinoma 36/56 (64%). See page 1100.
From Muranaka T, et al: *Acta Radiol* 31:483-488, 1990.

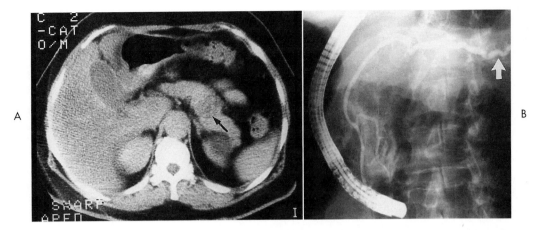

Fig. 32-50. A, CT shows an area of decreased density *(arrow)* within the gland that represents focal pancreatitis. **B,** ERCP shows enlargement of the duct *(arrow)* in the central part of the gland; enlargement is typical of pancreatitis.

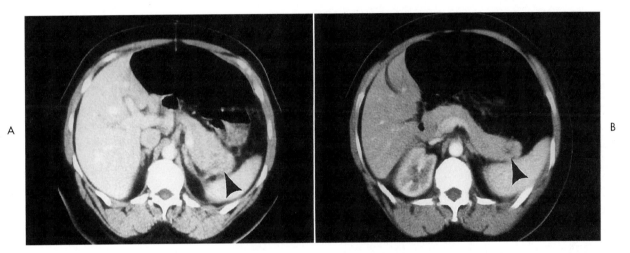

Fig. 32-51. A, CT scan shows focal enlargement of the tail *(arrowhead)* secondary to pancreatitis. **B,** After resolution, the gland returned to normal size *(arrowhead).*

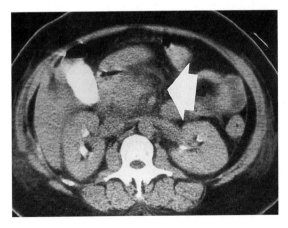

Fig. 32-52. Subtle inflammatory mass *(arrow)* of the head secondary to ERCP. Note the small amount of fluid next to the superior mesenteric artery.

cases, there may be no positive laboratory findings; the serum amylase and lipase levels may be normal.

The pancreas may increase or decrease in size, depending on the stage of inflammation (Fig. 32-51). The contour of the gland may change significantly, depending on the amount of fluid and edema enlarging the gland (Fig. 32-52). The anterior or posterior margins of the gland may be difficult to delineate because of the presence of edema or fluid in the immediate area of the gland. A slight amount of edema posteriorly makes the fat plane between the gland and vessels slightly denser, whereas a large amount of fluid may totally obscure the margins of the splenic vessels (Figs. 32-53 and 32-54). Edema anteriorly blurs the margin of the gland and may then extend along the anterior ligamentous pathways, such as the mesentary, hepatoduodenal ligament, or the

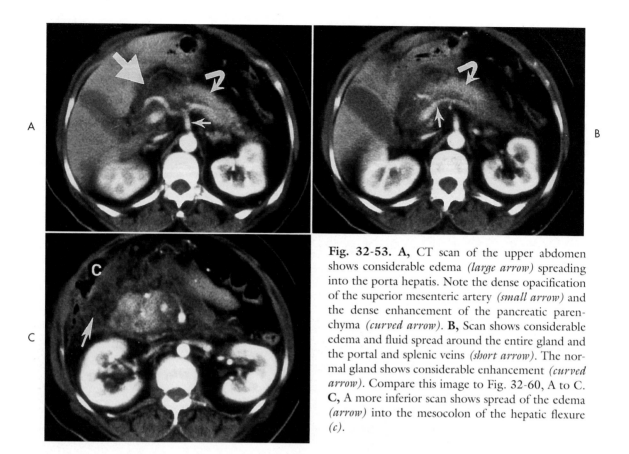

Fig. 32-53. A, CT scan of the upper abdomen shows considerable edema *(large arrow)* spreading into the porta hepatis. Note the dense opacification of the superior mesenteric artery *(small arrow)* and the dense enhancement of the pancreatic parenchyma *(curved arrow)*. **B,** Scan shows considerable edema and fluid spread around the entire gland and the portal and splenic veins *(short arrow)*. The normal gland shows considerable enhancement *(curved arrow)*. Compare this image to Fig. 32-60, A to C. **C,** A more inferior scan shows spread of the edema *(arrow)* into the mesocolon of the hepatic flexure *(c)*.

mesocolon.[226] With the mesocolon originating from the anterior surface of the pancreas, spread of the inflammation resulting in a sentinal loop is quite common in the hepatic, transverse, or splenic portions of the colon.

Further progression of the inflammation most commonly produces ascites, which can fill the adjacent peritoneal space, including the greater peritoneal cavity and lesser sac. Involvement of the general cavity produces ascitic fluid in the adjacent dependent spaces, such as the paracolic gutters and Morrison's pouch. The lesser sac being immediately anterior to the gland is the most common space involved by accumulation of fluid (Fig. 32-55). Fluid collections or subsequent pseudocysts can occur in either the inferior or the superior medial recesses of the lesser sac.

The second most common anatomical area involved by continued inflammation is the anterior perirenal fascia on either the right or left side depending on involvement of the head or the body of the gland. The fluid may extend either cephalad to involve the bare area behind the liver or spleen or caudad to involve the retroperitoneum down into the pelvis by the psoas muscle. The amount of the fluid can be so great it produces distention of the fascia, creating an elliptically shaped mass

(see Fig. 32-5, *B, C*). With the sparing of the perinephric fat, this appearance has been given the name the "halo sign" by Susman et al.[228]

Progressive inflammation and spread of edema can produce pronounced extension into contiguous organs or bowel.[164] Inflammatory involvement of the mesentery and mesocolon may produce sufficient edema to cause lymphatic and venous congestion to produce an ileus or sentinal loop of the adjacent bowel. Involvement of the stomach and edema can produce such severe thickening that they may simulate a mass (Fig. 32-56). Digestion of the enzymatic material along the vasculature of the ligaments or through fascia can result in direct involvement of the liver, spleen, or even the kidney and ultimately form pseudocysts in those organs.

One specific area of inflammatory spread that has been the source of some controversy has been the perivascular fat plane around the superior mesenteric artery. Traditional teaching has been that only tumors can produce this appearance of encasement, but it has been documented by Schulte et al[205] and others that the loss of the fat plane can also occur with pancreatitis in addition to neoplastic inflammation. This finding can be seen in both the acute and the chronic situation.

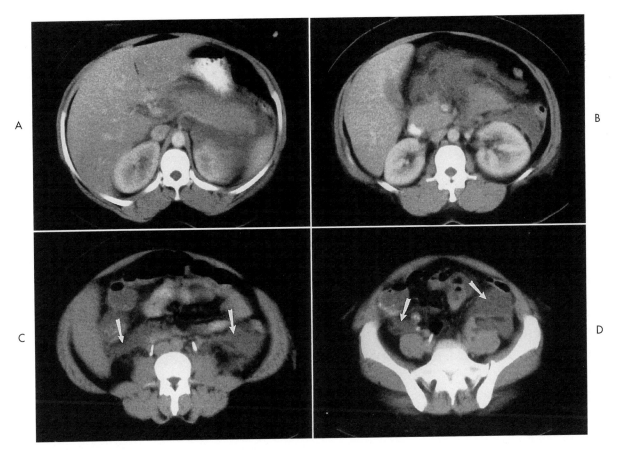

Fig. 32-54. A, Severe pancreatitis producing remarkable fluid and edema around the entire gland, left kidney, and hilum of spleen. **B,** Massive edema accumulating in the mesocolon anterior to the gland and spreading into the anterior fascia on the left around the descending colon. **C,** Edema at lower level extends into both the right and left anterior renal fascia *(arrows).* The descending colon is displaced anteriorly. **D,** Scan at a lower level shows further extension of the edema on the right behind the cecum and the sigmoid colon *(arrows).*

Evolution of inflammation

Inflammation has many different appearances as it evolves through various stages. In the earliest phases, the inflammation appears as a subtle increase in the density of the fat. As fluid accumulates, it may fill tissue spaces until it develops well-defined margins. Although no formal study correlating the appearance with fluid composition has been made, it has been my perception that if the process becomes more severe, the density of the fluid increases. If the inflammatory fluid remains low in density or changes from high density to low density, it seems that resolution soon follows. The resolution of the edema and fluid collections may be complete, but some may remain as residual collections of enzymatic material, thereby creating pseudocysts (Figs. 32-57).

Although observations about the extent and nature of fluid distribution are important, the most important diagnostic signs that should be sought are those re-

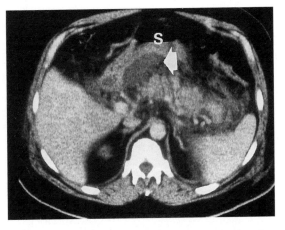

Fig. 32-55. CT scan performed after several weeks of severe inflammation shows progressive inflammation with fluid accumulation *(arrow)* in the lesser sac in front of the pancreas, behind the stomach *(S).*

lated to necrosis and possible infection. Both of these problems can have a devastating effect on patients if they are not treated promptly and correctly. A number of surgeons and clinicians, including Maier,[148] have stressed that both of these entities are accurate predictors of the ultimate outcome of severe pancreatitis and also have used them as indications for surgical intervention, as noted in the later section on necrosing pancreatitis.

Differentiating inflammatory mass from neoplasm. Thickening of the perirenal fascia is a nonspecific sign and can be associated with any entity that produces edema or obstructs the flow of lymphatics (e.g., masses,

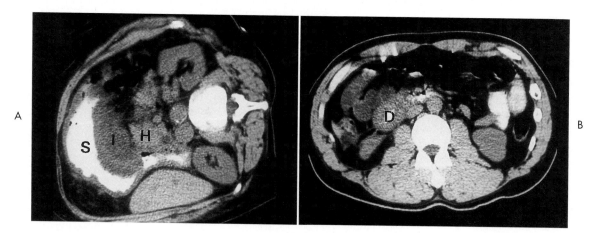

Fig. 32-56. A, CT scan of a patient in the decubitus position. Note the remarkable thickening of the posterior gastric wall *(I)* of the stomach *(S)* in front of the pancreas *(H)*. **B,** CT scan shows duodenum *(D)* with a thick wall owing to inflammatory edema.

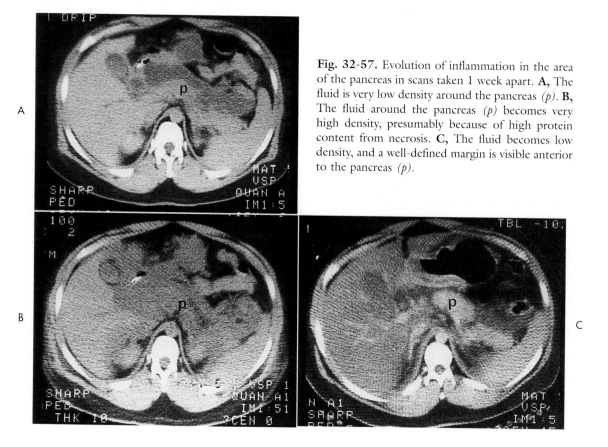

Fig. 32-57. Evolution of inflammation in the area of the pancreas in scans taken 1 week apart. **A,** The fluid is very low density around the pancreas *(p)*. **B,** The fluid around the pancreas *(p)* becomes very high density, presumably because of high protein content from necrosis. **C,** The fluid becomes low density, and a well-defined margin is visible anterior to the pancreas *(p)*.

infection). As a practical matter, however, thickening of the perirenal fascia is more common with inflammation in both the acute and chronic situation.[175] Published data have shown that thickening of the left perirenal fascia occurs infrequently in early pancreatic carcinoma. This is not an absolutely reliable finding because in occasional cases pancreatic cancer can be coexistent with inflammation. Another finding commonly confused as pathognomonic of neoplasm is loss of the perivascular fat plane; loss can occur with inflammation as well as neoplasm[131,136,170] (Fig. 32-58).

Differentiating tissue edema from fluid collection. When severe inflammation occurs, a large amount of edema occurs as well as the accumulation of fluid. Differentiation of these two entities can be made by looking for the presence of small "fat islands" within the fluid density. These areas represent intact areas of normal tissue and fat uninvolved with edema fluid, thereby distinguishing them from collections of liquefied tissue or fluid that may require drainage.

Spontaneous hemorrhage with acute pancreatitis. A sudden loss of blood sufficient enough to produce a sudden drop in a patient's hematocrit value can occur in an inflamed area. Such a sudden blood loss in the area of the pancreatic bed is easily detectable on CT as an increased density collection of material in the inflamed area (Fig. 32-59). This blood loss can result from a diffuse leakage of inflamed granulation tissue or a break in a vessel damaged by digestive enzymes. Hemorrhage associated with pancreatitis should not be confused with hemorrhagic pancreatitis, which has been used in the past to refer to severe or life-threatening pancreatitis.

From experience with CT procedures and surgical procedures, it is clear that virtually all fluid or inflammatory material obtained from an acute inflammatory process appears bloody regardless of the severity of the disease. The irrelevance of the hemorrhagic nature of inflammatory fluid was noted by both Isikoff et al[99] and Lawson and others.[132-134] They reported detecting high-density material believed to be blood in the inflammation associated with pancreatitis. Both authors noted that the finding was not consistently related to the severity of the disease, and Lawson stated, "There did not appear to be any correlation between the mortality, sever-

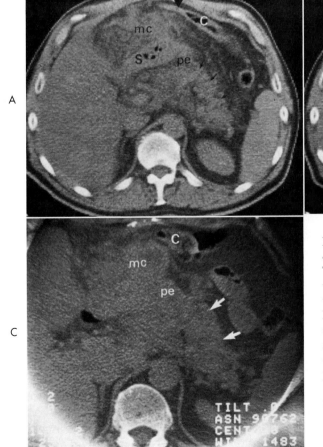

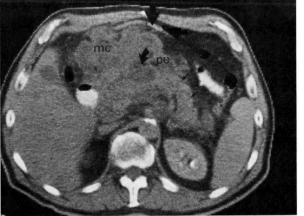

Fig. 32-58. **A,** Acute edematous pancreatitis produces significant edema in the peripancreatic fat *(pe)* and mesocolon *(mc).* The stomach *(S)* appears to be surrounded by the edema, and the colon *(C)* is narrowed *(large arrow)* where the inflammation is maximum. The pancreas is defined by the *small arrows.* **B,** Several weeks later, there is some resolution of the pancreatitis. Some edema has now decreased, and the inflammation in the mesocolon *(mc)* and peripancreatic area *(pe)* has now coalesced. Note the islands of fat *(curved arrow)* around the pancreas *(small arrows)* and the narrow colon *(large arrow).* **C,** In the last stages of resolution, the inflammation becomes a fibrotic mass in the mesocolon *(mc)* and peripancreatic area *(pe).* The pancreas is defined by *arrows.* The colon *(c)* has now resumed its normal caliber.

ity of the illness, or extent of retroperitoneal necrosis and the presence or absence of hemorrhage as observed at surgery."

Severe necrosing pancreatitis. Severe pancreatitis, regardless of the descriptive terms or the method of categorization, is a devastating disease with a reported

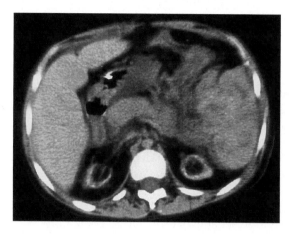

Fig. 32-59. Pancreatitis may be associated with severe spontaneous hemorrhage from simple granulation tissue or pseudoaneurysms. Note the large high-density hematoma in the left side of the abdomen.

mortality rate between 33% and 100%.[112,148,243] Before CT scanning, the objective assessment of the anatomical extent of pancreatic inflammation and the degree of involvement was difficult to confirm.[176]

Clinically, this entity has been virtually impossible to distinguish from severe edematous pancreatitis. Previously the most reliable method of assessing the severity of the disease was by carefully examining and correlating clinical signs and relevant serum laboratory tests, such as serum calcium, serum methemalbumin, and hematocrit. Paracentesis was occasionally performed to obtain fluid analysis. Data published by surgeons have shown that the standard clinical method for grading severity of disease, such as Ranson's criteria or the Apache II system, are neither good indicators for operative intervention nor for prognostication.

The most valuable diagnostic method for evaluating the status of the pancreas with severe inflammation is a good quality CT scan enhanced by adequate doses of intravenous contrast material, as noted in the technique section.[41,111,122,125] The normal gland shows considerable enhancement as a normal pancreatogram (Fig. 32-60). The devascularized or necrotic gland shows a lack of this enhancement in the focal area of necrosis. Furthermore, authors have shown that the larger the area

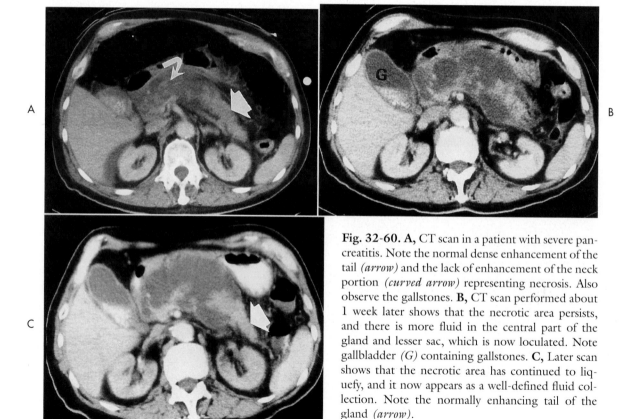

Fig. 32-60. A, CT scan in a patient with severe pancreatitis. Note the normal dense enhancement of the tail *(arrow)* and the lack of enhancement of the neck portion *(curved arrow)* representing necrosis. Also observe the gallstones. **B,** CT scan performed about 1 week later shows that the necrotic area persists, and there is more fluid in the central part of the gland and lesser sac, which is now loculated. Note gallbladder *(G)* containing gallstones. **C,** Later scan shows that the necrotic area has continued to liquefy, and it now appears as a well-defined fluid collection. Note the normally enhancing tail of the gland *(arrow)*.

of devascularized necrosis, the poorer the outcome of the patient, and there is a greater probability of secondary infection. The significance of this sign has been studied by several authors, but the importance of this finding was best demonstrated by Block and colleagues.[24] These authors studied the effectiveness of CT and ultrasound procedures versus clinical staging for identifying pancreatic necrosis. The authors studied 93 patients in a prospective fashion, who subsequently had surgical exploration. They found that CT with enhancement was superior for detection of pancreatic necrosis. Ninety percent of cases of severe necrosis and 79% of those of minor necrosis were demonstrated with enhanced CT. Ultrasound failed to be diagnostic in 24% because of the presence of meteorism. Other observations made by these authors are also noteworthy. They noted that even with CT, there is the risk that the area of necrosis may be larger and that occasionally an avascular area may be ischemic but not necrotic. Maier[148] reported that the contrast-enhanced CT evaluation for pancreatic necrosis was a better indicator for surgery than any of the currently accepted clinical methods for grading severity of disease.

Once the diagnosis is made, a diversity of therapeutic regimens is recommended, including conservative management, sump drainage, and pancreatectomy. Serious complications, such as pancreatic abscess, pseudocyst, fistula formation, and endocrine and exocrine deficiency, can result. Despite the fact that diverging opinions on the modes of therapy can be found, all authors agree that expeditious, accurate diagnosis of the problem is needed.[122,237] Morbidity and mortality rates of severe pancreatitis are still high.

Distinguishing infected and sterile necrosis. Bittner and colleagues[22] and others[20,24,148] pointed out the importance of differentiating pancreatic abscesses (well-marginated fluid collections) from pancreatic necrosis and infected pancreatic necrosis. The outcome of pancreatitis does not depend on the amount or degree of inflammation but rather the presence or absence of infection. Although abscesses can usually be drained by percutaneous methods, infected necrosis requires surgical evacuation of all infected material and insertion of postoperative lavage of the lesser sac. Necrosis tends to become infected, and it is of critical importance that the presence of infection be detected.

The inflammatory material with necrotic material, blood, and enzymes is a good culture medium and has a high susceptibility for secondary infection.[9] Unfortunately, it is not possible to detect any transition from necrosis to infection based on the scan. Serial aspiration samples for culture must be obtained if an infectious process is suspected or if any air is present. In such cases, it is absolutely imperative that the diagnostic aspiration be completely and technically precise, without contamination from intestinal material; passage through bowel negates the reliability of the culture because false-positive findings may result, and, more important, contamination with the gastrointestinal contents may introduce an inoculation, which can result in infection. (It might be hypothesized that one could distinguish between contami-

Table 32-2. Early prognostic signs of acute pancreatitis*

Admissions or diagnosis	Initial 48 hours
Over 55 years of age	Hematocrit falls more than 10%
White blood cell count over $16 \times 10^3/\mu l$ ($16 \times 10^9/L$)	Blood urea nitrogen level rises more than 5 mg/dl (1.79 mmol/L)
Blood glucose level over 200 mg/dl (11 mmol/L)	Serum calcium level falls below 8 mg/dl (2 mmol/L)
Serum lactic dehydrogenase level over 350 μ/ml	Arterial Po_2 below 60 mm Hg (7.98 kPa)
Serum glutamate oxaloacetate transminase level over 250 μ/ml	Base deficit greater than 4 mEq/L (4 mmol/L)
	Estimated fluid sequestration more than 6000 ml (6 L)

*Each sign counts as 1 for score.
From Balthazar EJ, et al: Acute pancreatitis: prognostic value of CT. *Radiology* 156:767, 1985.

Table 32-3. Relationship between prognostic signs and clinical course

No. of patients	Prognostic signs*	Average fasting days	Average days hospitalized	No. of abscesses	No. of deaths with abscess
56	0-2	16.4	24.6	7 (12.5%)	—
22	3-5	28.9	40.6	7 (31.8%)	2 (9.1%)
5	6-8	39.7	48.0	4 (80.0%)	3 (60%)

*See Table 32-2 for signs.
From Balthazar EJ, et al: Acute pancreatitis: prognostic value of CT. *Radiology* 156:767, 1985.

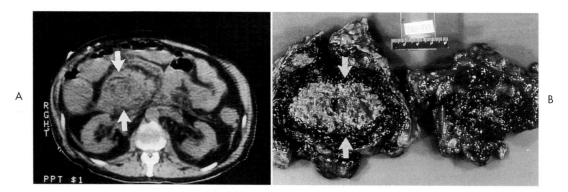

Fig. 32-61. A, Patient with fatal pancreatitis has a well-defined mass *(arrows)* with the appearance of a "capsule." **B,** Pathologic section shows a thick, edematous gland with a thick, inflammatory wall *(arrows).*

nation and infection in the culture results because of the mixed colonic flora obtained. This is incorrect because most authors believe the major source of infection is from small gastrointestinal fistulaes.)

Staging or predicting outcome. With the seriousness of pancreatitis and the difficulty in predicting the outcome, several authors have attempted to devise a method for predicting the outcome of patients with pancreatitis. One imaging approach developed by Balthazar and others[13-15] parallels the Ranson's criteria and has been somewhat useful for staging the inflammatory process in a slightly different fashion than the simple method of looking for necrosis.[13,15]

Balthazar et al devised the following grading system based on CT findings: A, normal pancreas; B, focal or diffuse enlargement of the gland (includes nonhomogeneous attenuation of gland, dilatation of duct, and foci of fluid within the gland, as long as there is no extrapancreatic edema); C, peripancreatic edema and intrinsic abnormalities of grade B; D, single ill-defined fluid collections or phlegmon; and E, two or more fluid collections or the presence of gas. Balthazar and associates found the hospital course corresponded closely to their findings. Abscess occurred in 21.6% of all patients and 80% of patients with grade E pancreatitis. The authors also point out the use of CT to pick up associated findings, such as gallstones and peritoneal and pleural fluid. All deaths occurred in grades C, D, and E, with the majority in grade E.

The authors also noted that the longer the hospital stay, the higher the grade. Patients with grade A stayed 13 days; grade B, 17 days; grade C, 25 days; grade D, 31 days; and grade E, 52 days. They also found a correlation between CT findings and the clinical prognostic signs previously described by Ransom; the signs are listed in Tables 32-2 and 32-3.

This information provides a mechanism for effec-

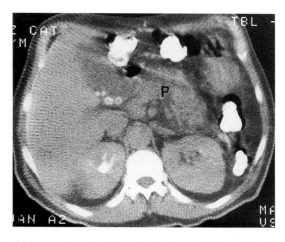

Fig. 32-62. Patient who died within 24 hours after admission and 8 hours after this study has minimal signs of inflammatory disease around the pancreas *(P),* despite the fact that the cause of death was pancreatitis.

tively communicating in a concise fashion the severity of a patient's inflammation. This system, however, does not always correctly predict the outcome.

Despite these attempts to predict and manage acute situations, the outcomes are remarkably different from expectations. Sometimes disease with fairly benign-appearing inflammation can have a precipitous course (Figs. 32-61 and 32-62). Conversely, individuals with more anatomically extensive disease can do well.

Presence of infection

Relative to infection, many authors have noted that no imaging method can differentiate the presence or absence of infection. The only effective way to determine the presence or absence of infection is to perform a diagnostic aspiration for culture, as discussed in Chapter 46. Several short comments are appropriate. CT is extremely well suited to perform these aspirations because of its ability to detect fluid collections and guide diagnostic aspirations accurately. During such procedures, several technical points are relevant. It is always prudent to perform an intense bolus injection to demonstrate any pseudoaneurysms that might be present. The trajectory planning of any diagnostic aspiration should be made to avoid intestinal loops because contamination of the needle could result in a spurious culture result or potentially a contamination of any fluid collection. Finally, one should realize that infection is a dynamic event and may occur during different phases of the pancreatic inflammation. Repeat diagnostic aspirations should be performed whenever there is a consideration of infection; spontaneous development of infection can occur at any time, so a negative prior aspiration is meaningless.

Once infection has been discovered, proper management is critical because it is a consensus among authors that the outcome of infected pancreatitis depends on effective drainage. In a limited number of cases, percutaneous methods may work if a fluid collection is well confined and contains very thin material. In many cases, patient survival is contingent on effective surgical drainage.[27,28,222]

Emphysematous pancreatitis

Emphysematous pancreatitis is a diagnostic term originating from plain-film radiography that describes a life-threatening pyogenic infection of the pancreas caused by gas-forming bacteria. When applied to CT imaging, however, the term describes a wide spectrum of pathological disorders, some of which are severe and some of which are benign and self-limited.

Gas-forming pyogenic infection superimposed on pancreatitis can result from a variety of causes, including spontaneous, hematogenously seeded colonization from gastrointestinal fistula or secondarily from surgical procedure (usually cystotomy). The most common organisms to produce gas are the *Escherichia coli, Enterobacter aerogenes,* and *Clostridia.* The most infamous of these bacteria are the *E. coli,* which classically produce emphysematous pancreatitis associated with a high mortality rate in diabetic patients. Because plain-film radiography has a much lower contrast resolution than CT, it is virtually impossible to detect gas in the pancreas in an early phase of development on plain-film radiography. Conversely, the slightest amount of gas can be detected with CT; the presence of gas caused by a multitude of disorders is thereby possible.

With the advent of CT with its superlative axial anatomical images and contrast resolution, the diagnosis of gas in the pancreas has become much easier from a detection standpoint but more complex because of the

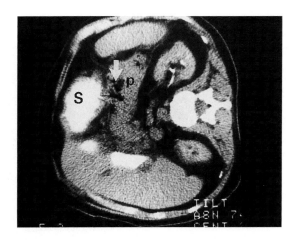

Fig. 32-63. Patient with air *(arrow)* in the pancreas *(p)* posterior to the stomach *(s)*. This was a benign form of emphysematous pancreatitis.

multitude of various entities that can be seen and must be differentiated.

A number of authors[162] have noted that there may be a discrepancy between the imaging appearance of the gland compared with the clinical appearance in many cases of emphysematous pancreatitis. A high percentage of cases of emphysematous pancreatitis have resolved without aggressive treatment by drainage (Fig. 32-63). In a smaller percentage, some cases have a disastrous outcome, regardless of adequate treatment (Fig. 32-64).

In most seriously ill patients with emphysematous changes, there are significant associated problems, such as a gastrointestinal fistula,[9,184] which may have developed because of an ulcer,[147] perforation, or another problem (Fig. 32-65). Such patients may do well temporarily, but most eventually develop sepsis and do poorly unless proper expeditious drainage and correction of the basic problem is made. In the case illustrated, the patient initially appeared well, and the clinical physicians were not convinced of his serious situation until he suffered cardiorespiratory collapse. While on a respirator and supported with vasopressive agents, the patient underwent percutaneous drainage, which effected a cure.

The cause of the gas in patients who do well is in question. Two plausible hypotheses explain these observations. The first explanation is that the gas is a byproduct of necrosis. The gas may be nitrogen or another gaseous material, not from gas-forming bacteria but from tissue necrosis. An alternate theory, which I propose, is that the gas is produced by gas-forming organisms or from a small gastrointestinal fistula that closed spontaneously that may or may not adversely affect the patient, depending on his or her immune status. I have scanned

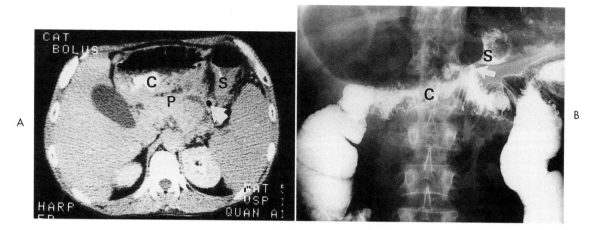

Fig. 32-64. A, Scan with gas *(arrow)* anterior to the pancreas *(P)*, posterior to the stomach *(S)*, and close to the colon *(C)*. Note also the fluid adjacent to the pancreas and the air. **B,** Barium enema shows a fistula *(arrow)* between the colon *(C)* and the stomach *(S)*.

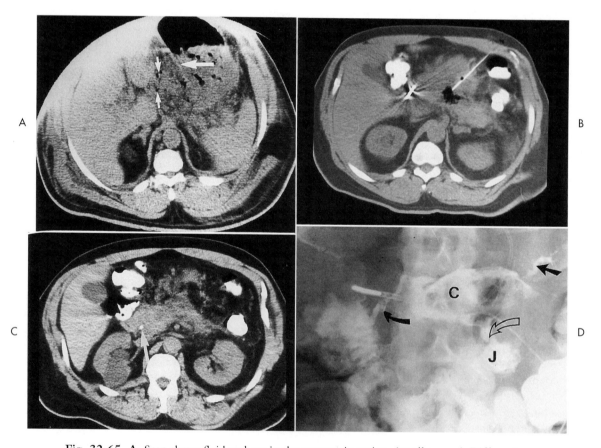

Fig. 32-65. A, Scan shows fluid and gas in the pancreatic region *(small arrows)*. Differentiation from gastric contents is best made by noting the location of the gastric wall *(large arrow)*. **B,** Follow-up scan after drainage shows a small collection of air that was aspirated under CT and injected with contrast material. **C,** Lower scan shows a calcification *(arrow)*, which retrospectively proved to be a calculus in the duct. **D,** Sinogram shows a fistula *(open arrow)* between the jejunum *(J)* and the cavity *(C)*. The dilated pancreatic duct *(arrow)* and the calculus in the proximal duct *(curved arrow)* can also be seen.

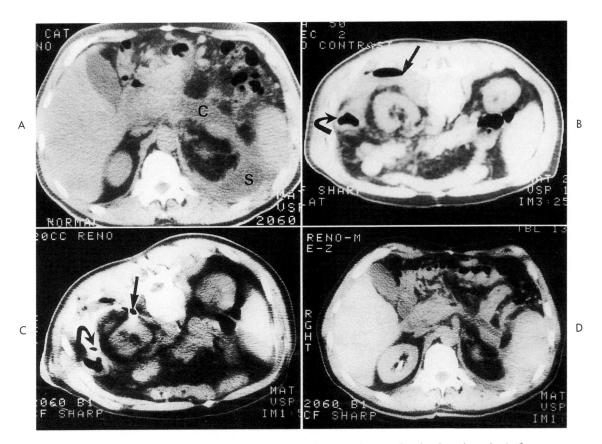

Fig. 32-66. A, Baseline CT scan of a patient with a pseudocyst who developed a colonic fistula. This scan shows a pseudocyst *(C)* with an extension to the splenorenal ligament *(S)*. **B,** Repeat scan 2 days later with the patient prone shows air *(arrow)* in the posterior fluid collection and fluid extending around the colon *(curved arrow)*. **C,** After diagnostic puncture, contrast injection goes to the medial side of the retroperitoneal cavity *(arrow)* and into the colon *(curved arrow)*. (Patient is prone.) Aspirated material was purulent, and culture was positive for mixed flora. Plain film showed fistula to colon. **D,** Follow-up study (with the patient supine) shows resolution of most fluid and all the air. The patient did well with short-term antibiotics and no drainage; long-term follow-up of several years confirmed resolution.

several patients with gas in the pancreas produced by pyogenic organisms who have recovered without surgery or antibiotics. The presence of pyogenic bacteria in both cases was proved by diagnostic aspiration, which was obtained by an aseptic method (avoiding bowel) (Fig. 32-66).

The outcome in these patients probably depends on their immune status. Some patients who have a competent immune system can handle a borderline colonization or infection from their own flora. Those who are immunocompromised or become debilitated are unable to mobilize or sustain the competence of the immune system to handle the infection. Such patients become severely ill and can even die.

Management. The management and disposition of patients who have emphysematous pancreatitis should be made based on clinical, laboratory, and imaging data. First, it is important to ensure clear communication between the internist, surgeon, and radiologist. Close cooperation ensures that all physicians are aware of any change in clinical status or imaging appearance so adjustment in patient care can be made without delay.

There does not appear to be any controversy about the best treatment for symptomatic patients with gas. These patients require early surgical or percutaneous drainage of infected areas around the pancreas. The methods for draining such areas are discussed in Chapter 46.

In asymptomatic patients, aspiration should be performed under CT guidance at the earliest time, with careful avoidance of intestinal loops or bowel (assuming that other causes of gas have been excluded) (see follow-

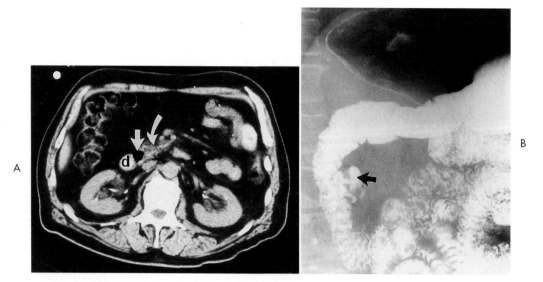

Fig. 32-67. A, Duodenal diverticulum *(straight arrow)* appears as a well-defined air collection adjacent to the duodenum *(d)*. In this example, the diverticulum is between the duodenum and the uncinate portion of the pancreas *(curved arrow),* but in other examples, it may appear intrapancreatic. **B,** Barium study shows the diverticulum *(arrow).*

ing section). Careful avoidance of bowel loops is important if the culture of the sample is to be valid. The sample obtained must be free of bowel contents. Second, enteric bacteria must not be introduced into a pancreatic fluid collection; such a contaminant could result in an abscess if the pyogenic bacteria grew.

Management of asymptomatic patients should be based on the results of the culture. If the culture is negative, observation and a repeat CT examination should be performed until the gas disappears. Any clinical or CT sign of deterioration should result in a re-evaluation, and surgery should be considered.

If resolution of the gas does not occur within 1 week, repeat aspiration should be performed to make sure there was not a sampling or handling error made on the first sample.

If the culture is positive, several separate courses of action can be taken. First, if the sample aspirated is culture positive, the proper antibiotic medication should be chosen and surgical drainage considered. If the patient is a poor surgical candidate (Fig. 32-65), a percutaneous procedure may be performed to stabilize the patient. This permits a decrease in the "toxic load" and, it is hoped, stabilization of homeostasis (e.g., nutrition, cardiovascular system). If the patient remains stable on antibiotic medications and the emphysematous appearance on the CT scan resolves, no further intervention is required. If the patient improves generally but the gas remains, further investigation is required to determine the origin of the infection (e.g., penetrating ulcer or gastrointestinal fistula).

Other causes of gas. One of most common benign causes of gas in the pancreas is a duodenal diverticulum. The air collection is usually single, well defined, and located just medial to the second portion of the duodenum or in the lower portion of the uncinate process just cephalad to the third portion of the duodenum (Fig. 32-67). The diverticulum may contain a fluid level or even barium if an oral contrast agent is given.

A penetrating ulcer has one of two appearances. If the ulcer penetration seals, only a single minute collection of gas in the pancreas just adjacent to the duodenal or stomach wall can usually be seen. In some cases, edema of the wall can be seen. If a large penetration has occurred and it is not sealed, there may be a large amount of air scattered throughout the omental bursa.

Gastrointestinal fistula also produces air in and adjacent to the pancreas. The gas is ill defined and closely related to the stomach, jejunum, duodenum, or colon. It is difficult to ascertain the origin of the fistula on the CT scan; contrast studies of the bowel and injection after drainage are most useful.

Other common causes for benign gas in the pancreas are iatrogenic and are usually the result of a recent or remote surgery or interventional procedure. Peustow procedures (enterostomy to the duct) or papillotomy can produce gas in the duct. Patients who have had internal drainage procedures on pseudocysts (e.g., cystogastrostomies) can have variable amounts of gas and fluid in the cavity (Fig. 32-68, *A*). Immunocompromised patients have a long delay in the healing of such cavities (Fig. 32-68, *B*). Occasionally, some asymptomatic elderly patients

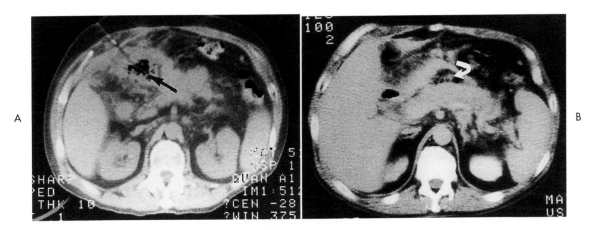

Fig. 32-68. A, Immunocompromised patients require a long period even after surgical drainage before the pseudocyst cavity closes well. The cavity contains a large amount of fluid and air *(arrow)* that could be mistaken for an abscess; sinogram showed enteric anastomosis as intact. **B,** Repeat study after removal of the internal drain shows a small residual cavity *(arrow)* containing minimal air and fluid.

have a patulous sphincter, and spontaneous reflux of air into the ductal system occurs.

PANCREATIC ABSCESS

Pancreatic abscesses are a severe, life-threatening problem if not correctly treated. As has been noted previously, the outcome of pancreatic inflammation occasionally depends on the presence or absence of infection. Pyogenic infection of the pancreas can be caused by a variety of organisms introduced by different mechanisms.

Virtually any organism can infect the pancreas,[50] but most are bacteria or fungi from the gastrointestinal tract. These include many gram-negative and gram-positive organisms and *Candida albicans.* Hurley and Vargish[97] showed a significant difference between those infections caused by different organisms. In their series, gram-negative infections were polymicrobial and had a high mortality, whereas those that were gram-positive were monomicrobial and had a low mortality. (In immunocompetent patients, primary infection from *Candida* probably does not occur; it is probably opportunistic initially after treatment with broad-spectrum antibiotics.) If the causative organism is not gas forming, the appearance of fluid on the CT study is industinguishable from a typical case of suppurative or hemorrhagic pancreatitis.[54] If there is any question of possible infection in a patient, a percutaneous diagnostic aspiration should be performed.

The mechanisms for introduction of the infection are the same as for emphysematous pancreatitis, and they include hematogenous seeding, lymphatic spread, gastrointestinal performation or fistula,[90] or an iatrogenic response from some type of procedure. Hematogenous seeding is most likely to occur superimposed on a gland that has some type of baseline problem, such as pancreatic necrosis. It is our impression that patients who have large amounts of fluid around the colon are at risk for infection because of possible lymphatic or venous seeding from enteric flora.

Iatrogenic causes of abscess can also occur after surgical drainage procedures, ERCP,[50] or percutaneous instrumentation. After an internal drainage procedure during which a stoma between a cyst and a loop of bowel has been created, colonization of the pseudocysts by enteric flora occurs. In most instances, this colonization does not create a problem, but if there is an anatomical region that does not freely communicate with the bowel, a local accumulation of material can result in an abscess. Considering the number of bacteria involved, it is actually surprising that more infections do not occur.

Abscesses caused by other pathogens

In addition to the typical bacteria that cause abscesses, fungi, tuberculosis,[38,218] parasites, and other pathogens[134] can also cause abscesses. In such patients, especially if percutaneous cultures are to be obtained, proper handling of the material for culture must be ensured. Experience shows that the appearance of abscesses is nonspecific except for *Echinococcus.* All abscesses appear as fluid collections with variable density depending on the amount of blood and debris. With echinococcal disease, daughter cysts should be visible.[7,249] Also, with acquired immunodeficiency syndrome (AIDS) patients, one can expect a variety of unusual opportunistic pathogens. Lederman[135] had a patient with toxoplasmosis microabscesses of the pancreas. Sarcoidosis of the pancreas has also been reported by Sagalow et al.[200]

PSEUDOCYSTS

Pseudocysts are a fluid collection consisting of necrotic material, proteinaceous debris, and enzymatic material that is confined by a fibrous capsule. The term *pseudocyst* notes the difference between it and other fluid collections within the pancreas that are true cysts (with an endothelial lining) or retention cysts (with a ductal cell lining).[201]

The exact pathogenesis is not well understood, especially the initiating process, but it is well known that a pseudocyst can result from any significant inflammatory process. It can result from either acute or chronic inflammation or acute injury such as trauma. Some authors believe that the fluid in such pseudocysts results from tissue damage, whereas others believe it results from the rupture of ductal elements that contribute significant amounts of pancreatic secretions. Obviously both processes must occur, and the cause has no impact on detection, therapy, or prognosis.

Pseudocysts are unique entities because of the protean manifestations they can produce, the many locations in which they can appear, and the many complications[19,25,28] with which they can be associated. The location and size of the cyst can produce symptoms and problems for the patient, but the complications can be life-threatening. With prompt adequate treatment, most pseudocysts can be treated effectively.

Symptoms associated with pseudocysts depend on the amount and degree of pancreatitis and the size and speed of their growth. Patients may have significant, ill-defined pain associated with pancreatitis and have small pseudocysts. Large pseudocysts can cause pain secondary to the inflammatory process, displacement of or effect on adjacent structures, or the amount of pressure within such pseudocysts.

Some patients show an evolution of pseudocysts over sequential examinations, first showing a large amount of edema in the area of the pancreas, which usually obscures the margin of the gland and extends into various adjacent areas (Fig. 32-69, *A*). As the inflammation resolves, the fluid may coalesce into a well-defined pseudocyst with a clearly defined wall (Fig. 32-69, *B*). In other patients, the pseudocyst appears to evolve from necrosis within the pancreas. The necrosis begins as a subtle area of low density and progresses to a well-defined cavity.

The administration of intravenous urographic contrast material enhances the margins of such collections and makes the central portion appear less dense. Because of the high-protein content of such pseudocysts, the density may appear high, and the appreciation of the cystic nature may not be apparent without intravenous contrast material.

Anatomical location

Pseudocysts are typically located in the pancreas and the immediate peripancreatic region. They can be associated with other severe or minimal findings of pancreatitis (Fig. 32-70). In some cases, however, pseudocysts may extend to more remote anatomical areas, by dissection along or through fascial planes, along areolar tissue around vessels (intermesenteric space according to a new concept of retroperitoneum; see Chapter 36), through capsules, or into the substance of solid organs.

The omental bursa is the second most common location of pseudocysts, according to Siegelman and associates.[211] The inflammation causes closure of Winslow's foramen, and the fluid fills the entire omental bursa or is confined to a local region of the bursa.[129]

When located in the inferior portion of the omen-

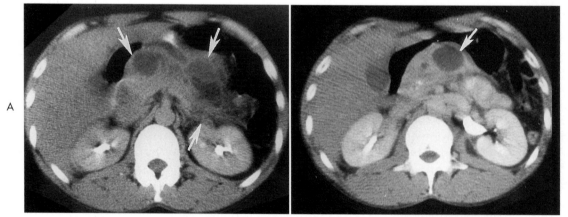

Fig. 32-69. A, CT scan performed early in the patient's course shows diffuse edema and fluid accumulation around the entire gland as defined by the arrows. **B,** CT scan performed at a later time shows resolution of most of the edema fluid, but there is a residual, well-defined fluid collection that has become a pseudocyst *(arrow).*

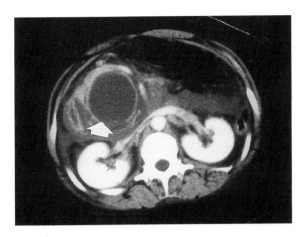

Fig. 32-70. Well-defined pseudocyst *(arrow)* in the head, which has increased enhancement in the wall.

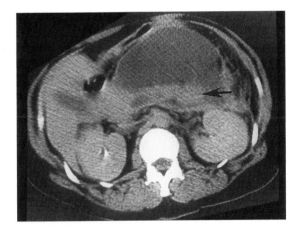

Fig. 32-71. Large pseudocyst that actually contains part of the pancreas *(arrow)*.

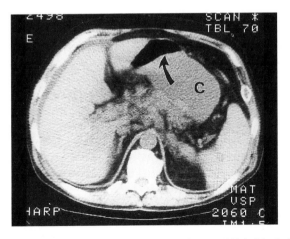

Fig. 32-72. Patient with a large pseudocyst *(C)* behind the stomach that was initially mistaken for fluid-filled fundus. The *arrow* points to an indentation of cyst on the posterior wall of the stomach; note that the level would be even if this were fluid in the stomach. The patient was too ill for oral contrast administration.

tal bursa, pseudocyts produce anterior displacement of the body and antrum of the stomach. When located in the splenic portion of the inferior recess, they produce anterior displacement of the fundus (Fig. 32-71). Those extending into the superior medial recess of the lesser sac lie adjacent to the caudate lobe of the liver. In such cases, it is important to use oral contrast material or the decubitus position because the pseudocyst can be mistaken for fluid-filled stomach or duodenum.

If the patient is too ill for these technique modifications, a large pseudocyst might be confused for the distended fundus of the stomach.[160] If adequate intravenous contrast material is given, the gastric wall enhances, permitting distinction from the wall of the pseudocyst. Pseudocysts located in splenic recess may reveal themselves by producing a circular interface with the air in the stomach rather than the normal level air-fluid interface (bezoar, retained food, or gastric mass may give similar appearance) (Fig. 32-72).

If a pseudocyst is large and has an aggressive behavior, it may erode from the lesser bursa into adjacent contiguous areas. Extending inferiorly, it may split the leaves of the omentum, producing a mass that projects below the surface of the stomach in an anterior position

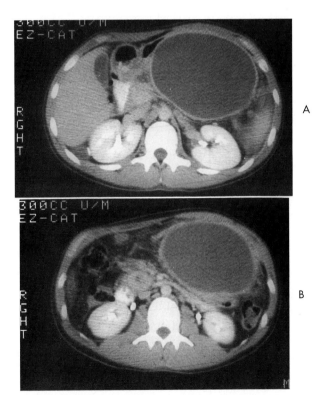

Fig. 32-73. A, Pseudocyst in the greater omentum begins at the margin of the stomach and projects caudally below the stomach. **B,** The pseudocyst below the stomach is located anteriorly within the abdomen rather than in the root of the mesentery.

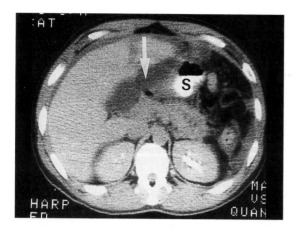

Fig. 32-74. Inflammatory fluid may digest through the bursal lining into the hepatogastric ligament and collect in the sub-capsular area of the left lobe *(arrow)*. Contrast-filled stomach *(S)* is anterior to the pancreas.

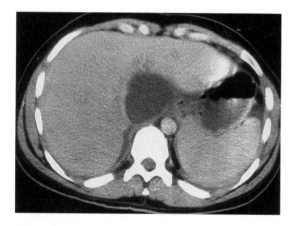

Fig. 32-75. Pseudocyst in the superior recess of the omental bursa. Note the left gastric artery adjacent to the stomach that demarcates the separation between the superior recess on the right and the remainder of the bursa.

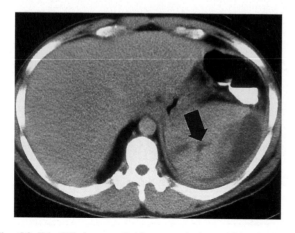

Fig. 32-76. CT shows a fluid accumulation within the hilum of the spleen *(arrow)*.

(Fig. 32-73). The inflammatory fluid may also digest through the lining of the omental bursa and dissect into the hepatogastric ligament and even beneath the capsule of the liver (Fig. 32-74). A pseudocyst may also proceed cephalad from the superior medial recess next to the caudate lobe into the posterior mediastinum[178] adjacent to the esophagus (Fig. 32-75).

As with the spread of material during the acute inflammatory phase, a pseudocyst may develop or digest through fascia[87,193] and capsules directly into a solid organ. This may occur in the spleen (Fig. 32-76), liver, or kidney (Fig. 32-77). Such pseudocysts can be diagnosed by knowing the patient's history or looking for signs of pancreatitis, but in many instances, diagnostic aspiration is required, as suggested by Baker and coworkers.[12]

Resolution

Spontaneous resolution of pseudocysts can occur simply from resorption of fluid or drainage into a loop of bowel. Both mechanisms are commonly observed. When evacuation into bowel occurs, there may be residual gas seen in the cyst or a small pathway between the cyst and the bowel loop (Figs. 32-78 and 32-79).

Beebe and colleagues[19] found that pseudocysts smaller than 4 cm in diameter were more likely to resolve spontaneously than those larger than 4 cm in diameter. Kolars and colleagues[124] studied pseudocysts and found that the outcome or recurrence did not depend on the size, multiplicity of pseudocysts, anatomical location, or communication with the pancreatic duct.

Complications

Pseudocysts must be treated because there are a number of severe complications that can occur. Pseudocysts can rupture into the peritoneum or a loop of bowel. Rupture into the peritoneum can be catastrophic, producing a generalized chemical peritonitis (Fig. 32-80, *A*). Rupture into a loop of bowel can be catastrophic or curative. The outcome probably depends on the loop of bowel that is entered, the degree of bacterial colonization, and the immune competence of the patient (Fig. 32-80, *B*). Rupture into colon is potentially more threatening than other bowel because of the nature of the gram-negative flora. Patients with an incompetent immune system or an overwhelming bacterial innoculum may succumb if prompt, effective treatment is not given.

Finally, hemorrhage can occur in association with a pseudocyst and can produce life-threatening loss of blood. Such bleeding may simply be from the inflamed wall, or pseudoaneurysms may occur in the wall as a result of enzymatic digestion (Figs. 32-81 and 32-82).

Pseudocysts with air: abscess or fistula

Gas in pseudocysts suggests the following possibilities: (1) fistula formation, (2) gas-forming infection,

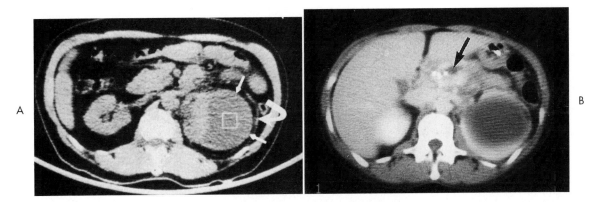

Fig. 32-77. A, Pseudocysts may cross the fascia into the perirenal space. This scan shows a large pseudocyst *(arrows)* in the perirenal space on the left side. **B,** Intrarenal pseudocyst is on the left. Note the associated calcification and duct dilatation in the pancreas *(arrow).*

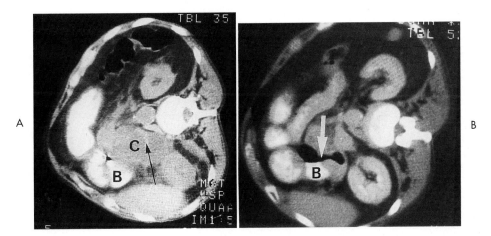

Fig. 32-78. A, Large retroperitoneal pseudocyst *(C)* around the vena cava *(arrow)*, which is located behind the duodenal bulb *(B)*. **B,** Follow-up study shows an "empty pseudocyst" containing air *(arrow)* beside the bulb *(B)*. Note the normal size of the vena cava.

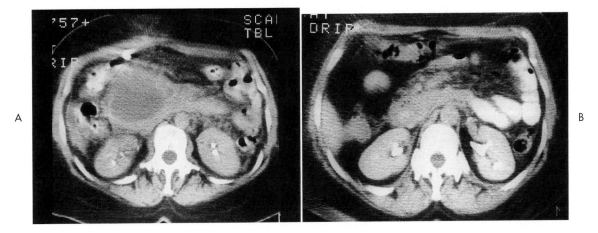

Fig. 32-79. A, CT scan shows a large pseudocyst in the head. **B,** Several weeks later, the pseudocyst has completely resolved, spontaneously. Hemachromatosis produces increased density of lymph nodes owing to retained iron *(arrow).*

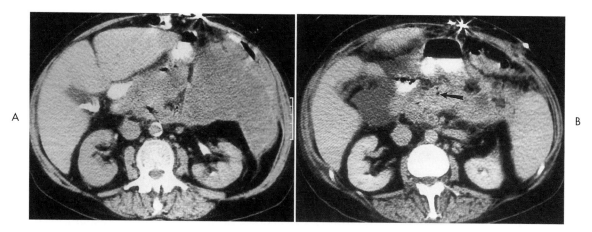

Fig. 32-80. **A,** CT scan showing large fluid collection in left side of abdomen after rupture of pseudocyst. **B,** Scan showing small gas bubble *(arrow)* within fluid collection in the pancreatic bed; aspiration subsequently showed this area to be infected.

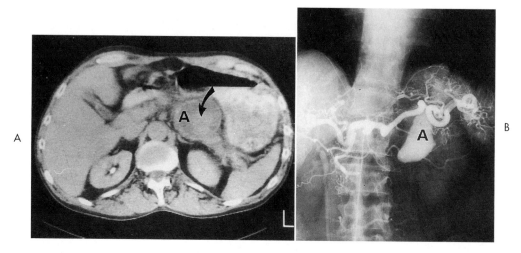

Fig. 32-81. **A,** CT scan shows a low-density mass *(A)* with a central, high-density region *(arrow)* that represents a pseudoaneurysm of the splenic artery. **B,** Angiogram shows the large pseudoaneurysm *(A)* coming from the splenic artery.

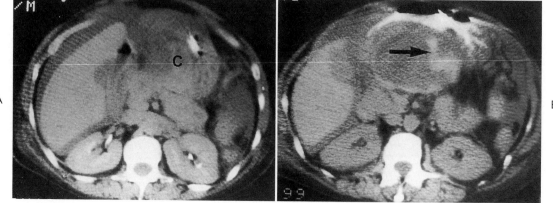

Fig. 32-82. **A,** Baseline scan of a patient who developed hemorrhage shows an ill-defined pseudocyst *(C)* behind the stomach. **B,** Emergency follow-up scan shows enlargement of cyst and hemorrhage *(arrow)* inside.

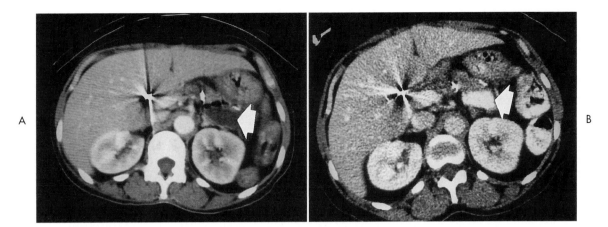

Fig. 32-83. A, Appropriate surgery for pseudocysts is gastrocystotomy. Scan shows fluid-filled and air-filled cavity *(arrow)* behind the stomach. **B,** Subsequent scan shows contrast material *(arrow)* filling the cyst cavity, indicating nature of cavity and communication with stomach. Note the high-density suture line between the stomach and cyst.

(3) surgically produced internal cystotomy (Fig. 32-83), and (4) any combination of these three.

There are several reports in the literature that provide useful insights into gas in pseudocysts. Torres et al,[235] Alexander et al,[3] and Petrushak et al[184] have reported seeing gas in pseudocysts from gastrointestinal fistulaes. A common observation is that patients who have gas in pseudocysts should be evaluated to determine the type, size, and nature of the fistula. In some patients, the fistula can be found before surgery by radiological methods, but in other patients it may be detectable only at surgery.

Depending on the site of the fistula, treatment may be easy or difficult. In most patients, a traditional bowel study using water-soluble iodinated contrast or a barium sulfate contrast suffices (i.e., upper or lower study). In other patients, it may be helpful to perform a percutaneous aspiration for a diagnostic sample, drainage, or sinogram (see Fig. 32-65).

Fistulaes occurring in the stomach or duodenum may drain a pseudocyst effectively, and surgical intervention may not be needed. In patients who have fistulaes in the colon, the prognosis is not so good because colonic pathogens are more likely to cause serious infections and sequelae; traditional surgical method requires immediate debridement and bowel diversion in this case. The circumstances of each patient must be considered, however, because rarely some may tolerate a colonic fistula and not require surgery (see Fig. 32-66). The following factors determine the outcome of such a problem: the immune status of the patient, the size and nature of the fistula, innoculum size, and virulence of the pathogens. Healthy immunocompetent patients may tolerate such events well, and immunocompromised patients may not.

Vascular problems

Pancreatitis and pseudocysts can cause a number of vascular problems, including vascular occlusion, pseudoaneurysms, and spontaneous hemorrhage.

Occlusion of many vessels but most commonly the splenic vein and artery can occur. In such cases, only the secondary effects, such as varice formation or shrinkage of the spleen, may be seen.

Pseudoaneurysms occur in pancreatitis in 10% of patients as a result of enzymatic digestion of the vessel wall. Proper diagnosis and treatment are important because hemorrhage is associated with bleeding 37% of the time.[23,181,227] Pseudoaneurysms can occur in any vessel in the peripancreatic area, but the most common vessel is the splenic, followed by the gastroduodenal[163] and branches of the pancreaticoduodenal arteries.[30,32,219] In some patients, diagnosis of a pseudoaneurysm is not made prospectively, but the patients have acute hemorrhage associated with a pseudocyst.

Sometimes a clearly definable pseudoaneurysm in the area of the pancreas can be confused with a pseudocyst.[137,210] Careful scrutiny of the CT scan shows a circular area of low density, which may correspond to a clot within the aneurysm. Because of the potential for such pseudoaneurysms, it is imperative that a dynamic intravenous study be performed before any interventional procedure[26] (Fig. 32-82).

Natural history of pseudocysts

The natural history of undisturbed pseudocysts has been extensively studied by several authors,[119] including Bradley and others[27,28] and Pollack and associates.[190] In their series, 54 patients had serial studies over many months; the authors were able to follow the outcomes accurately.

Of 54 patients who had serial, clinical, and sonographic evaluations, 10 (or 40%) had spontaneous resolution.[28] Five (20%) experienced complications, including abscess, rupture, and biliary obstruction. In patients with pseudocysts lasting 7 to 12 weeks, the number of spontaneous resolutions and the frequency of complications remained constant at 46% (6 of 13 cases). Spontaneous resolution did not occur in 12 patients observed between 13 and 18 weeks, but the rate of complication increased to 75% (8 of 12 cases). These complications included spontaneous rupture in five patients, secondary infection in one, obstructive jaundice with sepsis in another, and a spontaneous cystogastric fistula in another. This last patient died after massive gastrointestinal hemorrhage. Of five patients studied more than 19 weeks, three had complications and two did not complete follow-up. Seven deaths occurred as a direct result of the pseudocyst, and complications occurred on an average of 13½ weeks after initial development.

In another study by Pollack and associates,[190] similar findings were noted in a large group of 54 patients. The authors treated patients with nonoperative means until sepsis occurred or until the pseudocyst persisted more than 3 weeks. They found that 29 patients had elective surgery during the initial hospitalization, and 6 patients who did not undergo surgery developed abscesses and died.

Surgical treatment

Good information exists on selected surgical treatment based on pseudocyst evolution. Bradley and others[27,28] and Bodurtha and colleagues[25] have recommended that surgical intervention not be performed in the first 6 weeks because of the high incidence of spontaneous resolution. Furthermore, they recommend that treatment be deferred during this time because the inflammation usually does not have a well-defined fibrous wall that could hold sutures required for a cystogastrostomy. In such cases, external instead of internal drainage would be required. The external drainage has a high rate of infections, fistulae, and complications. Between 6 and 13 weeks, the pseudocyst wall becomes well defined; thus internal drainage is possible. If a pseudocyst is well defined and has a thick fibrous wall, internal drainage is indicated. Most authors concur that internal drainage by cystotomy is the preferred method of treatment because it has the greatest success rate and the lowest complication and recurrence rate. Waiting longer than 13 weeks creates a greater risk for spontaneous complications.

As one might anticipate, radiological procedure development paralleled the surgical experience. Initial methods of external drainage were used with some success, but these methods had problems similar to the surgical ones. More recently, certain radiological methods have had some successes.

Imaging follow-up of internal drainage

Patients who have an internal drainage procedure show a consistent pattern of resolution on CT scan. Initially the pseudocyst appears as a total fluid density, but immediately after surgery it contains air. As long as patency with the bowel exists, such cysts fill with gastrointestinal contrast material. With further resolution, the amount of air and fluid lessens (Fig. 32-83). Patients who do not promptly have resolution should be suspected of having an abscess caused by colonized bacteria that have sequestered a portion of the pseudocyst.

CHRONIC PANCREATITIS

Once the acute phase of pancreatitis has resolved, the pancreas may return to normal. Chronic changes may occur, however, resulting in persistent or permanent alterations in the pancreatic function or morphological features.

Pathologically, fibrosis and scarring may alter the morphological characteristics and density of the parenchyma and duct system.[153] The entire gland may be affected, but only a focal area may be involved. Focal changes may occur in the acinar or ductal portions and may involve the deposit of calcium salts.

Clinically the patient may have chronic symptoms of upper abdominal pain, back pain, steatorrhea, diabetes, or recurrent inflammation. Diagnosis of chronic pancreatitis is important because a plausible explanation for a number of clinical signs can be given if its presence can be documented on scanning. Furthermore, a more definite statement about the presence of new findings can be made if it is known that a patient has had previous pancreatitis. In such cases, comparison scans are important.

Diagnostic signs

In chronic pancreatitis, the overall size of the gland may be normal, enlarged, or reduced, depending on the amount of fibrosis, atrophy, and degree of activity of the inflammation.[56] Atrophy or reduction of the size of the gland, similar to the enlargement, can occur in either a diffuse or focal fashion (Fig. 32-84). In addition to these findings, the thickening of the renal fascia, which is seen in the acute form of the disease, may become chronic (Fig. 32-85, 32-86). Chronic fibrosis can produce loss of the fat plane around the vessels and can be mistaken for tumor encasement.[11,107,145] Chronic pancreatitis is usually associated with intermittent episodes of recurrent inflammation, which can produce alterations on the baseline appearance of a diseased gland.

Acute edema and swelling may be superimposed on the fibrotic gland and fluctuate with the activity of the disease. With resolution of the acute process, follow-up studies show a return to the baseline appearance. If reduction of the mass does not occur or if the

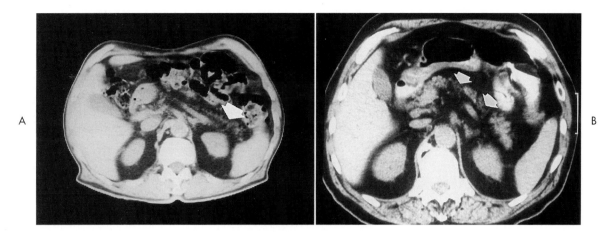

Fig. 32-84. A, Chronic inflammation may result in complete atrophy of the glandular elements so the only residual is a faint pattern of the ductal system *(arrow).* **B,** Atrophy of the glandular system may occur in segmental areas *(arrows)* rather than the entire gland.

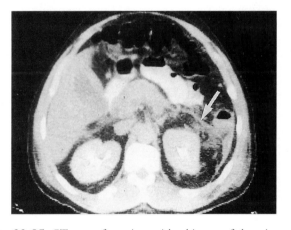

Fig. 32-85. CT scan of a patient with a history of chronic pancreatitis shows thickening of the renal fascia *(arrow).*

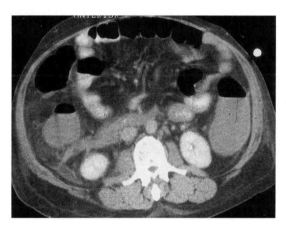

Fig. 32-86. CT scan shows thickening of right renal fascia secondary to subacute pancreatitis.

mass increases in size, a coexisting neoplasm must be considered. A percutaneous biopsy should be performed. If the biopsy is negative and follow-up studies show no definitive progress, one can accept the premise that the chronic inflammation is establishing a new baseline with an increased size.

Calcifications. The hallmark of chronic inflammation is the deposition of calcium.[202,239] With inflammation and necrosis in the pancreas, the local chemical changes produce the deposit of calcium carbonate and calcium phosphate. The deposit of calcium salts can be variable in location and amount. Most commonly, calcification first occurs in the head, but with continued inflammation, calcification occurs in the body and tail. Calcifications can occur within the parenchymal or ductal portions; either area can be involved first (Fig. 32-86). It is important to note whether the duct is involved be-

cause various surgeons believe that relieving pancreatic duct obstruction may be beneficial to some patients.

Although the typical pattern is one of progressive deposit, it is possible to observe the reverse decalcification[8] (Fig. 32-87). This is a rare phenomenon, but it has been observed on plain radiographs as well as CT scans. Initially, decalcification was thought to indicate the development of a neoplasm, but authors have refuted this point. To our knowledge, decalcification is neither good nor bad. One should not mistake the change in configuration for calcification that can occur with changes in size of the gland (Fig. 32-88).

CT is the most sensitive of all radiographic procedures for detection and accurate localization of calcifications. A number of processes other than inflammation can produce calcifications, and some materials can simulate calcium. First, a variety of tumors produce calcifica-

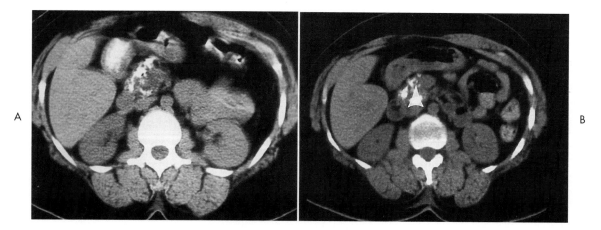

Fig. 32-87. A, Decalcification can occur rarely. This early scan shows dense calcium deposits within the head. **B,** Later scan demonstrates that the overall size of the gland has not changed, but the density of the anterior calcification *(arrow)* has decreased owing to decalcification.

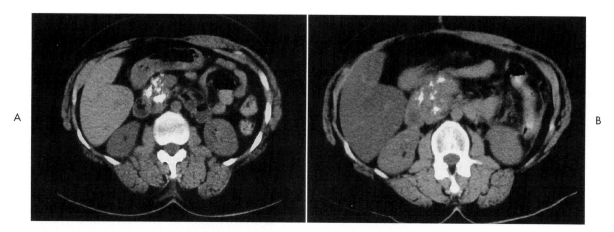

Fig. 32-88. A, CT scan before resumption of inflammation shows dense calcification within the head of the gland. **B,** Subsequent scan shows enlargement of the head of the gland, demonstrating that the calcifications have moved peripherally as the gland has enlarged.

tions in a large percentage of cases (see section on tumors). Second, the most common entity producing calcification in this area is probably arteriosclerotic changes in vessels or aneurysms. Finally, foreign bodies (swallowed objects, surgical sutures, catheters, or other devices) and iron-filled lymph nodes in hemachromatosis appear opaque and simulate calcification.

Pancreatic duct. The changes that occur in the pancreatic duct were discussed earlier. In summary, one can make some statement about the probability of malignancy or inflammation from the size and the configuration, but these relationships are not absolute. These factors depend on the benign or malignant nature of the process and the duration or completeness of the obstruction.

Frequency of signs in chronic disease. The frequency of these signs in pancreatitis has been extensively studied, but one of the better reviews of the findings related to chronic pancreatitis was by Luetmer and others.[145,146] These authors studied 56 consecutive patients with documented pancreatitis, without surgical intervention, who had contrast-enhanced CT scans. In their series, dilatation of the pancreatic duct was seen in 68% of the cases, pancreatic atrophy in 54%, pancreatic calcifications in 50%, fluid collections in 30%, focal enlargement in 30%, biliary dilatation in 29%, and fascial plane or perivascular fat changes in 16%. Although there has been some variation among the various reports in the frequency of these signs, the constellation of findings are all similar.

TRAUMA

Pancreatic trauma is common in patients with injury to the abdomen. The most common types of injury

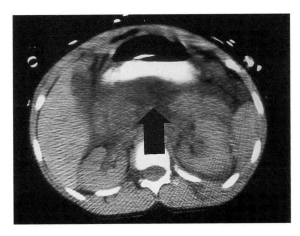

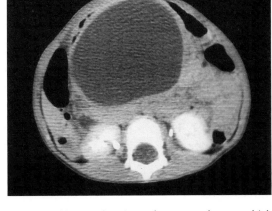

Fig. 32-89. Traumatic damage to the pancreas may be difficult to visualize. This scan shows a defect *(arrow)* in the midportion of the gland.

Fig. 32-90. CT scan showing a large pseudocyst, which has followed a severe injury to the gland.

include contusion, tear, or damage to the duct; late sequelae include pseudocysts, abscesses, or fistulaes. Because CT is a commonly used tool for early evaluation of abdominal injury, it is important to become familiar with its usefulness and limitations.[104,106-109,187]

The largest evaluation of the pancreas by CT was by Jeffrey and others.[106-109] In 13 cases, they found that CT was helpful for detecting some injury to the pancreas but was limited in determining the exact nature or extent of the problem (Fig. 32-89). They observed nonspecific thickening of the left anterior renal fascia in 8 of 11 cases. They were able to identify fracture or laceration of the gland in some cases, but the actual planes were not easy to visualize. ERCP is indicated if there is significant injury to the gland.

After acute injury to the pancreas and formation of a fluid collection with or without secondary infection, CT is well suited to detect and determine the extent of any such process (Fig. 32-90).

MISCELLANEOUS DISORDERS
Hereditary pancreatitis

Hereditary pancreatitis is relapsing pancreatitis among multiple family members. The symptoms, signs, and pathophysiological process of this type of pancreatitis are no different from the other types of pancreatitis discussed. It has been suggested but unproved that factors such as hyperlipidemia, hypercalcemia, and alcohol consumption may play a role in this disease. There are, however, two unique traits of the disease: (1) The onset is typically in children around the age of 10 years, and (2) there are usually calcifications within the gland in both the parenchyma and the duct system.[17,204,217] Reportedly calcification in the duct system occurs more commonly than parenchymal calcifications.

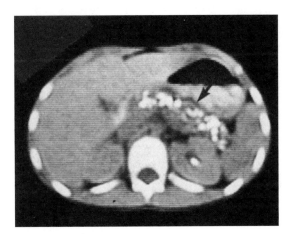

Fig. 32-91. Hereditary pancreatitis produces calcifications *(arrow)* in the pancreas of this 6-year-old child.

The majority of the patients seen with this entity have been those in the pediatric age group. Calcifications occurred in the parenchymal portion as much as the ductal portion (Fig. 32-91). They are the same types of inflammation and pseudocysts seen with adults. The best treatment has been obtained with pancreatectomy.

Hemachromatosis

Hemachromatosis results from excessive accumulation of iron in the body. The disease has a primary form, which is idiopathic, and a secondary form, which results from ingestion of exogenous iron or multiple transfusions.[53] CT characteristically shows an increased density in the pancreas and adjacent peripancreatic lymph nodes; similar findings have been reported by Long et al[144] and Mitnick et al.[166] Long et al did not find a correlation between the amount of increased density and the pancreatic dysfunction or insufficiency. Dense nodes in the porta hepatis and peripancreatic, periaortic, and perisplenic nodes should be noted (Fig. 32-92). These findings should not be confused with calcifications. Un-opacified vessels may give the spurious impression of a low-density mass in the pancreas in some cases. Intrave-nous contrast material eliminates any question of a pos-sible mass (Fig. 32-93).

Cystic fibrosis

Cystic fibrosis or mucoviscidosis is a hereditary generalized disease affecting all mucus-producing exo-crine glands of the body. The disease results in abnor-mally thick secretions that obstruct most exocrine glands, including the pancreas. Studies have shown that there is

an increased concentration of protein in the pancreatic fluids, which may account for increased viscosity. It is postulated that inspissation of the material can produce ductal ectasia. A variety of changes that can result in var-ied clinical situations with a variety of findings on CT scan can occur.

Most patients who have cystic fibrosis have prob-lems that are associated with exocrine function. The gland usually appears completely replaced with fat (Fig. 32-94). Presumably the gland has complete and long-term obstruction, which results in complete atropy of the acinar portions. The islet cells are not usually affected, and the endocrine functions remain intact, without de-velopment of diabetes or other problems. This process would seem to parallel studies with laboratory animals, which show complete autolysis and atrophy of the gland when the duct is ligated; the function of the islet cells is typically not affected.

Also reported and considered to be a different en-tity along the same spectrum is cystosis of the pan-creas.[92,186] Although this is an uncommon disorder, a number of large cysts scattered throughout the course of the pancreas can be observed. The cysts are typically thin walled and cannot be distinguished from pseudo-cysts (Fig. 32-95). In some patients, lesser variations are seen, which include presence of a fluid-filled duct or smaller cysts. The fluid has calcium and eosinophilic con-cretions. Antigenically, it is said to be identical to serum and contains increased amounts of inactive trypsinogen; this indicates that autodigestion has no major role in this process.

In another group of patients with a mild form of cystic fibrosis, the exocrine function of the gland may be preserved with or without any pulmonary symptoms. Pa-

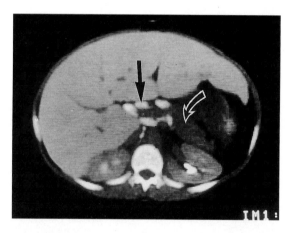

Fig. 32-92. Some patients with iron overload show increased density of lymph nodes *(arrow)* in the peripancreatic area and not in the gland *(open arrow)*.

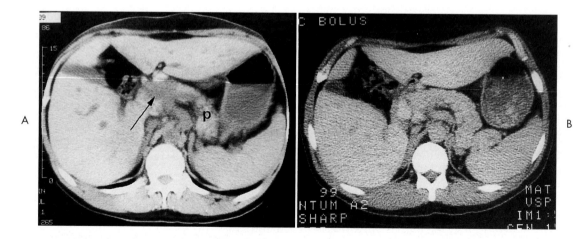

Fig. 32-93. A, A patient with iron overload shows increased density of the gland *(p)* and not the portal vein *(arrow)*. The vessels should not be mistaken for an intrapancreatic tumor. **B,** After intravenous contrast administration, the vessels are opacified, dispelling the question of a tumor.

tients with pulmonary problems who have a normal-appearing pancreas and no associated abdominal problems have been observed. Other patients who do not suffer from pancreatic insufficiency may develop recurrent, severe pancreatitis. The incidence of pancreatitis is said to be approximately 0.05% of all patients. Pancreatitis may develop in some patients who have a mild but undiagnosed form of cystic fibrosis without pulmonary symptoms. Masaryk and Achkar[157] reported several cases of patients with active clinical pancreatitis thought to originate from functional obstruction of the pancreatic duct. The diagnosis of cystic fibrosis had not even been considered until pancreatitis occurred. Although these authors did not postulate the etiological conditions, it seems logical to assume that inspissated pancreatic fluid creates partial obstruction of the duct. It is not sufficient to destroy the acinar portion but is sufficient to impair flow, which produces inflammation.

Fatty pancreas

A fat-density pancreas can be entirely normal (see section on normal variations), but there are a number of entities that have been reported to produce fat replacement of the gland.[183] These include pancreatic duct obstruction, malnutrition, Schwachman syndrome, hemachromatosis, viral infection, Cushing's syndrome, steroid therapy, and an unusual entity called lipomatous pseudohypertrophy of the pancreas. Specific reports on these entities have not yet appeared, but one would anticipate future reports on this topic.

BENIGN TUMORS
Cysts

True cysts of the pancreas differ from pseudocysts and retention cysts because of their origin, histologic appearance, and clinical significance. These cysts are believed to be anomalously developed from remnants of the embryological ductal systems. Histologically, they may have a lining of epithelial cells, but with pressure changes the lining may atrophy. In such cases, the wall may consist of smooth, fibrous tissue. Rarely, they may be complicated by infection or hemorrhage (not with the frequency of pseudocysts).

They can appear incidentally but most commonly occur with multicystic[209] or von Hippel-Lindau disease. Levine et al[139] reported on 31 patients with a history of von Hippel-Lindau disease. Five of the patients showed pancreatic cysts. The CT appearance of this entity is identical to that of any other well-defined cystic abnormality (Fig. 32-96).

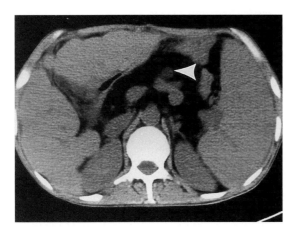

Fig. 32-94. Patients with cystic fibrosis with pancreatic atrophy typically have a pancreas *(arrow)* completely replaced with fat.

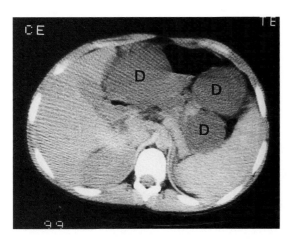

Fig. 32-95. Rarely, cystic fibrosis produces a massive cyst formation of residual ducts *(D)*, which are occluded. Such changes have been called *cystosis.*

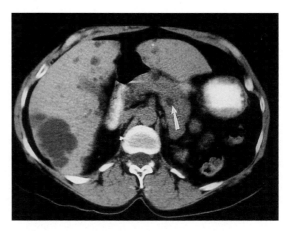

Fig. 32-96. True cysts of the pancreas *(arrow)* may occur with polycystic disease.

Lymphangioma

A single case of lymphangioma of the pancreas has been reported.[180] CT scan demonstrated a "cystic" mass that was indistinguishable from a cystadenoma; the diagnosis can be made only on pathological study.

Adenomas

A number of benign solid tumors, some of ductal and some of acinar cell origin, do occur, but no specific reports have appeared in the literature. We have encountered one case of adenoma of the pancreas that was palpated and examined by biopsy at surgery but did not show any morphological or density changes on CT scan that would distinguish it from a neoplasm (Fig. 32-97). Further experience must be reported before any generalizations of their CT appearance can be made.

Von Hippel-Lindau disease

Von Hippel-Lindau disease is a hereditary disease with a dominant trait. It can be associated with a number of abnormalities, including angiomas of the central nervous system and eye as well as neoplasms and cysts of the pancreas, kidney, adrenal glands, and epididymis.

Pancreatic involvement by this disease includes cysts, serous cystadenomas, solid nonfunctional islet cell tumors, and adenocarcinomas. The earliest signs are said to be small cysts, but calcifications are common. Progression of the disease can result in steatorrhea and diabetes. Solid tumors usually represent nonfunctional islet cell tumors or adenocarcinoma.

Periodic monitoring of diagnosed patients and screening for the disease in unaffected family members is appropriate. This permits genetic counseling for family planning. Also, early detection of high morbidity and mortality problems can permit earlier effective treatment.

Levine et al[139] and Choyke et al[40] have reported on screening of visceral problems. Choyke et al[40] found CT to be most accurate as compared with MRI and ultrasound. CT detected all pancreatic and renal abnormalities in a group of 14 patients, whereas ultrasound and MRI each missed abnormalities in three cases. These included two pancreatic masses that were seen only on CT.

Recommended choice for screening modality depended on the age of the patient. Choyke et al[40] recommended ultrasound and MRI for evaluation of the abdomen and central nervous system in patients younger than 11 years old. Contrast-enhanced CT was recommended for patients older than 16 years.

VASCULAR ABNORMALITIES

Because the pancreas lies in a location surrounded by vascular structures, a number of vascular entities occur in the region and can be associated or confused with pancreatic pathological conditions. Abnormalities can be related to inflammatory, arteriosclerotic, or neoplastic involvement of the vessels.

Splenic artery aneurysms and pseudoaneurysms

Splenic artery aneurysms are common and characteristic. Surgical repair of such aneurysms is required only when they are more than 3 cm in diameter or if they occur in women during child-bearing years or taking oral contraceptives. This latter group is at risk for spontaneous rupture. The aneurysms appear as circular soft tissue densities or curvilinear calcification in the area of splenic artery (Fig. 32-98). On some occasions, when there is no extensive calcification of the aneurysm, they may simulate focal masses. They can be definitively diagnosed

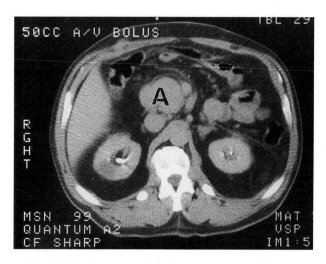

Fig. 32-97. Adenoma of the head of the pancreas *(A)*.

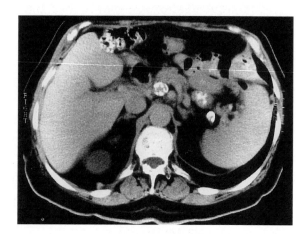

Fig. 32-98. Aneurysms of the hepatic artery and splenic artery may demonstrate calcified dilatations as noted in this case.

only by a dynamic bolus scan or an infusion of contrast material at a high rate (Fig. 32-99). Identification is important because of the possibility that they can be mistaken for a mass in the gland. Spontaneous hemorrhage into the pancreatic duct has been reported with a splenic aneurysm.

Other aneurysms

Aneurysms in the peripancreatic vessels can occur based on arteriosclerotic disease, but they are rare anomalies. They most commonly contain calcifications, and the diagnosis is best made by dynamic bolus scanning. Historically, these vessels are likely to rupture, so most authors recommend surgical correction in the ap-

propriate patients. The aneurysms may be seen in the gastroduodenal, hepatic, or other vessels.

Hepatic artery aneurysms. Hepatic artery aneurysms represent 19% of splanchnic aneurysms and are atherosclerotic, traumatic, or mycotic. Surgical treatment is recommended because 44% of these aneurysms rupture. Therapy consists of ligation of aneurysmectomy; the extensive collateral network provides an adequate blood supply.

On CT, the aneurysm is a mass of blood density, which enhances with bolus injection of contrast material. It may be adjacent to the artery or peripheral in the liver (Fig. 32-100).

Superior mesentery aneurysms. Superior mes-

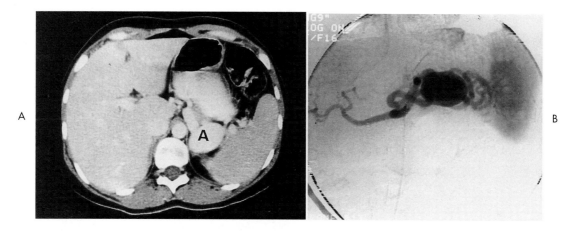

Fig. 32-99. A, Although the patient was referred because of suspected tumor, the correct diagnosis of noncalcified splenic artery aneurysm was made preoperatively. CT scan with bolus dynamic contrast injection shows a high-density mass *(A)* in the area of the splenic pedicle, suggestive of an aneurysm. Digital subtraction angiography (DSA) was performed to document it. **B,** DSA shows the large aneurysm.

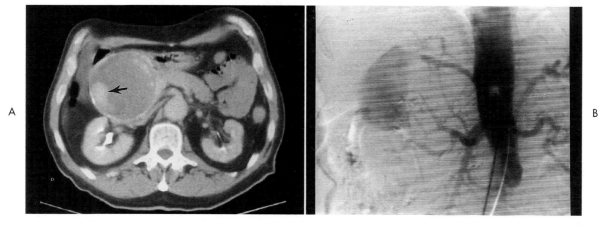

Fig. 32-100. Massive aneurysms or pseudoaneurysms may simulate fluid density pseudocysts. Note the large area of low-density clot surrounding the small area of high density representing flowing blood in this large aneurysm.

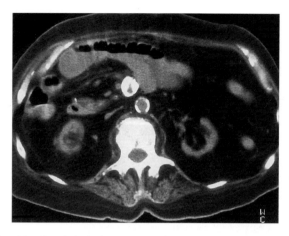

Fig. 32-101. Calcified aneurysm of the superior mesenteric artery.

entery aneurysms are the third most common splanchnic aneurysms, of which 63% are mycotic lesions, and most are associated with endocarditis on the left side. Most other causes are secondary to medial degenerative disease. Operative treatment is justified because of the common occurrence of rupture or arterial occlusion (Fig. 32-101)

Celiac artery aneurysms. Celiac artery aneurysms are uncommon and are mainly atherosclerotic in origin. Approximately 20% rupture. Surgical treatment is recommended and consists of resection or ligation.

Cavernous transformation of the portal vein

Cavernous transformation of the portal vein is a vascular anomaly that consists of multiple venous collaterals in the area of the portal vein. The incidence is small,

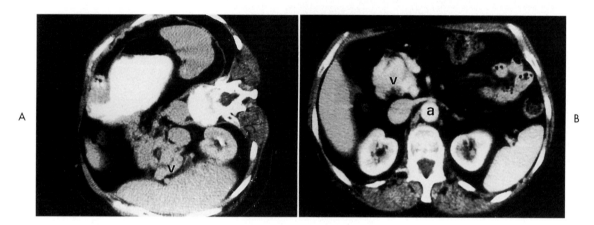

Fig. 32-102. **A,** CT scan shows a patient in right decubitus position with tubular structures (*v*) that resemble veins. This may be cavernous transformation of the portal vein. **B,** Bolus dynamic scan shows increased enhancement of the venous structures (*v*) consistent with cavernous transformation and the aorta (*a*).

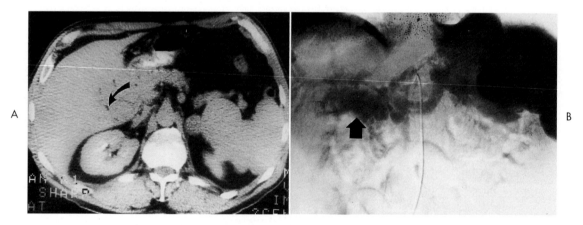

Fig. 32-103. **A,** The diagnosis of cavernous transformation is more difficult to make from this scan. There is, however, a multilobulated mass with interspersed fat that suggests the diagnosis (*arrow*). **B,** Angiogram was done to confirm the diagnosis. Note the diffusely enhancing venous channels (*arrow*) in the area where the portal vein should be.

and only one series of 16 cases has been reported by Mathieu et al[158] Although it was once thought to be a congenital problem, it is now thought to result from portal vein occlusion or compromise. Because the numerous vascular channels can occur in any portion of the porta hepatis, a network of vascular channels adjacent to the pancreatic head can simulate a pancreatic mass. Correct diagnosis depends, of course, on familiarity with the entity and appropriate scanning technique, which includes ample intravenous contrast enhancement.

The correct diagnosis can be easily made if the channels are large and the dynamic bolus scan has been done properly (Fig. 32-102). Diagnosis is more difficult when the vascular channels are not as well formed, smaller, and in the area of the portal vein. In such cases,

the diagnosis can sometimes be suggested by the presence of small amounts of fat irregularly interspersed within the porta hepatis region (Fig. 32-103). In difficult cases, an angiogram may be required. In our early experience before we were familiar with the appearance of this entity, we inadvertently performed biopsies using fine-needle aspiration on three patients with cavernous transformation, which was producing a pseudomass in the head of the gland. No ill effects or blood loss occurred.

Portal systemic collaterals and varices

Because of the close physical proximity to the pancreas and the possible effect of pancreatitis on adjacent structures, venous abnormalities of the portal vein

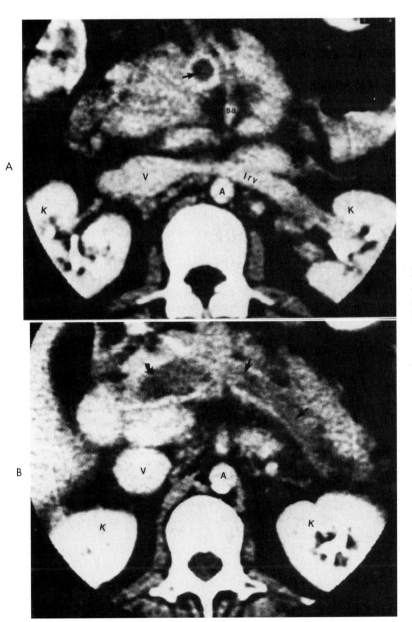

Fig. 32-104. A, Thrombosis of the superior mesenteric vein *(arrow)* in a patient with Hodgkin's disease who had a splenectomy. **B,** A more cephalad scan shows thrombosis of the splenic vein *(straight arrows)* and the portal vein *(curved arrow)*. *sa,* Superior mesenteric artery; *V,* vena cava; *A,* aorta; *K,* kidneys; *lrv,* left renal vein.

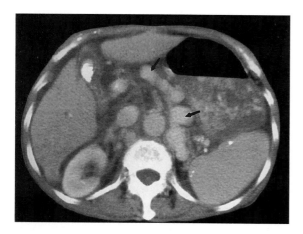

Fig. 32-105. CT scan shows extremely large varices in the retroperitoneum adjacent to the left adrenal gland, aorta, and superior mesenteric artery *(arrows)*.

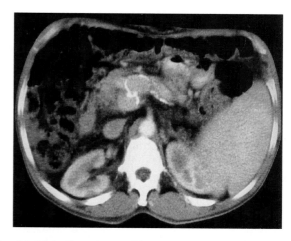

Fig. 32-106. Chronic portal hypertension may rarely produce calcifications in the walls of the portal vein and splenic vein, as noted in this scan.

and splenic vein are discussed. A patent, anatomically normal splenic or portal vein may be visualized in cases of massive splenomegaly; this occurs simply as a result of increased flow. Other entities, such as occlusion; thrombosis; or encasement of the splenic, superior mesenteric, or portal vein, result in portal hypertension and portal systemic collaterals.[156,220]

If thrombosis of the veins is suspected as the primary problem, administration of contrast material as a dynamic bolus study is essential. In instances of thrombosis of the portal or mesenteric vein, clot within the vessel is visualized as a filling defect (Fig. 32-104). If the clot extends into the intrahepatic portion of the liver, it may give the spurious impression of biliary dilatation.

When the obstruction to flow is intrahepatic, such as occurs with cirrhosis, dilatation of the portal, splenic, and other veins occurs.[154,159] Assessing enlargement of the portal and splenic vessels is subjective, but the appearance is usually obvious (Fig. 32-105). When portal pressure has been present for long periods, calcifications may occur in the wall (Fig. 32-106).

With portal hypertension, a number of portal systemic collaterals appear.[113,115] A common finding in such patients is recanalization of the umbilical vein in the falciform ligament, which can feed superficial periumbilical veins that form the classic caput medusae. There is dilation of the inferior mesenteric vein coming off of the splenic vein in some patients with portal systemic collaterals. In such cases, the dilated inferior mesenteric vein on the left side of the aorta, down to the perirectal hemorrhoidal veins.[98]

Large esophageal varices may be seen as a mass of serpiginous structures that enhance on bolus injection. Systemic collaterals forming a splenorenal shunt can be well seen as enhancing tubular structures in the splenorenal ligament. The collateral pathway is through small veins from the medial surface of the spleen, through the adrenal veins, and into the left renal vein. There may be a significant change in the caliber of the vena cava above and below the renal vessels probably because of the difference in blood flow at these two levels. We have seen these vessels persist in a patient with such a shunt, with even-flowing splenectomy. In this case, tumor was considered until a bolus-dynamic scan was performed.

The accuracy of detecting varices has not been defined, but a number of authors have discussed the CT appearances. Primary diagnosis is probably not as good as endoscopy or barium swallow, but varices should be recognized when they are present. Such information may be helpful as an additional clue for correct and complete interpretation and is a critical factor if a percutaneous interventional procedure is being considered.

MALIGNANT TUMORS

In contrast to some other cancers, the incidence of pancreatic carcinoma has increased in recent years. In the United States and the United Kingdom, it is now the fourth leading cause of cancer death in men and the sixth leading cause of cancer death of women. Contributing causes have not been well defined, and previous associations with pancreatitis and alcohol abuse have been disproved.[138] Some related factors may be smoking, high-fat diet, diabetes, industrial exposure, and perhaps coffee.

Tumors other than adenocarcinoma are rare, and no change in their incidence has been noted in recent years. The diagnosis of all tumors has been advanced in recent years as a result of laboratory, clinical, and imaging studies.

Clinical syndromes

Several syndromes that have specific symptoms have been associated with exocrine gland tumors. The most familiar sign is the association of adenocarcinoma neoplasms with migratory thrombophlebitis, called *Trousseau's sign*. The exact cause of Trousseau's sign is not clear, but the most commonly proposed mechanism is the release of tumor proteins from necrosis that act like tissue thromboplastin material. This material triggers the normal coagulation system to form thrombi in various veins.

A somewhat characteristic perineoplastic syndrome has been associated with acinar cell carcinoma. With this syndrome, there is peripheral fat necrosis, polyarthralgia, and eosinophilia. It is thought that the release of lipase and other active enzymes into the bloodstream produces digestion of fat in the marrow and other areas; this produces the symptoms of the syndrome.

The endocrine types of islet cell tumors produce clinical syndromes related to excessive secretion of their respective products. At least eight different cell lines in the islet of Langerhans and specific syndromes related to most of these cell lines have been reported. The endocrine products causing these syndromes include insulin, glucagon, gastrin, somatostatin, and vasoactive polypeptide; the signs and symptoms are discussed later.

Nonendocrine tumors

Pancreatic adenocarcinoma. Ductal cell adenocarcinoma constitutes 80% of the neoplasms of the pancreas and most commonly occurs in the head (65%). It is most common in the older age group and has a higher incidence among men. Patients frequently have weight loss, pain, and jaundice, but a variety of other symptoms related to the gastrointestinal tract or metastatic spread can occur.[25]

The treatment and outcome have not significantly changed in recent years. The overall long-term results from surgery and chemotherapy have not been good, but there is good reason for some optimism. With the availability of modern CT equipment, proliferation of medical information, and greater experience, two positive trends exist. At least with current technology, it has been possible to exclude inappropriate patients from needless surgery, which can have a high morbidity.[79-83] Similarly, because more appropriate patients are being taken to surgery, it is my belief that outcome data in the future will show an improvement in survivorship. Second, there are several new chemotherapeutic agents that have produced remarkable improvements in the short-term.

Diagnostic signs. Tumors may demonstrate one or a combination of the following diagnostic signs:[79-83,85,140,207,221]

1. Morphological and contour changes.

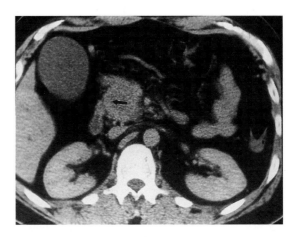

Fig. 32-107. Tumor in the head of the pancreas shows central decreased density, not the inner margin of the viable tumor *(arrow)*.

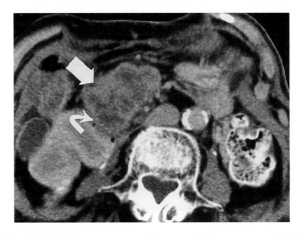

Fig. 32-108. Large pancreatic mass with some central decreased density *(arrow)*. Note the loss of the plane *(curved arrow)* between the mass and the duodenum, which is somewhat dilated.

2. Mass effect.
3. Density changes (i.e., low density or calcification).
4. Contrast enhancement.
5. Pancreatic duct changes.
6. Secondary signs.

Morphological and contour changes. The morphology of the normal gland has already been discussed. Complete familiarity with the variations of shape and contour is important if one is to diagnose subtle pancreatic tumors. In most cases, alteration in the morphology by the mass is so remarkable that it is hard to discern even the normal margins of the remaining gland. In other cases, the changes may be so subtle that only careful attention to detail reveals the nature of the problem.[34,140]

Masses of the head of the pancreas are usually obvious because of their size, but subtleties can occur that require attention to diagnostic details. Such masses may have smooth contours or a lobulated appearance (Figs. 32-107 and 32-108). Masses of considerable size produce displacement of adjacent structures, such as bowel and the vascular structures. If aggressive local invasion occurs, the margin of the adjacent bowel can be involved, and there may be encasement of vessels resulting in vascular compromise and collateral vessel formation. Vessel involvement is an indicator of unresectability (see later section).

When appreciation of a mass in the head is difficult, it may be helpful to note the presence of any dis-

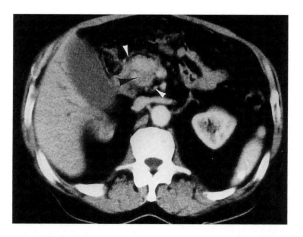

Fig. 32-109. A different patient with a tumor in the head. *Black arrowhead* shows an area of decreased density representing avascular tumor. The *white arrowheads* show small vascular collaterals anterior and posteriorly. In some cases, these enlarge as a result of vascular occlusion of the major vessels.

crepancy between the size of the head and the neck and tail. Although this was initially believed to be an early sign of malignancy, a study indicates that it is simply a frequent appearance and does not indicate the presence of early disease (Figs. 32-47, 32-109 and 32-110).

An extensive study of morphological changes was made by Muranaka et al,[169] who studied the overall size relationships of the head and body of the pancreas as well as the size and configuration of the pancreatic duct (Fig. 32-111). In this study, the authors classified the body of the gland as enlarged when it exceeded 2.2 cm and atrophic when it measured less than 1.0 cm (see Table 32-1). They classified the head of the pancreas into four grades depending on the anteroposterior measurement: T1, 0 to 2 cm; T2, 2.1 to 4 cm; T3, 4.1 to 6.0 cm; and T4, more than 6 cm. In their series of 72 patients, there were 11 patients with T1, 14 patients with T2, 20 patients with T3, and 11 patients with T4. They evaluated the size of normal and cancerous glands and assessed the ratio of the head and body to validate or refute earlier observations about size discrepancy.

Muranaka's results (Fig. 32-111) showed that the normal gland varied in size as follows: The head varied between 19.8 and 29.5 cm, and the body varied between 12.1 and 21.4 cm. Although the size decreased with age, the ratio of head and body remained constant at 1.45 ± 0.03. The ratio of the head and body in carcinoma patients was $3.4 + 0.9$. An interesting finding in this series was that contrary to the traditional thinking that a discrepancy between the head and body can be found in small tumors, Muranaka found that more than half of the patients with small tumors actually had a body greater in size than normal and that resulted in a ratio less than normal (between 1.0 and 1.5 cm). As the tumors increased in size, the increase in the pancreatic ratio oc-

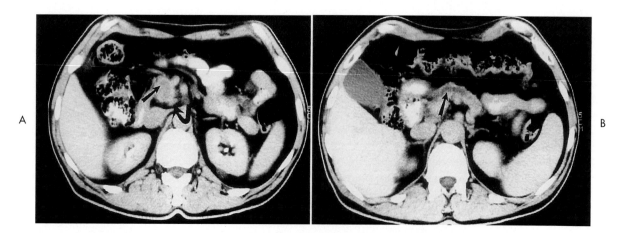

Fig. 32-110. A, CT scan shows a low-density mass in the head *(arrow).* The posterior pancreaticoduodenal vein is slightly enlarged *(curved arrow).* **B,** Higher scan shows a dilated pancreatic duct *(arrow).*

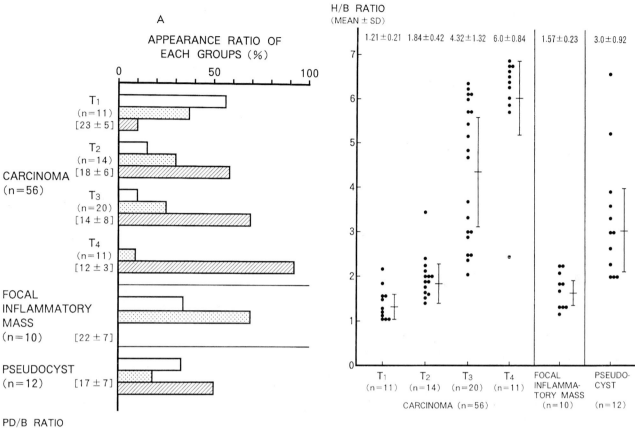

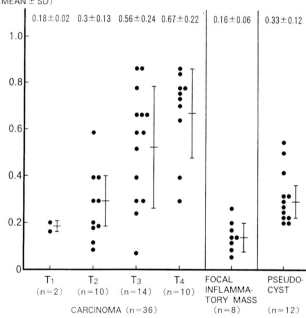

Fig. 32-111. **A,** Width of the pancreatic body in patients with a pancreatic head mass. The body was significantly larger in patients with a T-1 carcinoma than normal subjects ($P < 0.05$). Number in parentheses means mean width of the pancreatic body in each disease (mean ± SD mm). *Bars,* enlarged pancreatic body; *stippled bars,* normal pancreatic body; *striped bars,* atrophic pancreatic body. **B,** Pancreatic head-to-body width ratio (H/B ratio) in patients with a pancreatic head mass. The ratio in all patients with carcinoma was 3.4 ± 0.9 (mean ±). The difference between patients with carcinoma and normal subjects was significant ($P < 0.05$). **C,** Pancreatic duct caliber-to-pancreatic body width ratio (PD/B ratio) in patients with a pancreatic head mass. The ratio in all patients with carcinoma was 0.49 ± 0.12 (mean ± SD). The difference between the carcinoma group and others was significant ($P < 0.05$). (From Muranaka T, et al: *Acta Radiol* 31:483-488, 1990.)

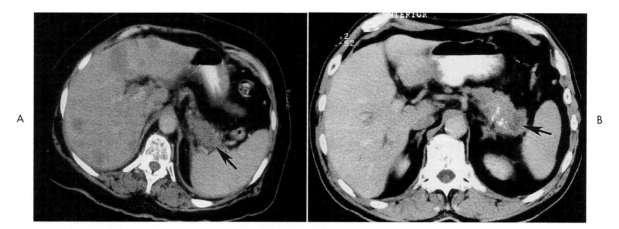

Fig. 32-112. A, Small adenocarcinoma *(arrow)* enlarging the contour of the tail and obscuring the fat planes around the vessels in the hilum. **B,** Different patient with adenocarcinoma of the tail *(arrow)*. Note the decreased density as well as the small calcifications in the tail. It is difficult to determine if the calcifications are related to the tumor or previous pancreatitis.

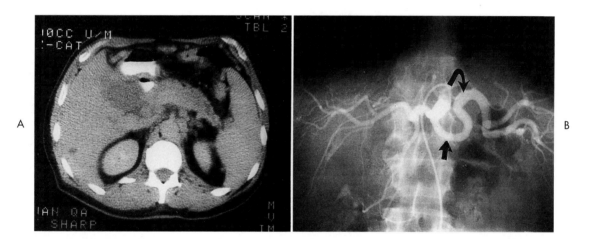

Fig. 32-113. A, Patient with a diffuse mass proven to be carcinoma. Because of the patient's young age, an angiogram was performed to document inoperability. **B,** Angiogram shows diffuse encasement of the proximal splenic artery *(arrow)* relative to the distal portion *(curved arrow)*.

curred as previously noted. These findings contrasted with the ratio as noted in patients with inflammation. The ratio with pancreatitis was close to normal despite the large size of any mass because of concomitant enlargement of the body.

Tumors of the neck and body commonly produce enlargement of the gland and local extension to the splenic pedicle (Fig. 32-112). When a mass is immediately adjacent to the stomach, it may be difficult to appreciate it unless there is adequate contrast material in the fundus. In such cases, it may be helpful to turn the patient in a decubitus position, which shifts the anatomy somewhat and clarifies the appearance. Although most

tumor enlargements occur in the plane of the axial slice (i.e., anterior, posterior, right or left sides), they may grow in a cephalad caudad direction and be difficult to identify as a pancreatic tumor.

Wittenberg et al[246] noted that carcinoma may appear as enlargement of almost the entire gland. They found that three or more portions of the gland (head, neck, body, and tail) were involved in 27% of cases, and they recommended that multiple biopsies might be required to differentiate between neoplastic and secondary inflammatory components (Fig. 32-113).

One of the most disappointing facts is that despite the remarkable evolution of the diagnostic equipment

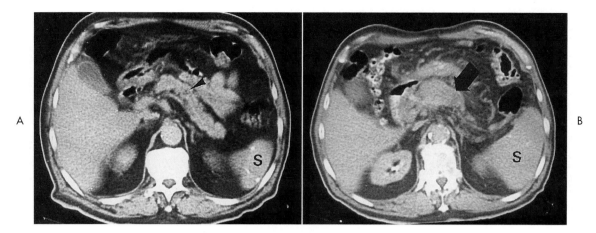

Fig. 32-114. A, CT scan performed early in the clinical course shows a subtle enlargement of the pancreatic duct and a tiny low-density area in the body *(arrowhead)*. Note the normal-sized spleen. Study was not read as abnormal. **B,** Repeat CT scan shows large mass in body of gland. There are numerous collateral vessels noted in the mesentery and enlargement of the spleen *(S)* indicating definite occlusion of the splenic vein.

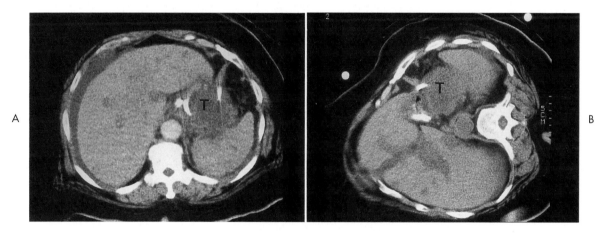

Fig. 32-115. A, When this patient was scanned in the supine position, there was the question of a subtle mass *(T)* in the tail adjacent to the stomach. **B,** Repeat study of the patient in the decubitus position shows the mass *(T)* better than on the decubitus study. Note the contrast material located anteriorly within the stomach.

and advanced experience level, carcinoma of the gland can occur without any distortion of the contour (Fig. 32-114). In such cases, the tumor may become manifest many months later.

Other problems simulating a pancreatic mass. A variety of problems can cause difficulties in interpreting a "mass" in the head of the gland. (See the section on normal variants and pseudomasses.) If there is not adequate contrast administration to opacify the venous structures, a prominent portal vein, or vena cava, an overall impression of "fullness" in the area of the pancreas may be noted. In such cases, restudy with adequate contrast ma-

terial or an ultrasound examination can clarify the findings. When a mass abuts against the stomach or duodenum, administration of oral contrast material and examining the patient in the decubitus position may be helpful (Fig. 32-115).

On other occasions, enlargement of the caudad lobe of the liver by cirrhosis or another problem may produce the spurious finding of a "mass." Another confusing abnormality is enlargement of lymph nodes in the retroperitoneum adjacent to the head of the pancreas. Finally, another unusual entity that can cause an apparent mass is a partial malrotation of the duodenum. Because

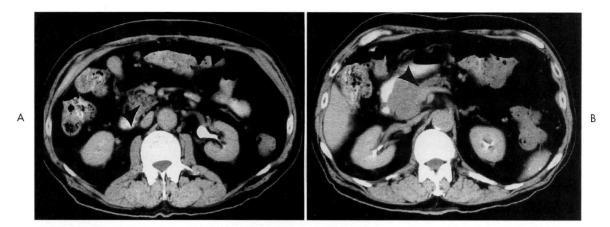

Fig. 32-116. A, This and the subsequent scan shows the paradoxical increased density of a neoplasm compared with the normal gland. Note the head has a low density owing to fat infiltration *(arrowhead)*. **B,** Slightly higher scan shows higher density mass in the head of the gland. *Arrowhead* shows the junction point with the neck and body, which is slightly atrophied and has a lower density owing to fat infiltration.

Treitz's ligament is in an abnormal location and the path of the bowel is redundant, the duodenum can produce a "clump" that looks like a mass. A fluid-filled duodenal diverticulum may also produce a "mass."

Density changes. Although early scanning devices did not demonstrate many density differences between tumor and normal gland, modern CT consistently shows decreased density in almost all non-islet-cell tumors, with contrast enhancement. Freeny and others[60-63] noted diminished density in 83% of patients with focal masses. Without intravenous contrast material, many adenocarcinomas have an almost isodense appearance (compared with the rest of the gland) on the unenhanced scan (see Fig. 32-107). This low density observed on the CT scan is thought to be due to decreased vascularity of the neoplasm compared with the normal gland. Necrosis or low-density fluid production may be visible in many tumors with or without contrast material;[116] this is common with mucinous adenocarcinomas, cystadenomas or cystadenocarcinomas, adenosquamous carcinomas, papillary adenocarcinoma, or any necrotic tumor resulting from necrosis or a mucin material.

A paradoxically unusual finding can occur in patients who have the normal variation of extensive fatty infiltration of the gland. Because the tumor does not contain the same amount of fat as seen in the parenchyma, it is higher in density than the normal gland (Fig. 32-116). Interestingly, one of the tumors we have observed became isodense with the rest of the gland after contrast administration. This is comparable to seeing lesions in a fat-density liver.

Another obvious change in the density of tumors is calcifications, which occur in a number of different tumor types in the de novo state. Typically, adenocarcinoma only rarely calcifies (see Fig. 32-112, *B*), and calcium is considered typical for other unusual pancreatic tumors. The nonfunctioning islet cell tumor is the most common. The configuration of the calcifications is not helpful because they may vary in both amount and size. Other more rare tumors[93] that may also contain calcifications are mucinous adenocarcinomas, cystadenomas, cystadenocarcinomas, papillary epithelial tumors, fibromas, and glucagonomas, which are discussed later. Dystrophic calcifications may occur in any type of tumor after treatment if necrosis has resulted. Dastur and Lewin[48] reported a case of adenocarcinoma that showed calcification in the primary tumor and metastases after chemotherapy.

Contrast enhancement. The effects of contrast enhancement vary according to the method of contrast administration: enhancement by generalized equilibration or dynamic bolus injection aided by mechanical injector. The optimal method as noted previously is enhancement with mechanical injection. With this type of enhancement, the relative decreased density of the tumor is better visualized as well as any vascular collaterals that may exist in the peripancreatic area (Figs. 32-117 and 32-118). When contrast material has been given as a single bolus or drip infusion, the contrast has equilibrated between the intravascular and extravascular spaces. (Experimental work indicates it takes only a few minutes for this to occur.) Direct arterial injection through arterial catheters has been performed in specific cases and can be helpful in finding a small vascular endocrine tumor.

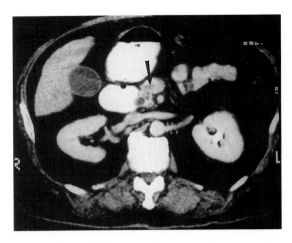

Fig. 32-117. CT scan shows small avascular tumor *(arrow)* within enhanced head of pancreas, which is adjacent to dilated common bile duct.

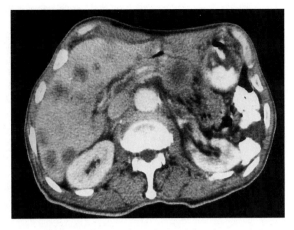

Fig. 32-118. Adenocarcinoma of the pancreas, which is producing vascular obstruction and collateral vessel formation. Note the decreased density of the mass and the multiple metastatic disease in the liver.

The importance of giving adequate contrast material was noted by Hosoki,[95] who discussed the benefit of dynamic bolus injection for the diagnosis of neoplasms. As others have noted, he noted that contrast material permitted better visualization of the pancreatic duct. He thought this procedure facilitated (1) correct evaluation of the tumor vascularity, allowing a differential diagnosis; (2) location of the boundary between tumor and nontumor tissue; (3) detection of small tumors; and (4) visualization of pancreatic invasion by peripancreatic tumors. He found that tumors were more likely to appear isodense compared with the normal gland if contrast material was given as a slow bolus before the scan, whereas they appeared hypodense compared with the normal gland if rapid contrast injection was given (Fig. 32-118). He also confirmed findings by other authors about the vascularity of cystic and islet cell tumors (see later section).

Ductal dilatation and cyst formation. Ductal dilatation can occur in either pancreatitis or neoplasm. Several observations based on the size and configuration of the pancreatic duct can be helpful. (See the section on the pancreatic duct.)

Dilatation occurs in patients who have obstruction of the duct by a neoplasm. As noted in earlier sections, visibility of the duct is improved by intravenous injection of contrast material, which highlights the density of the glandular tissue around the fluid density duct (Fig. 32-119). In most cases, the dilatation of the duct is uniform, but on occasion there may be some tortuosity or beading of the duct. In unusual cases, obstruction of the duct may produce ectasia and enlargement of a localized segment, producing a retention cyst or pseudo-

cyst distally (Fig. 32-120). (See earlier section on the pancreatic duct.)

Biliary obstruction. Biliary obstruction occurs with great frequency in patients who have a mass in the head of the gland. In these cases, the course of the dilated biliary system from the liver through the porta hepatis and down the length of the common bile duct should be followed[75,183] and the level of the obstruction determined. In most cases, the dilatation ends just above the level of the pathological condition (unless metastatic nodes are in the porta hepatis) (Fig. 32-120, *A*).

In such cases, the configuration of the common bile duct may have a characteristic finding that can help to distinguish between neoplastic and inflammatory narrowing of the duct. The complete details are noted in Chapter 31. In pancreatitis, sequential concentric narrowing of the distal duct occurs as it passes through the inflammatory mass. An abrupt end to the duct on sequential scans or an irregular margin of the dilated common bile duct is expected with neoplasm. These findings parallel those seen on cholangiography.

Local extension. Local invasion of adjacent structures can be easy or difficult to see, depending on the nature or degree of involvement. In most instances, the margins of the contiguous anatomical structures are displaced and distorted by an extension of the soft tissue mass (Figs. 32-121 and 32-122). In other cases, infiltration of the vascular planes around the superior mesenteric artery and vein or the portal venous system must be carefully sought. Acute obstruction of the portal system produces clinical symptoms and collateral vessels that are best seen with dynamic contrast studies.

Contiguous spread into adjacent organs occurs

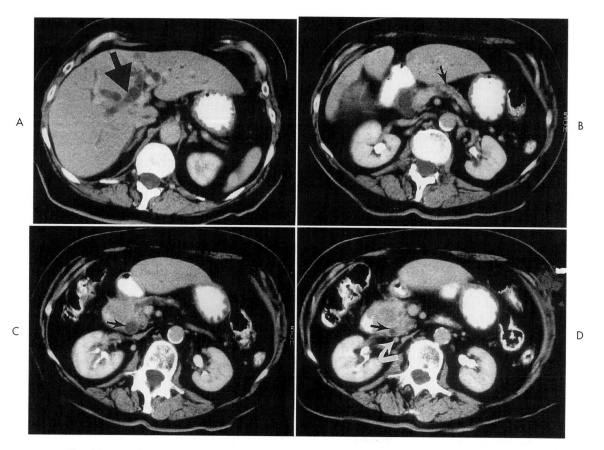

Fig. 32-119. A, Biliary dilatation shows low-density branching structure that converges centrally *(arrow)*. **B,** Slightly enlarged pancreatic duct *(arrow)*. **D,** This lower scan shows the abrupt tapering of the distal common bile duct, which suggests neoplasm (see Chapter 31). *Curved arrow* shows dilated posterior pancreaticoduodenal vein commonly seen with pancreatic cancer.

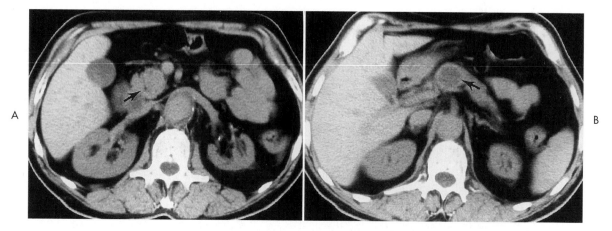

Fig. 32-120. A, This and the following scan shows retention cyst associated with a pancreatic tumor. This scan shows a mass in the head *(arrow)*. **B,** Lower scan shows a fluid density mass *(arrow)* in the neck of the gland, which represents a retention cyst.

commonly and is obvious most of the time. The tumor extension usually follows the areolar tissue, containing the vessels, lymph nodes, and lymphatic system with the various peritoneal reflections or ligaments. When the tumor invasion is subtle or there is associated inflammation, the appearance may be confused with edema, which can occur with pancreatitis.[238] Extension may occur along the lines of the splenic hilum and the splenorenal peritoneal reflection. It can produce focal areas of neoplasm or necrosis with the spleen (Fig. 32-122).

Invasion into the duodenum or stomach can produce a gastric or duodenal obstruction. In most instances, displacement and massive involvement occur, but in some cases, the infiltration can be so subtle that

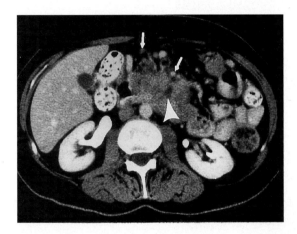

Fig. 32-121. Large tumor mass, with necrosis *(arrowhead)* in the area of the pancreatic head, which extends into the base of the mesentery and the left side of the retroperitoneum. Note the vascular collaterals *(arrows)* in the mesentery.

the bowel can be affected without any significant soft tissue mass.

Direct invasion into or from the bowel can occur along the mesocolon, especially at the hepatic or splenic flexures. If a fistula to the bowel is created, gas in the tumor may produce an appearance suggestive of an abscess. The amounts may be so remarkable that distinction from an abscess or infected pseudocyst may be difficult (Fig. 32-123). Comparison studies are helpful because such patients may be only slightly more ill when they are seen than other tumor patients.

Spread of the tumor along the margins of the vasculature[205] may result in narrowing or encasement of the arteries and veins (Fig. 32-124). In such cases, venous occlusion usually occurs first, and numerous venous collaterals can usually be seen in the adjacent tissues. When occlusion of the artery is complete, it may produce vascular compromise of the involved organ, such as the spleen, which shows characteristics changes. Several authors, including Megibow and colleagues[161] and Itai and others,[101-103] have studied encasement of vessels comparing CT and angiography and have found that the finding of the loss of the fat plane around arteries on CT is as accurate for encasement as the angiographic finding of narrowing (Figs. 32-124 and 32-125).

A corollary sign of tumor invasion of the venous system is the dilatation of the posterior superior pancreaticoduodenal vein reported by several authors. The essence of this sign is that with occlusion of the normal anterior venous pathways by tumor, there is increased flow through the posterior pancreaticoduodenal vein, which becomes more apparent[103] (Fig. 32-110, 32-119, D, and 32-126).

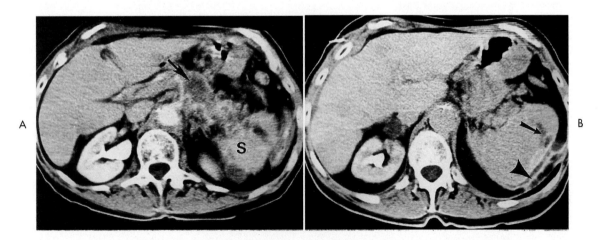

Fig. 32-122. A, CT scan shows low-density mass *(arrow)* in the body of the pancreas. Note the vascular collaterals and the low-density areas in the spleen *(S).* **B,** CT scan taken at a higher level shows a low-density peripheral area *(arrow)* and linear areas of increased density *(arrowhead),* which represents capillary collaterals. These findings would be consistent with "infarction."

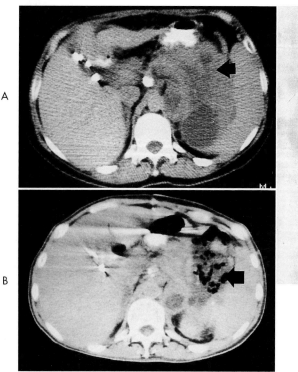

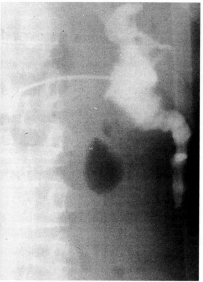

Fig. 32-123. A, Baseline scan of a patient with a tumor of the tail of the pancreas, producing a soft tissue mass *(arrow)* in the hilum. **B,** Later scan shows "air" within the mass *(arrow);* the origin of the air was not known. **C,** Percutaneous puncture followed by injection of contrast material shows a fistula to the colon.

Fig. 32-124. A, CT scan of pancreatic mass with encasement of the splenic artery *(large arrow),* which is producing low-density areas *(small arrows)* in the spleen. **B,** Scan taken at a later phase shows the splenic vein *(black arrow)* and collateral veins in the perisplenic area and the left gastric area *(white arrows).* **C,** Arteriogram showing encasement *(arrow)* of the origin of the splenic artery. **D,** Numerous venous collaterals in the perisplenic area *(arrow)* produced by occlusion of the splenic vein.

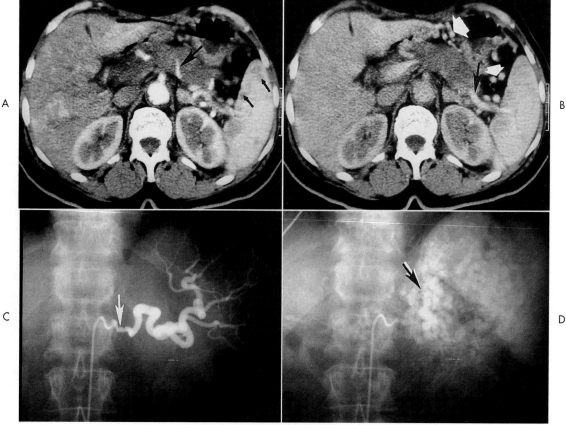

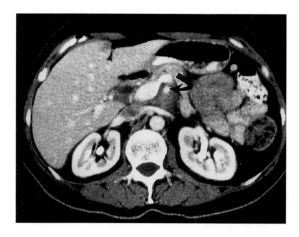

Fig. 32-125. Tumor infiltrating *(curved arrow)* into the fat planes around the superior mesenteric artery and behind the splenic vein.

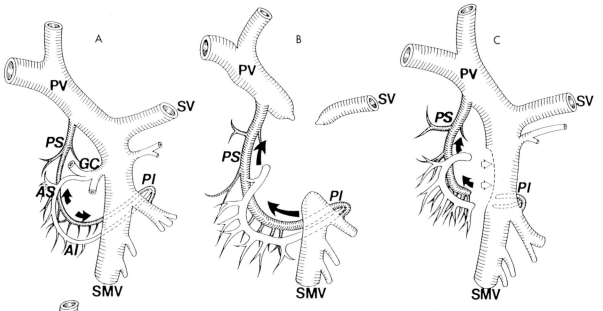

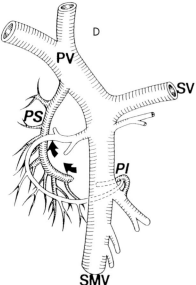

Fig. 32-126. A, Normal venous drainage of the pancreaticoduodenal veins. *PV,* portal vein; *SV,* splenic vein; *PS,* posterior-superior pancreaticoduodenal vein (PSPDV); *PI,* posterior-inferior pancreaticoduodenal vein (PIPDV); *AS,* anterior-superior pancreaticoduodenal vein (ASPDV); *AI,* anterior-inferior pancreaticoduodenal vein (AIPDV); *GC,* gastrocolic trunk. *Arrows* indicate direction of drainage of the posterior pancreaticoduodenal venous arcade. **B,** Occlusion of the confluence of the P-SMV by advanced cancer of the pancreas. The PSPDV dilates as a result of being one of the hepatopetal collateral veins. **C,** Tumor extension to the right lateral wall of the P-SMV *(open arrows)* with occlusion of the PIPDV. The AIPDV, ASPDV, and gastrocolic trunk may also be occluded. The PSPDV drains blood from the posterior pancreaticoduodenal arcade and probably also from the anterior pancreaticoduodenal arcade via anastomotic branches into the portal vein. **D,** Occlusion of the PIPDV with no tumor invasion of the P-SMV. The ASPDV and AIPDV may or may not be occluded. The PSPDV drains blood from the posterior pancreaticoduodenal arcade and, when the AIPDV is occluded, also from the anterior arcade. (From Mori et al: *Radiology* 181:793-800, 1991.)

Lymph node involvement. Lymph node involvement is common with tumors.[6] The first nodes to be involved are usually those around the vessels in the immediate peripancreatic and porta hepatis regions (Fig. 32-127). The lymph node pathways can be best appreciated by looking at the arteriogram in the early part of this chapter and remembering that the lymph channels follow the veins. Accordingly, these nodes are located in their prospective peritoneal reflections (e.g., hepatoduo-

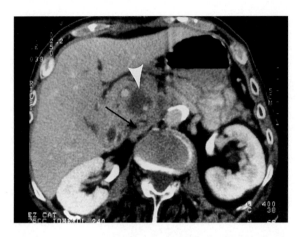

Fig. 32-127. Large low-density tumor *(arrowhead)* of the head of the pancreas with spread into the hepatoduodenal ligament. There is loss of the fat planes within the porta hepatis at this level. Note the enlarged pancreaticoduodenal vein *(arrow)* anterior to the cava.

denal area, root of the mesentery). Direct spread within the areolar tissue of the peritoneal reflection also occurs.

Liver metastases. Metastatic disease to the liver is common and does not have a specific appearance. Metastatic foci appear low density within the enhanced liver and may be well circumscribed or diffuse (see Fig. 32-118).

Operability and staging. In my experience, the only patients who are operable candidates for curative surgery of this disease are those with no significant enlargement of the gland or any evidence of invasion, spread, or metastasis.

The most likely candidates for surgery are those patients who have painless jaundice. Such patients may show obstruction only of the biliary system and pancreatic duct with no significant enlargement or other findings.

Staging. There are a number of staging methods[89,240] for pancreatic carcinoma, but the most widely accepted is the TNM classification for tumors. Use of this classification is appropriate because in recent years there has actually been progress in the treatment of pancreatic tumors with chemotherapy. The standard classification permits better coordination of large studies, which are so critical for assessing outcome of this devastating disease. This classification can be noted in Table 32-4. Staging is I, II, III, or IV depending on location, extension, and presence or absence of lymph nodes.

Several authors have directly addressed the issue

Table 32-4. Standard classification of tumors of the pancreas

Staging			
Stage I	T1	NO	MO
	T2	NO	MO
Stage II	T3	NO	MO
Stage III	Any T	N1	MO
Stage IV	Any T	Any N	M1

Primary tumor (T)	
TX	Primary tumor cannot be assessed
TO	No evidence of primary tumor
T1	Tumor limited to the pancreas
	T1a Tumor 2 cm or less in greatest dimension
	T1b Tumor more than 2 cm in greatest dimension
T2	Tumor extends directly to the duodenum, bile duct, or peripancreatic tissues
T3	Tumor extends directly to the stomach, spleen, colon, or adjacent large vessels

Regional lymph nodes (N)	
NX	Regional lymph nodes cannot be assessed
NO	No regional lymph node metastasis
N1	Regional lymph node metastasis

Distant metastasis (M)	
MX	Presence of distant metastasis cannot be assessed
MO	No distant metastasis
M1	Distant metastasis

of reliability of CT for determining operability. One article by Jafri and colleagues[105] compared the value of CT and angiography for assessing the resectability of pancreatic carcinoma. The authors looked at 27 patients with pancreatic carcinoma who had both CT and angiography before surgical exploration. They found that CT and angiography were about as accurate for detecting the presence of vascular encasement and inoperability (CT, 18 cases, and angiography, 19 cases). The CT sign used by the authors for vascular encasement was loss of the perivascular fat plane. The authors found that although both angiography and CT showed encasement, angiography tended to show encasement of the similar vessels better but would miss large vessel encasement. Conversely, CT was better at showing encasement of the celiac and superior mesenteric vessels. Other signs of inoperability included liver metastases, lymph node spread, or invasion of the anterior perirenal fascia. The authors recommended that both angiography and CT be used to screen patients for operability.

Similar information about 154 cases was presented by Freeny and associates,[61] who found that CT and angiography were essentially equivalent for the staging of operability. In a group of 40 patients considered inoperable by CT criteria, none was incorrectly staged. It is at least reassuring to know that salvageable patients are not inappropriately excluded from surgery. Itai and others[101-103] have reported on their experience with resectable pancreatic carcinoma. The authors retrospectively evaluated CT scans on patients and found the following criteria useful in determining resectability: a mass with a distinct contour (as if encapsulated), a low-density, area, and dilatation of the caudal portion of the main duct. Patients with involvement of large vessels, the liver, or lymph nodes should be excluded from surgery.

As a side note, the only patient I have observed who was cured had a large mass with well-defined contour (Fig. 32-128). (See section on adenosquamous carcinoma.) Certain chemotherapeutic agents have produced some initial success (Figs. 32-129 and 32-130).

Prognosis based on staging. One of the most complete studies of staging and prognosis was by Freeny and others,[62] who evaluated the accuracy of CT staging relative to operative findings and also looked at the overall outcome of their patients. They studied a series of 174 patients over a 6-year period. They judged patients as resectable if there was an isolated pancreatic mass with or without ductal dilatation or combined pancreatic-bile duct dilatation without an identifiable pancreatic mass. Patients were judged unresectable if one or more ancillary findings of carcinoma were present, including local tumor extension, contiguous organ invasion, metastases, ascites, or vascular involvement.

Relative to accuracy of diagnosis and staging, CT proved to be reliable. There were only 13 cases of false-positive scans (8%) for adenocarcinoma. The other diagnoses included two normal pancreas, four pancreatitis, one ampullary carcinoma, two metastases, two lymphomas, one islet cell, and one gastric carcinoma. There were two false-negative studies (1%) on patients who later proved to have carcinoma by ERCP. Thirteen patients had findings indicative of resectability by CT scan, and nine finally went to surgery for possible resection. At surgery, resection was performed in five patients, with two being inoperable by visual and manual inspection. Forty-two patients went to surgery for possible resection despite the CT diagnosis of unresectability; none of these patients was resectable.

Of this entire group, 12 patients had surgical resections, 7 judged resectable and 5 judged unresectable.

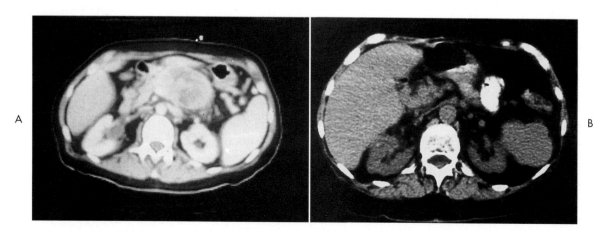

Fig. 32-128. A, Adenosquamous tumor of the pancreas appears well encapsulated. It was believed to be inoperable. **B,** After a palliative removal of the tumor, the patient died 6 years after surgery. There was no evidence of tumor at autopsy.

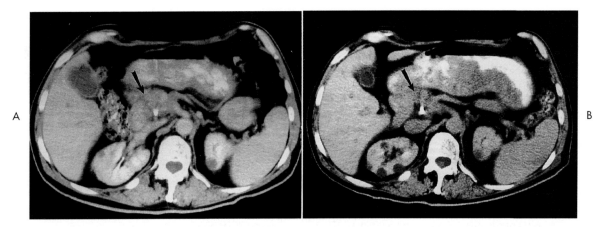

Fig. 32-129. A, Carcinoma in the head *(arrow)* that is infiltrating the fat planes and some anterior displacement of the stomach. **B,** CT scan of the same patient taken weeks after chemotherapy treatment. Note that the tumor mass has decreased in size *(arrow)*.

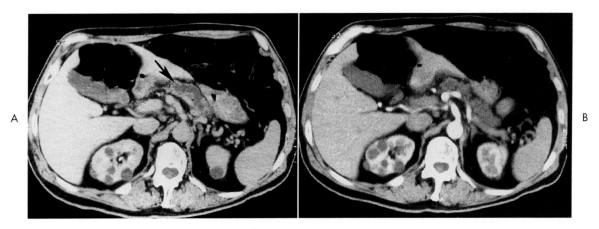

Fig. 32-130. A, Same patient as in Fig. 32-129 before treatment shows an enlarged pancreatic duct *(arrow)* that has a duct-to-glanddiameter ratio less than 0.5. **B,** After chemotherapy, the pancreatic duct returned to normal size.

Of these 12 patients, 11 have died. The average survival time was 17.2 months (range 6 to 31 months). There was no significant difference in the survivorship between those patients who had resections or not based on the CT findings, 19.5 months (range 6 to 27 months) compared with 14.6 months (range 6 to 27 months). Average time for tumor recurrence after surgery was 9.2 months.

The most optimistic prognosis of this disease was reported by Manabel et al.[150] who reported a 4-year survivorship of 37% for patients with small tumors less than 2 cm. Their positive results have yet to be confirmed by other groups.

Warshaw et al[242] reported a series of patients studied by CT, MRI, and angiography. They demon-

strated that 87% of all tumors were inoperable because of vascular invasion as shown by CT and angiography. Detection of small liver and peritoneal metastases was difficult by CT, with only 27% being identified. Laparoscopy evaluated a smaller group of 23 patients, but the accuracy for metastatic detection was 96%. MRI was almost equivalent but provided no additional benefit over CT.

Another prognostic factor emphasized by Kloppel and Maillet[123] is the tumor grade of the adenocarcinoma. The grading of the tumor has been classified into 1, 2, and 3 corresponding to well differentiated, moderately differentiated, and poorly differentiated. As one might expect, the more poorly differentiated tumors have the poorest prognosis. Virtually all patients with grade 3 have died within 15 months, whereas patients with grade 1 and 2 died within 30 months.

Although the data in the literature are discouraging about the current outcome of pancreatic carcinoma,[31,45,46,55] it clearly demonstrates that CT has a definitive role for diagnosing, staging, and predicting the outcome of surgical treatment. CT is and will be especially helpful for following the course of the disease during the development of study of new therapeutic regimens (Figs. 32-129 and 32-130). Further refinement of MRI may assist in these goals.

Distinguishing between carcinoma and pancreatitis. Most authors agree that it is difficult to make a distinction between carcinoma and pancreatitis based on only imaging studies.[131,136,170] Carcinoma can coexist with pancreatitis, even though there is no proof that a close relationship exists.

Several diagnostic points are helpful in distinguishing the two diseases. The most definitive method for distinguishing them is evidence for spread of malignancy, such as liver metastases or extensive local spread. Factors that would support pancreatitis are not as definite but may be suggestive. Pancreatitis is also more likely to produce diffuse changes in the gland and peripancreatic inflammation. The peripancreatic findings of thickened fascia occur in almost all cases of pancreatitic and only seldom in neoplasms. The appearance of the distal dilated common bile duct and the configuration of a dilated pancreatic duct may also be helpful. It is also true that loss of fat planes around arteries occurs most commonly in neoplasm, but it may be observed occasionally in pancreatitis.

In the final analysis, no imaging system is capable of absolutely differentiating carcinoma from inflammation or benign masses in the pancreatic area. Pathological confirmation is necessary.[81,100] CT and ultrasound currently provide remarkable assistance for percutaneous procedures, and MRI promises to provide the same capability.

CT combined with ERCP. Frick et al[64] reported on patients studied by CT immediately after injection of contrast material during ERCP. The authors did not specifically alter the ERCP study to optimize the CT study in any way. They found that the normal gland demonstrated diffuse homogeneous enhancement that persisted for several minutes on CT. Areas of pancreatitis showed irregular contrast distribution, presumably resulting from duct distortion. Obliteration of the duct by neoplasms resulted in absence of "stain" on the pancreatogram and clear delineation of the mass on the CT image.

Mucinous adenocarcinoma. Not much information is available on mucinous adenocarcinoma. Only a few cases have been encountered. A unique feature of

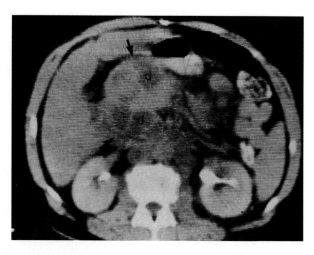

Fig. 32-131. Adenocarcinomas may on occasion produce a mucin-like material. This scan shows such a mucinous adenocarcinoma *(arrows),* with areas of lower density *(d).*

this tumor is that its density may be lower than that of ductal carcinoma, and it may appear almost cystic (Fig. 32-131). Mucinous adenocarcinomas can apparently calcify.

Ductal mucinous adenoma and carcinoma. An unusual mucin-producing tumor originates within the pancreatic duct. Initially reported by Itai et al,[101-103] it has been given the name duct ectatic adenoma and carcinoma and is typically located in the uncinate portion of the gland. There has been a single case report of this entity occurring in the body (Fig. 32-132). The number of cases reported is so limited that it is difficult to be certain of the outcome. The same caveat exists with this tumor as other cystic tumors. The mucin-producing epithelial cells of this entity have the same risk for malignant degeneration as other mucinous tumors.

The diagnostic key with this particular entity is the correlation of clinical factors with the imaging appearance. Agostini states,[1] "in the absence of chronic pancreatitis mucinous ductal ectasia should be suspected in cases with clusters of small void, thin-walled cysts."

Squamous or adenosquamous carcinoma. Squamous or adenosquamous carcinoma is a rare variant with some specific differential pathological and radiographic findings, but the outcome and prognosis are not much different from ordinary adenocarcinoma. In several large series, squamous or adenosquamous carcinoma occurred in less than 0.5% of all cases of carcinoma.

This carcinoma is said to occur predominantly in men. The clinical presentation and outcome are said to be no different from regular adenocarcinoma. The appearance is somewhat characteristic because the density of the tumor appears to be low, resulting from necrosis within the mass (Fig. 32-133).

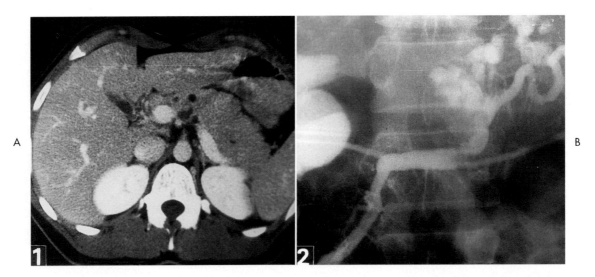

Fig. 32-132. Mucinous pancreatic duct ectasa. **A,** CT scan shows small cysts of different sizes in the body of the pancreas between the splenic and portal veins. **B,** Endoscopic retrograde pancreatogram shows dilated tips of side branches of the pancreatic duct. (From Agostini S, et al: Mucinous pancreatic duct ectasia in the body of the pancreas. *Radiology* 170:815-816, 1989.)

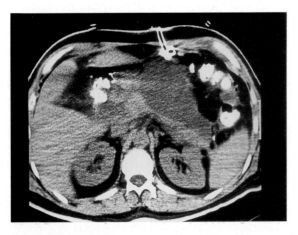

Fig. 32-133. Large soft tissue mass in pancreas is low in density and had the appearance of a fluid mass. This proved to be a necrotic squamous cell carcinoma.

Acinar cell tumors. Acinar cell tumors, which arise from acinar elements of the pancreas, are rare, occuring in 1% to 13% of all cases. An association with subcutaneous and intraosseous fat necrosis has occurred in only 20 cases.

Acinar cell tumors have a constellation of unique clinical signs. Symptoms are due to panniculitis or fat necrosis and consist of joint swelling, tenderness, and cutaneous nodules resembling erythema nodosum. Laboratory studies usually show leukocytosis, eosinophilia, and elevated lipase levels. Radiographs can show lytic areas involving medullary or cortical bone. These later changes are presumed to be due to a release of excessive amounts of lipase into the blood.

The prognosis of the disease is poor, the patient living 2 to 12 months. Most cases of the disease are not diagnosed until autopsy.

Radin et al[191] and Lim and Ko[141] have reported cases of acinar cell carcinoma. CT showed a well-circumscribed mass with some central necrosis (Figs. 32-134 and 32-135). The unique aspect of these cases is the presence of permeative lytic process, which may involve the phalanges of the hands and feet. A radionuclide bone scan also showed diffuse periarticular uptake around the peripheral joints.

Other tumors. A variety of other tumors can arise in the pancreas from connective or lymphatic tissue, including lymphoma, fibrosarcoma, leiomyosarcoma, fibrous histiocytoma, pancreatoblastoma, lymphangioma, and plasmacytomas.[69,180,229,244] Although they have no real distinguishing features, lymphomas may clinically be less symptomatic than other tumors; there also appears to be a more discrete appearance of lymph nodes in the area (Fig. 32-136) with lymphoma.

Cystadenoma and cystadenocarcinoma. Cystadenomas and cystadenocarcinomas are rare tumors thought to originate from the ductal epithelium. They are distinctly different in presentation, histological appearance, imaging characteristics, treatment, and prognosis. Several terms have been applied to them, but they are divided into two types, one thought to be a benign type, called *microcystic cystadenoma* (serous cystadenoma or glycogen-rich cystic tumor), and a premalignant or

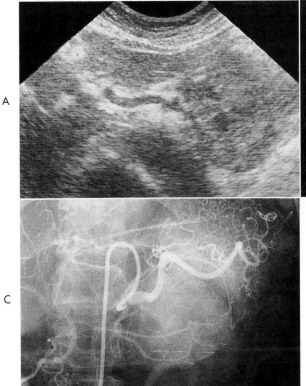

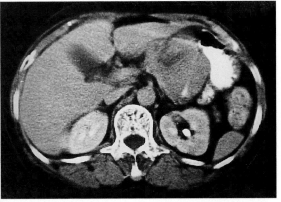

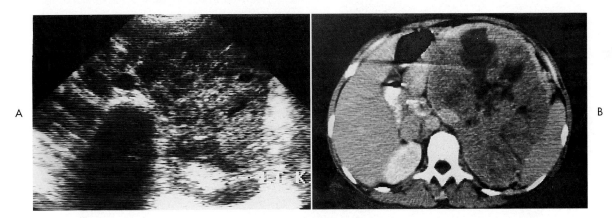

Fig. 32-134. Acinar cell carcinoma. **A,** Transverse sonogram show a well-demarcated solid tumor containing a necrotic area. **B,** CT scan obtained after injection of contrast material discloses a sharply circumscribed mass arising from body and tail of pancreas. The mass contains necrotic areas and a calcification. **C,** Splenic arteriogram shows a vascular mass with staining and vascular draping. (From Lim JH, et al: *Clin Imaging* 14:301-304, 1990.)

Fig. 32-135. Acinar cell carcinoma. **A,** Transverse sonogram discloses a large mass containing small anechoic spaces in pancreas body and tail. **B,** CT scan after injection of contrast material shows a well-defined large mass in left abdomen. The mass is covered by a thin enhancing capsule and contains small and medium-sized necrotic areas. (From Lim JH, et al: *Clin Imaging* 14:301-304, 1990.)

malignant type, called *macrocystic cystadenoma* (mucinous cystadenoma). Patients with these tumors usually have a gradually increasing tumor mass. They may or may not have symptoms of pain and weight loss.

Considerable attention has been focused on these two lesions and the methods to distinguish them. In 1962, Campbell and Cruickshank[35] observed that the two entities could be differentiated by pathological criteria. In the benign type they noted a relatively uniform population of cells without any evidence of malignant changes. In the other type, they noted a distinctly different pattern that showed malignant changes scattered throughout the tumor. Although they did not actually observe the transition in a patient, they postulated that malignant degeneration occurred in the latter type. Histologically, they found the benign tumor had cuboidal epithelium, with little secretion of mucus. The tumor with scattered changes of malignant tissue had tall, mucus-secreting epithelium and large, mucin-filled cystic spaces.

In 1978, Compagno and Oertel[43,44] clearly defined the histological difference between what they termed *benign microcystic* (glycogen-rich or serous) *cystadenomas* and *mucinous cystic neoplasms* (cystadenocarcinoma and cystadenoma) with overt and latent malignancy. They also noted distinct differences in the clinical data between the patients with the two distinctly different tumors.

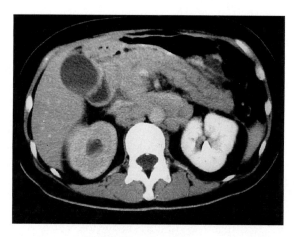

Fig. 32-136. Lymphoma involvement of the pancreas is not specific in its appearance. Note dilatation of the pancreatic duct and the enlarged lymph nodes in the retroperitoneum.

Microcystic adenomas occur more commonly in patients 60 to 70 years old and equally in men and women. Some patients were symptomatic with local pain or discomfort related to the mass, whereas others had no symptoms; some were incidentally found at autopsy. The tumors had a mean diameter of 10.8 cm and showed small cysts with glycogen but little or no mucin. They most commonly occurred in the head of the gland. Fatalities most commonly occurred from complications of surgery or obstruction of the gastrointestinal or biliary system.

Clinical data about mucinous cystic (macrocystic) neoplasms or cystadenocarcinoma differed greatly from the microcystic tumors. Mucinous cystic neoplasms occurred in a younger group of patients, most commonly female, with a mean and median age of 49 years. The symptoms were similar to the symptoms of microcystic cystadenomas but were more diffuse and severe. Patients had epigastric pain or discomfort, with some radiation of pain to the back. They had also anorexia, weakness, and weight loss. The tumors commonly appeared in the body and tail. Histologically the masses showed larger cystic areas that were lined with columnar, mucin-producing epithelium.

Imaging appearance. Although these tumors are fairly uncommon, a considerable experience has now been reported in the literature that characterizes the imaging appearance of these tumors.[18,65,110,126,182,198]

One of the first reports, by Friedman et al,[65] was published in 1983 on radiological and pathological correlation in 35 cases of cystic pancreatic neoplasms. CT and ultrasound findings paralleled closely the gross anatomical appearance of such tumors. Microcystic adenomas have a mixed variety of appearances that are similar

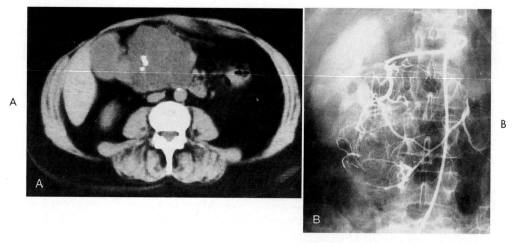

Fig. 32-137. A, Microcystic adenoma. Plain CT scan. Large, lobulated cystic mass with foci of central calcifications. **B,** Selective angiography. Enlarged pancreatic feeding arteries from the gastroduodenal artery. (From Mathieu D: *Radiol Clin North Am* 27:163-176, 1989.)

to the gross anatomical findings (Fig. 32-137). CT scan showed with contrast enhancement a mixture of connective tissue and fluid density. Sonography showed a mixed pattern; angiography showed hypervascularity (Figs. 32-137 to 32-139). Mucinous neoplasms showed large cystic changes on CT and sonography. Both types of cystic tumors showed calcifications.

Other authors, including Freeny et al[60-63] and Carroll and Sample,[36] have reported similar findings. Itai et al[102] reported that all tumors they studied appeared cystic in nature, with the major distinction being the number and size of the cystic areas. The macrocystic (mucinous) form was said to have larger and fewer cystic areas, compared with the microcystic form. Wolfman et al[247] reported several cases of the microcystic type appearing solid on the ultrasound and CT scans.

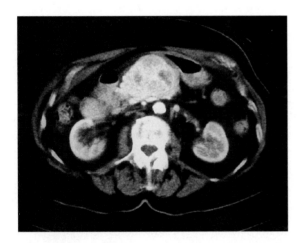

Fig. 32-138. Large soft tissue mass in the midabdomen shows intense enhancement with some areas of necrosis. Pathologically, this was a microcystic cystadenoma (glycogen-rich).

Two additional studies were informative relative to the appearance of these tumors. One study by Johnson et al[110] evaluated the various imaging criteria as applied by a number of blinded readers, and a second study by Warshaw et al[241] evaluated a large series of cystic tumors and made observations concerning the clinical, radiological, and pathological findings.

Johnson et al[110] studied 45 cystic tumors, which included 16 microcystic adenomas, 17 mucinous cystadenomas, and 12 mucinous cystadenocarcinomas. They evaluated the number of cysts, size of cysts, and presence of calcifications (Fig. 32-137). The authors concluded that one should use caution in using imaging studies for making the diagnosis of microcystic or mucinous tumors because there is considerable overlap with pseudocysts and other tumors, such as ductal adenocarcinoma, papillary and solid epithelial neoplasms, and pancreatic lymphangiomas. They did note that the typical appearances as described subsequently were present in 50% of the microcystic adenomas and about 90% of the mucinous cystadenomas and cystadenocarcinomas. Signs for the microcystic adenomas include multiple cysts smaller than 2 cm; the macrocystic adenomas were greater than 2 cm. Calcifications were present in either tumor.

Warshaw et al[241] made comments about the calcifications and noted that the calcifications were not specific, and only 2 of the 18 patients with microcystic adenomas showed the typical starburst configuration.

The latest study by Fugazzole et al[68] reconfirmed the findings of earlier authors on more current scanners. They noted that 7 of 11 tumors became partly or diffusely hyperdense after intravenous contrast administration as compared with normal pancreatic tissue. One of their patients showed a multiseptated mass with calcified walls. Calcifications were visible in three other cases. Me-

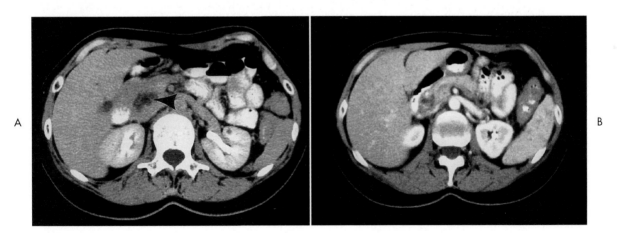

Fig. 32-139. A, Macrocystic adenoma *(arrowhead).* Low-density mass in head of pancreas was appropriately resected. **B,** Dynamic scan of the same mass shows increased enhancement of the cystic tumor.

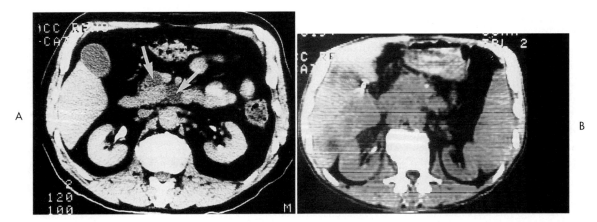

Fig. 32-140. **A,** Completely asymptomatic tumor with small cysts *(arrows)* measuring less than 2 cm; the tumor should be microcystic according to the criteria in the literature. The patient refused surgery. **B,** The patient showed widespread pancreatic carcinoma 6 months later (autopsy proven).

tastases from these tumors may or may not parallel the findings of calcifications and increased vascularity.

In my experience, the described findings apply in most cases, but several points should be clarified. These tumors are vascular with good contrast enhancement (Fig. 32-138). When the tumor size is small overall, it is difficult to characterize the cysts within the mass (Fig. 32-139). Furthermore, I am convinced that imaging appearance (CT or other) is not sufficiently characteristic to differentiate the two tumor types, as some authors imply. Using the imaging traits previously listed, I saw two cases that progressed contrary to what I would have predicted. These two cases should have been classified as microcystic based on the imaging appearance, yet both patients over the course of several years had growth of the tumor and subsequently died from carcinoma (Fig. 32-140). Several authors have reported on the benefits of percutaneous procedures for diagnosing the presence of cystadenocarcinoma, but even these authors recommend removal of these tumors regardless of the outcome of the cytological study.[68] I believe that all tumors should be surgically removed until definitive data appear indicating that a preoperative differentiation can be made by imaging or biopsy (see Chapter 46).

Papillary neoplasms. Papillary neoplasms (solid and papillary epithelial carcinoma, papillary carcinoma, papillary-cystic carcinoma) are unique because surgical resection is associated with a good prognosis.[39,66,185] The diagnosis, however, can be difficult to make preoperatively. In one case, the patient was healthy at the end of several years, and the original diagnosis of cystadenocarcinoma was changed retrospectively to papillary carcinoma (Fig. 32-141).

Demographically and histologically, papillary neoplasms vary significantly from other tumors. These tumors usually occur in young women around 26 years of

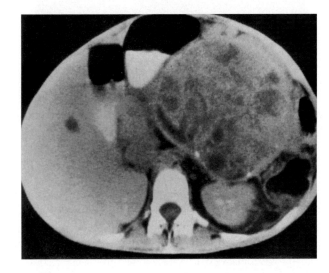

Fig. 32-141. Papillary epithelial tumor. This patient has a large mass with cystic areas and a well-encapsulated margin. The true nature of this lesion was not shown until the patient survived many years and a review of the pathological sections was made. Diagnosis was changed from cystadenocarcinoma to papillary epithelial tumor. (Courtesy of Dr. D.H. Stephens, Rochester, MN.)

age. The symptoms are related to vague abdominal symptoms, in turn related to the large size of the tumor; papillary neoplasms have even been found incidentally during surgery for other problems.

Pathologically, these tumors lack the microacinar patterns common to islet cell tumors and contain papillae as well as cysts of different sizes. The numerous small cysts and myxoid stroma may suggest microcystic adenomas, but they lack the glycogen. The nature of these tumors is not aggressive, and they seldom metastasize; surgical removal may produce good chances for survival.

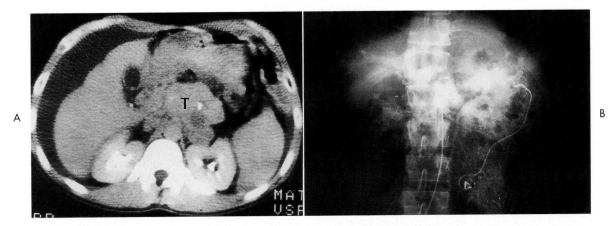

Fig. 32-142. A, Nonfunctioning islet cell tumor *(T)* shows necrotic areas and calcifications. **B,** Angiogram shows increased enhancement during celiac arteriogram.

The first report of CT findings was by Balthazar et al[14] in 1984. The characteristic CT findings were described as somewhat specific. They said the papillary neoplasm appeared as a sharply defined nonhomogeneous mass of uneven soft tissue density undergoing central necrosis. Contrast infusion produces no central enhancement and only slight peripheral enhancement. Although ill-defined cystic components should be expected, a sharply outlined, septate appearance, central scarring, or calcification would be unusual. Ultrasound showed a diffuse echogenic mass with no through transmission. Angiographically the vessels should be displaced and stretched but not encased.

Kim et al[120] reported a similar appearance on CT, but the sonographic findings differ from Balthazar et al;[14] the case studied by Kim et al showed a sonolucent rather than an echogenic mass.

Friedman et al[66] reported on nine cases from the Armed Forces Institute of Pathology, which provided imaging information on seven. The tumors were large, averaging 11.5 cm. CT showed mixed cystic-solid appearance in seven cases, and two tumors were chiefly cystic, with thick walls. In one patient, there was enhancement of the edge with contrast enhancement on the CT scan. The exact appearance on ultrasound was not specifically noted, other than saying that the findings paralleled the histological information. Choi et al[39] reported six additional cases, which confirmed the similar findings on CT.

Endocrine tumors

Islet cell tumors. Islet cell tumors differ from neoplasms of the acinar portion of the gland because they originate in the various cell lines of the islet of Langerhans.[47] The cell types and their corresponding products according to the Lausanne classification are A cell, glucagon; B cell, insulin; D cell, somatostatin; D1 cell, vasoactive intestinal polypeptide; EC cell, 5-hydroxytryptamine; G cell, gastrin; P cell, bombesin; and PP cell, pancreatic polypeptide.[73]

Depending on the tumor's degree of function, signs and symptoms may or may not be associated with endocrine secretion of these tumors. Tumors reported to cause syndromes include gluagonoma, insulinoma, gastrinoma, vipoma (watery diarrhea, hypokalemia, and anacidity), and somatostatinoma.[73,195] There have been reports relating to CT evaluation of these rare entities.

In addition to being isolated, there endocrine tumors can also be associated with the multiple endocrine neoplasia syndrome, specifically type I (Wermer's syndrome). Type I includes pituitary, pancreas, and parathyroid tumors; type II (Sipple's syndrome) includes thyroid, adrenal medulla, and parathyroid tumors; and type III includes thyroid, adrenal medulla, mucosal nerve, and ganglion cell tumors.[73,234]

Nonfunctioning islet cell tumors. There may be both benign and malignant tumors that do not function. Benign tumors seldom are seen because they do not produce hormones and do not grow large enough to appear as an abdominal mass. Patients with malignant tumors usually have vague abdominal symptoms produced by the large size of the tumor masses.[234] It is important to differentiate these malignant tumors from the typical adenocarcinoma of acinar origin because the prognosis and treatment vary considerably. In these tumors, special stains may demonstrate endocrine products; a clinical syndrome from excessive products may not occur.

As reported by Eelkema et al,[52] the typical CT appearance of this mass includes three specific findings: The tumors are typically large, contain calcification, and show increased enhancement with dynamic bolus arterial studies (Fig. 32-142). Slight differences between the different series were noted in the size and homogeneity of the mass. Stark et al[223,224] noted calcification in only one of five cases. Eelkema et al[51] in a report about 27 patients, noted that the soft tissue mass could have a variable density (i.e., either homogeneous or heterogeneous); when comparison was possible, most of these cases were isodense with the normal gland, and only a few were more or less dense than the normal gland. Finally, nonfunctioning islet cell tumors grow slowly, and they show minimal change over long periods of time, even years. In most cases, oncologists delay treatment until symptoms are present regardless of imaging appearance.

General localization of functioning islet tumors. Although absolute localization of the endocrine-producing tumors depends on imaging methods as described subsequently, an article by Howard et al[96] describes a general localization of the various tumors. Studying their data on endocrine tumors, they found there was a bimodal distribution of the various tumors. Considering the cluster 1, which included gastrinomas, pancreatic polypeptide-secreting tumors, and somatostatinomas, these occurred in 75% of the cases to the right of the superior mesenteric artery. In cluster 2, which included insulinomas and glucagonomas, 75% occurred to the right of the superior mesenteric artery. They further noted that the distribution paralleled the expected density of the various islet cell precursors in the gland. They finally speculated that the distribution might be a consequence of embryological development, with cluster 1 originating from the ventral bud and cluster 2 originating from the dorsal bud.

Insulinoma. When a tumor of the B cells develops, the patient usually has hypoglycemia and high serum insulin levels. Whipple's triad, a set of clinical features that should suggest the diagnosis, is as follows: (1) spontaneous hypoglycemia, followed by central nervous system and vasomotor symptoms; (2) repeated blood glucose levels below 50 mg/ml; and (3) relief of symptoms by administration of glucose.

These insulin-secreting tumors are generally small and usually less than 2.0 cm in diameter.[47] In 90% of the cases, they are solitary and benign, being malignant in only 15% of cases. They are multiple in 8% of cases and may present as a diffuse hyperplasia or microadenomatosis in 2% of cases. Most reports show a predilection for the head of the gland.

Because insulin produces such profound hormonal symptoms, the abnormality is usually diagnosed by clinical signs and serum hormonal assays. The role of imaging is not to diagnose the problem but rather to determine the number, location, and size of the abnormality. A variety of diagnostic methods have been used, including angiography, ultrasound, CT, percutaneous venous sampling for hormone, and intraoperative sampling

of glucose correlated with palpation. The vascular sampling techniques are usually used as a method of last resort if the other methods have failed so these techniques are not discussed here, but references are provided for additional information.

Angiography is an accurate method for detecting these tumors[179] before the refinement of CT and ultrasound. Insulinomas are well suited for this method because the tumors demonstrate hypervascularity that is clearly visualized during angiographic study. Historically, angiography has been accepted as the most accurate method, with accuracy varying between 29% and 91%, but authors such as Rossi et al[196,197] have shown that angiography and high-quality CT scanning are essentially equivalent for the detection of insulinoma. Most authors suggest that because of the invasive nature of angiography, this study should be deferred until other diagnostic methods have been used. A combination of CT and angiography was reported by Krudy et al[130] and Ahlstrom et al,[2] but this method has not gained acceptance[57] because current state-of-the-art scanners combined with dynamic contrast injection by mechanical injectors produce almost equivalent images (Fig. 32-143).

CT scanning combined with high-dose intravenous contrast material administration by mechanical injection has been demonstrated as quite accurate for the detection of insulinomas. Numerous authors have confirmed merits of CT for detecting this abnormality. Because these lesions tend to be small but hypervascular, the essential elements of an accurate examination include intense intravenous contrast enhancement and high-resolution scanning. Characteristically, these lesions are isodense with the normal unenhanced gland but show intense enhancement with contrast material, which may be uniform or "target"-like. The likelihood of detection also depends on the size, with tumors larger than 2 cm being detected between 90% and 100% of the time and tumors less than 1 cm being detected with an accuracy of 45% to 50%.

Unusual findings may include small calcifications, low density,[214] or a cystic appearance. Pograny et al,[189] reported an unusual cystic insulinoma.

Ultrasound. Before the development of high-quality real-time sonography, detection of insulinomas by ultrasound was unreliable. Several authors,[37,42,70,74,194,212] including Gunther et al[77,78] and Gorman et al,[72] using real-time ultrasound have reported favorable results for detecting insulinomas preoperatively. Using meticulous technique to ensure visualization of all parts of the gland, they reported accuracies of 60% and 63%. Most insulinomas are sonolucent in their appearance, but occasionally they are echogenic or isoechoic. When they are isoechoic, their detection is possible by observing the presence of a sonolucent "halo" (Fig. 32-143, *B*).

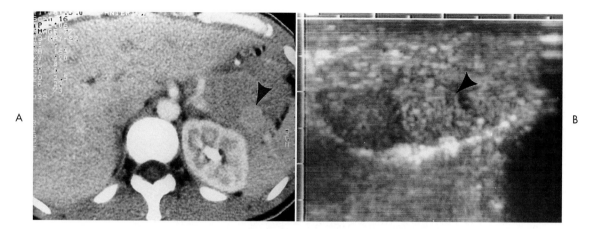

Fig. 32-143. A, CT scan with intense contrast enhancement shows considerable enhancement of small pancreatic insulinoma. **B,** Intraoperative ultrasound scan shows small echogenic mass with hypoechoic "halo" *(arrowhead).*

Although the transabdominal method[42] is comparable to the detection rate as reported by CT, there is no question that the experience with intraoperative ultrasound shows superiority of that method. The accuracy for intraoperative ultrasound varies between 86% and 100% and has been confirmed by numerous authors, including Ahlstrom et al,[2] Gorman et al,[72] Gunther et al,[77,78] and Norton et al.[177]

It is my opinion that diagnostic aspiration serves no purpose in patients with suspected endocrine tumors. The probability for a catastrophic event is high, and I think aspiration is not in the best interest of the patient. There has been one case report about percutaneous fine-needle aspiration performed on a patient with unsuspected insulinoma, and no problems were encountered (the lesion was "cystic"). Experience with other endocrine tumors, such as the adrenal gland, have resulted in some deaths.

Diagnostic algorithm. If one were to formulate a diagnostic algorithm based on the available data, it would be most reasonable to propose the following. For preoperative evaluation of insulinomas, one should perform either a high-resolution CT with thin section scans and dynamic contrast enhancement or a meticulous real-time ultrasound study. Choice between the methods depends on local expertise and body habitus of the patient (large patients examined by CT). At the time of surgery, final localization should be made by intraoperative ultrasound, which is the current "gold standard." Angiographic evaluation[2] or hormonal sampling should be reserved for problematic cases.[130,196]

Gastrinoma. Gastrinomas originate in the cells of the pancreas and are associated with a specific syndrome, known as the Zollinger-Ellison syndrome. This syndrome is associated with hypersecretion of stomach acid and associated multiple peptic ulcerations refractory to traditional treatment methods; removal of the tumor, which is the source of gastrin, is the most effective treatment.

The appearance reported in the literature is as follows: The masses are soft tissue density and may have a heterogeneous appearance because of necrosis. The lesions are vascular with dynamic bolus scanning or arterial enhancement (Fig. 32-144). Two of nine patients in the series had calcifications.

Krudy et al[130] reported on nine gastrinomas that were evaluated by CT, dynamic CT, angiography, venous sampling, and sonography. The gastrinoma was in the pancreas in only one case; this was a 1-cm lesion in the uncinate process. In the other eight cases, the gastrinoma was in lymph nodes adjacent to the pancreas or represented a recurrence. In five cases, the lesions were near the gland. Angiography detected six of the nine cases, routine CT detected five of the nine lesions, and dynamic CT detected two additional gastrinomas. Two lesions in small lymph nodes next to the gland were not seen by any method. Routine sonography detected two of the nine lesions. Percutaneous portal vein sampling was done in three cases and was helpful in two.

Krudy et al[130] found that all the lesions shown on dynamic scanning were demonstrated by angiography before CT (except one in the psoas). Angiography was used to identify the location for the dynamic scan. Although the lesions could have probably been found without CT, the surgeons found CT helpful in guiding the exploration. The limitation of the CT dynamic scan is that a large amount of contrast material for sequential bolus injection must be used; it is not practical to use CT in a primary study because of the number of boluses that would be required (Fig. 32-144).

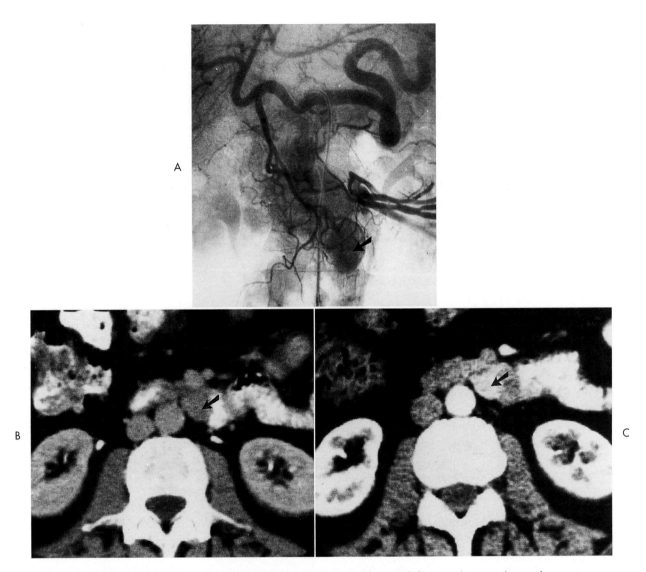

Fig. 32-144. A, Elevated gastrin levels in a 65-year-old man. Celiac arteriogram. A vascular mass *(arrow)* is near the origin of the superior mesenteric artery. **B,** Noncontrast CT scan. A gastrinoma *(arrow)* is indistinguishable from nonopacified bowel. **C,** Dynamic CT scan with intravenous bolus shows a brightly enhancing gastrinoma *(arrow)* behind the third part of the duodenum. At surgery, an extrapancreatic gastrinoma was found in the lymph node near Treitz's ligament.

Stark et al[223,224] reported a series of nine cases of gastrinoma. They found CT to be accurate for the detection and staging of gastrinomas. CT was accurate for showing the extent of the disease; in their series, four of nine patients were curable by surgery. Angiography detected only lesions larger than 2 cm, whereas CT detected 6 of 12 lesions smaller than 2 cm.

A report by London et al[143] defines the roles of CT, ultrasound, and angiography for detecting and staging gastrinomas. They found that ultrasound and CT were almost equal for the detection of hepatic gastrino-mas, but CT was slightly better than ultrasound for extrahepatic lesions. Angiography was superior to both ultrasound and CT for both of these areas.

A report by Tham et al[230,231] discussed the merits of CT and MRI for detection of gastrinomas. They found there was no clear advantage of MRI over CT in their series but also noted that MRI showed promise for future improvement. Because MRI showed increased intensity on T2-weighted images, they speculated that with future refinements related to motion compensation and imaging time, MRI might prove to be the modality of choice for the future (there were no consistent signal characteristics on T1-weighted images).

Considering the available data, it is clear that both CT and angiography are needed for the preoperative evaluation of gastrinoma. If these methods are unsuccessful in detecting a pancreatic lesion, intraoperative ultrasound will undoubtedly be useful for small lesion detection.

Glucagonoma. Tumors of the A islet cells result in a clinical syndrome consisting of a rash, diabetes mellitus, and weight loss. When benign, the lesion may be surgically extirpated, but when malignant, it responds favorably to chemotherapeutic agents.

The largest experience reported to date has been by Breatnach et al,[29] who reported on seven patients. Six cases had histological proof of glucagonoma, and one case had clinical proof. Five of the six cases with histological proof were malignant.

The size of the masses varied from 2.5 to 6 cm in size. Densities of the masses were less than those of the normal gland after the administration of intravenous contrast material. In most cases, there were clearly defined margins to the tumor (in contrast to infiltration of the planes, which occurs with adenocarcinoma). Calcifications occurred in three of the six cases. The authors did not comment on the use of dynamic bolus scanning in these patients.

All six patients underwent angiography, which demonstrated hypervascular lesions in all cases. Venous samplings were not mentioned.

Somatostatinoma. Somatostatinoma is the rarest of all islet cell tumors; only eight cases have been reported and only one case with CT findings. Somatostatinoma produces a hormone, somatostatin, that has some effect on insulin and glucagon, which may account for diabetes. It is a direct antagonist of cholecystokinin, which inhibits gallbladder contractility. The associated clinical findings with this entity are not as clearly defined as with other entities, but patients with this disorder have shown glucose intolerance and cholecystitis. Half have had diarrhea and weight loss.

The reported tumor size in this case and in the other cases was quite large, 3 to 10 cm. CT findings were nonspecific and showed only a soft tissue mass. No mention of vascularity or calcifications was made.[195]

It was the author's belief that CT should be capable of detecting such lesions because of the large size of the tumors.

Vipoma. Since the previous edition of this book, there has been a single report on CT and MRI imaging of a vipoma by Tham et al.[230,231] In their case report, they noted the tumor on CT was large, measuring 5 × 7 cm, and showed heterogeneous density with contrast enhancement. On MRI study, the tumor was isointense

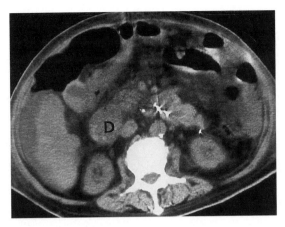

Fig. 32-145. Duodenal tumor *(D)* adjacent to the head of pancreas.

with T1-weighted images and hyperintense with T2-weighted images. There were no distinguishing features that would permit a preoperative diagnosis without the clinical information.

Percutaneous biopsy. I believe that percutaneous procedures are not prudent in patients who have endocrine-secreting tumors. It is not inconceivable that a surge of endocrine products that might threaten the patient or cause a bad result could be released. An aspiration was performed without difficulty in one patient with a cystic insulinoma. The authors were not aware of the diagnosis before the procedure.

Small bowel and metastatic tumors. Small bowel tumors are fairly common in the region of the third and fourth portion of the duodenum (Fig. 32-145). In such cases, careful attention to detail is necessary to ensure proper diagnosis. By the careful study of the normal anatomy around the uncinate process and Treitz's ligament, tumors in this region can successfully be identified because of the effacement of the contrast material.

Metastatic tumors in the pancreas are not uncommon.[169,199] The cell types that may occur include breast, lung (Fig. 32-146), colon, gastric, renal, pulmonary, ovarian, gallbladder, hepatoma, melanoma, lymphoma, angiosarcoma, and leiomyosarcoma. The most frequent are lung, breast, and lymphoma. Gastric, colon, or renal cells can contiguously spread through the adjacent ligaments. They have no distinguishing features except at times extension of the tumor margins from the stomach, colon, or kidney.

Postoperative evaluation

Two types of postoperative evaluation should be discussed: changes associated with displacement of the gland after surgery on adjacent organs and changes associated with surgery on the gland itself. In most patients

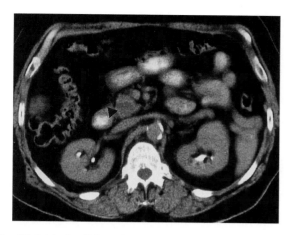

Fig. 32-146. Small low-density mass *(arrowhead)* in head of pancreas proved to be metastatic lung tumor.

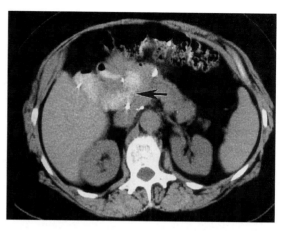

Fig. 32-147. CT scan of postoperative pancreas shows dilute barium in bowel adjacent to the pancreas *(arrow)*.

who have resection of the kidneys or the spleen, the pancreas changes location slightly and moves toward the area where the adjacent organ has been removed. Once movement has occurred, the position remains stable, and one must then simply monitor the appearance on any subsequent examinations.

After pancreatectomy, several findings can be seen, depending on the location and type of resection. Because some type of gastric bypass will have been performed, the appearance of the surgical anastomosis of the bowel must be monitored (Fig. 32-147). If motility of the bowel is excessive, it may be necessary to administer glucagon to immobilize the bowel, as suggested by Heiken et al.[88]

OVERALL DIAGNOSTIC ACCURACY

With the continued refinement of CT imaging and contrast enhancement techniques, CT scanning has continued to be the mainstay for diagnosing pancreatic pathology. In the early years of CT, considerable work was performed to assess the diagnostic accuracy as compared with ultrasound. These classic articles[10,16,114,168] showed the superiority of CT.

The largest and most comprehensive study about the pancreas evaluated the diagnostic accuracy of ultrasound and CT.[94] In this series, which included 279 patients (146 normal and 133 abnormal), the accuracy rate was evaluated using receiver operator curves (ROC). Hessel et al[94] found that CT was more accurate than ultrasound for determination of normal tissue, inflammation, or neoplasm. When 44 suboptimal ultrasound studies were excluded, CT proved to be better. In detecting a lesion as abnormal and identifying it as malignant or inflammatory, CT had a sensitivity level of 0.84 and ultrasound of 0.56.

For the evaluation of inflammatory processes, CT is superior to all other modalities. It is capable of determining the full extent of inflammatory processes and presence of complications and can determine the need for surgical debridement when pancreatic necrosis occurs. Furthermore, with the refinement of interventional techniques, CT offers a superior guidance method for diagnosing and treating pseudocysts and inflammatory processes.

Despite the fact that CT, ultrasound, and MRI have improved visualization of tumors, a positive effect on the outcome of the pancreatic tumors has not been found. The mortality rate and detection of resectable cases have not significantly changed. It does appear, however, that diagnoses are being made earlier, with fewer studies and greater ease for the patient.

In 1983, Savarino et al[203] reviewed the outcome of two groups of tumor patients, one evaluated before and the other after the development of angiography, ultrasound, and CT. Accuracy rates for resectable tumors were as follows for the different modalities: angiography, 85%; ERCP, 88%; ultrasound, 73%; and CT, 81%. The sensitivity levels for unresectable tumors were as follows: angiography, 88%; ERCP, 90%; ultrasound, 75%; and CT, 85%. There was no difference in the number of resections after the development of the newer imaging tests, but the number of exploratory laparotomies was reduced.

In the most recent review of the outcome and staging of pancreatic neoplasms by Freeny et al,[62] there was a high accuracy for detection and staging of tumors, but the outcome of the patients was uniformly poor (see earlier section on tumor staging and prognosis). It seems that for the foreseeable future, the role of imaging will be to prove inoperability of patients with tumors to prevent needless morbidity, mortality, and expense for treating incurable patients.

COST EFFICACY

CT has decreased the role of other diagnostic tests. This, of course, translates into monetary and emotional economy for the patient and the health care system. Freeny et al[61] looked at two groups of patients, one group of 278 studied before CT and the other group of 300 studied after. CT enabled the correct diagnosis without the aid of other studies in 74% of the cases. Additional studies required in the other cases are as follows: ERCP, 15%; angiography, 5%; and ERCP and angiography, 5%. The accumulative diagnostic accuracy rate, for normal tissue, pancreatitis, and neoplasm, was 99% for the pre-CT group and 97% for the post-CT group. For the post-CT group, CT reduced the use of ERCP by 68% and angiography by 54%; there was also an overall reduction in cost of radiological diagnosis by 47%. This was an absolute dollar-value change from $863 per case to $459.

Use of fine-needle biopsy combined with CT scanning has been described by Mitty et al.[167] They evaluated the total cost for initial diagnosis and palliation of pancreatic carcinoma in patients in whom radiological biopsy and drainage procedures were performed. They then compared it with the cost of standard surgical methods. For 53 patients, there was an overall cost savings of $169,800, mostly from avoidance of laparotomy and reduced hospitalization.

REFERENCES

1. Agostini S: Mucinous pancreatic duct ectasia in the body of the pancreas. *Radiology* 170:815-816, 1989.
2. Ahlstrom H, Magnusson A, Grama D, et al: Preoperative localization of endocrine pancreatic tumors by intra-arterial dynamic computed tomography. *Acta Radiol* 31:171-175, 1990.
3. Alexander ES, Clark RA, Federle MP: Pancreatic gas: indication of pancreatic fistula. *AJR* 139:1089, 1982.
4. Alfidi RJ, et al: Special report: new indications for computed body tomography. *AJR* 133:115, 1979.
5. Allibone G, Porter SC, Becker SN: Lipid granulomatosis causing lymph node enlargement: CT appearance. *AJR* 138:744, 1982.
6. Ammann R: Acute pancreatitis. In Bockus HL, editor: *Gastroenterology,* vol 3, Philadelphia, 1976, WB Saunders.
7. Andrew WK, Thomas RG: Hydatid cyst of the pancreatic tail. *S Afr Med* 59:235, 1981.
8. Andriole, et al: Spontaneous pancreatic calcification—case report. *J Comput Assist Tomogr* 7:534-535, 1983.
9. Arenholz DH, Simmons RL: Fibrin in peritonitis. I. Beneficial and adverse effects of fibrin in experimental *E. coli* peritonitis. *Surgery* 88:41, 1980.
10. Ariyama J, et al: Critical comparison of methods of examination for the diagnosis of pancreatic carcinoma. *ROFO* 133:6, 1980.
11. Baker ME, Cohan RH, Nadel SN, et al: Obliteration of the fat surrounding the celiac axis and superior mesenteric artery is not a specific CT finding of carcinoma of the pancreas. *AJR* 155:991-994, 1990.
12. Baker MK, Kopecky KK, Wass JL: Perirenal pancreatic pseudocysts: diagnostic management. *AJR* 140:729, 1983.
13. Balthazar EJ, Robinson DL, Megibow AJ, Ranson JHC: Acute pancreatitis: value of CT in establishing prognosis. *Radiology* 174:331-336, 1990.
14. Balthazar EJ, et al: Solid and papillary epithelial neoplasm of the pancreas. *Radiology* 150:39, 1984.
15. Balthazar EJ, et al: Acute pancreatitis: prognostic value of CT. *Radiology* 156:767, 1985.
16. Barkin J, et al: Computerized tomography, diagnostic ultrasound, and radionuclide scanning: comparison of efficacy in diagnosis of pancreatic carcinoma. *JAMA* 238:2040, 1977.
17. Bartholomew LG: Hereditary and familial pancreatitis. In Bockus HL, editor: *Gastroenterology,* vol 3, Philadelphia, 1976, WB Saunders.
18. Bastid C, Sahel J, Sastre B, et al: Mucinous cystadenocarcinoma of the pancreas. *Acta Radiol* 30:45-47, 1989.
19. Beebe DS, et al: Management of pancreatic pseudocysts. *Surg Gynecol Obstet* 195:562-564, 1984.
20. Beger HG, Maier W, Block S, Buchler M: How do imaging methods influence the surgical strategy in acute pancreatitis? In Malfertheiner P, Ditschuneit H, editors: *Diagnostic procedures in pancreatic disease,* Berlin, 1986, Springer-Verlag.
21. Berland LL, et al: Computed tomography of the normal and abnormal pancreatic duct: correlation with pancreatic ductography. *Radiology* 141:715, 1981.
22. Bittner R, Block S, Buchler M, Beger HG: Pancreatic abscess and infected pancreatic necrosis. Different local septic complications in acute pancreatitis. *Dig Dis Sci* 32:1082-1087, 1987.
23. Bivens BA, et al: Hemosulcus pancreaticus: gastrointestinal hemorrhage due to rupture of a splenic artery aneurysm. *Radiology* 129:276, 1978.
24. Block S, et al: Identification of pancreas necrosis in severe acute pancreatitis: imaging procedures versus clinical staging. *Gut* 27:1035-1042, 1986.
25. Bodurtha AJ, Dajee H, You CK: Analysis of 29 cases of pancreatic pseudocyst treated surgically. *Can J Surg* 23:432, 1980.
26. Borlaza GS, et al: Computed tomographic and angiographic demonstration of gastroduodenal artery pseudoaneurysm in a pancreatic pseudocyst. *J Comput Assist Tomogr* 3:612, 1979.
27. Bradley EL: Management of infected pancreatic necrosis by open drainage. *Ann Surg* 206:542-550, 1987.
28. Bradley EL, Clements JL, Gonzalez AC: The natural history of pancreatic pseudocysts: a unified concept of management. *Am J Surg* 137:135, 1979.
29. Breatnach ES, et al: CT evaluation of glucagonomas. *J Comput Assist Tomogr* 9:25, 1985.
30. Bretagne JF, et al: Pseudoaneurysms and bleeding pseudocysts in chronic pancreatitis: radiological findings and contribution to diagnosis in 8 cases. *Gastrointest Radiol* 15:9-16, 1990.
31. Brooks JR, Culebras JM: Cancer of the pancreas: palliative operation, Whipple procedure, or total pancreatectomy? *Am J Surg* 131:516, 1976.
32. Burke JW, et al: Pseudoaneurysms complicating pancreatitis: detection by CT. *Radiology* 161:447, 1986.
33. Callen PW, London SS, Moss AA: Computed tomographic evaluation of the dilated pancreatic duct: the value of thin-section collimation. *Radiology* 134:253, 1980.
34. Callen PW, et al: Carcinoma of the tail of the pancreas: an unusual CT appearance. *AJR* 133:135, 1979.
35. Campbell JR, Cruickshank AH: Cystadenoma and cystadenocarcinoma of the pancreas. *J Clin Pathol* 15:432, 1962.
36. Carroll B, Sample WF: Pancreatic cystadenocarcinoma: CT body scan and gray scale ultrasound appearance. *AJR* 131:339, 1978.

37. Charboneau JW, et al: Intraoperative real-time ultrasonographic localization of pancreatic insulinoma: initial experience. *Radiology* 151:853, 1984.

38. Cho KC, Lucak SL, Delany HM, et al: CT appearance in tuberculous pancreatic abscess. *J Comput Assist Tomogr* 14:152-154, 1990.

39. Choi BI, Kim KW, Han MC, et al: Solid and papillary epithelial neoplasms of the pancreas: CT findings. *Radiology* 166:413-416, 1988.

40. Choyke PL, et al: Von-Hippel-Lindau disease: radiologic screening for visceral manifestations. *Radiology* 174:815-820, 1990.

41. Clavien PA, Hauser H, Meyer P, Rohner A: Value of contrast-enhanced computerized tomography in the early diagnosis and prognosis of acute pancreatitis: a prospective study of 202 patients. *Am J Surg* 155:457-466, 1988.

42. Clyne CAC, Greene WJ, Paisey RB: Intra-operative ultrasound localization of an insulinoma undetected pre-operatively. *J Clin Ultrasound* 19:419-420, 1991.

43. Compagno J, Oertel JE: Microcystic adenomas of the pancreas (glycogen-rich cystadenomas): a clinicopathologic study of 34 cases. *Am J Clin Pathol* 69:289, 1978.

44. Compagno J, Oertel JE: Mucinous cystic neoplasms of the pancreas with overt and latent malignancy (cysadenocarcionma and cystadenoma): a clinicopathologic study of 41 cases. *Am J Clin Pathol* 69:573, 1978.

45. Cooperman AM, et al: *Pancreatoduodenal resection (PDR) and total pancreatectomy (TP): an institutional review.* New York, 1981, Departments of Surgery and Pathology, College of Physicians and Surgeons of Columbia University.

46. Crile G: The advantages of bypass operations over radical pancreatoduodenectomy in the treatment of pancreatic carcinoma. *Surg Gynecol Obstet* 130:1049, 1970.

47. Cubilla AL, Hajdu SI: Islet cell carcinoma of the pancreas. *Arch Pathol* 99:204-207, 1975.

48. Dastur KJ, Lewin JR: Computed tomography demonstration of tumor calcification after chemotherapy in a case of pancreatic carcinoma (abstract). *Radiology* 143:592, 1982.

49. Dembner AG, et al: A new computed tomographic sign of pancreatitis. *AJR* 133:477, 1979.

50. Doherty DE, et al: *Pseudomoas aeruginosa* sepsis following retrograde cholangiopancreatography. *Radiology* 145:266, 1982.

51. Eelkema EA, et al: CT features of nonfunctioning islet cell carcinoma. *AJR* 143:943, 1984.

52. Elechi EN, et al: The treatment of pancreatic pseudocysts by external drainage. *Surg Gynecol Obstet* 148:707, 1979.

53. Ertman R, Hausdorf G, Landbeck G: Pancreatic sonography in thallassemia major. *Klin Padiatr* 195:97, 1983.

54. Federle MP, et al: Computed tomography of pancreatic abscesses. *AJR* 136:879, 1981.

55. Feduska MJ, Dent TL, Lindenauer SM: Results of palliative operation for carcinoma of the pancreas. *Arch Surg* 103:330, 1971.

56. Ferrucci JR, et al: Computed body tomography in chronic pancreatitis. *Radiology* 130:175, 1979.

57. Fink IJ, et al: Demonstration of an angiographically hypovascular insulinoma with intraarterial dynamic CT. *AJR* 144:555, 1985.

58. Fishman A, et al: Significance of a dilated pancreatic duct on CT examination. *AJR* 133:225, 1979.

59. Foley WD, Lawson TL, Quiroz F: Sagittal and coronal image reconstruction: application in pancreatic computed tomography. *J Comput Assist Tomogr* 3:717, 1979.

60. Freeny PC: Portal vein tumor thrombus: demonstration by computed tomographic arteriography. *J Comput Assist Tomogr* 4:263, 1980.

61. Freeny PC, Marks WM, Ball TJ: Impact of high-resolution computed tomography of the pancreas on utilization of endoscopic retrograde cholangiopancreatography and angiography. *Radiology* 142:35, 1982.

62. Freeny PC, Marks WM, Ryan JA, Traverso LW: Pancreatic ductal adenocarcinoma: diagnosis and staging with dynamic CT. *Radiology* 166:125-133, 1988.

63. Freeny PC, et al: Cystic neoplasms of the pancreas: *new angiographic and ultrasonographic findings.* AJR 131:795, 1978.

64. Frick MP, et al: Pancreas imaging by computed tomography after endoscopic retrograde pancreatography. *Radiology* 150:191, 1984.

65. Friedman AC, Lichtenstein JE, Dachman AH: Cystic neoplasms of the pancreas. *Radiology* 149:45, 1983.

66. Friedman AC, et al: Solid and papillary epithelial neoplasm of the pancreas. *Radiology* 154:333, 1985.

67. Frucht H, et al: Gastrinomas: comparison of MR imaging with CT, angiography, and US. *Radiology* 171:713-717, 1989.

68. Fugazzola C, et al: Cystic tumors of the pancreas: evaluation by ultrasonography and computed tomography. *Gastrointest Radiol* 16:53-61, 1991.

69. Fukuya T, et al: Plasmacytoma of the pancreatic head. *Gastrointest Radiol* 14:226-228, 1989.

70. Galiber AK, et al: Pancreatic insulinoma localization: a comparison of preoperative and intraoperative US with angiography, CT and MR imaging. Scientific Program E394, presented at the Radiological Society of North America (RSNA) Conference, Chicago, 1986.

71. Gold RP, et al: Pancreas divisum with pancreatitis and pseudocyst. *AJR* 143:1343, 1984.

72. Gorman B, et al: Benign pancreatic insulinoma: preoperative and intraoperative sonographic localization. *AJR* 147:929-934, 1986.

73. Gould V, Delellis: The neuroendocrine system: its tumors, hyperplasia, and dysplasia. In *Principles and practice of surgical pathology,* New York, 1983, John Wiley & Sons.

74. Grant CS, et al: Insulinoma: the value of intraoperative ultrasonography. *Arch Surg* 123:843-848, 1988.

75. Greenberg M, et al: Computed-tomographic cholangiograhy: a new technique for evaluating the head of the pancreas and distal biliary tree. *Radiology* 144:363, 1982.

76. Gunn GD, Gibson RN: The left-sided pancreas. *Radiology* 159:713, 1986.

77. Gunther RW, Klose KJ, Ruckert K, et al: Localization of small islet-cell tumors. Preoperative and intraoperative ultrasound, computed tomography, arteriography, digital subtraction angiography and pancreatic venous sampling. *Gastrointest Radiol* 10:145-152, 1985.

78. Gunther W, et al: Islet cell tumors: detection of small masses with computed tomography and ultrasound. *Radiology* 148:485, 1983.

79. Haaga JR, Alfidi RJ: CT scanning of the pancreas. *J Belg Radiol* 59:281, 1976.

80. Haaga JR, Alfidi RJ: Computed tomographic scanning of the pancreas. *Radiol Clin North Am* 15:367, 1977.

81. Haaga JR, Alfidi RJ: Diagnostic procedures: computed tomography. In Cooperman AM, Hoerr SO, editors: *Surgery of the pancreas,* St. Louis, 1977, CV Mosby.

82. Haaga JR, Reich N: *Computed tomography of abdominal abnormalities,* St. Louis, 1978, CV Mosby.

83. Haaga JR, et al: Computed tomography of the pancreas. *Radiology* 120:589, 1976.

84. Hadar H, Gadoth N, Herskovitz P, Heifetz M: Short pancreas in polysplenia syndrome. *Acta Radiol* 32:299-301, 1991.

85. Haertel M, Zaunbauer W, WA: Computed tomographic morphology of pancreatic carcinoma. *ROFO* 133:1, 1980.

86. Hauser H, Battikha JG, Wettstein P: Computed tomography of the dilated main pancreatic duct. *J Comput Assist Tomogr* 4:53, 1980.

87. Havrilla TR, et al: Pseudocyst of the pancreas with perirenal extension: demonstration by computed tomography. *Comput Axial Tomogr* 1:199, 1977.

88. Heiken JP, et al: Radical pancreatectomy: postoperative evaluation by CT. *Radiology* 153:211, 1984.

89. Henrick AJ, Thomas CY, Friesen SR: Importance of pathologic staging in the surgical management of adenocarcinoma of the exocrine pancreas. *Am J Surg* 127:653, 1974.

90. Henderson JM, MacDonald JAE: Fistula formation complicating pancreatic abscess. *Br J Surg* 63:233, 1976.

91. Herman TE, Siegel MJ: Polysplenia syndrome with congenital short pancreas. *AJR* 156:799-800, 1991.

92. Heranz-Schulman et al: Pancreatic cystosis in cystic fibrosis. *Radiology* 158:629, 1986.

93. Hertzanu Y, Bar-Ziv J, Freund U: Computed tomography of unusual calcified pancreatic tumors. *J Comput Assist Tomogr* 13:75-76, 1989.

94. Hessel SJ, et al: A prospective evaluation of computed tomography and ultrasound of the pancreas. *Radiology* 143:129, 1982.

95. Hosoki T: Dynamic CT of pancreatic tumors. *AJR* 140:959, 1983.

96. Howard TJ, Stabile BE, Zinner MJ, et al: Anatomic distribution of pancreatic endocrine tumors. *Am J Surg* 159:258-264, 1990.

97. Hurley JE, Vargish T: Early diagnosis and outcome of pancreatic abscesses in pancreatitis. *Am Surg* 53:29-33, 1987.

98. Ishikawa T, et al: Venous abnormalities in portal hypertension demonstrated by CT. *AJR* 134:271, 1980.

99. Isikoff MB, et al: The clinical significance of acute pancreatic hemorrhage. *AJR* 136:679, 1981.

100. Isler RJ, et al: Tissue core biopsy of abdominal tumors with a 22 gauge cutting needle. *AJR* 136:725, 1981.

101. Itai Y, Moss AA, Goldberg HI: Pancreatic cysts caused by carcinoma of the pancreas: a pitfall in the diagnosis of pancreatic carcinoma. *Radiology* 147:309, 1983.

102. Itai Y, Moss AA, Ohtomo K: Computed tomography of cystadenoma and cystadenocarcinoma of the pancreas. *Radiology* 145:419, 1982.

103. Itai Y, et al: Computed tomographic appearance of resectable pancreatic carcinoma. *Radiology* 143:719, 1982.

104. Ivancev K, Kullendorff C-M: Value of computed tomography in traumatic pancreatitis in children. *Acta Radiol [Diagn] (Stockh)* 24:441, 1983.

105. Jafri SZH, et al: Comparison of CT and angiographic in assessing resectability of pancreatic carcinoma. *AJR* 142:525, 1984.

106. Jeffrey RB, Federle M, Crass RA: Computed tomography of pancreatic trauma. *Radiology* 147:491, 1983.

107. Jeffrey RB, Federle MP, Laing FC: Computed tomography of mesenteric involvement in fulminant pancreatitis. *Radiology* 147:185, 1983.

108. Jeffrey RB, Laing FC, Wing VW: Extrapancreatic spread of acute pancreatitis: new observations with real-time US. *Radiology* 159:707, 1986.

109. Jeffrey RB, et al: Early computed tomographic scanning in acute severe pancreatitis. *Surg Gynecol Obstet* 154:170, 1982.

110. Johnson CD, Stephens DH, Charboneau JW, et al: Cystic pancreatic tumors: CT and sonographic assessment. *AJR* 151:1133-1138, 1988.

111. Johnson CD, Stephens DH, Sarr MG: CT of acute pancreatitis: correlation between lack of contrast enhancement and pancreatic necrosis. *AJR* 156:93-95, 1991.

112. Jordan GL, Spjut HJ: Hemorrhagic pancreatitis. *Arch Surg* 104:489, 1972.

113. Juttner HU, et al: Ultrasound demonstration of portosystemic collaterals in cirrhosis and portal hypertension. *Radiology* 142:459, 1982.

114. Kamin PD, et al: Comparison of ultrasound and computed tomography in the detection of pancreatic malignancy. *Cancer* 46:2410, 1980.

115. Kane RA, Katz SG: The spectrum of sonographic findings in portal hypertension: a subject review and new observations. *Radiology* 142:453, 1982.

116. Kaplan JO, et al: Necrotic carcinoma of the pancreas: "the pseudo-pseudocyst." *J Comput Assist Tomog* 4:166, 1980.

117. Karasawa E, et al: CT pancreatogram in carcinoma of the pancreas and chronic pancreatitis. *Radiology* 148:489, 1983.

118. Kaye MD, et al: Gastric pseudotumor on CT scanning. *AJR* 135:190, 1980.

119. Kellokumpu-Lehtinen P, Huovinen R, Tuominen J: Pancreatic cancer. Evaluation of prognostic factors and treatment results. *Acta Oncol* 28:481-484, 1989.

120. Kim SY, Lim JH, Lee JD: Papillary carcinoma of the pancreas: findings of US and CT. *Radiology* 154:338, 1985.

121. Kivisaari L, Korman M, Rantakokko V: Contrast enhancement of the pancreas in computed tomography. *J Comput Assist Tomogr* 3:772, 1979.

122. Kivisaari L, et al: A new method for the diagnosis of acute hemorrhagic-necrotizing pancreatitis using contrast enhanced CT. *Gastrointest Radiol* 9:27-30, 1984.

123. Kloppel G, Maillet B: Classification and staging of pancreatic nonendocrine tumors. *Radiol Clin North Am* 27:105-119, 1989.

124. Kolars JC, Allen MO, Ansel H, et al: Pancreatic pseudocysts: clinical and endoscopic experience. *Am J Gastroenterology* 84:259-264, 1989.

125. Kolmannskog F, Kolbenstvedt A, Aakhus T: Computed tomography in inflammatory mass lesions following acute pancreatitis. *J Comput Assist Tomogr* 5:169, 1981.

126. Kolmannskog F, Schrumpf E, and Valnes K: Computed tomography and angiography in pancreatic apudomas and cystadenomas. *Acta Radiol [Diagn] (Stockh)* 23:365, 1982.

127. Kolmannskog F, et al: Computed tomography and ultrasound of the normal pancreas. *Acta Radiol [Diagn] (Stockh)* 23:443, 1982.

128. Kreel L, Sandin B: Changes in pancreatic morphology associated with aging. *Gut* 14:952, 1973.

129. Kressel HY, et al: CT scanning and ultrasound in the evaluation of pancreatic pseudocysts: a preliminary comparison. *Radiology* 126:153, 1978.

130. Krudy AG, et al: Localization of islet cell tumors by dynamic and venous sampling. *AJR* 143:585, 1984.

131. Lammer J, et al: Pseudotumorous pancreatitis. *Gastrointest Radiol* 10:59, 1985.

132. Lawson DW, et al: Surgical treatment of acute necrotizing pancreatitis. *Ann Surg* 4:605, 1970.

133. Lawson TL: Inflammatory disease of the pancreas: computed tomographic evaluation. Syllabus for Society of Computed Tomography, 1982.

134. Lawson TL: Acute pancreatitis and its complications: computed tomography and sonography. *Radiol Clin North Am* 21:495, 1983.

135. Lederman M: Personal communication, 1988.

136. Lee JKT, et al: Pancreatic imaging by ultrasound and computed tomography: a general review. *Radiol Clin North Am* 16:105, 1979.

137. Lee MJ, Saini S, Geller SC, et al: Pancreatitis with pseudoaneurysm formation: a pitfall for the interventional radiologist. *AJR* 156:97-98, 1991.

138. Legg M, Khettry: The pancreas and extrahepatic biliary system. In *Principles and practice of surgical pathology,* New York, 1983, John Wiley & Sons.

139. Levine E, et al: CT screening of the abdomen in von Hippel-Lindau disease. *AJR* 139:505, 1982.

140. Levitt RG, et al: Complementary use of ultrasound and computed tomography in studies of the pancreas and kidneys. *Radiology* 126:149, 1978.

141. Lim JH, Ko YT: Clonorchiasis of the pancreas. *Clin Radiol* 41:195-198, 1990.

142. Lindstrom E, Ihse I: Computed tomography findings in pancreas divisum. *Acta Radiol* 6:609-613, 1989.

143. London JF, et al: Zollinger-Ellison syndrome: prospective assessment of abdominal US in the localization of gastrinomas. *Radiology* 178:763-767, 1991.

144. Long JA, et al: Computed tomographic analysis of beta-thalassemic syndromes with hemochromatosis: pathologic findings with clinical and laboratory correlations. *J Comput Assist Tomogr* 4:159, 1980.

145. Luetmer PH, Stephens DH, Fischer AP: Obliteration of periarterial retropancreatic fat on CT in pancreatitis: an exception to the rule. *AJR* 153:63-64, 1989.

146. Luetmer PH, Stephens DH, Ward EM: Chronic pancreatitis: reassessment with current CT. *Radiology* 171:353-357, 1989.

147. Madrazo BL, et al: Computed tomographic findings in penetrating peptic ulcer. *Radiology* 153:751, 1984.

148. Maier W: Grading of acute pancreatitis by computed tomography morphology. In Malfertheiner P, Ditschuneit H, editors: *Diagnostic procedures in pancreatic disease,* Berlin, 1986, Springer-Verlag.

149. Mailberger E, Edoute Y, Nagler A: Rare complications after transabdominal fine needle aspiration. *Am J Gastroenterol* 79:458-460, 1984.

150. Manabe T, Miyashita T, Ohshio G, et al: Small carcinoma of the pancreas: clinical and pathologic evaluation of 17 patients. *Cancer* 62:135-141, 1988.

151. Marchal G, Baert AL, Wilms G: Intravenous pancreaticography in computed tomography. *J Comput Assist Tomogr* 3:727, 1979.

152. Markle B, et al: *Anomalies and congenital disorders: radiology of the liver, biliary tract, pancreas, and spleen,* Baltimore, 1987, Williams & Wilkins.

153. Marks IN, Bank S: Chronic pancreatitis, relapsing pancreatitis, calcifications of the pancreas. II. Clinical aspects. In Bockus HL, editor: *Gastroenterology,* vol. 3, Philadelphia, 1976, WB Saunders.

154. Marn CS, Glazer GM, Williams DM, Francis IR: CT-angiographic correlation of collateral venous pathways in isolated splenic vein occlusion: new observations. *Radiology* 175:375-380, 1990.

155. Martin EW, et al: Surgical decision-making in the treatment of pancreatic pseudocysts: internal versus external drainage. *Am J Surg* 138:821, 1979.

156. Marx M, Scheible W: Cavernous transformation of the portal vein. *J Ultrasound Med* 1:167, 1982.

157. Masaryk TJ, Achkar E: Pancreatitis as initial presentation of cystic fibrosis in young adults: a report of two cases. *Dig Dis Sci* 28:874, 1983.

158. Mathieu, et al: Portal cavernoma: dynamic CT features and transient differences in hepatic attenuation. *Radiology* 154:743-748, 1985.

159. McCain, et al: Varices from portal hypertension: correlation with CT and angiography. *Radiology* 154:63, 1985.

160. McCowin MJ, Federle MP: Computed tomography of pancreatic pseudocysts of the duodenum. *AJR* 154:1003, 1985.

161. Megibow AJ, et al: Thickening of the celiac axis and/or superior mesenteric artery: a sign of pancreatic carcinoma on computed tomography. *Radiology* 141:449, 1981.

162. Mendez et al: Significance of intrapancreatic gas demonstrated by CT: review of nine cases. *AJR* 132:59, 1979.

163. Mercer D, Ghent WR: Gastroduodenal artery aneurysm associated with chronic relapsing pancreatitis. *Can Med Assoc J* 126:1065, 1982.

164. Meyers MA, Evans JA: Effects of pancreatitis on the small bowel and colon: spread along mesenteric planes. *Department of Radiology, The New York Hospital Cornell University Medical Center* 119:151, 1973.

165. Minami M, et al: Cystic neoplasms of the pancreas: comparison of MR imaging with CT. *Radiology* 171:53-56, 1989.

166. Mitnick JS, et al: CT in β-thalassemia: iron deposition in the liver, spleen, and lymph nodes. *AJR* 136:1191, 1981.

167. Mitty HA, Efremidis SC, Yeh H-C: Impact of fine-needle biopsy on management of patients with carcinoma of the pancreas. *AJR* 137:1119, 1981.

168. Moss AA, et al: The combined use of computed tomography and endoscopic retrograde cholangiopancreatography in the assessment of suspected pancreatic neoplasm: a blind clinical evaluation. *Radiology* 134:159, 1980.

169. Muranaka T, et al: Computed tomography and histologic appearance of pancreatic metastases from distant sources. *Acta Radiol* 30:615-619, 1989.

170. Neff CC, et al: Inflammatory pancreatic masses: problems in differentiating focal pancreatitis from carcinoma. *Radiology* 150:35, 1984.

171. Neumann CH, Buttner CH: Pancreatic tail pseudotumor: CT demonstration of an anatomic variation of the pancreatic tail responsible for abnormal finding on conventional radiographic and ultrasonographic abdominal examinations. *CT-Sonographic* 3:80, 1983.

172. Neumann CH, Hessel SJ: CT of the pancreatic tail. *AJR* 135:741, 1980.

173. Nguyen KT, Pace R, Groll A: CT appearance of annular pancreas: a case report. *J Can Assoc Radiol* 40:322-323, 1989.

174. Nicholas DM, Li DK: Superior mesenteric vein rotation: a CT sign of midgut malrotation. *AJR* 141:707-708, 1983.

175. Nicholson RL: Abnormalities of the perinephric fascia and fat in pancreatitis. *Radiology* 139:125, 1981.

176. Nordestgaard AG, Wilson SE, Williams RA: Early computerized tomography as a predictor of outcome in acute pancreatitis. *Am J Surg* 152:127-132, 1986.

177. Norton JA, et al: Localization and surgical treatment of occult insulinomas. *Am Surg* 212:615-620, 1990.

178. Owens GR, et al: CT evaluation of mediastinal pseudocyst. *J Comput Assist Tomogr* 4:256, 1980.

179. Paivansalo M, Makarainen H, Siniluoto T, et al: Ultrasound compared with computed tomography and pancreatic arteriography in the detection of endocrine tumours of the pancreas. *Eur J Radiol* 9:173-178, 1989.

180. Pandolfo I, et al: Cystic lymphangioma of the pancreas: CT demonstration. *J Comput Assist Tomogr* 9:209, 1985.

181. Pantongrag-Brown L, Suwanwela N, Arjhansiri K, et al: Demonstration on computed tomography of two pseudoaneurysms complicating chronic pancreatitis. *Br J Radiol* 64:754-757, 1991.

182. Parienty RA, et al: Cystadenomas of the pancreas: diagnosis by computed tomography. *J Comput Assist Tomogr* 4:364, 1980.

183. Patel S, et al: Fat replacement of the exocrine pancreas. *AJR* 135:843, 1980.

184. Petruschak MJ, Haaga JR, Pardes JG: CT demonstration of spontaneous internal drainage of a pancreatic pseudocyst. *CT* 5:534, 1981.

185. Phillips GWL, Chou ST, Mulhauser J: Papillary cystic tumour of the pancreas: findings at computed tomography and ultrasound. *Br J Radiol* 64:367-369, 1991.

186. Phillips HE, et al: Pancreatic sonography in cystic fibrosis. *AJR* 137:69, 1981.

187. Pistolesi GF, et al: Computed tomography in surgical pancreatic emergencies. *J Comput Assist Tomogr* 2:165, 1978.

188. Pochhammer K-F, et al: The craniocaudad dimension [measurement] of the pancreatic head. *Digit Bilddiagn* 4:118, 1984.

189. Pograny AC, et al: Cystic insulinoma. *AJR* 142:951, 1984.

190. Pollack EW, Michas C, Wolfman EF Jr: Pancreatic pseudocyst management in fifty-four patients. *Am J Surg* 135:199, 1978.

191. Radin DR, et al: Pancreatic acinar cell carcinoma with subcutaneous and intraosseous fat necrosis. *Radiology* 158:67, 1986.

192. Ramming KP, Haskell CM, Tesler AS: Gastrointestinal tract neoplasms. In Haskell CM, editor: *Cancer treatment,* Philadelphia, 1980, WB Saunders.

193. Raptopoulos V, et al: Renal fascial pathway: posterior extension of pancreatic effusions within the anterior pararenal space. *Radiology* 158:367, 1986.

194. Rifkin MD, Weiss SM: Intraoperative sonographic identification of nonpalpable pancreatic masses. *J Ultrasound Med* 3:409-411, 1984.

195. Roberts L, et al: Somatostatinoma of the endocrine pancreas: CT findings. *J Comput Assist Tomogr* 8:1015, 1984.

196. Rossi P, et al: Multiple bolus techniques: single bolus or infusion of contrast medium to obtain prolonged contrast enhancement of the pancreas. *Radiology* 144:929, 1982.

197. Rossi P, et al: CT of functioning tumors of the pancreas. *AJR* 144:57, 1985.

198. Rubin GD, Jeffrey RB, Walter JF: Pancreatic microcystic adenoma presenting with acute hemoperitoneum: CT diagnosis. *AJR* 156:749-750, 1991.

199. Rumancik WM, et al: Metastatic disease to the pancreas: evaluation by computed tomography. *J Comput Assist Tomogr* 8:829, 1984.

200. Sagalow BR, Miller CL, Wechsler RJ: Pancreactic sarcoidosis mimicking pancreatic cancer. *J Clin Ultrasound* 16:131-134, 1988.

201. Sandy JT, et al: Pancreatic pseudocyst. *Am J Surg* 14:574, 1981.

202. Sarles H, et al: Chronic pancreatitis, relapsing pancreatitis, calcifications of the pancreas. I. Pathology. In Bockus HL, editor: *Gastroenterology,* vol 3, Philadelphia, 1976, WB Saunders.

203. Savarino V, et al: Failure of new diagnostic aids in improving detection of pancreatic cancer at a resectable stage. *Dig Dis Sci* 28:1078, 1983.

204. Schmidt H, Creutzfeldt W: Etiology and pathogenesis of pancreatitis. In Bockus HL, editor: *Gastroenterology,* vol 3, Philadelphia, 1976, WB Saunders.

205. Schulte SJ, et al: Root of the superior mesenteric artery in pancreatitis and pancreatic carcinoma: evaluation with CT. *Radiology* 180:659-662, 1991.

206. Semelka RC, et al: Pancreatic disease: prospective comparison of CT, ERCP, and 1.5-T MR imaging with dynamic gadolinium enhancement and fat suppression. *Radiology* 181:785-791, 1991.

207. Sheedy PF II, et al: Computed tomography in the evaluation of patients with suspected carcinoma of the pancreas. *Radiology* 124:731, 1977.

208. Sheflin JR, Lee CM, Kretchmar KA: Torsion of wandering spleen and distal pancreas. *AJR* 142:100, 1984.

209. Shirkhoda A, Mittel Staedt CA: Demonstration of pancreatic cysts in adult polycystic disease by computed tomography and ultrasound. *AJR* 131:1074, 1978.

210. Shultz S, Drury EM, Friedman AC: Common hepatic artery aneurysm: pseudopseudocyst of the pancreas. *AJR* 144:1287, 1985.

211. Siegelman SS, et al: CT of fluid collections associated with pancreatitis. *AJR* 134:1121, 1980.

212. Sigel B, et al: Localization of insulinomas of the pancreas at operation by real-time ultrasound scanning. *Surg Gynecol Obstet* 156:145-147, 1983.

213. Smith FW, et al: Low-field (0.08 T) magnetic resonance imaging of the pancreas: comparison with computed tomography and ultrasound. *Br J Radiol* 62:796-802, 1989.

214. Smith TR, Koenigsberg M: Low-density insulinoma on dynamic CT. *AJR* 155:995-996, 1990.

215. Soulen MC, et al: Enlargement of the pancreatic head in patients with pancreas divisum. *Clin Imag* 13:51-57, 1989.

216. Soulen MC, et al: Pancreatic divisum: CT scanning and ERCP correlation. *Radiology* 161:145, 1986.

217. Spencer JA, Lindsell DRM, Isaacs D: Hereditary pancreatitis: early ultrasound appearances. *Pediatr Radiol* 20:293-295, 1990.

218. Stambler JB, et al: Tuberculous abscess of the pancreas. *Gastroenterology* 83:922, 1982.

219. Stanley J: Splanchnic aneurysms. In Rutherford RB, editor: *Splanchnic artery aneurysms,* Philadelphia, 1977, WB Saunders.

220. Stanley P: Portal hypertension. In Stanley P, Miller J, editors: *Pediatric angiography,* Baltimore, 1982, Williams & Wilkins.

221. Stanley RJ, Sagel SS, Levitt RG: Computed tomography evaluation of the pancreas. *Radiology* 124:715, 1977.

222. Stanten R, Frey CF: Comprehensive management of acute necrotizing pancreatitis and pancreatic abscess. *Arch Surg* 125:1269-1275, 1990.

223. Stark DD, Moss AA, Goldberg HJ, Deveney CW: CT of pancreatic islet cell tumors. *Radiology* 150:491-494, 1984.

224. Stark DD, et al: CT of pancreatic islet cell tumors. *Radiology* 150:491, 1984.

225. Steiner E, Stark DD, Hahn PF, et al: Imaging of pancreatic neoplasms: comparison of MR and CT. *AJR* 152:487-491, 1989.

226. Strax R, Toombs BD, Rauschkolb EN: Correlation of barium enema and CT in acute pancreatis. *AJR* 136:1219, 1981.

227. Stuckman ML, et al: Major gastrointestinal hemorrhage from peripancreatic blood vessels in pancreatitis: treatment by embolotherapy. *Dig Dis Sci* 29:486, 1984.

228. Susman N, Hammerman AM, Cohen E: The renal halo sign in pancreatitis. *Radiology* 142:323, 1982.

229. Teefey SA, Stephens DH, Sheedy PF II: CT appearance of primary pancreatic lymphoma. *Gastrointest Radiol* 11:41, 1986.

230. Tham RTOTA, Falke THM, Jansen JBM, Lamers CBHW: CT and MR imaging of advanced Zollinger-Ellison syndrome. *J Comput Assist Tomogr* 13:821-828, 1989.

231. Tham RTOTA, et al: MR, CT, and ultrasound findings of metastatic vipoma in pancreas. *J Comput Assist Tomogr* 13:142-144, 1989.

232. Tham RTOTA, et al: Cystic fibrosis: MR imaging of the pancreas. *Radiology* 179:183-186, 1991.

233. Thoeni RF, Fell SC, Goldberg HI: CT detection of asymptomatic pancreatitis following ERCP. *Gastrointest Radiol* 15:291-295, 1990.

234. Tisell LE, Ahlman H: Treatment of the pancreatic disease of multiple endocrine neoplasia type 1 (MEN 1). *Acta Oncol* 28:415-417, 1989.

235. Torres WE, et al: Gas in the pancreatic bed without abscess. *AJR* 137:1131, 1981.

236. Tucker DH, Moore B: Vanishing pancreatic calcifications in chronic pancreatitis: a sign of pancreatic carcinoma. *N Engl J Med* 268:31-33, 1963.

237. Vernacchia FS, et al: Pancreatic abscess: predictive value of early abdominal CT. *Radiology* 162:435-438, 1987.

238. Ward E, et al: Computed tomographic characteristics of pancreatic carcinoma: analysis of 100 cases. *Radiographics* 3:547, 1983.

239. Warren KW: Chronic pancreatitis, relapsing pancreatitis, calcifications. III. Surgery. In Bockus HL, editor: *Gastroenterology,* vol 3, Philadelphia, 1976, WB Saunders.

240. Warren KW: Tumors of the pancreas: II to IV. Surgical aspects of exocrine tumors. In Bockus HL, editor: *Gastroenterology,* vol 3, Philadelphia, 1976, WB Saunders.

241. Warshaw AL, Compton CC, Lewandrowski K, et al: Cystic tumors of the pancreas: new clinical radiologic and pathologic observations in 67 patients. *Ann Surg* 212:432-445, 1990.

242. Warshaw AL, Gu Z-Y, Wittenberg J, et al: Preoperative staging and assessment of resectability of pancreatic cancer. *Arch Surg* 125:230-233, 1990.

243. White EM, et al: Pancreatic necrosis: CT manifestations. *Radiology* 158:343, 1986.

244. Wilson TE, Korobkin M, Francis IR: Pancreatic plasmacytoma: CT findings. *AJR* 152:1227-1228, 1989.

245. Wilverstein W, et al: Diagnostic imaging of acute pancreatitis: prospective study using CT and sonography. *AJR* 137:497, 1981.

246. Wittenberg J, et al: Non-focal enlargement in pancreatic carcinoma. *Radiology* 144:131, 1982.

247. Wolfman NT, Karstaedt N, Kawamoto EH: Pleomorphic carcinoma of the pancreas: computed-tomographic, sonographic, and pathologic findings. *Radiology* 154:329, 1985.

248. Yuh WTC, et al: Pancreatic transplants: evaluation with MR imaging. *Radiology* 170:171-177, 1989.

249. Zakari S, et al: Ultrasonographic features of hydatid cyst of the pancreas: report of 2 cases. *Radiology* 156:266, 1985.

250. Zeman RK, et al: Pancreas divisum: thin-section CT. *Radiology* 169:395-398, 1988.

33
The Spleen

KATHRYN GRUMBACH
RHONDA McDOWELL

Until the advent of cross-sectional imaging techniques, the spleen remained a poorly understood organ, relatively inaccessible to the radiologist. However, the availability of computed tomography (CT) and magnetic resonance imaging (MRI) allow us to image the spleen with ease and identify a large gamut of disease entities affecting it. Over the years, CT and MRI have proved to be the imaging modalities of choice in the evaluation of most types of splenic pathologic conditions, allowing the radiologist to play a key role in the diagnosis and management of patients with splenic disease.

NORMAL ANATOMY

The spleen lies obliquely in the left upper quadrant with its long axis parallel to the left lower posterior ribs. Its diaphragmatic surface is smooth and closely abuts the left hemidiaphragm. Its visceral surface is in apposition to the stomach, left kidney, splenic flexure of the colon, and the tail of the pancreas. Each of these organs indents the splenic surface, giving it an undulating visceral surface contour.[131,135] A prominent splenic lobulation often projects between the tail of the pancreas and the left kidney and may become even more pronounced as the spleen enlarges (Fig. 33-1). This lobulation may be present in the normal spleen and may be confused with a left renal, left adrenal, or pancreatic tail mass on other imaging studies.[41,105] The superior border of the spleen is interposed between the diaphragm and the stomach and may have several notches of varying depth. The inferior border lies between the diaphragm and the left kidney and parallels the course of the posterior left eleventh rib. The inferior splenic margin may also be notched. On axial CT sections these notches appear as clefts in the splenic parenchyma and should not be con-

fused with splenic lacerations or infarcts (Fig. 33-2). The posterior aspect of the spleen abuts the vertebral column, and the anterior surface is related to the splenic flexure of the colon and the phrenicocolic ligament.

The spleen is entirely surrounded by peritoneum, which closely adheres to its capsule. Several folds of the peritoneum act as suspensory ligaments.[74] The splenorenal (lienorenal) ligament connects the hilum of the spleen with the left kidney, and it contains the splenic artery and vein and the tail of the pancreas. The gastrosplenic ligament is formed by the union of two leaves of peritoneum of the greater and lesser sacs and connects the hilum of the spleen with the stomach; it contains branches of the short gastric and left gastroepiploic vessels between its two layers. The phrenicocolic ligament supports the inferior pole of the spleen as it passes from the splenic flexure of the colon to the diaphragm.[74,131]

The size of the spleen varies with the age and the size of the patient, as well as with the individual's nutritional state.[135] Average splenic dimensions are 12 cm in craniocaudal extent, 7 cm in width, and 3 to 4 cm in thickness. Mean splenic weight is approximately 150 g with a range of 50 to 250 g. Splenic volume is usually less than 175 cc. The spleen tends to decrease in size and weight with advancing age in the normal individual.[131,135] On CT, variation in section level with respiration makes assessment of true splenic size difficult. A maximum craniocaudad extent of 12 to 15 cm has been suggested as the upper limit of normal for splenic size in the adult. However, we find it more accurate to make a qualitative assessment of splenic size. As a rule of thumb, if the inferior margin of the spleen extends further caudally than the tip of the right lobe of the liver or if the anterior splenic border extends further medially than the midaxillary line, then the spleen is enlarged (Fig. 33-3). If a more quantitative evaluation of splenic size is necessary, splenic volume determination may be carried out. Using the electronic cursor, the volumes of contiguous, 1-cm thick splenic slices may be obtained and then simply added together to calculate total splenic volume. This is accurate to ±5% of the splenic volume[13,82] and may be useful in cases, such as in the assessment of distal splenorenal shunt patency,[50] where changes in splenic size are of clinical importance.

Accessory spleens are normal anatomic variants that are commonly encountered on CT scanning. They appear as aggregates of splenic tissue varying in size from a few millimeters to several centimeters in diameter and may enlarge dramatically after splenectomy (Figs. 33-4, 33-5).[6] Accessory spleens have identical attenuation values and contrast enhancement to normal spleen and are usually located in the gastrosplenic ligament near the splenic hilum (Fig. 33-4), although they may be found anywhere within the peritoneal cavity.[94,116] Their presence may be confirmed on technetium-99m sulfur colloid images of the spleen.

The spleen is invested in a fibroelastic capsule that gives rise to the trabecular framework of the splenic interior. The interstices of this collagenous framework are

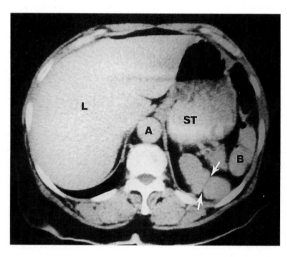

Fig. 33-2. Notched inferior splenic margin *(white arrows)* simulating splenic laceration. *L,* liver; *A,* aorta; *ST,* stomach; *B,* unopacified bowel. (From Friedman AC: *Radiology of the liver, biliary tract, pancreas and spleen,* Baltimore 1986, the Williams & Wilkins Co.)

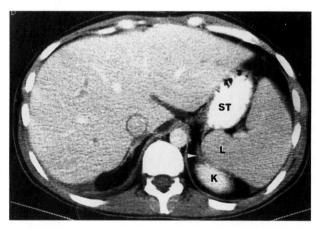

Fig. 33-1. Prominent medial splenic lobulation *(L)* interposed between left kidney *(K)* and stomach *(ST).* Left adrenal gland *(white arrow)* closely abuts the medial splenic lobulation.

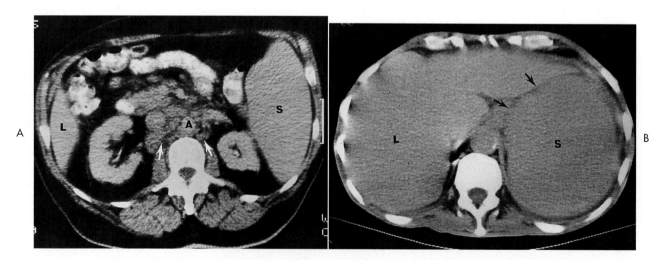

Fig. 33-3. A, Splenic tip *(S)* extends farther caudally than inferior margin of right hepatic lobe *(L)* in a patient with splenomegaly and retroperitoneal lymphadenopathy *(white arrows)* in diffuse histiocytic lymphoma. *A,* aorta. **B,** Anteromedial splenic border *(arrows)* extending medial to midaxillary line in a patient with splenomegaly and AIDS.

filled with the functional tissue of the spleen, the red and white pulp. The splenic artery divides into a variable number of branches (usually about five) within the splenorenal ligament as it enters the splenic hilum. Arteriolar branches of these splenic arteries ramify within the splenic trabeculae, lose their adventitial coat, and become ensheathed with lymphatic aggregates that constitute the splenic white pulp. These splenic lymphatic follicles are the site of the spleen's important immunologic and cytopoietic functions in the adult. The splenic arterioles continue to ramify and finally terminate in splenic cords that consist of reticular fibers to which macrophages are attached, in addition acting as a filter and regulator of blood flow. Blood then courses into numerous venous sinusoids, which are thin-walled vascular cavities conducting blood to the splenic trabecular veins. The splenic cords and sinusoids constitute the red pulp and are the site of erythrocyte storage and macrophage proliferation and differentiation within the spleen. The splenic trabecular veins drain the red pulp into five or more splenic vein branches, which emerge from the hilum and unite to form the splenic vein within the splenorenal ligament.[131,135]

COMPUTED TOMOGRAPHY
Technique of examination

The spleen is usually evaluated as part of a complete CT examination of the abdomen, especially in cases of abdominal trauma, metastatic carcinoma or lymphoma in which a survey of multiple abdominal structures is indicated. In our institution this routine survey consists of scans of 10-mm thickness obtained at 10-mm intervals from the dome of the diaphragm through the pelvis. If a specific splenic pathologic condition is suspected, narrower scan thickness and intervals of 5 mm to 10 mm

are used. Each image is obtained during the same phase of respiration to avoid changes in splenic position resulting from variations in diaphragmatic excursion and to more accurately assess splenic size. Opacification of adjacent gastrointestinal organs is achieved by the oral administration of a contrast agent, either diatrizoate meglumine (Gastrografin) diluted to a 2% solution in fruit juice or a 1% solution of barium sulfate (E-Z-CAT). This must be given in sufficient quantity (at least 500 ml) to distend the stomach and to opacify small bowel loops and the splenic flexure of the colon.

Intravenous contrast agents are usually necessary for the detection of splenic pathologic conditions because many splenic lesions may be isodense with the splenic parenchyma on precontrast scans. In most cases, the rapid administration of 100 to 150 cc of 60% water-soluble iodinated contrast (such as meglumine diatrizoate) or 70% iodinated nonionic contrast (such as Iohexol) in a total dose of 2 ml/kg in adults is sufficient to opacify the splenic parenchyma and to accentuate lower density hematomas, cysts, tumors, or abscesses. The contrast is best delivered in a single, rapid, intravenous bolus given at 2 cc/second. Scanning is begun 40 to 50 seconds after initiation of the bolus, and a rapid sequence of scans with a less than 3-second interscan delay is obtained. However, care must be taken not to initiate scanning too early in the bolus injection, since scanning in the arterial phase may lead to inhomogeneous splenic enhancement and the spurious diagnosis of a splenic pathologic condition (Fig. 33-6). Glazer et al found that 50% of patients with normal spleens displayed significant inhomogeneity of splenic enhancement if scans were obtained within 5 seconds of the termination of a rapidly administered contrast bolus (administered over 5 seconds). They postulated that this was due to variable rates of

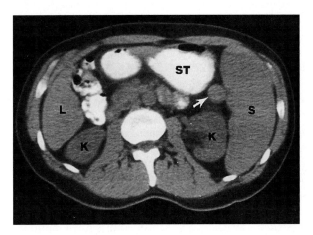

Fig. 33-4. Accessory spleen near the splenic hilum *(arrow)* in a patient with splenomegaly *(S)* and lymphoma. *ST,* stomach; *L,* liver; *K,* kidneys.

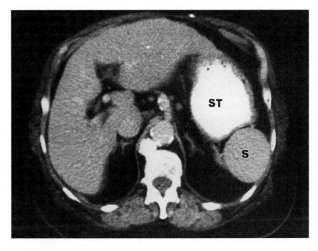

Fig. 33-5. Hypertrophied accessory spleen *(s)* in a patient after splenectomy. *ST,* stomach.

blood flow through the splenic red pulp.[38] A longer delay before the initiation of scanning may be necessary with ultrafast helical or spiral scanning, since there is no interscan delay with this technique.

Dynamic scanning during the arterial phase is helpful in several situations. It may be useful in distinguishing normal spleen from adjacent structures such as liver, left kidney, and pancreatic tail that have different temporal enhancement patterns.[38] In addition, rapid dynamic scanning through the splenic hilum may be useful in distinguishing accessory spleens from splenic hilar lymph nodes, varices, pancreatic tail masses, or a splenic artery aneurysm. Splenic varices enhance synchronously with the splenic vein, and a splenic artery aneurysm should show maximal enhancement at the same time as the aorta. Both of these vascular lesions show much higher peak CT numbers during enhancement than do accessory spleens, splenic hilar nodes, or pancreatic masses. Accessory spleens have an enhancement pattern similar to normal spleen, whereas splenic hilar lymph nodes rarely enhance to a significant degree.[38]

On nonenhanced scans, the spleen is slightly less dense than the liver, although the absolute attenuation value may vary with scanner type, calibration methods, beam-hardening artifacts over the spleen, kVp, and patient size and shape.[95] Because the spleen is a highly vascular organ with a single arterial blood supply, it reaches its peak level of contrast enhancement soon after the aorta. Since the liver has a dual blood supply that is 75% portal venous, it has a more delayed peak of contrast enhancement. If contrast is administered in sufficient quantity and concentration and if scanning is properly timed, peak splenic attenuation values of 100 to 150 Hounsfield units (HU) may be obtained during the arterial phase.

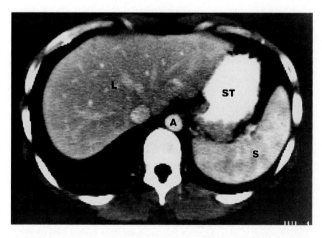

Fig. 33-6. Inhomogeneous splenic enhancement after rapid bolus injection in a normal patient. *S,* spleen; *ST,* stomach; *L,* liver; *A,* aorta.

If scans are obtained during or after the venous phase or if the contrast infusion rate is slow, splenic attenuation values will reach a lower peak (60 to 100 HU) and will be closer to that of liver. It should be noted that hypotensive patients may exhibit decreased splenic contrast enhancement relative to liver, resulting from sensitivity of the splenic vasculature to sympathetic stimulation in the hypotensive state. This should be remembered when interpreting CT examinations in traumatized patients, as hypotension alone may lead to decreased splenic enhancement without disruption of splenic circulation by direct injury.[8]

Experimental liver-spleen–specific CT contrast materials have been developed; the most popular of these is *EOE-13,* a liposoluble, iodinated agent.[75,121,126,128,129] Miller et al reported using this agent in 225 CT examinations.[75] EOE-13 causes large increases in normal splenic parenchymal attenuation (52 HU) but very little increase in tumor attenuation (3 HU), allowing identification of smaller lesions (1 to 1.5 cm in diameter) than with water-soluble contrast. The liver and spleen accumulate 80% of the iodine within 15 minutes of injection of EOE-13 and maintain a high concentration over the next 3 hours. Because of this organ specificity, examination may be performed with less than 10% of the iodine used with water-soluble contrast. Also, scanning may be performed at any time between 15 minutes and 3 hours after injection. EOE-13 easily differentiates spleen from surrounding structures such as the left kidney[126] and may be used to identify accessory spleens or splenic remnants after splenectomy.[127] Other liver-spleen–specific contrast agents, such as radiopaque liposomes and particulate iodipamide ethyl ester, have also been developed.[49,61,93] These agents all provide superior delineation of splenic pathology, but all, including EOE-13, remain classified as investigational and further proof of their diagnostic accuracy awaits further use.

Diffuse disease

Splenomegaly. When the diagnosis of splenomegaly is made clinically, CT is the radiologic examination of choice for further diagnostic investigation. A wide variety of disease entities lead to splenomegaly without evidence of focal masses on CT. These are caused by diffuse microscopic changes and are only reflected in changes in size or attenuation values of the spleen.[35]

A large number of infectious processes cause nonspecific splenomegaly without abscess formation. These include subacute bacterial endocarditis, infectious mononucleosis, cytomegalovirus infection, and parasitic diseases such as malaria and schistosomiasis.[35] Granulomatous diseases, including tuberculosis and histoplasmosis, may cause splenomegaly during the acute phase, but the most common CT finding is calcified granulomata in a normal-sized spleen indicating the residue of previous infection. These appear as punctate, high-density lesions within the splenic parenchyma and are common incidental findings on CT (Fig. 33-7). Splenomegaly is also a feature of acquired immune deficiency syndrome (AIDS), caused by the HIV virus. It is seen in the prodromal phase of the disease (AIDS-related complex) and in the full-blown syndrome of AIDS.[54] In addition, in AIDS patients splenomegaly may be related to superimposed infection by a wide variety of organisms or metastatic tumors.[55] A clue to the CT diagnosis of AIDS is the presence of generalized lymphadenopathy, soft-tissue infiltration of the perirectal fat, and masses within the gastrointestinal tract (Fig. 33-8). Splenic enlargement may also occur in AIDS-related lymphomas, and focal

splenic masses may be evident on CT in 10% to 26% of cases.[87]

Hematologic disease, particularly the myeloproliferative disorders, commonly cause diffuse splenic enlargement. These disease entities include chronic myelocytic leukemia, polycythemia vera, myelofibrosis, and myeloid metaplasia. Other forms of leukemia such as chronic lymphocytic leukemia also cause splenomegaly. In these disorders, the CT appearance is a homogeneously enlarged spleen of normal CT attenuation without focal masses. Nonneoplastic hematologic disorders that also cause splenomegaly include autoimmune hemolytic anemia, thrombocytopenic purpura, hereditary spherocytosis, and the hemoglobinopathies.[35] Patients with heterozygous sickle cell disease commonly demonstrate splenic enlargement on CT but may also have superimposed focal lesions such as infarcts, hematomas, or abscesses.[66] Patients with homozygous sickle cell disease may have enlarged spleens early in the course of the disease, but they invariably undergo autosplenectomy secondary to repeated infarction. On CT these end-stage spleens appear as small densely calcified organs with occasional low-density infarcts (Fig. 33-9).[66]

Congestive splenomegaly is usually caused by advanced hepatic cirrhosis with portal hypertension or by splenic vein occlusion or thrombosis.[35] The associated CT findings of nodular liver, enlarged caudate lobe, ascites, gastroesophageal varices, and collateral venous channels should suggest the diagnosis of portal hypertension. As previously mentioned, dynamic CT scanning may demonstrate a thrombosed or occluded splenic vein and may also suggest an underlying cause such as pancreatitis or pancreatic carcinoma.

Connective tissue disorders, including systemic lupus erythematosus and rheumatoid arthritis, may also

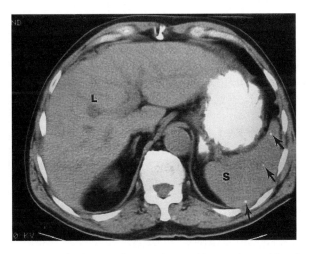

Fig. 33-7. Splenic granulomata *(arrows)* in a patient with prior exposure to histoplasmosis. *S,* spleen; *L,* liver.

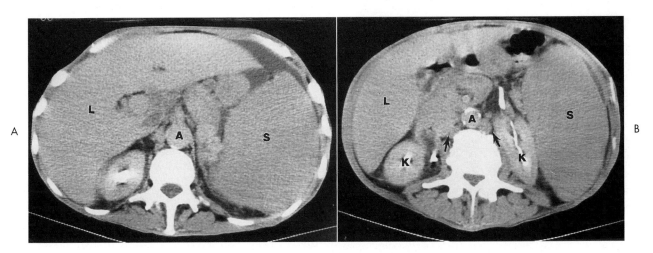

Fig. 33-8. A, Significant splenomegaly. **B,** Retroperitoneal lymphadenopathy *(arrows)* in a patient with AIDS. *S,* spleen; *L,* liver; *K,* kidneys; *A,* aorta.

lead to splenomegaly. Also, massive splenic enlargement is noted in a wide variety of metabolic disorders such as Gaucher's disease or Niemann-Pick disease.[35] Although clinical signs and symptoms are relied on for diagnosis of these disorders, CT is a useful method of follow-up of these patients, since change in splenic size may reflect success or failure of medical therapy.

Splenosis. The phenomenon of autotransplantation of splenic tissue within the peritoneal cavity results in splenosis. This most commonly follows traumatic rupture of the spleen and leads to rounded masses of splenic tissue anywhere within the abdomen with homogeneous enhancement similar to liver parenchyma.[36,72] These splenules rarely cause symptoms but are subject to the same abnormalities detected in normal spleens.[23] They provide immunologic function after the removal of a traumatized spleen and enlarge in size once vascularization of splenic tissue is established.

Polysplenia and asplenia. In polysplenia, the multiple right-sided splenic nodules are usually associated with midline or left-sided liver, equality in size of both hepatic lobes, azygous or hemiazygous continuation of the inferior vena cava, absent gallbladder, and malrotation of the bowel. The splenic nodules appear similar to accessory spleens, and no normally shaped aggregate of splenic tissue is noted in the upper abdomen.[24,111] CT plays an important role in identification of the abdominal anomalies seen in this syndrome. The syndrome of asplenia may also be identified on CT with absence of the spleen, total situs inversus or ambiguous abdominal situs, centrally located liver, and aorta and inferior vena cava located on the same side. Unlike polysplenia, this syndrome is commonly associated with congenital heart defects.[101]

Wandering spleen. This is an uncommon condition and is characterized by laxity or absence of the suspensory splenic ligaments, allowing the spleen to assume ectopic locations within the abdomen. Thus a wandering spleen may be confused with other abdominal masses, and radionuclide scintigraphy may be necessary to confirm the diagnosis.[26] Also, because of its long vascular pedicle, a wandering spleen may undergo torsion and infarction. This will present on CT as a nonenhancing heterogeneous mass anywhere within the abdomen, and no spleen will be evident in the left upper quadrant.[51,85,91]

Focal disease

Splenic trauma. The spleen is the most frequently injured organ in the upper abdomen secondary to blunt abdominal trauma.* CT has become the imaging modality of choice in the evaluation of hemodynamically stable patients after abdominal trauma, because it can image multiple organs simultaneously. It is quite sensitive in the diagnosis of traumatic lesions of the spleen, liver, and kidneys and is also accurate in the diagnosis of hemoperitoneum and retroperitoneal hemorrhage.[33,123] Jeffrey et al, in a series of 50 patients with suspected splenic trauma, found that CT correctly detected the presence or absence of splenic injury in 48 patients, with 21 of 22 true positives and 27 of 28 true negatives accurately diagnosed.[54] This accuracy of close to 100% has been confirmed by other prospective series.[59,136]

Traumatic lesions of the spleen include two broad categories: (1) subcapsular or intrasplenic hematoma, and (2) splenic laceration.[32,33,79,119,136] Subcapsular hematoma is easily diagnosed by CT and usually has a characteristic appearance of a crescentic, low-density fluid collection most commonly located along the lateral splenic margin.[60,83] Since the fluid collection is under tension within the splenic capsule, there is flattening of the normal convex lateral splenic surface. These hematomas commonly dissect around the medial and superior splenic margins, causing a similar flattening of the parenchymal borders in these regions (Figs. 33-10, 33-11). They may have a layered or "onion-skin" appearance, secondary to alternating layers of clotted and unclotted blood.[79] Intrasplenic extension may also occur, giving the hematoma a more irregular shape. In the acute phase, within 1 to 4 hours of injury, subcapsular hematomas may be isodense with splenic parenchyma on precontrast enhanced scans and may be visible only after contrast administration. Also, if CT scanning with intravenous con-

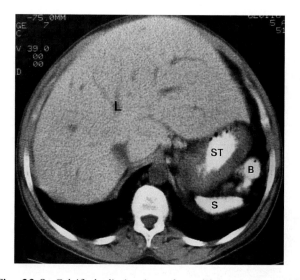

Fig. 33-9. Calcified, diminutive spleen *(S)* in a patient with homozygous sickle cell disease. Liver *(L)* is enlarged and of increased attenuation secondary to hemosiderosis. *ST,* stomach; *B,* bowel.

*References 32, 34, 54, 79, 119, 136.

trast is performed within 1 to 2 hours of injury, high-density material may be noted within a lower-density hematoma, representing continued leakage of blood with a high iodine content into the existing hematoma (Fig. 33-10). Both of these phenomena have been demonstrated in actual trauma patients and in experimental animals with surgically created subcapsular hematomas.[54,83]

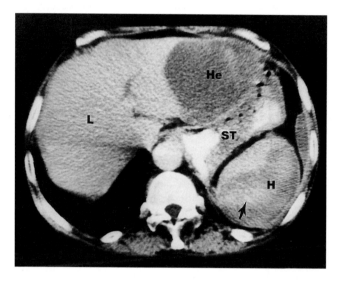

Fig. 33-10. Subcapsular hematoma of the spleen *(H)* containing high-density material *(arrow)* representing leakage of contrast into hematoma in a patient with acute, blunt abdominal trauma. A second, lower-density subcapsular hematoma of the liver *(He)* is also demonstrated. *L,* liver; *ST,* stomach. (From Friedman AC: *Radiology of the liver, biliary tract, pancreas and spleen,* Baltimore, 1986, the Williams & Wilkins Co.)

In the experimental group, subcapsular hematomas 7 days or older were readily apparent on CT even without intravenous contrast and showed a 25% to 55% reduction in CT number in the ensuing 7- to 28-day period posttrauma. Subacute and chronic hematomas more than 1 month of age may maintain their crescentic or oval shape, but because of lysis of clot and resorption of protein they have attenuation values approaching that of water.[83] The final sequelae of many splenic hematomas are thought to be false or non–epithelial-lined cysts that may remain unchanged in size for many years and may contain water-density cystic fluid[21,30] (see Fig. 33-15).

Splenic lacerations may be more subtle and variable in appearance on CT than subcapsular hematomas.[33,54,79] The findings on CT in splenic laceration include (1) indistinct splenic margins, (2) inhomogeneous splenic parenchyma, (3) linear, stellate, or rounded low density lacerations, (4) perisplenic clot, which may be higher in attenuation value than the splenic parenchyma, and (5) free fluid in left subphrenic space or elsewhere in the peritoneal cavity, which may be high density in acute splenic rupture[32,33,54] (Fig. 33-11). Splenic lacerations may be simulated by clefts in the splenic parenchyma (Fig. 33-2) or the splenic interface with an elongated left hepatic lobe (Fig. 33-12); however, these congenital variations will not be associated with perisplenic or subcapsular hematoma. As has been previously discussed, inhomogeneous enhancement of the normal spleen with rapid bolus injection may simulate splenic laceration, but again, no associated hematoma or hemoperitoneum will be visualized[38] (Fig. 33-6). Unopacified jejunal loops high in the left upper quadrant may simu-

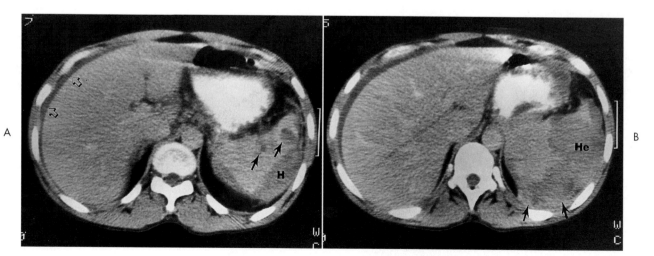

Fig. 33-11. A, Irregular and rounded, low-density splenic lacerations *(black arrows)* and subcapsular hematoma *(H)* in a patient after blunt abdominal trauma. There is fluid around the liver *(open arrows),* indicating hemoperitoneum. **B,** At a slightly lower level irregular, low-density subcapsular and intrasplenic hematomas are again demonstrated *(He)* with perisplenic extension of the fluid collection *(arrows).*

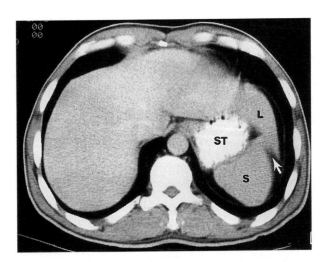

Fig. 33-12. Interface between extensive left hepatic lobe *(L)* and spleen *(S)* simulating splenic laceration *(white arrow)* in a normal patient. *ST,* stomach.

late splenic fragments; however, opacification of bowel, with oral contrast via nasogastric intubation if necessary, will clarify this situation. The intrasplenic hematomas that often accompany splenic lacerations have an irregular contour and inhomogeneous density. However even if a splenic laceration is not easily seen, the presence of perisplenic clot, subcapsular hematoma or free intraperitoneal blood should suggest the diagnosis of splenic trauma.[32,33,34,54,79] Artifacts caused by patient motion may mimic subcapsular or perisplenic hematoma; streak artifacts from IV lines, tubes or air-fluid levels may be confused with lacerations as may "beam-hardening" artifacts from adjacent ribs.[79] Careful scanning techniques should eliminate confusion of these artifacts with true splenic injuries.

CT now plays a major role in not only the diagnosis, but also in the management of patients with splenic trauma. Because of the risk of sepsis after splenectomy,[110,115] many surgeons opt for nonoperative management or splenic salvage procedures such as splenorrhaphy or splenic reimplantation in cases of splenic injury.[67,81] Thus follow-up CT scanning has become a common practice in patients managed without splenectomy and is important for the detection of delayed splenic rupture in such patients.* Several grading systems have been proposed in staging splenic injuries to determine which patients may need immediate surgery and which may be managed conservatively.[80,102,109,124] These systems depend heavily on the morphology of the splenic injury, the integrity of splenic vascular supply and the presence and size of the hemoperitoneum. Clinical

*References 25, 53, 80, 102, 109, 124.

factors such as hemodynamic status, transfusion requirements, peritoneal signs, or need for prolonged orthopedic or neurosurgical procedures precluding accurate physical examination all play an important role in management decisions.[80] If nonoperative management is elected, contrast-enhanced CT scans are usually performed 3 to 5 days and again 4 to 6 weeks after trauma if the patient is clinically stable.[25,79] Commonly, intrasplenic hematomas decrease in CT attenuation and initially increase in size as a result of dilution of clotted blood. Splenic lacerations develop smoother borders and often resolve as cystic masses within the splenic parenchyma. Large subcapsular hematomas may lead to fibrosis and thickening of the splenic capsule.[25,79] Occasionally the initial CT will fail to reveal significant splenic injury, but the spleen will go on to "delayed rupture" in the posttrauma period.[31,90,120] Therefore close clinical follow-up with repeat CT scanning with any hemodynamic deterioration is strongly recommended. In children, nonsurgical management of splenic injuries is more common than in adults because of decreased propensity to splenic rupture, and therefore CT plays a key role in follow-up of these children.[12] If posttraumatic splenectomy is necessary, CT is useful in detecting postsplenectomy complications such as left subphrenic hematoma or abscess, gastric wall or pancreatic lacerations.[79]

Splenic infarction. Splenic infarction is a relatively common process resulting from occlusion of a portion of the splenic arterial system, the most common etiology being emboli originating from mural thrombi in the heart. Local thrombosis of the splenic artery can occur in diseases affecting the arterial system, including atherosclerosis, polyarteritis nodosa and other arteritides, pancreatitis, pancreatic carcinoma, and splenic artery aneurysm. Thrombosis may also be caused by direct invasion of the arterial wall as in chronic myelocytic leukemia or by sludging of cells within the arterial lumen as in sickle cell disease and other hemoglobinopathies. Anatomic abnormalities such as splenic torsion also predispose one to local thrombosis. Septic infarcts are most commonly caused by bacterial endocarditis and may lead to splenic abscess formation.[4,19,44,69,113]

Splenic infarcts vary in size, but they rarely involve the entire organ. In the acute phase, they may cause mild splenomegaly, but as they heal by fibrosis, formation of multiple scars causes notching of the splenic contour and shrinkage of splenic mass. With global infarction of the spleen as seen in sickle cell disease, functional asplenia ensues, leading to a small, scarred, calcified organ[66] (Fig. 33-9).

Most splenic infarcts are asymptomatic and are often incidental findings at autopsy. When they do cause symptoms, they may present with left upper quadrant pain, friction rub over the upper abdomen, elevation of

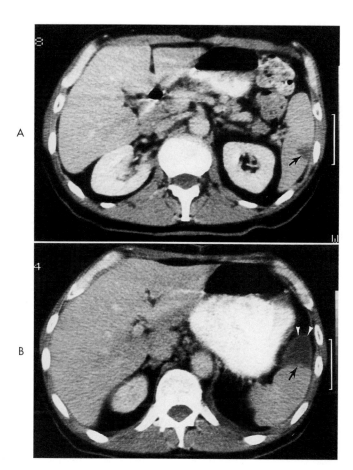

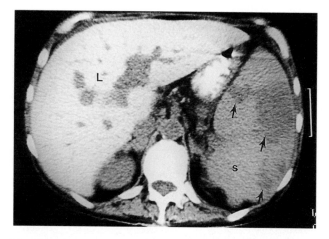

Fig. 33-14. Extensive, irregular-shaped, hypodense splenic infarcts *(arrows)* in a patient with splenomegaly *(S)*. The liver appears hyperdense secondary to hemosiderosis *(L)*. (From Friedman AC: *Radiology of the liver, biliary tract, pancreas and spleen,* Baltimore 1986, the Williams & Wilkins Co.)

Fig. 33-13. A, Characteristic peripheral, low-density, wedge-shaped splenic infarct *(arrow)* in a patient with a prosthetic heart valve, on contrast-enhanced CT. B, At a slightly higher level a second, low-density splenic infarct is demonstrated *(black arrow)* with residual enhancement of splenic capsule *(white arrowheads)*.

the left hemidiaphragm, or pleural effusion. The diagnosis of infarction is clinically important only to exclude other causes for left upper quadrant pain for which medical or surgical intervention is necessary. Such etiologies would include splenic rupture or abscess, perforated viscus, and ruptured aortic aneurysm. Except in the case of global infarction, splenic function is rarely compromised and requires no specific medical therapy.[4,113]

The widely accepted CT appearance of splenic infarcts is peripheral, wedge-shaped, low-density lesions without appreciable contrast enhancement (Fig. 33-13). However, Balcar et al have described two other CT patterns occurring in splenic infarction in humans.[4] These include multiple, heterogeneous, poorly marginated lesions (Fig. 33-14) and massive, poorly defined hypodense lesions that nearly replace the entire splenic parenchyma. In all of these patterns, detection of infarction is improved with the administration of intravenous contrast

material. There is tremendous overlap between these last two CT patterns and other splenic pathologic conditions such as tumor, hematoma, or abscess, but generally the clinical setting will help to differentiate among these etiologies. Global infarction, usually caused by major injury to or acute thrombosis of the main splenic artery trunk, also has a specific CT appearance. On contrast-enhanced scans in the acute phase the splenic parenchyma appears very low in density, presumably secondary to necrosis, whereas the splenic capsule enhances as a result of its alternate blood supply.[19] This ring of increased density around an infarcted organ resulting from capsular enhancement has been described in other organs such as the kidney.[39]

Infarction of the spleen has been described as a complication of transcatheter hepatic artery embolization in the treatment of primary and secondary hepatic neoplasms.[118] The embolic particles delivered into the hepatic artery cause increased resistance to hepatic blood flow and may be refluxed into the splenic artery, eventually lodging in the spleen. Of the five cases described by Takayasu et al all showed multiple small, rod- or wedge-shaped hypodense lesions and none showed evidence of global infarction.[118] Nonsuppurative gas formation within the spleen has also been demonstrated after transcatheter splenic infarction.[65]

Splenic cysts. Cysts of the spleen may be parasitic, epithelial-lined (true cyst) or non–epithelial-lined (false cyst).[21,30] Parasitic cysts are caused by infection with *Echinococcus granulosus,* and the spleen is affected in less than 5% of cases in endemic regions. The CT appearance of splenic hydatid cysts consists of well-defined

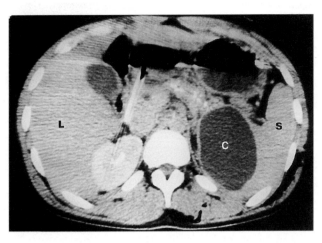

Fig. 33-15. False (non–epithelial-lined) cyst of the spleen *(C)* in a 30-year-old male with a remote history of abdominal trauma. *S,* spleen; *L,* liver. (From Friedman AC: *Radiology of the liver, biliary tract, pancreas and spleen,* Baltimore, 1986, the Williams & Wilkins Co.)

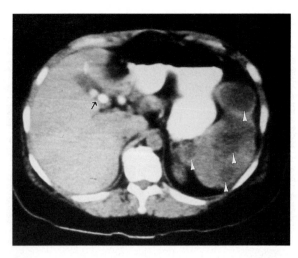

Fig. 33-16. Multiple, low-density, splenic masses *(white arrowheads)* in a 44-year-old woman with cystic lymphangiomatosis of the spleen. Incidental note is made of gallstones *(black arrow).*

single or multiple hypodense masses with characteristic multiple septae denoting daughter cysts. There is usually a thick cyst wall that enhances with intravenous contrast infusion. Clinically these patients have a history of exposure to *E. granulosus,* eosinophilia and positive serologic tests. The combination of characteristic CT findings and suggestive history and clinical presentation should suggest this diagnosis before any percutaneous or surgical manipulation that might prove dangerous.[30]

Nonparasitic splenic cysts are epithelial-lined or non–epithelial-lined.[3,21,30,112] Epithelial-lined cysts of the spleen constitute less than 20% of cystic lesions. They are distinguished from false cysts by their epithelial lining and are thought to be developmental in origin. Possible causes of true splenic cysts include (1) infolding of peritoneal mesothelium after rupture of the splenic capsule, (2) aggregates of peritoneal mesothelial cells trapped in splenic sulci, or (3) dilatation of normal lymphatic spaces.[21] Non–epithelial-lined cysts are thought to be secondary to previous splenic trauma, and it is proposed that they arise from encapsulation of subcapsular or intrasplenic hematomas. Over time the cellular and proteinaceous elements of the hematoma are resorbed, leaving a cavity with a thin, fibrous wall containing serous fluid.[21,30]

It is often impossible to distinguish true from false splenic cysts on CT. Both usually appear as thin-walled, unilocular, rounded, or oval intrasplenic masses of water density and typically display no contrast enhancement (Fig. 33-15). Cyst wall trabeculation and septation may occur in either type of cyst, but rim calcification is more common in false cysts. Debris or high-density material

may be noted within either type of cyst secondary to intracystic hemorrhage or in the case of false cyst residua of resolving hematoma.[21,30] Other cystic lesions that may mimic the appearance of true or false cysts are cystic lymphangiomas of the spleen.[20,97,98,100] These are rare benign neoplasms of the spleen, usually asymptomatic, which do not undergo malignant transformation. They may be single or multiple and are composed of thin-walled, endothelial-lined cysts containing lymph (Fig. 33-16). The only distinguishing feature of cystic lymphangioma is a slightly high CT number (15 to 33 HU) compared with true or false cysts.[98]

Pancreatic pseudocysts may be intrasplenic or perisplenic, and the diagnosis may be suggested in the presence of acute or chronic pancreatitis. Occasionally a pancreatic pseudocyst may be multiseptate and may literally engulf the spleen (Fig. 33-17). On cyst puncture a high amylase concentration in the cystic fluid is diagnostic of pancreatic pseudocyst.[130]

Splenic abscess. Splenic abscess is an uncommon disorder occurring in less than 1% of autopsies; however, it carries an alarmingly high mortality rate even in the antibiotic era.[17,18] Twenty to sixty percent of splenic abscesses are unsuspected until the time of surgery or autopsy.[17,18] Therefore cross-sectional imaging modalities, including CT, play an important role in the early diagnosis and the medical or surgical management of this condition.*

Splenic abscesses are more common in males during the first three decades of life, and a wide variety of

*References 5, 15, 27, 43, 56, 76, 77, 84, 125.

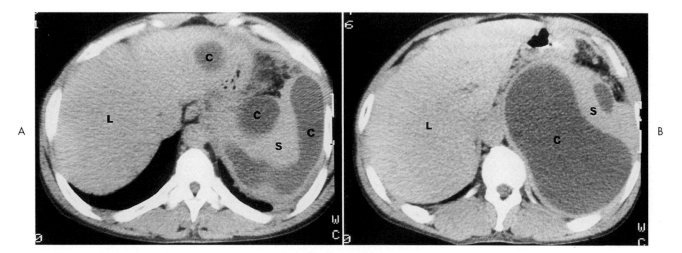

Fig. 33-17. A and **B,** Pancreatic pseudocysts *(C)* engulfing the spleen *(S)* and invaginating the left hepatic lobe. Because of the large size of the cystic masses, the remainder of the pancreas is compressed and poorly visualized. *L,* liver.

diseases predispose their development.[17,18] These predisposing factors include (1) pyogenic infections such as bacterial endocarditis and typhoidal or nontyphoidal salmonellosis, (2) splenic trauma, (3) bland splenic infarction, and (4) contiguous spread of infection from adjacent organs. Certain underlying diseases that commonly preexist in patients who develop splenic abscess include diabetes mellitus, hemoglobinopathies, immunosuppression, alcoholism, and intravenous drug abuse.[17,18] The pathogenesis of splenic abscess may follow several courses:

1. The spleen is directly infected via septic emboli from a distant source such as a heart valve.
2. Bland splenic infarction (as in sickle cell disease) acts as a nidus for hematogenous spread of organisms from elsewhere.
3. Contiguous spread of infection from adjacent organs leads to septic splenic arterial or venous thrombosis and thus results in septic embolization of the spleen.[18]

The most common causative organisms are streptococci, staphylococci, salmonella and other gram-negative organisms, and fungi. However, in the setting of hemoglobinopathies, salmonella is the most common causative organism.[18] The number of cases caused by gram-negative organisms has increased in the last 15 years as a result of improved survival of the critically ill, increased length of hospital stay, and the widespread use of antibiotics. Clinical findings may be nonspecific, although most patients will exhibit evidence of sepsis with fever and elevated white blood cell count. Blood cultures are positive in only about 60% of patients with splenic abscess. Plain radiographic findings are also nonspecific,

and findings such as elevated left hemidiaphragm, left pleural effusion, left basilar infiltrate or atelectasis, or left upper quadrant mass with medial displacement of the gastric air bubble can be seen in just about any type of splenic lesion.[17,18]

Although CT findings are not always specific for splenic abscess, taken with the history and clinical signs and symptoms an accurate diagnosis may be made. Solitary, centrally located or multiple, low-density lesions with rounded or irregular shape suggest the diagnosis of abscess. The abscess wall is usually thick and may enhance with intravenous contrast administration. Air within the cavity is pathognomonic of abscess[5,43,56] (Fig. 33-18). Associated perisplenic or subcapsular collections of fluid or pus are easily demonstrated by CT as is disease in adjacent organs from which the splenic infectious process may have originated.[5] In the proper clinical setting, multiple, small, low-density, rounded, splenic masses with ill-defined margins should suggest the diagnosis of fungal abscesses, such as those caused by *Candida albicans*[77,92,114] (Fig. 33-19). Multiple septic infarcts may lead to spontaneous splenic rupture with the striking CT appearance of significantly irregular splenic contour, intrasplenic fissures, and perisplenic fluid. This is a serious complication of splenic abscess and usually requires immediate splenectomy.[5]

Overlap does occur between the CT appearance of splenic abscess and the CT findings in other focal lesions of the spleen including hematoma, infarction, lymphoma, and metastatic tumor. If the CT features are nonspecific and the clinical presentation confusing, CT-guided fine-needle–aspiration biopsy may be performed for diagnosis. There are several cases reported in the lit-

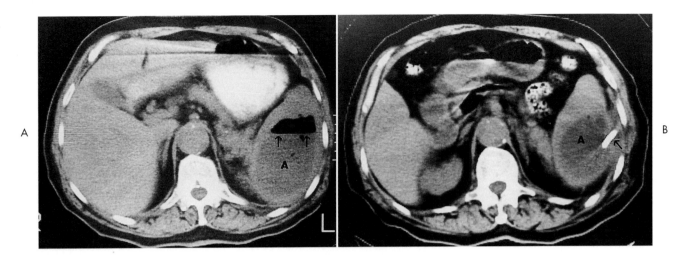

Fig. 33-18. A, Large intrasplenic abscess *(A)* with a thick enhancing rim and air-fluid level *(arrows)* caused by gram-negative organisms. **B,** Percutaneously placed drainage catheter within the abscess *(arrow)* was successful in draining the cavity, and splenectomy was avoided. (From Friedman AC: *Radiology of the liver, biliary tract, pancreas and spleen,* Baltimore, 1986, the Williams & Wilkins Co.)

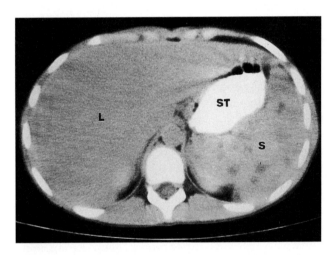

Fig. 33-19. Multiple, poorly defined, small hypodense splenic masses representing multiple candidal abscesses. *S,* spleen; *ST,* stomach; *L,* liver. (From Friedman AC: *Radiology of the liver, biliary tract, pancreas and spleen,* Baltimore, 1986, the Williams & Wilkins Co.)

erature of definitive treatment of splenic abscess by CT guided percutaneous drainage[7,62] (Fig. 33-18). This form of therapy may be necessary in patients who are poor surgical risks or who have dense splenic adhesions. The advantages of percutaneous drainage over surgery are (1) decreased morbidity in patients who are poor surgical risks, (2) preservation of splenic tissue and thus important splenic immunologic function, and (3) perhaps shorter length of hospital stay.[7]

Lymphoma. Lymphoma is the most common malignancy affecting the spleen. CT now plays an important role in the diagnosis, staging, and follow-up of patients with this disease, despite CT's variable rate of detection of involvement of solid organs such as liver and spleen.

Hodgkin's lymphoma is by far the most common form of lymphoma to involve the spleen, and laparotomy with splenectomy reveals clinically unsuspected splenic disease in 23% to 30% of patients.[117] With the introduction of CT, it was hoped that a more accurate preoperative diagnosis of splenic Hodgkin's disease would be possible. However, most published series show rather disappointing results in the assessment of the histologic state of the spleen.* In one of these series, CT did not detect splenic involvement in 20 of 24 spleens that contained tumor on histologic examination.[10] The reason for these poor results may be that although splenic involvement in Hodgkin's disease is usually macroscopically visible pathologically, the abnormal lymphoid aggregates are usually less than 1 cm in diameter and beyond the resolution of CT scanning.[117] Indeed, the only abnormality that may be visible on CT is mild splenomegaly, and low-density, focal masses are a rare occurrence (Fig. 33-20). In one series, only one of five cases with pathologically proven nodules larger than 1 cm in diameter showed focal lesions on CT.[117] The presence of splenomegaly alone does not establish the diagnosis of splenic involvement, since splenectomy series have

*References 2, 10, 11, 28, 29, 37, 103, 117.

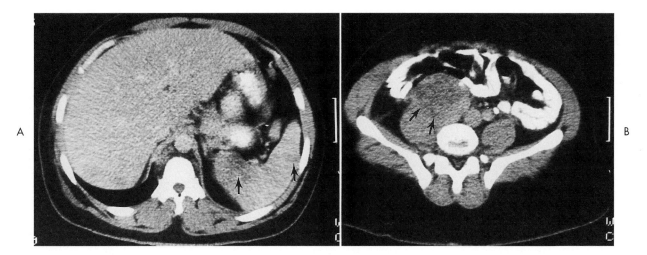

Fig. 33-20. A, Two ill-defined hypodense splenic lesions *(arrows)* in a patient with Hodgkin's lymphoma. Note the spleen is normal in size. **B,** Low-density retroperitoneal lymphadenopathy *(arrows)* in the same patient with Hodgkin's disease.

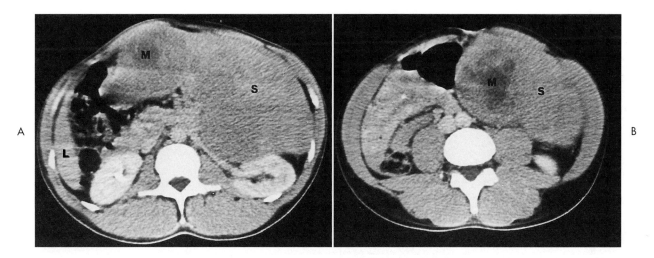

Fig. 33-21. A and **B,** Massive splenomegaly *(S)* and a focal hypodense splenic mass *(M)* in a 21-year-old male with histiocytic lymphoma. (From Friedman AC: *Radiology of the liver, biliary tract, pancreas and spleen,* Baltimore, 1986, the Williams & Wilkins Co.)

shown that one third of enlarged spleens are uninvolved in patients with Hodgkin's disease.[96,137] Also, one third of normal-sized spleens are involved with tumor in patients with Hodgkin's disease.[96] Because of these unreliable data, diagnostic laparotomy with splenectomy is still advocated in our institution for the clinical staging of Hodgkin's disease, if CT demonstrates no evidence of focal splenic or abdominal or retroperitoneal nodal involvement.

Splenic involvement by non-Hodgkin's lymphoma occurs in about 30% of cases, and the most common types to affect the spleen are lymphocytic and follicular.[48] As in Hodgkin's disease, focal, low-density masses represent the minority of CT presentations (Fig. 33-21), and homogeneous splenomegaly represents the majority.[14,73] Both AIDS-related Hodgkin's disease and AIDS-related non-Hodgkin's lymphoma have an increased incidence of focal splenic and hepatic lesions than is seen in the non-AIDS population. This rate of focal involvement is 10% for AIDS-related Hodgkin's and 26% for AIDS-related non-Hodgkin's lymphomas.[87] Primary splenic lymphoma without clinical evidence of nodal disease is even less common, occurring in 1% of all types of non-Hodgkin's lymphomas.[73] When it does occur, bulky, solitary, or multiple low-attenuation splenic masses are seen on CT, and these masses may transgress

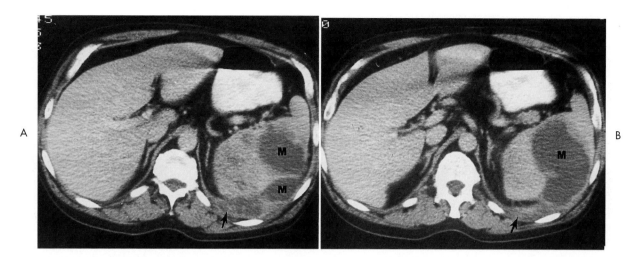

Fig. 33-22. A and **B,** Multiple low-density splenic masses *(M)* are well visualized after contrast bolus in a 47-year-old male with malignant lymphoma. Invasion of the perisplenic fat and diaphragm is noted *(arrows).*

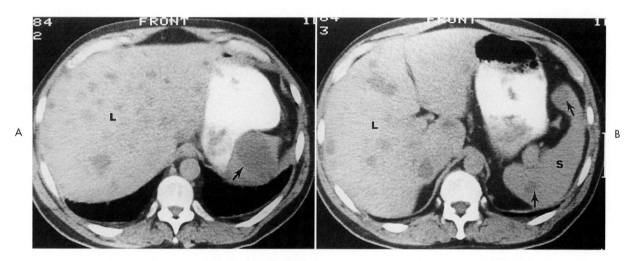

Fig. 33-23. A and **B,** Primary splenic angiosarcomas *(arrows)* presenting as multiple, hypodense masses. Numerous liver metastases are also demonstrated as hypodense mass lesions. *L,* liver; *S,* spleen.

the splenic capsule and involve adjacent organs such as diaphragm, stomach, pancreas, and abdominal wall[73] (Fig. 33-22).

Primary neoplasms. Primary neoplasms of the spleen are extremely rare lesions.[22] Among the benign tumors, splenic hamartoma, cavernous hemangioma, and adenoma are histologically similar masses consisting of an abnormal mixture of normal splenic pulp, large thin-walled endothelial vascular spaces, and fibrous tissue.[30] They appear as low-attenuation masses with variable degrees of contrast enhancement on CT.[30,63,86,89,106] Less common benign neoplasms, including dermoids, fibro-

mas, leiomyomas, osteomas, chondromas, and lipomas, are encountered in autopsies; their CT appearances have not been characterized.

Angiosarcoma is the most commonly encountered primary malignant splenic tumor, although only 55 cases are reported in the world literature.[16,22,64] This tumor has a poor prognosis with a 20% survival rate at 6 months. Seventy percent of cases develop liver metastases, and one third undergo spontaneous rupture with hemorrhage.[68] Just as in hepatic angiosarcoma, the primary splenic form of this tumor is also associated with thoratrast exposure.[64] Splenic angiosarcoma on CT ap-

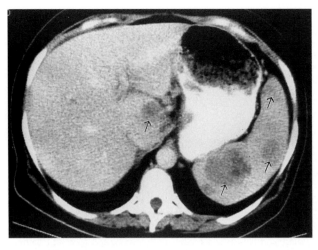

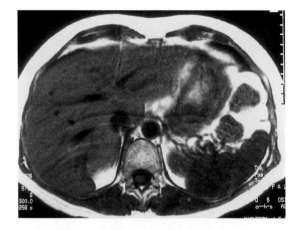

Fig. 33-25. T1-weighted MRI [605/10/2 nex] of normal spleen. Note that the normal spleen is slightly hypointense compared to the liver in this case.

Fig. 33-24. Metastatic poorly differentiated carcinoma involving the spleen and liver *(black arrows)* in a 71-year-old female. The primary site is unknown. Note low-density areas of tumor necrosis within the largest splenic mass.

pears as a low-density mass on CT that may have solid and cystic components and a variable enhancement pattern (Fig. 33-23). When this neoplasm occurs in a thoratrast-exposed patient, it appears as a low-density mass on a background of high-density splenic parenchyma as a result of thoratrast deposition.[64]

Metastases. Although the spleen acts as a hematologic filter and contains abundant lymphoid tissue, it is an uncommon site of metastatic carcinoma. Overall, splenic metastatic deposits are noted in 4% of patients with cancer and usually only occur in patients with widespread metastases.[9] The most common primary tumors to metastasize to the spleen include melanoma and lung, breast, pancreas, gastric, and colonic carcinoma. It is postulated that the majority of secondary splenic tumors are caused by hematogenous dissemination of tumor.[71] The CT appearance consists of rounded or irregularly shaped nodules with a variable degree of contrast enhancement. In bulky masses there is commonly a central low-density area of necrosis (Fig. 33-24). One third of splenic metastases observed at autopsy are microscopic aggregates of tumor and are not visible on CT. Metastatic breast carcinoma is the most common tumor to appear in this fashion and may cause splenomegaly, thickened splenic capsule, and splenic infarction, all of which may be visible on CT.[71] However, whether focal or diffuse, the CT characteristics of splenic metastases are nonspecific; when focal they are indistinguishable from primary neoplasms, abscesses, or infarcts. Only the presence of similar lesions in the liver or other abdominal organs suggests the diagnosis of metastatic disease.

MAGNETIC RESONANCE IMAGING
Technique of examination

The spleen is usually studied as part of a complete examination of the upper abdomen. T1- and T2-weighted spin-echo sequences in the transverse plane are routinely acquired.[45,134] Other pulse sequences such as short-time inversion recovery (STIR) or fat suppression may be used if necessary to enhance lesion detection. T1-weighted spin-echo sequences (TR <500, TE <30 msec) provide superior anatomic resolution and on these the spleen has a slightly lower signal intensity than does normal hepatic parenchyma (Fig. 33-25). On T2-weighted sequences (TR = 2000 to 3000, TE >60 msec) the spleen has a higher signal intensity than does normal liver, and solid or cystic lesions of the spleen become detectable. However, because of susceptibility to motion artifact, the anatomic resolution on T2-weighted images is generally inferior and may be improved with motion-suppression techniques, respiratory compensation, and cardiac gating.[45] Other imaging planes such as coronal or sagittal may be useful for evaluation of specific lesions along the diaphragmatic surface of the spleen, but these are rarely acquired routinely (Fig. 33-26).[45,132]

The use of contrast agents improves focal lesion detection and the differential diagnosis of splenomegaly. Superparamagnetic iron oxide (ferrite) particles are phagocytosed by the macrophages localized in normal splenic red pulp but are not taken up by tumor nodules.[45,133,134] These particles shorten the T2 relaxation time of normal spleen, and the MR signal intensity of normal spleen decreases significantly. Tumor nodules will remain unaffected and are more obvious because of decreased signal in surrounding splenic tissue.[133,134] Bolus injection of Gd-DTPA combined with rapid acquisition

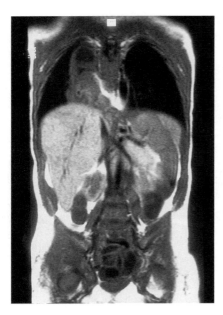

Fig. 33-26. Normal coronal MRI image demonstrating confluence of splenic with superior mesenteric veins.

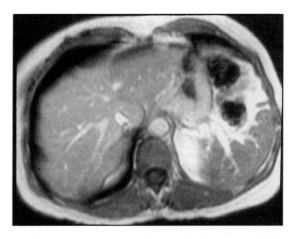

Fig. 33-27. Intense vascular enhancement is noted on this gradient echo image [143/4/1 nex], which was obtained following intravenous gadolinium administration.

spin-echo (RASE) MR imaging (T1-weighted sequences) also improves lesion detectability, compared with conventional T1- and T2-weighted images (Fig. 33-27).[47,78] Also, gadolinium-labeled liposomes have been used with some success to increase splenic MR contrast relative to pathologic masses.[58,122] The sensitivity of contrast-enhanced techniques in differentiating benign from malignant splenic disease, particularly in lymphoma, awaits further confirmation in experimental studies.

Diffuse disease

Splenomegaly. Benign causes of splenomegaly cannot be differentiated on the basis of MR signal characteristics. Congested spleens resulting from portal hypertension may show mild increase in signal intensity on T2-weighted imagines, but otherwise most enlarged spleens have signal intensities similar to normal spleen. The ability to distinguish benign from malignant splenomegaly (as in diffuse lymphomatous or leukemic infiltration) may be enhanced by injection of ferrite, as congested or hyperplastic spleens will take up ferrite normally and show decreased T2 signal, but diffusely malignant spleens will not take up ferrite to a significant degree.[46,133,132]

Iron overload. In many disease states resulting in hemolysis or requiring repeated blood transfusion, iron (hemosiderin and ferritin) is preferentially deposited in the liver and spleen. This causes shortening of T2 and reduces the MR signal intensity of the spleen on T2-

weighted pulse sequences.[1,40] Predominant deposition in the spleen is seen in hemoglobinopathies (such as sickle cell disease and thalassemia) and in individuals (such as those with renal failure) receiving repeated transfusion.[1,40,57,99] In hereditary hemochromatosis, the majority of the excess iron is deposited in the hepatocytes and the liver shows diminished T2 signal relative to spleen.[132]

Focal disease

Benign masses. Hemorrhage within the spleen or subcapsular space is distinguished from normal splenic tissue by its high T2 signal. The age of the hematoma dictates its appearance on MR images. Acute hemorrhage (<24 hours) is isointense with splenic parenchyma on T1- and T2-weighted images due to high oxyhemoglobin and deoxyhemoglobin concentrations. Subacute hematomas (3 to 14 days) become hyperintense on T1-weighted images as a result of methemoglobin formation. Chronic hematomas (>14 days) become significantly hyperintense on T1- and T2-weighted pulse sequences but may show a hypointense peripheral ring of hemosiderin.[45,132]

Splenic infarcts have been described as wedge-shaped, peripheral, hyperintense masses on T1- and T2-weighted images; they are most obvious in the setting of iron overload (such as sickle cell disease) resulting from the reduced signal within the splenic parenchyma. Infarcts are more difficult to detect on MRI in normal spleens because the splenic parenchyma is less hypointense.[46,52,132]

Splenic cysts and hemangiomas may be difficult to distinguish from one another because they usually present as well-circumscribed masses that are hypointense on T1-weighted spin-echo sequences and signifi-

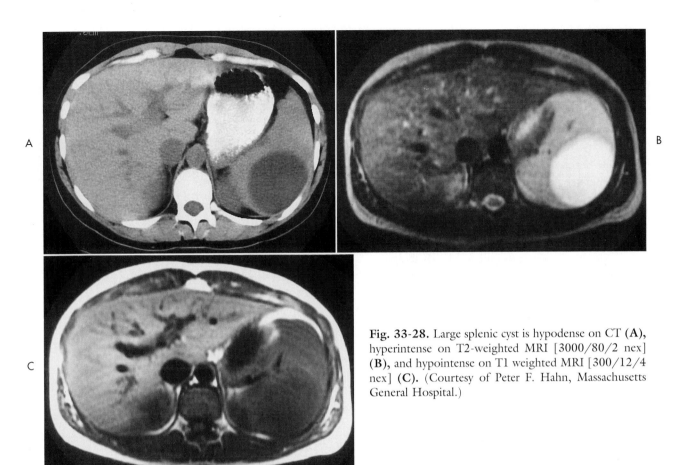

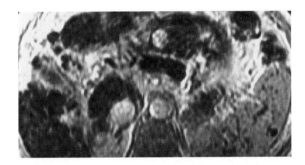

Fig. 33-28. Large splenic cyst is hypodense on CT **(A)**, hyperintense on T2-weighted MRI [3000/80/2 nex] **(B)**, and hypointense on T1 weighted MRI [300/12/4 nex] **(C).** (Courtesy of Peter F. Hahn, Massachusetts General Hospital.)

Fig. 33-29. Gradient echo MRI demonstrates marked hypointensity of multiple gamma gandy bodies throughout the spleen. These siderotic nodules are found in a patient with severe hemosiderosis and cirrhosis as demonstrated by an extremely hypointense, shrunken liver. (Courtesy of Peter F. Hahn, Massachusetts General Hospital.)

cantly hyperintense on T2-weighted images relative to normal spleen.[45,46,132] Dynamic scanning following a rapid bolus of Gd-DTPA may be necessary to show the typical peripheral puddling, late central enhancement, and prolonged contrast retention characteristic of cavernous hemangiomas. Cysts do not enhance significantly with Gd-DTPA and rarely show internal septations or fibrous strands commonly encountered in hemangiomas (Fig. 33-28, *A* to *C*).[45,63,132]

Gamna-Gandy bodies (siderotic nodules) are seen in the spleens of about 10% of patients with portal hypertension. They constitute localized areas of hemorrhage within the spleen and appear low in signal intensity on T2-weighted spin-echo or gradient-echo images because of hemosiderin deposition (Fig. 33-29).[70,107]

Malignant tumors. Conventional MR spin-echo imaging is relatively insensitive in detecting focal splenic tumor masses because of similarity of T1 and T2 relaxation times and proton densities of tumor and spleen.[45,52,88,104] Cystic or necrotic areas within tumor lengthen T2 signal, and tumor-associated hemorrhage shortens T1 signal, thus aiding in detection of focal tumor masses caused by metastases or primary lymphoma.

Iron overload in the underlying splenic parenchyma also enhances lesion conspicuity by shortening T2 signal in normal spleen surrounding focal masses.[45,46,132] The sensitivity of conventional MR imaging for detection of splenic lymphoma in a focal or diffuse pattern varies from

10% to 87% in the reported literature, reflecting the variability of this tumor in appearance on MR imaging.[46,52,88,104] Focal splenic lymphoma may appear as lesions of increased or decreased signal intensity on T1- and T2-weighted images.[88,104]

Contrast-enhanced MR imaging will likely increase lesion detection in malignant disease, but little experimental data are available on these agents at this time. Superparamagnetic iron oxide (ferrite) particles[133,134] and liposomal gadopentetate dimeglumine[58,122] are organ-specific contrast agents that increase detection of tumor masses and diffuse lymphomatous involvement of the spleen. However, these agents remain under investigation at this time and have not been approved for clinical use. Dynamic gadolinium-enhanced MR imaging allows for improved focal lesion detectability in the spleen, but it has not been shown to be sensitive in diffuse malignant involvement as in lymphoma. This technique is currently available, but its sensitivity is unproved.[78,108]

REFERENCES

1. Adler DD, Glazer GM, Aisen AM: MRI of the spleen: normal appearance and findings in sickle-cell anemia. *AJR* 147:843-845, 1986.
2. Alcorn FS, et al: Contributions of computed tomography in the staging and management of malignant lymphoma. *Radiology* 123:717-723, 1977.
3. Arnold J, McGahan JP, Stadalnik RC: Epidermoid cyst of the spleen: value of noninvasive imaging modalities in preoperative diagnosis. *J Comput Assist Tomogr* 6:836-838, 1982.
4. Balcar l, et al: CT patterns of splenic infarction: a clinical and experimental study. *Radiology* 151:723-729, 1984.
5. Balthazar EJ, et al: CT of splenic and perisplenic abnormalities in septic patients. *AJR* 144:53-56, 1985.
6. Beahrs JR, Stephens DH: Enlarged accessory spleens: CT appearance in postsplenectomy patients. *AJR* 135:483-486, 1980.
7. Berkman WA, Harris SA, Bernadino ME: Nonsurgical drainage of splenic abscess. *AJR* 141:395-396, 1983.
8. Berland LL, VanDyke JA: Decreased splenic enhancement on CT in traumatized hypotensive patients. *Radiology* 156:469-471, 1985.
9. Bernardino ME, et al: Diagnostic approaches to liver and spleen metastases, *Radiol Clin North Am* 20:469-485, 1982.
10. Blackledge G, et al: Computed tomography (CT) in the staging of patients with Hodgkin's disease: a report on 136 patients. *Clin Radiol* 13:143-147, 1980.
11. Breiman RS, et al: CT-pathologic correlation in Hodgkin's disease and non-Hodgkin's lymphoma. *Radiology* 126:159-166, 1978.
12. Brick SH, et al: Hepatic and splenic injury in children: role of CT in the decision for laparotomy. *Radiology* 165:643-646, 1987.
13. Brieman RS, et al: Volume determinations by computed tomography. *AJR* 138:329-333, 1982.
14. Burgener FA, Hamlin DJ: Histiocytic lymphoma of the abdomen: radiographic spectrum. *AJR* 137:337-342, 1981.
15. Caslowitz PL, et al: The changing spectrum of splenic abscess. *Clin Imaging* 13:201-207, 1989.
16. Chen KT, Bolles CG, Gilbert EF: Angiosarcoma of the spleen. *Arch Pathol Lab Med* 103:122-128, 1979.
17. Chulay JD, Lankerani MR: Splenic abscess: report of 10 cases and review of the literature. *Amer J Med* 61:513-522, 1976.
18. Chun CH, et al: Splenic abscess. *Medicine* 59(1):50-65, 1980.
19. Cohen BA, Mitty HA, Mendelson DS: Computed tomography of splenic infarction. *J Comput Assist Tomogr* 8(1):167-168, 1984.
20. Cornaglia-Ferraris P, et al: A pediatric case of cystic lymphangioma of the spleen. *J Comput Assist Tomogr* 5(3):449-450, 1981.
21. Dachman AH, et al: Nonparasitic splenic cysts: a report of 52 cases with radiologic-pathologic correlation. *AJR* 147:537-542, 1986.
22. Das Gupta T, Coombs B, Brasfield RD: Primary malignant neoplasms of the spleen. *Surg Gynecol Obstet* 120(5):947-960, 1965.
23. Delamarre J, et al: Splenosis: ultrasound and CT findings in a case complicated by an intraperitoneal implant traumatic hematoma. *Gastointest Radiol* 13:275-278, 1988.
24. DeMaeyer P, Wilms G, Baert AL: Polysplenia. *J Comput Assist Tomogr* 5:104-105, 1981.
25. Do HM, Cronan JJ: CT appearance of splenic injuries managed nonoperatively. *AJR* 157:757-760, 1991.
26. Dodds WJ, et al: Radiologic imaging of splenic anomalies. *AJR* 155:805-810, 1990.
27. Dubuisson RL, Jones TB: Splenic abscess due to blastomycosis: scintigraphic, sonographic and CT evaluation. *AJR* 140:66-68, 1983.
28. Earl HM, et al: Computerized tomography (CT) abdominal scanning in Hodgkin's disease. *Clin Radiol* 31:149-153, 1980.
29. Ellert J, Kneel L: The role of computed tomography in the initial staging and subsequent management of the lymphomas. *J Comput Assist Tomogr* 4:368-391, 1980.
30. Faer MJ, et al: RPC from the AFIP. *Radiology* 134:371-376, 1980.
31. Fagelman D, Hertz MA, Ross AS: Delayed development of splenic subcapsular hematoma: CT evaluation. *J Comput Assist Tomogr* 9:815-816, 1984.
32. Federle MP: CT of upper abdominal trauma. *Semin Roentgenol* 19(4):269-280, 1984.
33. Federle MP: CT of abdominal trauma. In Federle MP, Brant-Zawadzh M, editors: *Computed tomography in the evaluation of trauma*, Baltimore, 1986, Williams & Wilkins.
34. Federle MP, et al: Evaluation of abdominal trauma by computed tomography. *Radiology* 138:637-644, 1981.
35. Fefer A: Enlargement of the lymph nodes and spleen. In Petersdorf RG, et al, editors: *Harrison's principles of internal medicine*, ed 10, New York, 1983, McGraw-Hill.
36. Gentry LR, Brown JM, Lindgren RD: Splenosis: CT demonstration of heterotopic autotransplantation of splenic tissue. *J Comput Assist Tomogr* 5:1184-1187, 1982.
37. Gilbert T, Castellino RA, et al: The spleen in Hodgkin disease: diagnostic value of CT. *Invest Radiol* 21:437-439, 1986.
38. Glazer GM, et al: Dynamic CT of the normal spleen. *AJR* 137:343-346, 1981.
39. Glazer GM, et al: Computed tomography of renal infarction: clinical and experimental observations. *AJR* 140:721-727, 1983.
40. Gomori JM, Grossman RI, Drott HR: MR relaxation times and iron content of thalassemic spleens: an in vitro study. *AJR* 150:567-569, 1988.
41. Gooding GAW: The ultrasonic and computed tomographic appearance of splenic lobulations: a consideration on the ultrasonic differential of masses adjacent to the left kidney. *Radiology* 126:719-720, 1978.
42. Goodman PC, Federle MP: Splenorrhaphy: CT appearance. *J Comput Assist Tomogr* 4:251-252, 1980.
43. Grant E, Mertens MA, Mascatello VJ: Splenic abscess: comparison of four imaging methods. *AJR* 132:465-466, 1979.
44. Haft JI, et al: Computed tomography of the abdomen in the diagnosis of splenic emboli. *Arch Intern Med* 148:193-197, 1988.

45. Hahn PF, Stark DD, Glastad K: Biliary system, pancreas, spleen and alimentary tract. In Stark DD, Bradley WG, editors: *Magnetic resonance imaging*, St. Louis, 1992, Mosby-Year Book.

46. Hahn PF, et al: MR imaging of focal splenic tumors. *AJR* 150:823-827, 1988.

47. Hamed MM, et al: Dynamic MR imaging of the abdomen with gadopentetate dimeglumine: normal enhancement patterns of the liver, spleen, stomach and pancreas. *AJR* 158:303-307, 1992.

48. Harris NL, et al: Diffuse large cell (histiocytic) lymphoma of the spleen. *Cancer* 54:2460-2467, 1984.

49. Havron A, et al: Radiopaque liposomes: a promising new contrast material for computed tomography of the spleen. *Radiology* 140:507-511, 1981.

50. Henderson JM, et al: Measurement of liver and spleen volume by computed tomography. *Radiology* 141:525-527, 1981.

51. Herman TE, Siegel MJ: CT of acute splenic torsion in children with wandering spleen. *AJR* 156:151-153, 1991.

52. Hess CF, et al: Focal lesions of the spleen: preliminary results with fast MR imaging at 1.5T. *J Comput Assist Tomogr* 12:569-574, 1988.

53. Jeffrey RB: CT diagnosis of blunt hepatic and splenic injuries: a look to the future. *Radiology* 171:17-18, 1989.

54. Jeffrey RB, et al: Computed tomography of splenic trauma. *Radiology* 141:729-732, 1981.

55. Jeffrey RB, et al: Abdominal CT in acquired immunodeficiency syndrome. *AJR* 146:7-13, 1986.

56. Johnson JD, et al: Radiology in the diagnosis of splenic abscess. *Rev Infect Dis* 7:10-20, 1985.

57. Johnston DL, et al: Assessment of tissue iron overload by nuclear magnetic resonance imaging. *Am J Med* 87:40-47, 1989.

58. Kabalka G, et al: Gadolinium-labeled liposomes: targeted MR contrast agents for liver and spleen. *Radiology* 163:255-258, 1987.

59. Kaufman RD, et al: Upper abdominal trauma in children: imaging evaluation. *AJR* 142:449-460, 1984.

60. Korobkin M, et al: Computed tomography of subcapsular splenic hematoma. *Radiology* 129:441-445, 1978.

61. Lauteala L, Kormano M, Violante MR: Uptake and dissolution of particulate iodipamide ethyl ester in the spleen: a morphologic study. *Invest Radiol* 22:829-835, 1987.

62. Lerner RM, Spartaro M: Splenic abscess: percutaneous drainage. *Radiology* 153:643-645, 1984.

63. Levine E, Wetzel LH, Nett JR: MR imaging and CT of extrahepatic cavernous hemangioma. *AJR* 147:1299-1304, 1986.

64. Levy DW, et al: Thoratrast-induced hepatosplenic neoplasia: CT identification. *AJR* 146:997-1004, 1986.

65. Levy JM, Wasserman PL, Weiland DE: Nonsuppurative gas formation in the spleen after transcatheter splenic infarction. *Radiology* 139:375-376, 1981.

66. Magid D, Fishman EK, Siegelman SS: Computed tomography of the spleen and liver in sickle cell disease. *AJR* 143:245-249, 1984.

67. Mahon PA, Sutton JE: Non-operative management of adult splenic injury due to blunt trauma: a warning. *Am J Surg* 149:716-721, 1985.

68. Mahony B, Jeffrey RB, Federle MP: Spontaneous rupture of hepatic and splenic angiosarcoma demonstrated by CT. *AJR* 183:965-966, 1982.

69. Maier W: Computed tomography in the diagnosis of splenic infarction. *Eur J Radiol* 2:202-204, 1982.

70. Minami M, et al: Siderotic nodules in the spleen: MR imaging of portal hypertension. *Radiology* 172:681-684, 1989.

71. Marymont JH, Gross S: Patterns of metastatic cancer in the spleen. *Am J Clin Pathol* 40(1):58-66, 1963.

72. Mendelson DS, Cohen BA, Armas RR: CT appearance of splenosis. *J Comput Assist Tomogr* 6:1188-1190, 1982.

73. Meyer JE, et al.: Large-cell lymphoma of the spleen: CT appearance. *Radiology* 148:199-201, 1983.

74. Meyers MA: *Dynamic radiology of the abdomen*, New York, 1982, Springer-Verlag.

75. Miller DL, et al: CT of the liver and spleen with EOE-13: review of 225 examinations. *AJR* 143:235-243, 1984.

76. Miller FJ, et al: Clinical and roentgenographic findings in splenic abscess. *Arch Surg* 111:1156-1159, 1976.

77. Miller JH, Greenfield LD, Wald BR: Candidiasis of the liver and spleen in childhood. *Radiology* 142:375-380, 1982.

78. Mirowitz SA, et al: Dynamic gadolinium-enhanced MR imaging of the spleen: normal enhancement patterns and evaluation of splenic lesions. *Radiology* 179:681-686, 1991.

79. Mirvis SE, Dunham CM: Abdominal/pelvic trauma. In Mirvis SE, Young JW, editors: *Imaging in trauma and critical care*, Baltimore, 1992, Williams & Wilkins.

80. Mirvis SE, Whitley NO, Gens DR: Blunt splenic trauma in adults: CT-based classification and correlation with prognosis and treatment. *Radiology* 171:33-39, 1989.

81. Moore FA, et al: Risk of splenic salvage after trauma. *Am J Surg* 148:800-805, 1984.

82. Moss AA, Friedman MA, Brito AC: Determination of liver, kidney and spleen volumes by computed tomography: an experimental study in dogs. *J Comput Assist Tomogr* 5:12-14, 1981.

83. Moss AA, et al: Computed tomography of splenic subcapsular hematomas: an experimental study in dogs. *Invest Radiol* 14:60-64, 1979.

84. Moss ML, et al: CT demonstration of a splenic abscess not evident at surgery. *AJR* 135:159-160, 1980.

85. Nemcek AA, Miller FH, Fitzgerald SW: Acute torsion of a wandering spleen: diagnosis by CT, duplex doppler and color flow sonography. *AJR* 157:307-309, 1991.

86. Norowitz DC, Morehouse HT: Isodense splenic mass: hamartoma. *Comput Med Imaging Graph* 13:347-350, 1989.

87. Nyberg DA, et al: AIDS-related lymphomas: evaluation by abdominal CT. *Radiology* 159:59-63, 1986.

88. Nyman R, et al: An attempt to characterize malignant lymphoma in spleen, liver and lymph nodes with magnetic resonance imaging. *Acta Radiol* 28:527-533, 1987.

89. Pakter RL, et al: CT findings in splenic hemangiomas in the Klippel-Trenaunay-Weber syndrome. *J Comput Assist Tomogr* 11:88-91, 1987.

90. Pappas D, Mirvis SE, Crepps JT: Splenic trauma: false-negative CT diagnosis in cases of delayed rupture. *AJR* 149:727-728, 1987.

91. Parker LA, et al: Torsion of a wandering spleen: CT appearance. *J Comput Assist Tomogr* 8:1201-1204, 1984.

92. Pastakia B, et al: Hepatosplenic candidiasis: wheels within wheels. *Radiology* 166:417-421, 1988.

93. Payne NI, Whitehouse GH: Delineation of the spleen by a combination of proliposomes with water soluble contrast media: an experimental study using computed tomography. *Br J Radiol* 60:535-541, 1987.

94. Piekarski J, et al: Computed tomography of the spleen. *Radiology* 135:683-689, 1980.

95. Pierkarski J, et al: Difference between liver and spleen CT numbers in the normal adult: its usefulness in predicting the presence of diffuse liver disease. *Radiology* 137:727-729, 1980.

96. Pilepich MV: Contribution of computed tomography to the treatment of lymphomas. *AJR* 131:69-73, 1978.

97. Pistoia F, Markowitz SK: Splenic lymphangiomatosis: CT diagnosis. *AJR* 150:121-122, 1988.

98. Pyatt RS, et al: CT diagnosis of splenic cystic lymphangiomatosis. *J Comput Assist Tomogr* 5:446-448, 1981.

99. Querfeld U, et al: Magnetic resonance imaging of iron overload in children treated with peritoneal dialysis. *Nephron* 50:220-224, 1988.

100. Rao BK, et al: Cystic lymphangiomatosis of the spleen: a radiologic-pathologic correlation. *Radiology* 141:781-782, 1981.

101. Rao BK, et al: Dual radiopharmaceutical imaging in congenital asplenia syndrome. *Radiology* 145:805-810, 1982.

102. Raptopoulos V, Fink MP: CT grading of splenic trauma in adults: how the same statistics can be interpreted differently. *Radiology* 180:309-311, 1991.

103. Redman HC, et al: Computed tomography as an adjunct in the staging of Hodgkin's disease and non-Hodgkin's lymphomas. *Radiology* 124:381-385, 1977.

104. Richards MA, et al: Low field strength magnetic resonance imaging of the spleen: results from volunteers and patients with lymphoma. *Br J Cancer* 57:408-411, 1988.

105. Roa AKR, Silver TM: Normal pancreas and splenic variants simulating suprenal or renal tumors. *AJR* 126:530-537, 1976.

106. Ros PR, et al: Hemangioma of the spleen: radiologic-pathologic correlation in ten cases. *Radiology* 162:73-77, 1987.

107. Sagoh T, et al: Gamna-Gandy bodies of the spleen: evaluation with MR imaging. *Radiology* 172:685-687, 1989.

108. Saini S, et al: Advances in contrast-enhanced MR imaging. *AJR* 156:235-254, 1991.

109. Scatamacchia SA, et al: Splenic trauma in adults: impact of CT grading on management. *Radiology* 171:725-729, 1989.

110. Sekikawa T, Shatney CH: Septic sequelae after splenectomy for trauma in adults. *Am J Surg* 145:667-673, 1983.

111. Shadle CA, et al: Spontaneous splenic infarction in polysplenia syndrome. *J Comput Assist Tomogr* 6:177-179, 1982.

112. Shin MS, Ho K-J: Mesodermal cyst of the spleen: computed tomographic characteristics and pathogenetic considerations. *J Comput Assist Tomogr* 7:295-299, 1983.

113. Shirkohoda A, Wallace S, Sokhandan M: Computed tomography and ultrasonography in splenic infarction. *J Can Assoc Radiol* 36:29-33, 1985.

114. Shirkhoda A, et al: CT findings in hepatosplenic and renal candidiasis. *J Comput Assist Tomogr* 11:795-798, 1987.

115. Standage BA, Gross JC: Outcome and sepsis after splenectomy in adults. *Am J Surg* 143:545-548, 1982.

116. Stiris MG: Accessory spleen versus left adrenal tumor: computed tomographic and abdominal angiographic evaluation. *J Comput Assist Tomogr* 4:543-544, 1980.

117. Strijk SP, et al: The spleen in Hodgkin disease: diagnostic value of CT. *Radiology* 154:753-757, 1985.

118. Takayasu K, et al: Splenic infarction, a complication of transcatheter hepatic arterial embolization for liver malignancies. *Radiology* 151:371-375, 1984.

119. Taylor AJ, et al: CT of acquired abnormalities of the spleen. *AJR* 157:1213-1219, 1991.

120. Taylor AR, Rosenfield AT: Limitations of computed tomography in the recognition of delayed splenic rupture. *J Comput Assist Tomogr* 9:1205-1207, 1984.

121. Thomas JL, et al: EOE-13 in the detection of hepatosplenic lymphoma. *Radiology* 145:629-634, 1982.

122. Tilcock C, et al: Liposomal Gd-DTPA: preparation and characterization of relaxivity. *Radiology* 171:77-80, 1989.

123. Toombs BD, et al: Computed tomography in blunt trauma. *Radiol Clin North Am* 19:17-35, 1981.

124. Umlas SL, Cronan JJ: Splenic trauma: can CT grading systems enable prediction of successful nonsurgical treatment. *Radiology* 178:481-487, 1991.

125. van der Laan RT, et al: Computed tomography in the diagnosis and treatment of solitary splenic abscesses. *J Comput Assist Tomogr* 13:71-74, 1989.

126. Vermess M, Inscoe S, Sugarbaker PH: Use of liposoluble contrast material to separate left renal and splenic parenchyma on computed tomography. *J Comput Assist Tomogr* 4:540-542, 1980.

127. Vermess M, Javadpour N, Blayney DW: Post-splenectomy demonstration of splenic tissue by computed tomography with liposoluble contrast material. *J Comput Assist Tomogr* 5:106-108, 1981.

128. Vermess M, et al: Clinical trial with a new intravenous liposoluble contrast material for computed tomography of the liver and spleen. *Radiology* 137:217-222, 1980.

129. Vermess M, et al: Computed tomography of the liver and spleen with intravenous lipoid contrast material: review of 60 examinations. *AJR* 138:1063-1071, 1982.

130. Vick CW, et al: Pancreatitis-associated fluid collections involving the spleen: sonographic and computed tomographic appearance. *Gastrointest Radiol* 6:247-250, 1981.

131. Walls EW: The blood vascular and lymphatic systems. In Romanes GJ, editor: *Cunningham's textbook of anatomy,* London, 1972, Oxford University Press.

132. Weissleder R, Hahn PF, Stark DD: Spleen: magnetic resonance imaging. In Margulis AR, Burhenne HJ, editors: *Alimentary tract radiology,* St. Louis, 1989, Mosby-Year Book.

133. Weissleder R, et al: The diagnosis of splenic lymphoma by MR imaging: value of superparamagnetic iron oxide. *AJR* 152:175-180, 1989.

134. Weissleder R, et al: Superparamegnetic iron oxide: enhanced detection of focal splenic tumors with MR imaging. *Radiology* 169:399-403, 1988.

135. Williams PL, Warwick R, editors: In *Gray's anatomy,* ed 36, New York, 1980, Churchill Livingstone.

136. Wing VW, et al: The clinical impact of CT for blunt abdominal trauma. *AJR* 145:1191-1194, 1985.

137. Zadin ME, Glatstein E, Dorfman RF: Clinicopathologic studies of 117 untreated patients subjected to laparotomy for the staging of Hodgkin's disease. *Cancer* 27:1277-1294, 1971.

34
The Adrenal Glands

TIMOTHY J. WELCH
PATRICK F. SHEEDY II
ROBERT R. HATTERY

During the past 20 years, many techniques have been used to detect tumors of the adrenal gland. In our practice, these methods have included excretory urography with tomography, bolus nephrotomography, adrenal angiography, adrenal venography and venous sampling, radionuclide scanning, ultrasonography, and computed tomography (CT). Since the mid-1970s, CT scanning has gradually displaced all other methods for adrenal gland imaging. Paralleling this increased use of CT has been an increased frequency of accurate preoperative localization of pathological conditions of the adrenal gland. A review documenting trends of adrenal surgery during the 1970s[18] indicated that accurate preoperative localization occurred in 50% of patients in the early 1970s, 80% of patients in the mid-1970s, and 98% of patients in the late 1970s. The improvement during the mid-1970s reflects the success of radionuclide scanning, nephrotomogtraphy, and arteriography, but improvement in the late 1970s is due to the success of CT.

When CT scanning of the body was introduced into the clinical practice of radiology at the Mayo Clinic in October, 1975, we did not anticipate that it would have a great value in evaluating the adrenal gland compared with its potential in other organs, such as the liver, pancreas, and kidney. Several early examination, however, revealed large masses in the upper abdomen that were subsequently identified at surgery as being adrenal lesions. It soon became clear that normal adrenal glands could be seen in almost all patients who were properly examined using CT; even small tumors could be identified. By the end of 1976, experience with 74 cases of patients with adrenal gland disease indicated that CT would be valuable in the detection of adrenal tumors.

Currently 2% to 3% of all patients referred for CT body scans have a clinical indication of adrenal gland pathological conditions. More than 50% of patients scanned have had positive results, with an entire spectrum of pathological conditions demonstrated. As might be expected, the most diagnostic adrenal gland scans are obtainable on equipment that provides the shortest scan times and highest resolution. With the opportunity to use late-generation CT scanning, it rarely is necessary to proceed to other methods of adrenal imaging. Angiography is used only occasionally to evaluate the blood supply to large masses when the organ of origin remains obscure after CT scanning. Venography and venous sampling are helpful in selected patients with suspected primary hyperaldosteronism or a pheochromocytoma when biochemical evidence is strong and the CT scan is negative. Ultrasonography is used to confirm the fluid characteristics of lesions that appear to be cysts on CT. Iodocholesterol radionuclide scanning is used in selected, difficult diagnostic problems with primary hyperaldosteronism and Cushing's disease. MIBG (I^{131} metaiodobenzyl guanidine) has become an excellent imaging modality in the detection of pheochromocytomas, especially in ectopic locations.

Success of CT has not eliminated the value of other imaging methods for detection of adrenal masses. In many patients referred for CT of the adrenal gland, tumors have been previously discovered with plain films of the abdomen, excretory urography, sonography, or even arteriography. In this group of patients, CT either confirms the presence of a tumor or reveals normal glands and provides a specific anatomical explanation for the "pseudomass" identified on another imaging method.

NORMAL ANATOMY

The right adrenal gland is located in the area just above the right kidney, medial to the right lobe of the liver, lateral to the crus of the right hemidiaphragm, and posterior to the inferior vena cava. Its shape is variable and may resemble an elongated comma lying in the

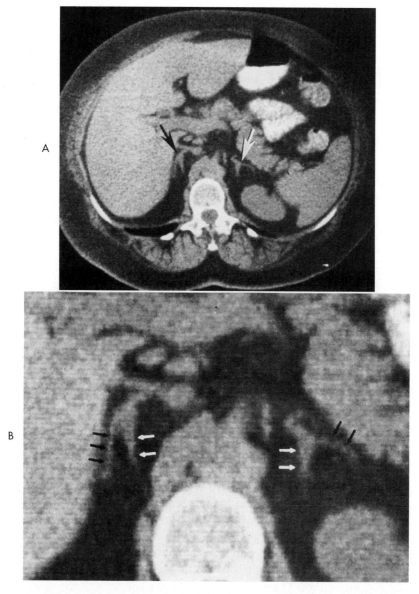

Fig. 34-1. Normal adrenal glands. **A,** A typical location and appearance for the right gland *(black arrow)*, which is shaped like an upside-down letter V. On the left, the gland is located in a triangle bounded by the pancreas, aorta, and kidney. It is shaped like an upside-down letter Y *(white arrow)*. **B,** Magnification view of the same scan shows the medial *(white arrows)* and lateral *(black arrows)* limbs of the gland to better advantage. Note that the limbs are thinner than the apex of the gland.

crease between the liver and the crus of the diaphragm (Fig. 34-1). Also, it may be shaped like an inverted letter V or Y. The lateral limb of the gland lies close to the right lobe of the liver and sometimes cannot be separated from the liver.

The left adrenal gland is located above and extending anterior to the upper pole of the left kidney in a triangle formed by the left lateral margin of the aorta, posterior surface of the body and tail of the pancreas, and

superoanteromedial surface of the upper pole of the left kidney (Fig. 34-2). The left gland is shaped like an inverted letter V or Y or an inverted and reversed letter L. It may also be triangular in shape.

The right gland is usually in a clearly suprarenal location, whereas the left gland frequently lies in front of the anterior surface of the left kidney. The superoinferior length of the gland is variable but can extend from 2 to 6 cm. The right gland maintains a constant rela-

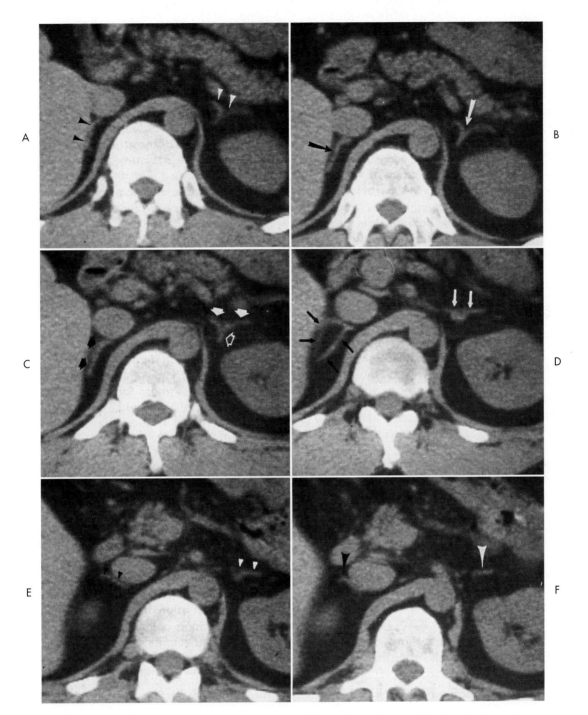

Fig. 34-2. Normal adrenal glands. Scans at six different levels (5 mm thick slices) reveal variability in the size, shape, and configuration of right *(black arrows and arrowheads)* and left gland *(white arrows and arrowheads)* at different levels in the same patient. For instance, the medial limb of the right gland extends superiorly **(A to C).** On the right *(black arrows),* both medial and lateral limbs are visible at only one level **(D).** The lateral limb extends inferiorly **(E** and **F,** *black arrowheads).* On the left, both limbs are visible on the upper three scans **(A to C,** *white arrows and white arrowheads).* The lateral limb only is visible on the lower three scans **(D to F,** *white arrows and arrowheads).*

tionship to the posterior surface of the inferior vena cava. Its lateral limb tends to extend more inferiorly than the medial limb. The superior portion of the left gland, behind the pancreas, often abuts the splenic vessels, and its inferior margin extends to the superior aspect of the left renal vein.

The apparent thickness of both glands depends on their orientation relative to the plan of the transaxial scan. It appears thicker if obliquely oriented and thinner if vertically oriented. Measurements of thickness have been offered as a guideline. Rarely does the thickness of a normal gland exceed 10 mm, and more commonly the gland is 5 to 6 mm thick.

The adrenal glands lie within the cone of renal fascia and are embedded in fat. This location within fat permits their clear visualization in most patients. If body fat content is sparse, such as in children or thin or cachectic patients, the glands may be difficult to see.

The normal gland varies in appearance from patient to patient because of differences in relative abdominal fat content, different degrees of orientation of the gland with respect to a plane of the scan, and minor differences in locations of the gland. A variable appearance at different scan levels in the same patient is due to the prominence of either the medial or lateral limb of the gland at a particular level. Both glands appear slightly thicker superiorly and anteriorly where the medial and lateral limbs fuse. They often appear thinnest inferiorly where the lateral limb commonly extends more inferiorly than the medial limb.

In our practice, absolute measurements are not relied on to determine whether glands are normal or enlarged. The overall size, shape, configuration, and smooth appearance of the margins and the lack of nodularity or marginal irregularity are more important than thickness alone in estimating the normality of the gland.

Artifacts that cause difficulties in visualization of the adrenal glands are usually due to respiratory motion during the scan, residual barium in the gastrointestinal tract, and metallic surgical clips adjacent to the adrenal glands.

Normal glands are difficult to see in patients after surgical procedures, especially a nephrectomy, because other organs fall into the renal fossae and can obscure the glands. On the right side, this rearrangement of normal structures is commonly due to the medial displacement of the right lobe of the liver and posterior displacement of loops of small intestine and colon. On the left side after a nephrectomy, the tail of the pancreas and bowel loops move into the renal fossa and may make adrenal gland identification difficult.

In patients with congenital renal anomalies, the adrenal glands are typically different from the normal appearance. Kenney et al[25] studied 30 patients with renal anomalies and found that the normal gland could be identified in 83% on the ipsilateral side of the anomaly and that it differed in configuration. In these patients, the adrenal gland appeared linear in shape and had a disk shape on coronal reconstruction; this correlates with the autopsy data that were previously reported.

CT EXAMINATION TECHNIQUES

Differences in equipment require a modification of scanning technique best suited to the available scan times and slice thicknesses. In general, shorter scan times and thinner sections produce the most satisfactory results.

Thickness of slice and scanning increment

Usually scans performed with a 1 cm slice thickness at 1 cm contiguous increments are satisfactory. If a small mass is suspected or if the initial findings are equivocal, however, repeat scans (using a thinner slice and scanning at closer or overlapping intervals) yield better results. On scanners with a fixed slice thickness, overlapping scans can be performed to improve the detectability of small lesions. Often the mere performance of a few repeat scans at a given level serves to confirm or exclude a lesion.

Intravenous contrast enhancement

It is possible to obtain diagnostic scans of the adrenal glands without use of intravenous contrast material. The administration of contrast material, however, assists in the differentiation of the adrenal gland from tortuous segments of the splenic artery or vein on the left side. Contrast material assists in the characterization of an adrenal cyst, which does not enhance as do most tumors. Enhancement may be uniform throughout the tumor or irregular because of the presence of hemorrhage, necrosis, or zones of avascularity. Contrast material can assist in the identification of metastases from malignant tumors to other sites, such as the liver.

Oral contrast material

The use of contrast material is helpful for adrenal examination because unopacified bowel loops can be a source of confusion. This especially occurs after a nephrectomy when bowel loops fall into the renal fossae or in those patients who are being examined for an ectopically located tumor, such as a pheochromocytoma, in which case the tumor may lie anywhere in the retroperitoneum or pelvis and be close to bowel loops.

Extent of examination

It is critical that examinations of the adrenal glands begin at a level above them and extend to a level below them. Serial, contiguous, or overlapping scans from above, entirely through, and to a level below the glands are required for a complete examination. Failure to detect small, eccentrically located tumors that project from the apex or inferiorly from a limb may occur if the examination is incomplete. Portions of a gland containing a small tumor may appear normal at any individual level above or below the tumor.

Postoperative patient

Scanning for pathological conditions of the adrenal gland after an adrenalectomy or nephrectomy poses a special problem because artifact and rearrangement of normal anatomical structures result in confusing images. In this situation, narrow collimation and oral and intravenous contrast enhancement as well as meticulous attention to scanning technique are necessary.

INDICATIONS FOR ADRENAL GLAND SCANNING

The most common reasons for referral of patients for adrenal examination have been (1) biochemical diagnosis of a hyperfunctioning adrenal gland tumor, (2) discovery of a possible adrenal mass on another imaging examination, and (3) screening of the adrenals for metastasis in patients with tumors that have a high predilection to metastasize to this gland. Less common reasons for referral have been for patients with signs or symptoms of pathological conditions in the adrenal gland accompanied by either negative or equivocal biochemical findings. The least common indications for referral are asymptomatic patients with no biochemical evidence of tumor but who have a clinical syndrome or a family history associated with an increased incidence of adrenal tumor.

General diagnostic signs

The full spectrum of adrenal gland disease is visible on CT. With the exception of hyperplasia, pathological conditions of the adrenal gland as seen on CT scans appear as a mass lesion.

Large masses (those greater than 4 to 5 cm in diameter), such as carcinomas, neuroblastomas, and some pheochromocytomas, appear as upper abdominal masses, and based on the scan appearance alone, it may be difficult to predict the exact origin of the mass. These large tumors obliterate any semblance of the normal gland configuration and displace adjacent organs. Of course, biochemical evidence of adrenal hyperfunction indicates the possibility of adrenal tumor, but if the lesion is nonfunctioning, it can be difficult to determine whether the lesion is adrenal, renal, pancreatic, hepatic, or primary retroperitoneal in origin. The smallest tumors (1 or 2 cm in diameter), such as aldosterone-producing adenomas, appear as subtle masses arising from a portion of an oth-

erwise normal-sized gland and may project from either limb or from the apex of the gland. Intermediate-size tumors (2 to 5 cm in diameter) usually obliterate the normal configuration of the gland but are found exactly in the expected location of the adrenal glands and so are more reliably identifiable as adrenal in origin.

Attenuation characteristics of tumors are helpful in masses such as cysts and myelolipomas. The CT attenuation value of fluid in cysts or fat in myelolipomas often permits accurate tissue characterization. Some other attenuation features of tumors can be used as hints, but they occur infrequently and cannot be considered characteristic. Such findings might include low density of an aldosterone-producing adenoma with a high cholesterol content, eccentric calcification in malignant tumors, or a central area of decreased density (more apparent after injection of intravenous contrast material) in pheochromocytomas. Such distinguishing features are not the rule, and each type of adrenal gland tumor may appear exactly as any other.

Adrenal cortex carcinoma

Carcinoma of the adrenal cortex usually appears as a large mass on CT examinations. The organ of origin may not be clear because of invasion or displacement of contiguous organs, whereas evidence of adrenal hyperfunction implicates the adrenal gland. Reliance on such associations usually permits a correct diagnosis, but there are exceptions.

CT findings that suggest adrenal origin in large nonfunctioning tumors include anterior displacement of the inferior vena cava, pancreas, and splenic artery and vein. Scans made after administration of intravenous contrast material can improve the visibility of tissue planes between; adjacent displaced organs, such as the kidney, liver, or pancreas; and the adrenal mass. Occasionally it is possible to exclude adrenal origin of large tumors if the normal adrenal gland is seen in a displaced location. In some cases, an angiographic study is needed to identify the organ of origin precisely by identifying the artery that supplies it with blood.

All adrenal cortex carcinomas identified in our experience have been visible on CT. Occasionally confusion arises in patients with both lung and adrenal lesions that have a similar histological appearance. It may be difficult to be certain, even after biopsy, which is the primary tumor and which represents the metastasis.

Neuroblastomas

Neuroblastoma is the most common solid neoplasm in the abdomen in childhood. Only leukemia, lymphoma, and central nervous system tumors are more common in childhood. The adrenal medulla is a common site of these tumors owing to the neurocrest origin

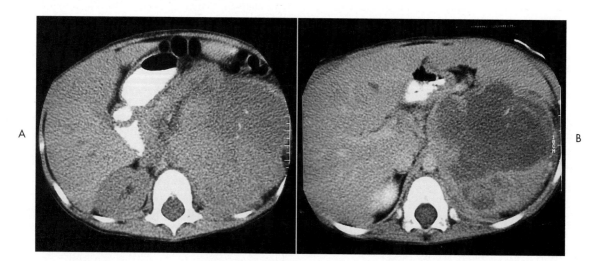

Fig. 34-3. A 3-year-old boy with neuroblastoma. **A,** Large inhomogeneous mass with calcification on noncontrast CT. **B,** After contrast administration, the large neuroblastoma demonstrates mild contrast enhancement with a large amount of necrosis present.

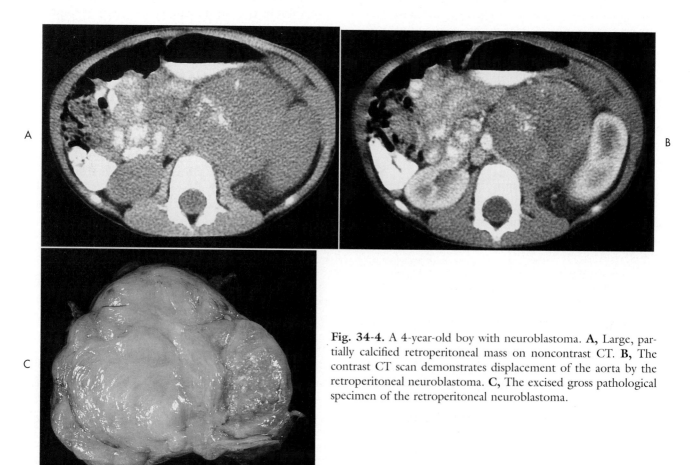

Fig. 34-4. A 4-year-old boy with neuroblastoma. **A,** Large, partially calcified retroperitoneal mass on noncontrast CT. **B,** The contrast CT scan demonstrates displacement of the aorta by the retroperitoneal neuroblastoma. **C,** The excised gross pathological specimen of the retroperitoneal neuroblastoma.

of those tumors. Neuroblastoma usually presents under 2 years of age. The most common presentation is a palpable abdominal mass. Varied presentation can occur owing to the ability of the tumor to be neurosecretory. Evans et al[12] has defined a staging system for neuroblastomas, which is the most common staging system in use today:

> Stage 1: Tumor is confined to the organ of origin.
>
> Stage 2: Tumor extends beyond the organ and involves surrounding lymph nodes.
>
> Stage 3: Tumor crosses the midline or involves contralateral lymph nodes.
>
> Stage 4: Distant metastases are present.
>
> Stage 4S: A subgroup of patients is seen with skin, liver, and bone marrow spread but not affecting the osseous bone itself.

Stage 4S usually presents in the youngest age group. In general, the more advanced the stage, the worse the prognosis for cure. An exception to this is stage 4S, which depending on the circumstances, can carry a better prognosis.

CT scanning is the primary imaging modality used in evaluating patients with suspected neuroblastomas (Fig. 34-3).* Neuroblastomas appear as solid masses on CT with frequent areas of inhomogeneity owing to necrosis or hemorrhage. Calcification can also frequently be seen in these tumors and as an important marker in differentiating these tumors from other abdominal masses in children. Contrast enhancement is not marked in these tumors (Fig. 34-4). Important points to recognize in performing a CT scan on a patient with suspected neuroblastoma is the presence of nodal involvement, the presence of liver involvement, and if the tumor crosses the midline because these are important factors in staging the tumor.

Radionuclide imaging with MIBG is being used to diagnose and in some cases for treatment of neuroblastoma lesions. This is an area of rapid advance, and the exact role MIBG scanning plays in the diagnosis and treatment of neuroblastoma is yet to be fully defined.

Mesenchymal tumors

The most common masses arising from the stroma of the adrenal gland are the myelolipoma and the adrenal cyst.[23] These two masses are characterizable because of their attenuation values. Most often they are discovered incidentally on CT scans of the upper abdomen carried out for other reasons.

Cysts are recognized as sharply circumscribed, smooth-margined, low-density (approximately water density) masses with identifiable thin walls (Fig. 34-5).

*References 2, 5, 27, 33, 36, 37.

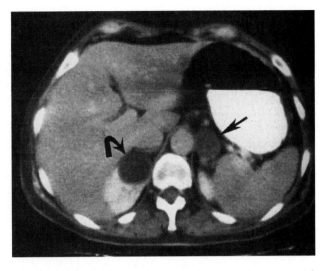

Fig. 34-5. Adrenal and renal cysts. Oval low-density mass with a thin wall in the left adrenal gland *(arrow)*. The density of the left adrenal cyst is slightly greater than the density of the cyst in the upper pole of the right kidney *(curved arrow)*, but the attenuation value is compatible with diagnosis of a cyst.

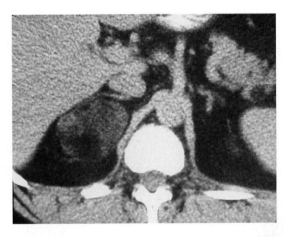

Fig. 34-6. Incidentally discovered right adrenal myelolipoma. Inhomogenous right adrenal mass with large fatty component within the mass.

In those cases in which the attenuation values are not strictly those of a cyst, ultrasonography may be necessary to confirm the diagnosis. Low-density adenomas may simulate the appearance of a cyst, but they can be differentiated by administration of intravenous contrast material. The adenoma enhances, and the cyst does not.

Adrenal myelolipomas are common incidental autopsy findings (Fig. 34-6). These tumors are benign and are composed of mature fat cells with focal areas of myeloid tissue. CT scans of these tumors show a low attenuation value because of the high fat content. The tumors may be homogeneous and composed almost entirely of fat, or they can be interlaced with fibrous strands and septations that produce a nonhomogeneous CT appearance.

Pheochromocytomas

Patients with a pheochromocytoma arising from the adrenal medulla commonly have characteristic signs and symptoms. Clinical syndromes lead to biochemical testing, which establishes the diagnosis. This is turn leads to a need for accurate preoperative localization of the functioning tumor. CT scanning is the most accurate method for preoperative localization of an intra-adrenal pheochromocyoma (Figs. 34-7 and 34-8).[29,38]

The signs and symptoms of pheochromocytomas almost always result from excessive production and release of catecholamines. They most commonly occur in patients with hypertension that is difficult to control with the usual antihypertensive measures. The blood pressure is often unusually labile, and the symptoms are paroxysms of hypertension and tachyarrhythmia. The episodic spells often are associated with headache and palpitations. Other clinical clues include accelerated hypertension, hypermetabolism with weight loss, abnormal carbohydrate metabolism, and a pressor response to induction of anesthesia or to any antihypertensive drug. The diagnosis of pheochromocytomas is confirmed by abnormalities in catecholamine biochemistry. The determina-

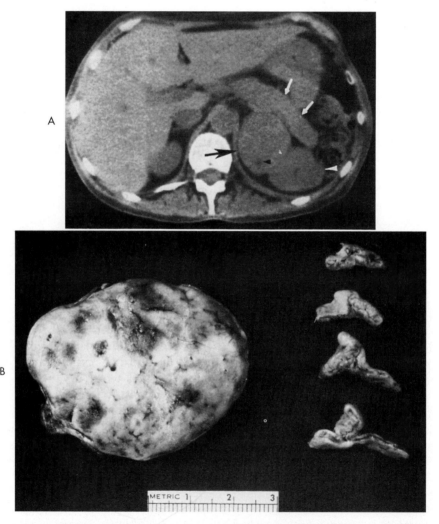

Fig. 34-7. Left adrenal gland pheochromocytoma. **A,** Scan without contrast material demonstrating 5×5 cm in diameter left adrenal tumor *(black arrow)* indenting the posterior aspect of the pancreas *(white arrows)* and touching the anteromedial surface of the left kidney *(white arrowhead)*. Small areas of decreased density within the tumor *(black arrowhead)* suggest cystic degeneration. **B,** Gross specimen.

tion of total urinary metanephrine is the most desirable choice for a screening test because it has yielded the fewest false-negative results.

A pheochromocytoma may occur at any age, but the peak incidence occurs in the fourth and fifth decades. Pheochromocytomas are extra-adrenal in location in approximately 10% of the cases, multicentric in about 10%, and bilateral in 5%. Of the unilateral lesions, 60% occur in the right gland and 40% in the left gland. Of the pheochromocytomas found in ectopic locations, 90% occur in the abdomen, and the most common sites are the organ of Zuckerkandl; retroperitoneal para-aortic and paracaval areas, particularly medial to the kidneys; and in the region of the bladder.

Chromaffin cells in a pheochromocytoma are found not only in the normal adrenal medulla but also in the paraganglial locations of the carotid, aortic, and jugular bodies. Because of this, pheochromocytomas can be found anywhere from the base of the brain down to the epididymus. Malignant pheochromocytomas occur in 14% of the cases. In general, extra-adrenal tumors are more commonly malignant.

When a patient with a suspected pheochromocytoma is referred for localization, the initial CT examination is of the adrenal glands. If a unilateral intra-adrenal tumor is discovered, we usually do not extend the examination to other intra-abdominal or thoracic locations because of the relative infrequency of multicentricity. If the initial CT examination of the adrenal glands fails to reveal a tumor, radionuclide MIBG scanning is then performed for tumor localization. CT can play a complementary role with MIBG scanning for anatomical localization.[1,28,34,35]

We have had occasion to examine patients who have had previous resections of a pheochromocytoma and have symptoms and biochemical findings suggesting recurrence. In these patients, the operative site, contralateral adrenal gland, and other potential sites of ec-

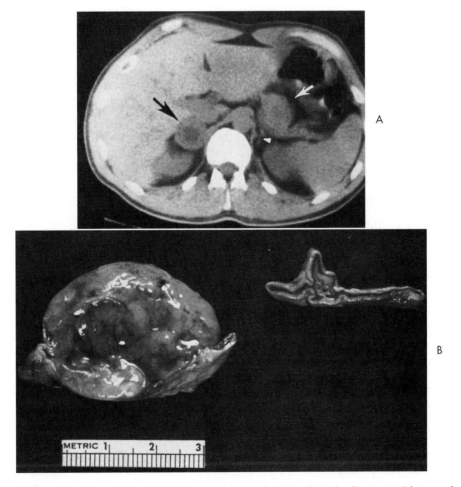

Fig. 34-8. Right adrenal gland pheochromocytoma. **A,** Mass 3 cm in diameter with central low density *(black arrow)*. The normal left adrenal gland *(arrowhead)* is located behind a bulbous-appearing pancreas *(white arrow)* that was normal at surgery. **B,** Gross specimen.

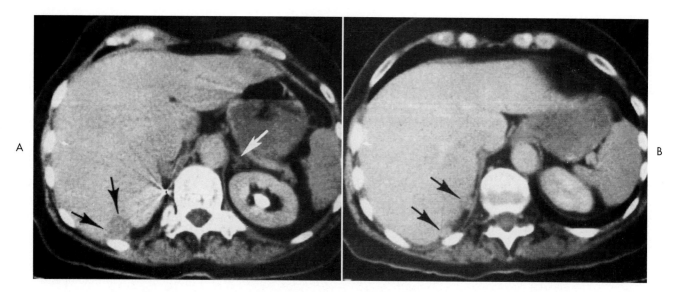

Fig. 34-9. Recurrent pheochromocytoma. CT examination was carried out to evaluate the left adrenal gland in a patient with recurrent biochemical evidence of a pheochromocytoma. The original tumor had been removed several years previously. **A,** Scan at one level shows normal left adrenal gland *(white arrow)* but also reveals a 1.5 cm in diameter low-density mass in the operative site *(black arrows)*. **B,** A scan at a slightly higher level shows two additional nodules *(arrows)* between the right lobe of the liver and the diaphragm. At surgery, these were found to be three nodules of pheochromocytoma "rests."

topic tumor location are examined. MIBG scanning, however, has largely replaced CT for detection of pheochromocytoma recurrences. This is due to the increased accuracy of MIBG scanning in this clinical setting (Fig. 34-9).

The CT characteristics of a pheochromocytoma are variable, reflecting the variability of the gross pathological conditions found in this tumor. Most unilateral intra-adrenal pheochromocytomas appear as round or oval, discrete, sharply circumscribed masses that measure from 2 to 4 cm in diameter. Their CT density can be homogeneous and usually slightly less than the density of the adjacent liver or pancreas. Often there is nonhomogeneous density and a tendency for the periphery of the tumor to be more dense than the central portion. This is because of central necrosis of cystic degeneration. Pheochromocytomas increase in density after the injection of contrast material, and often the periphery enhances to a greater degree than the central, less vascular area. There is an increased occurrence of central low density with larger tumors. Calcification occasionally occurs within these tumors and can be located in the middle or periphery of the mass. As with other adrenal tumors, the organ of origin of large pheochromocytomas may be difficult to determine if adjacent organs are displaced and contiguous with the tumor.

The literature contains many references indicating the accuracy of CT in the assessment of pheochromocytomas. The best results have been in detection of the unilateral intra-adrenal tumors. Ectopic lesions, multicentric lesions, and recurrent tumors have been identified, but the accuracy rate of detecting tumors in unusual locations is less than for the usual intra-adrenal lesions.

Our experience indicates that CT is the most accurate technique for preoperative localization in patients with a suspected intra-adrenal pheochromocytoma. Most pheochromocytomas should be visible on CT scans carried out on suitable equipment, with proper scanning techniques, and by an experienced examiner. It is clear, however, that in ectopic locations or in recurrence cases, MIBG scanning is the imaging method of choice.

Adrenal gland hyperplasia

The appearance of diffuse bilateral adrenal gland enlargement on CT has occurred most frequently in patients referred for an attempted localization of a tumor responsible for either Cushing's syndrome or primary aldosteronism (Fig. 34-10).

It is clear that hyperfunction of the adrenal glands does not always equate with hyperplasia and that hyperfunctioning glands may appear normal in size on CT. Accurate assessment of size may be difficult because of variation in the superoinferior and anteroposterior dimensions. Also, the appearance of the thickness of the

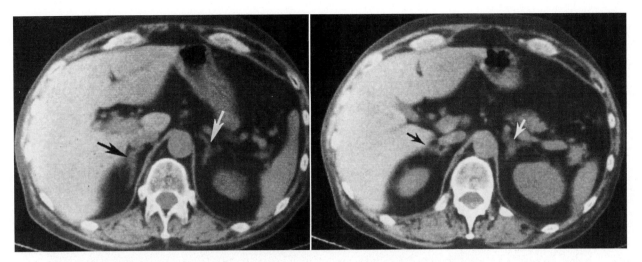

Fig. 34-10. Adrenal gland hyperplasia. Scans at two levels in a patient with Cushing's disease and pituitary tumor demonstrate increased size and thickness of both the right *(black arrows)* and the left *(white arrows)* glands.

gland depends on its orientation relative to the plane of the scan. The incidence of patients with Cushing's disease and hyperplasia exceeds that of primary aldosteronism and hyperplasia. We do not ordinarily scan patients with pituitary tumors in an effort to identify enlarged glands; however, when the question of pituitary hyperfunction is not clear, adrenal CT examination is often carried out to exclude or diagnose a primary adrenal tumor. We have also examined several patients with Cushing's disease in whom the biochemical investigation has suggested the presence of an autonomously functioning adrenocorticotropic hormone (ACTH) source. In our experience, adrenal hyperplasia was usually evident, and in some of these patients, the tumor responsible for the syndrome was discovered. Other authors who reported their experience have noted that the majority of their cases had normal-appearing adrenals.

In patients with primary aldosteronism, hyperplasia is the cause less often than the tumor. In this group of patients, the hyperfunctioning glands are often normal in size on CT examinations. Most patients who have primary aldosteronism, without clear evidence of an adrenal tumor, do not generally undergo adrenalectomy, particularly if they respond to suitable medical therapy.

Adrenal adenomas

The three most common adenomas are (1) nonfunctioning adenomas, (2) adenomas associated with Cushing's disease, and (3) adenomas associated with primary hyperaldosteronism.

A patient with Cushing's disease in which an adenoma is discovered is perhaps the most clear-cut situation in CT adrenal scanning (Figs. 34-11, 34-12, and 34-13). In our overall experience, there has been near 100% accuracy in the identification of such adenomas, and there have been no false-negative or false-positive results. They have all been unilateral, appearing as round or slightly oval, smooth, sharply circumscribed masses ranging between 2 and 5 cm. They may obliterate the entire gland, or sometimes a remnant of normal-appearing adrenal tissue may protrude from one of the margins of the tumor. The presence of this hyperfunctioning tumor often is associated with atrophy in the contralateral gland or even atrophy of the visible remnant of the ipsilateral gland. Baert et al[3] have cautioned that it is hazardous to speak of hypoplasia of the contralateral gland in a patient with Cushing's disease. Nevertheless, in our experience with a unilateral adrenal adenoma associated with Cushing's disease, the contralateral gland has almost always appeared atrophic. This contralateral atrophy is most common when the adenoma is autonomic and independent of the hypothalamic-hypophyseal control circuit.

The density of the adenoma is usually less than the adjacent organs, such as the liver, spleen, and kidneys. It also usually is less than the adjacent aorta and inferior vena cava, presumably because of the high lipid content of adrenocortical tumors. The low density of some adenomas can create confusion in differentiating them from cysts, but intravenous contrast enhancement usually allows this distinction to be made with certainty. Differential diagnosis in patients with Cushing's disease and unilateral adrenal tumors is rarely difficult.

The second most common benign functioning

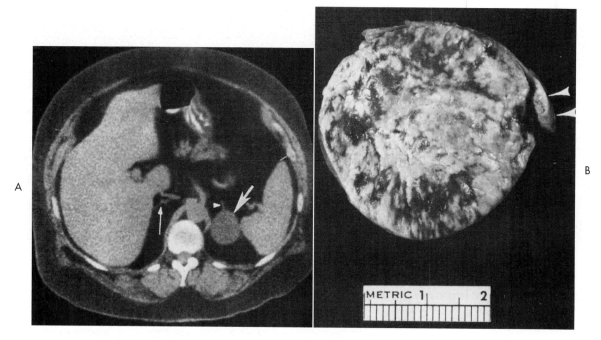

Fig. 34-11. Left adrenal gland adenoma in a patient with Cushing's disease. **A,** Mass 2.5 cm in diameter in the left adrenal gland *(large white arrow)* is present. Also visible is a hypoplastic remnant of the left gland *(arrowhead)*. The right adrenal gland *(small white arrow)* is hypoplastic. **B,** The gross specimen includes the hypoplastic gland remnant *(arrowheads)*.

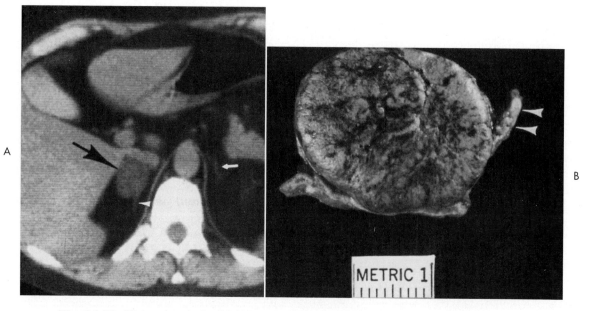

Fig. 34-12. Right adrenal gland adenoma in patient with Cushing's disease. **A,** A tumor 2 cm in diameter in the right gland *(black arrow)* associated with a hypoplastic ipsilateral remnant *(arrowhead)*. The left gland is also hypoplastic *(white arrow)*. **B,** The gross specimen includes the hypoplastic remnant *(arrowheads)*.

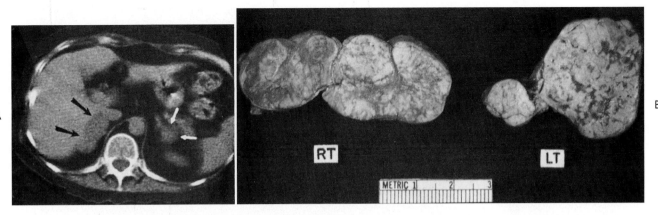

Fig. 34-13. Bilateral adrenal gland masses in patient with Cushing's disease. **A,** Scan at a single level shows lobulated enlargement of the right adrenal gland *(black arrows)* and a round mass in the left adrenal gland *(white arrows)*. **B,** The CT appearance suggested bilateral tumors, but pathological assessment of the resected organs indicated nodular hyperplasia of the adrenal glands.

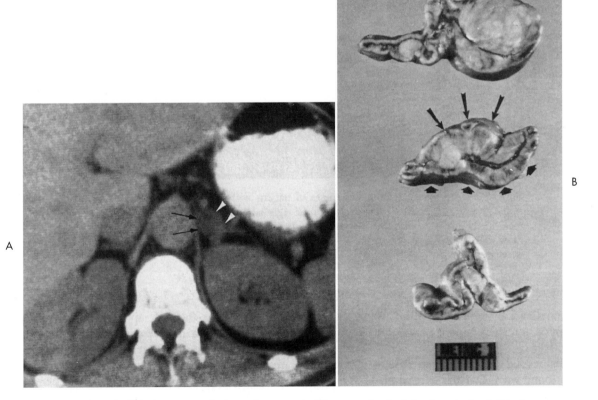

Fig. 34-14. Aldosterone-producing adenoma. **A,** Tiny mass in the left adrenal gland *(black arrows)* preserves the configuration of the left adrenal gland but indents the central portion of the gland *(arrowheads)*. **B,** Inspection of the gross specimen reveals both a tumor *(arrows)* and a portion of the normal glands *(arrowheads)*.

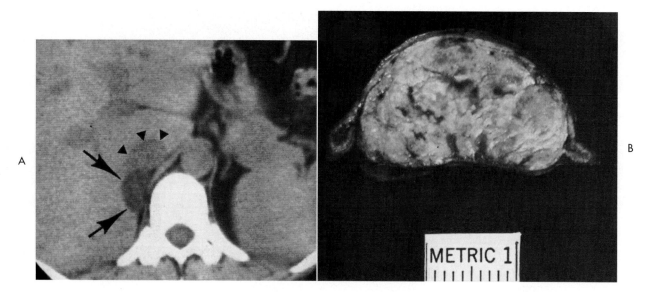

Fig. 34-15. Aldosterone-producing adenoma. **A,** A mass 1.5 cm in diameter in the right adrenal gland *(arrows)* is located posterior to and is lower in density than the inferior vena cava *(arrowheads).* **B,** Examination of the gross specimen revealed a high cholesterol content.

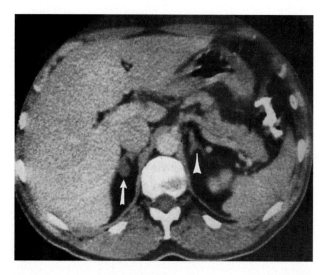

Fig. 34-16. Aldosterone-producing adenoma. An adenoma 1 cm in diameter arises from the lateral limb of the right adrenal gland *(arrow).* The left adrenal gland *(arrowhead)* is normal.

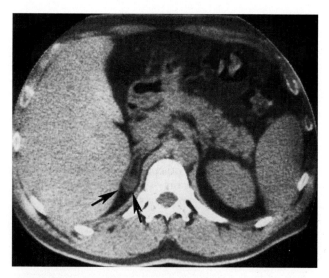

Fig. 34-17. Aldosterone-producing adenoma. An adenoma in the right adrenal gland *(black arrows)* 1.2 cm in diameter arises from the tip of either the medial or lateral limb but is in contact with both limbs.

adenoma found on CT of the adrenal gland is the tumor responsible for primary aldosteronism (Conn's syndrome) (Figs. 34-14, 34-15, 34-16, and 34-17). Primary aldosteronism occurs in hypertensive patients who have persistent hypokalemia, elevated plasma and urine levels of aldosterone, and suppressed plasma renin activity. Of patients with primary aldosteronism, 75% have a benign adenoma that causes autonomous secretion of aldoste-

rone. In 25% of the cases, the syndrome is associated with hyperplasia of the zona glomerulosa. Aldosterone-producing adenomas are generally small tumors, and in an early series,[5] 85% of the tumors measured less than 3 cm in diameter. Clinically, it is important to distinguish between primary aldosteronism resulting from a functioning adenoma and from that due to hyperplasia. This differentiation can be done occasionally by biochemical

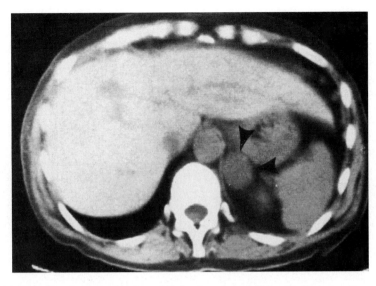

Fig. 34-18. Nonfunctioning adenoma. A left adrenal mass 3 cm in diameter *(arrowheads)* in a patient who had no evidence of adrenal hyperfunction and no history of a primary neoplasm. The adrenal tumor did not explain the patient's symptoms but was the only positive finding and was removed at surgery.

means, but often the biochemical findings are inconclusive. If they are diagnostic, localization of the tumor is often necessary. If diagnostic uncertainty exists, clinicians are reluctant to recommend surgery to these patients because bilateral adrenal nodular hyperplasia would require an adrenalectomy followed by long-term adrenal inefficiency. Accurate detection and localization of these small tumors with CT scanning play a significant part in planning a unilateral adrenalectomy.[8,9,17,19]

Patients with hypersecretion of aldosterone associated with CT evidence of normal-sized glands or even large glands are given medical therapy. Even though adenomas causing primary aldosteronism are small, our experience and that of others indicate that CT can readily detect them. It appears that CT has been responsible for an increased frequency of detection and surgical removal of aldosterone-producing adenomas. Improvements in CT instrumentation with faster scan times and thinner collimation have increased the visibility of these small tumors. Our experience with aldosterone adenomas is similar to that of White et al,[39] in which 12 of 16 patients with unilateral intra-adrenal aldosterone-producing tumors had positive CT scans. In one of those patients, the tumor was only 1 cm in diameter. Of the eight tumors discovered during the 18-month period in our series, the mean diameter of the tumor was 2 cm with a range from 1 to 3 cm.

We and others agree that CT should be considered as the initial diagnostic imaging method for the detection of aldosterone-producing adenomas. Adrenal venous sampling and adrenal scintiphotography are reserved for those patients with biochemical evidence of an adenoma in whom the CT scan is normal, equivocal, or indeterminate.

An aldosterone-producing adenoma appears on CT as a small tumor, generally 1 to 3 cm in diameter. It is round or oval and sometimes less dense than the adjacent visible remnant of the adrenal gland. The low density has been said to be due to a high cholesterol content. The small tumors often arise eccentrically in the adrenal gland and project from one of the limbs of the gland. The unaffected portions of the gland have a normal appearance. Ease of detection of aldosterone-producing adenomas has improved with the use of thin-section, high-resolution scanners with fast scan times.

A nonfunctioning adenoma is the most common benign adenoma of the adrenal gland (Fig. 34-18). It is discovered most often in patients who are referred for CT scanning after a suggestive or equivocal finding on another imaging method, or it is discovered in patients who are referred for CT scanning for problems unassociated with the adrenal gland. Occasionally, they are found to be the cause of a calcification first discovered with conventional radiography.

In general, we believe that if a small mass is discovered in the adrenal gland in a patient who has no signs or symptoms of adrenal hyperfunction, no biochemical evidence of a functioning tumor, and no evidence of primary carcinoma, the lesion most likely is a benign nonfunctioning adenoma.[10]

Several other syndromes can result from the functioning adenomas. These include the adrenogenital syndrome, the feminizing syndrome, and the various mixed syndromes. These syndromes are rare and can be caused by hyperplasia, adenomas, or carcinoma, but they are more often associated with malignant tumors.

Adrenal gland metastases

Metastases in the adrenal gland occur often in the advanced stage of many malignancies.[16,20,32] Adrenal metastases appear as mass lesions of the adrenal gland that are not necessarily distinguishable on CT scan appearance from other types of adrenal masses (Figs. 34-19

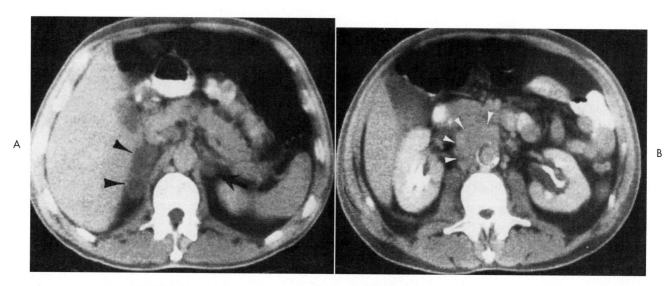

Fig. 34-19. Adrenal gland metastasis. **A,** Elongated oval mass in the right adrenal gland *(arrowheads)* and round mass in the medial limb of the left adrenal gland *(arrow)* are seen. **B,** The adrenal masses are associated with a retroperitoneal mass *(arrowheads)* found at another scan level, posterior to the head of the pancreas and anterior to the aorta and inferior vena cava. These findings occurred in a patient with known prostatic carcinoma and are presumed to be prostatic metastases.

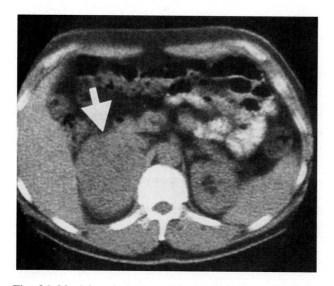

Fig. 34-20. Adrenal gland metastasis. A large round mass in the region of the right adrenal gland *(arrow)* found in a patient with a known metastatic melanoma. Tissue for diagnosis was obtained from another metastatic site.

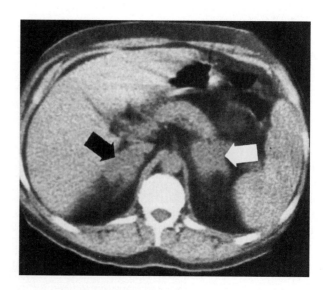

Fig. 34-21. Adrenal gland metastasis. Irregular mass in the right adrenal gland *(black arrow)* and in the left adrenal gland *(white arrow)* in a patient with known primary lung carcinoma. Adrenal gland masses were presumed to be metastasis.

to 34-21). They do occur in patients with known primary tumors in other locations. We have not recognized any particular distinguishing features among the various primary cell types. Often tissue confirmation of the nature of a mass believed to be an adrenal metastasis is not obtained because adrenal metastasis represents just one manifestation of disseminated carcinomatosis or because another site of metastasis is more accessible for biopsy. When it appears that an adrenal mass is the only site of possible metastasis in a patient with a known primary tumor, CT guidance has been used for biopsy and histological confirmation of adrenal metastasis.

Review of our CT experience with adrenal metastases indicates that the left adrenal gland is involved slightly more often than the right. Even though histo-

logical confirmation of the nature of all adrenal metastases was not obtained, the most common primary tumor was lung carcinoma, representing 33% of the metastases, followed by primary tumors in the genitourinary tract (renal, prostatic, and bladder), representing 25%. Gastrointestinal malignancy accounted for 15% of the metastases, and miscellaneous lesions, such as breast carcinoma and melanoma, accounted for 5%. Of the presumed metastases, 22% occurred in patients with demonstrated carcinomatosis but no known primary tumor.

The adrenal glands may also be involved in patients with lymphomas and have been involved by direct extension of neoplasms arising in adjacent organs such as the kidneys.[22]

Adrenal gland metastases are usually discovered

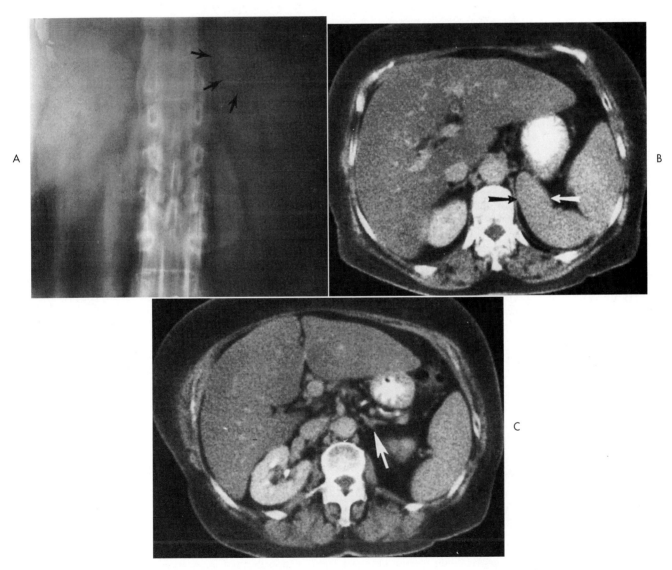

Fig. 34-22. Adrenal gland pseudotumor. Apparent suprarenal mass on conventional tomogram (**A,** *arrows*) was shown to be a prominent medial lobulation of the spleen (**B,** *arrows*) located above a normal left adrenal gland (**C,** *arrow*).

on CT scans that are performed as part of a staging examination in patients with known primary neoplasms or in the evaluation of patients with known metastases at other sites when looking for a primary tumor. Sometimes they are found on CT examinations being done for another nonadrenal indication. The discovery of bilateral adrenal gland masses in the patient with a known pri-

mary tumor and in the absence of any evidence of adrenal hyperfunction certainly suggests metastasis. In a patient with a known malignancy, a unilateral adrenal mass could be a solitary metastasis, a carcinoma, or an adenoma. Percutaneous biopsy is then undertaken to make the differentiation.

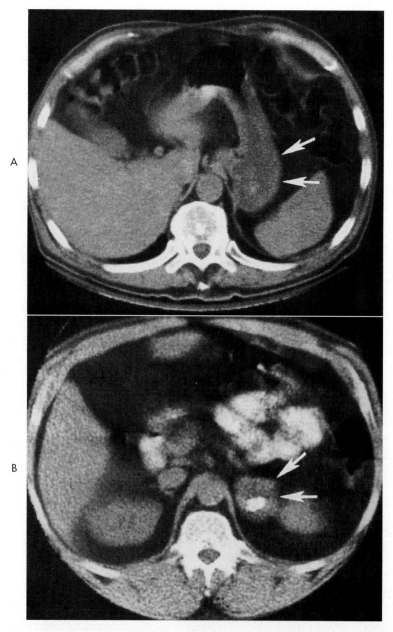

Fig. 34-23. Adrenal gland pseudomass. **A,** Scan in patient with possible left adrenal mass revealed that the gastric fundus *(arrows)* had simulated an adrenal tumor on a conventional abdominal examination. **B,** Comparison of the appearance of the gastric fundus with the scan of another patient with a proven, centrally calcified pheochromocytoma *(arrows)* indicates how the prominent gastric fundus might simulate an adrenal tumor.

Differentiation of masses

Considerable work has been done trying to assess how well CT can distinguish between neoplastic benign, and functioning tumors. In this regard, Hussain et al[21] evaluated 43 adrenal masses and assessed three parameters: size, contrast enhancement, and consistency. In their study, larger tumors were more likely to be malignant. Contrast enhancement was more likely in malignant lesions. Benign lesions had a regular consistency. A number of authors have noted that tumors such as aldosterone tumors or other hyperfunctioning cortical tumors may show decreased density because of an accumulation of lipid material; this is somewhat inconsistent.

Adrenal gland pseudotumors

CT examination clearly demonstrated normal adrenal glands and in almost all cases identified a specific structure that had been responsible for the apparent adrenal mass on the other method (Figs. 34-22 and 34-23).[6,30] Prominent lobulations of the spleen, the gastric fundus, tortuous splenic vessels, and occasionally the tail of the pancreas were responsible for the pseudomass on the left. On the right, abundant suprarenal fat, a fluid-filled duodenum, or a prominent lobulation of the right lobe of the liver suggested an adrenal mass. In addition, exophytic upper pole renal cysts and carcinomas occasionally simulate adrenal masses, as did a splenic artery aneurysm, a liver cyst, and nonadrenal retroperitoneal metastases.

Incidental discovery of tumors

With the increased use of CT scanning, adrenal gland masses are being discovered in increasing frequency in patients being examined for problems not related to the adrenal gland. The most common of these have been incidental discovery of a adrenal cysts or benign tumors, such as myelolipomas or nonfunctioning adenomas. Most adrenal lesions incidentally discovered on CT are nonfunctioning adenomas.

Nonfunctioning adenomas occur in autopsy populations ranging from 0.5% to 3% (Figs. 34-24 and 34-25). These lesions have an increasing incidence in age as well. Lesions on CT appearance are usually smooth, round, lower density, and less than 6 cm in size. Calcification within these lesions can occur but is unusual. Criteria favoring a benign, incidentally discovered adrenal

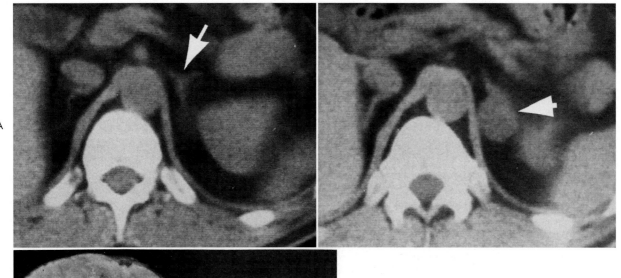

Fig. 34-24. Nonfunctioning adenoma. CT scans show a normal-appearing upper left adrenal gland (**A,** *arrow*) but at a level 1.5 cm below there is a left adrenal tumor (**B,** *arrowhead*). The scans were obtained in a patient with hypertension and were suggestive of but did not provide diagnostic biochemical evidence for, pheochromocytoma. The tumor (**C),** removed at surgery, was a benign adenoma and not a pheochromocytoma. The patient's hypertension was not cured.

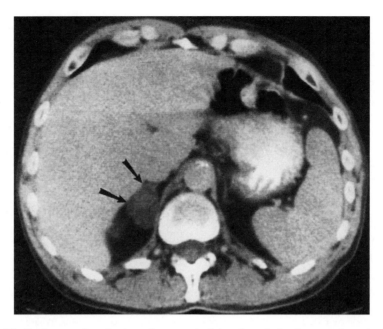

Fig. 34-25. Benign nonfunctioning adenoma. A right adrenal gland tumor 3 cm in diameter *(arrows)* was discovered in a patient being scanned for a nonadrenal indication. The adrenal mass did not seem to explain the patient's vague signs and symptoms. There was no biochemical evidence of hyperfunction or evidence of primary tumor in another location. Follow-up CT examination will be carried out in an effort to detect an increase in size. The diagnosis of a nonfunctioning adrenal adenoma is a tentative one.

lesion are homogeneous attenuation, round or oval shaped, maintenance of the normal configuration of the adrenal gland, and smaller size. If any question as to malignancy develops, either follow-up scanning or percutaneous biopsy is advisable. Articles have suggested that magnetic resonance imaging (MRI) may be able to differentiate benign nonfunctioning adenomas from other adrenal lesions. Although this work appears promising, there has not been a large study done with long-term follow-up yet to document this.

Adrenal biopsy

Percutaneous biopsy of adrenal masses has become a standard diagnostic procedure in evaluating adrenal pathology (Figs. 34-26 and 34-27).[4,7,24] The most common indication for adrenal biopsy is in patients with a known malignancy to exclude metastasis. Other biopsy indications would be for the diagnosis of primary adrenal tumors, infectious disease of the adrenal, or adrenal hemorrhage.

The technique of adrenal biopsy should include the largest size biopsy device that can be used safely. In our experience, 18-gauge biopsy devices have a higher degree of accuracy in adrenal biopsy with no difference in complication rate as compared with smaller gauge de-

vices. Adrenal biopsies are largely performed under CT guidance owing to its excellent advantages as an imaging modality of the adrenals compared with ultrasonography or MRI. The advent of automated biopsy devices or biopsy guns has enabled physicians to obtain material for both cytology and histology in adrenal biopsy. It is important to obtain both cytology and histology when performing biopsy because in up to 10% of cases, only one of either the cytology or histology is positive. Accuracy rates for percutaneous biopsy of the adrenal glands are generally greater than 90% in most published series. The complication rate for major complications is less than 1%, and in our experience, in more than 300 adrenal biopsies, there have been no deaths or tumor seeding from these procedures.

The approach to biopsy of the right adrenal gland can be made through either a posterior or a transhepatic route. We have found no difference in accuracy or complication rate from either route when the pleura is not transversed. The left adrenal can be a more difficult biopsy owing to the surrounding organs. In our experience, either a posterior or left lateral decubitus approach is most often successful. Various anterior approaches can be used if anatomical locations permit.

The use of percutaneous adrenal biopsy for the

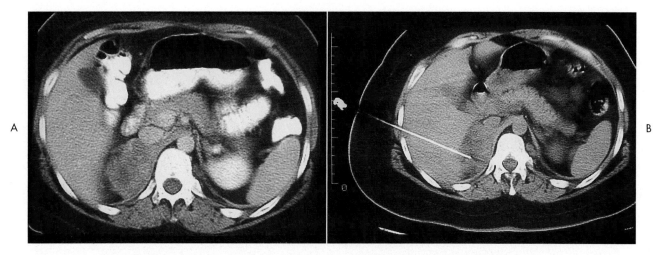

Fig. 34-26. A 66-year-old patient with question of adrenal metastases. **A,** Large infiltrating right adrenal mass. **B,** Transhepatic biopsy specimen of the right adrenal metastases.

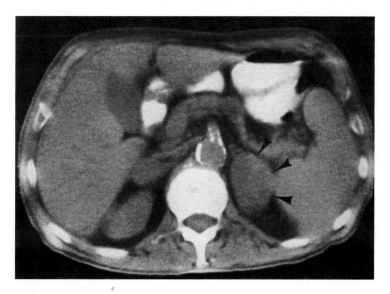

Fig. 34-27. Adrenal gland histoplasmosis. Left adrenal mass *(arrowheads)* discovered in a patient with known histoplasmosis. Examination of material obtained by CT-guided biopsy permitted diagnosis of adrenal involvement with histoplasmosis.

diagnosis of adrenal pathology has been an important step in the care of the affected patient population. It has reduced the use of other more invasive procedures for evaluating adrenal pathology. Percutaneous adrenal biopsy will continue to play an important role as further technological developments make the procedure safer and more accurate.

Inflammatory processes

Inflammatory processes of the adrenal gland are relatively uncommon except for granulomatous pro-

cesses, such as tuberculosis and histoplasmosis (Fig. 34-28).[41,42] According to Wilson et al[42] the appearance of these processes can be varied and may include minimal enlargement with faint flecks of calcium, moderate enlargement with focal low attenuation nodules, and massive enlargement with large areas of necrosis or dense calcification. In their group, five of seven patients had adrenal insufficiency. In such cases, CT-guided biopsy may be used for diagnostic confirmation if the cause is in question.

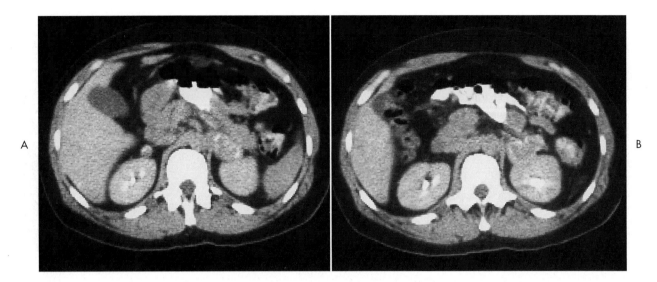

Fig. 34-28. A 60-year-old man with adrenal insufficiency secondary to tuberculosis. **A** and **B,** CT scan with contrast enhancement of the adrenals demonstrating bilateral calcified adrenal masses.

Adrenal hemorrhage

Adrenal hemorrhage can occur in both adult and pediatric populations. In the adult population, several clinical and pathological conditions are associated with adrenal hemorrhage (Figs. 34-29 and 34-30).[26,43] The first of these is anticoagulation or coagulopathies, which predispose to hemorrhage. The other is acute medical or surgical illness that results in a high level of corticotropin stimulation of the adrenal glands. Clinical examples of this latter group would include surgical stress, shock, and other major medical illnesses. The clinical presentation of adrenal hemorrhage is nonspecific. It may, however, be associated with abdominal pain, fever, or hypotension. Adrenal insufficiency can be absent in some cases or if present attributed to other illnesses. CT plays an important role in the early diagnosis of adrenal hemorrhage and the identification of those high-risk patients in whom prompt steroid replacement should be instituted.

The CT appearance of acute adrenal hemorrhage in adults is usually bilateral adrenal masses that appear high density on noncontrast scans. These gradually decrease in size over time, and the associated density of the masses likewise decreases as would be expected in a hemorrhage. An unusual complication of adrenal hemorrhage is abscess formation. This may occur in those patients in whom the hemorrhage is secondary to overwhelming sepsis in which infection has been superimposed on the bleed. Also, rarely, metastatic neoplasms can cause adrenal hemorrhage.

Adrenal hemorrhage is the most common adrenal mass in infancy. Although it does not commonly occur, infant adrenal hemorrhage does not have a clear cause in most cases. Possible predisposing conditions include a traumatic delivery, neonatal bradycardia, or asphyxia. In contrast to adults, in whom hemorrhage is more common bilaterally, in children it is more common unilaterally, and it is most often entirely asymptomatic. The appearance on CT again can be of a unilateral high-density mass if noncontrast scans are performed. Again, these masses usually decrease in size over the next several months in most patients.

MAGNETIC RESONANCE IMAGING

The rapid development of MRI in the past several years has led to its investigation in identifying adrenal pathology.[11,13-15,31,40] The adrenal glands can be readily visualized on any of the many varied imaging sequences available on modern MRI scanners. The identification of pathology on MRI of the adrenals appears to be nearly equivalent to that of CT scanning. CT, however, has the advantages of being less expensive and more readily available and has larger clinical experience with adrenal pathology imaging and the ability to perform biopsy procedures readily.

The areas of major study in MRI of the adrenal glands have been in pheochromocytoma and identification of benign nonfunctioning adenomas of the adrenal (Figs. 34-31 and 34-32). Pheochromocytomas have a characteristic high intensity signal on T2-weighted images. This has proved a reliable indicator of this tumor.

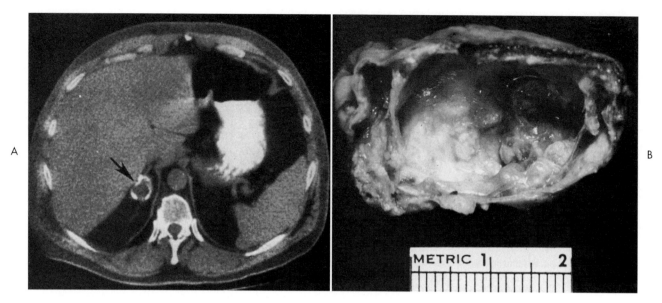

Fig. 34-29. Adrenal gland hematoma. **A,** CT scan shows a peripherally calcified right adrenal mass *(arrow)*. The calcification had originally been discovered on plain films of the abdomen. **B,** Inspection and pathological examination of the gross specimen revealed a partially calcified ancient adrenal hematoma.

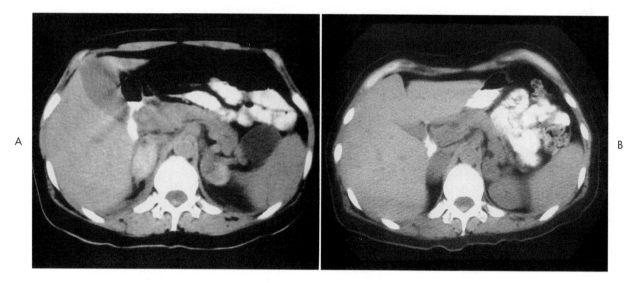

Fig. 34-30. A 53-year-old woman with adrenal insufficiency secondary to adrenal hemorrhage postsurgically. **A,** Noncontrast CT scan demonstrates bilateral high-density adrenal masses. **B,** Noncontrast CT scan 6 weeks later demonstrates that the mass has decreased in both size and density.

There has also been much study of identification of benign nonfunctioning adenomas on MRI. Although much promising work has been done in this area, there has as yet been no large prospective study to document the results in identification of these lesions. MRI does not appear to have as good a spatial resolution as current body MRI techniques, and therefore CT may be more accurate in detecting masses smaller than 1 cm in the adrenal glands. The use of MRI in defining adrenal pathology is a area of active study and the exact nature of the relationship of CT and MRI in evaluating adrenal disease will continue to evolve.

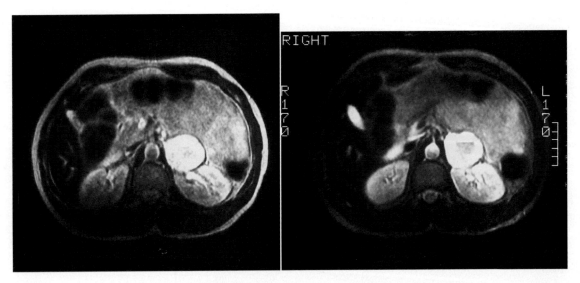

Fig. 34-31. "Snapshot" MRI images illustrating a left intraadrenal pheochromocytoma.

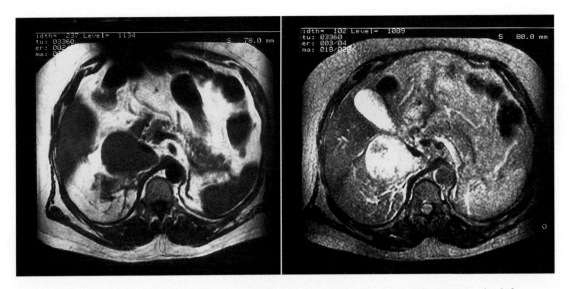

Fig. 34-32. T2-weighted MRI images demonstrate a high signal intensity mass in the left adrenal gland compatible with an intraadrenal pheochromocytoma.

REFERENCES

1. Ackery D, Tippett P, Condon B, et al: New approach to the localization of phaeochromocytoma: Imaging with 131 I-MIBG. *Br Med J* 288:1587, 1984.
2. Amundson GM, Trevensen CL, Mueller DL, et al: Neuroblastoma: A specific sonographic tissue pattern. *AJR* 148:943, 1987.
3. Baert AL, Wachenheim A, Jeanmart L: Abdominal computed tomography. In Wachenheim A, et al, editors: *Atlas of pathological computed tomography,* vol. 2, New York, 1980, Springer-Verlag.
4. Bernardino ME, Walther MM, Phillips VM, et al: CT-guided adrenal biopsy: Accuracy, safety, and indications. *AJR* 144:67-69, 1985.
5. Boechat MI, Ortega J, Hoffman AD, et al: Computed tomography in stage III neuroblastoma. *AJR* 145:1283, 1985.
6. Brady TM, Gross BH, Glazer GM, Williams DM: Adrenal pseudomasses due to varices: Angiographic-CT-MRI-pathologic correlations. *AJR* 145:301-304, 1985.
7. Charboneau JW, Reading CC, Welch TJ: CT and sonographically guided needle biopsy: Current techniques and new innovations. *AJR* 154:1-10, 1990.
8. Conn JW, Conn ES: Primary aldosteronism versus hypertensive disease with secondary aldosteronism. *Rec Prog Horm Res* 17:389-414, 1961.
9. Conn JW, Morita R, Cohen EL, et al: Primary aldosteronism: Pho-

toscanning of tumors after administration of [131]iodocholesterol. *Arch Intern Med* 129:417, 1972.

10. Copeland PM: The incidentally discovered adrenal mass. *Ann Intern Med* 98:940-945, 1983.

11. Davis PL, Hricak H, Bradley WG: Magnetic resonance imaging of the adrenal glands. *Radiol Clin North Am* 22:891, 1984.

12. Evans AE: Staging and treatment of neuroblastoma. *Cancer* 45:1799-1802, 1980.

13. Falke THM, teStrake L, Sandler MP, et al: Magnetic resonance imaging of the adrenal glands. *Radiographics* 7:343, 1987.

14. Falke THM, te Strake L, Shaff MI, et al: MR imaging of the adrenals: Correlation with computed tomography. *J Comput Assist Tomogr* 10:242-253, 1986.

15. Glazer GM, Woolsey EJ, Burrello J, et al: Adrenal tissue characterization using MR imaging. *Radiology* 158:73-79, 1986.

16. Greene KM, Brantly PN, Thompson WR: Adenocarcinoma metastatic to the adrenal gland simulating myelolipoma: CT evaluation. *J Comput Assist Tomogr* 9:820-821, 1985.

17. Gross MD, Shapiro B, Grekin RJ, et al: The scintigraphic localization of the adrenal lesion in primary aldosteronism. *Am J Med* 77:839, 1984.

18. Hamburger B, et al: Adrenal surgery: Trends during the seventies. *Am J Surg* 144:523-526, 1982.

19. Horton R, Finck E: Diagnosis and localization in primary aldosteronism. *Ann Intern Med* 76:885-890, 1972.

20. Huebener K-H, Treugut H: Adrenal cortex dysfunction: CT findings. *Radiology* 150:195-199, 1984.

21. Hussain S, et al: Differentiation of malignant from benign adrenal masses: Predictive indices on computed tomography. *AJR* 144:61-65, 1985.

22. Jafri SZH, Francis IR, Glazer GM, et al: CT detection of adrenal lymphoma. *J Comput Assist Tomogr* 7:254-256, 1983.

23. Johnson CD, Baker ME, Dunnick NR: CT demonstration of an adrenal pseudocyst. *J Comput Assist Tomogr* 9:817-819, 1985.

24. Katz RL, Shirkhoda A: Diagnostic approach to incidental adrenal nodules in the cancer patient. Results of a clinical, radiologic, and fine-needle aspiration study. *Cancer* 55:1995-2000, 1985.

25. Kenney PJ, et al: Adrenal glands in patients with congenital renal anomalies: CT appearance. *Radiology* 155:181-182, 1985.

26. Ling D, Korobkin M, Silverman PM, Dunnick NR: CT demonstration of bilateral adrenal hemorrhage. *AJR* 141:307-308, 1983.

27. Lopez-Ibor B, Schwartz AD: Neuroblastoma (reviews). *Pediatr Clin North Am* 32:755-778, 1985.

28. Lynn MD, Shapiro B, Sisson JC, et al: Improved visualization of pheochromocytomas and normal adrenal medullae with ^{123}I-MIBG scintigraphy. *Radiology* 156:789, 1985.

29. Quint LE, Glazer GM, Francis IR, et al: Pheochromocytoma and paraganglioma: Comparison of MR imaging with CT, and I-131 MIBG scintigraphy. *Radiology* 165:89, 1987.

30. Rao AKR, Silver TM: Normal pancreas and splenic variants simulating suprarenal and renal tumors. *AJR* 126:530-537, 1976.

31. Schultz CL, Haaga JR, Fletcher BD, et al: Magnetic resonance imaging of the adrenal glands: A comparison with computed tomography. *AJR* 143:1235-1240, 1984.

32. Shah HR, Love L, Williamson MR, et al: Hemorrhagic adrenal metastases: CT findings. *J Comput Assist Tomogr* 13:77-81, 1989.

33. Siegal MJ, Sagel SS: Computed tomography as a supplement to urography in the evaluation of suspected neuroblastoma. *Radiology* 142:435, 1982.

34. Sisson JC, Frager MS, Valk TW, et al: Scintigraphic localization of pheochromocytoma. *N Engl J Med* 305:12, 1981.

35. Sisson JC, Shapiro B, Beierwaltes WH, et al: Radiopharmaceutical treatment of malignant pheochromocytoma. *J Nucl Med* 25:197, 1984.

36. Stark DD, Brasch RC, Moss AA, et al: Recurrent neuroblastoma: The role of CT and alternative imaging tests. *Radiology* 148:107, 1983.

37. Stark DD, Moss AA, Braasch RC, et al: Neuroblastoma: Diagnostic imaging and staging. *Radiology* 148:101, 1983.

38. Welch TJ, Sheedy PF, VanHeerden JA, et al: Pheochromocytoma: Value of computed tomography. *Radiology* 148:501-503, 1983.

39. White EA, et al: Use of computed tomography in diagnosing the cause of primary aldosteronism. *N Engl J Med* 303:1503-1506, 1980.

40. White EM, Edelman RR, Stark DD, et al: Surface coil MR imaging of abdominal viscera. Part II. The adrenal glands. *Radiology* 157:431-436, 1985.

41. Wilms GE, Baert AL, Kint EJ, et al: Computerized tomographic findings in bilateral adrenal tuberculosis. *Radiology* 146:729-730, 1983.

42. Wilson DA, Muchmore HG, Tisdal RG, et al: Histoplasmosis of the adrenal glands studied by CT. *Radiology* 150:779-783, 1984.

43. Wolverson MK, Kannegiesser H: CT of bilateral adrenal hemorrhage with acute adrenal insufficiency in the adult. *AJR* 142:311-314, 1984.

35

The Kidney

ERROL LEVINE

Computed tomography (CT) is a rapid, easily performed, and safe diagnostic imaging technique that provides valuable information about a wide spectrum of renal disorders. CT is highly accurate for determining the nature and extent of renal masses and plays a valuable role in assessing patients with renal cystic disease, renal trauma, renal infections, renal blood flow disturbances, and hydronephrosis of unknown cause. The recent introduction of helical (spiral) CT shows promise of providing even more rapid assessment of the kidneys and a higher accuracy in the evaluation of renal masses and of the renal blood vessels than is currently provided by conventional CT. The technology of magnetic resonance imaging (MRI) has also advanced rapidly, and MRI is now almost equivalent to CT in detecting and characterizing renal masses. However, since CT is less expensive, quicker, and more generally available, renal MRI is mainly used for evaluating patients in whom CT findings are equivocal or in whom contrast-enhanced CT is contraindicated because of previous reactions to intravenous iodinated contrast medium or the presence of renal failure. This chapter will address and analyze the important roles of CT and MRI in uroradiologic diagnosis.

NORMAL CT ANATOMY

The kidneys are surrounded by perinephric fat, which, in turn, is enveloped by a dense connective tissue sheath called the renal fascia (Fig. 35-1). The anterior renal fascia (Gerota fascia) covers the kidney anteriorly, while the posterior renal fascia (Zuckerkandl fascia) covers the kidney posteriorly (Fig. 35-1). The renal fascial layers divide the general retroperitoneal space into three compartments extending from the diaphragm to the pelvic brim, namely, the anterior pararenal, perinephric, and posterior pararenal spaces (Fig. 35-1).[124] Because it differentiates between fat and fascial tissue, CT usually shows the renal fascia and major extraperitoneal compartments (Fig. 35-2).

Perinephric space

The perinephric space contains the kidney, adrenal gland, inferior vena cava, the lower aorta, renal pelvis, proximal ureter, renal blood vessels, renal capsular vessels, and perinephric fat (Fig. 35-1).[124] It is bound by the anterior and posterior renal fascial layers and is demarcated by their sites of fusion. Above the adrenal glands, the two fascial layers fuse and adhere firmly to the diaphragmatic fascia, while laterally they fuse behind the ascending or descending colon to form the lateroconal fascia (Fig. 35-1). Medially, the anterior renal fascia blends into the connective tissue near the midline (Fig. 35-1).[50,124] Medially, the posterior renal fascia fuses with the psoas or quadratus lumborum fascia. The renal fascial cone extends inferior to the kidney, forming a caudal extension of the main perinephric space containing the proximal ureter and gonadal vessels (Fig. 35-1).[124]

The perinephric space is divided into multiple compartments by fibrous lamellae, the bridging septa (Fig. 35-3).[93] Some arise from the renal capsule and extend to the anterior and posterior renal fascia. Others are attached only to the renal capsule and are arranged nearly parallel to the renal surface (Fig. 35-3). One of the more constant of these is the posterior renorenal bridging septum. It arises from the renal capsule at its posteromedial aspect and runs nearly parallel to the posterior surface of the kidney, inserting into the posterolateral aspect of the renal capsule. Still other bridging septa directly connect the anterior and posterior leaves of the renal fascia.[93] The bridging septa determine the distribution of blood, pus, or urine collections in the perinephric space.[93]

Kidneys

On CT, the transverse contour of the kidney is smooth and oval, with an anteromedial break in the renal outline at the hilus where the vascular pedicle enters (Fig. 35-4). The renal sinus is a potential space contained by the renal parenchyma. The space is filled with fatty tissue and contains the renal arteries, veins, lymphatics,

1176

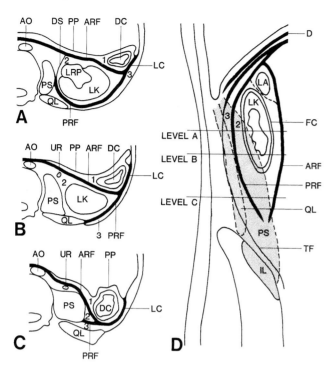

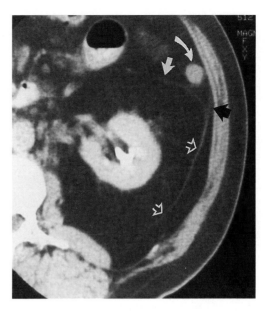

Fig. 35-1. Transverse **(A to C)** and parasagittal **(D)** sections of the left flank. Sections **A to C** show the cross-sectional anatomy at the three levels indicated in **D**—the level of the renal hilus **(A),** lower renal pole **(B),** and above the iliac crest **(C).** In **D,** the approximate positions of the psoas and quadratus lumborum muscles (stippled areas) are indicated by dashed lines. *AO* = aorta; *PS* = psoas muscle; *QL* = quadratus lumborum muscle; *LK* = left kidney; *LRP* = left renal pelvis; *UR* = ureter; *PP* = parietal peritoneum; *ARF* = anterior renal fascia; *PRF* = posterior renal fascia; *LC* = lateroconal fascia; *DS* = deeper stratum of renal fascia; *DC* = descending colon; *1* = anterior pararenal space; *2* = perinephric space; *3* = posterior pararenal space; *D* = diaphragm; *LA* = left adrenal; *FC* = fibrous capsule of kidney; *TF* = transversalis fascia; *IL* = iliacus muscle. (From Feldberg MAM, Koehler PR, van Waes PFGM: *Radiology* 148:505, 1983.)

Fig. 35-2. Normal CT anatomy. The posterior renal fascia *(open arrows)* separates the perinephric and posterior pararenal spaces. The anterior renal fascia *(straight white arrow)* separates the perinephric and anterior pararenal spaces. The lateroconal fascia *(black arrow)* extends lateral to the descending colon *(curved arrow).*

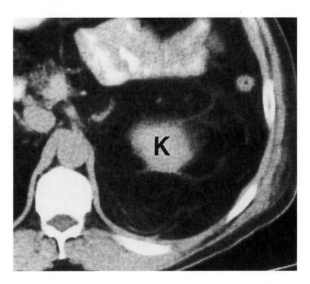

Fig. 35-3. Bridging septa in perinephric space. Multiple delicate fibrous bridging septa traverse the upper part of the left perinephric space. *K* = kidney.

and pelvicalyces. The renal sinus fat is directly continuous with the perinephric fat through the renal hilus. On unenhanced CT scans, the normal renal parenchyma has an attenuation value of 30 to 50 HU, depending on patient hydration, and the cortex and medulla show no visible density differences. After a rapid, intravenous injection of contrast medium, dynamic CT scanning often shows a cortical nephrogram in which there is clear demarcation of the renal cortex and columns of Bertin from the renal medulla (Fig. 35-5). However, the cortical nephrogram phase is transient and a homogeneous tubular nephrogram rapidly develops (Fig. 35-5).[17]

The renal veins are usually densely opacified during dynamic CT scanning and are shown anterior to the renal pelvis as tubular structures joining the inferior vena cava. However, during dynamic scanning the inferior vena cava often shows significantly less contrast enhancement than the renal veins; this is due to mixing of opacified renal vein blood and unopacified blood from the

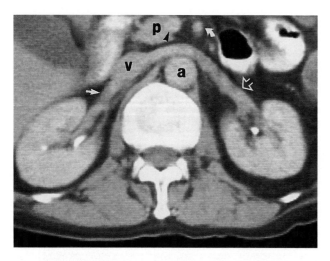

Fig. 35-4. Normal CT renal anatomy. The longer left renal vein *(open arrow)* passes between the aorta *(a)* posteriorly and the superior mesenteric artery *(curved arrow)* and vein *(arrowhead)* anteriorly. It joins the inferior vena cava *(v)* at the level of the uncinate process of the pancreas *(p).* The right renal vein *(arrow)* is shorter.

A

B

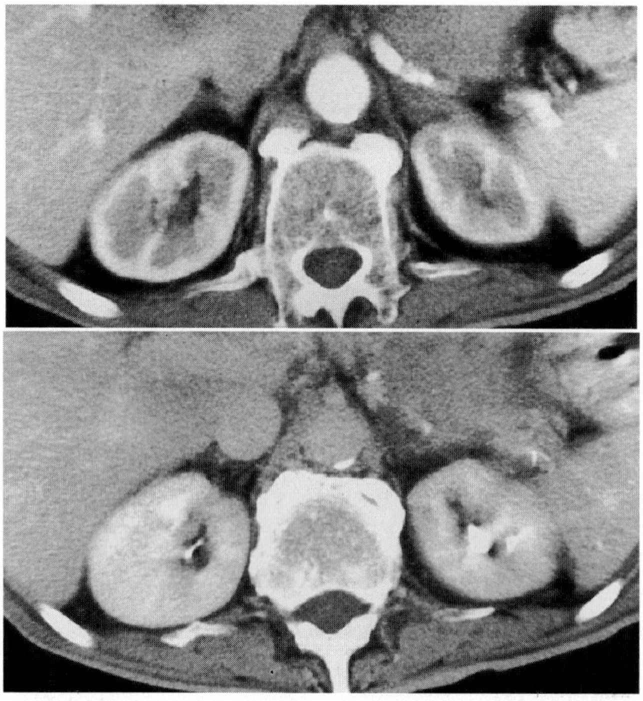

Fig. 35-5. Normal CT nephrogram. **A,** The cortical nephrogram is characterized by symmetrical corticomedullary differentiation on dynamic sequential CT after a rapid intravenous bolus injection of contrast medium. The columns of Bertin appear as high-density structures. **B,** After a brief delay the tubular nephrogram is manifested by a homogeneously dense appearance of the renal parenchyma. The calyces are now opacified.

lower extremities (Fig. 35-6). This appearance should not be mistaken for vena caval thrombosis or tumor extension. The longer left renal vein crosses the retroperitoneum between the aorta posteriorly and the superior mesenteric vessels anteriorly, and joins the inferior vena cava at the level of the uncinate process of the pancreas. The right renal vein usually has a shorter, more oblique course (Figs. 35-4, 35-6). The renal arteries are located posterior to the renal veins and are usually smaller. Normal renal arteries are usually not well shown on dynamic CT scanning but can be shown by helical (spiral) CT performed during breath-holding using narrow scan collimation.[152]

Developmental renal anomalies and minor anatomic variants are commonly encountered and are usually readily evaluated by excretory urography. However, CT is sometimes necessary for further evaluation when urographic findings are confusing (Figs. 35-7, 35-8). Renal sinus lipomatosis may masquerade as a mass lesion in the renal sinus on excretory urography. CT reveals the benign nature of the process by showing that the renal sinus is occupied by tissue with a fat-attenuation value. Normal variants, such as a dromedary hump in the left kidney and prominent columns of Bertin, may simulate renal masses on excretory urography. These are easily recognized by CT since they enhance to the same degree as normal renal parenchyma after intravenous administration of contrast medium.

CT TECHNIQUE

CT may be used as the primary method of kidney evaluation or patients may be referred for CT after a renal abnormality is discovered by excretory urography or sonography. The technique should be tailored accord-

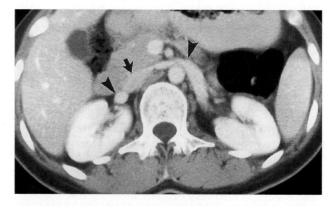

Fig. 35-6. Normal renal veins. On dynamic sequential bolus-enhanced CT the renal veins *(arrowheads)* are densely opacified. The inferior vena cava *(arrow)* appears less dense because of mixing of opacified renal vein blood and unopacified blood from the lower extremities. This appearance should not be confused with vena caval thrombus.

ing to the specific clinical problem involved. However, there are some aspects common to all dedicated renal CT studies. Since unopacified bowel loops may simulate perinephric masses and retroperitoneal adenopathy, patients undergoing renal CT should receive oral contrast medium. Flavored dilute barium sulfate suspensions specially manufactured for CT are most suitable for this purpose. About 450 ml are administered about 30 minutes before the CT scan, and a further 225-ml dose is given 5 to 10 minutes before scanning begins.

In dedicated renal CT, unenhanced scans should always be performed. In general, contiguous 10-mm-thick CT sections are obtained unless there is a known small renal lesion, when 5-mm-thick scans should be performed. Scans are usually acquired during suspended respiration. Unenhanced scans permit contrast enhancement of a renal lesion to be measured and also ensure that renal parenchymal calcifications, renal calculi, renal and perinephric hemorrhage and fat and calcification in a renal mass will not be obscured by contrast medium.[22] Unenhanced scans are also useful for evaluating the liver for metastases in patients with renal cell carcinoma.

Administration of intravenous contrast medium is a fundamental requirement for CT evaluation of most renal lesions. Enhancement of a mass indicates that the lesion is vascular and is therefore possibly a neoplasm. Contrast medium should be administered rapidly with a mechanical injector via an antecubital vein as a 150-ml bolus containing 40 to 45 g of iodine at a rate of 1.5 to 2 mL per second. The scanning protocol depends on the nature of the clinical problem. If the patient has a suspected renal cell carcinoma, evaluation of the renal veins and of the liver for metastases is important.[186] Using a conventional CT scanner, dynamic sequential scanning is begun about 50 seconds after the start of contrast administration. Renal scans obtained in this way usually show good opacification of the renal veins (Fig. 35-6) and a cortical nephrogram (Fig. 35-5). However, because of the relative lack of medullary enhancement, small masses can be overlooked. Because of this concern the kidneys are rapidly examined by conventional axial scanning after completion of the dynamic scan. The nephrogram is then usually homogeneous (Fig. 35-5). If the purpose of the CT study is to evaluate the nature of a benign renal disease, the dynamic phase of the study may be omitted and conventional axial CT scanning of the kidneys can be started about 50 seconds after the beginning of rapid intravenous contrast administration.

A somewhat different protocol is required for helical (spiral) CT scanning of the kidneys.[187] Unenhanced scans are first obtained. About 120 to 150 ml of contrast medium are then injected at a rate of 1.5 to 2 mL per second, and scanning is performed during breath-holding with 5- or 10-mm collimation during a 30-second helical exposure. Helical scanning is begun about

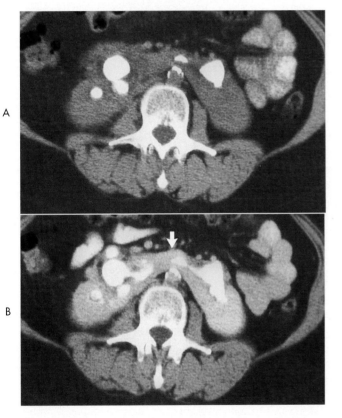

Fig. 35-7. Horseshoe kidney. **A,** Unenhanced scan shows staghorn calculi involving both elements of a horseshoe kidney. **B,** Contrast-enhanced CT scan shows malrotation of both kidneys with the renal pelves directed anteriorly. The kidneys are joined by an isthmus *(arrow)* of functioning renal parenchyma.

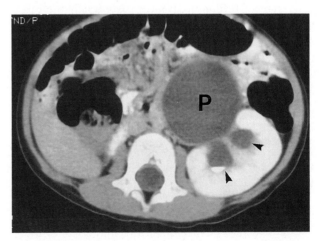

Fig. 35-8. Agenesis of the right kidney and congenital left ureteropelvic junction obstruction in an infant. The left renal pelvis *(P)* is markedly dilated, and there is also calyceal dilatation *(arrowheads)*.

70 seconds after the start of contrast administration.[187] This technique results in a cortical nephrogram and good opacification of the renal vessels. The kidneys are then rapidly rescanned using conventional axial CT scanning. This provides renal images that show a homogeneous nephrogram.[187] Helical CT can show renal lesions smaller than 1 cm because of lack of registration artifacts and the ability to reconstruct overlapping sections from the volumetric CT data acquisition.[187]

When CT diagnoses are based on the presence or absence of contrast enhancement in a renal lesion, it is important to ensure that accurate attenuation values have been obtained. Attenuation value measurements are necessary in all regions of the lesion. Unless a mass occupies the entire thickness of the CT section, partial volume averaging with the normal adjacent renal parenchyma increases the displayed attenuation value of the lesion. Mass size and section thickness should therefore be correlated when contrast enhancement is assessed. Careful attention should also be paid to streak artifacts resulting from such factors as surgical clips and patient obesity, since these can significantly affect attenuation values and therefore give a false indication of enhancement.[24] The same peak kilovoltage, milliampere-second setting, section thickness, and field of view should be used for both precontrast and postcontrast scans when small renal masses are being evaluated.[24] The accuracy of attenuation values should also be tested by measuring the attenuation value of the gallbladder contents before and after intravenous contrast administration. Apparent enhancement of the gallbladder contents suggest that apparent mild enhancement of a renal mass may be spurious.[24]

MRI TECHNIQUES AND ANATOMY

Recent technical advances have greatly increased the accuracy of MRI in evaluating renal lesions.[45,160,161] Dynamic gadolinium-enhanced gradient-echo imaging achieves coverage of the entire kidney during breath holding, thereby reducing respiratory-induced phase artifacts.[160] Gadolinium-enhanced fat-suppressed T1-weighted spin-echo technique images the kidneys with significantly fewer artifacts than does conventional spin-echo imaging.[161] Recent studies using these techniques indicate that MRI is now about equal to CT for detecting and characterizing even small renal masses.[160,161] However, despite these advances the role of MRI in evaluating renal masses remains uncertain.[43] Contrast-enhanced CT is highly accurate in detecting and characterizing renal masses, including those in the 1.5- to 3-cm size range.[24] Accordingly, since CT is generally available, quicker, and less expensive than MRI, it is usually preferred to MRI for evaluating patients with suspected renal masses.

However, MRI is valuable in determining the ce-

phalic extent of intracaval tumor in patients with renal cell carcinoma, when this is not adequately documented by CT.[68,84,150] MRI may also assume a primary role in evaluating renal lesions in patients in whom contrast-enhanced CT is contraindicated because of previous major reactions to contrast medium or preexisting renal failure.[149] Other uses for renal MRI include differentiation between hemorrhagic renal cysts and renal neoplasms,[104] and characterization of small renal masses that are indeterminate on CT or sonography.[24] MR angiography has considerable potential for evaluating diseases of the renal arteries.[53]

The MR pulse sequences and the precise imaging parameters used depend on the nature of the available MRI equipment and on the clinical problem. Conventional spin-echo sequences may be used for evaluating

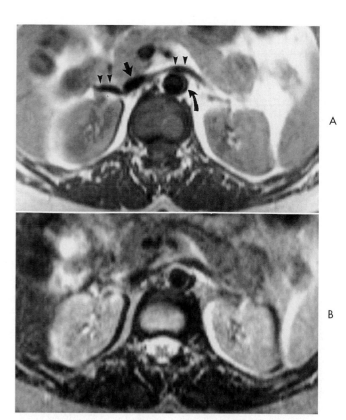

A

B

Fig. 35-9. Normal kidneys shown by MRI (1.5-T field strength). **A,** Axial T1-weighted (500/15) spin-echo image. The renal medulla has a lower intensity than does the renal cortex. The perinephric fat emits a strong signal. The renal veins *(arrowheads)*, inferior vena cava *(arrow)*, and aorta *(curved arrow)* are free of intraluminal signal. **B,** T2-weighted (2200/90) spin-echo image shows increased signal intensity throughout the renal parenchyma, with loss of corticomedullary differentiation. A band of high signal intensity along the medial aspect of the left kidney and a band of low signal intensity along the medial aspect of the right kidney are due to chemical-shift artifact.

the kidneys. Usually both T1- and T2-weighted images are acquired in the axial plane, although both the coronal and sagittal planes are sometimes helpful. T1-weighted images usually show good corticomedullary differentiation (Fig. 35-9).[82] On T2-weighted images the renal cortex and medulla increase in signal and become isointense (Fig. 35-9). The renal arteries, renal veins, aorta, and inferior vena cava are seen as tubular structures that are free of intraluminal signal (Fig. 35-9), although flow-related artifacts may cause high-signal areas in these blood vessels.[82] Fat-suppressed T1-weighted spin-echo images are useful in evaluating the kidneys. Precontrast images show striking corticomedullary differentiation (Fig. 35-10). Images obtained after gadolinium injection show a homogeneous nephrogram. Fat-suppressed images are characterized by high contrast resolution, and minimal phase or chemical shift artifact.[160,161]

Gradient-echo fast low-angle shot [FLASH] images are helpful for evaluating renal masses. The images are acquired during breath-holding in the axial, sagittal or coronal planes.[160,161] Precontrast images of the kidneys are first obtained (Fig. 35-11). Gadopentetate dimeglumine is then injected intravenously by hand in a dose of 0.1 mmol/kg over 5 seconds with the patient positioned in the bore of the magnet. Imaging is started during breath-holding at 20 to 30 seconds after a rapid saline flush of the intravenous catheter has been performed. These images show striking corticomedullary differentiation and also significant enhancement of the renal vein blood (Fig. 35-11). FLASH images obtained after a slight delay show a homogeneous tubular nephrogram.

Unenhanced gradient-echo images of the vena cava and renal veins are helpful in confirming or excluding venous tumor extension in patients with renal cell carcinoma.[150] With this technique, flowing venous blood has a significantly increased signal intensity and appears white, whereas tumor thrombus has a medium signal intensity and appears as an intravenous filling defect (Fig. 35-12).[150] The renal arteries can be evaluated with sequential two-dimensional or three-dimensional time-of-flight MR angiography or with phase-contrast techniques (Fig. 35-13).[41,53,89] Appropriate presaturation slabs are needed to eliminate signal in the renal veins and inferior vena cava.[53]

RENAL CYSTS

Renal cysts usually represent notably dilated nephrons or collecting ducts.[59] A cystic kidney is a kid-

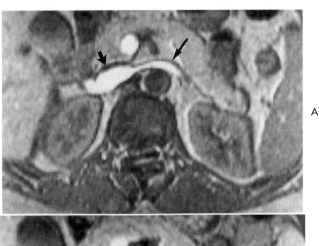

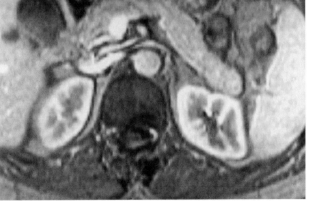

Fig. 35-11. Normal kidneys shown by gradient-echo imaging (1.5-T field strength). **A,** Dynamic gradient-echo (FLASH) image (168/6; flip angle = 75°) performed during suspended respiration. The renal cortex has a higher intensity than the medulla. Blood in the left renal vein (*long arrow*) and inferior vena cava (*short arrow*) has a high signal intensity. **B,** Gradient-echo (FLASH) image repeated after an intravenous bolus injection of gadolinium-DTPA. There is significant corticomedullary differentiation and the columns of Bertin are prominently opacified.

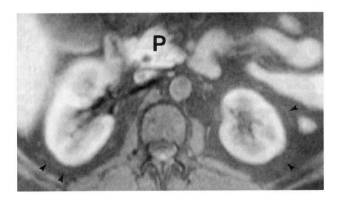

Fig. 35-10. Normal kidneys. T1-weighted (500/15) fat-suppressed spin-echo image (1.5-T field strength) shows a high signal intensity in the renal cortex, whereas the medulla has a medium signal intensity. The signal in the perinephric fat is suppressed and the renal fascia (*arrowheads*) is seen. P = pancreatic head.

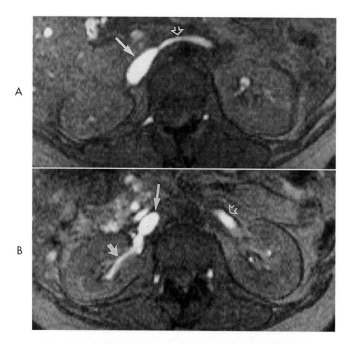

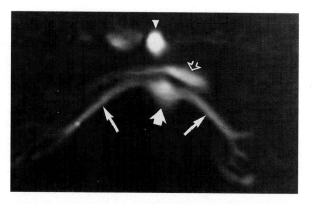

Fig. 35-13. Normal renal arteries *(long arrows)* shown in axial projection by cine phase-contrast MR angiography. The aorta *(short arrow)*, left renal vein *(open arrow)*, and superior mesenteric artery *(arrowhead)* are also shown. (Courtesy of Richard L. Ehman, M.D., Rochester, Minn.)

Fig. 35-12. Normal renal veins. Gradient-echo (29/8; flip angle = 35°) MR images performed during suspended respiration show: **A** and **B,** the left renal vein *(open arrow)*, the inferior vena cava *(long arrow)*, and right renal vein *(short arrow)* appear as structures with high signal intensity. Signal from the viscera is suppressed and aortic signal is eliminated by a presaturation band placed over the liver.

ney with 3 to 5 or more cysts. The term renal cystic disease refers to any disorder that results from the presence of multiple renal cysts.

Simple cysts

Simple cysts are the most common renal masses. Most are clinically insignificant and are discovered incidentally at autopsy or on imaging studies. Their frequency increases with age, with only rare examples reported in children.[136] Although the cause of renal cysts is unknown, their frequent occurrence in older patients suggests that they are acquired lesions.[136] Although most simple cysts are asymptomatic, they occasionally cause pressure symptoms because of their large size, and cyst hemorrhage or infection may cause pain and hematuria. Simple renal cysts may be solitary or multiple and are frequently bilateral. Sonography is usually considered the most appropriate next investigation for further evaluation of a presumed renal cyst discovered by excretory urography. However, renal cysts are currently often found on abdominal CT performed for nonrenal complaints. Such cysts may vary in size from less than 1 cm to 10 to 15 cm (Figs. 35-14, 35-15).

CT features. The accuracy of CT diagnosis of a simple renal cyst approaches 100% if a renal mass strictly fulfills the following well-established criteria: (a) sharp margination and demarcation from surrounding renal parenchyma, (b) a smooth, thin wall, (c) a homogeneous, water-density content with an attenuation value of 0 to 20 HU, and (d) no enhancement after intravenous administration of contrast medium (Fig. 35-14).[22,121] If a renal mass fulfills these CT criteria no further evaluation is necessary.[22,121]

In routine CT, performed for nonrenal complaints, usually only intravenous-contrast enhanced scanning is performed and the presence or absence of contrast enhancement in renal masses, therefore, often cannot be determined.[22] A simple cyst can usually be diagnosed even without this information, however, if the other CT criteria listed above are fulfilled (Fig. 35-15).[22] If CT findings are atypical or if the patient is referred because of symptoms such as hematuria, then nonenhanced scans should also be obtained. This permits contrast enhancement to be measured and also precludes nonenhancing high-density renal cysts from being confused with solid renal masses.[22]

Although CT is accurate in diagnosing simple renal cysts, there are potential pitfalls that should be avoided when interpreting CT findings. Small renal cysts may be volume-averaged with normal renal tissue, causing spuriously high attenuation values,[121] or falsely high attenuation values may be caused by streak artifacts.[24] In these circumstances, sonography should be performed to determine whether the lesion is a cyst or a neoplasm. If sonographic findings are indeterminate, dedicated renal CT should be repeated with special attention to the lesion (see CT technique).[22]

MRI features. The use of gadolinium-enhanced MRI, particularly with gradient-echo imaging techniques

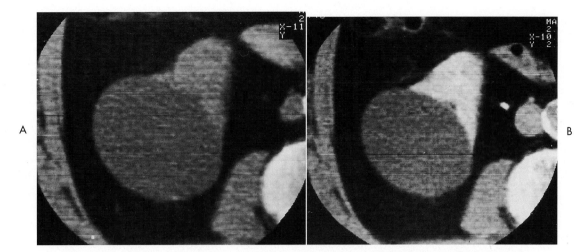

Fig. 35-14. Simple renal cyst. Unenhanced **(A)** and contrast-enhanced *(B)* CT images show that the mass is round, with a smooth margin and distinct margination from adjoining renal parenchyma. It has a homogeneous water density and does not enhance (precontrast and postcontrast attenuation value = 7 HU) and has no discernible wall thickness.

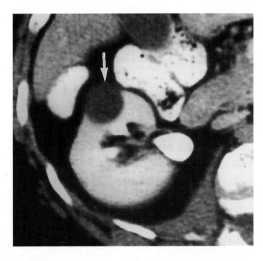

Fig. 35-15. Simple renal cyst. Lesion *(arrow)* has attenuation value of 9 HU and was detected during survey CT scan performed only with intravenous contrast enhancement. Even though an unenhanced scan is unavailable, the diagnosis of a cyst can be made with confidence because of the low-attenuation value, smooth-rounded shape, sharp margination, and demarcation from surrounding renal parenchyma and thin wall where the lesion projects beyond the renal outline.

applied during breath-holding, is helpful in evaluating renal cystic lesions in patients with contraindications to iodinated intravenous contrast medium, such as chronic renal failure or previous contrast reactions.[149,161] Even a small simple renal cyst can be diagnosed on contrast-enhanced MRI if it fulfills the following criteria: *(a)* sharp margination and demarcation from surrounding renal parenchyma, *(b)* a smooth, thin wall, *(c)* homogeneous contents with signal characteristics of water (such lesions have a low signal intensity on T1-weighted spin-echo images and a high signal intensity on T2-weighted spin-echo images), and *(d)* no enhancement after intravenous injection of gadolinium-DTPA (Fig. 35-16).[161]

Atypical cysts and cystic neoplasms

Many renal cystic lesions do not fulfill the criteria for simple cysts outlined above. Such lesions vary from minimally complicated simple cysts that usually do not require surgery to cystic renal neoplasms that generally require resection. Complicated cysts often result from bleeding in a simple cyst. Bosniak has suggested categorizing cystic renal masses using CT and sonographic criteria in an attempt to separate lesions requiring surgery from those that do not.[22] The application of Bosniak's classification is most useful in evaluating and managing cystic renal lesions.[5]

In Bosniak's classification, *Category I* lesions are classic simple cysts as described above (Figs. 14 to 16).[22] They require no further evaluation or management. *Category II* lesions are minimally complicated cysts that also usually do not require surgery. Occasional thin ($\leq$1 mm), smooth septa, or small, smooth plaques of fine linear calcification in the cyst wall or septa, occur in these lesions (Fig. 35-17). Also included in category II are high-density cysts (Fig. 35-18). These lesions have attenuation values ranging from 40 to 100 HU on unenhanced CT scans and usually result from previous hemorrhage.[103] Most high-density renal cysts are benign and

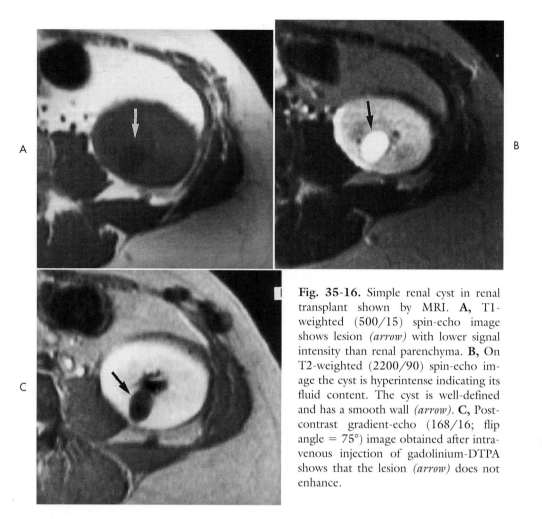

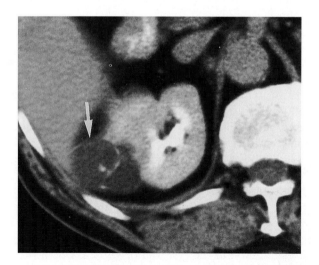

Fig. 35-16. Simple renal cyst in renal transplant shown by MRI. **A,** T1-weighted (500/15) spin-echo image shows lesion *(arrow)* with lower signal intensity than renal parenchyma. **B,** On T2-weighted (2200/90) spin-echo image the cyst is hyperintense indicating its fluid content. The cyst is well-defined and has a smooth wall *(arrow)*. **C,** Post-contrast gradient-echo (168/16; flip angle = 75°) image obtained after intravenous injection of gadolinium-DTPA shows that the lesion *(arrow)* does not enhance.

Fig. 35-17. Minimally calcified benign cyst *(arrow)*; category II lesion. A contrast-enhanced CT scan reveals fine linear calcification in the cyst wall and septa. The lesion shows a thin wall, and no focal nodules or areas of enhancement. The fluid in the cyst measured 12 HU.

can simply be followed by serial imaging provided that the following CT criteria are fulfilled: *(a)* the lesion must be perfectly smooth, round, sharply marginated, and homogeneous; *(b)* the lesion should not enhance with intravenous contrast medium; *(c)* at least one fourth of the lesion's circumference should extend outside the kidney so that the smoothness of some of the wall can be evaluated; and *(d)* the lesion should be less than 3 cm in diameter.[24] Although most lesions showing these findings are benign hemorrhagic cysts,[25] cystic renal cell carcinoma may rarely show similar CT findings.[76]

MRI may also help in characterizing high-density renal cysts that do not fulfill all the above CT criteria or that show internal echoes on sonography. Hemorrhagic cysts appear on MRI as sharply marginated, smooth, round, homogeneous lesions. They have high signal intensities on both T1- and T2-weighted spin-echo images,[104] and they do not enhance after intravenous administration of gadolinium-DTPA. In addition, hemorrhagic cysts often show fluid-iron levels on MRI prob-

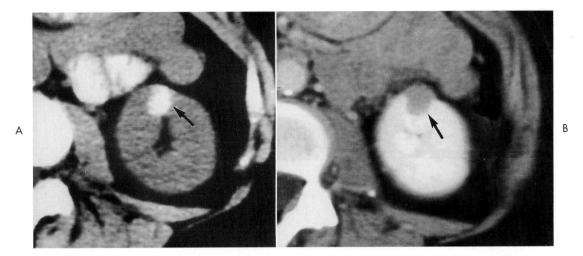

Fig. 35-18. Hyperdense benign renal cyst; category II lesion. Unenhanced CT scan **(A)** shows a high-density mass (92 HU) *(arrow)* located anteriorly in the kidney. On contrast-enhanced CT scan **(B)**, the lesion *(arrow)* did not enhance; it is homogeneous and reveals a smooth margin where it projects beyond the renal outline.

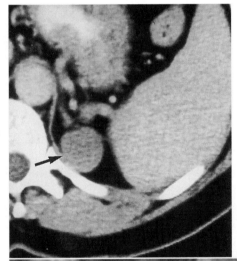

Fig. 35-19. Hemorrhagic cyst in upper pole of left kidney. **A,** A contrast-enhanced CT scan shows a well-defined mass *(arrow)* in the upper pole of the left kidney. The lesion had a precontrast and postcontrast attenuation value of 45 HU. **B,** Gradient-echo (168/16; flip angle = 75°) MR image shows fluid-iron level in cyst with high-intensity methemoglobin sediment located posteriorly *(arrow)* and lower intensity cyst fluid located anteriorly. **C,** T2-weighted (2200/90) spin-echo image reveals that anteriorly located cyst fluid is hyperintense, whereas dependent sediment *(arrow)* has a lower signal intensity.

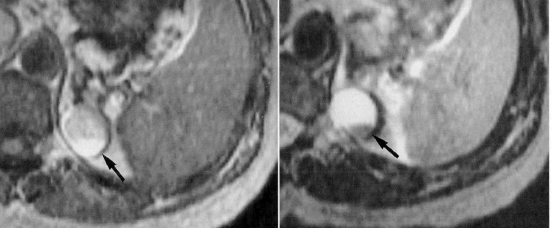

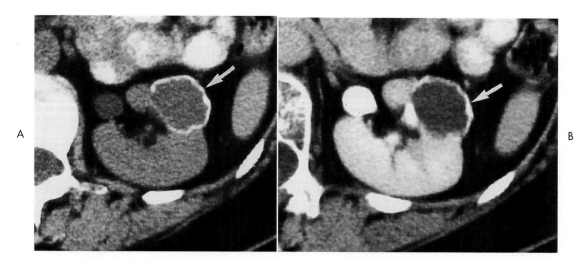

Fig. 35-20. Hemorrhagic benign renal cyst; category III lesion. The lesion *(arrow)* shows thick, irregular mural calcification. The lesion has an attenuation value of 12 HU on an unenhanced CT scan **(A)** and showed no enhancement after contrast administration **(B).** The kidney was explored, and a local resection of the lesion was performed.

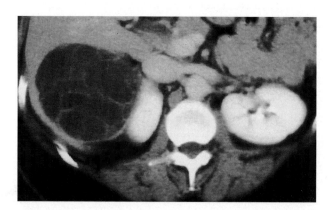

Fig. 35-21. Multilocular cystic renal cell carcinoma; category III lesion. A contrast-enhanced CT scan reveals a well-defined, mainly fluid-containing mass in the right kidney. Enhancing septa are seen throughout the lesion. A right nephrectomy was performed.

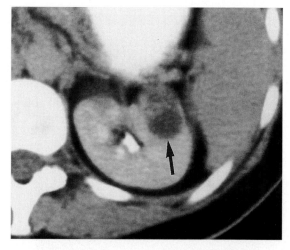

Fig. 35-22. Cystic renal cell carcinoma; category IV lesion. Contrast-enhanced CT scan shows a cystic mass *(arrow)* with irregular and enhancing solid elements located anteriorly.

ably because of dependent settling of methemoglobin-containing sediment (Fig. 35-19).[104] Since methemoglobin is paramagnetic, the T1 relaxation time of the sediment is shortened and it is therefore more intense than cyst fluid on T1-weighted images. On T2-weighted images, the relative intensities of the two cyst layers reverse because of the greater T2 relaxation time of cyst fluid. The accuracy of these MR features in differentiating hemorrhagic cysts from cystic neoplasms is currently unknown.[161]

Category III lesions are more complicated cystic lesions. These lesions exhibit some findings seen in malignant lesions. These findings include thick, irregular mural or septal calcification (Fig. 35-20), numerous or thick (>1 mm), irregular septa (Fig. 35-21), and uniform or slightly nodular wall thickening.[22] Some of these lesions are benign (e.g., multilocular cystic nephromas and hemorrhagic renal cysts); others are cystic renal cell carcinomas (Fig. 35-21). All these cases should be explored surgically, unless contraindicated because of the

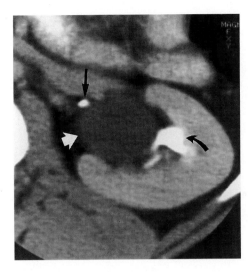

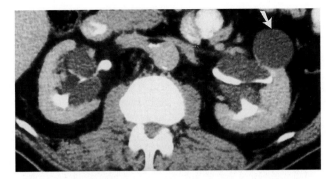

Fig. 35-24. Bilateral renal sinus cysts. The cysts cause displacement and attenuation of the opacified collecting systems. A simple renal cyst is also present anteriorly in the left kidney *(arrow)*.

Fig. 35-23. Renal sinus (parapelvic) cyst. A contrast-enhanced CT scan reveals that the cyst *(white arrow)* is surrounded by a halo of renal sinus fat, indicating its extrarenal origin. The nondilated collecting system *(curved arrow)* and ureter *(long arrow)* are displaced by the cyst.

patient's advanced age or poor general medical condition.[22] *Category IV* lesions are clearly malignant lesions with large cystic components; they should be resected.[22] They may show marginal irregularity or solid vascular elements (Fig. 35-22).

Renal sinus cysts

Renal sinus (parapelvic) cysts are benign extraparenchymal cysts located in the renal sinus.[77] They are not true renal cysts, but are probably lymphatic in origin.[77] They may be unilocular or multilocular and are often bilateral (Figs. 35-23, 35-24).[77] They do not communicate with the renal collecting system. Most renal sinus cysts are asymptomatic and are discovered incidentally by imaging studies.[77] They may in rare cases cause hypertension, hematuria or hydronephrosis, or they may become secondarily infected.

Renal sinus cysts display the same CT features as simple renal parenchymal cysts.[77] They have attenuation values in the water range (0 to 20 HU) and are difficult to distinguish from dilated or extrarenal pelves on unenhanced CT scans. After intravenous contrast administration, the cysts remain of water density and cause displacement of the renal pelvis and calyces (Fig. 35-24). Differentiation from hydronephrosis is thus readily made by contrast-enhanced CT.[77] On CT, the characteristic feature of a renal sinus cyst is a surrounding halo of renal sinus fat, indicating its extrarenal origin (Fig. 35-23).[35] CT easily distinguishes between a renal sinus cyst and renal sinus lipomatosis, which causes a similar deformity of the collecting system on excretory urography.[77] In renal sinus lipomatosis, the attenuation value of the tissue is in the fat range. Solid masses in the renal sinus, such as lymphoma and invasive transitional cell carcinoma, are readily differentiated from renal sinus cysts because they have soft-tissue attenuation values.

RENAL CYSTIC DISEASE

Renal cystic diseases include a wide variety of disorders. Although imaging studies help greatly in evaluating renal cystic diseases, they are seldom diagnostic per se because many types of cystic kidneys show similar imaging findings. Imaging findings should therefore always be interpreted with knowledge of patient age, family history, symptoms, clinical findings, and renal functional status.[105]

Multicystic dysplastic kidney

Multicystic dysplastic kidney (MDK) is the most common form of cystic disease in infants, usually presenting as an asymptomatic flank mass. The disorder is associated with intrauterine ureteral obstruction or atresia.[156] Two types of MDK may be shown by imaging.[170] The classic type (pelvo-infundibular atresia) shows no discernible renal pelvis on imaging.[155] The kidney may be small, normal in size, or enlarged and contains multiple variable-sized noncommunicating renal cysts (Fig. 35-25).[135,155] There is no perfusion of the affected kidney on renal scintigraphy, and contrast-enhanced CT shows no evidence of contrast excretion by the affected kidney.[170]

The hydronephrotic form of MDK is characterized by dilatation of the renal pelvis and calyces. Differentiation of this type of MDK from simple hydronephrosis is based on the imaging demonstration of parenchymal cysts that do not communicate with the collecting

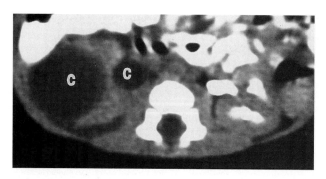

Fig. 35-25. Multicystic dysplastic kidney in a neonate. The right kidney was replaced by cysts *(c)*, one of which was larger than the others. The right kidney did not excrete contrast medium. The left kidney is normal.

system.[135,155] Significant contralateral hydronephrosis occurs in about 10% of cases of MDK.[175] Most patients with MDK are currently managed nonsurgically and are followed by serial sonography.[175] The affected kidney may remain unchanged, but it frequently undergoes spontaneous regression.[135,175] MDK may occasionally first be detected in adults when imaging studies show a small kidney with calcified cysts (Fig. 35-26).

Polycystic kidney disease

Hereditary polycystic kidney disease may be transmitted as an autosomal recessive or autosomal dominant trait.

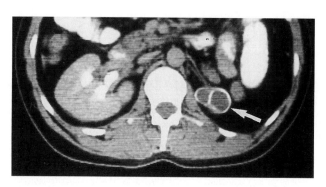

Fig. 35-26. Multicystic dysplasia of left kidney in a 27-year-old man with microscopic hematuria. The left kidney is small and composed of cysts with mural calcification *(arrow)*. There is compensatory hypertrophy of the right kidney.

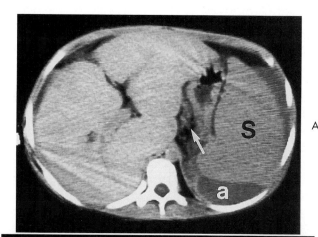

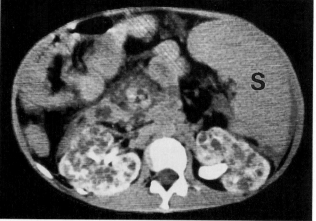

Fig. 35-28. Autosomal recessive polycystic kidney disease in a 14-year-old female with normal renal function. **A,** The liver contour is irregular as a result of congenital hepatic fibrosis. The spleen *(S)* is enlarged because of portal hypertension. Ascites *(a)* is present, and there is an enlarged left gastric vein *(arrow)* in the hepatogastric ligament. **B,** A more caudal scan shows mild nephromegaly and multiple medullary cysts with relative preservation of the renal cortex. (From Levine E: *CRC Crit Rev Diagn Imaging* 24:91, 1985.)

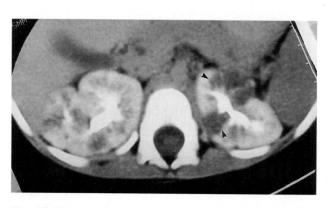

Fig. 35-27. Autosomal recessive polycystic kidney disease in a 30-month-old infant with normal renal function. A contrast-enhanced CT scan shows dilated collecting ducts in the renal medulla bilaterally and relative preservation of the renal cortex. Occasional macroscopic cysts *(arrowheads)* are present in the left kidney.

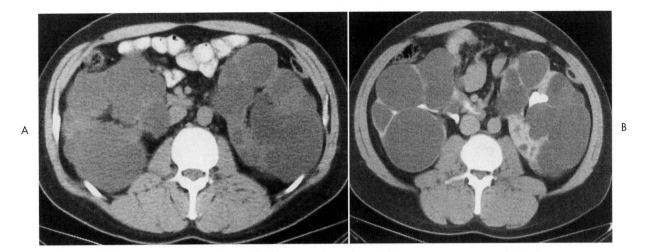

Fig. 35-29. Autosomal dominant polycystic kidney disease in a 39-year-old man with hypertension and mildly impaired renal function. Unenhanced CT scan (**A**) shows bilateral nephromegaly. Contrast-enhanced CT scan (**B**) reveals large renal cysts with enhancing residual parenchyma between the cysts.

Autosomal recessive polycystic disease. Autosomal recessive polycystic kidney disease (ARPKD) is characterized by ectasia of the renal collecting tubules and ducts, and variable degrees of portal hepatic fibrosis (congenital hepatic fibrosis) often causing portal hypertension.[29] A severe form of the disease is seen in the neonatal period and is associated with a high mortality due to pulmonary and renal insufficiency. This is best evaluated by sonography.[21] Patients with milder renal involvement may present at any age from infancy to early adulthood. The severity of renal and liver involvement in these patients is inversely related. If renal function is normal, contrast-enhanced CT may be performed and shows collecting duct ectasia confined mainly to the renal medulla with only occasional macrocysts. The renal cortex is less severely affected (Fig. 35-27).[122] CT may also show evidence of congenital hepatic fibrosis and portal hypertension. The liver contour is often irregular, and dilated intrahepatic bile ducts, ascites, splenomegaly, and enlarged portal-systemic collateral veins may be seen (Fig. 35-28). Liver cysts are not usually evident. However, some patients show large liver cysts of biliary origin due to the presence of Caroli's disease.[39]

Autosomal dominant polycystic disease. Autosomal dominant polycystic kidney disease (ADPKD) is the most common genetic disease.[58] Most cases are due to an abnormal gene located on the short arm of chromosome 16.[58] Although multiple bilateral cysts that involve both the renal cortex and medulla are the most important manifestation, ADPKD is really a systemic disease and may be associated with intracranial aneurysms, cardiac valvular abnormalities, liver cysts, and colonic diverticula.[58] Although the disorder usually presents in

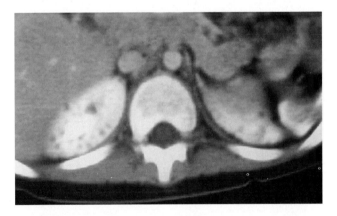

Fig. 35-30. Autosomal dominant polycystic kidney disease in an asymptomatic 14-year-old boy whose father has the disease. A contrast-enhanced CT scan shows multiple, tiny bilateral renal cysts.

adults (Fig. 35-29), it may be diagnosed during infancy and childhood.[58] Patients with fully developed ADPKD often show dramatic CT findings (Fig. 35-29). CT is slightly more sensitive than sonography for detecting small renal cysts in asymptomatic progeny of patients with ADPKD (Fig. 35-30).[58]

Flank pain and macroscopic hematuria are the most common symptoms of ADPKD and may be due to cyst hemorrhage, calculi, or renal infection.[103] Cyst hemorrhage is a common cause of pain in ADPKD and can be detected by CT in about 69% of patients.[103] Hemorrhagic cysts have attenuation values of 40 to 100 HU on unenhanced scans, do not enhance after intravenous contrast administration and are homogeneously hyper-

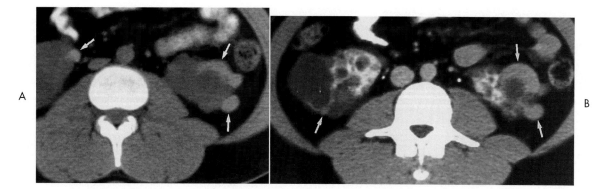

Fig. 35-31. Hemorrhagic renal cysts in autosomal dominant polycystic kidney disease. **A,** Unenhanced CT scan shows bilateral subcapsular high-density cysts *(arrows).* **B,** After IV contrast enhancement, the high-density cysts *(arrows)* are hypodense relative to enhanced residual renal parenchyma. Many fluid-density cysts are present. The high-density cysts had an average attenuation value of 70 HU on both precontrast and postcontrast scans.

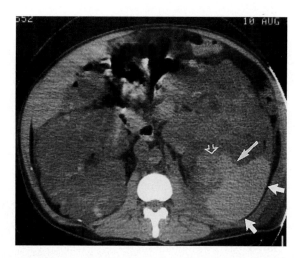

Fig. 35-32. Autosomal dominant polycystic kidney disease with perinephric hemorrhage. Unenhanced CT scan reveals bilateral nephromegaly and multiple cysts. A posterior perinephric hematoma *(short arrows)* causes anterior displacement of the left kidney. A ruptured hemorrhagic cyst *(open arrow)* communicates *(long arrow)* with the hematoma. (From Levine E, Grantham JJ: *J Comput Assist Tomogr* 11:108, 1987.)

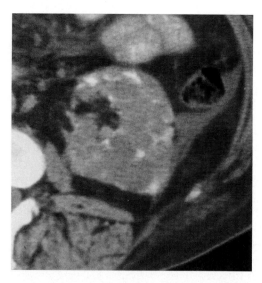

Fig. 35-33. Autosomal dominant polycystic kidney disease with multiple curvilinear calcifications in cyst walls.

dense and well defined (Fig. 35-31). They may rupture into the perinephric space, causing large hematomas (Fig. 35-32).[104] Hemorrhagic cysts often develop mural calcification (Fig. 35-33).

Renal calculi occur in 20% to 36% of patients with ADPKD, and they commonly cause flank pain.[106,174] About 57% of calculi in ADPKD are composed predominantly of uric acid and are therefore radiolucent on conventional tomography.[174] Such calculi are best evaluated

by CT (Fig. 35-34).[106] Acute pyelonephritis occurs commonly in patients with ADPKD and may cause cyst infection. Cyst infection is difficult to diagnose on CT; it is suggested by a cyst larger than surrounding cysts with thickening and irregularity of its wall, increase in attenuation value of its contents, and localized thickening of the adjacent renal fascia (Fig. 35-35).[105] Radionuclide scanning using gallium-32 citrate or indium-111–labeled white blood cells may help confirm the diagnosis of cyst infection by showing increased tracer activity at the cyst periphery.[105,157]

The presence of liver cysts strongly suggests the diagnosis of ADPKD. They are found by CT in as many

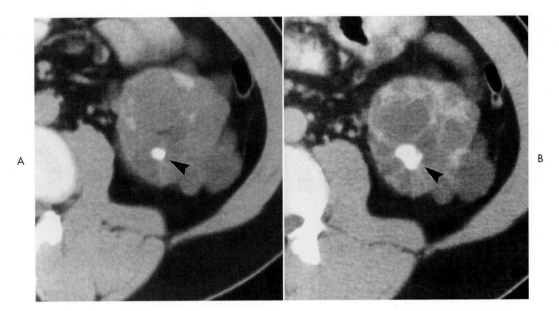

Fig. 35-34. Autosomal dominant polycystic kidney disease with a calculus in the lower pole of the left kidney. **A,** An unenhanced CT scan shows a small, rounded calcification *(arrowhead)*. **B,** A contrast-enhanced CT scan reveals that the calcification is located in an opacified calyx *(arrowhead)*. (From Levine E, Grantham JJ: *AJR* 159:77, 1992.)

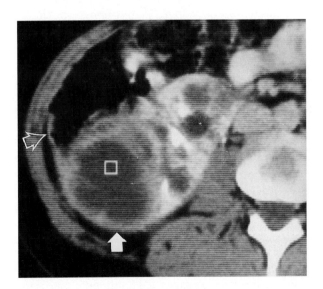

Fig. 35-35. Acute pyelonephritis complicated by cyst infection in autosomal dominant polycystic kidney disease. A lower pole cyst *(solid arrow)* is larger than adjacent cysts and shows an irregular, thickened wall and adjacent renal fascial thickening *(open arrow)*. The patient responded to antibiotic therapy and a follow-up sonogram showed absence of the large cyst, suggesting rupture into the collecting system. (From Levine E, Grantham JJ: *AJR* 159:77, 1992.)

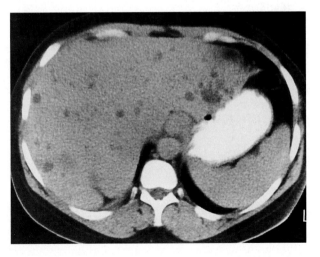

Fig. 35-36. Multiple small liver cysts in autosomal dominant polycystic kidney disease.

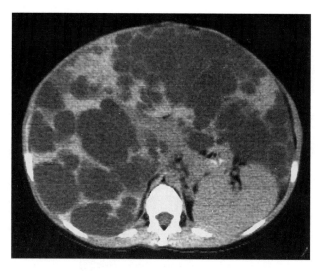

Fig. 35-37. Significant hepatomegaly caused by liver cysts in a 45-year-old woman with autosomal dominant polycystic kidney disease. (From Levine E, Cook LT, Grantham JJ: *AJR* 145:229, 1985.)

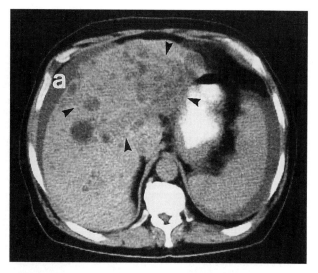

Fig. 35-38. Autosomal dominant polycystic kidney disease complicated by cholangiocarcinoma in a 69-year-old man complaining of abdominal pain and weight loss. Liver function tests were notably abnormal. CT shows several cysts in the right lobe of the liver. A poorly defined, low-density mass *(arrowheads)* involves the left lobe and part of the anterior segment of the right lobe. Ascites *(a)* is present. The neoplasm was not resectable, and the patient died from metastatic disease. (From Levine E, Cook LT, Grantham JJ: *AJR* 145:229, 1985.)

as 57% of patients, varying from occasional small cysts (Fig. 35-36) to multiple, large cysts that cause hepatomegaly (Fig. 35-37).[102] Liver cysts are usually asymptomatic and are associated with normal liver function tests even when extensive. Abnormal liver function tests suggest the development of such complications as common hepatic duct compression by cysts, cyst infection, and cholangiocarcinoma arising from the cyst lining (Fig. 35-38).[102,173]

Unilateral (localized) renal cystic disease

In unilateral renal cystic disease (URCD), also known as localized renal cystic disease, most of one kidney is replaced by multiple cysts and the contralateral kidney is normal. There is usually no family history of renal cysts, and the condition is not related to autosomal dominant polycystic kidney disease.[109] Liver cysts and renal failure do not occur. Affected patients range in age from childhood to the sixth decade and may have hypertension, flank pain, or hematuria.[109] On CT, the cysts are separated by enhancing bands of normal renal parenchyma so that no distinct encapsulated renal mass is found (Fig. 35-39). The affected kidney may be enlarged and shows normal contrast excretion. Although the cysts may predominate in one part of the affected kidney, careful assessment of the CT scan usually shows multiple smaller cysts elsewhere in the renal parenchyma.[109]

Although the absence of cysts in the contralateral kidney on CT in adults usually excludes the diagnosis of ADPKD, caution is necessary before making a definitive diagnosis of URCD in children. In ADPKD, renal cysts

develop slowly during childhood and may become apparent earlier in one kidney.[140] Accordingly, in children follow-up CT should be performed after an appropriate interval before a final diagnosis of URCD is made.

Uremic acquired renal cystic disease

Uremic acquired renal cystic disease (ARCD) is characterized by the development of multiple renal cysts in patients with chronic renal failure due to a variety of noncystic primary renal disorders. Cyst formation begins in renal failure before dialysis is started and progresses during dialysis.[105] About 40% of all dialysis patients show the disorder, although ARCD develops eventually in almost all patients treated with dialysis for 10 years or more.[115] The condition is usually asymptomatic but may be associated with serious complications such as retroperitoneal hemorrhage and renal neoplasms.[115]

The radiologic diagnosis of ARCD is best established by contrast-enhanced CT, although sonography and MRI are useful for evaluating patients with end-stage renal disease not treated with dialysis.[100,114] The diagnosis is confined to those patients with bilateral renal involvement and five or more cysts per kidney. The affected kidneys are usually small (Fig. 35-40). However, ARCD is a progressive disorder, and nephromegaly may eventually develop (Fig. 35-40).[115] On MRI, renal cysts in

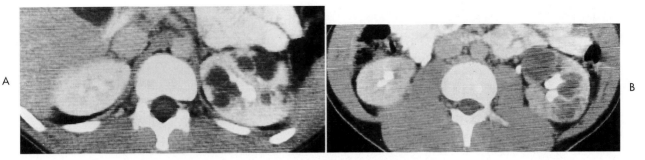

Fig. 35-39. Unilateral renal cystic disease in a 15-year-old male with intermittent gross hematuria starting at 5 years of age. Contrast-enhanced CT scans **(A** and **B)** show partial replacement of the left kidney by many cysts that are separated by enhancing bands of normal parenchyma. The right kidney is free of cysts, and a follow-up CT scan 7 years later showed no change.

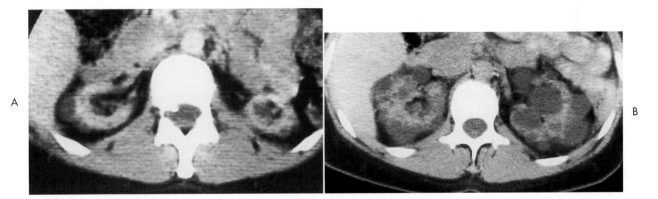

Fig. 35-40. Acquired renal cystic disease in a 45-year-old man on long-term hemodialysis. **A,** CT scan after 4 years of dialysis shows bilateral small cysts in shrunken kidneys. **B,** A follow-up CT scan 4 years later shows enlargement of cysts and kidneys.

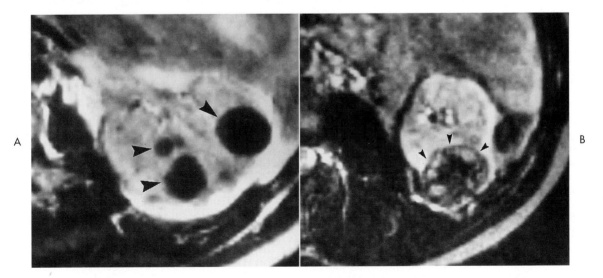

Fig. 35-41. Acquired renal cystic disease and left renal cell carcinoma in 34-year-old man with azotemia not treated with dialysis. **A,** T1-weighted (500/17) spin-echo MR image after gadolinium-DTPA administration shows several well-defined cysts *(arrowheads)* of low signal intensity in the left kidney. **B,** T2-weighted (2100/90) image without gadolinium administration reveals a heterogeneous, 3.5-cm lower-pole carcinoma *(arrowheads)*.

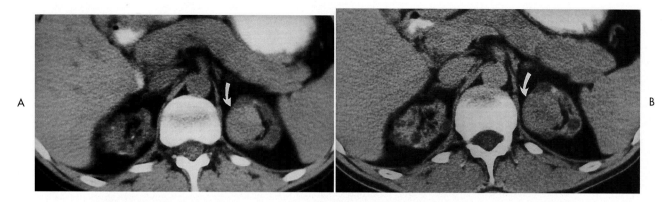

Fig. 35-42. Acquired renal cystic disease with cyst hemorrhage in a 41-year-old man with gross hematuria. **A,** An unenhanced CT scan shows a 3.8-cm high-density (44 HU) mass *(arrow)* in the upper pole of the left kidney. **B,** After contrast enhancement, the attenuation value of the mass *(arrow)* was 43 HU. Multiple bilateral fluid-density cysts are also present. The mass resolved completely on a follow-up CT scan 3 months later, suggesting a hemorrhagic cyst that had ruptured into the collecting system. (From Levine E, Slusher SL, Grantham JJ, et al: *AJR* 156:501, 1991.)

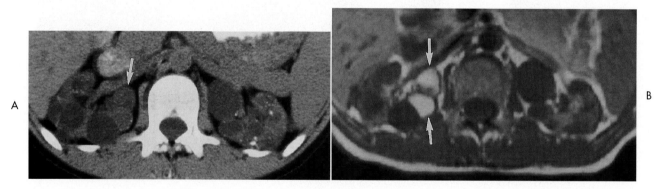

Fig. 35-43. Hemorrhagic cysts in acquired renal cystic disease. **A,** Unenhanced CT scan shows multiple bilateral fluid-density cysts with cyst wall calcifications. An area *(arrow)* located medially in the right kidney was considered suspicious for a neoplasm. **B,** T1-weighted (500/15) spin-echo MR image shows that most cysts have low signal intensity. However, two lesions *(arrows)* located medially in the right kidney have a high signal intensity, which persisted on T2-weighted images (not shown) consistent with cyst hemorrhage.

ARCD are best shown on gadolinium-enhanced images (Fig. 35-41).

Hemorrhagic cysts occur in about 50% of patients with ARCD and sometimes attain a large size.[115] On CT, hemorrhagic cysts present as well-defined masses with attenuation values ranging from 40 to 100 HU on unenhanced CT scans (Fig. 35-42). Differentiation of these lesions from renal neoplasms on CT is suggested by lack of contrast enhancement and a homogeneous appearance on contrast-enhanced CT scans (Fig. 35-42).[115] Sonography may help in establishing the cystic nature of hemorrhagic cysts by showing anechoicity, posterior acoustic enhancement, and a smooth wall. On MRI, hemorrhagic cysts often show high signal intensities on both T1- and T2-weighted images and do not enhance after gadolinium administration (Fig. 35-43). Subcapsular and perinephric hematomas occur in as many as 13% of patients with ARCD and are usually due to rupture of hemorrhagic cysts (Fig. 35-44).[107,115]

The incidence of invasive renal cell carcinoma in dialysis patients is 3 to 6 times greater than in the general population (Fig. 35-45).[100,115] Small renal neoplasms (≤3 cm in diameter) are significantly more common than large carcinomas and occur in about 7% of dialysis patients (Fig. 35-46).[71] Most such lesions remain unchanged on prolonged follow-up. However, some

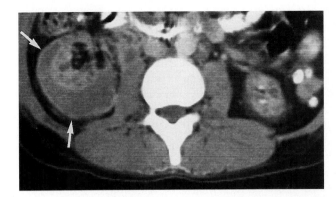

Fig. 35-44. Acquired renal cystic disease and a right perinephric hematoma *(arrows)* in a long-term dialysis patient. (From Levine E, Grantham JJ, Slusher SL, et al: *AJR* 142:125, 1984.)

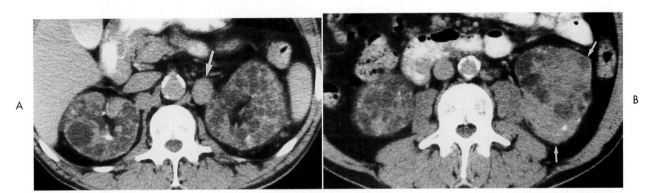

Fig. 35-45. Acquired renal cystic disease and metastatic renal cell carcinoma in a 46-year-old man treated with hemodialysis for 120 months. **A,** Contrast-enhanced CT scan shows multiple bilateral renal cysts and nephromegaly. The enlarged left renal hilar lymph node *(arrow)* is due to a metastasis. **B,** A caudal CT scan reveals two solid, heterogeneous masses *(arrows)* with irregular contours and focal calcifications in the lower pole of the left kidney. The masses enhanced by 30 HU. (From Levine E, Slusher SL, Grantham JJ, et al: *AJR* 156:501, 1991.)

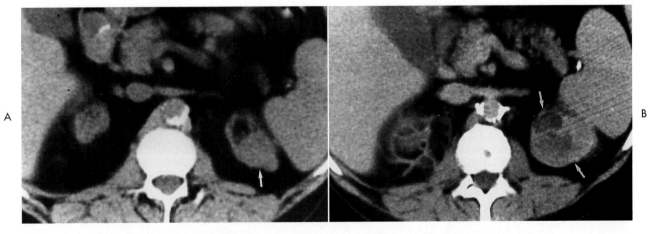

Fig. 35-46. Growth of renal cell carcinoma in a hemodialysis patient with acquired renal cystic disease. **A,** The first CT scan shows a small mass *(arrow)* in the upper pole of the left kidney. **B,** A CT scan performed 18 months later during an episode of gross hematuria reveals that the left renal mass *(arrows)* has enlarged and become heterogeneous, suggesting renal cell carcinoma. On pathologic examination, the lesion had invaded the renal capsule. Linear strands related to the right kidney resulted from perinephric hemorrhage. (From Levine E, Grantham JJ, MacDougall ML: *AJR* 148:755, 1987.)

gradually enlarge and may become locally invasive or even metastasize (Fig. 35-46).[107] Because of their propensity to develop malignant renal neoplasms, dialysis patients should have CT evaluation of their native kidneys if they develop flank pain or hematuria. Annual imaging of the native kidneys in asymptomatic dialysis patients should be restricted to those with a good general medical condition and a good life expectancy.[115]

Hereditary syndromes

Von Hippel-Lindau disease. Von Hippel-Lindau disease (VHLD) is caused by a genetic defect in the short arm of chromosome 3 and is characterized by an autosomal dominant pattern of inheritance. Manifestations include retinal angiomas, central nervous hemangioblastomas, pancreatic cysts and tumors, pheochromocytomas, and renal cysts and tumors. The abdominal lesions are best detected by CT.[31,113] Renal cysts, which are usually multiple and bilateral, are the most common manifestation of VHLD, occurring in more than 70% of patients (Fig. 35-47).[113] Most remain stable on long-term CT follow-up and transformation from typical simple cysts to solid lesions is rare.[32] However, complex lesions with both cystic and solid elements may transform into solid lesions and therefore require careful imaging follow-up.[32]

Renal cell carcinomas occur in about 36% of patients with VHLD and are often multifocal and bilateral.[112,113] Most carcinomas arise de novo and are not initially cystic.[32] Once solid renal lesions develop, they grow at rates similar to those of sporadic renal cell carcinomas (Fig. 35-48).[32] Selective renal angiography has a low sensitivity for detecting small carcinomas in VHLD.[125] Its role is therefore limited to providing a vascular map before partial nephrectomy or tumor enucleation.[125] The pancreas is commonly involved in VHLD, with pancreatic cysts occurring in about 30% of patients (Fig. 35-49).[31] Solid pancreatic lesions including non-functional islet cell tumor and ductal carcinoma occur less commonly in VHLD.[31] Pheochromocytomas occur in about 10% of all individuals with VHLD and may be unilateral or bilateral (Fig. 35-50).[113]

Screening in families affected by VHLD permits timely genetic counseling and early identification of potentially life-threatening lesions. Abdominal CT should first be performed late in the second decade in at-risk individuals (i.e., primary relatives of patients with the diagnosis). The frequency of imaging thereafter depends on the initial findings. Patients with suspicious renal lesions may require annual CT evaluation.

Tuberous sclerosis. Tuberous sclerosis may be inherited as an autosomal dominant trait or may occur sporadically. It is characterized by mental retardation, seizures, and cutaneous lesions.[105] Renal angiomyolipomas, which are usually multiple and bilateral, occur in about 67% of patients.[105] However, renal cystic disease also occurs in tuberous sclerosis and may sometimes be the earliest and only clinical manifestation of the disorder in infancy and childhood.[129] The kidneys are often significantly enlarged in such patients and are replaced by multiple cysts of varying sizes (Fig. 35-51). The cysts usually involve the renal cortex and medulla diffusely, and the findings are similar to those of autosomal dominant polycystic kidney disease (Fig. 35-51).[126]

Careful study of the kidneys with thin-section CT may show occasional small fat-containing angiomyolipomas in addition to cysts (Fig. 35-51).[126] The combination of renal cysts and angiomyolipomas is strongly suggestive of tuberous sclerosis.[126] If no renal angiomyolipomas are found, cranial CT may help establish the diagnosis of tuberous sclerosis by showing small, high-attenuation paraventricular nodules (Fig. 35-52). Renal biopsy may also help establish the diagnosis because the cysts in tuberous sclerosis are lined by a typical hyperplastic epithelium.[168]

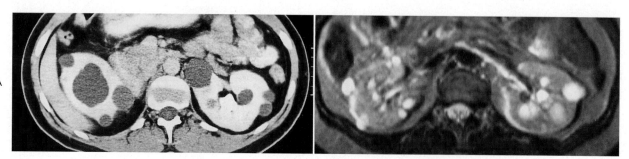

Fig. 35-47. Multiple renal cysts in two different patients with von Hippel-Lindau disease. **A,** Contrast-enhanced CT scan shows multiple bilateral renal cysts. **B,** T2-weighted (2200/90) spin-echo MR image shows multiple cysts with high signal intensities involving both kidneys.

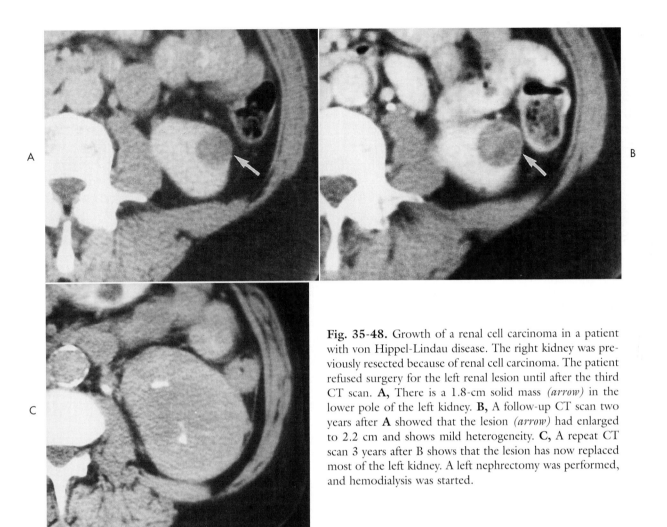

Fig. 35-48. Growth of a renal cell carcinoma in a patient with von Hippel-Lindau disease. The right kidney was previously resected because of renal cell carcinoma. The patient refused surgery for the left renal lesion until after the third CT scan. **A,** There is a 1.8-cm solid mass *(arrow)* in the lower pole of the left kidney. **B,** A follow-up CT scan two years after **A** showed that the lesion *(arrow)* had enlarged to 2.2 cm and shows mild heterogeneity. **C,** A repeat CT scan 3 years after B shows that the lesion has now replaced most of the left kidney. A left nephrectomy was performed, and hemodialysis was started.

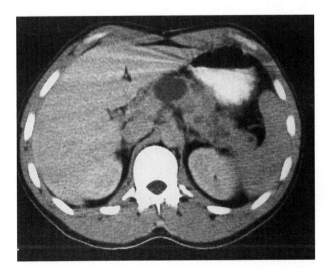

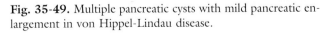

Fig. 35-49. Multiple pancreatic cysts with mild pancreatic enlargement in von Hippel-Lindau disease.

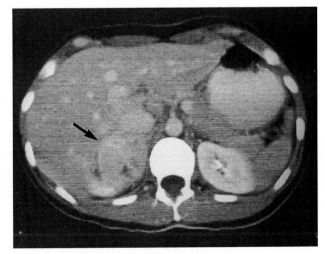

Fig. 35-50. Right adrenal pheochromocytoma *(arrow)* in von Hippel-Lindau disease.

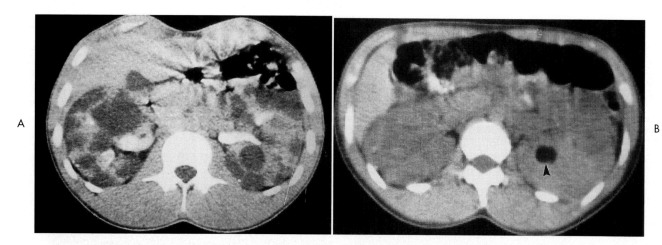

Fig. 35-51. Tuberous sclerosis with renal cystic disease in a 15-year-old female. **A,** Contrast-enhanced CT scan shows enlarged kidneys with multiple fluid-density cysts. The appearances closely resemble autosomal dominant polycystic kidney disease. **B,** Unenhanced CT scan shows a 1.9-cm rounded lesion *(arrowhead)* in left kidney with fat-attenuation value of 110 HU. The findings indicate an angiomyolipoma and strongly suggest tuberous sclerosis. (From Mitnick JS, Bosniak MA, Hilton S, et al: *Radiology,* 147:85, 1983.)

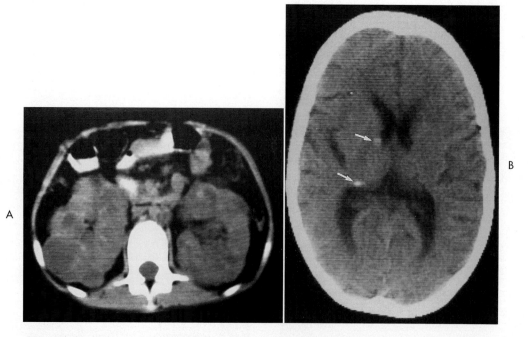

Fig. 35-52. Tuberous sclerosis with renal cystic disease in a 14-year-old female. **A,** Unenhanced CT scan displays kidneys containing multiple cysts. No fat-containing angiomyolipomas were detected. **B,** A cranial CT scan reveals paraventricular calcifications *(arrows)*, indicating diagnosis of tuberous sclerosis and permitting differentiation from autosomal dominant polycystic kidney disease.

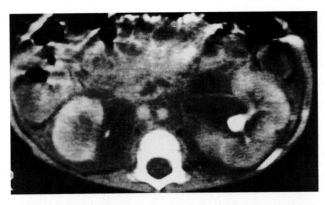

Fig. 35-53. Renal lymphangiectasia in a 10-month-old boy with abdominal masses on routine physical examination and normal renal function. A contrast-enhanced CT scan reveals nephromegaly and many renal sinus, perinephric and central retroperitoneal lymphatic cysts. (From Blumhagen JD, Wood BJ, Rosenbaum M: *J Ultrasound Med*, 6:487, 1987.)

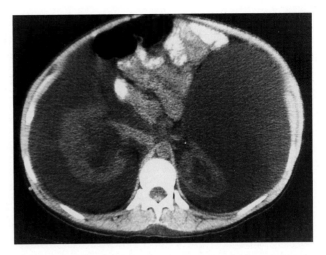

Fig. 35-54. Renal lymphangiectasia in a 25-year-old woman who developed severe abdominal distension during pregnancy. An unenhanced CT scan shows large bilateral perinephric lymph collections and renal sinus lymphatic cysts. (From Meredith WT, Levine E, Ahlstrom NG, Grantham JJ: *AJR*, 151:965, 1988.)

Renal lymphangiectasia

Renal lymphangiectasia is probably due to developmental obstruction of the larger lymphatics draining the kidney through the renal pedicle.[20,118,137] The condition is usually bilateral and is characterized on imaging studies by large lymphatic cysts in the renal sinuses, perinephric tissues, and central retroperitoneum, as well as diffuse intrarenal lymphangiectasia (Fig. 35-53).[20,123] The condition is usually discovered clinically because of abdominal masses due to nephromegaly.[20,137] Renal lymphangiectasia may be complicated during pregnancy by large perinephric lymph collections and ascites (Fig. 35-54).[123] These findings may be secondary to lymphatic rupture due to increased renal lymph flow during pregnancy in the presence of lymphatic obstruction.[123]

RENAL PARENCHYMAL NEOPLASMS
Malignant neoplasms

Malignant renal parenchymal neoplasms may be either primary or secondary. Renal cell carcinoma is the most common primary renal cancer, accounting for about 86% of all primary malignant renal parenchymal neoplasms. Of the remainder, 12% are Wilms' tumors and 2% are renal sarcomas.[99] Secondary neoplasms of the renal parenchyma include malignant lymphoma and metastases.

Renal cell carcinoma. Renal cell carcinoma is a common urologic malignant lesion in adults, accounting for about 3% of adult malignancies.[99] Although renal cell carcinoma may occur at any age, including childhood,[97] patients most commonly present between the ages of 50 and 70 years.[99] Current imaging techniques have had a notable effect on tumor detection. Small low-stage carcinomas are now commonly identified during abdominal CT or sonography performed for nonrenal complaints (Fig. 35-55).[110] Indeed, almost as many new renal cell carcinomas are currently being detected incidentally as are being found in patients investigated because of hematuria or flank pain.

CT is generally used as the primary imaging technique for evaluating suspected renal cell carcinoma. MRI assumes a primary role in tumor detection and staging in those patients in whom contrast-enhanced CT scanning is contraindicated because of either previous major reactions to contrast material or renal failure.[43,149] MRI may be used as a supplement to CT in those patients who have renal carcinoma and venous tumor extension and in whom the status of the vena cava is not clearly established.[43,45,68]

The precontrast CT appearances of renal cell carcinomas vary considerably, depending on their gross pathologic features. Neoplasms may be hypodense, isodense (Fig. 35-55), or hyperdense (Fig. 35-56) as compared with normal renal parenchyma on unenhanced CT scans.[185] Tumor calcification occurs in as many as 31% of cases and may take the form of amorphous internal calcification (Figs. 35-56, 35-57) or curvilinear calcification (Fig. 35-58), which may be peripheral or central.[185] After intravenous contrast administration, most renal cell carcinomas enhance, but usually to a lesser extent than normal renal parenchyma (Figs. 35-55, 35-56). Enhancement is often heterogeneous because of tumor

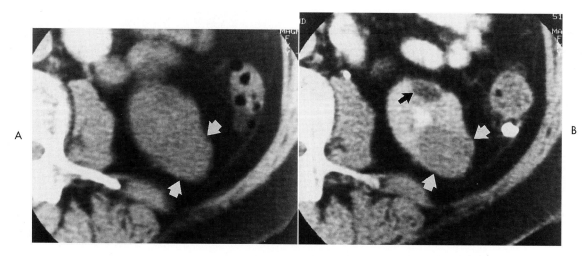

Fig. 35-55. Renal cell carcinoma. **A,** The neoplasm *(arrows)* has a similar density to normal renal parenchyma on an unenhanced CT scan. **B,** A contrast-enhanced CT scan shows a homogeneous 2.3-cm mass *(white arrows)* with a slightly irregular outline. The attenuation value increased from 37 to 87 HU. A small renal cyst *(black arrow)* is seen anteriorly.

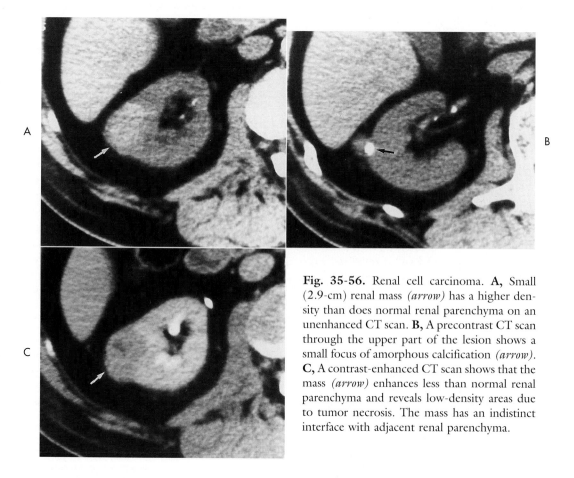

Fig. 35-56. Renal cell carcinoma. **A,** Small (2.9-cm) renal mass *(arrow)* has a higher density than does normal renal parenchyma on an unenhanced CT scan. **B,** A precontrast CT scan through the upper part of the lesion shows a small focus of amorphous calcification *(arrow)*. **C,** A contrast-enhanced CT scan shows that the mass *(arrow)* enhances less than normal renal parenchyma and reveals low-density areas due to tumor necrosis. The mass has an indistinct interface with adjacent renal parenchyma.

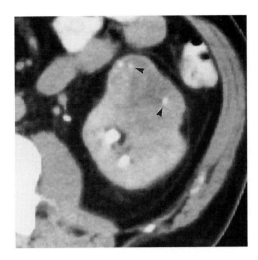

Fig. 35-57. Renal cell carcinoma. Small foci of amorphous calcification *(arrowheads)* are present in a left renal carcinoma. The mass has an indistinct interface with adjacent renal parenchyma, and it is heterogeneous.

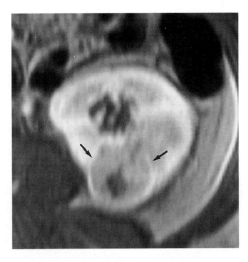

Fig. 35-59. Renal cell carcinoma. Gradient-echo (168/6; flip angle = 75°) MR image obtained during breath-holding after intravenous gadolinium injection shows a 3.6-cm left renal tumor *(arrows)* with areas of necrosis.

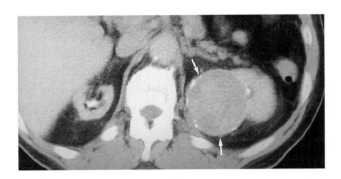

Fig. 35-58. Renal cell carcinoma. Left renal carcinoma *(arrows)* shows peripheral curvilinear calcification. The right kidney is small because of renal artery stenosis.

hemorrhage or necrosis (Figs. 35-56, 35-57).[99] The mass often shows an indistinct interface with the surrounding parenchyma and frequently has a lobulated or irregular outer margin (Figs. 55 to 57). Small renal carcinomas, however, often have distinct, smooth margins.[99,185]

The appearance of renal cell carcinoma on unenhanced MR spin-echo images varies depending on whether the neoplasm is homogeneous or contains areas of hemorrhage or necrosis.[84] In the absence of hemorrhage or necrosis, renal cell carcinomas are usually homogeneous in appearance and their signal intensity is similar to that of normal renal parenchyma on both T1- and T2-weighted images. Tumors smaller than 3 cm in diameter are detected in only 63% of unenhanced sequences.[84] Tumors containing areas of hemorrhage and

necrosis often appear heterogeneous on unenhanced spin-echo images. The use of intravenous gadolinium enhancement with either conventional or fat-suppressed T1-weighted spin-echo imaging or with gradient-echo imaging usually greatly increases tumor conspicuity.[160,161] Solid renal cell carcinomas often show significant contrast enhancement and may reveal irregular, ill-defined margins and heterogeneity (Fig. 35-59). Tumor calcification is difficult to appreciate on almost all MR pulse sequences.

Staging of renal cell carcinoma. The prognosis of patients with renal cell carcinoma depends mainly on histologic tumor grade and the extent or stage of the disease when first seen. Renal cell carcinoma is most commonly staged according to the system of Robson et al.[148] Stage I consists of tumor confined within the renal capsule, stage II of perinephric extension (yet contained by the renal fascia), stage IIIA of venous invasion (renal vein that may extend into the inferior vena cava), stage IIIB of regional lymph node metastases, and stage IIIC of both venous tumor extension and regional lymph node metastases. Stage IVA neoplasms extend through the renal fascia to involve adjacent organs (other than the ipsilateral adrenal), and stage IVB neoplasms have distant metastases.

Radiologic staging of renal cell carcinoma has an important influence on patient management. Small stage I neoplasms are sometimes managed by partial nephrectomy.[141] A radical nephrectomy is usually required for patients with large stage I tumors or stage II disease. Detection of venous tumor thrombus is important preoperatively, because a more extensive surgical procedure is required to remove intravascular tumor, particularly as the thrombus propagates cephalad towards the right atrium. Debulking of enlarged lymph nodes can also be planned if nodal metastases are identified. Treatment of stage IV disease differs from center to center. Some surgeons perform a radical nephrectomy in nearly all patients, while others do so only in symptomatic patients. In advanced disease, percutaneous biopsy to document a distant metastasis is all that may be required before starting chemotherapy or immunotherapy.[177]

CT has an overall accuracy of about 90% in the abdominal staging of renal cell carcinoma.[86,186] The accuracy of CT staging is enhanced by the use of dynamic scanning with a rapid intravenous bolus injection of contrast medium.[186] CT and MRI achieve approximately equal accuracy in the local staging of renal cell carcinoma.[161] Perinephric invasion is suggested by a perinephric soft-tissue mass at least 1 cm in diameter (Fig. 35-60), but lesser degrees of perinephric involvement are difficult to diagnose by CT or MRI (Fig. 35-61)[86,111,179,186] Perinephric soft-tissue stranding is an unreliable indicator of perinephric tumor invasion. Venous tumor invasion can only be definitely diagnosed on CT if there is identifiable thrombus in the renal vein (Figs. 35-62, 35-63) or inferior vena cava (Fig. 35-63) with or without venous enlargement.[186] Ipsilateral renal vein enlargement on CT without identifiable tumor thrombus is not a reliable sign of venous tumor extension (Fig. 35-64). Although it may reflect the presence of tumor thrombus, it more frequently results from increased blood flow due to a hypervascular tumor (Fig. 35-64).[186] Errors in diagnosis of venous tumor extension on CT often occur when large right-sided tumors cause notable distortion of the ipsilateral renal vein and inferior vena cava.[86,111]

MRI is particularly useful in detecting venous tumor involvement when CT findings are indeterminate (Figs. 35-65, 35-66).[68,150] Tumor thrombus in the renal vein and vena cava may be suspected on T1-weighted spin-echo pulse sequences if the signal void of flowing blood is replaced by relatively high signal as a result of tumor thrombus (Fig. 35-65). Tumor thrombi emit signal with an intensity similar to that of the primary neo-

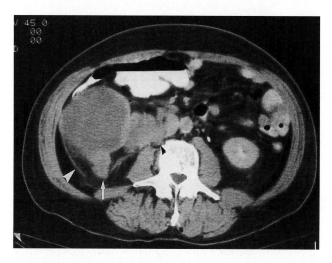

Fig. 35-60. Renal cell carcinoma. A right-sided tumor has invaded the perinephric fat posteriorly *(arrow)* and medially *(black arrowhead).* The medial perinephric mass indents the inferior vena cava. The renal fascia *(white arrowhead)* is thickened.

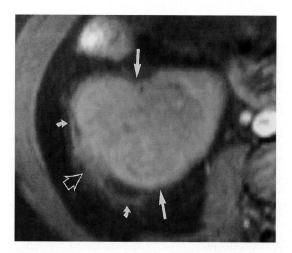

Fig. 35-61. Renal cell carcinoma with early perinephric extension. Unenhanced fat-suppressed T1-weighted MR image (600/15) shows a large neoplasm *(straight arrows)* in the lower pole of the right kidney. There is early extension into the perinephric fat *(open arrow)* and associated renal fascial thickening *(curved arrows).*

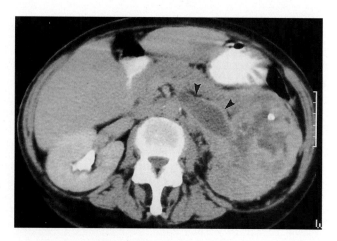

Fig. 35-62. Left renal cell carcinoma with venous extension. The proximal part of the left renal vein is enlarged *(arrowheads)* and occupied by low-density tumor.

plasm (Fig. 35-65). The use of venous presaturation pulses is necessary to reduce the occurrence of flow-related artifacts. Gradient-echo images are also useful for detecting venous tumor extension.[53,150] Flowing blood with this technique has a significantly increased signal intensity and appears white, whereas tumor thrombus has a medium signal intensity and appears as an intravenous filling defect (Fig. 35-67).[53,150] Tumor extension to the level of the hepatic veins or into the right atrium may require surgical exposure of the intrathoracic vena cava and cardiopulmonary bypass.[68,99] Accordingly, if CT shows vena caval tumor extension but the cephalad extent of tumor cannot be determined, MRI may be performed. MRI has largely replaced inferior vena cavography for this purpose.[68] Sagittal or coronal MRI accurately evaluates the superior extent of caval thrombus

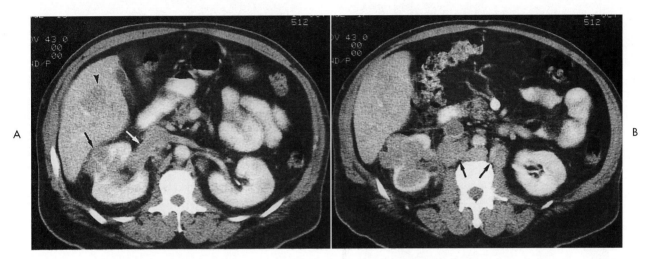

Fig. 35-63. Renal cell carcinoma with venous extension and regional lymph node metastases. **A,** Contrast-enhanced CT scan shows a right renal mass *(black arrow).* The right renal vein *(white arrow)* is enlarged and occupied by tumor, which has also extended into the inferior vena cava. There is a metastasis *(arrowhead)* in the right lobe of the liver. **B,** Multiple enlarged, central retroperitoneal lymph nodes *(arrows)* were due to metastatic disease.

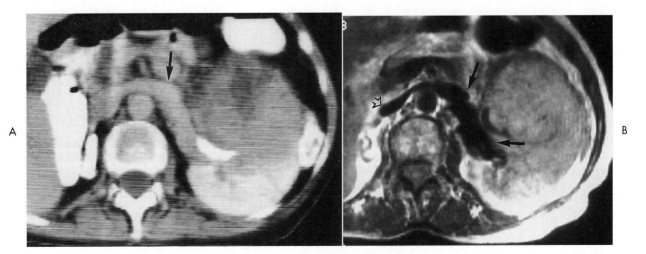

Fig. 35-64. Left renal cell carcinoma with renal vein enlargement *(arrow)* on contrast-enhanced CT scan **(A).** The right kidney is atrophic. On MRI **(B)** (spin-echo, 2100/30) the left renal vein *(arrows)* is enlarged but shows a normal signal void indicating that venous enlargement is probably due to increased blood flow rather than tumor extension. The inferior vena cava *(open arrow)* is also normal.

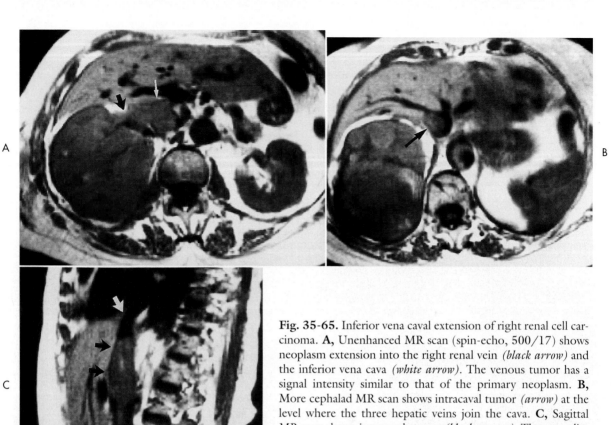

Fig. 35-65. Inferior vena caval extension of right renal cell carcinoma. **A,** Unenhanced MR scan (spin-echo, 500/17) shows neoplasm extension into the right renal vein *(black arrow)* and the inferior vena cava *(white arrow)*. The venous tumor has a signal intensity similar to that of the primary neoplasm. **B,** More cephalad MR scan shows intracaval tumor *(arrow)* at the level where the three hepatic veins join the cava. **C,** Sagittal MR scan shows intracaval tumor *(black arrows)*. The supradiaphragmatic part of the cava *(white arrow)* is not affected.

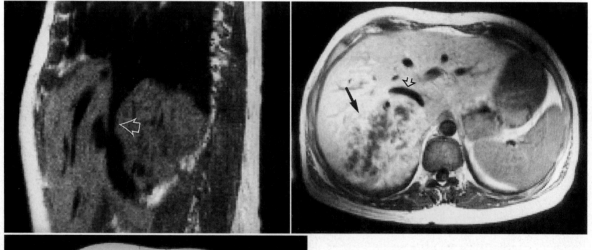

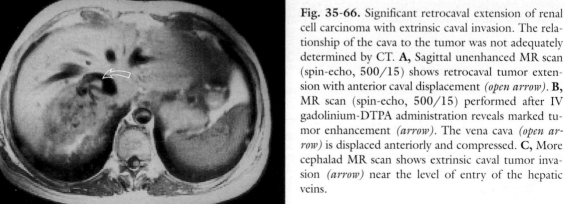

Fig. 35-66. Significant retrocaval extension of renal cell carcinoma with extrinsic caval invasion. The relationship of the cava to the tumor was not adequately determined by CT. **A,** Sagittal unenhanced MR scan (spin-echo, 500/15) shows retrocaval tumor extension with anterior caval displacement *(open arrow)*. **B,** MR scan (spin-echo, 500/15) performed after IV gadolinium-DTPA administration reveals marked tumor enhancement *(arrow)*. The vena cava *(open arrow)* is displaced anteriorly and compressed. **C,** More cephalad MR scan shows extrinsic caval tumor invasion *(arrow)* near the level of entry of the hepatic veins.

relative to the diaphragm, hepatic veins, and right atrium (Figs. 35-65, 35-66).[68,150]

Regional lymph nodes are considered to be involved by tumor if they are at least 1 cm in diameter. However, lymph nodes 1 to 2 cm in diameter may be due to reactive hyperplasia as well as to metastases.[86] Lymph nodes larger than 2 cm in size are almost always due to metastases (Fig. 35-63).[86,111] Adjacent organ invasion is diagnosed only if there is enlargement of and/or a density change in an adjacent structure (Fig. 35-68). The loss of a fat plane between the tumor and an adjacent organ is not reliable evidence of tumor invasion (Fig. 35-68).[86] CT may detect metastases in the adrenal glands, contralateral kidney, liver, and lumbar vertebrae (Fig. 35-63).

Postnephrectomy evaluation. Renal bed recurrence of neoplasm occurs in about 5% of patients after radical nephrectomy, as detected by follow-up CT.[143] Patients with large, invasive stage III and IV tumors have a higher risk of local recurrence than those with small low-stage tumors.[1] Renal bed recurrence is most likely to occur within 2 years of nephrectomy.[143] If asymptomatic neoplasm recurrence is detected at an early stage, it may be amenable to local surgery, which will result in improved survival.[130] CT may detect neoplasm recurrence in the renal fossa by showing a soft-tissue mass.[16] However, normal structures migrate into the renal fossa after nephrectomy and may simulate recurrent tumor. The liver, ascending colon, second part of duodenum, pancreatic head, and small bowel migrate into the right renal fossa. The pancreatic tail, spleen, and large and small bowel migrate into the left renal fossa.[143] Interpretational errors can be avoided by ensuring adequate bowel opacification with oral contrast medium. Postoperative scarring in the renal fossa is distinguished from neoplasm recurrence if the area shows no change on serial CT examinations.[1]

Local neoplasm recurrence may also be suggested by enlargement or irregularity of the psoas muscle on the

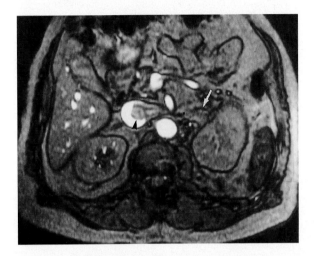

Fig. 35-67. Inferior vena caval extension of left renal cell carcinoma. A gradient-echo MR image (60/12; flip angle = 60°) shows tumor extension along the left renal vein *(arrow)* and into the inferior vena cava. Flowing blood in the cava appears white and the tumor is shown as a filling defect *(arrowhead)*. (Courtesy of Richard L. Ehman, M.D., Rochester, Minn.)

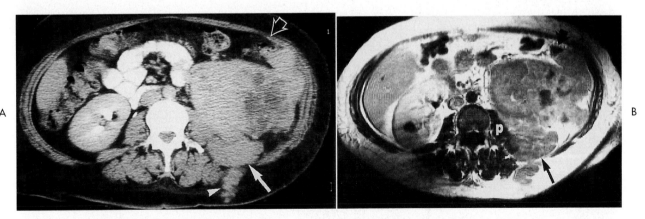

Fig. 35-68. Left renal cell carcinoma with extension beyond the renal fascia. **A,** The tumor invades the abdominal wall in the region of the left quadratus lumborum muscle *(arrow)*. Tumor has grown along a needle-biopsy track in the subcutaneous tissues *(arrowhead)*. There is tumor invasion of the descending colon *(open arrow)* that was confirmed at surgery. Although the neoplasm abuts the left psoas muscle, there was no actual muscle invasion. **B,** Contrast-enhanced MR scan (spin-echo, 500/15) reveals that the neoplasm does not invade the psoas muscle *(p)*. However, there is abdominal-wall invasion *(long arrow)* and colon invasion *(short arrow)*.

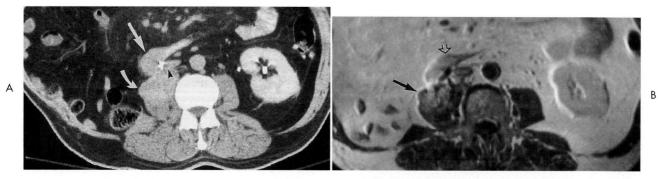

Fig. 35-69. Local recurrence of renal cell carcinoma 7 years after nephrectomy for right renal cell carcinoma. Patient presented with upper gastrointestinal bleeding. **A,** An enhancing mass *(curved arrow)* causes enlargement of the right psoas muscle. The third part of the duodenum *(straight arrow)* and the inferior vena cava *(arrowhead)* are adherent to the mass. **B,** MRI (spin-echo, 500/15) performed after IV injection of gadolinium-DTPA shows an enhancing mass *(arrow)* involving the right psoas muscle. Endoscopy with biopsy showed clear cell carcinoma invading the third part of the duodenum *(open arrow)*.

side of the nephrectomy (Fig. 35-69), although this appearance may also be caused by postoperative scarring.[16] CT may also detect tumor recurrence in the retroperitoneal lymph nodes, in the inferior vena cava, and around the aorta and inferior vena cava. Liver metastases, adrenal metastases, and metastases in the opposite kidney are also easily identified by CT.[1,16] Ideally, all patients managed by radical nephrectomy or partial nephrectomy for renal cell carcinoma should have a baseline postoperative CT scan and later scans at regular intervals. This is particularly important in patients with large invasive tumors.[1]

Wilms' tumor. Wilms' tumor accounts for 87% of pediatric renal neoplasms.[9] The tumor occurs most often during the first 7 years of life, with a peak incidence at 3.5 years.[92] Occasional cases are encountered during adult life.[54] Most patients present because of an enlarging abdominal mass.[92] Less frequent presenting symptoms include abdominal pain, fever, and microscopic or gross hematuria.[92] The lung is the most frequent site of metastatic disease, and the liver is less frequently involved. With appropriate therapy about 95% of patients with Wilms' tumor can be cured.[178] Tumor histology and stage are the most useful predictors of patient outcome and also help determine the nature of therapy. Although all Wilms' tumors require surgical resection, preoperative imaging helps determine tumor stage and resectability, therefore influencing decisions about preoperative chemotherapy or radiation therapy.[36,92,178]

Sonography is the most common method for initial diagnosis of Wilms' tumor. However, CT and more recently MRI have been found to be more accurate than ultrasound in tumor staging.[13,36,144] Chest and abdominal CT may be performed during the same examination,

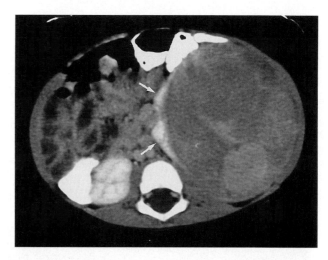

Fig. 35-70. A large heterogeneous Wilms' tumor is present in the left kidney. The residual renal parenchyma is displaced medially *(arrows)*.

thereby determining the presence or absence of lung metastases.[36] Adequate CT requires a rapid scanner (preferably 1 second), adequate sedation, and IV contrast enhancement.[36]

On CT, a Wilms' tumor usually presents as a large, spherical, intrarenal mass often with a well-defined rim of compressed renal parenchyma or pseudocapsule surrounding the tumor (Fig. 35-70). Tumors that arise in the peripheral cortex may grow in an exophytic manner with most of the tumor mass outside the kidney.[54] The tumor is less dense than normal renal parenchyma on contrast-enhanced CT scans and often shows extensive necrosis (Fig. 35-71).[54,144] About 13% of Wilms' tu-

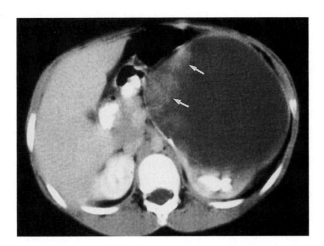

Fig. 35-71. Left Wilms' tumor with extensive necrosis. A contrast-enhanced CT scan shows that the tumor has a mainly fluid density. Solid and enhancing tumor elements are present medially *(arrows)*.

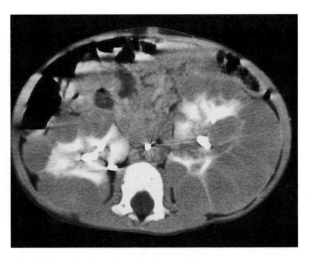

Fig. 35-72. Multicentric and bilateral Wilms' tumors. The tumors have a low density, and they compress residual enhancing renal tissue.

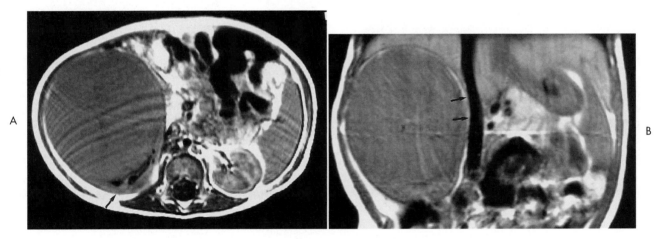

Fig. 35-73. Wilms' tumor of right kidney shown by MRI (spin-echo, 600/15). **A,** An axial scan reveals that the mass is well defined and displaces normal renal tissue *(arrow)* posteriorly. **B,** A coronal scan shows that the mass indents the inferior vena cava *(arrows)*, but there is no intracaval tumor extension.

mors contain calcifications[54] as seen on unenhanced CT scans, and occasional tumors contain fat.[51,54] About 10% of patients show poor or absent function of the involved kidney because of either venous tumor extension, compression of the collecting system, or extensive tumor infiltration throughout the kidney.

Perinephric tumor extension thickens the renal fascia and obliterates the perinephric fat, but subtle perinephric extension may be missed by CT. Central retroperitoneal adenopathy may be detected by CT, although distinction is usually not possible between nodes en-

larged as a result of metastases and those enlarged because of reactive changes.[36,144] Renal vein and inferior vena caval tumor extension are best shown after an intravenous bolus injection of contrast medium. The thrombus may be seen as a low-density intraluminal filling defect. CT may also identify bilateral Wilms' tumors (Fig. 35-72), present in about 7% of patients,[9] and liver and pulmonary metastases.[36,144]

On MRI, Wilms' tumor appears as a large, well-defined mass with relatively distinct margins (Fig. 35-73).[13] It has a low signal intensity on T1-weighted images and a high signal intensity on T2-weighted images. The tumor often appears heterogeneous because of hemorrhage and necrosis.[13] Hemorrhage produces areas of high signal intensity on T1-weighted images, while necrotic areas result in high-signal areas on T2-weighted images.[13] MRI has a low accuracy in predicting capsular tumor invasion.[13] Although MRI is sensitive for detecting regional lymph node enlargement, it cannot predict the cause of enlargement.[13] Currently, CT and MRI appear equivalent in staging Wilms' tumor. However, MRI shows venous extension better than does CT because it can distinguish caval displacement from intracaval tumor extension (Fig. 35-73).[13]

Nephroblastomatosis. Nephrogenesis is normally complete by 34 to 35 weeks of gestation. However, metanephric blastema may persist into infancy and childhood. Foci of persistent metanephric tissue are designated as nephrogenic rests.[11] The presence of multiple nephrogenic rests is termed *nephroblastomatosis*.[11] Nephrogenic rests are seen in almost 1% of infants at autopsy.[11] They occur significantly more frequently in children with Wilms' tumor, being found in about 41% of children with unilateral Wilms' tumor and in about 99% of children with synchronous bilateral Wilms' tumor.[11] There is wide acceptance of nephroblastomatosis as a precursor lesion to Wilms' tumor.[176] Hyperplastic nephrogenic

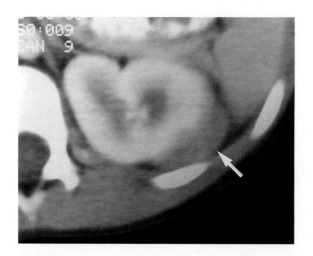

Fig. 35-74. A hyperplastic intralobar nephrogenic rest presents as a low-density subcapsular mass *(arrow)* on a contrast-enhanced CT scan.

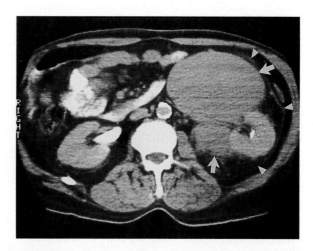

Fig. 35-75. Undifferentiated liposarcoma *(arrows)* arising in the perinephric fat. The neoplasm is confined within the renal fascia *(arrowheads)*. The left kidney is displaced laterally, but there is no renal parenchymal tumor invasion.

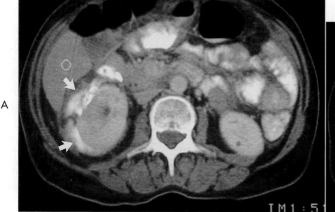

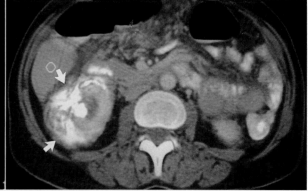

Fig. 35-76. Renal osteosarcoma. A densely ossified mass *(arrows)* arises peripherally in the lower pole of the right kidney. (Courtesy of Clive Levine, M.D., Columbia, Mo.)

rests are macroscopic and plaque-like (Fig. 35-74). Any macroscopic nephrogenic rest that is nodular and enlarges over time is considered neoplastic.[176]

CT is the technique of choice in the evaluation of suspected nephroblastomatosis.[176] It is particularly useful for evaluating the contralateral kidney in children with Wilms' tumor, for renal screening in children with syndromes associated with Wilms' tumor, and for follow-up of patients with known nephroblastomatosis to detect neoplastic change.[52,176] The hallmark of neoplastic transformation of a benign nephrogenic rest is enlargement on serial CT scans.[176]

Renal sarcoma. Renal sarcomas account for fewer than 2% of malignant renal parenchymal neoplasms.[47] Leiomyosarcoma is the most common renal sarcoma, accounting for about 58% of all sarcomas.[47] Hemangiopericytoma and liposarcoma each account for about 20% of renal sarcomas.[47] Renal rhabdomyosarcoma and osteogenic sarcoma occur rarely. Capsular localization is a feature of more than 50% of these tumors[47] and should suggest the diagnosis on CT (Figs. 35-75, 35-76). When these neoplasms arise in the renal parenchyma, however, they are indistinguishable from renal cell carcinoma on CT.[99]

Renal liposarcomas usually arise in the renal capsule or perinephric fat (Fig. 35-75).[47] On CT, liposarcomas cause compression without invasion of the renal parenchyma and show a variety of appearances correlating closely with their gross and histologic features.[94] Tumors containing a large amount of mature fat show negative attenuation values. Myxoid liposarcomas contain little mature fat, and their predominant fluid and connective tissue composition results in attenuation values nearer those of water.[94] On CT, undifferentiated liposarcomas are indistinguishable from other types of sarcomas.

coma (Fig. 35-75). The diagnosis of renal osteogenic sarcoma is suggested on CT by a peripherally located renal mass containing dense ossification (Fig. 35-76).[184]

Malignant lymphoma. Because the kidney normally does not contain lymphoid tissue, primary lymphoma arising in the kidney is very rare.[33] However, secondary renal involvement occurs commonly from either generalized hematogenous dissemination of lymphoma or by direct extension of retroperitoneal disease.[33] Bilateral renal involvement occurs three times more frequently than does unilateral disease.[99] Renal involvement occurs significantly more commonly in non-Hodgkin's lymphoma than in Hodgkin's disease.[99] With the extensive use of abdominal CT for lymphoma staging, renal lymphoma is now recognized by CT in about 8% of patients with lymphoma.[33] Multiple renal nodules are the most common CT manifestation of renal lymphoma, occurring in about 59% of cases (Fig. 35-77).[33,145] The nodules are less dense than normal renal parenchyma on contrast-enhanced CT scans and typically show homogeneous appearances. As multiple renal nodules grow, coalesce, and replace nephrons, the kidneys are almost diffusely replaced by lymphoma (Fig. 35-78). However, the multinodular nature of the disease process usually remains apparent.[99] Retroperitoneal lymph node enlargement is not visible on CT in a significant percentage of patients with renal lymphoma not due to direct spread of retroperitoneal tumor (Fig. 35-78).[33,145]

Renal involvement from retroperitoneal lymphoma commonly occurs either by invasion through the renal capsule or extension through the renal sinus (Fig. 35-79). This pattern accounts for about 28% of patients with renal lymphoma.[33,145] Retroperitoneal adenopathy is invariably present, and many patients show obstructive hydronephrosis. Rarely, a solitary mass in one kidney is the only CT manifestation of renal lymphoma (about 3% of cases) (Fig. 35-80). Some patients (about

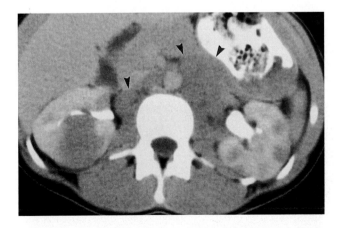

Fig. 35-77. Non-Hodgkin's lymphoma with bilateral multiple renal masses. There is extensive retroperitoneal adenopathy *(arrowheads)*.

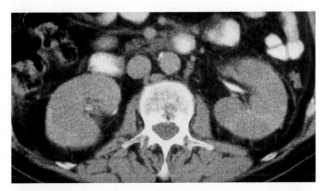

Fig. 35-78. Bilateral renal replacement and mild nephromegaly in non-Hodgkin's lymphoma. There is no enlargement of retroperitoneal lymph nodes.

10%) show a predominance of perinephric disease without extensive parenchymal or retroperitoneal disease (Fig. 35-81).[33] The role of MRI in evaluating renal lymphoma has yet to be defined.

Metastases. Renal metastases occur two to three times as frequently as primary renal neoplasms in autopsy series.[99] The kidney is the fifth most common site of metastases in the body after lung, liver, bone, and adrenals, most metastases reaching the kidney via the hematogenous route.[127] The three neoplasms with the highest frequency of renal metastases are lung carcinoma, breast carcinoma, and carcinoma of the opposite kidney. Renal metastases also occur commonly in patients with malig-

nant melanoma and sometimes present as large solitary renal masses simulating renal cell carcinoma.[166]

Renal metastases are usually discovered incidentally during abdominal CT performed for tumor staging. However, some patients have hematuria and flank pain.[127] Most patients have small renal lesions that are multiple and bilateral.[30] These are best seen on contrast-enhanced CT scans. Although metastases are usually homogeneous on CT, larger lesions may show central necrosis.[127] Occasionally, patients with metastases have solitary renal masses.[30] If the patient has other areas of metastatic disease and a current known primary neoplasm, such solitary renal lesions can usually be safely assumed to be metastases, and pathologic proof of their nature is unnecessary (Fig. 35-82).[30,127] However, if there are no other metastases, it is difficult to determine whether the renal lesion is a synchronous renal cell car-

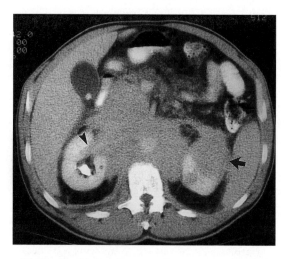

Fig. 35-79. Renal involvement from retroperitoneal non-Hodgkin's lymphoma. There is extensive central retroperitoneal adenopathy causing lateral displacement of the kidneys. The upper pole of the left kidney *(arrow)* is invaded through the renal capsule. Tumor extends into the right kidney via the renal sinus *(arrowhead)*.

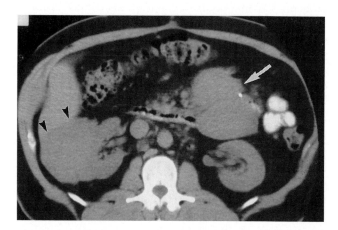

Fig. 35-81. Right perinephric mass *(arrowheads)* shown on unenhanced CT scan in patient with non-Hodgkin's lymphoma. There is a large nodal mass *(arrow)* involving the small bowel mesentery.

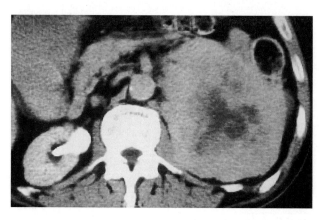

Fig. 35-80. Hodgkin's disease with solitary heterogeneous left renal mass.

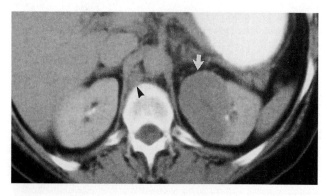

Fig. 35-82. Left renal metastasis *(arrow)* and retrocrural adenopathy *(arrowhead)* in patient with small cell lung cancer. A follow-up scan after 3 weeks of chemotherapy showed complete resolution of the renal mass and adenopathy.

cinoma or a renal metastasis (Fig. 35-83).[30,127] In these circumstances further investigation is necessary, particularly if there has been an apparent remission of the primary neoplasm. Urine cytology is especially useful in detecting metastases from squamous cell carcinoma of the lung;[30] the urine should be examined for melanin in patients with a history of malignant melanoma.[166] If such tests are negative, percutaneous biopsy is necessary for diagnosis and may obviate the need for nephrectomy (Fig. 35-83).[127,166]

Benign neoplasms

Adenoma. During the last decade, there has been a significant increase in detection of asymptomatic renal tumors 3 cm or smaller in diameter by sonography and CT (Fig. 35-84).[110,164] Most are neoplasms of tubular origin. In the past such lesions were often classified as renal adenomas, because they rarely metastasize.[12] However, serial imaging shows that they often gradually enlarge (Fig. 35-85)[18,110] and that even small tumors may metastasize (Fig. 35-86).[164] Indeed, such lesions are histologically indistinguishable from larger carcinomas more commonly encountered in the kidneys, and they often have histologic grades indicating a definite potential for malignant behavior.[2,15,110,164] Accordingly, most investigators believe that these lesions should be regarded as carcinomas in an early stage of evolution and should not be classified as adenomas.[15,18,110] On CT these small renal tumors are usually well defined and homogeneous in appearance (Fig. 35-84).[110,164] Less commonly, they show marginal irregularity, heterogeneity, or central calcification (see Fig. 35-56),[110] findings that may suggest pathologically high-grade tumors.[24]

The management of small renal neoplasms detected by imaging is controversial.[18,19] Some believe that these lesions may remain clinically occult for the patient's lifetime and that they therefore may not require surgical management.[19] Support for this argument derives from the finding that renal "adenomas" are observed incidentally in the kidneys of about 15% of autopsied cases.[181] However, the future behavior of any individual tumor cannot be predicted; surgical resection is therefore usually favored.[131] Some urologists believe that these lesions are best managed by partial nephrectomy,[141] while others recommend radical nephrectomy.[131] Follow-up by serial imaging may be the best approach in elderly patients who are unfit for surgery.[18]

Oncocytoma. Oncocytomas are composed of large, regular cells with abundant granular eosinophilic cytoplasm. They do not usually show necrosis, nuclear anaplasia, or mitotic activity.[108] Lesions with such features are designated as grade I tumors and behave in a benign fashion. However, occasional lesions show nuclear anaplasia (grade II tumors) and may cause metastases.[116] Most oncocytomas are small tumors discovered incidentally during CT performed for nonrenal complaints.[108,110] However, occasional patients have large oncocytomas and present with hematuria and palpable abdominal masses.

On CT, oncocytomas are typically well-defined masses with smooth, rounded margins (Fig. 35-87).[108,110] Tumor calcification occurs rarely, and oncocytomas are sometimes multiple and bilateral.[37,80] Small oncocytomas are usually homogeneous in appearance on contrast-enhanced CT scans, although they are occasionally heterogeneous due to the presence of central scars (Fig. 35-88). On CT small oncocytomas are usually indistinguishable from slowly growing small renal cell carcinomas that lack hemorrhage or necrosis.[38,110] A cen-

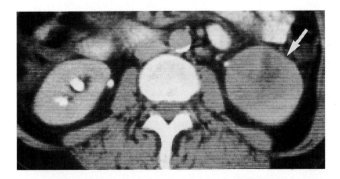

Fig. 35-83. Solitary renal metastasis from squamous cell carcinoma of the lung. The patient underwent a left upper lobectomy. Two years later, he developed left flank pain and hematuria. CT shows a heterogeneous left renal mass *(arrow)*. No other lesions were found. A renal cell carcinoma was suspected, but percutaneous biopsy revealed metastatic squamous carcinoma.

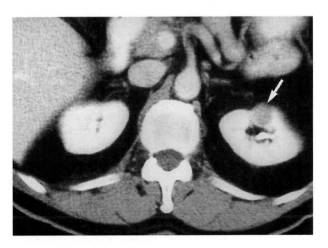

Fig. 35-84. Small (1.8-cm) renal cell carcinoma *(arrow)* detected incidentally by CT.

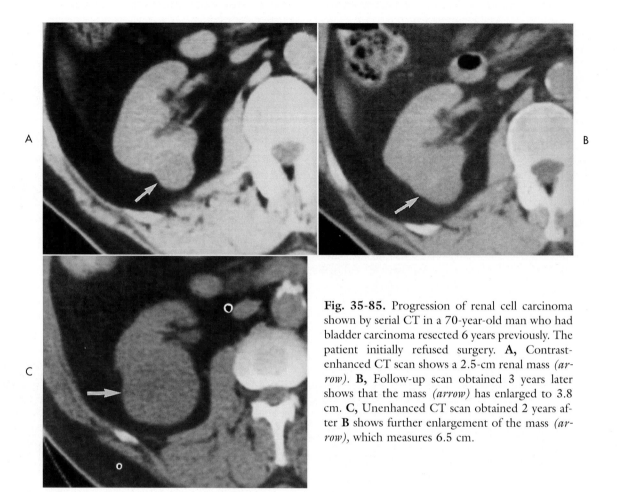

Fig. 35-85. Progression of renal cell carcinoma shown by serial CT in a 70-year-old man who had bladder carcinoma resected 6 years previously. The patient initially refused surgery. **A,** Contrast-enhanced CT scan shows a 2.5-cm renal mass *(arrow)*. **B,** Follow-up scan obtained 3 years later shows that the mass *(arrow)* has enlarged to 3.8 cm. **C,** Unenhanced CT scan obtained 2 years after **B** shows further enlargement of the mass *(arrow)*, which measures 6.5 cm.

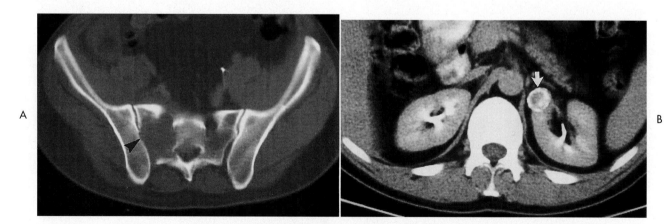

Fig. 35-86. Small renal cell carcinoma with sacral metastasis. The patient was a 42-year-old man who complained of low back pain. **A,** A lytic metastasis *(arrowhead)* is present in the right sacral ala. **B,** CT performed to search for a primary neoplasm shows a small mass *(arrow)* with dense peripheral calcification in the left kidney. Histologic examination revealed a high-grade left renal cell carcinoma.

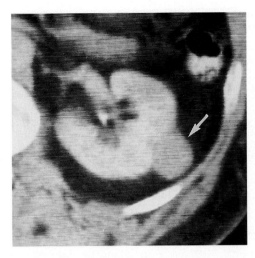

Fig. 35-87. Left renal oncocytoma. A contrast-enhanced CT scan shows a homogeneously enhancing, well-circumscribed, exophytic renal mass *(arrow)*.

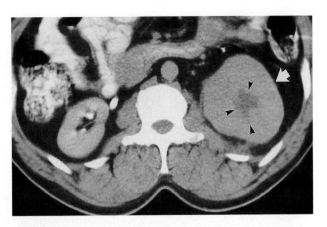

Fig. 35-89. Large left renal oncocytoma *(arrow)*. The centrally placed, sharply defined, stellate area of low attenuation *(arrowheads)* suggests the diagnosis of oncocytoma.

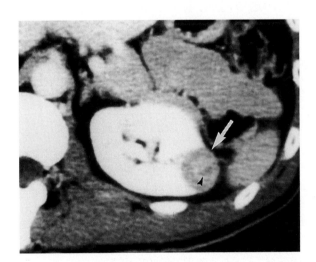

Fig. 35-88. Left renal oncocytoma *(arrow)* with eccentric scar *(arrowhead)*. Distinction from a small renal cell carcinoma is not possible by CT.

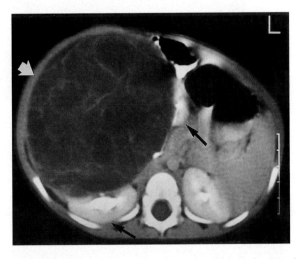

Fig. 35-90. Multilocular cystic nephroma *(white arrow)* in the right kidney in an infant. Multiple septa separate the fluid-containing locules. The renal parenchyma is displaced medially and posteriorly *(black arrows)*.

tral, sharply defined stellate scar (Fig. 35-89) is present in 25% to 33% of large oncocytomas and strongly suggests the diagnosis.[142] However, CT criteria are usually poor discriminants in distinguishing between oncocytoma and renal cell carcinoma, regardless of tumor size.[38,110] If the diagnosis of oncocytoma is suspected preoperatively, small tumors may be treated by partial nephrectomy because of their excellent prognosis. Larger tumors may require nephrectomy.[142]

Juxtaglomerular neoplasm. Renin-producing tumors of juxtaglomerular cells (reninomas) are a rare, but curable, cause of hypertension.[44] They occur most frequently in young adults and affect women more frequently than men. The plasma renin and aldosterone levels are usually elevated. None of the reported neoplasms has been invasive or has metastasized. Reninomas are usually well shown on contrast-enhanced CT scans in which they show a smooth outline and sharp margination. Small foci of hemorrhage may cause a heterogeneous tumor appearance. Because of their benign nature, these tumors may be managed by partial nephrectomy.[44]

Multilocular cystic nephroma. Multilocular cystic nephroma (MLCN) is a well-encapsulated, multilocular, noninfiltrating cystic renal tumor. It presents in

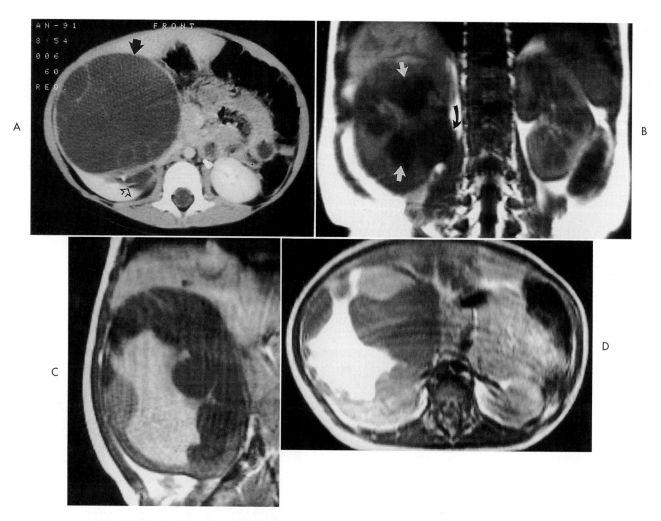

Fig. 35-91. Multilocular cystic nephroma occurring in the right kidney in an infant. **A,** CT shows fine septa in well-defined cystic renal mass *(arrow)*. Hydronephrosis *(open arrow)* was due to herniation of the tumor into the right renal pelvis. **B,** Coronal MRI (spin-echo, 350/15) obtained posteriorly through the right kidney shows dilated calyces *(white arrows)* and renal pelvis *(curved arrow)*. **C,** Coronal T1-weighted MR scan (spin-echo, 350/15) shows that the tumor has a heterogeneous appearance with area of high signal intensity probably due to hemorrhage or high protein content in cyst fluid. **D,** Axial proton-density weighted MR image (2000/22) shows that fluid locules have significantly variable signal intensities.

young children (usually boys) as an asymptomatic abdominal mass, and in adults (usually women) with abdominal pain and hematuria.[120] The lesion may represent a partially differentiated Wilms' tumor at least in children.[10] Most lesions are benign, although occasionally foci of Wilms' tumor or sarcoma are found in the septal stroma separating the cysts.[120] On CT, MLCN presents as a well-defined encapsulated mass containing multiple cysts separated by septa (Fig. 35-90). The septa may be as thick as several millimeters, but they do not display significant nodularity. Calcification may be found in the wall of the tumor or in the septa.[120] Contrast ex-

cretion by the affected kidney is usually normal. However, the lesion frequently protrudes into the renal pelvis causing a filling defect and sometimes obstructive calycectasis (Fig. 35-91). MRI does not add much information to that provided by CT (Fig. 35-91). MLCN may be indistinguishable on imaging from other cystic renal neoplasms, particularly cystic Wilms' tumor in infancy and multilocular cystic renal cell carcinoma in adults (see Fig. 35-21). Accordingly, surgical resection is always necessary.[120]

Angiomyolipoma. Angiomyolipomas, also called renal hamartomas or choristomas, contain blood vessels,

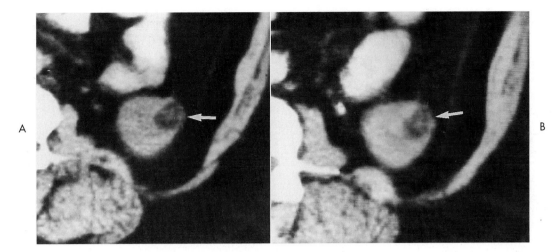

Fig. 35-92. Small renal angiomyolipoma. **A,** Unenhanced CT scan shows a low-density mass *(arrow)* in the lower pole of the left kidney. Attenuation values as low as −42 HU, indicating the presence of fat, were found in the lesion using small regions of interest. **B,** On a contrast-enhanced CT scan the attenuation values of the lesion *(arrow)* were in the soft-tissue range.

smooth muscle, and fatty tissues, although one or two of these elements may predominate.[169] Angiomyolipomas occur as solitary renal masses usually in women older than 40 years.[169] They also occur in more than 70% of patients with tuberous sclerosis, in whom they are frequently multiple and bilateral.[169] These tumors are usually asymptomatic and are often discovered incidentally during abdominal imaging. However, patients sometimes present with flank pain or hematuria due to intratumoral or perinephric hemorrhage.[169]

Angiomyolipomas are seen on CT as well-circumscribed renal masses. They vary in size from tiny renal nodules to large tumors (Fig. 35-92). Patients with tuberous sclerosis often show extensive bilateral renal involvement by these lesions (Fig. 35-93). The presence of intratumoral fat is almost diagnostic of angiomyolipomas,[27] although in rare cases fat has been reported in Wilms' tumor in children[134] and in renal oncocytomas.[37] The presence of fat is best shown by CT. MRI may also detect the presence of fat in renal angiomyolipomas. The fat has a similar signal intensity to perinephric fat on spin-echo and gradient-echo pulse sequences, and the fat signal is suppressed on images obtained with fat-saturation techniques.[161]

Problems in diagnosis occur when angiomyolipomas are composed predominantly of muscle or vascular tissue and contain only minimal amounts of fat.[27] Such small amounts of fat can be easily overlooked unless searched for carefully in the CT study. Careful sampling of low-density regions within such masses should be performed using small regions of interest, because a large

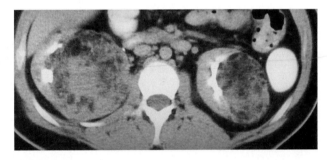

Fig. 35-93. Tuberous sclerosis with multiple bilateral renal angiomyolipomas. The lesions contain low-density areas consistent with fat.

region of interest may produce an average attenuation value in the soft-tissue range. Measurements should be made on unenhanced 5-mm sections to avoid partial volume effects from adjacent enhancing renal parenchyma (Fig. 35-92). Fatty tissue is considered to be present in a tumor if a region-of-interest measurement of −10 HU or lower is found within the tumor.[27] Lesions without detectable fat cannot be distinguished by imaging from other renal neoplasms (Fig. 35-94). Extensive intratumoral hemorrhage may also obscure the presence of fat.

Angiomyolipomas are always benign in that no deaths from metastatic disease have been documented.[169,172] However, the tumors may exhibit extrarenal extension. Large perinephric tumor components may be found (Fig. 35-95), and angiomyolipomas may extend into the renal vein and inferior vena cava, as

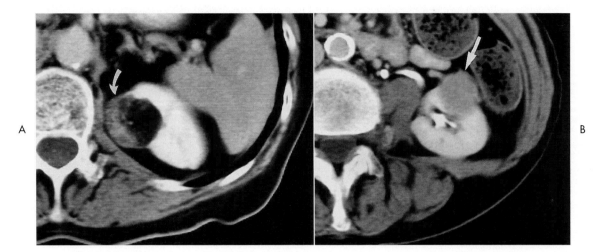

Fig. 35-94. Two left renal angiomyolipomas in a patient without tuberous sclerosis. **A,** A lesion *(curved arrow)* in the upper pole of the left kidney contains fat indicating the diagnosis of angiomyolipoma. **B,** A mass *(arrow)* in the midregion of the kidney contained no detectable fat and was therefore indistinguishable from a renal cell carcinoma. Nephrectomy revealed that both lesions were angiomyolipomas, although the lesion shown in **B** had only a minimal fat content.

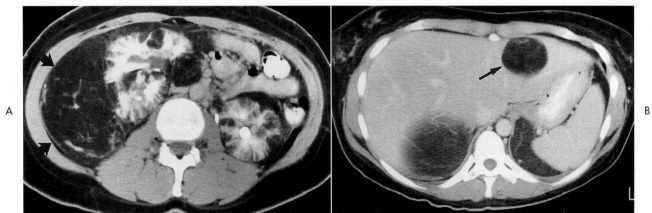

Fig. 35-95. Tuberous sclerosis with renal and liver involvement. **A,** The kidneys show multiple fat-containing lesions. On the right side, there is extensive involvement of the perinephric space by an angiomyolipoma *(arrows)* containing fat and prominent blood vessels. The right kidney is displaced anteromedially. **B,** A fat-containing mass *(arrow)* is present in the left lobe of the liver. (Courtesy of Randi W. Hart, M.D., Waukesha, Wis.)

shown by CT.[4] Regional lymph node involvement may also occur in patients with and without tuberous sclerosis.[153,172] Coincident renal cell carcinoma and renal angiomyolipomas may occur in tuberous sclerosis, and the renal cell carcinomas may sometimes metastasize.[73,172] However, there is no definite evidence that patients with tuberous sclerosis show a greater prevalence of renal cell carcinoma than the general population.

Surgery and biopsy are rarely needed in asymptomatic patients with typical imaging findings of angiomyolipoma. Patients with extensive intratumoral or perinephric hemorrhage can usually be managed conservatively (Fig. 35-96). However, if bleeding continues, percutaneous arterial tumor embolization may be used if the bleeding is arterial and if the bleeding site can be identified angiographically.[119,169] Surgery may rarely become

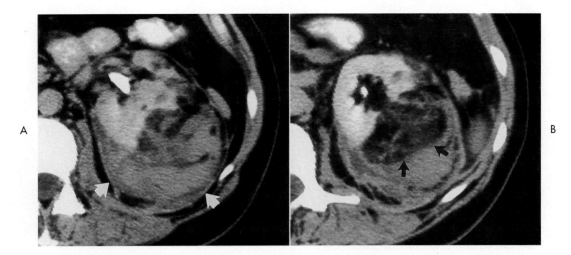

Fig. 35-96. Extensive left perinephric hematoma due to hemorrhage from a renal angiomyolipoma. **A,** The hematoma *(arrows)* is partially contained by the posterior renorenal bridging septum. **B,** A more cephalad scan shows a fat-containing angiomyolipoma *(arrows)* closely related to the hematoma. The bleeding responded to conservative management.

necessary in patients in whom bleeding does not respond to conservative management.[172]

PELVICALYCEAL AND URETERAL NEOPLASMS

Primary neoplasms of the renal pelvis, calyces, and ureter are relatively uncommon. CT plays a limited but often important role in the diagnosis and staging of these tumors.

Pelvicalyceal neoplasms

About 90% of pelvicalyceal cancers are transitional cell carcinomas, about 9% are squamous cell carcinomas, and less than 1% are adenocarcinomas.[70,96] Occupational exposure to industrial dyes, phenacetin abuse, cigarette smoking, prior cyclophosphamide therapy, and urinary stasis associated with horseshoe kidneys predispose an individual to the development of transitional cell carcinoma.[96,101,136] Squamous cell carcinoma of the renal pelvis is commonly associated with chronic irritation secondary to renal calculi and chronic infection. Transitional cell carcinoma has a peak frequency in the sixth and seventh decades of life, and about 68% of affected patients are men.[136] About 90% of patients present with painless hematuria.[136] Transitional cell carcinoma of the renal pelvis is frequently multicentric with either synchronous or metachronous tumor involvement of the ureter, bladder, and contralateral renal pelvis.[136]

CT diagnosis. Imaging findings in urothelial cancer include a calyceal or renal pelvic filling defect, hydronephrosis with a nonfunctioning kidney, and extensive renal parenchymal infiltration.[96] Although the diagnosis

of pelvicalyceal cancer is usually established by various combinations of excretory urography, retrograde pyelography, urine cytologic analysis, retrograde brush biopsy and ureteroscopy, and biopsy,[177] these techniques may not be definitive and CT may help distinguish between urothelial cancer and other causes of these imaging findings.[96]

CT evaluation of pelvicalyceal filling defects of unknown nature shown by excretory urography or retrograde pyelography requires a series of 5- or 10-mm-thick contiguous unenhanced scans of the kidneys. A repeat series of similar scans is obtained after rapid intravenous administration of contrast material. Small pelvicalyceal neoplasms may be difficult to detect on precontrast scans, although occasional neoplasms show coarse, punctate calcification.[42] After intravenous contrast injection, pelvicalyceal neoplasms are detected as collecting system filling defects with smooth, lobulated, or irregular margins (Fig. 35-97).[7] Precontrast attenuation values of pelvicalyceal cancers range from 20 to 46 HU.[133] Although characteristically hypovascular on angiography, pelvicalyceal tumors often show mild enhancement on CT after intravenous contrast administration. Postcontrast attenuation values range from 64 to 84 HU.[133] Contrast enhancement differentiates pelvicalyceal neoplasms from other filling defects that occur in the collecting system.

Radiolucent renal calculi are usually composed predominantly of uric acid and are shown by CT as densities with attenuation values greater than 200 HU on unenhanced CT scans (Fig. 35-98).[49,159] The attenuation values of recent pelvicalyceal blood clots on unen-

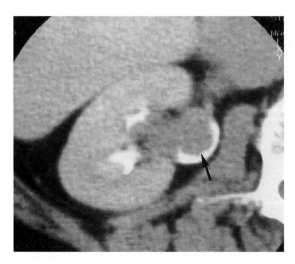

Fig. 35-97. Polypoid transitional cell carcinoma *(arrow)* of the right renal pelvis. The lesion invaded to but not beyond the muscularis. As compared with the unenhanced CT scan, the lesion enhanced by 36 HU.

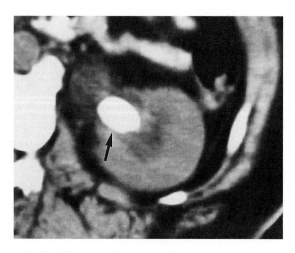

Fig. 35-98. Urate calculus *(arrow)* in the left renal pelvis. Excretory urography showed a pelvic filling defect, but the lesion was radiolucent on conventional tomography. The stone has an attenuation value of 458 HU.

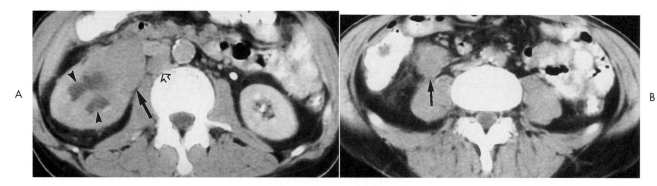

Fig. 35-99. Hydronephrosis due to transitional cell carcinoma of the right renal pelvis. **A,** A soft-tissue mass *(arrow)* fills the right renal pelvis. Dilated calyces *(arrowheads)* are seen in the right kidney. An enlarged retrocaval lymph node *(open arrow)* was involved by metastatic disease. **B,** The tumor also involved the upper half of the right ureter *(arrow)*.

hanced CT scans range from 45 to 75 HU; this is higher than that of urothelial cancer and lower than that of urate calculi.[96] Moreover, blood clots do not show contrast enhancement and follow-up studies show disappearance of blood clots with time.[96] Recognition that an apparent intrinsic pelvic filling defect is produced by extrinsic compression of the renal pelvis by renal sinus lipomatosis, renal sinus cysts, renal cell carcinomas, and lymphoma is readily attained by CT.

The hydronephrotic form of urothelial cancer with a nonfunctioning kidney is due to ureteropelvic junction obstruction and may present a diagnostic problem on excretory urography.[96] Although retrograde py-

elography may suggest the diagnosis, CT sometimes provides a definitive diagnosis (Fig. 35-99).[158] An enhancing soft-tissue mass at the apex of a dilated renal pelvis or diffuse thickening of the renal pelvic wall on CT indicates a tumor causing ureteropelvic junction obstruction. The proximal ureter may be thickened and filled from invasion by the neoplasm (Fig. 35-99).[96] Most cases of ureteropelvic junction obstruction are congenital in origin, and on CT a dilated renal pelvis with a smooth wall and a smooth transition at the ureteropelvic junction to the collapsed proximal ureter is seen.[158] A calculus impacted at the ureteropelvic junction is easily shown by CT. Extrinsic lesions causing ureteropelvic

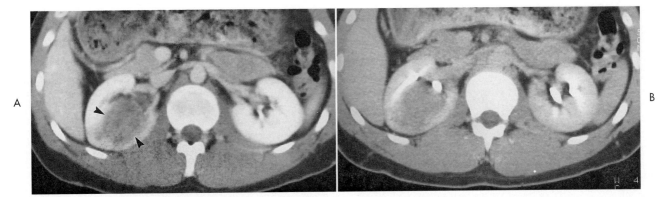

Fig. 35-100. Transitional cell carcinoma of the right renal pelvis in a 20-year-old man associated with cyclophosphamide therapy 6 years earlier. **A,** Dynamic CT scan obtained immediately after bolus injection of contrast material shows an enhancing mass (*arrowheads;* attenuation value = 71 HU) in the right renal pelvis. The precontrast attenuation value was 43 HU. The mass obliterates and invades the renal sinus fat. A poorly defined margin between the tumor and the renal parenchyma indicates parenchymal invasion. **B,** A CT scan obtained 5 minutes after **A** shows displacement of the opacified collecting system. (From Levine E: *AJR* 159:1027, 1992.)

junction obstruction (e.g., enlarged lymph nodes or retroperitoneal neoplasms) are also easily diagnosed by CT.[158]

Another presentation of urothelial cancer is that of extensive parenchymal infiltration of the kidney.[96] Urothelial cancer is centrally located, and its pattern of renal invasion differs from the eccentric origin and invasion of the renal sinus seen in renal cell carcinoma.[96] Urothelial cancers do not usually distort the shape of the kidney.[96] A central mass that is less dense than normal renal parenchyma and shows minimal tumor enhancement strongly suggests a urothelial cancer (Fig. 35-100).[96] The renal sinus fat may be obliterated, and there is often a poorly defined margin between the tumor and the renal parenchyma.[96] The calyces may be displaced, compressed, or dilated.

Tumor Staging. In the past, preoperative determination of the extent of pelvicalyceal neoplasms was of limited importance because radical nephroureterectomy with resection of a cuff of bladder was almost always performed because of the tumor's tendency to recur locally.[177] However, because of the multicentricity of these tumors, a trend toward renal-conserving procedures for low-grade and/or low-volume lesions has developed in recent years.[177] This approach is also particularly useful in patients with solitary kidneys or previous urothelial tumors at other sites.[7] When conservative surgery is planned, CT is helpful for tumor staging.[177] Patients with high-grade and/or high-volume pelvicalyceal cancers have a high frequency of metastases, primarily to regional lymph nodes, lung, bones, and liver in decreasing

order of frequency.[177] Abdominal and chest CT scans are most helpful in these cases. If metastases or local extension into adjacent organs are documented, the prognosis is extremely poor, and nonsurgical treatment may then be appropriate.[177]

Although CT cannot determine the depth of tumor invasion in the renal pelvic wall (Fig. 35-97), it can determine whether the tumor has extended beyond the muscularis into the renal sinus fat.[7] Renal sinus fat invasion is suggested by obliteration of the peripelvic fat stripe, which is the renal sinus fat separating the anterior and posterior cortical hilar lips from the renal pelvic adventitia (Fig. 35-100).[7] Invasive renal pelvic tumors may become attached to the aorta and inferior vena cava and may invade the psoas muscle (Fig. 35-101). Tumor extension into the renal vein and inferior vena cava may in rare cases be shown by CT.[61] CT may also show regional lymph node metastases (Fig. 35-102), although CT sometimes understages tumors with metastases in normal-sized central retroperitoneal lymph nodes.[7] MRI is not used frequently in the diagnosis and management of urothelial tumors. However, it may help determine local tumor extent.

Ureteral neoplasms

Transitional cell carcinoma accounts for about 93% of ureteral neoplasms. Of the remainder, 5% are squamous cell carcinomas, and 2% are adenocarcinomas.[136] The age and gender distribution, symptoms, and causes are similar to those for pelvicalyceal carcinoma. Tumors have a predilection for the mid and distal ure-

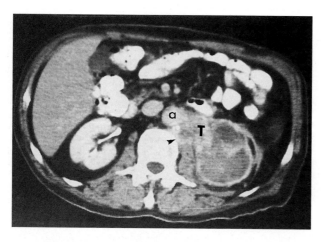

Fig. 35-101. Invasive transitional cell carcinoma of the left renal pelvis. The tumor *(T)* causes left hydronephrosis. It extends through the wall of the renal pelvis and is attached to the aorta *(a)* and the left psoas muscle *(arrowhead)*. Complete resection was not possible.

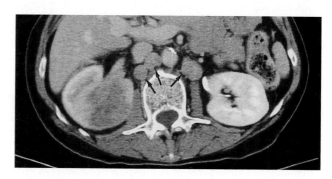

Fig. 35-102. Transitional cell carcinoma of the right renal pelvis with extensive parenchymal invasion and regional nodal metastases *(arrows)*.

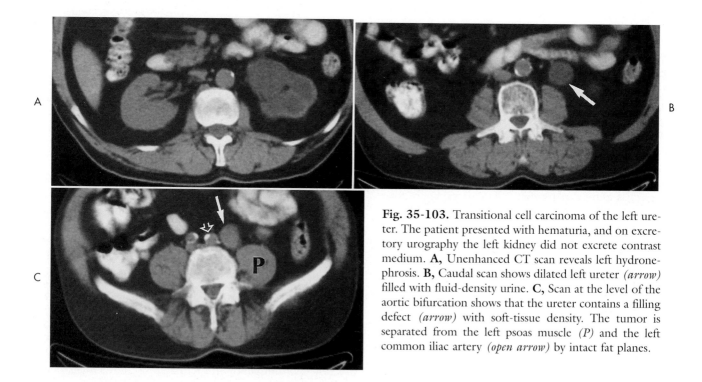

Fig. 35-103. Transitional cell carcinoma of the left ureter. The patient presented with hematuria, and on excretory urography the left kidney did not excrete contrast medium. **A,** Unenhanced CT scan reveals left hydronephrosis. **B,** Caudal scan shows dilated left ureter *(arrow)* filled with fluid-density urine. **C,** Scan at the level of the aortic bifurcation shows that the ureter contains a filling defect *(arrow)* with soft-tissue density. The tumor is separated from the left psoas muscle *(P)* and the left common iliac artery *(open arrow)* by intact fat planes.

ter.[136] The diagnosis of ureteral carcinoma is usually readily established using a combination of excretory urography and retrograde pyelography. However, CT may help by confirming that a ureteric filling defect represents a neoplasm and not a radiolucent calculus or blood clot. Ureteral neoplasms present on CT as soft-tissue intraluminal filling defects (Fig. 35-103), often with ureteral widening or thickening of the ureteral wall.

These are findings that can also occur in inflammatory conditions and ureteral metastases.[96] CT also helps determine whether a ureteral neoplasm has extended outside the muscularis to involve the retroperitoneal fat (Fig. 35-103) and surrounding structures, or whether it has metastasized to regional lymph nodes.

An important use of CT is in determining whether ureteral obstruction is due to an intrinsic neoplasm or extrinsic disease, when excretory urography and retrograde pyelography are indeterminate.[26] CT is particularly useful in detecting such causes of extrinsic ureteric obstruction as idiopathic and malignant retroperitoneal fibrosis, inflammatory aortic aneurysm, and lymphomatous and metastatic retroperitoneal adenopathy.[26]

RENAL INFECTIONS

Acute bacterial renal infection

Acute bacterial renal infection in adults frequently causes fever, chills, flank pain, leukocytosis, pyuria, and bacteriuria. It occurs significantly more commonly in women than in men. Vesicoureteric reflux is sometimes an important predisposing factor in children, but it is only rarely found in adults with acute pyelonephritis. Acute renal infection may be due to ascending infection from the bladder or may result from hematogenous dissemination of organisms.[128,165] Most infections are caused by gram-negative organisms such as *Escherichia coli*, but gram-positive organisms such as *Staphylococcus aureus* may sometimes be responsible.[128,165] The diagnosis of acute bacterial renal infection is usually made clinically, and antibiotic therapy is started. About 95% of patients with uncomplicated infections treated with appropriate antibiotics become afebrile in 48 hours, and nearly 100% do so in 72 hours.[165] Such patients do not need renal imaging.

However, imaging studies are valuable in patients with severe refractory renal infections. Imaging is needed to determine if there are complications requiring prolonged antibiotic therapy or surgical intervention (e.g., renal and perinephric abscess or pyonephrosis). Imaging is also useful for excluding abnormalities such as nephrolithiasis or ureteric obstruction that predispose to refractory infections. CT is a useful imaging technique for both diagnosis and treatment in patients with refractory acute bacterial renal infections.[66,67,79,165] As shown by CT, acute bacterial renal infection spans a continuum of severity from uncomplicated acute pyelonephritis through progressively worsening stages of tubulo-interstitial inflammation to frank abscess formation.[66,67]

Acute pyelonephritis. In acute pyelonephritis inflammatory cells in the renal tubules and interstitial edema cause obstruction of the tubules and compression and spasm of the local vasculature.[66,67] The involved parenchyma is affected as a group of lobules or an entire renal lobe. Kidneys with clinically mild and uncomplicated acute pyelonephritis often appear normal on CT. However, with more severe infection, a variety of abnormalities may be noted on CT; these may be unilateral or bilateral. Some patients with acute pyelonephritis show diffuse renal involvement on CT. This is manifest by poor renal contrast enhancement, delayed to absent excretion of contrast medium, and global renal enlargement (Fig.

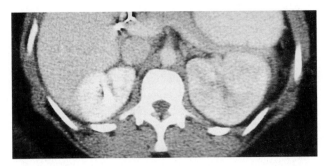

Fig. 35-104. Acute pyelonephritis with diffuse renal involvement. The affected left kidney shows diminished contrast enhancement, global enlargement, and delayed contrast excretion. The right kidney is normal.

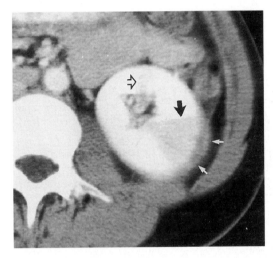

Fig. 35-105. Acute pyelonephritis. The kidney shows a wedge-shaped zone *(black arrow)* of decreased attenuation. The lesion exhibits straight borders, radiates from the collecting system to the renal capsule, and is widest at the kidney periphery. There is inflammatory change in the adjacent perinephric fat and localized renal fascial thickening *(white arrows)*. A similar but smaller zone of inflammation *(open arrow)* is present anteriorly.

35-104).[66,67] Other patients show unifocal or multifocal renal abnormalities with extensive areas of apparently uninvolved renal parenchyma.[67] These abnormalities are seen on contrast-enhanced CT scans as wedge-shaped zones of decreased attenuation (Fig. 35-105). They often manifest straight borders, radiate from the collecting system to the renal capsule, and are widest at the periphery of the kidney.[66,67] A small percentage of patients with acute pyelonephritis show hemorrhage into these regions, evident on unenhanced CT scans as wedge-shaped zones of high attenuation.[147]

Severe tubulo-interstitial inflammation may progress to form a hypodense mass or masses with rounded or irregular contours and bulging of the renal surface (Fig. 35-106).[66,67] If treated too late or inadequately, such lesions may develop single or multiple small areas of liquefaction (i.e. small abscesses).[66,67] These areas are often irregular and of near-water attenuation (20 to 30 HU); they do not enhance after intravenous administration of contrast medium (Fig. 35-107). Small abscesses often eventually heal with long-term antibiotic therapy (6 to 8 weeks). Areas of severe tubuloin-terstitial inflammation can be followed, if necessary, by serial CT. Ultimately, the kidney may return to normal, or scarring of the affected regions of the kidney as well as papillary necrosis and global parenchymal loss may occur.[66]

Renal and perinephric abscesses. If inadequately treated, small abscesses in areas of severe tubulointerstitial inflammation may coalesce to form macroabscesses. On contrast-enhanced CT scans, renal abscesses usually have attenuation values of about 30 H; this distinguishes them from fluid-density renal cysts.[165] Their contents do not enhance. They may have distinct, rounded margins and thick enhancing walls (Figs. 35-108 and 35-109).[98,165] Alternatively, abscesses may be ill-defined and surrounded by zones of decreased parenchymal enhance-

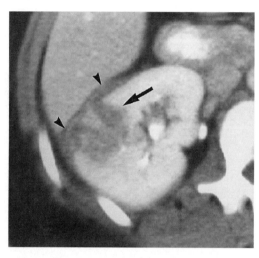

Fig. 35-106. Acute pyelonephritis with focal mass formation. The kidney shows a rounded, heterogeneous mass *(arrow)* with a poorly defined margin. Inflammatory changes in the adjacent perinephric fat and renal fascial thickening *(arrowheads)* are also present.

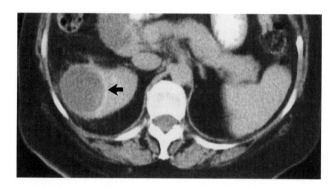

Fig. 35-108. Right renal abscess *(arrow)* shows a thick wall and low-density (30 HU). Inflammatory stranding is present in the perinephric fat.

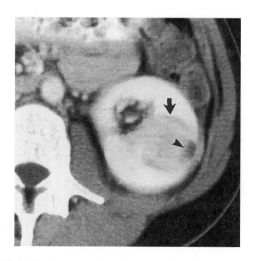

Fig. 35-107. Acute pyelonephritis with early abscess formation. The inflammatory mass *(arrow)* shows a small, peripheral area of liquefaction *(arrowhead)*.

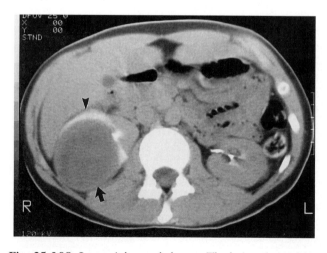

Fig. 35-109. Large right renal abscess. The lesion *(arrow)* has an attenuation value of 36 HU and shows a thick wall. High-density renal parenchyma on its anteromedial aspect *(arrowhead)* is probably due to retention of contrast medium in compressed and obstructed renal tubules on the periphery of the abscess.

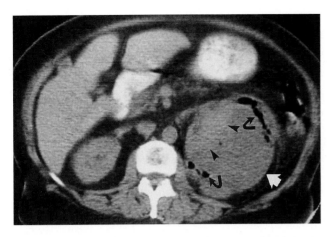

Fig. 35-110. Unenhanced CT scan shows a perinephric abscess *(white arrow)* complicating acute pyelonephritis in a diabetic patient. Gas collections *(curved arrows)* are present in the abscess, and the left kidney *(arrowheads)* is displaced anteriorly.

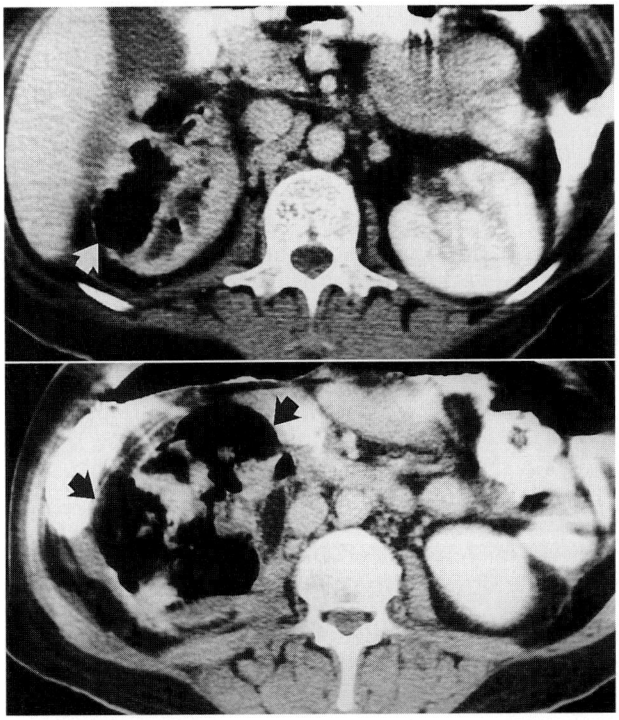

ment, representing inflammation that has not yet progressed to necrosis.[165] Gas is occasionally found in renal abscesses.[128] Focal thickening of the adjacent renal fascia and stranding in the adjacent perinephric fat are common CT findings.[79,98] A perinephric abscess may ultimately result if the infection extends through the renal capsule (Fig. 35-110).[67,165] Although small renal abscesses may respond to antibiotic therapy alone,[66,98] percutaneous drainage is usually the treatment of choice in patients with larger renal abscesses. Perinephric abscesses always require drainage.[128] Abscesses can be drained using a combination of sonographic and fluoroscopic guidance.[154]

Emphysematous Pyelonephritis. Emphysematous pyelonephritis is a diffuse gas-forming parenchymal infection. It is a serious complication of acute pyelonephritis and occurs typically in diabetic patients secondary to *Escherichia coli* infection. CT is the most sensitive method for establishing the diagnosis and can also distinguish among gas in the collecting system, parenchymal gas, and gas in the perinephric tissues (Fig. 35-111).[66] Gas in the renal pelvis or calyces alone does not qualify as emphysematous pyelonephritis (Fig. 35-112).[66]

Pyonephrosis. Pyonephrosis is the accumulation of pus in an obstructed pelvicalyceal system. It may occur when urinary tract infection occurs in patients with ureteric obstruction due to calculi, strictures, developmental ureteric anomalies, or malignant disease.[183] Pyonephrosis is often associated with severe urosepsis. It represents a true urologic emergency requiring either urgent percutaneous nephrostomy or passage of a ureteral stent to bypass the obstruction (Fig. 35-113). Sonography is the imaging method of choice for diagnosis of pyonephrosis.[85] However, sonography often cannot distinguish between simple hydronephrosis and pyonephrosis.[85] Accordingly, sonographically guided diagnostic

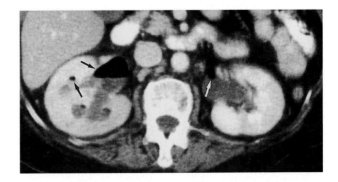

Fig. 35-112. Emphysematous pyelitis in a diabetic patient. Gas is present in both collecting systems *(arrows)*, but the right kidney is more significantly involved. The renal parenchyma is uninvolved, and the infection responded to antibiotic therapy.

Fig. 35-111. Emphysematous pyelonephritis in a diabetic patient. There is extensive destruction of the right kidney (**A** and **B**), which is largely replaced by gas *(arrow)*. Gas is also present in the perinephric space *(arrows)* (**B**). A right nephrectomy was performed.

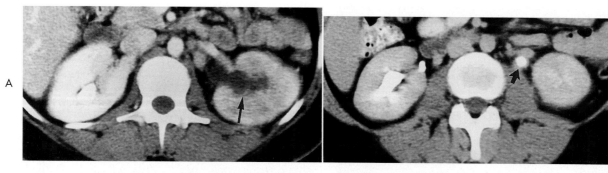

Fig. 35-113. Pyonephrosis and severe urosepsis due to an obstructing left ureteric urate calculus not visible on plain films. **A,** There is decreased enhancement of the left renal parenchyma, and the left renal pelvis is dilated with delayed contrast excretion *(arrow)*. **B,** An obstructing calculus *(arrow)* is present in the proximal ureter. Differentiation between simple hydronephrosis and pyonephrosis could not be made by CT. However, the diagnosis of pyonephrosis was suggested by clinical findings. The patient responded rapidly to percutaneous nephrostomy.

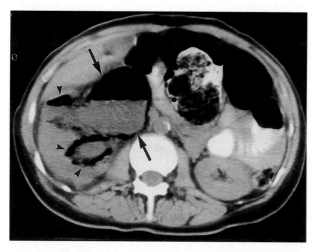

Fig. 35-114. Pyonephrosis complicating congenital ureteropelvic junction obstruction in a diabetic patient. The significantly dilated right renal pelvis *(arrows)* shows a gas fluid level, and gas is also present in dilated calyces *(arrowheads)*.

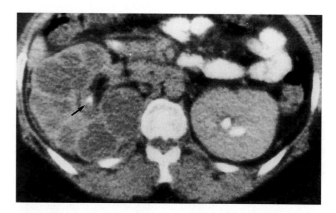

Fig. 35-115. Xanthogranulomatous pyelonephritis. The right kidney is globally enlarged, shows no contrast excretion, and is replaced by multiple, rounded, fluid-density areas. A calculus *(arrow)* is present in a nondilated renal pelvis with a thickened wall. (Courtesy of David S. Hartman, M.D., Hershey, Pa.)

needle aspiration may be required in patients with urosepsis and significant hydronephrosis. On CT, patients with pyonephrosis may show increased pelvic wall thickness, inflammatory changes in the perinephric fat, and in rare cases, layering of intravenously injected contrast material anterior to the pus in the dilated renal pelvis.[56,183] Pelvicalyceal system gas in the absence of a history of urinary tract instrumentation, although uncommon, is a strong diagnostic indicator of pyonephrosis (Fig. 35-114).[56] However, CT usually cannot reliably distinguish between infected and uninfected hydronephrosis (Fig. 35-113). The presence of clinical signs of infection in the presence of hydronephrosis is an indica-

tor more sensitive than CT findings of pyonephrosis. CT may show the site and cause of urinary tract obstruction (Fig. 35-113).[183]

Chronic renal infections

Xanthogranulomatous pyelonephritis. *Xanthogranulomatous pyelonephritis* is a chronic granulomatous disorder of the kidney associated with indolent bacterial infection. The inflammatory process begins in the renal pelvis and later extends into the medulla and cortex, which are gradually destroyed and replaced by lipid-laden macrophages (xanthoma cells).[69] The disease is usually diffuse, but may be focal. Patients are typically middle-aged women.[69] Systemic symptoms include malaise, fever, chills, and weight loss. Nonspecific urinary

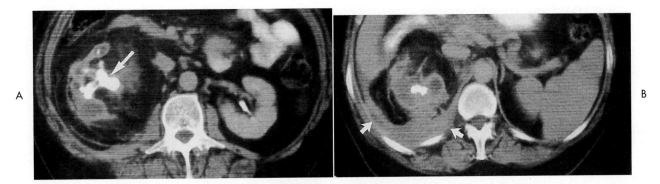

Fig. 35-116. Xanthogranulomatous pyelonephritis with a contracted kidney. **A,** A staghorn calculus *(arrow)* is present in the right renal pelvis. The right kidney is small and replaced by oval, fluid-density areas. **B,** A more cephalad scan shows extensive chronic inflammatory change *(arrows)* in the posterior pararenal space.

symptoms include flank pain, increased frequency of micturition, dysuria, and nocturia. *Proteus* and/or *Escherichia coli* organisms are commonly cultured from the urine. CT is valuable in diagnosis and preoperative planning.[69] Nephrectomy is usually required particularly in the diffuse form of the disease.[88]

On CT, diffuse xanthogranulomatous pyelonephritis is usually characterized by a globally enlarged, nonfunctioning kidney (Fig. 35-115). Less commonly a small, contracted kidney with replacement lipomatosis is found (Fig. 35-116).[69] Often, there is a staghorn calculus in a nondilated, encased renal pelvis (Fig. 35-116).[69] Multiple fluid-density rounded areas almost completely replace the renal parenchyma (Fig. 35-115). Pathologically, these represent either dilated calyces or focal areas of parenchymal destruction filled with pus and/or debris.[69] Histologically, these cavities are lined by xanthoma cells.[69] Rim enhancement of the low-density areas often occurs.[69] Extrarenal extension of the inflammatory process is common and may involve the perinephric space, pararenal spaces, ipsilateral psoas muscle, flank muscles, diaphragm, and skin (Fig. 35-116).[69] Perinephric and psoas abscesses often occur. In the focal form of xanthogranulomatous pyelonephritis, CT shows a poorly enhancing mass adjacent to a calyx or in one pole of a kidney with a duplicated collecting system.[162] Associated calculi may be found. The focal form may be misdiagnosed as a renal neoplasm.[162] Associated involvement of the perinephric and pararenal spaces may occur.[88]

Malacoplakia. Malacoplakia is a rare granulomatous inflammatory disease associated with chronic *Escherichia coli* infection. Affected patients are usually middle-aged women with recurrent urinary tract infections.[88] Malacoplakia is attributed to abnormal monocyte function, and the monocytes in the granulomatous masses contain oval basophilic inclusions called

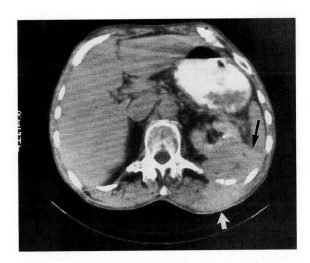

Fig. 35-117. Renal parenchymal malacoplakia. CT shows a nonspecific soft-tissue mass *(black arrow)* extending from the left kidney and invading the perinephric space and the left flank *(white arrow).* (Courtesy of David S. Hartman, M.D., Hershey, Pa.)

Michaelis-Gutmann bodies. Renal parenchymal malacoplakia is usually unilateral and multiple poorly defined hypodense cortical masses may be shown by CT. Nephromegaly and perinephric extension of disease may occur.[88] The CT findings are nonspecific, and renal parenchymal malacoplakia may be indistinguishable from a neoplasm (Fig. 35-117).

Tuberculosis. Renal tuberculosis usually results from hematogenous dissemination of a pulmonary infection. The diagnosis is usually best made by excretory urography, which shows typical calyceal and ureteric abnormalities. CT may show a variety of abnormalities, many of which are nonspecific. Obstruction of a single major calyx or of a group of minor calyces often occurs

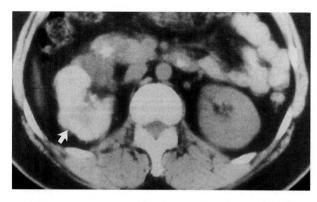

Fig. 35-118. Renal tuberculosis with diffuse parenchymal calcification involving most of the right kidney *(arrow)* as shown on an unenhanced CT scan. (Courtesy of David S. Hartman, M.D., Hershey, Pa.)

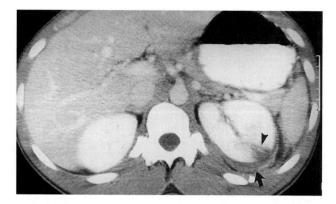

Fig. 35-120. Category I renal trauma. There is a small cortical laceration *(arrowhead)* involving the left kidney. An associated small perinephric hematoma is present *(arrow)*.

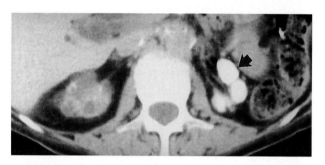

Fig. 35-119. Renal tuberculosis. The left kidney shows large, oval, dense calcifications *(arrow)* representing calcified caseating material in medullary cavities and dilated calyces (tuberculous autonephrectomy). Low-density areas in the right kidney probably represent foci of caseous necrosis.

because of scarring. The obstructed calyces are dilated and show no excretion of contrast medium, and thinning of the overlying renal parenchyma occurs.[88] Tuberculosis of the renal pelvis is manifested either by hydronephrosis secondary to ureteropelvic junction obstruction or diffuse pelvic contraction with fibrosis extending down a thickened ureter. Low-density parenchymal lesions probably representing areas of caseous necrosis may be seen.[88] Fine diffuse parenchymal calcification, often in a lobar distribution, may be found (Fig. 35-118). In a tuberculous "putty kidney," large, round or oval, dense renal calcifications representing calcified caseating material in medullary cavities and dilated calyces are found. This condition is also called tuberculous autonephrectomy and is due to the superimposition of ureteral obstruction on renal parenchymal tuberculosis (Fig. 35-119).

RENAL TRAUMA

Renal trauma may be caused by both blunt and penetrating abdominal injuries. Blunt trauma is responsible for most renal injuries. Such injuries are usually mild and heal without specific therapy.[48] Serious renal injury is often associated with damage to other structures such as the liver, spleen, bowel, pancreas, or chest. Multiorgan involvement occurs in about 80% of patients with penetrating injuries and in about 20% of those with blunt trauma.[48]

Imaging classification and management

Categorization of renal injuries according to severity provides a helpful guide to patient management. Renal injuries are classified into four categories based on imaging findings.[48] Category I lesions (75% to 85% of cases) are clinically insignificant; they include contusions and small corticomedullary lacerations that do not communicate with the collecting system (Fig. 35-120). They are managed nonoperatively.[138,182] Category II lesions (10% of cases) are more serious and consist of corticomedullary lacerations that communicate with the collecting system, as manifested by urine extravasation (Fig. 35-121). Many of these lesions are managed nonoperatively. However, surgery is sometimes required in patients with extensive hemorrhage or urinary extravasation and a large amount of nonviable renal tissue.[48] Category III lesions (5% of cases) are catastrophic and consist of shattered kidneys and injuries to the renal pedicle (Figs. 35-122, 35-123). The rare entities of ureteropelvic junction avulsion and laceration of the renal pelvis are designated as Category IV lesions. Category III and IV renal trauma usually require surgical intervention.[138,182] Subcapsular and perinephric hematomas may occur in any of the categories of renal trauma.[163] Although an image-based classification of renal trauma is useful in guiding man-

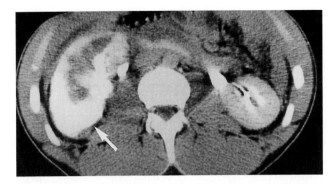

Fig. 35-121. Category II renal trauma. A renal laceration (not shown) involved the collecting system, resulting in contrast extravasation into the right perinephric space *(arrow)*. The lesion responded to conservative management.

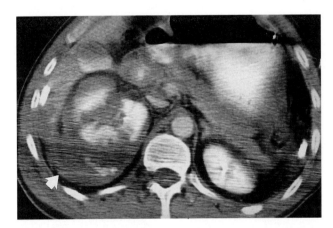

Fig. 35-122. Category III renal trauma—shattered kidney. There are multiple right renal lacerations with the fragments separated by blood clot. An associated perinephric hematoma *(arrow)* is present. A right nephrectomy was performed.

agement, treatment is often ultimately determined by the patient's clinical status.

Imaging of renal trauma

Gross hematuria is the most reliable indication of potentially serious renal damage.[167] Patients who sustain deceleration injuries in motor vehicle accidents or who fall from a height should be considered at risk for renal pedicle injuries regardless of the presence or absence of hematuria.[48] CT should be the primary study for evaluating suspected renal trauma when multiple abdominal injuries are suspected, when a severe renal injury is suspected, or when CT is already being performed to evaluate head or chest trauma.[138]

However, excretory urography is an appropriate alternative in stable, asymptomatic patients clinically evaluated to have only minor, exclusively renal inju-

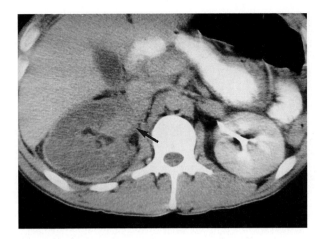

Fig. 35-123. Category III renal trauma—occlusion of the right main renal artery. The right kidney shows absence of contrast enhancement except for a subcapsular rim of renal tissue perfused via capsular collateral vessels. Aortography showed occlusion of the main right renal artery. A hematoma *(arrow)* is present around the renal vascular pedicle.

ries.[138] Most of these patients have normal findings at excretory urography, all but ruling out significant renal damage. CT is used as a secondary procedure when urography suggests a severe renal parenchymal injury or when deterioration of the patient's condition occurs.[138] Unilateral absence of contrast excretion at urography may be secondary to renal artery or vein occlusion, severe laceration, subcapsular hematoma, or to preexisting renal disease or renal agenesis.[138] Immediate CT should be performed because renal artery occlusion requires urgent surgical management if the kidney is to be salvaged.

Contrast-enhanced CT is the most accurate imaging technique for categorizing renal trauma and for detecting associated abdominal visceral injuries.[48] The three basic types of renal injury demonstrable by CT are contusions, lacerations, and infarcts, any of which may be further complicated by intrarenal or extrarenal hematomas or by urine extravasation.[138] The mildest form of renal injury is the contusion, characterized by an amorphous, interstitial extravasation of blood and edema. On unenhanced CT scans, the affected kidney zones may show focal swelling and irregular infiltrates of high-density fresh blood. After IV contrast material administration, small interstitial accumulations of contrast medium and areas of diminished perfusion are seen on the affected areas.[48,138]

Superficial lacerations are limited to the renal cortex (Fig. 35-120); deep ones extend into the medulla (Fig. 35-124) where they may enter the collecting system and/or transect the kidney.[138] Contrast extravasation is often seen in the perinephric space (Fig. 35-121).

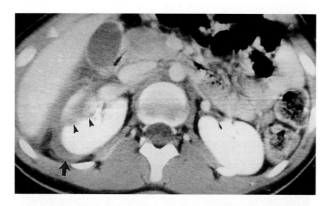

Fig. 35-124. Deep renal laceration *(arrowheads)* extending into the renal medulla without involvement of the collecting system. A small perinephric hematoma *(arrow)* is present.

In patients with multiple lacerations (shattered kidney), the fragments are separated and surrounded by blot clot (Fig. 35-122).[138] Renal infarcts are due to arterial injury and may be either focal or global (Fig. 35-125). Posttraumatic bleeding is commonly associated with all injuries to the kidney. Hematomas may be intrarenal or subcapsular, or may involve the perinephric or pararenal spaces.[163] Main renal artery injuries can be diagnosed by CT employing the criteria of absent renal contrast enhancement and excretion associated with "rim" cortical perfusion (Fig. 35-123). Other findings that suggest the diagnosis of pedicle injury include a hematoma surrounding the renal hilus (Fig. 35-123) and abrupt cutoff of the contrast-filled renal artery.[48] CT has a high sensitivity in detecting traumatic renal artery occlusion, although angiography is occasionally needed for diagnosis.[95] Acute renal vein occlusion may be suspected if the kidney is enlarged, and shows rim enhancement and thrombus in the renal vein.[46]

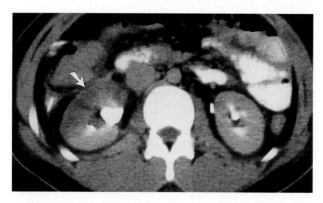

Fig. 35-125. Focal renal infarction after blunt trauma. The nephrogram is absent anteriorly *(arrow)* in the right kidney. "Rim" cortical perfusion of the infarct is present.

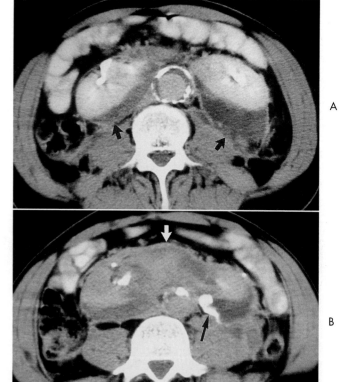

Fig. 35-127. Injury of horseshoe kidney. **A,** Bilateral perinephric hematomas *(arrows)* are present. **B,** A caudal scan shows a hematoma *(white arrow)* involving the isthmus connecting the two kidneys. There is contrast extravasation *(black arrow)* from the left collecting system because of a laceration.

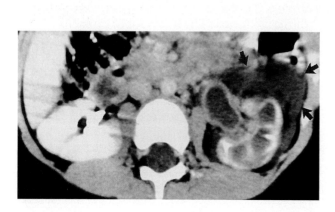

Fig. 35-126. Left perinephric urinoma *(arrows)* secondary to blunt trauma to a hydronephrotic left kidney. Hydronephrosis was due to congenital ureteropelvic junction obstruction.

Abnormal kidneys, including hydronephrotic kidneys (Fig. 35-126), ectopic, and horseshoe kidneys (Fig. 35-127), as well as kidneys containing neoplasms or cysts, may sustain injury secondary to minor trauma.[146] CT is an accurate method for detecting underlying abnormalities in the injured kidney.

MRI is not widely used in the evaluation of renal trauma, because of problems in using life-support systems in a strong magnetic field. However, MRI using fast scanning, gadolinium-DTPA enhancement, and angiographic techniques has the potential for showing most lesions that may result from renal injury.

RENAL BLOOD FLOW DISORDERS
Renal hemorrhage

CT is the most valuable examination in the evaluation of patients with suspected acute renal hemorrhage since it accurately diagnoses the presence and location of such hemorrhage and often shows the underlying cause.[14] Renal hemorrhage may be suburothelial, intraparenchymal, subcapsular, perinephric, or pararenal in location or may involve the renal sinus.[55,91,93]

Causes. The most common cause of renal hemorrhage is trauma either blunt or penetrating (Figs. 35-122, 35-127, 35-128). Extracorporeal shock wave lithotripsy for nephrolithiasis is another form of renal trauma not infrequently associated with parenchymal and perinephric hemorrhage (Fig. 35-129).[132] Spontaneous (nontraumatic) renal hemorrhage may be caused by anticoagulation, blood dyscrasias (Fig. 35-130), renal infarction, polyarteritis nodosa (Fig. 35-131), renal aneurysms and arteriovenous malformations, renal cell carcinoma, renal angiomyolipoma (see Fig. 35-96), renal abscess, renal vein thrombosis, and rupture of hemorrhagic solitary cysts (Fig. 35-132) or of hemorrhagic

cysts in renal cystic disease (see Figs. 35-32, 35-44).[14,40,57,104,107] Some cases are idiopathic.[14] Renal cell carcinoma is probably the most common cause of spontaneous subcapsular and perinephric hemorrhage.[14]

CT findings. Recent renal hemorrhage is characterized by high-attenuation blood (50 to 90 HU) best shown by unenhanced CT scans (Fig. 35-129). Postcontrast scans should also be obtained to facilitate identification of disorders such as small neoplasms causing spontaneous renal hemorrhage. Suburothelial hemorrhage is characterized on CT by thickening of the wall of the renal pelvis and upper ureter by blood that has a high attenuation value on unenhanced scans.[91] Spontaneous hemorrhage into the renal sinus is characterized by a

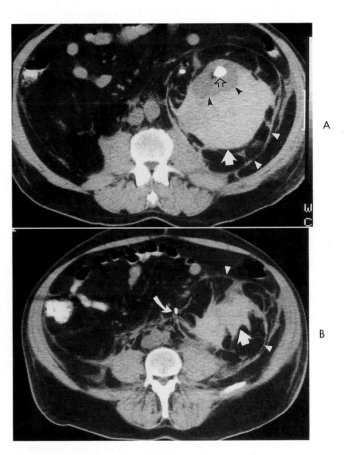

Fig. 35-129. Left perinephric hematoma secondary to extracorporeal shock wave lithotripsy. **A,** An unenhanced CT scan reveals anterior displacement of left kidney *(black arrowheads)* by high-density hematoma *(arrow)*. There is a calculus *(open arrow)* in the collecting system. The hematoma is limited posteriorly by the posterior renorenal bridging septum, which separates it from the thickened posterior renal fascia *(white arrowheads)*. **B,** The hematoma *(white arrow)* extends into the infrarenal fascial cone *(arrowheads)*. Infrarenal extension confirms the perinephric location of the hematoma and distinguishes it from a subcapsular hematoma. The left ureter *(curved arrow)* contains a stent and is displaced anteriorly.

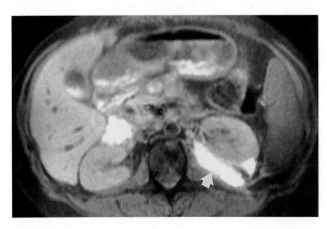

Fig. 35-128. Fat-suppressed T1-weighted MRI (600/17) shows a high-intensity left perinephric hematoma *(arrow)* due to a renal biopsy performed 2 weeks earlier. Loss of corticomedullary differentiation is due to chronic renal disease.

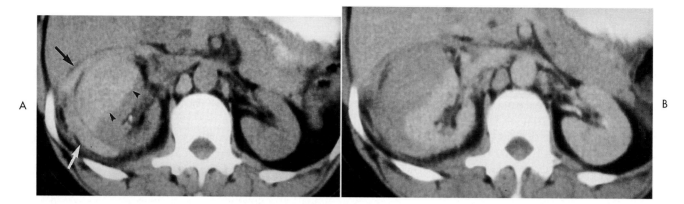

Fig. 35-130. Right subcapsular and perinephric hemorrhage associated with idiopathic thrombocytopenia. **A,** An unenhanced CT scan shows indentation of the lateral border *(arrowheads)* of the right kidney by a denser subcapsular hematoma. A smaller perinephric hematoma *(arrows)* is also present. **B,** A contrast-enhanced CT scan shows that the hematoma is less dense than the enhanced renal parenchyma. (From Levine E, Grantham JJ, MacDougall ML: *AJR* 148:755, 1987.)

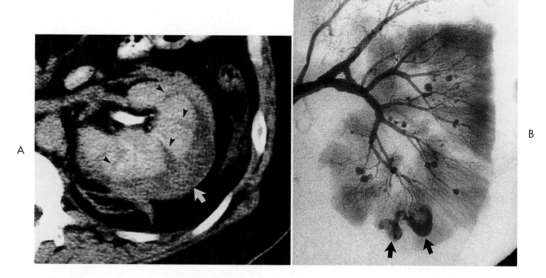

Fig. 35-131. Multiple renal infarcts and perinephric hemorrhage complicating polyarteritis nodosa. **A,** A left perinephric hematoma *(arrow)* is contained by the posterior renorenal bridging septum. There are several wedge-shaped infarcts *(arrowheads)* involving the renal parenchyma. **B,** A left selective renal arteriogram shows multiple small aneurysms arising from interlobar arteries. Active contrast extravasation *(arrows)* in the lower pole indicates bleeding from a ruptured aneurysm. The patient responded to selective embolization of the feeding artery. (Courtesy of James Bergh, M.D., Overland Park, KS.)

high-density blood collection in the renal sinus with displacement of the renal pelvis (Fig. 35-133).[55] Renal sinus hematomas usually resolve spontaneously, as shown by follow-up CT. Both suburothelial and renal sinus hemorrhage occur most commonly in anticoagulated patients or in those with bleeding or coagulation disorders.[55,91]

On an unenhanced CT scan, a recent subcapsular hematoma is characterized by a mass of higher attenuation value than that of adjacent renal parenchyma (Fig. 35-130). Pressure on the underlying renal parenchyma characteristically causes flattening of the kidney, elevation of the renal capsule, and medial displacement of the collecting system (Fig. 35-130). Sometimes, subcapsular

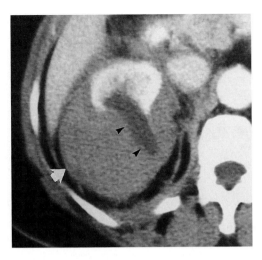

Fig. 35-132. Right perinephric hematoma *(arrow)* probably due to rupture of a simple renal cyst. The cyst *(arrowheads)* is flattened by the hematoma.

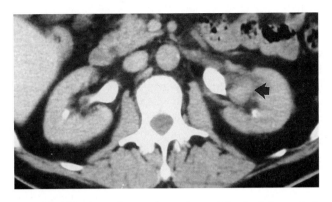

Fig. 35-133. Acute hemorrhage *(arrow)* in the left renal sinus associated with anticoagulant therapy displaces the renal pelvis.

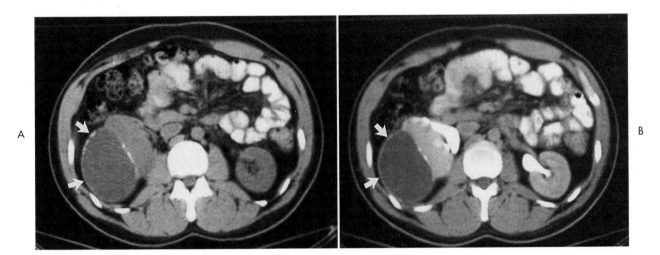

Fig. 35-134. Chronic calcified subcapsular hematoma in a hypertensive man. The low-density (17 HU) posterolateral mass with peripheral calcification *(arrows)* causes anteromedial displacement of the right kidney as seen on unenhanced **(A)** and contrast-enhanced **(B)** CT scans.

hematomas fail to resolve, causing chronic fluid collections that compress the renal parenchyma (Fig. 35-134). This, in turn, may cause hypertension by reducing renal blood flow, thereby triggering the renin-angiotensin-aldosterone system. This clinical entity is called the *Page kidney.*[28] The walls of chronic subcapsular hematomas may eventually calcify (Fig. 35-134).

Perinephric hematomas involve the fat between the renal capsule and the renal fascia. The configuration of such hematomas is determined largely by the bridging septa in the perinephric fat.[93] When a hematoma is confined by the posterior renorenal bridging septum, it

may compress and indent the renal surface, and because it is separated from the renal fascia, it may simulate a subcapsular hematoma (Figs. 35-129, 35-131).[93] However, while subcapsular hematomas are confined to the kidney by the renal capsule, perinephric hematomas often extend caudally below the kidney into the cone of renal fascia (Fig. 35-129).

CT often shows the cause of spontaneous subcapsular and perinephric hematomas.[14] Renal cell carcinomas or angiomyolipomas associated with such hematomas may be suspected on CT from the presence of a distinct mass clearly different in character from the surrounding hemorrhage (see Fig. 35-96).[14] Renal cell carcinomas present as heterogeneous, enhancing solid masses or as cystic masses, while an angiomyolipoma is suggested by the presence of tumor fat (see Fig. 35-96).[14] CT may show that hemorrhage originated in either a solitary renal cyst (Fig. 35-132)[40] or a cyst associated with hereditary or acquired renal cystic disease (see Figs. 35-32, 35-44).[104,107] If no cause for hemorrhage is shown by CT, renal angiography may help in showing underlying disorders such as angiitis, renal aneurysms, arteriovenous malformations, and polyarteritis nodosa (Fig. 35-131).[14]

Management. CT is valuable in the follow-up and management of renal hemorrhage whether due to trauma or occurring spontaneously. Patients with renal cell carcinomas complicated by hemorrhage are managed by nephrectomy, whereas patients with underlying hemorrhagic renal cysts, renal infarcts, or angiomyolipomas can usually be managed conservatively.[14,107] In those cases in which the bleeding is extensive and the patient is unstable, renal angiography with embolization (Fig. 35-131) or occasionally surgery may be necessary to stop the bleeding.[23,107] Patients with spontaneous renal hemorrhage who have no demonstrable cause for bleeding or for whom the diagnosis of the cause of the hemorrhage is in doubt should also be managed conservatively.[14,23] However, such patients should be followed by serial CT until the hematoma completely resolves to exclude an underlying renal cell carcinoma.[14,107] This approach avoids unnecessary nephrectomy in patients with spontaneous renal hemorrhage with benign renal disease or no underlying disease.[14,23]

Renal infarction

Renal infarction may be due to renal artery thrombosis or embolism, vasculitis as in polyarteritis nodosa, trauma, sickle cell disease, and aortic dissection.[139,180] CT findings depend on both the extent and age of infarction.[63] CT scans obtained without IV contrast enhancement usually show no abnormality in the presence of renal infarction, unless there is associated perinephric hemorrhage. However, occasionally renal infarcts are hemorrhagic and show a higher attenuation value than does normal renal parenchyma on enhanced CT scans.[14] On contrast-enhanced CT scans, acute renal infarcts present as zones of low attenuation due to both hypoperfusion of the infarcted tissue and tissue edema.[74] The size and shape of a renal infarct is determined by the size of the occluded artery. If the main renal artery is occluded, global infarction of the kidney occurs (Fig. 35-123). On contrast-enhanced CT scans, the affected kidney shows lack of enhancement, apart from a high-density cortical rim reflecting perfusion of the preserved outer rim of the cortex by collateral vessels (Fig.

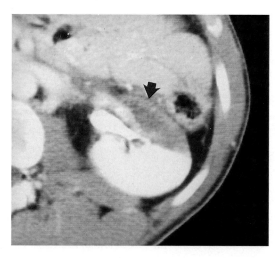

Fig. 35-135. Focal renal infarct associated with emboli from a prosthetic mitral valve. The lesion *(arrow)* presents as a wedge-shaped zone of low attenuation. The base of the wedge is contiguous with the renal capsule, and the apex is directed towards the renal hilus. There is a straight, sharp margin between the infarct and normal renal tissue. A rim of perfused tissue is seen on the capsular margin of the infarct.

35-123).[62,63,180] The renal collateral circulation is supplied via renal capsular vessels, peripelvic vessels, and periureteric vessels.

If a major renal artery branch is occluded, an acute focal infarct results and presents as a wedge-shape low-attenuation renal parenchymal lesion on a contrast-enhanced CT scan. The base of the wedge is contiguous with the renal capsule and the apex is directed towards the renal hilus.[62,74,180] There is usually sharp margination between infarcted tissue and the adjacent normal nephrogram (Fig. 35-135). A rim sign is often seen on the capsular margin of the infarct. Emboli and vasculitis cause multiple, often bilateral, focal renal infarcts (Fig. 35-131).[180] Unilateral infarcts are often the result of renal trauma, which is also a common cause of global renal infarction (Figs. 35-123, 35-125).[180] When smaller intrarenal arteries are occluded, the CT findings are less specific and consist of multiple low-attenuation defects that are scattered throughout the nephrogram though usually peripherally located. Vascular thrombosis in sickle cell disease causes multiple foci of "slit-like" areas of low attenuation.[180]

Both acute focal and global infarcts may be associated with subcapsular or perinephric blood or fluid collections and thickening of the renal fascia (Fig. 35-136).[180] A focal mass occurs infrequently in renal infarction, most likely due to edema.[180] Old infarcts present on CT as renal cortical scars or as a small, shrunken kidney (Fig. 35-137).[62,74,180]

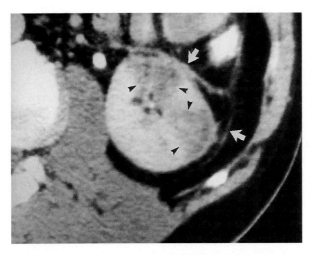

Fig. 35-136. Left renal infarcts *(arrowheads)* associated with fibrodysplastic occlusions of branches of the renal artery. Both lesions show subcapsular rims of perfused tissue, and there is associated thickening of the anterior and posterior renal fascia *(arrows).*

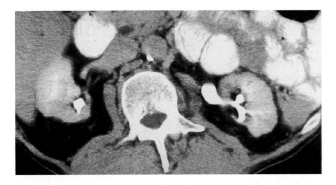

Fig. 35-137. Bilateral renal scarring due to old infarcts in a hypertensive patient.

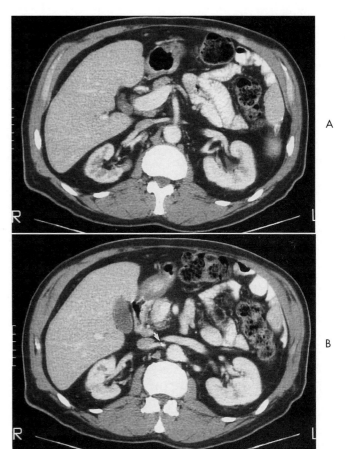

Fig. 35-138. Right renal artery stenosis. **A,** Dynamic CT scan after a rapid intravenous contrast injection shows prolonged corticomedullary differentiation in the right kidney as compared with the left kidney where the nephrogram is almost homogeneously dense. The right kidney also shows global atrophy. **B,** A contiguous caudal image reveals a calcified atherosclerotic plaque *(arrow)* at the origin of the right renal artery. (From Birnbaum BA, Bosniak MA, Megibow AJ: *Urol Radiol* 12:173, 1991.)

The main CT differential diagnosis of acute renal infarction is acute pyelonephritis because both conditions often show wedge-shaped, low-attenuation renal lesions on CT and because both often present with an acute onset of flank pain and fever. A cortical "rim" sign should strongly suggest the diagnosis of renal infarction (Fig. 35-136) because it is usually not seen in acute pyelonephritis.[180] Small renal infarcts may also be confused with focal lymphomatous lesions or metastases on CT.

Renal artery stenosis

Hypertension due to diseases of the major renal arteries (i.e., renovascular hypertension) accounts for about 3% to 5% of all cases of hypertension.[78] Atherosclerosis and the fibrodysplastic stenoses are the most common causes of significant renal artery narrowing.[78] Although there are several tests for evaluating patients with suspected renovascular hypertension, the standard for imaging the renal arteries is catheter angiography.[78] However, recent advances in technology suggest that CT and MR angiography may, in the future, play a useful role in the noninvasive diagnosis of renal artery stenosis.

Computed tomography. The renal arteries are not always well shown by conventional CT. However, significant renal artery stenosis or long-standing renal artery occlusion may be suspected on conventional dynamic CT scans if the affected kidney shows prolonged corticomedullary differentiation in comparison with the normal side (Fig. 35-138).[17] This finding results from a decrease in glomerular filtration rate secondary to reduced renal blood flow on the affected side (Fig. 35-138).[17] Global loss of renal parenchyma, if present, may be ancillary evidence of chronic arterial stenosis or occlusion (Fig. 35-138).[17]

The development of helical (spiral) CT with the ability to perform multiple contiguous 1-second tube rotations, coupled with continuous patient transport, allows volumetric acquisitions to be obtained during a single breath hold.[152] The advantage of this technique is that it can acquire contiguous patient data; this eliminates the respiratory misregistration that often degrades the image quality of three-dimensional displays in conventional CT scanning.[152] A further advantage is that as many as 30 3-mm-thick scans can be obtained during the vascular phase of a study performed with rapid intravenous iodinated contrast-medium injection. A single CT angiogram obtained with this technique permits three-dimensional depiction of the renal arteries in an infinite number of projections, whereas conventional arteriography is limited to one projectional view per injection.[151] Preliminary data suggest that intravenous helical CT angiography has a high sensitivity and specificity for diagnosing main renal artery stenoses greater than 50%.[151]

MR angiography. The role of MR angiography (see MRI technique) in the diagnosis of renal artery stenosis is currently a subject of active debate (Fig. 35-139).[53] Variable results regarding the sensitivity and specificity of MR angiography for detecting proximal renal artery stenosis have been reported by different investigators.[41,53,89] Both time-of-flight and phase-contrast imaging exaggerated anatomic stenoses because of flow disturbances distal to narrowed segments, and they may not detect branch stenoses.[53] Because MR angiography cannot detect distal or intrarenal stenoses, it is not recommended when fibrodysplastic stenosis is suspected.[53] Currently, MR angiography is best reserved for noninvasive screening in elderly patients who are poor candidates for angiography and for those with a low index of suspicion for disease.[53] In patients with abnormal MR angiographic studies, digital intra-arterial subtraction arteriography may then be performed to confirm the diagnosis and may be combined with angioplasty if a significant renal arterial lesion is found.[53]

Acute cortical necrosis

Acute cortical necrosis is a rare cause of acute renal failure in which the renal medulla is spared but in which most of the renal cortex undergoes necrosis.[6,65,87] The most common cause is hemorrhage in the third trimester of pregnancy, most often associated with placental abruption. Other causes include severe trauma with shock, transfusion reaction, severe dehydration, certain toxins including snake venom, the hemolytic-uremic syndrome, and acute aortic dissection.[65,87] Some of these conditions appear to act by producing renal cortical vasoconstriction, causing necrosis of the renal cortex.[65] The condition is usually bilateral, but it may occasionally be unilateral.[87]

Contrast-enhanced CT shows a distinctive nephrographic pattern characterized by a zone of nonenhanced cortex between a rim of enhancing subcapsular cortex and the enhancing juxtamedullary cortex and medulla (Fig. 35-140).[6,65,87] These CT findings correlate well with the pathologic features, which include necrosis of all cell types in the cortex, medullary congestion, and preserved rims of subcapsular and juxtamedul-

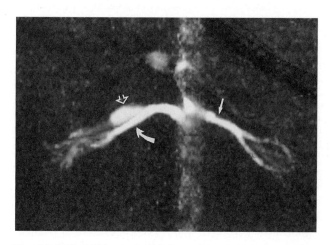

Fig. 35-139. Mild proximal left renal artery stenosis *(arrow)* shown by cine phase-contrast MR angiography. The right renal artery *(curved arrow)* appears normal. A part of the right renal vein *(open arrow)* is also shown. (Courtesy of Richard L. Ehman, M.D., Rochester, Minn.)

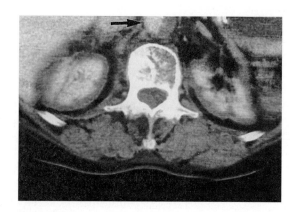

Fig. 35-140. Bilateral acute renal cortical necrosis complicating aortic dissection *(arrow)*. There is no enhancement of the renal cortex apart from a thin subcapsular rim perfused by capsular collateral vessels. Enhancement of the renal medulla is preserved. (From Badiola-Varela CM, *Urol Radiol* 14:159, 1992.)

lary cortex.[65] Eventually, dense linear calcification develops at the interfaces between viable and necrotic renal cortex, causing so-called "tram-line" calcification. Global atrophy of the kidneys occurs within a few months leading to small, smooth kidneys. Contrast-enhanced CT is rarely performed in patients with suspected acute cortical necrosis because of the presence of renal failure. However, if CT is performed for reasons unconnected with the kidneys (e.g., for evaluation of trauma), the appearance of acute cortical necrosis on contrast-enhanced CT is specific and easily recognized (Fig. 35-140).

Renal artery aneurysm and arteriovenous fistula

Renal artery aneurysms may be saccular or fusiform and may be congenital, traumatic, inflammatory, or atherosclerotic in cause, or they may be associated with renal artery stenosis in the fibrodysplastic stenoses.[78] Aneurysms of the main renal artery or its major branches may show rimlike calcification (Fig. 35-141) and significant enhancement on dynamic CT scans or appear as regions of signal void on MRI.[78] Demonstration of small intrarenal aneurysms requires selective renal arteriography.

Renal arteriovenous fistulae may be developmental when they are called arteriovenous malformations. Acquired fistulae may result from penetrating trauma or rupture of renal artery aneurysms or pseudoaneurysms.[78] Small intrarenal arteriovenous fistulae or malformations are best diagnosed by selective renal arteriography. However, larger lesions may be calcified and occur in the renal sinus where they may be confused with other renal masses (Fig. 35-142). These vascular lesions are best assessed by dynamic contrast-enhanced CT. A nonthrombosed lesion enhances to the same extent as does the adjacent aorta. A thrombosed lesion shows no contrast enhancement (Fig. 35-142). In an arteriovenous fistula, visualization of an enlarged feeding renal artery and draining renal vein confirms the nature of the lesion (Fig. 35-142).

Renal vein occlusion

Renal vein occlusion may be categorized into five groups: *(a)* extrinsic occlusion of the renal vein by an adjacent neoplasm, e.g., pancreatic carcinoma or lymphoma;[117] *(b)* direct renal vein extension of renal cell carcinoma or adrenal neoplasms;[86] *(c)* renal vein thrombosis associated with primary renal disease. About 20% of patients with the nephrotic syndrome due to such causes as membranous glomerulonephritis, lupus erythematosus and amyloidosis have renal vein thrombosis, which may be acute or chronic;[60] *(d)* secondary renal vein occlusion or thrombosis may occur when the inferior vena cava is thrombosed after caval extension of thrombus from pelvic or leg veins; and *(e)* renal vein thrombosis may occur as a primary phenomenon in infants with a history of maternal diabetes, sickle cell disease, hemoconcentration states such as diarrhea and sepsis, and hypoxia in cyanotic congenital heart disease.[72] Adults with hypercoagulable states may also develop renal vein thrombosis.

The clinical and imaging findings in renal vein thrombosis depend on the severity of occlusion, rapidity of onset, the location of the thrombus, and the cause.[179] Patients with acute renal vein occlusion resulting from sudden, complete thrombosis of the main renal vein usually have acute flank or abdominal pain, flank tenderness, hematuria, and increasing hematuria.[60] Patients with chronic renal vein occlusion are usually asymptomatic.[60]

Contrast-enhanced CT is an excellent method for the noninvasive diagnosis of renal vein thrombosis provided that renal function is normal. CT permits differentiation between acute renal vein thrombosis and conditions that have similar clinical presentations, such as acute pyelonephritis, acute renal infarction, and acute renal obstruction.[64] Early diagnosis is important since systemic anticoagulation and fibrinolytic therapy may avert permanent renal damage in patients with renal vein thrombosis and reduce the frequency of thromboembolic complications.[34,60]

Renal vein thrombosis is generally unilateral.[60] In acute and subacute cases, an enlarged, swollen kidney is seen on CT. The nephrogram in the affected kidney is initially diminished because of impaired renal perfusion.[60] However, once the nephrogram develops it persists for a prolonged period and there is often prolonged enhancement of the renal cortex relative to the renal medulla (Fig. 35-143).[17,60,64] A patchy nephrogram may also occur.[34] Calyceal opacification is often delayed, diminished or absent in the affected kidney.[60] Stranding of the perinephric fat due to edema and thickening of the renal fascia may occur. Enlarged perirenal collateral

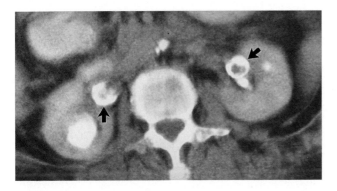

Fig. 35-141. Bilateral atherosclerotic renal artery aneurysms *(arrows)* with peripheral calcification.

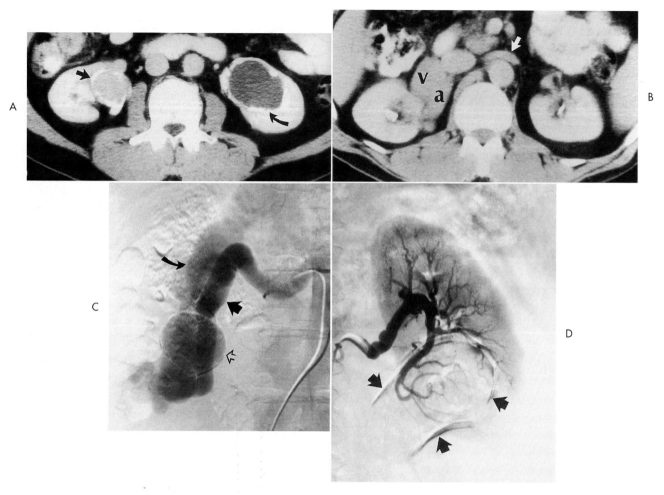

Fig. 35-142. Bilateral renal artery pseudoaneurysms in a patient with a history of previous trauma. **A,** Contrast-enhanced CT scan shows an enhancing mass with peripheral calcification *(arrow)* in the lower part of the right renal hilus. There is also a nonenhancing mass with peripheral calcification *(curved arrow)* in the lower part of the left renal hilus. **B,** Cephalad scan reveals significant enlargement of the right renal artery *(a)* and vein *(v)*, indicating an arteriovenous fistula. The left renal vein *(arrow)* is normal in size. **C,** Right selective renal arteriogram reveals enlargement of the right renal artery *(arrow)* and vein *(curved arrow)*. The calcified pseudoaneurysm is opacified *(open arrow)*. **D,** The left renal artery pseudoaneurysm *(arrows)* does not opacify due to thrombosis.

veins are often noted.[64,179] Perinephric hemorrhage may occur.[34,64] On CT the renal vein is often enlarged and may show a filling defect because of thrombus (Fig. 35-143).[18,34,64] Thrombosis of the inferior vena cava at or near the renal vein orifices occurs in about 40% to 50% of patients with renal vein thrombosis (Fig. 35-144).[60] Demonstration of venous thrombus is facilitated by scanning during the peak phase of vascular opacification after bolus injection of contrast medium and by obtaining 5-mm–thick sections (Fig. 35-143). Infarction of the affected kidney may occur, and long-term follow-up by CT may reveal severe atrophy and poor function in the affected kidney.[64]

Chronic renal vein thrombosis is often a silent complication of the nephrotic syndrome.[60] CT frequently shows the presence of venous thrombus (Fig. 35-144). Such patients show normal or only mildly abnormal patterns of renal parenchymal and calyceal opacification.[60] The affected kidney may be small.[60] Patients with chronic renal vein occlusion due to adjacent retroperitoneal tumors often develop an extensive network of collateral veins in the perinephric space.[117] This is particularly evident on the left where the left gonadal, left inferior phrenic, and left inferior adrenal veins drain directly into the left renal vein.[117]

Although MRI is widely used for detecting renal

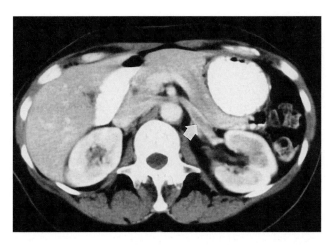

Fig. 35-143. Renal vein thrombosis. Dynamic CT scan shows a low attenuation clot *(arrow)* in a partially thrombosed left renal vein. There is prolonged corticomedullary differentiation in the left kidney as compared with the right kidney, which exhibits a homogeneous nephrogram. (From Birnbaum BA, Bosniak MA, Megibow AJ: *Urol Radiol* 12:173, 1991.)

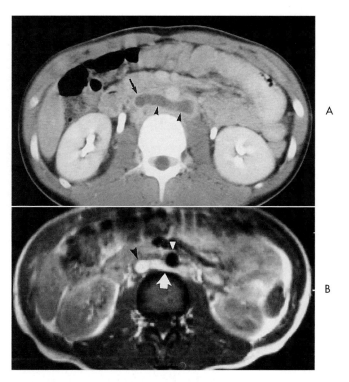

Fig. 35-144. Renal vein thrombosis associated with the nephrotic syndrome. **A,** Low-density thrombus is present in a retroaortic left renal vein *(arrowheads)* and in the adjacent inferior vena cava *(arrow)*. **B,** Spin-echo MR scan (650/30) shows high signal thrombus in the retroaortic left renal vein *(arrow)* and in the adjacent inferior vena cava *(black arrowhead)*. The aorta *(white arrowhead)* shows normal blood flow.

vein extension of renal cell carcinoma,[68,150] the technique has only been used occasionally in the evaluation of nonneoplastic renal vein thrombosis.[90] Contrast-enhanced CT remains the primary method of diagnosis for most patients, but MRI is most useful for evaluating patients with significant renal functional impairment and symptoms suggesting renal vein thrombosis. Renal vein thrombus may be shown on T1-weighted spin-echo pulse sequences when the signal void of flowing blood in the renal vein is replaced by high signal due to thrombus (Fig. 35-144). Gradient-echo technique shows thrombus as a medium signal intensity filling defect replacing the high signal of flowing blood (see Fig. 35-67). Coronal MR images help determine the extent of vena caval involvement. MRI in patients with acute renal vein thrombosis may also show loss of corticomedullary differentiation on T1-weighted spin-echo images, increased signal in the affected kidney on T2-weighted images,[90] renal fascial thickening, and renal enlargement.

URINARY OBSTRUCTION

CT may play a valuable role in diagnosis in patients with urinary obstruction of unknown cause and may be useful in evaluating complications of urinary obstruction such as urinomas.

CT of ureteric obstruction

Diagnosis of the presence and cause of unilateral or bilateral ureteral obstruction is usually readily made by various combinations of excretory urography, sonog-

raphy, retrograde pyelography, and antegrade pyelography. However, CT may help when these techniques fail to determine the cause of ureteral obstruction.[26] Unenhanced CT scans should be performed first to determine the approximate level of ureteral obstruction. The dilated, urine-filled ureter is a reliable guide to the point of obstruction and is followed by sequential CT images until a change of caliber is seen (see Fig. 35-103). The unenhanced CT scan allows recognition of a radiolucent urate calculus that may otherwise be obscured by contrast medium (see Fig. 35-113). In the absence of significant renal functional impairment, contrast-enhanced CT should be performed for further evaluation of the retroperitoneum and the site of ureteric obstruction. An intraluminal ureteric lesion with soft-tissue density suggests a urothelial carcinoma (see Fig. 35-103).[26]

CT is particularly helpful in evaluating patients with ureteric obstruction secondary to retroperitoneal fibrosis.[3] Retroperitoneal fibrosis may be due to a variety of causes. About 70% of cases are idiopathic (Fig. 35-145). Other causes include various drugs (especially methysergide), previous abdominal surgery or radiation

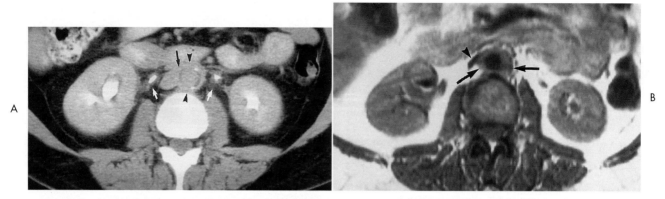

Fig. 35-145. Idiopathic retroperitoneal fibrosis. **A,** A rim of fibrous tissue *(arrowheads)* surrounds the aorta, which contains calcified atherosclerotic plaques. The fibrous tissue obscures the plane between the aorta and vena cava *(black arrow)*. Fibrous tissue strands *(white arrows)* extend laterally to surround the ureters, which contain stents. There is bilateral calyceal dilatation. **B,** Proton-density weighted MR image (spin-echo, 1800/15) obtained 6 months after bilateral ureterolysis reveals a periaortic rim of fibrous tissue *(arrows)* with a signal intensity higher than that of muscle. The inferior vena cava *(arrowhead)* is patent but is attached to the fibrous tissue.

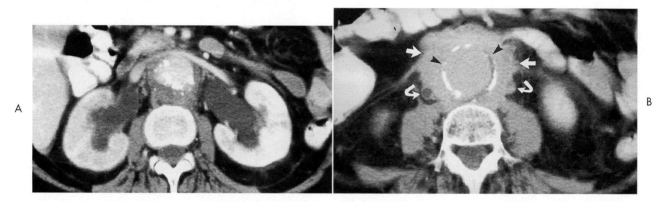

Fig. 35-146. Retroperitoneal fibrosis and ureteric obstruction due to an inflammatory aortic aneurysm. **A,** There is bilateral hydronephrosis. **B,** Caudal scan shows a calcified atherosclerotic aortic aneurysm *(arrowheads)* surrounded by thick fibrous tissue *(arrows)* that entraps the ureters *(curved arrows)*.

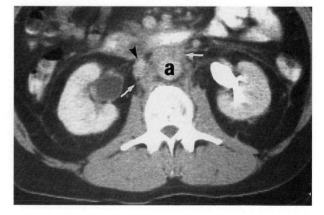

Fig. 35-147. Malignant retroperitoneal fibrosis due to metastatic gastric carcinoma. There is bilateral hydronephrosis with no contrast excretion on the right. The contrast-enhanced aorta *(a)* is surrounded by an ill-defined mantle of tissue *(arrows)* that displaces the vena cava *(arrowhead)* to the right. There is bilateral renal fascial thickening.

therapy, inflammatory aortic aneurysm (Fig. 35-146), and inflammatory bowel diseases. Retroperitoneal fibrosis may also be caused by a desmoplastic reaction secondary to retroperitoneal spread of some neoplasms, notably lymphomas, and carcinomas of the breast, stomach, lung, colon and bladder (Fig. 35-147).[3] CT-guided periureteral biopsy may help distinguish between idiopathic and malignant retroperitoneal fibrosis, when there is no known primary neoplasm.[26]

Urinoma

Continued leakage of urine from the collecting system in the presence of urinary obstruction may cause

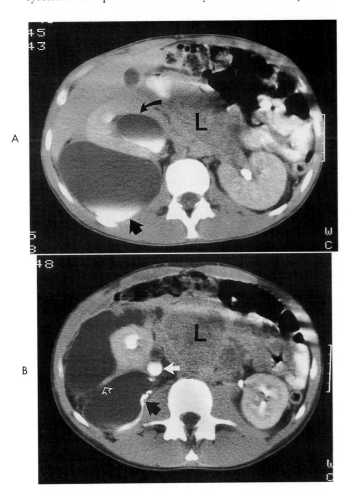

an encapsulated retroperitoneal urine collection usually called a urinoma. Urinomas may be associated with ureteropelvic junction obstruction; retroperitoneal fibrosis; retroperitoneal malignancy; cancer of the renal pelvis, ureter or bladder; and a variety of conditions causing bladder outlet obstruction.[171] Urinomas may also occur in patients who have experienced penetrating abdominal trauma, renal surgery, or urinary tract instrumentation.[171]

On CT, a urinoma is usually confined to the perinephric space by the cone of the renal fascia and often extends into the infrarenal part of the space. Most urinomas occur posterior to the kidney, which is displaced upward anteriorly and sometimes laterally (Figs. 35-148, 35-149).[171] They often show a thickened wall, which may contain dystrophic calcification (Fig. 35-149). Urinomas usually contain fluid of uniform water density.

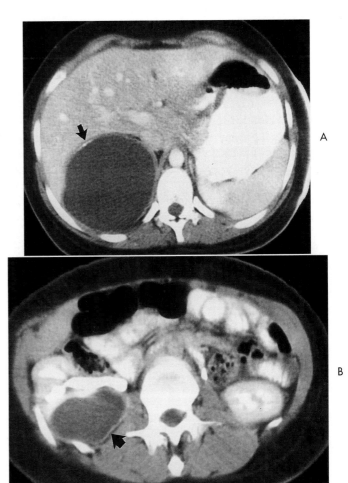

Fig. 35-148. Right perinephric urinoma secondary to ureteric obstruction caused by lymph node metastases from a testicular carcinoma. **A,** Perinephric fluid collection causes anterior displacement of the right kidney. Contrast material *(arrow)* is present posteriorly in the perinephric space. The right renal pelvis *(curved arrow)* is dilated. Enlarged retroperitoneal lymph nodes *(L)* are evident. **B,** Caudal scan exhibits contrast material *(black arrow)* tracking posteriorly from dilated and obstructed right ureter *(white arrow)*. There is a bridging septum *(open arrow)* between the renal capsule and posterior renal fascia.

Fig. 35-149. Chronic asymptomatic urinoma secondary to renal surgery during childhood. **A,** A fluid-density mass with peripheral calcification *(arrow)* extends above the right kidney. **B,** A caudal scan reveals that the mass *(arrow)* extends posterior to the kidney in the perinephric space.

Hydronephrosis is usually present and is aggravated by ureteric compression because of the urinoma (Fig. 35-148). The nature of a urinoma may be confirmed by contrast-enhanced CT, which sometimes shows layering of contrast medium in the dependent part of the urinoma (Fig. 35-148). Management of urinomas due to urinary obstruction consists of overcoming the obstruction and excision or drainage of the urinoma.[171]

RENAL TRANSPLANTS

Radiologic evaluation of suspected surgical complications and of kidney dysfunction in patients with renal transplants is best achieved by renal scintigraphy and sonography. Peritransplant fluid collections, including hematomas, lymphoceles, abscesses, and urinomas are readily assessed by sonography. Nonenhanced CT and MRI are reserved for cases in which sonography fails either because of lack of access due to a recent surgical incision or because the transplant area is obscured by intestinal gas. Contrast-enhanced CT should be avoided because of the potential for nephrotoxicity.

MRI is sometimes used for differentiating between acute transplant rejection and cyclosporine nephrotoxicity.[81] Excellent anatomic detail can be obtained in renal transplants with the use of surface coils.[8] The normal kidney shows good corticomedullary differentiation on conventional or fat-suppressed T1-weighted spin-echo images and good penetration of renal vessels into the parenchyma.[8] MR manifestations of acute rejection include an increase in transplant size, loss of corticomedullary differentiation on T1-weighted spin-echo images and a decrease in the degree of vessel penetration into the renal parenchyma.[8] However, none of these features is highly sensitive or specific in diagnosing acute rejection.[8,75,81,83] Transplant kidneys affected by cyclosporine toxicity appear normal on MRI and maintain excellent corticomedullary differentiation.[81,83] However, renal transplant dysfunction is more commonly assessed by radionuclide imaging, sonography, and renal biopsy than by MRI.[75] Solid and cystic masses involving transplant kidneys are well shown by gadolinium-enhanced MRI (see Fig. 35-16).

REFERENCES

1. Alter AJ, Uehling DT, Zwiebel WJ: Computed tomography of the retroperitoneum following nephrectomy. *Radiology* 133:663-668, 1979.
2. Amendola MA, et al: Small renal cell carcinomas: resolving a diagnostic dilemma. *Radiology* 166:637-641, 1988.
3. Amis ES: Retroperitoneal fibrosis. *AJR* 157:321-329, 1991.
4. Arenson AM, et al: Angiomyolipoma of the kidney extending into the inferior vena cava: sonographic and CT findings. *AJR* 151:1159-1161, 1988.
5. Aronson S, et al: Cystic renal masses: usefulness of the Bosniak classification. *Urol Radiol* 13:83-90, 1991.
6. Badiola-Varela CM: Acute renal cortical necrosis: contrast-enhanced CT and pathologic correlation. *Urol Radiol* 14:159-160, 1992.
7. Baron RL, et al: Computed tomography of transitional-cell carcinoma of the renal pelvis and ureter. *Radiology* 144:125-130, 1982.
8. Baumgartner BR, et al: MR imaging of renal transplants. *AJR* 147:949-953, 1986.
9. Beckwith JB: Pathological aspects of renal tumors in childhood. In Broecker BH, Klein FA, editors: *Pediatric tumors of the genitourinary tract,* New York, 1988, Alan R. Liss.
10. Beckwith JB, Kiviat NB: Multilocular renal cysts and cystic renal tumors. *AJR* 136:435-436, 1981 (editorial).
11. Beckwith JB, Kiviat NB, Bonadio JF: Nephrogenic rests, nephroblastomatosis, and the pathogenesis of Wilms' tumor. *Pediatr Pathol* 10:1-36, 1990.
12. Bell ET: *Renal disease,* ed 2, Philadelphia, 1950, Lea & Febiger.
13. Belt TG, et al: MRI of Wilms' tumor: promise as the primary imaging method. *AJR* 146:955-961, 1986.
14. Belville JS, et al: Spontaneous perinephric and subcapsular renal hemorrhage: evaluation with CT, US, and angiography. *Radiology* 172:733-738, 1989.
15. Bennington JL: Renal adenoma. *World J Urol* 5:66-70, 1987.
16. Bernardino ME, et al: Computed tomography in the evaluation of postnephrectomy patients. *Radiology* 130:183-187, 1979.
17. Birnbaum BA, Bosniak MA, Megibow AJ: Asymmetry of the renal nephrograms on CT: significance of the unilateral prolonged cortical nephrogram. *Urol Radiol* 12:173-177, 1991.
18. Birnbaum BA, et al: Observations on the growth of renal neoplasms. *Radiology* 176:685-701, 1990.
19. Black WC, Dwyer AJ: Renal cell carcinoma: earlier discovery and increased detection. *Radiology* 174:280, 1990 (letter).
20. Blumhagen JD, Wood BJ, Rosenbaum DM: Sonographic evaluation of abdominal lymphangiomas in children. *J Ultrasound Med* 6:487-495, 1987.
21. Boak DK, Teele RL: Sonography of infantile polycystic kidney disease. *AJR* 135:575-580, 1980.
22. Bosniak MA: The current radiological approach to renal cysts. *Radiology* 158:1-10, 1986.
23. Bosniak MA: Spontaneous subcapsular and perirenal hematomas. *Radiology* 172:601-602, 1989.
24. Bosniak MA: The small (≤3.0 cm) renal parenchymal tumor: detection, diagnosis and controversies. *Radiology* 179:307-317, 1991.
25. Bosniak MA: Difficulties in classifying cystic lesions of the kidney. *Urol Radiol* 13:91-93, 1991.
26. Bosniak MA, et al: Computed tomography of ureteral obstruction. *AJR* 138:1107-1113, 1982.
27. Bosniak MA, et al: CT diagnosis of renal angiomyolipoma: the importance of detecting small amounts of fat. *AJR* 151:497-501, 1988.
28. Chamorro HA, et al: Multiimaging approach in the diagnosis of Page kidney. *AJR* 136:620-621, 1981.
29. Chilton SJ, Cremin BJ: The spectrum of polycystic disease in children. *Pediatr Radiol* 11:9-15, 1981.
30. Choyke PL, et al: Renal metastases: clinicopathologic and radiologic correlation. *Radiology* 162:359-363, 1987.
31. Choyke PL, et al: von Hippel-Lindau disease: radiologic screening for visceral manifestations. *Radiology* 174:815-820, 1990.
32. Choyke PL, et al: The natural history of renal lesions in von Hippel-Lindau disease: a serial CT study in 28 patients. *AJR* 159:1229-1234, 1992.
33. Cohan RH, et al: Computed tomography of renal lymphoma. *J Comput Assist Tomogr* 14:933-938, 1990.
34. Coleman CC, Saxena KM, Johnson KW: Renal vein thrombosis in a child with the nephrotic syndrome: CT diagnosis. *AJR* 135:1285-1286, 1980.
35. Crummy AB, Madsen PO: Parapelvic renal cyst: the peripheral fat sign. *J Urol* 96:436-438, 1966.

36. Cushing B, Slovis TL: Imaging of Wilms' tumor: what is important! *Urol Radiol* 14:241-251, 1992.

37. Curry NS, et al: Intratumoral fat in a renal oncocytoma mimicking angiomyolipoma. *AJR* 154:307-308, 1990.

38. Davidson AJ, et al: Renal oncocytoma and carcinoma: failure of differentiation with CT. *Radiology* 186:693-696, 1993.

39. Davies CH, et al: Congenital hepatic fibrosis with saccular dilatation of intrahepatic bile ducts and infantile polycystic kidneys. *Pediatr Radiol* 16:302-305, 1986.

40. Davis JM, McLaughlin AP: Spontaneous renal hemorrhage due to cyst rupture: CT findings. *AJR* 148:763-764, 1987.

41. Debatin JF, et al: Imaging of the renal arteries: value of MR angiography. *AJR* 157:981-990, 1991.

42. Dinsmore BJ, Pollack HM, Banner MP: Calcified transitional cell carcinoma of the renal pelvis. *Radiology* 167:401-404, 1988.

43. Dunnick NR: Renal lesions: great strides in imaging. *Radiology* 182:305-306, 1992.

44. Dunnick NR, et al: The radiology of juxtaglomerular tumors. *Radiology* 147:321-326, 1983.

45. Eilenberg SS, et al: Renal masses: evaluation with gradient echo Gd-DTPA-enhanced dynamic MR imaging. *Radiology* 176:333-338, 1990.

46. Fanney DR, Casillas J, Murphy BJ: CT in the diagnosis of renal trauma. *Radiographics* 10:29-40, 1990.

47. Farrow GM, et al: Sarcomas and sarcomatoid and mixed malignant tumors of the kidney in adults—Part I. *Cancer* 22:545-550, 1968.

48. Federle MP: Evaluation of renal trauma. In Pollack HM, editor: *Clinical urography: an atlas and textbook of urological imaging*, Philadelphia, 1990, WB Saunders Co.

49. Federle MP, et al: Computed tomography of urinary calculi. *AJR* 136:255-258, 1981.

50. Feldberg MAM, Koehler PR, van Waes PFGM: Psoas compartment disease studied by computed tomography: analysis of 50 cases and subject review. *Radiology* 148:505-512, 1983.

51. Fernbach SK, et al: Fatty Wilms' tumor simulating teratoma: occurrence in a child with a horseshoe kidney. *Pediatr Radiol* 18:424-426, 1988.

52. Fernbach SK, et al: Nephroblastomatosis: comparison of CT with US and urography. *Radiology* 166:153-156, 1988.

53. Finn JP, Goldmann A, Edelman RR: Magnetic resonance angiography in the body. *Magn Reson Q* 8:1-22, 1992.

54. Fishman EK, et al: The CT appearance of Wilms tumor. *J Comput Assist Tomogr* 7:659-665, 1983.

55. Fishman MC, et al: Radiographic manifestations of spontaneous renal sinus hemorrhage. *AJR* 142:1161-1164, 1984.

56. Fultz PJ, Hampton WR, Totterman SMS: Computed tomography of pyonephrosis. *Abdom Imaging* 18:82-87, 1993.

57. Funston MR, Levine E, Stables DP: Spontaneous renal hemorrhage. *Urology* 6:610-617, 1976.

58. Gabow PA: Autosomal dominant polycystic kidney disease—more than a renal disease. *Am J Kidney Dis* 16:403-413, 1990.

59. Gardner KD: Cystic kidneys. *Kidney Int* 33:610-621, 1988.

60. Gatewood OMB, et al: Renal vein thrombosis in patients with nephrotic syndrome: CT diagnosis. *Radiology* 159:117-122, 1986.

61. Geiger J, Fong Q, Fay R: Transitional cell carcinoma of the renal pelvis with invasion of renal vein and thrombosis of subhepatic inferior vena cava. *Urology* 28:52-54, 1986.

62. Glazer GM, London SS: CT appearance of global renal infarction. *J Comput Assist Tomogr* 5:847-850, 1981.

63. Glazer GM, et al: Computed tomography of renal infarctions: clinical and experimental observations. *AJR* 140:721-727, 1983.

64. Glazer GM, et al:Computed tomography of renal vein thrombosis. *J Comput Assist Tomogr* 8:288-293, 1984.

65. Goergen TG, et al: CT appearance of acute renal cortical necrosis. *AJR* 137:176-177, 1981.

66. Gold RP, McClennan BL: Acute infections of the renal parenchyma. In Pollack HM, editor: *Clinical urography: an atlas and textbook of urological imaging*, Philadelphia, 1990, WB Saunders Co.

67. Gold RP, McClennan BL, Rottenberg RR: CT appearance of acute inflammatory disease of the renal interstitium. *AJR* 141:343-349, 1983.

68. Goldfarb DA, et al: Magnetic resonance imaging for assessment of vena caval tumor thrombi: a comparative study with venacavography and computerized tomography scanning. *J Urol* 144:1100-1104, 1990.

69. Goldman SM, et al: CT of xanthogranulomatous pyelonephritis: radiologic-pathologic correlation. *AJR* 141:963-969, 1984.

70. Grabstald H, Whitmore WF, Melamed MR: Renal pelvic tumors. *JAMA* 218:845-854, 1971.

71. Grantham JJ, Levine E: Acquired cystic disease: replacing one kidney disease with another. *Kidney Int* 28:99-105, 1985.

72. Greene A, Cromie WJ, Goldman M: Computerized body tomography in neonatal renal vein thrombosis. *Urology* 20:213-215, 1982.

73. Guiterrez OH, Burgener FA, Schwartz S: Coincident renal cell carcinoma and renal angiomyolipoma in tuberous sclerosis. *AJR* 132:848-850, 1979.

74. Haaga JR, Morrison SC: CT appearance of renal infarct. *J Comput Assist Tomogr* 4:246-247, 1980.

75. Halasz NA: Differential diagnosis of renal transplant rejection: is MR imaging the answer? *AJR* 147:954-955, 1986.

76. Hartman DS, et al: Cystic renal cell carcinoma: CT findings simulating a benign hyperdense cyst. *AJR* 159:1235-1237, 1992.

77. Hidalgo H, et al: Parapelvic cysts: appearance on CT and sonography. *AJR* 138:667-671, 1982.

78. Hillman BJ: Disorders of the renal arterial circulation and renal vascular hypertension. In Pollack HM, editor: *Clinical urography: an atlas and textbook of urological imaging*, Philadelphia, 1990, WB Saunders Co.

79. Hoddick W, et al: CT and sonography of severe renal and perirenal infections. *AJR* 140:517-520, 1983.

80. Honda H, et al: Unusual renal oncocytomas: pathologic and CT correlations. *Urol Radiol* 14:148-154, 1992.

81. Hricak H, Terrier F, Demas BE: Renal allografts: evaluation by MR imaging. *Radiology* 159:435-441, 1986.

82. Hricak H, et al: Nuclear magnetic resonance imaging of the kidney. *Radiology* 146:425-432, 1983.

83. Hricak H, et al: Post-transplant renal rejection: comparison of quantitative scintigraphy, US and MR imaging. *Radiology* 162:685-688, 1987.

84. Hricak H, et al: Detection and staging of renal neoplasms: a reassessment of MR imaging. *Radiology* 166:643-649, 1988.

85. Jeffrey RB, et al: Sensitivity on sonography in pyonephrosis: a reevaluation. *AJR* 144:71-73, 1985.

86. Johnson CD, et al: Renal adenocarcinoma: CT staging of 100 tumors. *AJR* 148:59-63, 1987.

87. Jordan J, Low R, Jeffrey RB: CT findings in acute renal cortical necrosis. *J Comput Assist Tomogr* 14:155-156, 1990.

88. Kenney PJ: Imaging of chronic renal infections. *AJR* 155:485-494, 1990.

89. Kim D, et al: Abdominal aorta and renal artery stenosis: evaluation with MR angiography. *Radiology* 174:727-731, 1990.

90. Koch KJ, Cory DA: Simultaneous renal vein thrombosis and bilateral adrenal hemorrhage: MR demonstration. *J Comput Assist Tomogr* 10:681-683, 1986.

91. Kossol J, Patel SK: Suburothelial hemorrhage: the value of preinfusion computed tomography. *J Comput Assist Tomogr* 10:157-158, 1986.

92. Kramer SA, Kelalis PP: Pediatric urologic oncology. In Gillenwater JY, Grayhack JT, Howards SS, Duckett JW, editors: *Adult and pediatric urology,* Chicago, 1987, Year Book Medical Publishers.

93. Kunin M: Bridging septa of the perinephric space: anatomic, pathologic, and diagnostic considerations. *Radiology* 158:361-365, 1986.

94. Lane RH, Stephens DH, Reiman HM: Primary retroperitoneal neoplasms: CT findings in 90 cases with clinical and pathologic correlation. *AJR* 152:83-89, 1989.

95. Lang EK, Sullivan J, Fretz G: Renal trauma: radiological studies. Comparison of urography, computed tomography, angiography and radionuclide studies. *Radiology* 154:1-6, 1985.

96. Leder RA, Dunnick NR: Transitional cell carcinoma of the pelvicalyces and ureter. *AJR* 155:713-722, 1990.

97. Levine C, Levine E: Small pediatric renal neoplasms detected by CT. *J Comput Assist Tomogr* 14:615-618, 1990.

98. Levine E: Computed tomography of renal abscesses complicating medullary sponge kidney. *J Comput Assist Tomogr* 13:440-442, 1989.

99. Levine E: Malignant renal parenchymal tumors in adults. In Pollack HM, editor: *Clinical urography: an atlas and textbook of urological imaging,* Philadelphia, 1990, WB Saunders Co.

100. Levine E: Renal cell carcinoma in uremic acquired renal cystic disease: incidence, detection, and management. *Urol Radiol* 13:203-210, 1992.

101. Levine E: Transitional cell carcinoma of the renal pelvis associated with cyclophosphamide therapy. *AJR* 159:1027-1028, 1992.

102. Levine E, Cook LT, Grantham JJ: Liver cysts in autosomal dominant polycystic kidney disease: clinical and computed tomographic study. *AJR* 142:229-233, 1985.

103. Levine E, Grantham JJ: High-density renal cysts in autosomal dominant polycystic kidney disease demonstrated by CT. *Radiology* 154:477-482, 1985.

104. Levine E, Grantham JJ: Perinephric hemorrhage in autosomal dominant polycystic kidney disease: CT and MR findings. *J Comput Assist Tomogr* 11:108-111, 1987.

105. Levine E, Grantham JJ: Radiology of cystic kidneys. In Gardner KD, Bernstein J, editors: *The cystic kidney,* Dordrecht, 1990, Kluwer Academic Publishers.

106. Levine E, Grantham JJ: Calcified renal stones and cyst calcifications in autosomal dominant polycystic kidney disease: clinical and CT study in 84 patients. *AJR* 159:77-81, 1992.

107. Levine E, Grantham JJ, MacDougall ML: Spontaneous subcapsular and perinephric hemorrhage in end-stage kidney disease: clinical and CT findings. *AJR* 148:755-758, 1987.

108. Levine E, Huntrakoon M: Computed tomography of renal oncocytoma. *AJR* 141:741-746, 1984.

109. Levine E, Huntrakoon M: Unilateral renal cystic disease: CT findings. *J Comput Assist Tomogr* 13:273-276, 1989.

110. Levine E, Huntrakoon M, Wetzel LH: Small renal neoplasms: clinical, pathologic, and imaging features. *AJR* 153:69-73, 1989.

111. Levine E, Lee KR, Weigel J: Preoperative determination of abdominal extent of renal cell carcinoma by computed tomography. *Radiology* 132:395-398, 1979.

112. Levine E, et al: Computed tomography in the diagnosis of renal carcinoma complicating Hippel-Lindau syndrome. *Radiology* 130:703-706, 1979.

113. Levine E, et al: CT screening of the abdomen in von Hippel-Lindau disease. *AJR* 139:505-510, 1982.

114. Levine E, et al: CT of acquired cystic kidney disease and renal tumors in long-term dialysis patients. *AJR* 142:125-131, 1984.

115. Levine E, et al: Natural history of acquired renal cystic disease in dialysis patients: a prospective longitudinal CT study. *AJR* 156:501-506, 1991.

116. Lieber MM, Tomera KM, Farrow GM: Renal oncocytoma. *J Urol* 125:481-485, 1981.

117. Lien HH, Lund G, Talle K: Collateral veins in left renal vein stenosis demonstrated via CT. *Europ J Radiol* 3:29-32, 1983.

118. Lindsey JR: Lymphangiectasis simulating polycystic disease. *J Urol* 104:658-662, 1970.

119. Lingeman JE, et al: Angiomyolipoma: emerging concepts in management. *Urology* 20:566-570, 1982.

120. Madewell JE, et al: Multilocular cystic nephroma: a radiographic pathologic correlation of 58 patients. *Radiology* 146:309-321, 1983.

121. McClennan BL, et al: CT of the renal cyst: is cyst aspiration necessary? *AJR* 133:671-675, 1979.

122. Melson GL, et al: The spectrum of sonographic findings in infantile polycystic kidney disease with urographic and clinical correlations. *J Clin Ultrasound* 13:113-119, 1985.

123. Meredith WT, et al: Exacerbation of familial renal lymphangiomatosis during pregnancy. *AJR* 151:965-966, 1988.

124. Meyers MA: *Dynamic radiology of the abdomen. Normal and pathologic anatomy,* ed 3, New York, 1988, Springer-Verlag.

125. Miller DL, et al: von Hippel-Lindau disease: inadequacy of angiography for identification of renal cancers. *Radiology* 179:833-836, 1991.

126. Mitnick JS, et al: Cystic renal disease in tuberous sclerosis. *Radiology* 147:85-87, 1983.

127. Mitnick JS, et al: Metastatic neoplasm to the kidney studied by computed tomography and sonography. *J Comput Assist Tomogr* 9:43-49, 1985.

128. Morehouse HT, Weiner SN, Hoffman JC: Imaging in inflammatory disease of the kidney. *AJR* 143:135-141, 1984.

129. Moss JG, Hendry GMA: The natural history of renal cysts in an infant with tuberous sclerosis: evaluation with ultrasound. *Br J Radiol* 61:1074-1076, 1988.

130. Murphy GP, Moore RH, Kenny GM: Current results from primary and secondary treatment of renal cell carcinoma. *J Urol* 104:523-527, 1970.

131. Novick AC, et al: Conservative surgery for renal cell carcinoma: a single-center experience with 100 patients. *J Urol* 141:835-839, 1989.

132. Papanicolaou N, et al: Significant renal hemorrhage following extracorporeal shock wave lithotripsy: imaging and clinical features. *Radiology* 163:661-664, 1987.

133. Parienty RA, et al: Diagnostic value of CT numbers in pelvocalyceal filling defects. *Radiology* 145:743-747, 1982.

134. Parvey LS, et al: CT demonstration of fat tissue in malignant renal neoplasms: atypical Wilms' tumor. *J Comput Assist Tomogr* 5:851-854, 1981.

135. Pedicelli G, et al: Multicystic dysplastic kidneys: spontaneous regression demonstrated with ultrasound. *Radiology* 160:23-26, 1986.

136. Petersen RO: *Urologic pathology,* ed 2, Philadelphia, 1992, JB Lippincott Company.

137. Pickering SP, et al: Renal lymphangioma: a cause of neonatal nephromegaly. *Pediatr Radiol* 14:445-448, 1984.

138. Pollack HM, Wein AJ: Imaging of renal trauma. *Radiology* 172:297-308, 1989.

139. Pope TL, et al: CT features of renal polyarteritis nodosa. *AJR* 136:986-987, 1981.

140. Porch P, Noe HN, Stapleton FB: Unilateral presentation of adult-type polycystic kidney disease in children. *J Urol* 135:744-746, 1986.

141. Provet J, et al: Partial nephrectomy for renal cell carcinoma: indications, results and implications. *J Urol* 145:472-476, 1991.

142. Quinn MJ, et al: Renal oncocytoma: new observations. *Radiology* 153:49-53, 1984.

143. Ramchandani P, et al: CT evaluation after radical nephrectomy for renal cell carcinoma. *Radiology* 181(P):125, 1991 (abstract).

144. Reiman TAH, Siegel MJ, Shackelford GD: Wilms' tumor in children: abdominal CT and US evaluation. *Radiology* 160:501-505, 1986.

145. Reznek RH, et al: CT in renal and perirenal lymphoma: a further look. *Clin Radiol* 42:233-238, 1990.

146. Rhyner P, Federle MP, Jeffrey RB: CT of trauma to the abnormal kidney. *AJR* 142:747-750, 1983.

147. Rigsby CM, et al: Hemorrhagic focal bacterial nephritis: findings on gray-scale sonography and CT. *AJR* 146:1173-1177, 1986.

148. Robson CJ, Churchill BM, Anderson W: The results of radical nephrectomy for renal cell carcinoma. *J Urol* 101:297-301, 1969.

149. Rofsky NM, et al: Renal lesion characterization with gadolinium-enhanced MR imaging: efficacy and safety in patients with renal insufficiency. *Radiology* 180:85-89, 1991.

150. Roubidoux MA, et al: Renal carcinoma: detection of venous extension with gradient-echo MR imaging. *Radiology* 182:269-272, 1992.

151. Rubin GD, et al: Spiral CT angiography of renal artery stenosis: comparison with arteriography. *Radiology* 185(P):163, 1992 (abstract).

152. Rubin GD, et al: Three-dimensional spiral CT angiography of the abdomen: initial clinical experience. *Radiology* 186:147-152, 1993.

153. Rumancik WM, et al: Atypical renal and pararenal hamartomas associated with lymphangiomyomatosis. *AJR* 142:971-972, 1984.

154. Sacks D, et al: Renal and related retroperitoneal abscesses: percutaneous drainage. *Radiology* 167:447-451, 1988.

155. Sanders RC, Hartman DS: The sonographic distinction between neonatal multicystic kidney and hydronephrosis. *Radiology* 151:621-625, 1984.

156. Sanders RC, Nussbaum AR, Solez K: Renal dysplasia: sonographic findings. *Radiology* 167:623-626, 1988.

157. Schwab SJ, Bander SJ, Klahr S: Renal infection in autosomal dominant polycystic kidney disease. *Am J Med* 82:714-718, 1987.

158. Schwartz JM, et al: The use of computed tomography in the diagnosis of carcinoma of the renal pelvis causing ureteropelvic junction obstruction. *Urol Radiol* 9:204-209, 1988.

159. Segal A, et al: Diagnosis of nonopaque calculi by computed tomography. *Radiology* 129:447-450, 1978.

160. Semelka RC, et al: Combined gadolinium-enhanced and fat-saturation MR imaging of renal masses. *Radiology* 178:803-809, 1991.

161. Semelka RC, et al: Renal lesions: controlled comparison between CT and 1.5-T MR imaging with nonenhanced and gadolinium-enhanced fat-suppressed spin-echo and breath-hold FLASH techniques. *Radiology* 182:425-430, 1992.

162. Shah M, Haaga JR: Focal xanthogranulomatous pyelonephritis simulating a renal tumor: CT characteristics. *J Comput Assist Tomogr* 13:712-713, 1989.

163. Siegel MJ, Balfe D: Blunt renal and ureteral trauma in childhood: CT patterns of fluid collections. *AJR* 152:1043-1047, 1989.

164. Smith SJ, et al: Renal cell carcinoma: earlier discovery and increased detection. *Radiology* 170:699-703, 1989.

165. Soulen MC, et al: Bacterial renal infection: role of CT. *Radiology* 171:703-707, 1989.

166. Spera JA, et al: Metastatic malignant melanoma mimicking renal cell carcinoma. *J Urol* 131:740-742, 1984.

167. Stalker HP, Kaufman RA, Stedje K: The significance of hematuria in children after blunt abdominal trauma. *AJR* 154:569-571, 1990.

168. Stapleton FB, et al: The cystic renal lesion in tuberous sclerosis. *J Pediatr* 97:574-579, 1980.

169. Stillwell TJ, Gomez MR, Kelalis PP: Renal lesions in tuberous sclerosis. *J Urol* 138:477-481, 1987.

170. Stuck KJ, Koff SA, Silver TM: Ultrasonic features of multicystic dysplastic kidney: expanded diagnostic criteria. *Radiology* 143:217-221, 1982.

171. Talner LB: Urinary obstruction. In Pollack HM, editor: *Clinical urography: an atlas and textbook of urological imaging*, Philadelphia, 1990, WB Saunders Co.

172. Taylor RS, et al: Renal angiomyolipoma associated with lymph node involvement and renal cell carcinoma in patients with tuberous sclerosis. *J Urol* 141:930-932, 1989.

173. Telenti A, et al: Hepatic cyst infection in autosomal dominant polycystic kidney disease. *Mayo Clinic Proc* 65:933-942, 1990.

174. Torres VE, et al: The association of nephrolithiasis and autosomal dominant polycystic kidney disease. *Am J Kidney Dis* 11:318-325, 1988.

175. Vinocur L, et al: Follow-up studies of multicystic dysplastic kidneys. *Radiology* 167:311-315, 1988.

176. White KS, Kirks DR, Bove KE: Imaging of nephroblastomatosis: an overview. *Radiology* 182:1-5, 1992.

177. Williams RD: Renal, perirenal and ureteral neoplasms. In Gillenwater JY, Grayhack JT, Howards SS, Duckett JW, editors: *Adult and pediatric urology*, vol 1, Chicago, 1987, Year Book Medical Publishers, Inc.

178. Wilms' tumor: status report, 1990. National Wilms' tumor study committee. *J Clin Oncol* 9:877-887, 1991.

179. Winfield AC, Gerlock AJ, Shaff MI: Perirenal cobwebs: a CT sign of renal vein thrombosis. *J Comput Assist Tomogr* 5:705-708, 1981.

180. Wong WS et al: Renal infarction: CT diagnosis and correlation between CT findings and etiologies. *Radiology* 150:201-205, 1984.

181. Xipell JM: The incidence of benign renal nodules (a clinicopathologic study). *J Urol* 106:503-506, 1971.

182. Yale-Loehr AJ, et al: CT of severe renal trauma in children: evaluation and course of healing with conservative therapy. *AJR* 152:109-113, 1989.

183. Yoder IC, et al: Pyonephrosis: imaging and intervention. *AJR* 141:735-740, 1983.

184. Zagoria RJ, Dyer RB: Computed tomography of primary renal osteosarcoma. *J Comput Assist Tomogr* 15:146-148, 1991.

185. Zagoria RJ, et al: CT features of renal cell carcinoma with emphasis on relation to tumor size. *Invest Radiol* 25:261-266, 1990.

186. Zeman RK, et al: Renal cell carcinoma: dynamic thin-section CT assessment of vascular invasion and tumor vascularity. *Radiology* 167:393-396, 1988.

187. Zeman RK, et al: Helical (spiral) CT of the abdomen. *AJR* 160:719-725, 1993.

36

The Peritoneum and Mesentery

JOHN R. HAAGA

As experience with imaging within the abdomen has accumulated, it has become apparent that computed tomography (CT) and magnetic resonance imaging (MRI) are useful for the diagnosis of the many peritoneal and mesenteric problems. Even if a primary peritoneal problem does not exist, many secondary signs that can add valuable insights about other disorders may be observed.

This chapter discusses the normal anatomy and physiology of the peritoneum and mesentery as well as the wide spectrum of pathological disorders that affect the area. I have also included information on the retroperitoneum as it interrelates to the peritoneum. Inclusion of this material permits a more comprehensive understanding of abdominal problems.

EMBRYOLOGY

The gastrointestinal tract is formed when the entoderm develops in a tube within the coelomic cavity. It acquires a single-layer covering of the mesodermal cells, which evolve from the space between the ectoderm and the endoderm (Fig. 36-1, A). The dorsal or posterior mesoderm forms the dorsal mesentery, which eventually composes the visceral peritoneum of the abdomen (the pericardium and pleura in the chest) (Fig. 36-1, A).

The anterior splanchnic mesoderms fuse to form the ventral (anterior) mesentery and later completely disappear, leaving the falciform ligament of the liver as the only remnant (Fig. 36-1, B and C). Within the transverse septum (from which the diaphragm evolves), the liver forms and moves into the coelomic cavity, carrying an investment of peritoneum. The only attachments of the liver to the transverse septum are small portions of the peritoneum, which become the triangular and coronary ligaments (behind which are the bare areas of the liver).

The blood vessels (e.g., lymphatics) to the various developing viscera course the posterior or dorsal mesentery. The anterior attachment of the mesentery between the liver and the stomach, esophagus, and duodenum become the lesser omentum with two portions, the gastrohepatic and the gastroduodenal ligaments (Fig. 36-1, B and C).

The relationships of the pancreas to the omental bursa can be best understood by considering the rotation of the bowel and changes in the dorsal mesentery. The pancreas forms from entodermal buds of the duodenum, the (ventral) anterior portion being slightly caudad but close to the common bile duct and the (dorsal) posterior portion bud being directly opposite to it. As the C loop of the duodenum rotates, the two pancreatic buds come together, and fusion occurs at the level of the head. The ventral segment remains as the uncinate and head portion. The spleen forms in the (dorsal) posterior mesentery and is carried laterally as the omental bursa forms. The dorsal mesentery containing the pancreas fuses with the posterior abdominal peritoneum (Fig. 36-1, D). The multiple layers of the embryological mesentery as it relates to the retroperitoneum, pancreas, and colon can be seen (Fig. 36-1, D).

The lesser omentum and the omental bursa are formed by the rotation of the stomach and duodenum and posterior movement of the pancreas (Fig. 36-1, B and C). The anterior aspect of the bursa consists of the lesser omentum, composed of the hepatoduodenal and the gastroduodenal ligament, the posterior wall of the stomach, the gastrocolic ligament, and the mesocolon. The posterior wall is bounded by the peritoneum over the top of the pancreas. (This peritoneum was on the right side of the dorsal mesentery, which is on the anterior surface of the pancreas). The lateral wall consists of the gastrocolic, gastrosplenic, and splenorenal ligaments (Fig. 36-1, C). The other boundaries of the omental bursa are described under the adult configuration.

As the bowel and the colon rotate, the mesentery of the mesocolon fuses posteriorly with the covering of the retroperitoneum (Fig. 36-1, E). If the fusion is complete, the spaces remain intact and conform to the traditional anatomical concepts of the retroperitoneum and

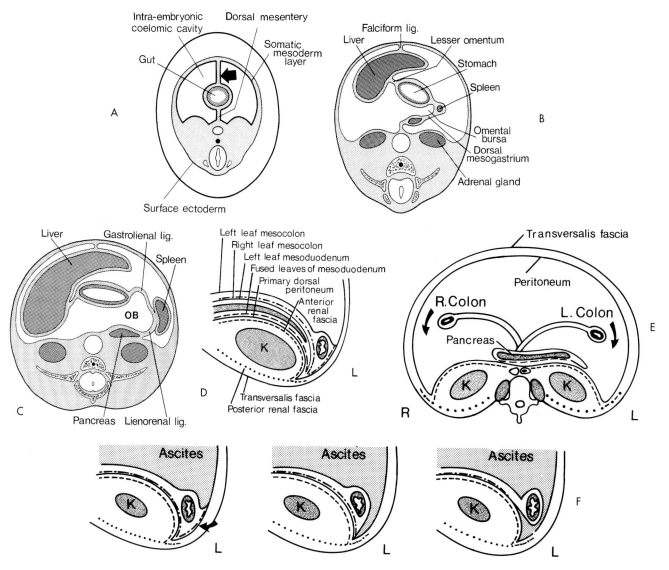

Fig. 36-1. A, Diagram shows the embryological formation of the gut as the entodermal canal within the layers of the mesoderm and ectoderm. The entoderm is attached posteriorly by the dorsal mesentery and anteriorly by the ventral mesentery *(arrow).* The coelomic cavity (later to be peritoneal cavity) is lined by mesodermal cells (later to be the peritoneum). **B,** A later stage in the embryo shows the liver having formed in the anterior or ventral mesentery. This mesentery persists as the falciform ligament and the lesser omentum between the liver and the stomach. The spleen and dorsal pancreas form in the posterior or dorsal mesentery. A folding of the posterior mesentery and mesogastrium forms the omental bursa. The adrenal gland is located in the rectoperitoneum. (According to Dodds et al the space within the mesentery is and should continue to be called the intermesenteric space, regardless of any changes in configuration.) **C,** This diagram approximates the adult configuration, with the liver having moved to the right. The rotation of the stomach, spleen, lienorenal ligament, and pancreas produces the margins of the omental bursa. **D,** Adult retroperitoneal spaces at the level of the left kidney. The primary retroperitoneum is divided by the anterior renal fascia *(dashed lines)* and the posterior renal fascia *(dotted lines)* into perirenal and posterior pararenal spaces. The fusion of the anterior renal fascia to the primary dorsal peritoneum eliminates any anterior pararenal space. Ventral to primary retroperitoneum, a secondary retroperitoneum forms, consisting of a pancreaticoduodenal space overlying a retroperitoneal colonic space. These secondary spaces are demarcated by folded, laminated leaves of mesentery that fuse with one another or the primary dorsal peritoneum. *K,* Kidney; *L,* left. **E** and **F,** Schematic of retroperitoneal colonic space. *K,* Kidney; *R,* right; *L,* left. Right leaf of the mesocolon, *long and short dashes;* anterior perirenal fascia, *short dashes;* posterior perirenal fascia, *dots;* and lateral fascia, *dots and dashes.* **E,** Axial section through the pancreas of a 14-week-old human fetus. During colonic rotation *(arrows),* the left and right colon swing toward the flanks so their dorsal mesentery, or mesocolon, lies flat against the posterior abdominal wall. At this stage, the mesentery of the duodenum and pancreas has already fused with the posterior peritoneum to form the pancreaticoduodenal space. Thus bilateral retroperitoneal colonic spaces come to lie ventral to pancreaticoduodenal space but extend more caudad. (**D** and **E** from Dodds WJ, et al: The retroperitoneal spaces revisited: Pictorial essay. *AJR* 147:1155, copyright by American Roentgen Ray Society, 1986.)

the peritoneum (i.e., the peritoneal space is the anterior space and has a number of different compartments).[61] Traditionally the retroperitoneum is divided into three parts: the anterior pararenal, posterior pararenal, and perirenal spaces. After extensive CT experience, it has become apparent that the traditional concept does not always explain some observations. Dodds et al[18,19] have reviewed the embryological formation of the retroperitoneum and proposed a new concept that reconciles some inconsistent observations.

PERITONEUM

The peritoneum is a serous membrane covered with a single layer of mesothelial cells that envelops all portions of the abdomen. The total surface area is about 1.7 mm², but the functional area (physiological conditions described in the next section) is only 1 m².[41] The cavity is closed except for the fallopian tubes and contains 50 to 75 ml of clear fluid, which has a specific gravity of 1.016, and fewer than 3000 cells/mm². The cells are lymphocytes, macrophages, eosinophils, mast cells, and rare free mesothelial cells. The peritoneum is normally sterile and free of bacteria.

Peritoneal function

The function of the peritoneum can be separated into fluid dynamics and particle clearance. The peritoneal membrane is a passive, semipermeable membrane that permits bidirectional diffusion of water and solutes. Fluid and solute exchange are related to membrane area and permeability. The permeability and transfer of material depend on blood flow, vasoactive compounds, and tonicity of the peritoneal fluid (or osmotic pressure of blood).[64,108] Hyperosmotic fluid, inflammation, chemical irritants (bile, gastric acid, pancreatic fluid), or vascular agents can cause a net flow of water as high as 300 to 500 ml/hour into the cavity.[42,57]

Although the passive exchange of fluids and solutes occurs over the entire surface, the clearance of particulate material (e.g., bacteria, cellular metastases) is restricted to the diaphragmatic surface of the peritoneum.[3,4,64] Through stomata between mesothelial cells, particulate material and fluid can be absorbed into specialized lymphatic vessels called *lacunae*.[3,4,100,101] The material is transported through retrosternal and anterior mediastinal lymphatic vessels to the right thoracic duct; reverse flow is prevented by lymphatic valves.[10,45] The stomata have been shown to accommodate particles smaller than 20 μm in size (using polystyrene beads); the size varies with respiratory movement. In conjunction with the active flow of fluid through the diaphragm, respiratory motion of the diaphragm, gravitational pull on the liver, and normal peristalsis of the bowel enhance the flow of fluid cephalad. Normal peristalsis displaces fluid to the lateral gutters where the upward flow occurs. The respiratory movement of the diaphragm creates a negative subphrenic pressure, which enhances upward flow (Fig. 36-2, *A*). Also the gravitational pull on the liver creates a negative pressure above the liver that enhances the flow upward. The sum of these influences is generally an upward movement of fluid toward the diaphragm. The net result and influence can be seen in Fig. 36-3, *A* and *B*.

Anything that alters the normal pattern of respiratory motion or affects motility of the bowel inhibits this normal flow. An ileus created by a laparatomy or other problem delays a clearance time of the peritoneum. Positive pressure ventilation, increased intra-abdominal pressure, or phrenic neurectomy impairs normal clearance.

Gravity also plays an important role in the flow of fluid and particulate material.[7,75,104] The in vivo effects of gravity on particle distribution were studied by looking at clearance of contrast material injected into peritoneal cavities after routine appendectomy and cholecystectomy. Material injected into the ileocecal region goes preferentially to the pelvis, right paracolic area, and right subhepatic area. A smaller amount passes to the left pericolic gutter and the left subhepatic space. Material injected into the right subhepatic space next to the duodenum spreads to the right subphrenic space, the left infrahepatic space, the right pericolic gutter, and the pelvis. The infracolic spaces were not involved in either case, even when contrast material was injected into the ileocolic region.

Response to infection

There are two effective defensive mechanisms against pyogenic infections in the peritoneum: the mechanism of particulate clearance[64,74,108] and the typical immune response (involving antibodies and white cells) (see Fig. 36-2, *B*). Absorption of bacteria into the diaphragmatic lymphatic system permits eradication of the bacteria by the systemic defense mechanisms of fixed tissue macrophages, reticuloendothelial cells, and polymorphonuclear leukocytes.[35,36] Laboratory models have shown that bacteria begin to disappear from the peritoneum, even before the influx of phagocytic cells. In such cases, bacteria have been isolated from mediastinal lymph channels within 6 minutes from the time of peritoneal injection.

The attraction of phagocytes, which can lyse bacteria, into the peritoneum[95] occurs by chemotaxis (see Fig. 36-2, *C*). Chemotaxis occurs after activation of various complement components and attraction of phagocytes.[7] Killing of the bacteria with intracellular chemicals occurs after phagocytosis. Ingestion by phagocytes may occur unaided, but at times opsonization by complement

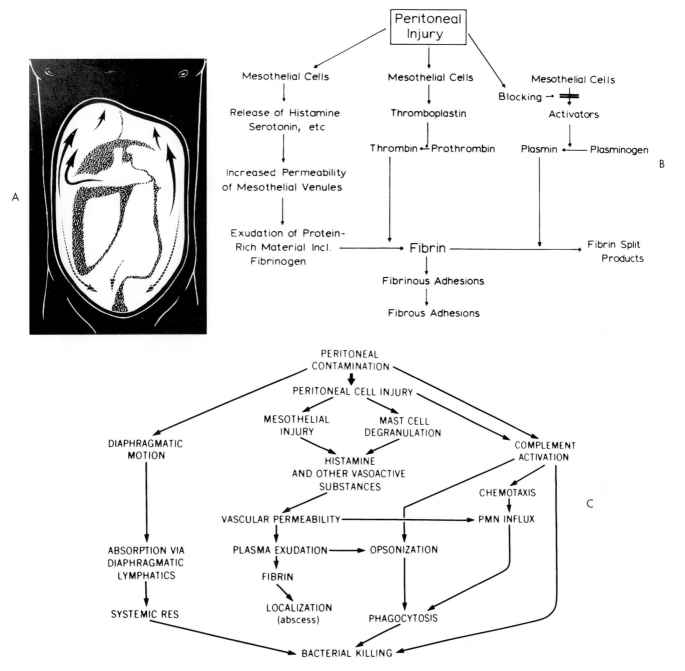

Fig. 36-2. A, Diagram showing the directions of fluid flow and clearance within the peritoneum. The relative size of the arrows indicates the relative contribution from each area. **B,** Pathogenesis of peritoneal adhesions. **C,** Diagram of bacterial interaction with the immune systems and their clearance mechanisms.

(C3) or immunoglobulin G (IgG) may be required with encapsulated organisms.[96]

Fibrin also serves as a local defense mechanism, which is useful in one regard but detrimental in others. With peritoneal injury, a release of histamine and other permeability factors that may permit leakage of a protein-rich material containing fibrinogen occurs. This material, combined with tissue thromboplastin, causes the polymerization of fibrin. Normally, fibrin may be split and removed as needed by the activation of plasminogen to plasmin, but when injury to the mesothelium or peritonitis occurs, no fibrinolytic activity takes place.[39,108]

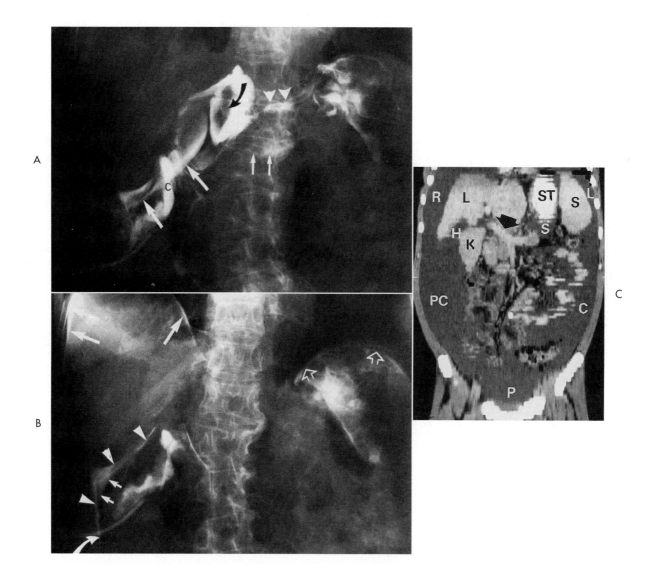

Fig. 36-3. A, This radiograph was taken after the injection of contrast material through a T-tube tract *(C)*, which was displaced from the common bile duct and into the subhepatic recess. The edge of the right lobe of the liver *(large arrows)* is seen. The falciform ligament *(curved arrow)* is surrounded by contrast material. Contrast flows to the left side into the anterior portion of the left subdiaphragmatic space *(arrowheads)* adjacent to the stomach. Some material has entered the omental bursa *(small arrows)* through Winslow's foramen. (The patient is rotated because of scoliosis.) **B,** In this later radiograph, contrast material is better seen in the subhepatic recess (Morison's pouch) *(arrowheads)*. It flowed cephalad into the right subdiaphragmatic space *(large arrows)*. The impression of the kidney on the subhepatic recess is seen *(small arrow)*. (The space appears to be located more medially because of the patient's rotation.) The left subdiaphragmatic space is also seen *(open arrows)*. **C,** This reconstructed coronal image from CT scans shows the general relationship of all of the peritoneal spaces. The right subphrenic space, *R*, extends over the cephalad surface of the liver and communicates inferiorly with the right subhepatic space, *H*, and the right paracolic space, *PC*, which continues into the pelvis. The left subphrenic space, *L*, extends over the surface of the spleen, inferiorly to the left paracolic space, *C*, and into the pelvis. Note the portal vein *(arrow)*, which lies in the margin of the hepatoduodenal ligament, at the orifice of the lesser sac. The splenic recess, *white S,* is behind the stomach, *ST.*

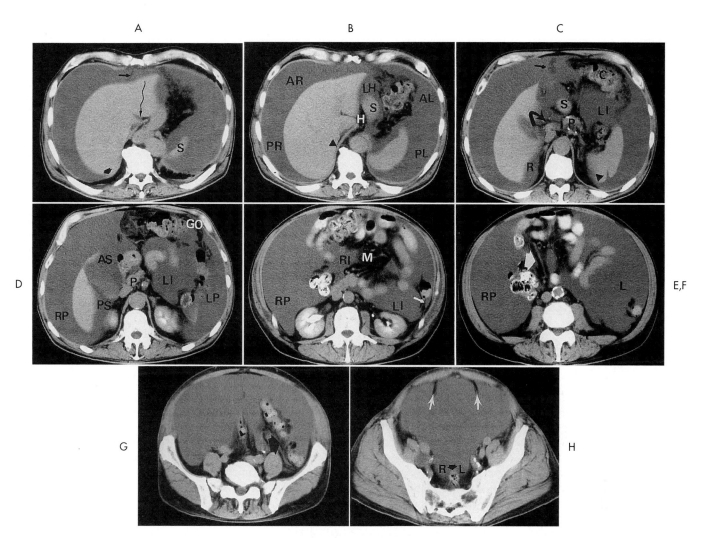

Fig. 36-4. This scan and the following scans demonstrate the various peritoneal spaces distended with ascitic fluid. **A,** Scan taken in the upper abdomen shows the fluid in the supracolic perihepatic spaces (see **B**) around the liver and the spleen, *s.* Note the posterior margin *(wide arrow)* of the right subdiaphragmatic space corresponding to the coronary hepatic ligaments. The falciform ligament *(horizontal arrow)* attaches to the anterior abdominal wall and diaphragm. The superior recess of the omental bursa (lesser sac) *(wavy arrow)* is located around the caudate lobe of the liver. **B,** Slightly lower scan shows the perihepatic spaces, including the anterior right *(AR)* subphrenic, posterior right *(PR)* subphrenic, anterior left *(AL)* subphrenic, posterior left *(PL)* subphrenic, and left subhepatic *(LH)* (gastrohepatic space). The stomach, *S,* is located adjacent to the gastrohepatic ligament, *H.* Note the "bare area" containing fat behind the right lobe of the liver *(arrowhead).* **C,** Next level caudad shows different boundaries. The posterior portion of the midportion of the left subphrenic space *(arrowhead)* ends by the spleen. The right subhepatic space, *R,* is behind the right lobe. Note the left infracolic space, *LI,* behind the colon, *C.* The hepatoduodenal ligament *(curved arrow)* containing the portal vein, hepatic artery, and the common bile duct extends from the margin of the foramen of Winslow beside the pancreas, *P,* to the liver. The stomach, *S,* and the falciform ligament *(horizontal arrow)* is located anteriorly. **D,** The greater omentum, *GO,* is located anteriorly. Other spaces include the left infracolic, *LI,* anterior right subhepatic, *AS;* posterior subhepatic, *PS;* right paracolic, *RP;* and left paracolic, *LP.* Note the pancreas which is medial to the left infracolic space. The paracolic spaces are continuous with the lower portion of both subphrenic spaces. **E,** The small bowel with its mesentery, *M,* floats in the midabdomen. Note the right infracolic space, *RI,* and the left infracolic space, *LI;* the right infracolic space is confined at its inferior margins, whereas the left space opens into the pelvis space. The right paracolic space, *RP,* is much larger than the left paracolic space *(arrow).* **F,** The right paracolic space, *RP,* is lateral to cecum. Note the insertion of the mesentery *(arrow)* close to the ileocecal area, which is the bottom of the right infracolic space and may serve as a point of metastatic implant. The left side of the lower abdomen communicates with the pelvis below and the left infracolic space above (see **E**). **G,** Lower scan shows the large amount of fluid in the pelvis; note the mesentery of the sigmoid colon *(arrow).* **H,** Scan through the pelvis shows fluid anterior to the rectum *(black arrow).* Note the inferior epigastric arteries anteriorly *(white arrows).* The right, *R,* and left, *L,* pararectal spaces are noted on each side of the rectum.

Although fibrin localizes the pathogens to a nearby area instead of permitting them to spread, it impairs eradication of the bacteria.[61,108] Fibrin hinders the clearance of bacteria into the lymphatic system. Fibrin also protects the bacteria from phagocytic activity and impairs exposure to antibiotics.[36-38,76] This latter problem is being addressed in percutaneous abscess drainages by the use of fibrinolytic agents (see abscess section).

An abscess occurs when further tissue destruction results from enzyme release from the phagocytes and bacteria. Further growth of the bacteria and mobilization of the immune system may rarely eradicate the abscess, or it may progress with more inflammation and destruction. Once a large inoculum of bacteria is established, a low oxidation potential results[36] and impairs phagocytosis and antibiotic activity. In most cases, drainage is required.

Normal peritoneal anatomy

Because of the extensive work and educational efforts by Meyers[75] and Whalen,[104] knowledge of the specific areas has become widespread among the radiological community. I have relied heavily on these sources for the information in this chapter, but I have also drawn on additional physiological data and clinical experience. The main method of display in this chapter is by axial CT scans and reconstructed sagittal CT scans. The general orientation of the anatomy can also be appreciated by studying radiographs with contrast injection delineating the perihepatic spaces[86] (see Fig. 36-3, A and B) and the reconstructed coronal image of the abdomen (see Fig. 36-3, C).

Supracolic and infracolic spaces

The peritoneal spaces are potential spaces that are not normally visualized, unless they are distended with fluid or unless the fascia is thick.

The abdomen can be divided into the supracolic, infracolic, pericolic (pericolonic), and pelvic spaces. The supracolic and the infracolic spaces are separated by the transverse colon. Anteriorly the greater omentum is located between the peritoneal wall and the bowel (Fig. 36-4, D).

The supracolic spaces include the perihepatic spaces and the omental bursa. The infracolic space is divided into the right and left spaces by the root of the mesentery, which extends right to left from Trietz's ligament to the ileocecal area. Laterally the pericolonic gutters communicate with the perihepatic spaces and the pelvic region.

Perihepatic spaces. The perihepatic spaces consist of the subphrenic (subdiaphragmatic) spaces and subhepatic spaces. There are right, left, anterior, and posterior spaces in each area.

The right subphrenic space is continuous with the right subhepatic space and the right pericolic space. The right subphrenic space lies adjacent to the lateral and superior portion of the liver between the diaphragm and body wall (Figs. 36-4 to 36-9). On axial images, the posterior margin of the subphrenic space ends at the anterior edge of the coronary ligaments (which encompasses the "bare area" of the liver against the posterior surface of the abdominal cavity) (see Fig. 36-4, A and B).

The right subphrenic space is limited medially by the falciform ligament (see Fig. 36-4, A and C) in the upper portion of the abdomen. Because of variability in size, the ligament may not serve as an effective barrier to the spread of material to the left side.

The left subphrenic space is beneath the left diaphragm and surrounds the fundus of the stomach anteriorly, the spleen, and the space between the liver and the stomach (see Fig. 36-4, A and B). Fluid can also be localized into various areas of the space (e.g., anterior, posterior). The left subhepatic space (see Fig. 36-4, B) is immediately continuous with the anterior part of the left subphrenic space. The lateral perisplenic portion is immediately continuous with the left pericolic space (see Fig. 36-4, B and D). Although it is traditionally taught that the phrenicolic ligament restricts flow of material from the left pericolic space to the left subphrenic space, in reality, it seldom is an effective barrier. The CT scan demonstrates the real situation, however, which may or may not conform to the traditional teachings of anatomy.

The subhepatic spaces consist of a right subhepatic and a left subhepatic space (see Figs. 36-3, C, 36-4, B and D, and 36-5). The right subhepatic space is adjacent to the gallbladder and extends posteriorly back to the anterior surface of retroperitoneum over the right kidney (see Figs. 36-4, D, 36-5, C, 36-6, A). It is immediately adjacent to the duodenum and Winslow's foramen, whose anterior edge consists of the edge of the lesser omentum, which contains the hepatic artery, portal vein, common bile duct, and lymph nodes (virtually all nodes from the perihepatic area—except the lower portion of the colon—converge at this area). In unusual cases, the uppermost extent of Morison's pouch can be high and can appear adjacent to the bare area and the vena cava. (See later section on specific abscesses.)

The left subhepatic space is the space immediately beneath the left lobe of the liver and is continuous with the anterior part of the left subphrenic space (see Fig. 36-4, B). It is bounded posteriorly by the lesser omentum and on the sides by the capsular surface of the left liver lobe and the stomach.

The omental bursa[18] is behind the stomach and anterior to the pancreas (see Figs. 36-5, B and C, 36-42, and 36-43). The left margin is the gastrolineal (gas-

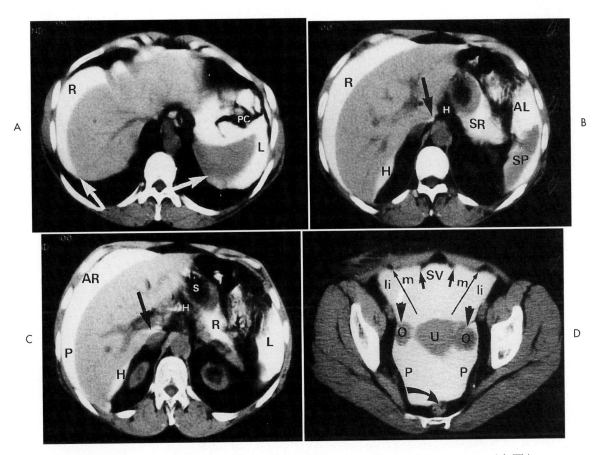

Fig. 36-5. A, The peritoneal spaces are seen in this scan with injected contrast material. This high scan shows the right *(R)* and the left subphrenic spaces *(L)*. The phrenicocolic ligament *(PC)* is also seen. Note that the posterior margins of both subphrenic spaces are limited posteriorly at the bare areas of the liver and spleen *(arrows)*. **B,** The right subphrenic *(R)* and the right subhepatic spaces *(black H)* are seen. The right subhepatic space is somewhat high in this patient. The superior recess *(arrow)* is adjacent to the gastrohepatic ligament *(white H)*. The splenic pouch *(SR)* of the inferior recess is behind the stomach. The left subhepatic space extends around the spleen *(SP)* and anteriorly *(AL)*. **C,** The subphrenic spaces, including the right anterior *(AR)*, the right posterior *(P)*, and the left subphrenic *(L)*, are seen. The right subhepatic space *(black H)* communicates with the right subphrenic space. The omental bursa includes the inferior recess *(R)* behind the stomach *(S)* and the superior recess *(arrow);* the two are separated by the left gastric artery in the gastrohepatic ligament *(white H)*. **D,** This low scan through the pelvis shows the pelvic peritoneal spaces. The anterior fossa is divided into five components by small reflections over the anterior parietal peritoneum that includes the area of the inferior epigastric arteries *(long arrows)* and the reflections over the obliterated umbilical arteries *(small arrows)*. The spaces include the supravesicular fossa *(SV)* between the vestigial umbilical arteries, the right and left medial inguinal spaces *(m)* between the umbilical and inferior epigastric arteries, and the right and left lateral inguinal spaces *(li)* lateral to the inferior epigastric arteries. The uterus *(U)*, ovaries *(O)*, broad ligaments *(arrowheads)*, and rectum *(curved arrow)* are seen.

trosplenic) ligament, and the upper margin is the gastrohepatic ligament; the right margin is the medial surface of the coronary ligament, which is the boundary of the superior recess. The caudad boundary of the omental bursa is the gastrocolic reflection and the mesocolon. The greater omentum extends caudally from the anterior edge of the fundus of the stomach and the gastrocolic ligament. It contains a potential space in the fused membranes that may be split into a true space by an active process (i.e., bleeding or infection). The omental bursa can be divided into an inferior and superior recess of the omental bursa by the reflection over the left gastric artery (see Fig. 36-42).

The superior recess is a potential space in the right side of the omental bursa and is seldom seen in patients with a transudative effusion. In cases of pseudocysts, infection, or processes that incite a pressure phenomenon, it may be visualized. The margins of these spaces are variable from one patient to another and may extend high beside the caudate lobe, vena cava, and into the porta hepatis (see Figs. 36-4, *A*, 36-44, and 36-45). The space designated as the superior recess is usually not as high as the upper portion of the inferior recess, which goes behind the stomach anterior to the spleen (the splenic recess of the omental bursa).

Pericolic spaces. The right and left pericolic spaces are spaces that are contiguous with the pelvic region and the subphrenic spaces (see Figs. 36-3, *C,* and 36-4, *D* and *E*). These spaces receive flowing fluid displaced from around the small bowel and are bounded laterally by the peritoneum of the abdominal wall and medially by the peritoneum over the colon. The depth and configuration of these spaces may vary depending on the completeness of the fusion of mesentery in the embryological state (see Fig. 36-4, *E*). The pericolic space may in such cases extend posteriorly, adjacent to the kidney.[89] The posterior extension occurs most commonly on the right side, which accounts for the observation that the right paracolic space is deeper than the left. This common variation has prompted new theories about the retroperitoneal spaces (see under new concepts of retroperitoneum and peritoneum).

In cases in which a portion of the colon, such as the splenic flexure, is not in the normal location, the configuration of such spaces may be difficult to predict. Regardless of the anatomical variation, however, one can be

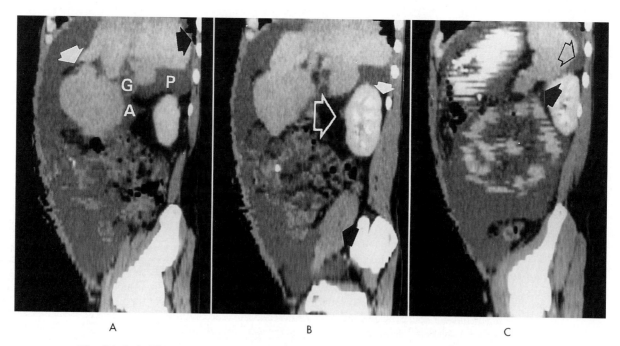

A   B   C

Fig. 36-6. A, This sagittal reconstruction through the lateral right side of the abdomen shows a portion of the falciform ligament anteriorly *(white arrow)* and the coronary ligament posteriorly *(black arrow)*. The anterior, *A,* and posterior, *P,* subhepatic spaces are noted beneath the liver in their relationships to the gallbladder *(G)*. **B,** This more medial section through the kidney shows the relationship of the anterior pararenal space *(open arrow)* and the posterior pararenal space *(white arrow)*. Note the psoas muscle *(black arrow)* in the lower retroperitoneum. **C,** Sagittal scan taken through the left side shows the relationship of the splenorenal ligament *(black arrow)* and the posterior lateral left subphrenic space *(open arrow)*.

confident that CT accurately displays the precise pathological anatomy (even if there is some controversy about the nomenclature).

Infracolic spaces. The right and left infracolic spaces are separated by the mesentery, which extends from Trietz's ligament in the left upper quadrant to the ileocecal region in the right lower quadrant (see Fig. 36-4, *C* to *F*). The left infracolic space communicates with the lower portions of the abdomen, but the right infracolic space is confined by the mesocolon, ascending colon, and the posterior attachment of the mesentery.

Pelvis

The right pericolic, left pericolic, and left infracolic spaces have pathways into the pelvis. On the left side, the mesentery of the sigmoid provides a surface on which neoplastic or inflammatory processes may center (see Fig. 36-4, *G*). In addition, the broad ligaments of the uterus create a surface on which processes become involved (see Fig. 36-5, *D*).

From an anatomical standpoint, the pelvis can be subdivided into an anterior portion, which has certain fossae common to both men and women, and a posterior portion, which has some differences between men and women. The anterior divisions are less consistently visualized, depending on individual anatomy (see Fig. 36-5, *D*).

The anterior pelvis is divided into several smaller fossae by peritoneal ligaments over certain vestigial remnants. These include the supravesical fossa in the midline, bounded laterally by reflections over the closed umbilical arteries (see Fig. 36-5, *D*). The medial umbilical fold, which reflects over the vestigial remnant of the urachus, is in the midline of this space. Immediately lateral to these reflections, the medial inguinal fossa can be seen

on the right and left; they are bounded laterally by the reflection over the inferior epigastric arteries. Lateral to these are the lateral inguinal fossae, which are lateral to the inferior epigastric arteries (see Fig. 36-5, *D*). There is little clinical significance of knowing these spaces except to distinguish between direct inguinal hernias, which are lateral to the epigastric artery, and indirect inguinal hernias, which are medial to the epigastric artery.

The posterior pelvic space is divided into areas that are determined by gender. In women, there is a space between the uterus and the bladder called the vesicouterine space. The rectouterine space is between the uterus and the rectum (see Fig. 36-5, *D*). The spaces on each side of the rectum are called the right and left pararectal spaces (see Figs. 36-4, *H*, and 36-5, *D*). Some have also designated an ovarian fossa adjacent to the ovaries.

Men have fewer spaces in the pelvis, the rectovesicular space, and the right and left pararectal spaces. There is no space associated with the prostate, which is below the bladder.

In women, the ovarian fossae and vesicouterine space vary according to the size, configuration, and angulation of the uterus (see Fig. 36-5, *D*). The right and left pararectal spaces may also vary in size. In some patients, the right side may predominate with no space on the left. In other patients, the pararectal spaces may extend posteriorly around the rectum and extremely low, almost to the level of the coccyx.

Retroperitoneum

Traditionally the retroperitoneum is said to have different compartments, depending on the level. At the level of the kidney, the space behind the peritoneum can be divided into the anterior pararenal, the perirenal, and

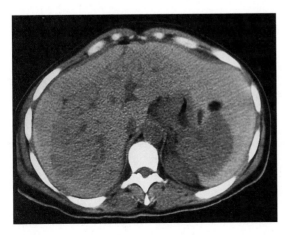

Fig. 36-7. Patient showing distention of the peritoneal spaces by high-density blood, which makes visualization of the liver margin difficult.

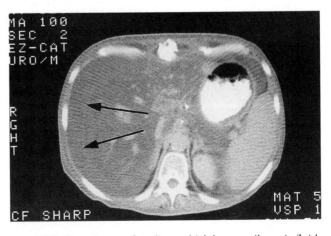

Fig. 36-8. Scan shows a fatty liver, which has a perihepatic fluid collection. It is difficult in some such cases to see the adjacent fluid next to the liver capsule (*arrows*).

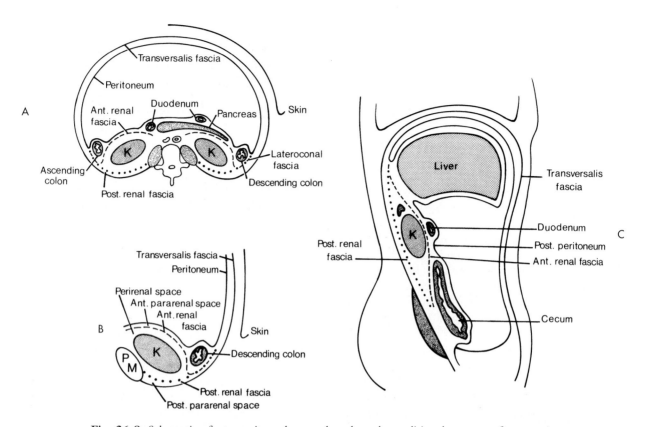

Fig. 36-9. Schematic of retroperitoneal spaces based on the traditional concept of retroperitoneal anatomy. *K,* Kidney; *PM,* psoas muscle. Anterior *(dashed)* and posterior *(dotted)* perirenal fascia join to form lateroconal fascia *(dot-dashed).* These fasciae divide the retroperitoneum into (1) the anterior pararenal space that contains the duodenum, pancreas, and right and left colon; (2) the perirenal space that contains the kidney and adrenal gland; and (3) the posterior pararenal space that contains fat. **A,** Axial section of the pancreas. **B,** Axial section of the left upper quadrant just caudal to the pancreatic tail. The anterior pararenal space is subtended ventrally by the posterior peritoneum and dorsolaterally by the anterior renal fascia and lateroconal fascia. The posterior pararenal space is demarcated ventrally by the posterior perirenal fascia and lateroconal fascia and dorsolaterally by transversalis fascia. **C,** Parasagittal section through the right kidney. The bare area of the liver is in continuity with the anterior pararenal space. The posterior pararenal space communicates with the anterior pararenal space in the iliac fossa, below the perirenal space. See Fig. 36-1, *D* to *F,* for an explanation of the newer concept. (**B** from Dodds WJ, et al: The retroperitoneal spaces revisited: A pictorial essay. *AJR* 147:1155, copyright by American Roentgen Ray Society, 1986.)

the posterior pararenal spaces (see Figs. 36-1, *E* and 36-6, *A* to *C*). The division of this space is made based on the perirenal fascia. Gerota's fascia is the posterior portion, and Zuckerkandl's is the anterior one. The anterior pararenal space is bordered anteriorly by the peritoneum on the retroperitoneum, posteriorly by the anterior perirenal fascia, and laterally by the lateroconal fascia. The perirenal space is the space around the kidney bordered anteriorly by the renal fascia and the posterior renal fascia. The posterior pararenal space is bordered anteriorly by the posterior renal fascia and posteriorly by the fascia over the psoas muscle, which is continuous with transversalis fascia.

Below the level of the kidneys, the retroperitoneal spaces are a single space with direct contiguity between the anterior and the posterior portions.

The cephalad and caudad relationships of the spaces should also be discussed. The perirenal space is the shape of an inverted cone (open at the bottom and closed at the top). The cone is attached superiorly to the diaphragm, whereas the open end of the cone is open to the pelvis (Figs. 36-9, *B,* and 36-10, *A* to *C*). Both the anterior and the posterior pararenal spaces extend into the pelvis and cephalad to the level of the diaphragm (Figs. 36-11 and 36-12). On the right side, the upper extent of this space is the bare area of the liver, and on

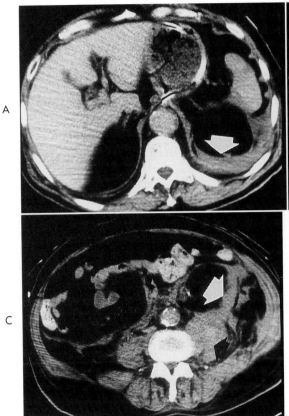

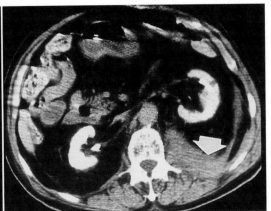

Fig. 36-10. **A,** This and the subsequent images show the overall configuration of the renal "cone" and the appearance of the posterior pararenal space. This scan shows blood *(arrow)* in the posterior pararenal space as it borders on the top of the perirenal fat. **B,** Scan through the midportion shows the blood in the posterior pararenal space *(arrow)*, which is contiguous with the psoas muscle. **C,** This lowest scan shows blood in the lowest portion *(arrow)* of the perirenal fascia. Correlate these images with Fig. 36-9.

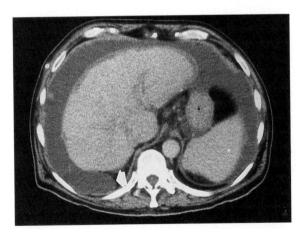

Fig. 36-11. This scan shows a large amount of fluid distending the peritoneal spaces. Especially interesting is how the coronary ligament posteriorly *(arrow)* is stretched in a concave fashion. Note the fat density bare area of the liver behind the arrow.

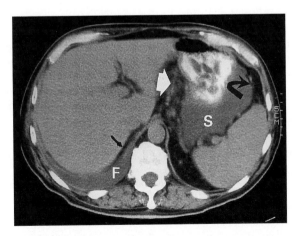

Fig. 36-12. Another scan showing the relationship of pleural fluid to the diaphragm. Pleural fluid, *F,* can be clearly identified in the chest by noting its posterior location, behind the fat density bare area *(small arrow)*. The distended splenic recess, *S,* of the inferior portion of the omental bursa is noted. This space is bounded by the peritoneal reflection over the left gastric artery *(white arrow)* and the gastrosplenic ligament *(curved arrow)*.

the left, it is the bare area of the spleen (see Fig. 36-4, *A* to *C*). With certain pathological processes, the mediastinum can communicate with either of these areas (see Fig. 36-50).

New concepts of retroperitoneum and peritoneum

With the extensive experience gained with CT over the years, it has become apparent that the traditional description of the retroperitoneum and the posterior portions of the peritoneum does not fit some observations that have been made.

The inconsistencies of the traditional approach have related predominantly to the relationship of the anterior pararenal space to the retroperitoneum and the peritoneum.[19,85] Authors have noted that the lateroconal fascia is not constant in its location and does not really function as a barrier to the spread of fluid or inflammation. Fluid from the pancreas region does not always spread to the margins of the colon, which are supposedly in the same space.

After reviewing the embryological information, Dodds et al[18,19] came to several conclusions that were different from the traditional description. During embryological development, the gut and its derivatives form in the intermesenteric space; they remain in this space regardless of any migration, folding, or fusion. Communication between the various components of the intermesenteric space follows the areolar connective tissue (the course of which can be followed by noting the vasculature) (see Fig. 36-1, *B* to *D*). Communication between the retroperitoneum and the intermesenteric space is therefore only by means of spaces along the vessels predominantly at the root of the mesentery. A number of rotations and fusions occur before the adult form results. With the rotation of the bowel, the ventral pancreas and dorsal pancreata come to fuse and, with the duodenum, lie against the embryological peritoneum. Fusion of the left side of the dorsal mesentery and the retroperitoneal embryological peritoneum occurs at a line that the traditionalists have called the *anterior renal fascia* (see Fig. 36-1, *D* and *E*), which Dodds et al[19] have called the *retropancreatic peritoneal recess*. It has been given this name because it represents a potential space that can be "split" by certain pathological processes in the area.[9]

At about this time, the colon rotates, and the mesocolon fuses to the mesentery over the pancreaticoduodenal space and laterally to the posterior parietal peritoneum (see Fig. 36-1, *E*). Most commonly the fusion is complete and extends from the ascending colon and the cecum on the right to the descending colon by the sigmoid on the left (see Fig. 36-1, *A* to *G*). If fusion is complete, the right and left colon are "sandwiched" between the flattened pancreaticoduodenal space and the retroperitoneum. If the fusion is not complete, a variation in the spaces results.

Without complete fusion, the colon has a mesentery (cecum or right colon in 10% to 20% of cases), and there is no colonic retroperitoneal space. When this occurs in some cases, the splenic flexure can occasionally be located medial to the spleen (see Fig. 36-4, *C*). In the adult, the distribution of ascitic fluid in the paracolic gutter depends on the shape of the recess and the extent of fusion of the mesocolon with the retroperitoneum. Without fusion, fluid or bowel can go posterior to the kidney by the psoas muscles.

Using this approach, the compartments of retroperitoneal spaces differ. The anterior renal fascia fuses with the primordial peritoneum over the retroperitoneum (so there is no anterior pararenal space). The posterior renal fascia fuses posteriorly with the fascia over the psoas and quadratus lumborum muscles. Laterally, it fuses with the peritoneum, which extends anteriorly inside the properitoneal fat.

The cephalad and caudad boundaries also differ in the new concept. First, below the level of the renal fascia, there are two separate spaces (anterior and posterior), which are different areas of the intermesenteric space and do not communicate directly. The anterior space contains the vessels of the sigmoid and ascending colon. The posterior space contains the retroperitoneal structures. The cephalad relationships also change. The anterior renal fascia is said not to extend above the adrenal glands; the bare area of the liver and spleen would then correspond to the posterior pararenal space.

A brief description of the new approach can be summarized as follows: The previously designated anterior pararenal space is called the intermesenteric space, which is separated into two compartments, one for the colon and one for the pancreas and the duodenum. Communication between the different components, such as the pancreaticoduodenal and the colonic intermesenteric space, is along the vessels. When fusion of the mesothelium is not complete, there may be separation of the potential spaces by pathological processes. With pancreatitis, for example, the primordial space splits with inflammatory fluid (which looks like the splitting of what was previously called the *anterior pararenal space*.[9,74] The depth of the paracolonic spaces can vary posteriorly, and the position of colic mesentery can vary depending on fusion of mesentery. The retroperitoneum above and below the cone of Gerota's fascia varies from the traditional viewpoint because there is only a posterior pararenal space (no anterior spaces).

Peritoneal reflections or ligaments

The various "ligaments" of the peritoneum are actually peritoneal reflections over tissue containing areolar tissue, arteries, veins, lymphatics, vessels, and lymph nodes. The margins of the ligaments are not definable except when the edges of the peritoneum are seen because of fluid or contrast material.

Understanding the reflections is important because they serve as boundaries to the peritoneal spaces and also possible conduits for the contiguous spread of inflammation or neoplasms. These ligaments have been discussed under the category of the subperitoneum at various material meetings.

Coronary and triangular ligaments. The coronary and triangular ligaments represent attachments between the liver and the parietal peritoneum over the abdominal wall. The coronary ligaments are contiguous with the capsule of the liver and attach the right lobe of the liver to the posterior abdominal wall (see Fig. 36-4, A and B). The triangular ligaments are extensions of Glisson's capsule and attach the left lobe to the diaphragm. Although they are typically called *suspensory ligaments,* it is not clear what mechanical support they really provide. The triangular ligaments are virtually never seen on CT scans, unless air is in the peritoneum, which highlights their margins. Although typically one thinks of the peritoneum and its spaces as completely constant, congenital variations may also occur. Authors have noted considerable variation in the size and position of the triangular ligaments.

Both sets of ligaments have little involvement with intra-abdominal processes except that they provide boundaries for the subphrenic and the right subhepatic spaces. When a retroperitoneal process occurs on the right side, it may extend into the bare area of the liver behind the right coronary ligaments or cross from one side to the other (see Fig. 36-50).

Falciform ligament. This is a vestigial remnant that represents a peritoneal reflection (see Fig. 36-4, A

to C) over the closed umbilical vein, which remains as the ligamentum teres. In inflammatory disease of the pancreas, inflammation can extend along the fascial tissues around the porta hepatis, around the ligamentum teres, and to the abdominal wall. In patients with portal hypertension, the ligamentum teres may recanalize resulting in a patient umbilical vein, which courses to the abdominal wall. Finally, in the presence of tumors, such as ovary, stomach, colon, and pancreas, the falciform ligament may be a site of peritoneal seeding or extension. The normal ligament is not seen on CT scan unless free air within the abdomen provides better visualization (Fig. 36-13).

Gastrohepatic, gastrosplenic (gastrolineal), and gastrocolic ligaments. These ligaments are in direct contiguity with the margins of the stomach. They provide the peritoneal boundaries of the omental bursa in conjunction with the peritoneal surfaces of the hilum of the liver,[8] the posterior wall of the stomach, and the parietal peritoneum over the retroperitoneum. Because they contain the arteries, veins, lymphatics, vessels, and lymph nodes, they are conduits for the contiguous spread of disease.

A neoplasm beginning in the stomach can spread through any of these pathways into the lymph nodes along corresponding vessels (Fig. 36-14). Spreading may occur along the left gastric artery and coronary vein in the gastrohepatic ligament (Fig. 36-15), along the celiac trunk and base of the hepatic artery in the hepatoduodenal ligament (see Fig. 36-4, C), along the gastroepiploic and short gastric vessels in the gastrosplenic ligament, and along the gastroepiploic vessels in the gastrocolic ligament.

Tumor involvement in the gastrohepatic ligament produces impression or impingement on the lesser curvature of the stomach. Involvement of the gastroduode-

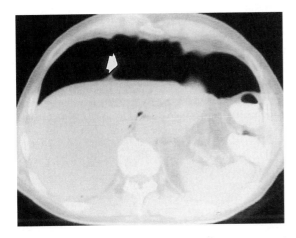

Fig. 36-13. Falciform ligament *(arrow)* is noted anteriorly in an abdomen that is distended with gas.

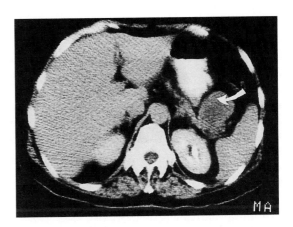

Fig. 36-14. Scan of a patient with a single metastatic deposit in the gastrosplenic ligament *(arrow).*

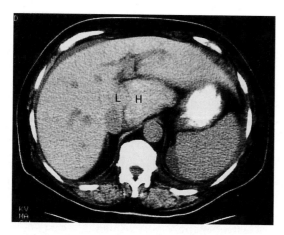

Fig. 36-15. Patient with a bleeding coagulopathy shows a large hematoma *(H)*, which has dissected within the gastrohepatic ligament adjacent to the caudate lobe of the liver *(L)*.

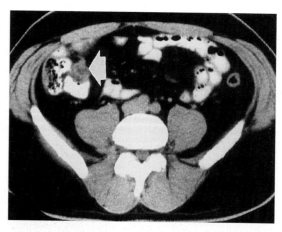

Fig. 36-16. Patient with carcinoma of the pancreas has metastatic implant *(arrow)* adjacent to the ileocecal valve by the cecum.

nal ligament produces impingement on the stomach antrum. Gastrosplenic involvement shows pressure on the greater curvature of the stomach, and gastrocolic involvement produces changes on the upper portion of the colon.

Conversely, processes that begin in the colon can spread to the stomach by these pathways. Processes from the duodenum or pancreas can spread along the hepatoduodenal ligament.

Extension within these various ligaments can also occur in some cases of pancreatitis or hemorrhage. The fluid may dissect within the ligaments and even extend to the subcapsular areas.

Phrenicocolic ligament and mesocolon. The mesocolon attached on the anterior surface of the pancreas has a lateral attachment on the left side called the *phrenicocolic ligament.* The mesocolon containing the various colic vessels and lymph nodes can also serve as a pathway for disease. Spread of inflammation or neoplasms from the colon to the pancreas is possible by either of these paths.

Splenorenal (lienorenal) ligament. The splenorenal ligament is the connection between the spleen and the kidney (see Fig. 36-6, *C*). It contains the tail of the pancreas, the splenic vessels, and small vessels to the retroperitoneum. They are of little significance except as a landmark to distinguish between peritoneal and pleural fluid. Tumor can spread, and systemic portal collaterals can develop in this space.

Ileocolic ligament. Mesentery at the ileocolic region may serve as a site for tumor implantation. Occurrence of this is infrequent (Fig. 36-16).

Sigmoid mesentery. The mesentery of the sigmoid colon in the left lower quadrant acts as a barrier or

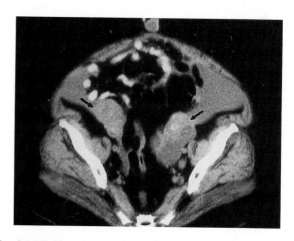

Fig. 36-17. Two metastatic implants *(arrow)* on the right and left side of the sigmoid mesentery.

a margin along which processes can collect. At times, it serves as a medial or caudad boundary for the spread of material down the left pericolic space (Fig. 36-17).

Broad ligaments and cul-de-sac. The broad ligaments and cul-de-sac represent two low peritoneal reflections that border the lower portions of the cavity (see Fig. 36-5, *B*). Tumors within the peritoneal cavity can seed to either location; most commonly, ovary, colon, or gastric tumors involve these areas.

Mesentery

The small bowel mesentery containing the superior mesenteric vessels extends from the left upper quadrant at Treitz's ligament to the right lower quadrant at the ileocecal valve (see Fig. 36-4, *F*). It serves as a dividing point between the right and the left infracolic spaces.

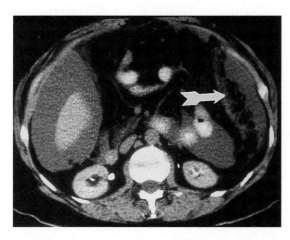

Fig. 36-18. Scan shows fat density greater omentum *(arrow)* in the anterior portion of the left abdomen.

Specific areas of the mesentery should be noted because they show changes with pathological processes. These areas are the neurovascular bundles, root of the mesentery, and the margin of the small bowel. Normally the neurovascular bundles are quite thin and are barely perceptible as thin lines within the fat density mesentery (see Fig. 36-4, *F*). The mesentery as a whole is fat density and normally extends quite high into the abdomen, permitting the small bowel loops to appose themselves closely to the anterior abdominal peritoneum.[93] The margins of the fat on the inner surface of the small bowel are typically poorly defined because the course of the bowel is quite irregular and overlapping. When pathological processes occur, the bowel dilates, the wall thickens, and the peristaltic motion lessens. Because the margins are more tubelike, they are better defined, and the junction between the mesentery and the bowel wall is better seen (see sections on inflammatory processes). Retroperitoneal, mesenteric and peritoneal processes can produce changes along the mesentery.[105]

Greater omentum

The greater omentum originates along the margin of the greater curvature of the stomach and can cover a broad expanse of the anterior abdominal wall. The function and role of the greater omentum is not really defined, but removal does not produce any adverse effects in peritoneal function.

The normal omentum is usually imperceptible on routine scan. It is visualized only when fluid is present (see Figs. 36-18 and 36-4, *D*) or it is pathologically involved. Two signs that can be helpful are the density of the omentum and the location of small bowel loops. The normal omentum is fat density and not seen; when it has infectious processes or neoplasms, it increases in density

and becomes thicker and therefore can produce a mass effect on the small bowel loops (see Fig. 36-77).

PERITONEAL FLUID AND PERITONITIS

Ascitic fluid occurs whenever there is active formation of peritoneal fluid or interference with its removal. It can be caused by anything that produces inflammation, venous obstruction, lymphatic obstruction, or albumin deficiency, including liver failure, caval or portal vein obstruction, infection, and neoplasms. Ascitic fluid can be detected quite well with CT, and with certain diseases, some specific ancillary findings may be provided to suggest the origin of the ascitic fluid. For example, in patients with cirrhosis, there may be associated findings in the liver. Similarly, with pancreatitis, there may be enlargement of the gland and thickening of the perirenal fascia.[9] If neoplasms of the liver, pancreas, lymph nodes, or ovaries are present, the tumor masses may be noted.

The distribution and progression of ascitic fluid can be easily visualized with CT. In early ascites when the fluid is free moving and small in amount, it localizes in the cul-de-sac or pericolic gutters or the subhepatic space. Gravity causes the fluid to collect in the pelvis or the right subhepatic space. Negative pressure beneath the diaphragm "pulls" fluid beneath the diaphragm. Fluid can loculate in unusual locations when the distribution is altered by adhesions or fibrinous material. When ascitic fluid becomes massive, it distends the peritoneal spaces (see Fig. 36-4, *A* to *G*).

Some individuals have attempted to characterize the density of ascitic fluid in the disease processes,[13,15,49] but this has not been consistent. Some authors have asserted that purulent ascites has a higher density than transudative fluid. Although it is true that the higher the protein content of the fluid, the higher the attenuation number, I have not found the high density specific enough to be uniformly helpful except in the presence of intraperitoneal bleeding (Fig. 36-7). One important diagnostic point about detecting small amounts of fluid should be made. Intravenous contrast material is helpful because it permits opacification of normal structures, which enhance compared with fluid (Fig. 36-19).

Rather than using the density as a critical factor, I have found the mobility of fluid and the presence of effacement more helpful (Figs. 36-20 and 36-21). If intraperitoneal fluid is localized to a single area, I place the patient in a decubitus position to see if the fluid moves. In a patient who is not immunosuppressed, infected fluid does not move, whereas sterile fluid usually shifts (Fig. 36-21). In an immunosuppressed patient, this has not been a useful sign.

Another useful finding is effacement of adjacent

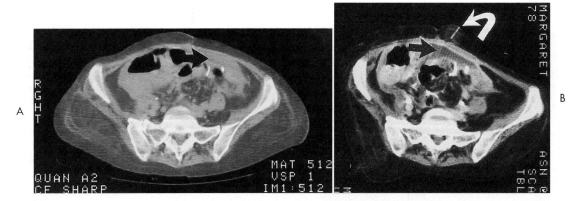

Fig. 36-19. A, Ascitic fluid, which has a high protein content, may have a density identical to bowel. Note that no demarcation between bowel and fluid can be seen. Although this fluid was high density, it was sterile (aspiration proved). **B,** After the intravenous administration of contrast material, the bowel enhances and the ascites *(arrow)*, which cannot equilibrate quickly with the vascular space, appears low density. Note the aspiration needle *(curved arrow)*.

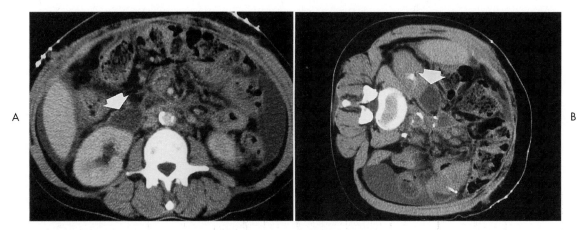

Fig. 36-20. A, CT scan shows a fluid collection *(arrow)* anterior to the right kidney. Differentiation of sterile and infected fluids is not possible based on its appearance. **B,** Differentiation can sometimes be made by changing the patient position. This scan shows the patient in the decubitus position; the fluid collection does not change *(arrow)*, indicating it is loculated.

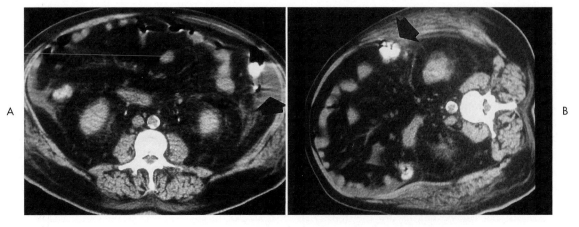

Fig. 36-21. A, Another scan shows fluid collection *(arrow)* adjacent to colon. **B,** Repeat scan in decubitus position shows the fluid has dispersed. There is no longer a fluid collection adjacent to colon *(arrow)*.

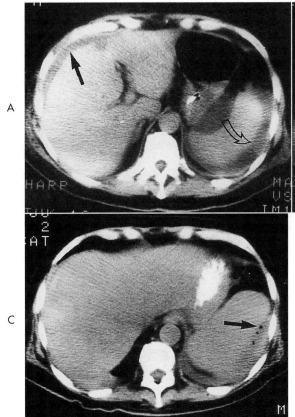
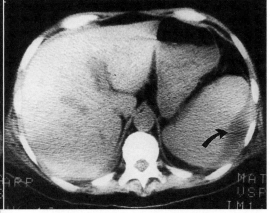

Fig. 36-22. A, Scan of a patient with generalized ascites who developed a single loculation of infection. On the initial scan, there is a small amount of fluid over the right lobe *(arrow)* and symmetrical fluid around the spleen *(open arrow).* **B,** A later scan shows that the fluid on the right side has resolved; however, there is now a "pressure" effect on the spleen *(arrow).* Aspiration at this time showed scattered colonies of gram-negative organisms. **C,** A later scan shows air *(arrow)* in the same area. Aspiration sample showed many gram-negative organisms.

anatomy by fluid. This can be best illustrated by a patient who developed a focal abscess after an episode of ascites (Fig. 36-22). This case was especially interesting because multiple aspirations were performed at the time of each scan, and the cultures changed during the clinical course: The cultures were sterile (Fig. 36-22, *A*), grew a few mixed colonies (Fig. 36-22, *B*), and grew many colonies (Fig. 36-22, *C*).

Although the finding of focal displacement or effacement of organs may suggest infection, this sign has limitations with loculated ascites. Any active process, inflammatory, neoplastic, or other, can produce fibrous margins to a space so active production of fluid can be quite confusing. Based on the CT image alone, it is virtually impossible to distinguish loculated ascites, abscess, or loculated neoplastic fluid. The only way to clarify the diagnosis is by percutaneous aspiration to inspect and culture the fluid.

If the pyogenic peritonitis is produced by intestinal perforation or there are gas-forming organisms, free gas can be seen within the peritoneum.[43,66,95] In a rare but deadly type of peritonitis produced by gas-forming organisms such as clostridia, the amount and distribution of gas may be so extensive and diffuse that it is hard to

determine the extraluminal nature. I misdiagnosed one case of clostridial peritonitis in a patient with an extensive sarcoma because I mistakenly thought the free "gas" around clumps of tumor was the gas in the bowel being compressed by a large mass.

Tuberculous and granulomatous peritonitis

Tuberculous peritonitis is said to occur in 3.5% of patients with pulmonary tuberculosis.[34,69] It is a rare disease that is a result of disseminated miliary tuberculosis of the bowel and peritoneum. It is thought to be a result of hematogenous spread or local spread from gastrointestinal involvement (penetration of involved bowel or lymph nodes draining into the peritoneum).[43,44]

Classically, it is divided into a "wet" form, with large exudates, and a "dry" form,[69,105,109] which has large amounts of inflammation caused by fibrinous exudates and tubercules.

There have been several reports about tuberculous peritonitis. Soft tissue densities produce thickening of the mesentery, omentum, and bowel wall. The lymph nodes in the mesentery and retroperitoneum may be increased in number and size (Fig. 36-23). The findings are not specific, and this entity cannot be diagnosed

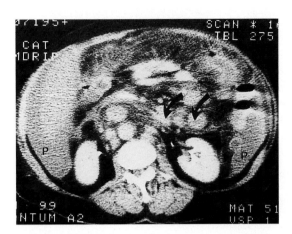

Fig. 36-23. Scan of a patient with intra-abdominal tuberculosis. There is fluid in the pericolic spaces *(p)* and large lymph nodes *(arrows)* in the retroperitoneum and mesentery.

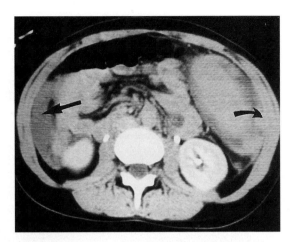

Fig. 36-25. Patient with mononucleosis and splenomegaly suffered a splenic laceration. There is fluid-density material *(arrow)* in the right paracolonic gutter from lysed blood and "clot" around the spleen *(curved arrow)*, which indicates recent, severe bleeding that has not had sufficient time to lyse.

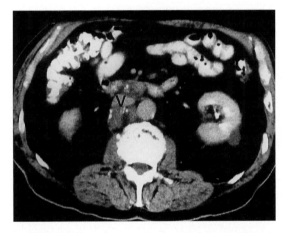

Fig. 36-24. CT scan shows enlarged lymph nodes beside the aorta and behind the vena cava, *V,* owing to histoplasmosis.

without a high index of clinical suspicion. On occasion, histoplasmosis may involve the abdomen and produce lymph node enlargement in the abdomen (Fig. 36-24).

Hemorrhage

With hemorrhage into the peritoneum, the blood can be visualized quite easily. When the earliest signs of hemorrhage are sought, the organ and the adjacent peritoneal spaces should be looked at quite carefully. The right subhepatic space, pericolic spaces, pelvis, and renal fascia should be examined. When splenic injury is suspected, the most posterior portion of the pericolic space or the anterior renal fascia should be examined.

In contrast to other areas of the body where the breakdown of blood and density changes over a period of days or weeks, the density changes are much more

rapid within the peritoneum. Because of the fibrinolytic activity of the peritoneum and rapid influx of fluid, the density changes occur quickly over a matter of hours. Such lysed blood has a low density, similar to any other fluid (Fig. 36-25). When the hemorrhage is recent or the bleeding is rapid, the peritoneum does not have sufficient time to lyse the clots, and blood appears as a high-density collection in the peritoneum or adjacent to the injured organ.

If a high-density "blood clot" is seen, it does not mean that the bleeding is stabilized, but the bleeding has been recent or rapid. It indicates that careful observation or intervention is needed (Fig. 36-25).

In cases of massive extraperitoneal bleeding, there may initially be some difficulty in defining the extraperitoneal location of the blood. With careful inspection, the proper location can usually be defined by noting the peritoneum displaced inwardly. In the pelvis, the anterior extraperitoneal space indents the peritoneum posteriorly and may extend caudally below the cul-de-sac and above the bladder and rectum.

Hematomas in the abdomen go through the same evolution in density as other body areas. Early a hematoma shows a homogeneous soft tissue density and then changes to a mixed appearance of high-density clot and serous fluid. Next, it usually evolves to a fluid density and then lessens in size until it is resorbed. In some unusual cases, the hematoma may simply shrink as a soft tissue mass.

ABSCESSES

Intra-abdominal abscesses are uniformly fatal if untreated and usually curable if properly treated.[5] CT has

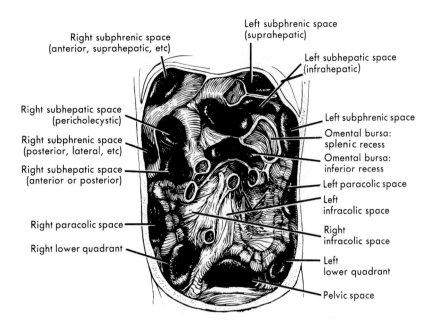

Right subphrenic space
(anterior, suprahepatic, etc)

Left subphrenic space
(suprahepatic)

Left subhepatic space
(infrahepatic)

Right subhepatic space
(pericholecystic)

Left subphrenic space

Omental bursa:
splenic recess

Right subphrenic space
(posterior, lateral, etc)

Omental bursa:
inferior recess

Right subhepatic space
(anterior or posterior)

Left paracolic space

Left
infracolic space

Right paracolic space

Right
infracolic space

Right lower quadrant

Left
lower quadrant

Pelvic space

Fig. 36-26. The various anatomical spaces that may have abscesses (for correlation with the axial scans and plain films). The splenic recess of the omental bursa is behind the fundus of the stomach and cannot be seen in this diagram.

proved useful in the detection and treatment of this entity.

Clinical presentation

Normal immune system. Patients with a normal immune system and an abscess have a typical clinical presentation. They have fever, tachycardia, leukocytosis, and localized symptoms to the area of the abscess. The localization of symptoms depends on the location of the abscess (Fig. 36-26). Pain from the visceral peritoneum is carried by the splanchnic nerves and is poorly localized. When the parietal peritoneum is involved, the pain is more precisely localized. In such patients, the typical appearance of abscesses, which consist of well-defined fluid collections producing effacement of any adjacent anatomy, can be seen.

Immunocompromised patients. Immunocompromised patients are a unique group that should be considered separately because of the lack of clinical signs and symptoms that may occur as a result of the altered immune system. Such patients may not exhibit fever or leukocytosis or discomfort by clinical examination.

Immunosuppression can be caused by a large number of factors, including corticosteroid medication, immunosuppressive agents, acquired immunodeficiency syndrome (AIDS), chemotherapy, or radiotherapy; patients with chronic diseases, such as hepatic cirrhosis, chronic renal failure, or malnutrition, may be immunocompromised. Some immunocompetent patients with

abscesses initially appear to be handling an infection well, but after a short time they may unexpectedly decompensate. Fry et al[20] found clinical signs in only 7% of 143 immunocompromised patients.

CT is important because it can detect subtle abscesses, even if immunocompromised patients lack localizing symptoms. In some such cases, a fluid collection may have the typical findings of an abscess, but in other patients, little fluid may be seen, and it may not produce the typical pressure effacement. The fluid in an immunocompromised patient may not loculate, but it may be widely disseminated throughout all of the peritoneal spaces. In such cases, the only practical way to assess the significance of the fluid collection is to sample it by needle aspiration.

An abscess is an isolated collection of purulent material and is the result of an unsuccessful attempt by the body to eradicate organisms from a focus of infection. Before the development of an abscess, the inoculation of a bacterium or yeast occurs, and the body responds with antibodies and leukocytes to eliminate the infection. At this stage, there is a focal inflammation, phlegmon, or cellulitis. If the body defenses prevail, the cellulitis clears;[37,38,94] if the organisms prevail and the focus of infection continues, a collection of purulent material results. With CT, it is usually not possible to find an infection before it forms a fluid collection, but in some cases, the process can be observed in evolution. This concept of abscess formation can be best demonstrated by several cases I have encountered. For example, 3 days after an operation, a fever developed in one patient; the patient was scanned, but no abnormality was noted. At 9 days after the operation, a repeat scan that showed the abscess was performed. In retrospect, I could see the area of edema and inflammation in the first scan. At that time, however, there was only an inflammatory process with no collection of fluid; thus it would not be likely that CT or ultrasonography would delineate an abscess at this stage.

Another good example of this dynamic process is the evolution of an infection in the kidney or liver. An early focal infection of the kidney produces focal interstitial nephritis, which has the appearance of a soft tissue mass. It may further evolve to an area of necrosis and

finally a fluid collection, producing an abscess. I have observed the evolution of an abscess in the liver in some cases. In the early scan, there was an area of edema, which was later developed into a large, typically appearing abscess (Figs. 36-27 and 36-28).

An understanding of this evolution is especially important because of the widespread use of CT for abscess drainage. If an infection is in the stage of inflammation that has no fluid to be drained, surgical or percutaneous drainage is not indicated. Attempts to drain such phlegmons fail and may lead to complications, such as hemorrhage.[29]

An abscess may occasionally be treated effectively with antibiotic medications and require no drainage (Fig. 36-29). I still recommend some type of drainage proce-

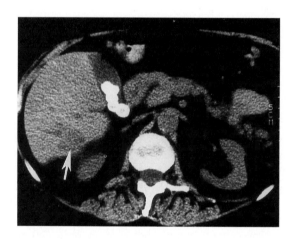

Fig. 36-27. Evolving abscess in right lobe of liver shows a nonspecific decreased density *(arrow)*. This was later surgically proved.

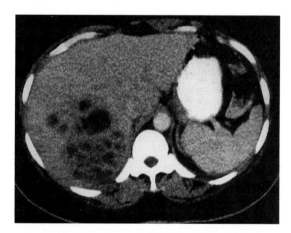

Fig. 36-28. Hepatic abscess with further development shows multiple small fluid loculations.

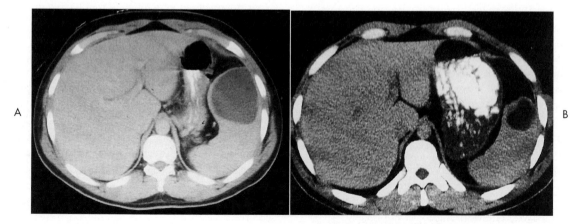

Fig. 36-29. A, Splenic abscess appearing as a well-defined fluid collection recurred after percutaneous abscess drainage. **B,** After antibiotic treatment, the abscess further resolved. No drainage was required.

dure for all abscesses, but as a matter of interest, I have observed the resolution of some abscesses with antibiotics alone.

Imaging appearance

The CT appearance of an abscess is quite characteristic. An abscess appears as an area of fluid density with well-defined or irregular margins, and it may contain multiple septations in the cavity (Fig. 36-28). Depending on the amount of debris, blood, or proteinaceous material, the attenuation value of that material may be the same as that of water or somewhat higher. Abscesses may contain gas, which appears in the CT scan as black densities. Gas may be abundant and produce an air-fluid level, or it may be scattered throughout the fluid-density area as small microbubbles. Approximately one third of abscesses contain gas (Fig. 36-30), which may be the result of a gastrointestinal fistula or gas-forming organisms (the most common of which are *Escherichia coli, Enterobacter aerogenes,* and *Klebsiella* and *Clostridium* organisms). In some cases, there may be no well-defined fluid collections, or small pockets of gas may be the only sign of infection.

The most common example of gas as the only sign of infection is the presence of small gas bubbles around an infected aortic graft or emphysematous pyelonephritis. One diagnostic caveat is that extremely small gas bubbles that may not measure − 1000 HU because of the partial volume effect; such bubbles may measure only − 200 to − 300 HU. The nature of such gas bubbles, however, can easily be confirmed by adjusting the window center until the adjacent fat appears gray. Any structure darker than the gray fat represents gas (Fig. 36-31).

CT and MRI are capable only of detecting a fluid or gas density but cannot determine if such densities represent infection. For example, low-density fluid masses can be produced not only by abscesses, but also by old hematomas, lobulated ascites, lymphoceles, necrotic tumors, mucinous tumors, and benign cysts. Thus aspiration may be necessary for diagnosis in these cases (see interventional).

Although free air within the peritoneum may be due to abscesses, it also may be secondary to surgery or to a perforated bowel. In fact, parenchymal gas can occur after any surgical or percutaneous procedure, such as embolization that introduces minute amounts of air by tissue necrosis [63,66] (Fig. 36-32). The gas appears on the scan, but there may be the spurious diagnosis of infection. When there is a large number of free, small gas bubbles, it may be the result of a perforated ulcer without any drainable purulent material.

The fluid densities of virtually all abscesses are identical in appearance, whether the causative organism is bacteria, yeast, or parasites. The only exception is when tuberculosis or echinococcosis may occasionally be associated with calcification.

Technical factors

When examining for an intra-abdominal abscess, several technical factors should be remembered. First, it is important to administer intravenous urographic contrast material in all instances (Fig. 36-33). Second, oral contrast material in either an iodinated or a barium solution should always be administered for opacification of the bowel. This is especially important for the evaluation of abscesses in the left subdiaphragmatic space, omental bursa, or the interloop region.

Abscesses in each of the organ systems and anatomical areas have some unique clinical characteristics and appearances on CT. In addition, each of the anatomical areas has some potential false-positive findings associated with the variants of normal and other abnor-

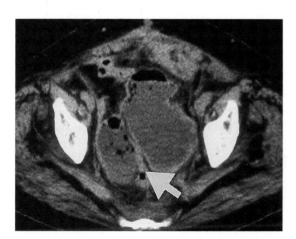

Fig. 36-30. Two large abscesses filled with fluid and air, compressing the sigmoid colon *(arrow)* on both sides.

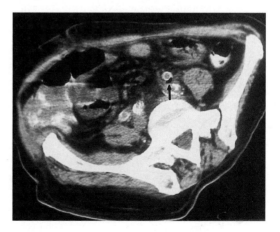

Fig. 36-31. Infection of vascular grafts may show small air collections. *Arrow* shows small gas pocket adjacent to the high-density vascular graft.

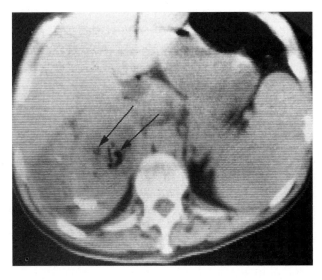

Fig. 36-32. Air *(arrows)* can be introduced after embolization procedures, as in this renal tumor.

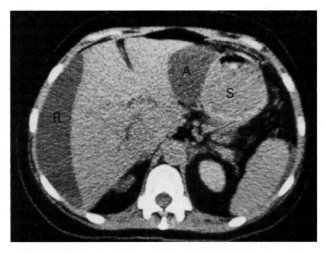

Fig. 36-34. This abscess, *A*, is in the left subhepatic recess between the stomach, *S*, and liver; this space is an anterior compartment of the left subdiaphragmatic space. There is also an abscess in the right subdiaphragmatic space, *R*.

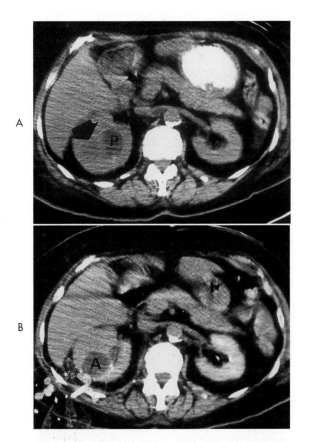

Fig. 36-33. A, Low-density area *(arrow)* in kidney adjacent to dilated collecting system, *P,* is difficult to see without contrast enhancement. **B,** After administration of contrast material, the abscess, *A,* is better visualized.

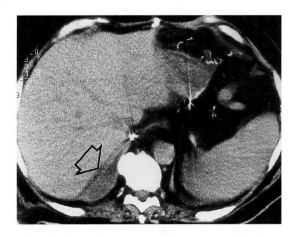

Fig. 36-35. Pleural fluid can be differentiated from subphrenic fluid because it is located behind the fat density *(arrow)* bare area of liver.

malities, which should be looked for to avoid an incorrect diagnosis of intra-abdominal abscesses.

Right subdiaphragmatic abscesses

Abscesses in the right subdiaphragmatic space are caused by a variety of disorders because this area has open access from the right pericolic gutter and right subhepatic recess. Virtually any inflammatory process in the abdomen can reach this area. The most common cause of an abscess, however, is appendicitis or a perforated viscus, gallbladder, or ulcer. The whole abscess may be of fluid density, or it may contain gas (Fig. 36-34).

The most important diagnostic point is that the

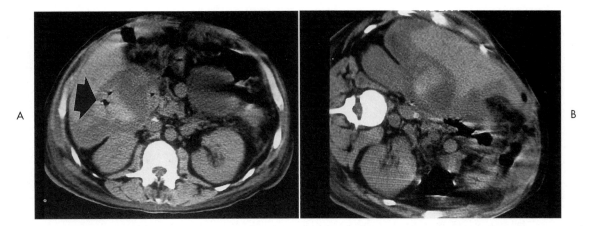

Fig. 36-36. A, Large fluid density *(arrow)* in subhepatic space containing high-density clot and air. **B,** With patient in decubitus position, the fluid collection remains in the same location.

peritoneal space ends at the coronary ligaments immediately lateral to the bare area of the liver (Fig. 36-35). A pleural effusion should not be mistaken for a subdiaphragmatic abscess. If the fluid of abscess is behind the fat that is posterior to the bare area of the liver, it represents a pleural effusion and not a subdiaphragmatic abscess. Any fluid or gas within the fat of this bare area is in the superiormost portion of the pararenal space. If both a pleural effusion and a subdiaphragmatic abscess exist, a decubitus view may permit the pleural fluid to move and confirm the diagnosis. In some unusual cases, a bolus injection of contrast material with dynamic scanning may have to be used to visualize the diaphragm, which enhances because of its rich blood supply. Any fluid in the subdiaphragmatic space can resemble an abscess, whether it be bile, blood, necrotic tumor, or loculated ascites.

Right subhepatic or hepatorenal abscesses

The right subhepatic space is located between the right lobe of the liver and the anterior surface of the kidney. It has been divided into anterior and posterior (Morison's pouch) compartments, a functional division based on etiological conditions (Fig. 36-6, *A*). The most common cause of abscesses in the anterior portion is a perforated gallbladder that borders immediately on this area. The posterior portion of the space is a dependent area within the peritoneum that can collect fluid from the paracolic gutters; subphrenic space; or direct extension from the duodenum, liver, or bowel.

Because this is such a common site for fluid collection, even with ascites, a distinction may have to be made between ascites and purulent material. In such cases, it is best to place the patient in a decubitus position to let the fluid move out of the space. Ascites moves,

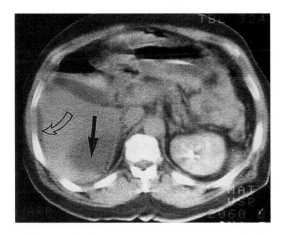

Fig. 36-37. CT scan on a different patient demonstrates a large fluid collection *(arrow)*, which is "apparently" surrounded by liver. This is not a hepatic abscess, however, but a "partial volume" of the uppermost part of a right subhepatic abscess. There is also a subphrenic abscess *(open arrow)*.

whereas inflammatory collections (in the immunocompetent patient) do not; this is a good differential point to mark the need for aspiration in some patients (Fig. 36-36).

Another uncommon problem is that sometimes the cephalad extent of this space is high. When an axial scan is taken above the typical location of the space in such cases, it may give the spurious impression of an intrahepatic abscess (Fig. 36-37).

Left subdiaphragmatic abscesses

An abscess in the left subdiaphragmatic space can be caused by a number of abnormalities. It has traditionally been said that access to this anatomical area is lim-

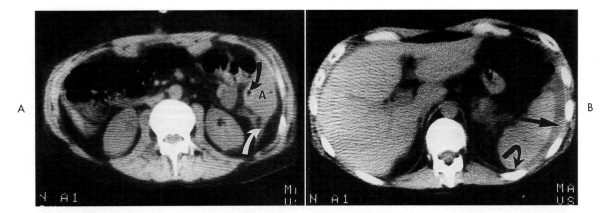

Fig. 36-38. A, CT scan of a patient with a left pericolic abscess, *A,* adjacent to the descending colon *(black arrow).* The fluid extends posteriorly *(white arrow)* because of incomplete fusion of the ligament. (See section on new concepts.) **B,** Higher scan shows an abscess in the left subphrenic space *(arrow)* lateral to the spleen. This occurred by direct extension of abscess below. Note the posterior limit *(curved arrow)* of the abscess at the upper portion of the splenorenal ligament.

ited from other peritoneal spaces because of the phrenicocolic and falciform ligaments. The typical origin is the stomach or colon, secondary to a gastric ulcer; postoperative leaks; or a perforated neoplasm, left colon, or esophagus. In some cases of a perforated esophagus, the inflammatory process usually involves the retroperitoneal space rather than the subdiaphragmatic space; if a portion of the stomach is involved, however, the subdiaphragmatic space is also involved.

Most abscesses can involve the entire diaphragmatic space, but they also may loculate in an anterior or posterior segment. Although it is traditionally taught that a process cannot extend from the left pericolic space or the right subphrenic space, experience has shown that, depending on individual anatomical variations or the nature of inflammatory processes, the falciform ligament and phrenicocolic ligaments may not serve as effective barriers to the spread of infection (Fig. 36-38).

To detect a small abscess in the left subdiaphragmatic space, oral contrast material must always be administered to fill the stomach. At times, a fluid-filled stomach may resemble an abscess or vice versa. The contrast material clearly defines the stomach and eliminates any question of the diagnosis.

Left-sided pleural effusion should not be mistaken for a left subdiaphragmatic abscess. The region between the upper pole of the left kidney and the spleen, which contains the splenic pedicle and tail of the pancreas, represents the splenorenal ligament. This region located behind the fat is within the pleural space and not the subdiaphragmatic peritoneal space (Fig. 36-39).[32] Any fluid within this area is in the superiormost area of the retroperitoneum rather than in the left subdiaphragmatic

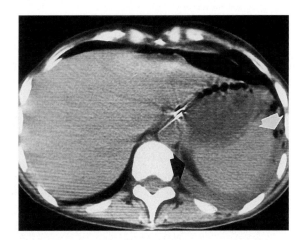

Fig. 36-39. Pleural fluid appears behind the fat density *(black arrow)* bare area of the spleen. Also note several small bubbles of gas beneath the left diaphragm *(white arrow).*

space. Above the level of the splenorenal ligament, fluid can surround the spleen entirely and become interposed between the diaphragm and spleen. (See sections of pararenal space abscesses). Any problems of distinguishing pleural effusions from subphrenic collections can be overcome by putting the patient in the decubitus position (Fig. 36-40).

One of the most difficult problems to differentiate from a subphrenic abscess is inversion of the diaphragm by a large pleural effusion. In these cases, a large pleural effusion is seen adjacent to the diaphragm (Fig. 36-41, *A*). On first glance, it is difficult to distinguish a pleural effusion from a subphrenic collection, but if one

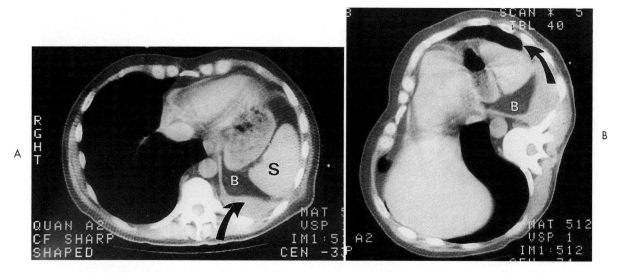

Fig. 36-40. A, Scan of a patient in the supine position shows a fluid collection *(arrow)* behind the bare area, *B,* of the spleen, *S.* This relationship indicates that the fluid is pleural, but in some cases the findings may still be questionable. **B,** Turning the same patient on the right side permits the fluid *(arrow)* to flow in the pleural space and clarify the position of the fluid behind the bare area, *B.*

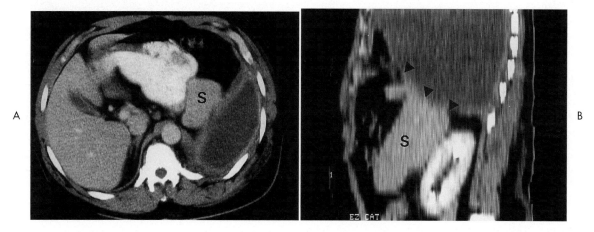

Fig. 36-41. A, Inverted diaphragm produces displacement of the spleen, *S,* anteriorly by the loculated chest fluid. **B,** Sagittal view of the inverted diaphragm *(arrowheads)* shows anterior and caudad displacement of the spleen, *S.*

looks carefully, the fluid is behind the spleen and the bare area of the spleen. A decubitus view or sagittal reconstruction may clarify the nature of the inversion (Fig. 36-41, *B*).

Left subhepatic abscesses

Abscesses in the left subhepatic space are caused by the same processes as those causing the subphrenic abscesses. They may spread from the right side, beneath the falciform ligament, or from other portions of the left subphrenic space (see Fig. 36-34).

Omental bursa abscesses

Abscesses in the omental bursa may be secondary to a process extending through Winslow's foramen, inflammation from the pancreas, a penetrating ulcer, or a tumor from the stomach or duodenum. The inferior recess of the omental bursa is anterior to the pancreas and is most commonly involved through penetrating ulcers or a pancreatic process. A small amount of air may be the only sign of a perforated ulcer. As was noted previously, the splenic recess of the omental bursa is located directly behind the fundus of the stomach (Figs. 36-42

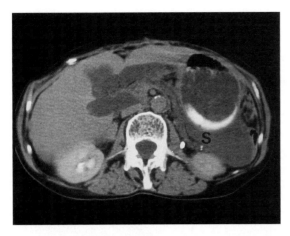

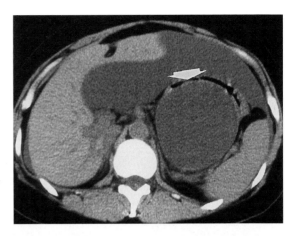

Fig. 36-42. This scan shows a large fluid collection in the inferior recess of the lesser sac and the splenic recess of the inferior recess, *S,* behind the stomach.

Fig. 36-43. Large fluid collection in splenic recess of the lesser sac, which is compressing the stomach *(arrow)* anteriorly. Note the fluid anteriorly, which is in the anterior left subphrenic space and the left subhepatic space.

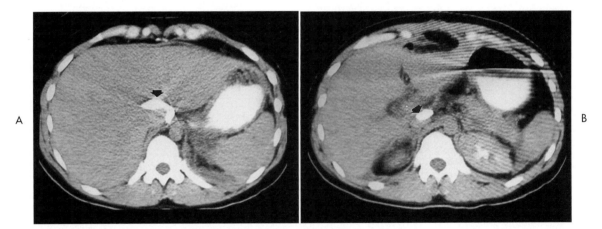

Fig. 36-44. A, This and the subsequent scan shows a dense catheter adjacent to the caudate lobe *(arrow)* in the superior medial recess of the omental bursa. **B,** This lower scan shows the location of the foramen of Winslow occupied by an opaque catheter *(arrow),* which was placed surgically.

and 36-43). The medial superior recess extends cephalad adjacent to the caudate lobe and vena cava (Figs. 36-44 and 36-45).

It is important to administer oral contrast material to see the posterior wall of the stomach and to distinguish it from an abscess in the splenic recess of the omental bursa (Figs. 36-42 and 36-43). Air may remain in the omental bursa for several days after a surgical procedure and should not be mistaken for an abscess.

Pericolic and interloop abscesses

Pericolic abscesses can occur as a result of virtually any inflammatory process within the abdomen, such as a perforated colon or bowel, appendicitis, or a rup-

tured gallbladder because the physiological movement of fluid is into the pericolic space (see earlier section on peritoneal function). Such abscesses are usually associated with a subhepatic or subdiaphragmatic abscess. On CT, a pericolic abscess appears as a mass of fluid density bordered on the lateral surface by the parietal peritoneum and medially by the serosa of the colon (Fig. 36-46, *A*). Such abscesses may spread into the right subhepatic or subdiaphragmatic space.

Interloop abscesses can be caused by the same etiological conditions as any abscess but are more commonly associated with fistulae from the bowel (Fig. 36-46, *B*).

Interloop abscesses can occur between isolated

loops of bowel or within the infracolic spaces. In such cases, it is best to give ample amounts of contrast material to try to opacify the bowel, but many times there is sufficient contrast enhancement of the bowel wall and the contents (Fig. 36-46, *B*) to distinguish the abscesses. At times with an abscess present, bowel adjacent to the

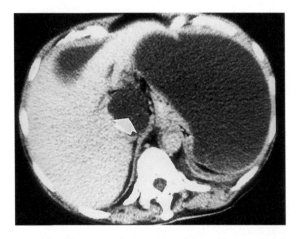

Fig. 36-45. CT scan in the upper abdomen shows a fluid collection *(arrow)* in the superior medial recess of the omental bursa, adjacent to the caudate lobe.

inflammation is paralytic and may not carry the contrast. In such cases, a fluid-filled or gas-filled abscess can be distinguished from the normal bowel because the wall of the abscess is smooth and lacks the irregular contour of the bowel wall produced by typical haustra or valvulae (Fig. 36-46, *C*). Moreover, the fluid in the bowel has a varied appearance with different densities, whereas an abscess is completely homogeneous.

Pelvic abscesses

The pelvis, the lowest point in the abdomen and the area to which exudates gravitate, is one of the most common locations for intra-abdominal abscesses. Abscesses in this area may result from diverticulitis, appendicitis, a perforated viscus, peritonitis, or trauma (Fig. 36-47).

On CT, the abscess has a typical appearance, being low in density and well margined; it may or may not contain gas. It is important to administer both intravenous and urographic contrast material to opacify the rectum and colon (see Fig. 36-30). Administration of both contrast materials should eliminate any false-positive results, especially in patients with ascites; the ascitic fluid in the pelvis may produce an area of fluid density on the image, which may be confusing.

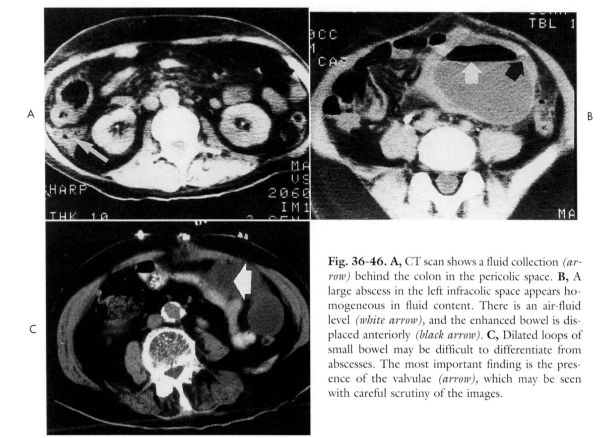

Fig. 36-46. A, CT scan shows a fluid collection *(arrow)* behind the colon in the pericolic space. **B,** A large abscess in the left infracolic space appears homogeneous in fluid content. There is an air-fluid level *(white arrow)*, and the enhanced bowel is displaced anteriorly *(black arrow)*. **C,** Dilated loops of small bowel may be difficult to differentiate from abscesses. The most important finding is the presence of the valvulae *(arrow)*, which may be seen with careful scrutiny of the images.

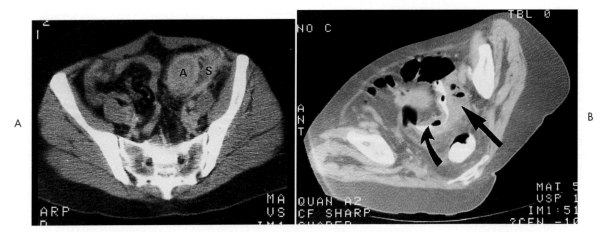

Fig. 36-47. A, CT scan through the upper portion of the pelvis shows an abscess, *A,* adjacent to the sigmoid colon, *S.* **B,** A scan of a different patient shows an abscess with an air-fluid level *(arrow)* next to a loop of sigmoid *(curved arrow).*

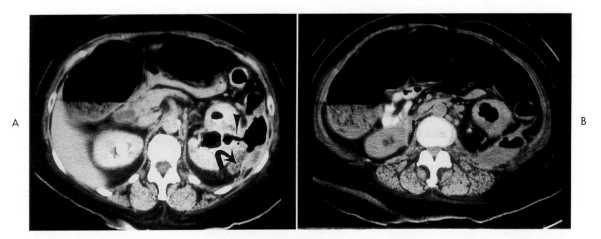

Fig. 36-48. A, Scan showing fistula *(arrowhead)* from the colon into the left kidney. Note the abscess extension *(curved arrow)* into the posterior pararenal space. **B,** This lower scan shows air within the left kidney and the air-fluid level in to the pararenal space.

Posterior pararenal space abscesses

The posterior pararenal space is bounded posteriorly by the transverse fascia and anteriorly by the posterior renal fascia (Fig. 36-48). This space extends caudad to the pelvis and cephalad to the diaphragm. Although most clinicians are familiar with the posterior pararenal space in the area of the kidneys, the pararenal space in the area adjacent to the diaphragm is not as familiar. In the space between the medial portion of the spleen and upper pole of the kidney is the splenorenal ligament, which represents the farthest extension of the pararenal space on the left side. There is an analogous space in the right side in the bare area of the liver. It has been my experience that both the anterior and posterior pararenal spaces communicate into these areas on the right and left sides, although this is not the traditional teaching.

Inflammatory processes in the posterior pararenal space usually result from a ruptured aortic aneurysm, pancreatitis, osteomyelitis from the rib or spine, intestinal or esophageal perforation, or trauma (Fig. 36-49). Abscesses may remain localized laterally within the pararenal space or become confluent with the psoas muscles. Processes from the aorta or spine may spread laterally. In addition to the abscess collection, there is concomitant thickening of the fascial planes. A psoas abscess produces enlargement of the psoas muscles;[84] in cases of bilateral psoas abscesses associated with destruction of the vertebral body, tuberculosis should still be considered.

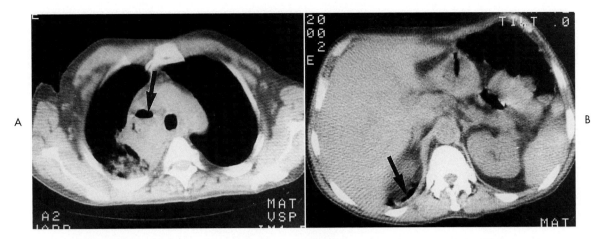

Fig. 36-49. A, CT scan of the mediastinum shows air *(arrow)* from an esophageal perforation. **B,** A scan through the upper portion of the abdomen shows air *(arrow)* in the bare area of the liver, which communicates with the anterior and posterior pararenal spaces.

Although little information is available in the literature, there are several cases indicating that the posterior pararenal space communicates with the posterior mediastinum (Fig. 36-49). Esophageal perforations or problems may extend caudally into the right or left posterior pararenal spaces, or vice versa.

Anterior pararenal space abscesses

The anterior pararenal space is bounded anteriorly by the posterior parietal peritoneum and posteriorly by the anterior renal fascia; this space is bounded laterally by the lateroconal fascia (which is the fused anterior and posterior perirenal fasciae). This compartment contains several alimentary organs, including the pancreas and ascending and descending colon. (This anatomical discussion is based on the traditional viewpoint; a new concept of the retroperitoneum proposes that there is no free communication between the space around the pancreas and the colon but that they are interconnected only through the attachment of the mesentery. In addition, the new concept no longer uses the term *anterior pararenal space* but considers these areas the *intermesenteric spaces.* (See section in this chapter on new concepts.)

Most inflammatory processes in this area originate from the colon, appendix, pancreas (see Fig. 36-7), or duodenum as a result of perforations from tumors, diverticulitis, inflammatory bowel disease, or trauma. Perforations of the bowel can produce gas, abscesses, or both, depending on the site of involvement. A localized perforation of the colon may occur in the retroperitoneal area and remain confined to the anterior pararenal space. If the process occurs below Gerota's fascia, it can move superiorly into both the anterior and the posterior pararenal spaces. The most cephalad extension of the

pararenal spaces on the right is the retroperitoneum behind the bare area of the liver, and on the left is the retroperitoneum medial to the spleen (Fig. 36-50).

Another sign I have found to be valuable in cases of inflammation is thickening of the renal fascia. For example, in some cases, it may be difficult to distinguish a loop of bowel with the density of fluid from an abscess; with an abscess, the renal fascia is thickened.

Liver abscesses

Pyogenic hepatic abscesses usually occur as a result of intra-abdominal infection, such as appendicitis, suppurative cholangitis, hematogenous dissemination by the portal vein draining the bowel, or hematogenous spreading from a distant focus.[48,81] The most common pyogenic organisms include gram-negative organisms, especially *Escherichia coli;* less commonly, anaerobes, such as *Clostridium* or *Bacteroides* organisms, also may be involved. Antibiotic therapy and drainage, either surgical or percutaneous, are indicated. The typical CT appearance of a hepatic abscess is a circumscribed mass with the density of fluid (Fig. 36-51). Amebic abscesses and echinococcosis are also types of hepatic abscesses (see following sections).

Two potential false-positive findings are commonly associated with the liver. The first is the partial volume effect produced by the upper pole of the right kidney. The space between the two is not clearly visualized but appears lower in density as a soft tissue mass; this may simulate a perirenal collection on the right side. The key to differentiating this partial volume error from a real perirenal collection is that there is ipsilateral thickening of perirenal fascia if an abscess is present. The second potential false-positive trait is a high hepatic flexure

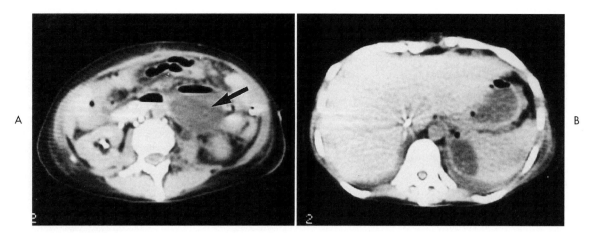

Fig. 36-50. A, Scan shows an abscess in the anterior pararenal space of the left side *(arrow).* **B,** The abscess extends cephalad behind the bare area of the spleen.

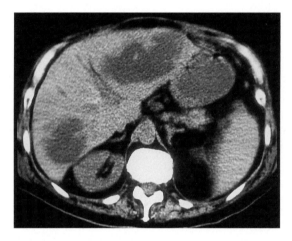

Fig. 36-51. Irregular large fluid collections in the right and left lobe, representing abscesses.

of the colon entering the porta hepatis. The course of the transverse colon to the hepatic flexure of the colon should be carefully traced; at times, a decubitus view may be required to confirm the diagnosis.

Amebic abscesses

Amebic abscesses are a complication of colonic infestation by *Entamoeba histolytica.* The disease is produced when material contaminated with ameba is ingested. Amebae reach the liver either by the portal drainage or by the lymphatic vessels from the bowel.[48] Once in the liver, the amebae release autolytic enzymes, and inflammation progresses until an abscess is produced. Such abscesses can become secondarily infected by pyogenic organisms, which may or may not be gas producing. The treatment of amebic abscesses consists of antibiotic therapy or surgical drainage, or both. Total reso-

lution of the amebic abscess can occur without complete drainage with proper medical therapy consisting of metronidazole. (The material aspirated from such amebic abscesses has the appearance of anchovy pate and consists of autolyzed liver tissue.) Surgical drainage may be required in some abscesses that have become superinfected with pyogenic organisms. The CT appearance of an amebic abscess is identical to that of a pyogenic abscess.[55] It appears as well-delineated masses of fluid density within the liver substance (Fig. 36-52).

Fungal infections

A number of different fungal infections can cause focal infections, with *Candida* being the most common. With most fungi, the early foci may appear low density and poorly defined, but they may liquefy into well-marginated fluid collections (Fig. 36-53).

Echinococcosis

Echinococcosis, or hydatid disease of the liver, is a parasitic abscess caused by the larvae of *Echinococcus multilocularis* (alveolaris) or *Echinococcus granulosus.* The dog is the host, and sheep are the intermediate hosts; humans may become intermediate hosts by ingesting food contaminated by the ova. The pathophysiological conditions follow: After ingestion of the ova, the embryo, which penetrates the intestinal wall and is transported to the liver by the portal system, is released. (Although echinococcosis can occur virtually anywhere in the body, the liver is the most common organ involved.) Once in the liver, the larva establishes itself, and inflammation proceeds. The hepatic cyst produced is composed of the endocyst, comprising the parasitic elements of the germinal membrane and daughter cysts, and the surrounding percyst, which is the compressed hepatic pa-

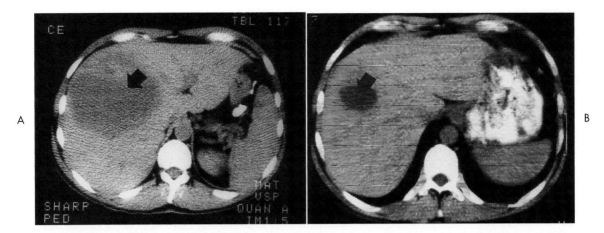

Fig. 36-52. A, A large amebic abscess *(arrow),* which looks similar to other abscesses. **B,** Resolution of the amebic abscess occurred over a number of months after administration of antibiotic medications.

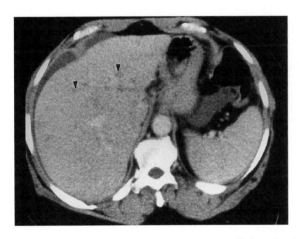

Fig. 36-53. Fungal granulomas appear as small low-density masses *(arrowheads)* in the right and left lobes of the liver.

renchyma and inflammatory reaction. Pathologically the two types of *Echinococcus* organisms differ. *Echinococcus granulosus* may have (1) a unilocular cavity, which is usually fertile, or (2) a multilocular cavity with irregular edges, which does not metastasize. Calcifications may indicate sterility. *Echinococcus multilocularis* produces small numerous cysts that multiply by exogenous budding to produce the malignant hydatid cyst, which can become confluent throughout the liver or metastasize to other organs.

Treatment of an echinococcal abscess historically has been possible only by surgical drainage,[21] but medical and drainage methods have improved. There are several chemical agents that have been shown to be effective. Percutaneous drainage can be performed if "killing" solution is injected and meticulous technique is used to prevent spillage. Drainage, however, should not be performed unless significant symptoms or complications exist. Surgical drainage consists of complete removal of the intact cyst after a "killing" solution of 10% povidone-iodine (Betadine), 20% sodium chloride or ethyl alcohol has been injected into the cyst (formalin has been abandoned because of adverse effects). The greater omentum is usually sutured over the remaining cavity in the liver to preclude any spillage of residual fluid or cysts into the peritoneal cavity.

The CT follow-up of such cases is informative because of the clear visualization of the anatomy. Before surgical treatment, the large mother cysts containing the daughter cysts are clearly seen (Fig. 36-54). With some of the new chemotherapeutic agents available, temporary improvement in the cysts can occasionally be seen, as evidenced by some dissolution of the walls of the daughter cysts. Whether such medical treatment will be effective in the long term is not known.

After surgery, the residual cavity can clearly be distinguished from the evacuated cyst and the fat density of the omentum, which is used to seal the cavity (Fig. 36-54, *D*). For several weeks, the size of the cavity reduces, and the amount of fat seen decreases as the fibrosis of healing continues.

In some cases, there may be secondary infection of daughter cysts by colonization from a biliary fistula. In such cases, air may be seen within the cysts from either pyogenic bacteria or a biliary fistula, which usually accompanies the infection. On some occasions, the pyogenic organisms can actually destroy the daughter cysts by enzymatic digestion (Figs. 36-54, *B* and *C*). Diagnostic aspiration should be avoided because of potential spillage of the daughter cysts and anaphylaxis from the

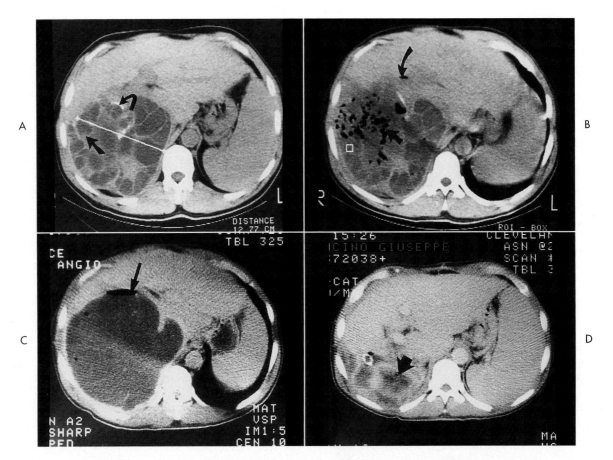

Fig. 36-54. A, CT scan of echinococcal cysts shows calcification in the wall *(curved arrow)* and daughter cysts *(arrow)* within the mother cyst. **B,** After secondary infection, air can be seen within a cyst. This scan shows multiple air pockets within the cyst and air within the biliary system *(curved arrow)*. **C,** With persistent infection, dissolution of the daughter cysts can be seen. Note the air *(arrow)* in the upper portion of the cyst and the absence of daughter cysts. **D,** After surgery, the cavity, filled with fat density omentum, can be seen.

foreign protein. Sensitization of the patient from the protein is necessary for anaphylaxis to occur; this usually follows a previous spillage of material, although it may occur without such an event.

Complications associated with the disease include rupture of the mother cyst and spillage into the peritoneum or adjacent structures. In approximately 10% of cases, secondary infection may occur because of erosion into the bowel or the biliary system.

Since the early report of the CT appearance of echinococcosis,[79] two articles discussing the CT detection and appearance of echinococcal cysts of the liver have appeared. Scherer et al[91] reported on the CT evaluation of 13 cases of echinococcosis and noted two distinct appearances. In six of eight cases involving *Echinococcus granulosus,* the cysts appeared as masses of fluid density (3 to 30 HU) with a radiodense rim. In six of eight cases, there was calcification, and in five of those cases, the calcifications were either crescent or ring

shaped. Daughter cysts were visible in the larger cyst in six cases. In five patients infected by *Echinococcus multilocularis,* the lesions were seen as low-density masses (14 to 38 HU) without a well-defined membrane. In four of five cases, there were small nodular calcifications present (never ring shaped). Gonzalez et al[27] reported on the accuracy of detecting hepatic echinococcosis with CT. They reported that CT diagnosis was correct in 19 of 19 cases. They noted that CT was the preferred modality because it "clearly and precisely shows the existence, number, size, and location of cysts and also yields data allowing assumption as to their vitality."

Splenic abscesses and splenitis

Splenic involvement directly or indirectly by infection is quite common. In addition to abscesses, a wide spectrum of inflammatory changes can occur with pyogenic or granulomatous disease.

Pyogenic systemic infections can cause diffuse

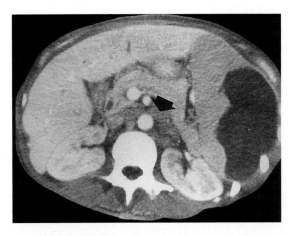

Fig. 36-55. Patient with AIDS. CT scan shows large, irregular abscess in the spleen. Also, note the numerous lymph nodes *(arrow)* in the retroperitoneum.

acute splenitis or focal fluid density abscesses. Pathologically, small septic infarcts with systemic sepsis, which have been called "milk-flecked," may be seen. These small collections may be below the level of resolution of the CT scanner, so they can be missed. With larger amounts of inflammation and infection, the typical intrasplenic abscesses, which are associated with endocarditis, AIDS, or intravenous drug abuse, can be seen (Fig. 36-55). Granulomatous processes, such as tuberculosis and histoplasmosis, are quite easily seen as clearly delineated calcium deposits. From gross pathology, it is known that granulomatous processes are associated with infarcts. There is no significant information available on this point, but I have noted the association of infarctlike areas in the spleen with such patients. In one patient with mature-appearing granulomas, I could see small cystic areas adjacent to the granulomas. In a patient with recently diagnosed tuberculosis, I noted the evolution of a typical infarct in association with the disease (Fig. 36-56), which changed with treatment. From my limited experience, it seems that CT scans will show the different stages of infarct evolution in association with these processes; such findings need not suggest a different process.

Nonspecific splenomegaly without splenitis can occur with a variety of systemic disorders, including parasitic infestations, systemic sepsis, and AIDS-related disease. In many cases of patients with myeloproliferative disorders, such splenomegaly may be associated with the underlying disease or borderline infection.

Renal abscesses

Renal abscesses may be caused by hematogenous "seeding," in which the organism is usually *Staphylococcus*, or a urinary tract infection, in which the organism is usually *Escherichia coli, Proteus mirabilis,* or *Enterobacter aerogenes.* An intrarenal abscess is low in density and well

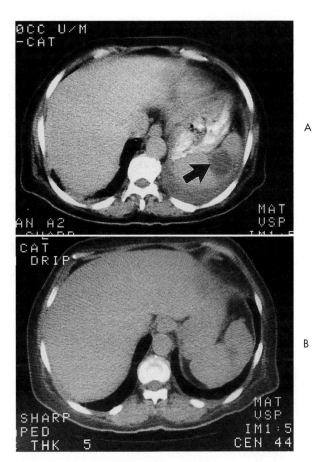

Fig. 36-56. A, CT scan shows a low-density area *(arrow)* in the spleen, believed to be early changes of tuberculosis. **B,** A follow-up scan shows resolution of the area several months after the institution of antituberculous therapy.

marginated and may resemble a renal cyst (see Fig. 36-33). More commonly, an abscess has a more irregular margin and higher density and produces unilateral thickening of the renal fascia (Fig. 36-57), whereas cysts seldom do this. When the infection is still an inflammatory phlegmon and not a fluid collection, there may be a focal area of enlargement that is isodense with a normal enhanced kidney but low in density with intravenous contrast enhancement. This area of localized inflammation and focal enlargement is the focal nephritis, or nephronia[88] (Fig. 36-58). If the infection resolves, the kidney may return to normal; if it progresses, an abscess may form. Emphysematous pyelonephritis is an uncommon disease produced by gas-forming organisms and usually occurs in patients with diabetes. On CT, the kidney may show small gas densities within the parenchyma, or the kidney may appear as a gas-filled structure barely recognizable as a kidney. A spurious finding of "gas" can be produced by embolization or infarction.[106]

An earlier form of the disease in the infectious spectrum shows even more subtle, temporary changes in the kidney. With diffuse pyelonephritis, a "striated" appearance or focal areas of decreased enhancement can be seen. These areas usually resolve with adequate therapy.

Polycystic renal disease associated with an abscess is a difficult clinical problem. By looking at the CT image, one cannot distinguish an infected cyst from the multitude of other cysts within the kidney. In such cases, a gallium scan is most helpful in finding an infected cyst among the other cysts of fluid density.

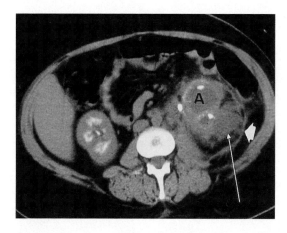

Fig. 36-57. Abscess, *A,* in the anterior portion of the left kidney. There is extension of the purulent material into the perinephric space *(long arrow)* and thickening of the perirenal fascia *(small arrow).*

Perirenal space abscesses

Abscesses of the perirenal space, confined by the renal fascia, are usually caused by spread of renal infection. The most common infecting organisms are *Escherichia coli, Enterobacter aerogenes,* and *Proteus mirabilis.*

The cross-sectional CT findings of a perirenal abscess are an area of fluid density surrounding the kidneys bounded by the renal fascia. In all cases, there is concomitant thickening of the renal fascia (Fig. 36-57). The partial volume effect associated with the right kidney and medial margin of the liver should not be mistaken for a perirenal collection. In the normal case, a "double density" can be perceived. One can be certain that this is not a perirenal collection because there should be associated fascial plane thickening if a true abscess exists.

Other considerations

One of the greatest advantages of CT is its ability to image all areas completely. This accurate localization is especially important for the preoperative evaluation of abscesses to facilitate their drainage. With CT, it is possible to determine the full extent of an inflammatory process and to detect multiple concurrent abscesses. This latter point is especially important because one must always be concerned about the occurrence of multiple concurrent abscesses. This information is especially important for patients who are to undergo surgical procedures, but

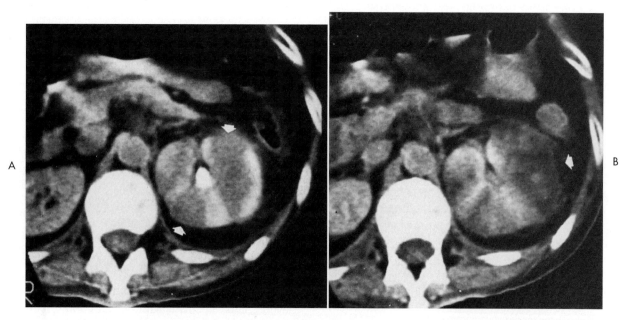

Fig. 36-58. Progression of multifocal bacterial nephritis to a frank abscess. **A,** Post–contrast-enhanced image of the kidney demonstrates the typical defects of multifocal bacterial nephritis *(arrow).* Pre–contrast-enhanced images were normal. **B,** Post–contrast-enhanced image 1 week later demonstrates more severe changes of bacterial nephritis and liquefaction *(arrow),* with extension beyond the renal capsule. Surgery revealed an abscess in a "dead" kidney.

it is absolutely critical if percutaneous drainage is considered.[23,28-31] For accurate localization of abscesses before percutaneous drainage procedures, the consensus in the literature is that CT is superior to other imaging systems and is the modality of choice.[56] Given equal availability of the instrumentation, CT should be used as the initial diagnostic modality when percutaneous aspiration drainage of an intra-abdominal abscess is anticipated.

Finally, another important advantage of CT is its ability to determine the initiating cause of abscesses. Entities such as appendicitis, diverticulitis, cholecystitis, and penetrating ulcers can sometimes be suspected or recognized. With appendicitis, the diagnosis is suggested by a fluid collection adjacent to the cecum or edema in the retroperitoneal fascia. With diverticulitis, the air-filled diverticuli adjacent to the abscess, which is of fluid density, can be recognized. Penetrating ulcers cannot be seen, but because of gas adjacent to the duodenum or in the omental bursa, the diagnosis should be suspected. In other cases, CT may not provide this information, and other radiological procedures or investigators are needed.

Mycotic aneurysms. Mycotic aneurysms of native vessels are a rare event. It is believed that such infection must be superimposed on a diseased vessel and that it occurs as a result of hematogenous or direct spread. In cases of non–gas-forming organisms, there may only be a fluid collection in direct proximity to the vessel. In patients with a gas-forming infection, small bubbles of gas can be seen.

Infected synthetic grafts. Infection of synthetic grafts is a disastrous complication of vascular reconstructive surgery. The incidence of graft infections is as high as 6%, and they are associated with a high rate of mor-

bidity and mortality. The potential causes of the infection are contamination, small gastrointestinal fistulae, or hematogenous seeding. Gram-positive organisms that can cause the infection of grafts include *Staphylococcus epidermidis, Staphylococcus,* and *Streptococcus faecalis.* The gram-negative organisms commonly encountered in such graft infections include *Escherichia coli* and *Klebsiella, Enterobacter, Proteus, Pseudomonas,* and *Bacteroides* organisms; the most common of this group is *Escherichia coli.* Before CT, the diagnosis of graft infections depended on such standard radiographic techniques as gastrointestinal studies or angiography. By the time such studies discovered the infection, however, the patient was often beyond the point of cure, even with proper surgical therapy. With CT, it is now possible to detect accurately fluid and gas collections that may indicate infection in and around synthetic grafts.

The typical findings of infected aortic grafts depend on the type of organism involved. A gram-positive cocci that does not produce gas produces a fluid collection in the aneurysm bed or adjacent to the graft itself. When the infecting organism is gas forming, such as *Escherichia coli,* or there is a small enteric fistula (Fig. 36-59), there are small microbubbles of gas in and around the graft. There are several possible causes of false-positive findings in such cases. If a significant amount of blood or old hematoma is around the graft in the aneurysm, it too appears to be an area of fluid density (Fig. 36-60). Normal postoperative gas may also be present within the aneurysm bed adjacent to the graft 7 to 10 days after surgery.[87] Because of the high mortality rate associated with this defense, radiologists have now adopted an aggressive approach for confirming the presence or absence of infection. In any case of a possible infected aortic graft, we now think that a CT-guided as-

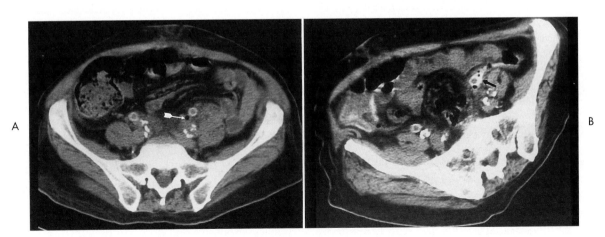

Fig. 36-59. A, Scan shows a small air collection *(arrow)* adjacent to the left iliac limb of a prosthetic graft. **B,** Communication with the colon is verified by leakage of contrast material *(arrow)* from the bowel to the graft.

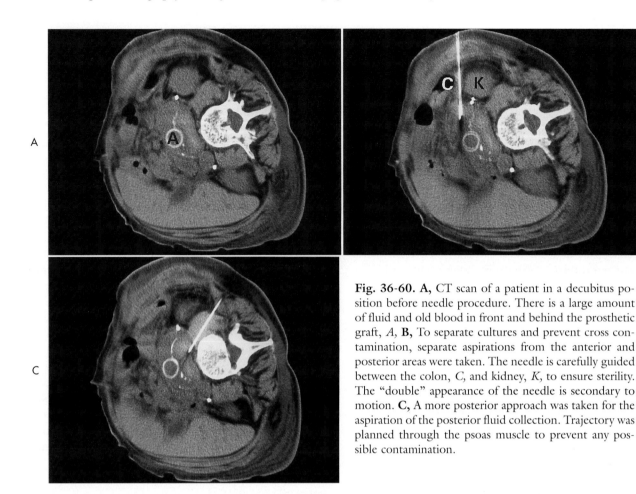

Fig. 36-60. A, CT scan of a patient in a decubitus position before needle procedure. There is a large amount of fluid and old blood in front and behind the prosthetic graft, **A, B,** To separate cultures and prevent cross contamination, separate aspirations from the anterior and posterior areas were taken. The needle is carefully guided between the colon, *C*, and kidney, *K*, to ensure sterility. The "double" appearance of the needle is secondary to motion. **C,** A more posterior approach was taken for the aspiration of the posterior fluid collection. Trajectory was planned through the psoas muscle to prevent any possible contamination.

piration through the retroperitoneum is imperative to obtain a culture of the material around the aneurysm directly and determine whether infection is present (Fig. 36-60, *B* and *C*). This is important because in infected patients, expeditious surgical treatment consisting of removal of the graft and an axillofemoral bypass is typically performed. When aspiration results are normal, an extensive, complicated, and difficult surgical procedure may be avoided. With the improved diagnostic accuracy of CT and the more potent antibiotics, some surgeons are now deferring surgery if the infectious area is not adjacent to the anatomical site. Advances with urokinase enhancement of percutaneous drainage may improve the outcome of percutaneous treatment in such cases.[54,83]

Accuracy in relation to other modalities

Since the introduction of CT, several articles have discussed its usefulness for detecting abscesses. The first such article by our group[30] reported a correct diagnosis in 20 of 22 abscesses. Since this first report, numerous others, including Callen,[14] Gerzof et al,[22] Aronberg et al,[6] Korobkin et al,[53] Levitt et al,[59] Wolverson et al,[10] and Knochel et al,[52] have confirmed the high detection rate of CT for abscesses. There are only sparse data, but some comparative information is available about other imaging systems, such as ultrasound and gallium-67 citrate. In our initial report, CT was correct for 20 of 22 abscesses, gallium was correct in 6 of 9 abscesses, and ultrasound was correct in 1 of 2 abscesses. Korobkin et al[53] reported CT correct in 9 of 9 abscesses, gallium in 9 of 12, and ultrasound in 12 of 12. Levitt et al,[59] found CT to be correct in 6 of 6 abscesses and gallium correct in 9 of 9. More recently, Knochel et al[52] presented larger numbers by which to compare CT and ultrasound, but they did not include gallium isotope scanning. In their series, CT was the most accurate modality, with a sensitivity rate of 97.5% and a specificity rate of 95%, whereas ultrasound had a sensitivity rate of 82% and a specificity rate of 94.5%. In the literature and at meetings, there is always a controversial debate as to whether use of CT is justified when ultrasound is also good and only 10% to 13% less accurate. Proponents of ultrasound argue that it is less expensive and does not use radiation. CT advocates point out that abscesses are curable, and therefore the 10% increased accuracy is worth the additional expense and radiation.

I have formulated an approach to these modalities based on several principles. According to the guideline about medical decision making, set by McNeil et al,[72] any false-negative results must be minimized with a curable disease, and therefore significant costs and efforts to find and treat such a disease are justifiable. Based on this reasoning, I can rationalize using CT for all patients. Realistically, however, a CT device is a limited resource; thus one must maximize the diagnostic return and not overuse it improperly. I believe that CT, ultrasound, and gallium scanning are complementary in that the patient can best be cared for by taking into account the advantages and disadvantages of each modality. An acutely ill patient does not have the luxury of waiting hours or even days for the results of an isotope test.[68] Therefore, I prefer using an immediate imaging system, such as CT or ultrasound. Considering the various anatomical areas within the abdomen and technical considerations of each modality, the best-suited method for each case can be selected. Thus, if the patient is acutely ill and has focal symptoms in the right upper quadrant, retroperitoneum, or pelvis, ultrasound should be the modality of choice. If the ultrasound results are normal in these areas and the patient is toxic, examination with CT is appropriate. If the patient has focal symptoms in the left upper quadrant, pancreatic area of midabdomen, CT is the preferred modality. If the patient is acutely ill or immunocompromised with general symptoms and no focal signs, CT is the modality of choice because it can evaluate all areas without difficulty. Finally, if the acutely ill patient has drains, wounds, or external appliances, CT is better suited immediately after surgery because it does not require a coupling agent to the skin. If the patient is chronically ill, a gallium scan should be performed to locate the potential area of infection. Depending on the region of uptake, one should use ultrasound (in the right upper quadrant, pelvis, and flank) or CT (in the left upper quadrant, pancreas, and abdomen).

PERITONEAL AND MESENTERIC ABNORMALITIES

Only a limited number of benign and malignant tumors affect the mesentery and peritoneum. The most common of these abnormalities are neoplastic diseases, but less commonly benign abnormalities of the mesentery can be seen.

Peritoneal cysts

Peritoneal cysts are unusual cystic masses that may be attached to the mesentery or peritoneum. The origin of these abnormalities is poorly understood, but some believe they are related to lymphatic abnormalities that produce sequestered secondary cysts. They are typically lined with endothelium. The cysts may be unilocular or

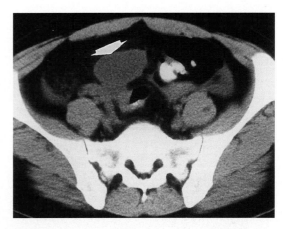

Fig. 36-61. CT scan shows a well-defined, low-density mass *(arrow)* in the midpelvis, which has the appearance consistent with a peritoneal cyst but later proved to be an abscess.

multilocular. Clinically, they produce the same symptoms as an abdominal mass; surgical treatment is curative.

On CT, these cysts appear as large, low-density masses with clearly demarcated fibroconnective tissue walls (Fig. 36-61). No unique imaging features distinguish these cysts from other low-density masses, such as mucinous metastases, abscesses, or hematomas. In such cases, the clinical history is important, and if indicated, a percutaneous puncture for cytological or bacteriological study can be performed (Fig. 36-62).

Desmoid fibromas

Desmoid fibromas are unencapsulated infiltrating fibromas occurring predominantly in women and in any part of the body, including the abdomen.[65] There is a high association of fibromas of the abdominal wall and peritoneum with familial polyposis syndrome,[71] and fibromas are one of the classic signs composing Gardner's syndrome. In one series of 44 intra-abdominal desmoid fibromas, 41 occurred within the mesentery.[71] The main clinical problem that arises with such desmoid fibromas is distinguishing these tumors from neoplastic masses resulting from colonic carcinoma. Pathologically the tumor is benign but difficult to distinguish from a low-grade fibrosarcoma; however, there have been no reported metastases. Occasionally the lesion may cavitate and enlarge quickly by the imbibition of fluid. The treatment is surgical excision, but unless complete meticulous resection is performed, recurrence is the rule.

On a CT scan, it appears as a mass of soft tissue density within the peritoneum, displacing other intra-abdominal organs (Fig. 36-63). No unique imaging traits distinguish these from neoplastic masses, such as lymphomas and metastatic disease, or even from other benign masses, such as hematomas or high-density peritoneal cysts.

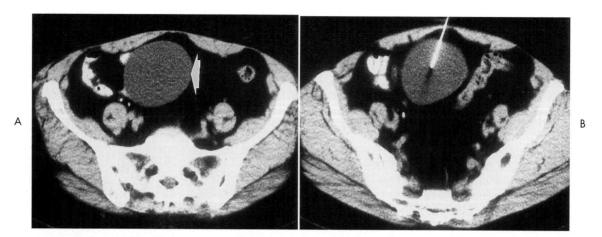

Fig. 36-62. A, CT scan shows a similar-appearing mass *(arrow)* which proved to be a mesenteric cyst. Compare with Fig. 36-61. **B,** CT-guided procedure proved the true nature of the mass. The trajectory chosen avoids any loops of bowel, thereby preventing the possibility of contamination.

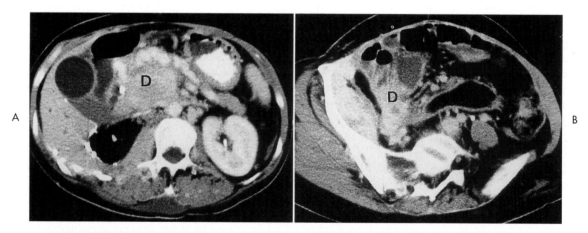

Fig. 36-63. A, Desmoid fibroma, *D,* involving the pancreas, which simulates a neoplastic tumor. Infiltration into the biliary system and portal hepatis is occurring and producing benign, aggressive extension with almost "malignant" properties. **B,** Lower scan taken through the pelvis shows an ill-defined mass behind the cecum and adjacent to the psoas.

Retractile mesenteritis

Retractile mesenteritis is an unusual disorder of the mesentery consisting of diffuse inflammatory thickening of the mesenteric fat.[17,51] The cause of the abnormality is unknown. Pathologically, there is fibrosis, inflammation, and fatty infiltration. Retractile mesenteritis is the term used when fibrosis predominates. The process originates in the root of the mesentery and then can extend diffusely throughout the mesenteric fat. The disease process is confined to the mesentery, and there are no abnormalities of the intestines or vessels.[51] With CT, the mesentery does not appear to be of normal fat density but appears as an area of soft tissue density (Fig. 36-

64). The bowel is not in its normal anterior location but is retracted posteriorly. One group[25] reports calcifications in some unusual cases of retractile mesenteritis and some resolution of the mesenteritis after treatment with steroids. In unusual cases, narrowing and rigidity of the colon with thumbprinting or displacement of bowel by mesenteric masses may be seen.[97] Han et al[33] reported a case involving the colon that produced transmural thickening of the colon.

Inflammatory processes

A number of inflammatory processes associated with the bowel, peritoneum, and mesentery produce cer-

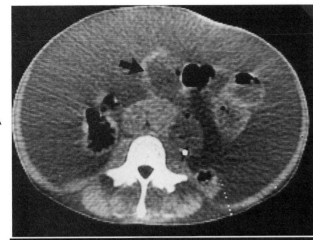

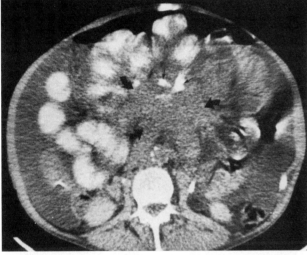

Fig. 36-64. A, Retractile mesenteritis produces a thickening of the mesentery *(arrow),* which may retract loops of the bowel posteriorly. Compare the posterior location of these bowel loops with those pictured in Fig. 36-71. **B,** A mass *(curved arrows)* with calcifications *(small arrows)* caused by retractile mesenteritis. (**B** Courtesy Dr. Richard Palmer Gold, Columbia-Presbyterian Medical Center, New York.)

tain predictable changes on CT scan. The findings of edema, bowel wall thickening, fluid distention, and fibrosis are nonspecific.

Crohn's disease causes transmural inflammation of the bowel, which produces fairly typical findings. Characteristically, thickening of the bowel wall associated with soft tissue density, edema, and fibrous reaction is seen. On occasion an increased amount of fat separating several loops of bowel is seen; it has been said that this represents proliferation of fat, but the cause of such fat accumulation is not known.

Ulcerative colitis produces only thickening of the bowel wall without producing the changes within the mesentery. There also is dilatation of the colon and some loss of the haustral markings.

Pseudomembranous colitis produces thickening of the colonic wall and changes in the lateroconal fascia and the perirenal fascia. The entire colon usually is involved, but there may also be segmental involvement.

Diverticulitis consistently shows changes recognizable on the CT scan.[43,62] First, small air pockets that represent air-filled diveritucli are seen on the wall of the colon. Inflammation from the diverticulitis produces edema in the fat adjacent to the bowel.

Appendicitis produces edema and inflammation adjacent to the end of the cecum. The normal appendix can be located in the peritoneum, pelvis, or retrocecal region. With inflammation, there is edema and thickening of the adjacent fascial planes.

Whipple's disease

A single report exists in the literature about Whipple's disease of the small bowel.[60] Clinically the disease is associated with abdominal pain, malabsorption, and diarrhea. There may also be some arthralgias associated. In a report by Li and Rennie,[60] the specific diagnostic points included enlarged lymph nodes in the 2 to 3 cm range in the mesentery and retroperitoneum. In addition, abnormal changes in the small bowel pattern similar to the findings noted on traditional barium studies were noted. The lymph nodes were low in density because of fat content. Some had necrosis within the center.

Amyloidosis

Systemic amyloidosis consists of systemic deposition of amyloid throughout organs and tissues. Gastrointestinal involvement is said to occur in 70% of primary and 55.5% of the secondary amyloidosis.[2]

A single report exists in the literature about the findings of secondary amyloidosis of the mesentery. In the case reported by Allen et al,[2] there was diffuse thickening of the mesentery and encasement of the mesenteric vessels, having the appearance of diffuse carcinomatosis. Diagnosis can be established only by biopsy.

AIDS

AIDS is becoming more significant because of its almost uncontrolled spread among designated risk groups.[12,47] It is caused by the human immunodeficiency virus (HIV). Identified risk factors include homosexuality, drug abuse, Haitian ancestry, or heterosexual exposure to prostitution.

These patients are at great risk for the development of any infectious process, including many opportunistic infections. In addition, such patients are predisposed to the development of a number of malignancies, including Kaposi's sarcoma and a severe form of large cell lymphoma.

Jeffrey et al[47] wrote an excellent article about AIDS within the abdomen. A review of this excellent article is highly recommended for more specific details.

AIDS-related complex is a constellation of symptoms and signs that predate the development of AIDS. Symptoms include fever, weight loss, diarrhea, malaise, and night sweats. There is associated lymphadenopathy in the mesentery and retroperitoneum secondary to reactive lymphoid hyperplasia (Fig. 36-55). The triad of CT findings previously reported for this entity are lymphadenopathy, splenomegaly, and perirectal thickening (presumably owing to venereal infection). The lymph nodes in this state are seldom larger than 1.5 cm in diameter; any enlargement beyond this should suggest neoplasm or infection and probably warrants a CT-guided biopsy.

Opportunistic infections with AIDS are common and can consist of many forms, including *Candida* esophagitis and small bowel or colon infection with *Cryptosporidium*, cytomegalovirus, herpes simplex, or *Mycobacterium avium–intracellulare*. These problems cause nonspecific changes in those portions of the gastrointestinal tract. Both tuberculosis and *Mycobacterium avium–intracellulare* can produce enlargement of mesenteric and retroperitoneal lymph nodes.[80,99]

The two most common malignancies associated with AIDS include Kaposi's sarcoma and non-Hodgkin's lymphoma. Kaposi's sarcoma can show lymphadenopathy or gastrointestinal involvement in the form of wall thickening. It may involve virtually any abdominal organ and may produce many unusual intra-abdominal lesions, which may be easily amenable to CT procedures.

The lymphoma associated with AIDS usually is a non-Hodgkin type (Hodgkin's disease occasionally occurs), which typically has increased incidence of extranodal involvement. Sites of occurrence may include brain, bone marrow, viscera, and mucocutaneous sites. The lymphoma is especially aggressive, and response to treatment has been generally poor.

NEOPLASTIC LESIONS
Peritoneal mesotheliomas

Peritoneal mesothelioma is a rare neoplasm arising in the peritoneal lining of the abdomen. The disease is believed to be associated with exposure to asbestos. Pathologically, it occurs in several forms: sarcoma, polygonal cell type, and tubular papillary type. All types have a uniformly poor prognosis, with most patients dying within 2 years of the diagnosis. In my experience, the appearance of the tumor coincided with those cases reported in the literature (Figs. 36-65 and 36-66). On CT examination,[16] it appears as an area of soft tissue den-

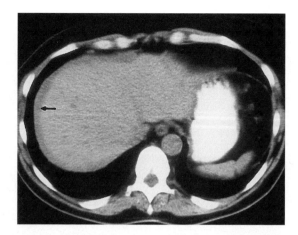

Fig. 36-65. Mesothelioma on the undersurface of the diaphragm *(arrow)*, which is producing a uniform thickening around the capsule of the liver.

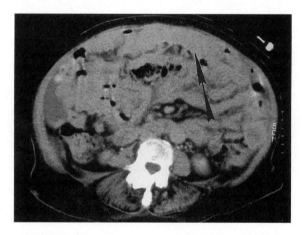

Fig. 36-66. Extensive soft tissue thickening in the anterior abdomen. The tumor is infiltrating throughout the mesentery in an irregular pattern.

sity within the abdomen. It may conform to the contour of the liver or produce a mass effect on adjacent structures. No features distinguish it clearly from other types of benign or malignant tumor with a benign fibrotic reaction. Whitley[105] has recommended signs for suggesting the diagnosis of mesothelioma.

Primary papillary tumors of the peritoneum

Since 1976, primary papillary tumor of the peritoneum has been recognized as a separate entity. For a time, this tumor was thought to be related to either mesothelioma or ovarian tumors, but it is now accepted by some as a distinct entity.[50]

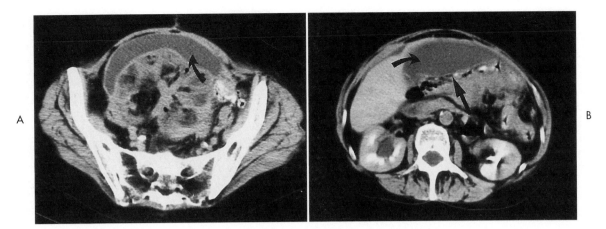

Fig. 36-67. CT scans of a patient with primary papillary carcinoma of the peritoneum. There is a fluid density anteriorly *(arrow)*, which represents a neoplastic loculation.

The tumor is thought to originate from mesothelial cells of the peritoneum, which are somewhat similar to ovarian cells. Clinical presentation of the patients is related to the involvement of multiple areas of the peritoneum. It is not possible to distinguish a metastatic focus from a localized origination point; the possibility of multicentric origin has been suggested.[50] The disease in patients having these tumors is consistently more extensive than in patients of the same age who have ovarian tumors.

Treatment of the disease is similar to that of disseminated ovarian tumor. The outcome has not been good.

CT findings of this disease are nonspecific. Scans may show discrete tumor mass over the peritoneum or simply collections of located fluid (Fig. 36-67).

Lymphomas

According to Goffinet et al,[24] 61% of the non-Hodgkin lymphomas involve the mesentery, whereas only 5% of Hodgkin's lymphomas do so. When involved, the mesentery contains a mass of soft tissue density, which may extend from the bowel loops to the root of the mesentery and the retroperitoneum (Fig. 36-68).[24,90] The normal mesenteric vessels are not clearly seen in such cases. In other cases, there may be localized masses within the mesentery adjacent to loops of bowel. To diagnose small mass lesions, it is important to attempt total opacification of the bowel loops with either iodine or dilute barium solution. Even if this opacification is not total, such lesions can be distinguished in a normal bowel by a sufficiently characteristic appearance with fluid and gas.

After treatment, the tumor shrink gradually, but they may leave residual fibrous tissue. Such tissue may be prominent but should not be confused for active tu-

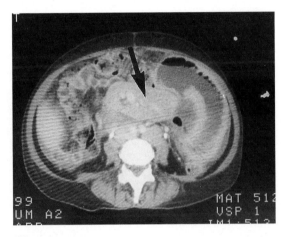

Fig. 36-68. CT scan shows a large soft tissue mass *(arrow)* in the root of the mesentery. The tumor extends to the wall of the small bowel, which is quite thick. Note that even when the bowel is distended, the mucosal markings can be seen.

mor. Treatment of such masses is usually continued until no interval shrinkage occurs in the mass.

Primary mesenchymal tumors

A variety of tumors that have no specific traits except liposarcoma originate from mesenchymal origin. Virtually all such tumors are soft tissue density without any distinguishing features. Well-differentiated liposarcoma can have a fat density, which is indistinguishable from normal fat (Figs. 36-69 to 36-71).

Metastatic disease

Metastatic involvement of the omentum and mesentery is quite common with neoplasms,[11] the most common being from the ovary, stomach, pancreas, and colon.[46] Spread within the peritoneum can be along the

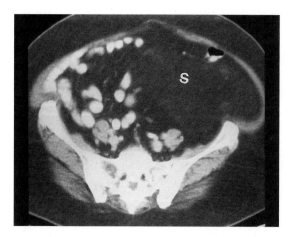

Fig. 36-69. Mesenchymal tumors may have a variable appearance, but liposarcomas are somewhat typical, as can be seen in the following scans. The well-differentiated liposarcomas, *S*, appear low in density similar to that of the normal mesenteric fat.

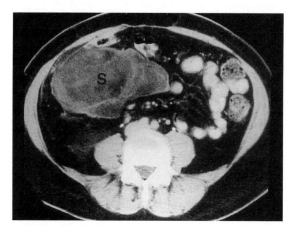

Fig. 36-70. This scan shows a well-defined, higher density tumor, *S*, which has an intermediate differentiation.

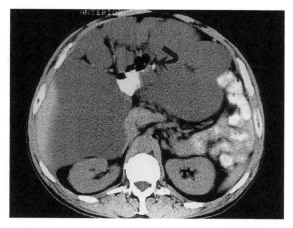

Fig. 36-71. This scan shows a poorly differentiated liposarcoma, with myxoid changes. It is producing a pseudomyxomatous invasion of the peritoneum. Note that the small bowel loops *(curved arrow)* are compressed centrally by the low-density tumor, which almost appears like fluid. The bowel does not float as with normal ascites, and note the contrast-filled small bowel, which is compressed posteriorly on the left.

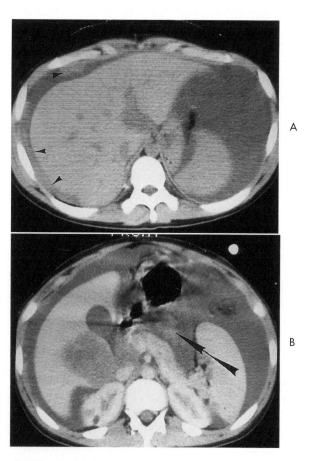

Fig. 36-72. A, Solid tumors that produce surface metastases may produce high-density implants. CT scan shows a small plaque lesions anteriorly and a broad soft tissue density posteriorly *(arrowheads).* **B,** Lower scan taken in the same patient shows mass *(arrow)* in omental bursa behind the stomach.

surface of the peritoneum or within the ligaments (Fig. 36-72) (areolar tissue surrounded by peritoneum), which contain the lymph nodes draining a specific area. Lymphatic spread can occur along the neurovascular muscular bundles within the intermesenteric space. When fibrosis is associated with the lesions, there may be retraction in the mesentery.

When metastatic lesions are on the peritoneal surface, several findings may be noted. First, if they are larger than 10 mm in size, they may be seen as discrete nodular lesions (Fig. 36-73). If the tumor is of mucinous origin, such as ovary or colon, it may be soft tissue or fluid density. When the size of the lesions are below the resolving power of CT, collections of fluid indistinguishable from any other fluid may be produced. The meta-

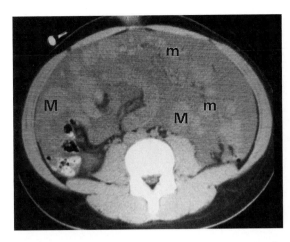

Fig. 36-73. Numerous round large masses, *M,* are implanted adjacent to the retroperitoneum. Many small masses, *m,* are noted on the greater omentum.

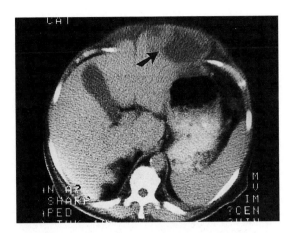

Fig. 36-75. Certain tumors, such as ovary and stomach, are said to have a propensity for the falciform ligament *(arrow).*

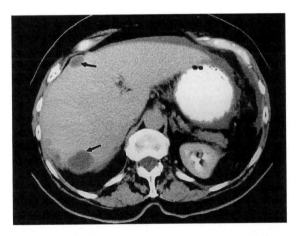

Fig. 36-74. Fluid density metastases occur from mucinous tumors, such as ovary, colon, and urachal tumors. Small masses are noted on the surface of the liver *(arrows).*

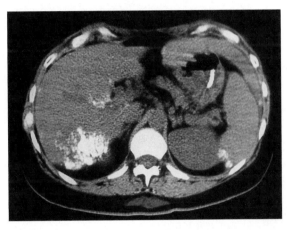

Fig. 36-76. On occasion, mucinous or necrotic tumors may calcify because of dystrophic calcifications. Note the high-density material on posterior right hepatic lobe, porta hepatis, and posterior spleen.

static sites of the ovarian tumor can be completely fluid in appearance.[73] In such cases, the tumors may have the appearance of subcapsular collections (Figs. 36-74 and 36-75).

Regardless of size, mucinous or other treated tumors can produce small calcifications throughout the peritoneum (Fig. 36-76).[82] Mitchell et al[78] reported a series on 15 patients with carcinoma of the ovary and found calcifications in six peritoneal sites of implant, perihepatic calcifications in five sites, and lymph node calcifications in one.

Making the diagnosis of a peritoneal metastasis can be difficult at times if the mass is not big enough to cause displacement of the bowel and if total opacification of the bowel has not been achieved.[102] The normal

bowel, however, does have a characteristic appearance that shows small amounts of fluid and gas in a diffuse pattern. Sometimes, even after administration of contrast material, there may be a problem distinguishing an adynamic loop of bowel from a mass. In such cases, intravenous administration of contrast material may be helpful because the wall of the bowel enhances well, or placing the patient in a decubitus position permits moving "gas" to reveal the true nature of a loop of bowel.

Omental changes

The thickened omentum produced by "caking" appears asa large soft tissue mass with poorly defined edges. The fat plane between the anterior abdominal wall and the intestinal loops may be obscured. When the

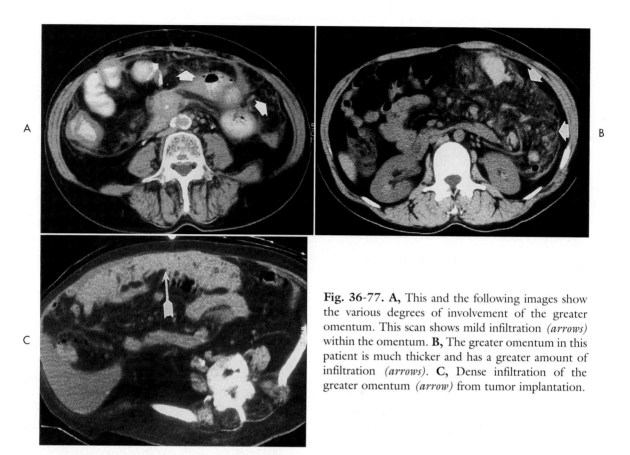

Fig. 36-77. **A,** This and the following images show the various degrees of involvement of the greater omentum. This scan shows mild infiltration *(arrows)* within the omentum. **B,** The greater omentum in this patient is much thicker and has a greater amount of infiltration *(arrows)*. **C,** Dense infiltration of the greater omentum *(arrow)* from tumor implantation.

omentum is not thick, soft tissue masses within or on the omentum, which is of fat density, may be seen (Fig. 36-77).

Sites of implants

It has been suggested in some works that the ligaments at the reflection of the sigmoid colon, the ileocolic region, and broad ligaments are the first location of implantation with malignancy.[75,104] Data have shown, however, that for the earliest detection of peritoneal seeding (at least with ovarian neoplasms) biopsy of the diaphragmatic areas are more likely to show early peritoneal involvement.[26] This is presumably due to the circulation of peritoneal fluid. Common metastases of ovarian or gastric cancers to the falciform ligament may also be a result of this normal upward flow toward the diaphragm (see Fig. 36-75).

General diagnostic signs

Whitley[105] has evaluated a group of 370 patients who had mesenteric tumors and recommended some diagnostic signs that are helpful in approaching mesenteric disease. The following diagnostic signs depend on characterizing the lesions according to their appearance: rounded, cakelike, ill-defined, and stellate.

Rounded masses were caused by non-Hodgkin disease in 33 of 41 cases, leukemia in 2 of 26 cases, and ovarian tumor in 3 of 38 cases. Whitley also noted a 30% occurrence in the nodes of the small bowel mesentery. Other authors have noted an overall occurrence of 50% if nodes at the root of the mesentery are included.[105]

Ill-defined masses, the next most common type of involvement, occurred in 27 patients. Of this group, the non-Hodgkin and ovarian carcinomas were the most common type of involvement, followed by colon, pancreas, stomach, and other masses (Fig. 36-77, *A* and *B*).

Cakelike masses of the mesentery occurred with ovarian tumors, non-Hodgkin lymphoma, and leukemia (Fig. 36-77, *C*).

Stellate infiltration of the neurovascular bundles of the mesentery occurred with all types of metastatic disease except lymphomas and leukemia. The stellate pattern is produced by the infiltration along the inner margins of the mesentery.

Levitt et al[58] reported the detection of metastases in 18 of 27 cases. They noted that CT did not show microscopic lesions, masses smaller than 1 cm, or omental metastases, such as pancreatic and gastric carcinomas that are immediately adjacent to primary masses.

An article by Goldhirsch et al[26] indicates that CT

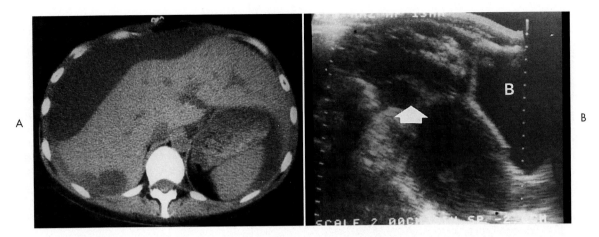

Fig. 36-78. A, Pseudomyxoma peritonei produced by mucinous tumor of the urachus. Note the posterior effacement of the liver by the mucinous tumor. **B,** Ultrasound scan of the patient shows a multiloculated tumor *(arrow)* cephalad to the bladder, *B*.

was not as accurate as second-look surgical exploration. A positive CT scan is a useful guide for the surgeon, but a negative study does not obviate the need for second-look surgical procedure.

Early authors used contrast peritoneography to demonstrate the normal peritoneal spaces.[86] More recently, workers have used positive contrast as a method of clearly defining small peritoneal implants especially close to the diaphragm.[98]

Pseudomyxoma peritonei

Pseudomyxoma peritonei is a rare disease resulting from the diffuse dissemination of mucinous material derived from neoplasms. Typically the neoplasms producing the peritoneal seeding are mucinous cystadenocarcinomas of either the ovary or appendix, but it may occur unusually with tumors of the urachus, uterus, or omphalomesenteric duct. The disease is quite indolent, and massive deposition of material may occur before it is noticed. On CT, this seems to have two appearances.[67,70,73,92,103] It may appear as discrete, low-density cystic masses located in multiple anatomical spaces. In other cases, the peritoneum is completely filled and resembles ascitic fluid, sometimes producing mass effects on adjacent organs (Fig. 36-78). Calcifications may occur following chemotherapy.[77]

Carcinoid tumors

A carcinoid is a serotonin-producing tumor commonly involving the terminal ileum; it can produce changes within the mesentery, creating a desmoplastic fibrotic reaction. If the tumor is small or microscopic, no abnormality is seen on the scan. If a significant desmoplastic reaction occurs, however, there may be thicken-

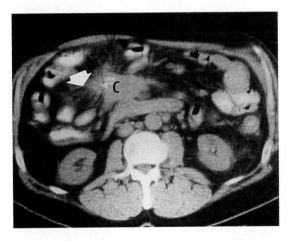

Fig. 36-79. Scan showing soft tissue density carcinoid tumor, *C,* producing reactive fibrosis *(arrow)* in the mesentery.

ing of the mesentery with areas of soft tissue density (Fig. 36-79). By the time the disease is first seen, there are liver metastases, which also may be an associated finding on CT.

REFERENCES

1. Ahrenholz DH, Simmons RL: Fibrin in peritonitis. I. Beneficial and adverse effects of fibrin in experimental E. Coli peritonitis. *Surgery* 88:41, 1980.
2. Allen HA, et al: Diffuse mesenteric amyloidosis: CT, sonographic, and pathologic findings. *J Comput Assist Tomogr* 9:196, 1985.
3. Allen L: The peritoneal stomata. *Anat Rec* 67:89, 1936.
4. Allen L, Weatherford, T: Role of fenestrated basement membrane in lymphatic adsorption from the peritoneal cavity. *Am J Physiol* 197:551, 1959.
5. Altemeier WA, et al: Intra-abdominal abscesses. *Am J Surg* 125:70, 1973.

6. Aronberg DJ, et al: Evaluation of abdominal abscess with computed tomography. *J Comput Assist Tomogr* 2:384, 1978.

7. Autio V: The spread of intraperitoneal infection. *Acta Chir Scand* 321(Suppl):1, 1964.

8. Balfe DM, et al: *Radiology* 150:485, 1984.

9. Balthazar EJ, et al: Acute pancreatitis: Prognostic value of CT. *Radiology* 156:767, 1985.

10. Bercovici B, et al: Antimicrobial activity of human peritoneal fluid. *Surg Gynecol Obstet* 141:885, 1975.

11. Bernardino ME, Jing BS, Wallace S: Computed tomography diagnosis of mesenteric masses. *AJR* 132:33, 1979.

12. Brody JM, et al: Gastric tuberculosis: Manifestation of acquired immunodeficiency syndrome. *Radiology* 159:347, 1986.

13. Bydder GM, Kreel L: Attenuation values of fluid collections within the abdomen. *J Comput Assist Tomogr* 4:145, 1980.

14. Callen PW: Computed tomographic evaluation of abdominal abscesses. *Radiology* 131:171, 1979.

15. Callen PW, Marks WM, Filly RA: Computed tomography and ultrasonography in the evaluation of the retroperitoneum in patients with malignant ascites. *J Comput Assist Tomogr* 3:581, 1979.

16. Dach J, et al: Peritoneal mesothelioma: CT, sonography and gallium-67 scan. *AJR* 135:614, 1980.

17. Day DL, Sane S, Dehner LP: Inflammatory pseudotumor of the mesentery and small intestine. *Pediatr Radiol* 16:210, 1986.

18. Dodds WJ, et al: Anatomy and imaging of the lesser peritoneal sac. *AJR* 144:567, 1985.

19. Dodds WJ, et al: The retroperitoneal spaces revisited: A pictorial essay. *AJR* 147:1155, 1986.

20. Fry DE, et al: Determinants of death in patients with intraabdominal abscess. *Surgery* 88:517, 1980.

21. Galematis B, Delikaris P: Treatment of echinococcal cyst. In Nyhus L, Baker R, editors: *Mastery of Surgery*, Boston, 1984, Little, Brown & Co., Inc.

22. Gerzof SG, Robbins AH, Birkett DH: Computed tomography in the diagnosis and management of abdominal abscesses. *Gastrointest Radiol* 3:287, 1978.

23. Gerzof SG, et al: Percutaneous catheter drainage of abdominal abscesses guided by ultrasound and computed tomography. *AJR* 133:1, 1979.

24. Goffinet DR, et al: Staging laparotomies in unselected previously untreated patients with non-Hodgkin's lymphomas. *Cancer* 32:672, 1973.

25. Gold R: Personal communication, 1983.

26. Goldhirsch A, et al: Computed tomography prior to second-look operation in advanced ovarian cancer. *Radiology* 152:861, 1984.

27. Gonzalez LR, et al: Radiologic aspects of hepatic echinococcosis: Value of the intravenous viscerogram and computed tomography. *Radiology* 130:21, 1979.

28. Haaga JR, Alfidi RJ: Precise biopsy localization by computed tomography. *Radiology* 118:603, 1976.

29. Haaga JR, Weinstein AJ: CT-guided percutaneous aspiration and drainage of abscesses. *AJR* 135:1187, 1980.

30. Haaga JR, et al: CT detection and aspiration of abdominal abscesses. *AJR* 138:465, 1977.

31. Haaga JR, et al: Interventional CT scanning. *Radiol Clin North Am* 15:449, 1977.

32. Halvorsen RA Jr, et al: Ascites or pleural effusion? CT differentiation: Four useful criteria. *Radiographics* 6:135, 1986.

33. Han SY, et al: Retractile mesenteritis involving the colon: Pathologic and radiologic correlation (case report). *AJR* 147:268, 1986.

34. Hanson RD, Hunter TB: Tuberculosis peritonitis: CT appearance. *AJR* 144:931, 1985.

35. Hau T, Ahrencholz DH, Simmons RL: Secondary bacterial peritonitis: The biological basis of treatment. *Curr Probl Surg* 16:1, 1979.

36. Hau T, Hoffman R, Simmons RL: Mechanisms of the adjuvant effect of hemoglobin in experimental peritonitis. I. In vivo inhibition of peritoneal leukocytosis. *Surgery* 83:223, 1978.

37. Hau T, Nishikawa RA, Phuangsab A: Treatment of peritonitis with systemic antibiotics. *Clin Pharmacol Ther* 29:251, 1981.

38. Hau T, Nishikawa RA, Phuangsab A: The effect of bacterial trapping by fibrin on the efficacy of systemic antibiotics in experimental peritonitis. *Surg Gynecol Obstet* 156:252, 1983.

39. Hau T, Payne WD, Simmons RL: Fibrinolytic activity of the peritoneum during experimental peritonitis. *Surg Gynecol Obstet* 148:415, 1979.

40. Hauser H, Gurret JP: Miliary tuberculosis associated with adrenal enlargement: CT appearance. *J Comput Assist Tomogr* 10:254, 1986.

41. Henderson LW: The problem of peritoneal membrane area and permeability. *Kidney Int* 3:409, 1973.

42. Henderson LW, Nolph KD: Altered permeability of the peritoneal membrane after using hypertonic peritoneal dialysis fluid. *J Clin Invest* 48:992, 1969.

43. Hulnick DH: Computed tomography in the evaluation of diverticulitis. *Radiology* 152:491, 1984.

44. Hulnick DH, et al: Abdominal tuberculosis: CT evaluation. *Radiology* 157:199, 1985.

45. Illig L: *Die terminale Strombahn*, Berlin, 1961, Springer-Verlag.

46. Jeffrey RB Jr: CT demonstration of peritoneal implants. *AJR* 135:323, 1980.

47. Jeffrey RB Jr, et al: Abdominal CT in acquired immunodeficiency syndrome. *AJR* 146:7, 1986.

48. Jeffries GH: The hepatic diseases. In Besson PB, McDermott W, editors: *Cecil-Loeb Textbook of Medicine,* Philadelphia, 1971, WB Saunders Co.

49. Jolles H, Coulan CM: CT of ascites: Differential diagnosis. *AJR* 135:315, 1980.

50. Kannerstein M, et al: Papillary tumors of the peritoneum in women: Mesothelioma or papillary carcinoma. *Am J Obstet Gynecol* 127:306, 1977.

51. Kipfer RE, Moertel CG, Dahlin DC: Mesenteric lipodystrophy. *Ann Intern Med* 80:582, 1974.

52. Knochel JQ, et al: Diagnosis of abdominal abscesses with computed tomography, ultrasound, and ^{111}In leukocyte scans. *Radiology* 137:425, 1980.

53. Korobkin M, et al: Comparison of computed tomography, ultrasonography, and gallium-67 scanning in the evaluation of suspected abdominal abscesses. *Radiology* 129:89, 1978.

54. Lahorra, JR, et al:

55. Landya MJ, et al: Hepatic and thoracic amebiasis. *AJR* 135:449, 1980.

56. Laing RK, et al: Abdominal abscess drainage under radiologic guidance: Causes of failure. *Radiology* 159:329, 1986.

57. Leak LV, Just EE: Permeability of peritoneal mesothelium: A TEM and SEM study. *J Cell Biol* 70:423, 1976.

58. Levitt RG, Sagel SS, Stanley RJ: Detection of neoplastic involvement of the mesentery and omentum by computed tomography. *AJR* 131:835, 1978.

59. Levitt RG, et al: Computed tomography and ^{67}Ga citrate radionuclide imaging for evaluating suspected abdominal abscesses. *AJR* 132:529, 1979.

60. Li DKB, Rennie CS: Abdominal computed tomography in Whipple's disease. *J Comput Assist Tomogr* 5:249, 1981.

61. Lieberman JM, Haaga JR: Duodenal malrotation (case report). *J Comput Assist Tomogr* 6:1019, 1982.

62. Lieberman JM, Haaga JR: Computed tomography of diverticulitis. *J Comput Assist Tomogr* 7:431, 1983.

63. Long JA, Dunnick NR, Doppman JL: Non-inflammatory gas formation following embolization of adrenal carcinoma. *J Comput Assist Tomogr* 3:840, 1979.

64. MacCallum WG: On the mechanism of adsorption of granular materials from the peritoneum. *Bull Johns Hopkins Hosp* 14:105, 1903.

65. Magid D, et al: Desmoid tumors in Gardner syndrome: Use of computed tomography. *AJR* 142:1141, 1984.

66. Marks WM, Filly RA: Computed tomographi demonstration of intraarterial air following hepatic artery ligation. *Radiology* 135:665, 1979.

67. Masaryk TJ, Chilcote WA: CT of pseudomyxoma peritonpei: Case report. *Radiology* 152:861, 1984.

68. Mathews AW, et al: The use of combined ultrasonic and isotope scanning in the diagnosis of amoebic liver disease. *Gut* 14:50, 1973.

69. Mathieu D, et al: Periportal tuberculous adenitis: CT features. *Radiology* 161:713, 1986.

70. Mayes BG, Chuang VP, Fisher RGL: CT of pseudomyxoma peritonei. *AJR* 136:807, 1981.

71. McAdam WAF, Goligher JC: The occurrence of desmoids in patients with familial polyposis coli. *Br J Surg* 57:618, 1970.

72. McNeil B, Keeler E, Adelstein FJ: Primer on certain elements of medical decision making. *N Engl J Med* 293:211, 1975.

73. Megibow AJ, et al: Ovarian metastases: Computed tomographic appearances. *Radiology* 156:161, 1985.

74. Mendez G, Isikoff MB, Hill MC: Retroperitoneal processes involving the psoas demonstrated by computed tomography. *J Comput Assist Tomogr* 4:78, 1980.

75. Meyers MA: *Dynamic Radiology of the Abdomen: Normal and Pathological Anatomy*, ed 2, New York, 1976, Springer-Verlag.

76. Miles AA, Miles EM, Burke J: The value and derivation of defense reactions of the skin to the primary lodgement of bacteria. *Br J Exp Pathol* 38:79, 1957.

77. Miller DL, Udelsman R, Sugarbaker PH: Calcification of pseudomyxoma peritonei following intraperitoneal chemotherapy: CT demonstration. *J Comput Assist Tomogr* 9:1123, 1985.

78. Mitchell DG, et al: Serous carcinoma of the ovary: CT identification of metastatic calcified implants. *Radiology* 158:649, 1986.

79. Newmark H, et al: Echinococcal cyst of the liver seen on computed tomography. *J Comput Assist Tomogr* 2:231, 1978.

80. Nyberg DA, et al: Abdominal CT findings of disseminated mycobacterium avium-intracellulare in AIDS. *AJR* 145:297, 1985.

81. Ochsner A: Pyogenic abscess. In Bockus HL, editor: *Gastroenterology*, Philadelphia, 1976, WB Saunders Co.

82. Pandolfo I, et al: Calcified peritoneal metastases from papillary cystadenocarcinoma of the ovary: CT features. *J Comput Assist Tomogr* 10:545, 1986.

83. Park, Jung, et al:

84. Ralls PW, et al: CT of inflammatory disease of the psoas muscle. *AJR* 134:767, 1980.

85. Raptooulos V, et al: Renal fascial pathway: Posterior extension of pancreatic effusions within the anterior pararenal space. *Radiology* 158:367, 1986.

86. Robb LW, et al: Computed tomographic positive contrast peritoneography. *Radiology* 131:699, 1979.

87. Rhodes R: Personal communication, 1988.

88. Rosenfield AT, et al: Acute focal bacterial nephritis (acute lobar nephronia). *Radiology* 132:553, 1979.

89. Rubinstein WA, et al: Posterior peritoneal recesses: Assessment using CT. *Radiology* 156:461, 1985.

90. Runyon BA, Hoefs JC: Peritoneal lymphomatosis with ascites: Characterization. *Arch Intern Med* 156:887, 1986.

91. Scherer U, et al: Computed tomography in hydatid disease of the liver: A report of 13 cases. *J Comput Assist Tomogr* 2:612, 1978.

92. Seshol MB, Coulam CM: Pseudomyxoma peritonei: Computed tomography and sonography. *AJR* 136:803, 1981.

93. Silverman PM, et al: Computed tomography of the normal mesentery. *AJR* 143:953, 1984.

94. Silverman PM, et al: CT appearance of diffuse mesenteric colon. *J Comput Assist Tomogr* 10:67, 1986.

95. Steinberg B: *Infections of the Peritoneum*, New York, 1944, Paul Hoeber, Inc.

96. Talley FP: Determinants of virulence in anaerobic bacteria. *Microbiology* 34:219, 1979.

97. Thompson GT, Fitzgerald ER, Somers SS: Retractilie mesenteritis of the sigmoid colon. *Radiology* 157:565, 1985.

98. Tipaldi L, Giunta L: Personal communication, 1987.

99. Vincent ME, Robbins AH: Mycobacterium avium-intracellulare complex enteritis: Pseudo-Whipple disease in AIDS. *AJR* 144:921, 1985.

100. von Recklinghausen FT: Zur Fettresorption. *Arch Pathol Anat Physiol* 26:172, 1983.

101. Wang N-S: The performed stomas connecting the pleural cavity and the lymphatics in the parietal pleura. *Am Rev Respir Dis* 111:12, 1975.

102. Warde P, et al: Computed tomography in advanced ovarian cancer: Inter- and intraobserver reliability. *Invest Radiol* 21:31, 1986.

103. Weigert F, Lindner P, Rohde U: Computed tomography and magnetic resonance of pseudomyxoma peritonei. *J Comput Assist Tomogr* 9:1120, 1985.

104. Whalen J: *Radiology of the Abdomen*, Philadelphia, 1976, Lea & Febiger.

105. Whitley NO: Mesenteric disease. In Meyers MA, editor: *Computed Tomography of the Gastrointestinal Tract: Including the Peritoneal Cavity and Mesentery*. New York, 1986, Springer-Verlag.

106. Wilms G, Baert AL, Bruneel M: CT demonstration of gas formation after renal tumor embolization. *J Comput Assist Tomogr* 3:838, 1979.

107. Wolverson MK, et al: CT as a primary diagnostic method in evaluating intraabdominal abscesses. *AJR* 133:1089, 1979.

108. Zinsser HH, Pryde AW: Experimental study of physical factors, including fibrin formation influencing the spread of fluids and small particles within and from the peritoneal cavity of the dog. *Ann Surg* 136:818, 1952.

109. Zirinsky K, et al: Computed tomography, sonography and MR imaging of abdominal tuberculosis. *J Comput Assist Tomogr* 9:961, 1985.

37

The Retroperitoneum

RICHARD H. COHAN
N. REED DUNNICK

THE RETROPERITONEUM

The retroperitoneum is that portion of the abdomen located posterior to the peritoneal cavity. It extends from the diaphragm to the pelvic inlet and includes portions of the colon, duodenum, pancreas, kidneys, adrenals, abdominal aorta, inferior vena cava, lymph nodes, fat, and much of the abdominal wall musculature.[79]

Cross-sectional imaging, particularly with computed tomography (CT) has had a profound effect on the diagnosis and treatment of retroperitoneal diseases. This chapter presents the CT and magnetic resonance imaging (MRI) appearance of normal retroperitoneal anatomy. CT and MRI manifestations of abnormalities involving the retroperitoneal spaces, inferior vena cava, aorta, lymph nodes, and psoas muscles are described and illustrated. Disease processes confined to the retroperitoneum, including primary retroperitoneal tumors and retroperitoneal fibrosis, are also discussed.

RETROPERITONEAL SPACES
Normal anatomy

The retroperitoneum is commonly divided into three spaces by the anterior and posterior renal fascia.[104] The anterior pararenal space is bordered anteriorly by the parietal peritoneum, posteriorly by the anterior renal fascia, and posterolaterally by the lateral continuation of the renal fasciae and the lateroconal fascia. This space contains the pancreas, retroperitoneal portions of the duodenum, and ascending and descending colon[141] (Fig. 37-1). The perirenal space, the largest retroperitoneal compartment, lies within the anterior and posterior renal fascia and contains the kidneys, adrenals, proximal renal collecting systems, and renal hilar vessels. There is a large amount of perirenal fat in the perirenal space, which is subdivided by bridging septae. These septae serve to confine some perirenal processes to portions of the perirenal space.[110] The perirenal fasciae fuse medially and blend with the retroperitoneal fat surrounding the great vessels and adjacent lymph nodes. Recent studies suggest that the perirenal spaces may communicate with one another across the midline via a narrow potential space anterior to the caudal aspects of the aorta and the inferior vena cava.[108] Usually, the perirenal fasciae do not completely fuse inferiorly, thereby allowing all three retroperitoneal spaces to communicate with each other caudal to the kidneys.[108]

Pathologic conditions

Identification of the retroperitoneal spaces on CT and MRI often is useful in elucidating the etiologies of various fluid collections or masses. The anterior and posterior renal and lateroconal fasciae are identified on CT and MRI as pencil-thin, linear soft-tissue densities enveloping the perirenal fat and extending toward the lateral abdominal wall.[36,108] This visualization permits definition of the three retroperitoneal compartments in most patients.

Inflammatory and neoplastic processes initially can cause subtle thickening of the retroperitoneal fasciae. This response is nonspecific and in patients with an adjacent malignancy does not necessarily indicate infiltration of these layers with tumor cells.

Anterior pararenal space fluid collections often result from pancreatitis, colonic or duodenal perforations, appendical abscesses, or hematomas (Fig. 37-2). Although these frequently involve only one side of the retroperitoneum, they may spread across the midline. This is true particularly for patients with pancreatitis.

Fluid in the perirenal space often results in obliteration of the borders of the upper half of the psoas muscle and of the ipsilateral kidney on plain film, CT, and MRI.[127] Abscesses, hematomas, urinomas, and neoplasms can all develop in the perirenal space. In most cases, these are due to abnormalities of the kidneys, adrenals, or proximal collecting systems. Perinephric space hemorrhage is usually due to blunt trauma, ruptured ab-

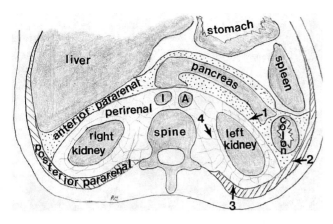

Fig. 37-1. Anatomy of the retroperitoneum. *1* = anterior perirenal fascia, *2* = lateral conal fascia, *3* = posterior perirenal fascia, *4* = bridging septa in the perirenal space.

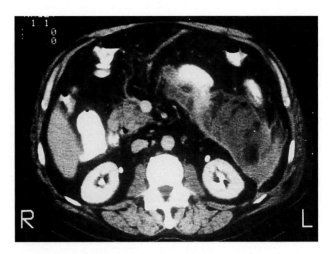

Fig. 37-2. Intravenous *(IV)* contrast media enhanced CT demonstrates a peripancreatic phlegmon in the left anterior pararenal space.

dominal aortic aneurysms, or bleeding from a renal mass.[108] In a study by Belville and co-workers, renal masses (renal adenocarcinomas and a single angiomyolipoma) accounted for spontaneous perinephric and subcapsular hematomas in 17 of 18 patients.[14]

Traditionally, it was believed that subcapsular fluid collections caused distortion of the renal parenchyma, while perinephric collections did not. It has been recently noted that when a perinephric fluid collection develops between the renal capsule and the posterior renorenal septum (one of the bridging perinephric septa), the renal parenchyma may be compressed and the CT appearance may be indistinguishable from that of a subcapsular hematoma.[108]

Fluid may accumulate in the posterior pararenal space as a result of adjacent infection or neoplasm. In a minority of patients, peripancreatic fluid or phlegmon may spread through or around the fascial layers into the posterior from the anterior pararenal space. Collections in the posterior pararenal space may obliterate the border of the lower half of the psoas muscle on plain-film, CT, and MRI in many patients, because the inferior margin of this muscle no longer abuts posterior pararenal space fat.

Localization of retroperitoneal fluid is sometimes difficult. This is no more apparent than in the retrorenal region. Retrorenal collections may reside within any of the intraabdominal compartments.[126] Occasionally, the paracolic gutters of the peritoneal cavity may extend posterolateral to the kidney. In some patients the anterior renal fascia, posterior renal fascia, and lateroconal fascia meet in a more dorsal location, and this also results in a portion of the anterior pararenal space lying posterior to the kidney. Also, perirenal fluid can layer in front of or behind the kidney. Since the anterior, posterior, and lateroconal fasciae often do not represent three distinct layers but rather a multilayered complex, fluid may migrate within the leaves of this fascial network.[164] Some processes, such as pancreatitis with its proteolytic enzymes and neoplasms, can destroy fascial barriers, further complicating attempts at fluid localization.

AORTA

Normal anatomy

The aorta extends from the diaphragmatic hiatus to the level of the umbilicus or fourth lumbar vertebral body where it bifurcates into the two common iliac arteries. The normal aorta is located just to the left of midline and is surrounded by retroperitoneal fat. It measures less than 3 cm in maximum diameter and decreases in size after giving rise to the major visceral branches.

Technique

The aorta can be identified on CT scans performed with or without intravenous contrast material. When evaluation of aneurysms, dissections, or grafts is required, however, bolus intravenous dynamic studies are most helpful. If possible, scans should be performed after oral contrast medium has been administered. Most patients can be imaged at 10-mm intervals. Patients with known aneurysms who are being evaluated for surgical repair should have thin (5-mm) contiguous section scans through the renal hila. When this is done, the main renal arteries can be visualized in 95% to 98% of patients.[71]

Aortic aneurysms

Abdominal aortic aneurysms (AAA) occur in 1% to 4% of the older population.[68,169,174] While they most commonly result from atherosclerosis, there are many other causes, such as trauma, infection, cystic medial necrosis, Marfan's syndrome, and syphilis.[115] AAAs are often asymptomatic, although patients may present with a pulsatile abdominal mass.[72] Surgical repair is recommended once aneurysms exceed 5 cm in maximal diameter because the tendency to rupture increases dramatically once they reach this size. In three recent series, the incidence of aortic rupture for unrepaired aneurysms 5 cm or greater in size ranged between 20% and 25%.[74,125,150] Although there have been isolated reports of ruptures occurring in smaller aneurysms,[170] this is unusual. In two current studies, none of the patients whose aneurysms were 4 cm or smaller in maximal diameter developed leaks.[68,125]

Patients with small aneurysms should be followed by serial ultrasound studies. The ultrasound examination can be repeated every 6 months, since small aneurysms expand relatively slowly (0.2 to 0.5 cm/year).[125,150]

Preoperative assessment of large abdominal aortic aneurysms is valuable for delineation of their proximal and distal extent, as well as for determination of maximum diameter. Although 95% of aneurysms are infrarenal, demonstration of renal artery involvement is crucial. Subsequent surgery will be much more complicated. In addition, iliac artery dilatation or stenosis may indicate the need for a "Y" (rather than a simple aortic) graft.[119]

Ultrasound is not recommended as the sole imaging procedure for patients about to undergo aneurysm repair. Ultrasound can often only interpret the relationship of the aneurysm to the renal arteries, because the latter are not consistently visualized.[52,59] (The superior mesenteric artery [SMA] originates in close proximity to the renal vessels; thus an aneurysm is most likely infrarenal if it begins over 1 cm caudad to the SMA.) Most radiologists and surgeons now advocate preoperative aneurysm assessment with CT. At some institutions, CT has even replaced angiography as the imaging study of choice before aneurysm repair. Todd and colleagues performed CT scans as the only preoperative radiographic study in 81 of 100 patients. They found that none of these patients was adversely affected by not having had angiography.[191] While CT missed five findings (two accessory renal arteries and three common iliac artery aneurysms) that might have been detected angiographically, it detected seven abnormalities (four cases of perianeurysmal fibrosis, two retroaortic renal veins, and one horseshoe kidney), at least six of which would not have been visualized during aortography. The remaining 19 patients in this study were also referred for arteriograms because aneurysms were thoracoabdominal (7), juxtarenal (2), or because there was concern about mesenteric or renal vascular disease.

Abdominal aortic aneurysms are easily visualized on CT. The aortic wall is calcified in nearly every patient in whom atherosclerosis is the etiology of the aneurysm.[68,131] CT is better able to define aneurysm size than is arteriography. Angiography demonstrates only the contrast-containing blood-flowing lumen of an aneurysm. Thrombus, which is detected by CT in nearly 90%

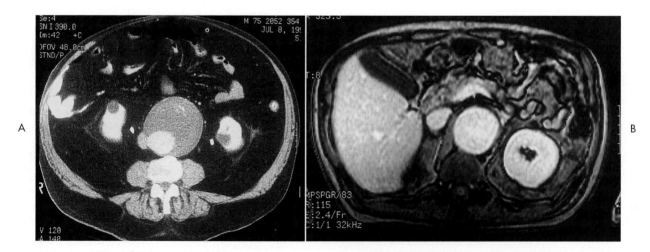

Fig. 37-3. Abdominal aortic aneurysm. **A,** Dynamic IV contrast-enhanced CT demonstrates a large amount of thrombus within the aneurysm. Note that some of the thrombus is calcified. An arteriogram on this patient would significantly underestimate the size of the aneurysm, since only the patient part of the lumen containing flowing blood would be opacified. **B,** Fat-suppressed limited flip angle MRI scan of a patient with a suprarenal abdominal aortic aneurysm. There is no thrombus in this aneurysm.

of aneurysms,[131] cannot be seen. Thus there is a tendency to underestimate aneurysm size when only angiography is performed (Fig. 37-3, *A*).

CT-detected mural thrombus is most often circumferential but may be crescentic and can be occasionally confused with a thrombosed false lumen in a patient with a chronic aortic dissection. Aneurysm thrombus may partially calcify, and this appearance can also be confused with displaced intima in a dissection.[81,131]

Aortic aneurysms are surrounded by increased soft-tissue stranding in 5% to 10% of cases.[68] This represents perianeurysmal fibrosis, believed by many to represent a form of idiopathic retroperitoneal fibrosis (Fig. 37-4).

MRI can be used in place of CT for evaluating patients with abdominal aortic aneurysms (see Fig. 37-3, *B*). The renal arteries are more easily identified and patients can be imaged in coronal, sagittal, or axial planes.[119] The patent aortic lumen can be reliably identified by the relative absence of signal emitted from flowing blood on spin-echo sequences, although increased turbulence will often result in some intraaortic signal at the level of the aneurysm. Since MRI may be more time-consuming and is usually more expensive, it has generally been reserved for patients in whom CT studies are not adequate and for patients in whom intravascular iodinated contrast media is contraindicated.

Small aorta

In rare instances, the aorta may actually be smaller than normal in caliber. This can be secondary to atherosclerotic occlusive disease (Leriche syndrome) or due to severe hypotension (Fig. 37-5). Shin Berland and Ho found the mean abdominal aortic diameter to be 17 mm ± 15 mm at a level 1 cm caudal to the origin of the superior mesenteric artery in normal young patients.[176]

In six hypotensive patients, the aorta caliber decreased to 10 to 12 mm, presumably secondary to vasoconstriction.

Retroperitoneal hemorrhage

Aneurysmal leak or rupture is a catastrophic event. If untreated, mortality is 50% to 90%. Thus, emergency surgery must be performed on any patient who survives long enough to be admitted to the hospital, although even here most patients will die (in a recent series only 30% of postoperative patients were still living at 30 days[96]).

A patient presenting with abdominal or back pain, a pulsatile mass (suspected of being an aortic aneurysm), and severe hypotension should proceed directly to surgery. CT is recommended only for evaluation of hemodynamically stable patients. Although there are some dissenting opinions,[23] it is generally believed that the delay imposed by obtaining an emergency CT in these patients does not adversely affect patient morbidity or mortality.[111] CT is quite sensitive in detecting aortic ruptures; it can also identify other causes of abdominal pain. In a recent study only 18 of 65 stable patients with clinically suspected aneurysm leaks had abdominal aortic aneurysm ruptures confirmed by CT.[111]

When imaged on CT, aneurysm ruptures are often extensive and easy to diagnose. Acute extraluminal blood is of soft-tissue attenuation. It has a vermiform, finger-like appearance as it infiltrates between fascial planes in the retroperitoneum.[35,87] Most often, blood accumulates in the perinephric space,[169] although leaks into other retroperitoneal compartments, the duodenum, psoas muscle, inferior vena cava, and even into the peritoneal cavity have been observed[62,68] (Fig. 37-6).

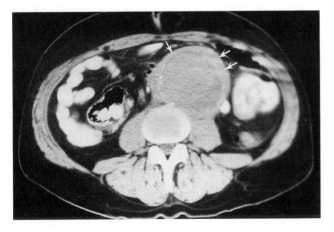

Fig. 37-4. Perianeurysmal fibrosis. A rind of soft tissue *(arrows)* surrounds the anterior and lateral aspects of a large abdominal aortic aneurysm (unenhanced scan).

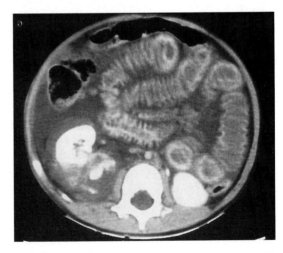

Fig. 37-5. Small aorta and slit-like IVC are noted on this dynamically enhanced CT of a severely hypotensive pediatric patient. Note the right renal laceration, enhancing bowel, and hemoperitoneum.

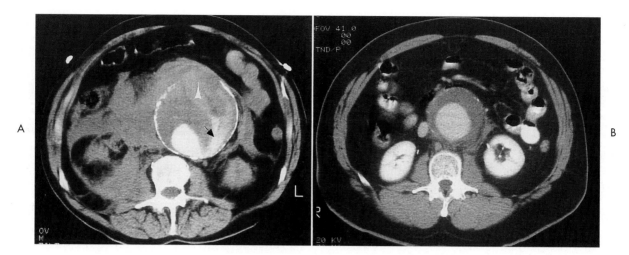

Fig. 37-6. Ruptured abdominal aortic aneurysms. **A,** Dynamic enhanced CT demonstrates active intravasation of blood into the extensive aneurysm thrombus *(black arrow)*. Blood is also extravasating into the retroperitoneum through a large defect in the anterior wall of the aorta *(white arrowhead)*. Note the disruption of the aortic calcification. **B,** A small "contained" rupture is visualized along the left posterolateral aspect of this aneurysm (dynamic IV contrast media injection).

The exact site of aortic rupture can often be suspected on discovery of a focal disruption in aortic wall calcification or an area of indistinctness where the fat between the aneurysm and the periaortic hematoma is obliterated (Fig. 37-6). In the series by Rosen et al, localization of the area of rupture was possible in four of six cases.[169] Detection of this area was helpful to the surgeon in his or her attempt to establish hemostasis.

Occasionally, areas of rupture may be small, and detection of extraluminal blood may be difficult or even impossible.[35] These may represent subacute, warning, or sentinel bleeds, all of which are at risk of rupturing massively at any time.[62] Greatorex and colleagues encountered one symptomatic patient who developed easily visualized massive retroperitoneal hemorrhage on CT recuts obtained 28 minutes after the initial images had failed to detect any extraluminal blood.[73] Obviously, patients with large aneurysms and abdominal pain should be closely monitored even if the CT is negative, because such "impending" or even delayed ruptures may occur.

Treatment of these two groups of patients can differ, however. While emergency surgery is recommended for patients with CT-diagnosed ruptures, hemodynamically stable patients with large symptomatic aneurysms but no CT evidence of rupture can usually safely undergo semi-elective aneurysm repair (within 24 to 48 hours). Operative mortality falls from between 35% and 50% to 17% when the patient can be prepped and when surgery is performed semi-electively.[35]

False-positive CT scans for aneurysm rupture can be minimized if the radiologist is aware of certain potential pitfalls. Asymmetric aneurysm thrombus can be confused with small ruptures in some instances. If not opacified with oral contrast material, the third and fourth portions of the duodenum can sometimes be confused with periaortic hemorrhage. Rarely, retroperitoneal lymphadenopathy can be mistaken for blood (Fig. 37-7).

Aortic ruptures have been rarely encountered in the absence of aneurysmal dilatation. These have been reported after blunt abdominal injury[130] and in a patient with nonaneurysmal bacterial aortitis.[134]

There are many other etiologies of retroperitoneal hemorrhage. Other spontaneous causes include blood dyscrasias, vasculitides, renal infections, retroperitoneal neoplasms, anticoagulant therapy, chronic hemodialysis, and hypertension.[33,146] Nonspontaneous causes include trauma, translumbar aortography, and renal biopsy.[33] Once in a while, a large retroperitoneal hemorrhage can develop in a patient who fortuitously happens to have a large abdominal aortic aneurysm. Usually, the lack of relationship between the hematoma and the aneurysm can be delineated. The fat planes between the aorta and the surrounding hematoma are preserved. There is no disruption in aneurysm-wall calcification, and the aortic wall is not indistinct (Fig. 37-8).

Aortic dissection

Aortic dissections are relatively rare, accounting for only one in 10,000 hospital admissions.[85] Mortality

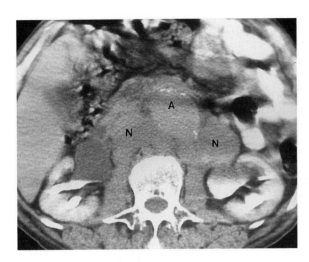

Fig. 37-7. Lymphadenopathy *(N)* mimicking retroperitoneal hemorrhage in a patient with an abdominal aortic aneurysm *(A)* and metastatic prostate cancer. Note that the retroperitoneal nodes are rounded and well defined (nondynamic enhanced scan).

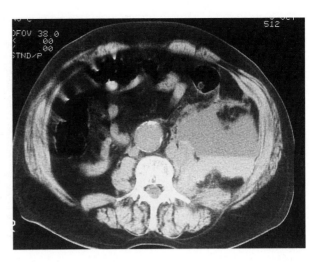

Fig. 37-8. Retroperitoneal hematoma in an anticoagulated patient with a small abdominal aortic aneurysm. Patient developed sudden flank pain soon after cardiac catheterization. Note that the hematoma is separated from the aneurysm by uninfiltrated fat (unenhanced scan).

of untreated dissection is extremely high, approaching 25% at 24 hours, 50% at 1 week, and 75% at 1 month.[6] Generally, a dissection involving only the descending aorta (Debakey type III or Stanford type B) may be treated medically. If the ascending aorta is involved (Debakey types I and II, or Stanford type A), surgery is required.

When dissections involve the abdominal aorta, they almost always have originated in the thorax. An aortic dissection that originates in the abdominal aorta is usually produced iatrogenically (i.e., retrograde intimal tears produced by arteriographic catheters, guidewires, or intra-aortic balloon pumps), or it develops secondary to blunt trauma.

Dynamic bolus CT is extremely sensitive in identifying the intimal flap and true and false lumens in both the chest and abdomen of most patients with aortic dissections.[155,157,189] Distinction of an abdominal aortic aneurysm from a chronic dissection with a clotted false lumen may be difficult, since thrombus may have a similar appearance in both instances.[67,200] Heiberg et al compared CT scans of 36 patients with aneurysms to those of 24 patients with dissections.[81] Linear peripheral calcifications were more common in patients with aneurysms (70%) than in patients with dissections (20%), although neither the appearance nor the location of the aortic calcifications was completely specific. Increased density of a thickened aortic wall on precontrast scans was seen in only one patient with an aneurysm, but it was seen in 44% of patients with dissections. The residual lumen was round in 94% of patients with aneurysms but was round

in only 29% of those with thrombosed dissections.

Medically treated aortic dissections may evolve with time. Yamaguchi et al demonstrated that serial CTs showed changes in false lumen size or the degree of thrombus in 7 of 13 patients with type III dissections.[200] All three of their patients with initially completely thrombosed false lumens showed disappearance or shrinkage of the false lumen 1 to 2 months after the first scan. Thus, serial CTs may prove helpful in confusing cases in which a type III or B dissection is suspected and treated, when the initial CT appearance is not diagnostic.

MRI is sensitive in detecting aortic dissections, in one series detecting intimal flaps in each of 13 patients.[5] Differences in flow rate between true and false lumens, and hence in signal intensities, may facilitate correct identification of a dissection. Limited flip-angle techniques are often extremely helpful. The intimal flap is easily identified, outlined by the high signal emitted when there is flowing blood in the true and false lumens (Fig. 37-9). In some instances, however, differences in flow may result in confusion between slow-flowing blood and hematoma or aneurysm thrombus. As with CT, thrombosed dissections can be difficult to distinguish from aneurysms.

Since severely ill patients (often including those with suspected acute dissections) are harder to manage and observe in most MRI suites than in most CT rooms, we advocate initial use of either CT or arteriography if intravenous contrast media can be safely administered. If either of these studies is nondiagnostic, the other can be obtained. Use of MRI is reserved primarily for problem

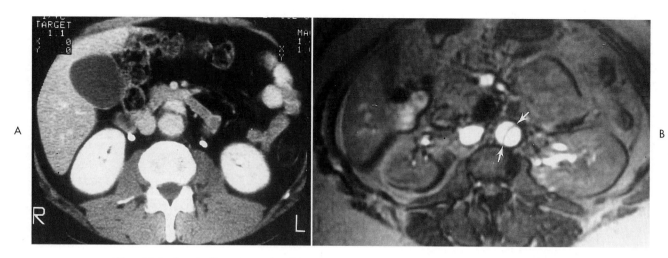

Fig. 37-9. Aortic dissections. **A,** CT scan of a patient with an aortic dissection originating distal to the origin of the left subclavian artery. Scan easily demonstrates the intimal flap between the anterior true and posterior false lumen (enhanced scan). **B,** MRI on another patient (limited-flip angle image) demonstrates the intimal flap *(arrows)* between the bright signal in the true and false lumina.

cases (when the CT or arteriogram are equivocal, or when the patient cannot tolerate iodinated radiographic contrast media because of allergy or renal failure).

Penetrating ulcers of the aorta

Recently, Kazerooni et al described 16 patients with irregular penetrating atherosclerotic ulcers of the aorta, an abnormality that leads to intimal displacement and creation of a "false aortic lumen."[105] Although these ulcers could conceivably develop anywhere along the course of the aorta, all of the ulcers detected by Kazerooni and colleagues occurred in the descending thoracic aorta. Treatment of penetrating ulcers (which are usually visualized on CT as irregular outpouchings, extending off the aortic lumen) is controversial, although a conservative (nonsurgical) approach appears to be effective in hemodynamically stable patients.

The normal postoperative aorta

Prosthetic grafting of the abdominal aorta is performed frequently for patients with aortic aneurysms or occlusions. Three types of aortic grafts are commonly employed. The end-to-side grafts are anastomosed to the anterior aspect of the abdominal aorta and continue caudad just anterior to the still patent aorta. When an aortoiliac or aortofemoral graft is required, the graft bifurcates several centimeters above the native aortic bifurcation and reanastomoses with the iliac or femoral vessels in an end-to-side manner (Fig. 37-10). Commonly, the portion of native aorta between both ends of the graft will eventually completely thrombose.[68,102]

Many surgeons prefer an end-to-end graft anastomosis because blood-flow patterns are less turbulent.[102] In this case the aorta is transected proximally, and the graft is anastomosed in an end-to-end manner. The proximal aortic aneurysm stump is oversewn. The distal ends of a bifurcation graft usually are attached to the iliac or femoral vessels end-to-side. The distal end of a simple aortic graft is anastomosed in an end-to-end fashion.

The preferred surgical treatment of simple abdominal aortic aneurysms is currently proximal, and distal end-to-end anastomoses with endoaneurysmorrhaphy. Here, the proximal and distal ends of the graft are attached to uninvolved portions of the aorta, after resection of the anterior wall of the aneurysm. The remaining aneurysm sac is then wrapped loosely around the graft and sutured closed. This approach is thought to lessen the incidence of injury to the vena cava, iliac veins, and lumbar vessels. Persistence of the aneurysm shell around the graft provides an additional protective layer between the graft and the overlying duodenum,[68,102] decreasing the frequency of postoperative aortoenteric fistulae (Fig. 37-11).

Aortic aneurysm grafts with endoaneurysmorrhaphy may have a CT appearance strikingly similar to that of aortic aneurysms. Initially, thrombus in the wrap-around aneurysmal sac may look like thrombus around a centrally opacified blood-containing lumen in an aneurysm, although the lumen of the aortic graft is usually smooth and circular, while the patient lumen of an aneurysm is irregular.[102] The graft itself may be of higher

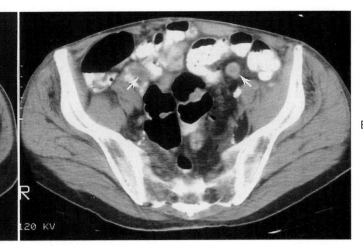

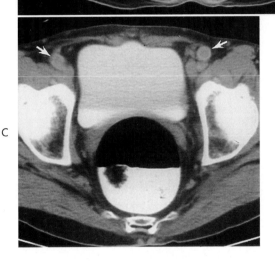

Fig. 37-10. End-to-side aortioiliofemoral graft. **A,** The proximal end of the graft is visualized just anterior to heavily calcified native distal abdominal aorta. **B,** The iliac limbs *(arrows)* are located anterior and slightly medial to the native iliac arteries. **C,** The femoral portions of the "Y" graft are easily identified anterior to the native femoral vessels, just cephalad to the distal anastomosis *(arrows)*. Note that on these unenhanced scans the graft has a higher attenuation than the flowing blood within it.

attenuation than the aortic lumen on unenhanced scans and thus may be identifiable. After contrast enhancement, however, this distinctive feature is not apparent.[68] On immediate postoperative scans it is not unusual to see some perigraft fluid and air.

With time, the space between the aneurysm wrap and the graft should diminish. Low et al noted that the space between the wrap and the graft was 5 mm or less in all 19 of their normal patients who were imaged *after* the immediate postoperative period.[128] All postoperative perigraft air should disappear by 3 weeks and all perigraft fluid by 3 months. A minimal amount of perigraft soft tissue may be seen several months after aortic repair; this likely corresponds to perigraft fibrosis.

Complications of abdominal aortic aneurysm repair

Complications of abdominal aortic graft surgery include graft infections (2% to 6%),[87] aortoenteric fistulae (1% to 5%),[175] false aneurysms (up to 5%),[68] occlusions, and hemorrhage. Surgical repair, usually with graft

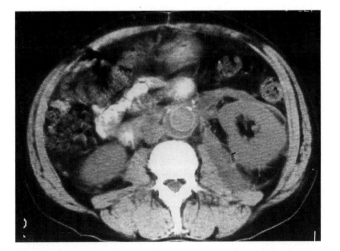

Fig. 37-11. Endoaneurysmorrhaphy in a patient who has had a recent aneurysm rupture. The partially calcified wall of the native aorta surrounds thrombus and/or perigraft fluid, which in turn surrounds the aortic graft. Note that the aortic graft is of higher attenuation than is blood in the aortic lumen of this unenhanced scan. There is extensive persistent hematoma in the retroperitoneum on the left.

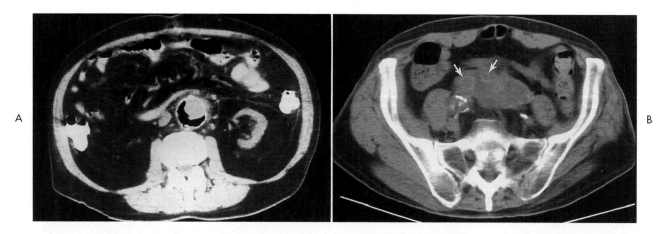

Fig. 37-12. Infected aortic grafts. **A,** Air has accumulated within the space between the graft and the surrounding native aorta in this patient who is status-post endoaneurysmorrhaphy. **B,** In another patient a large amount of fluid attenuation material surrounds the iliac limbs *(arrows)* of a "Y" graft. In this case (and in other instances), the infecting organism was not gas-producing. The perigraft fluid was found to be grossly purulent at surgery (unenhanced scans).

resection, is indicated in any patient in whom intra-abdominal extension of graft infection, aortoenteric fistulae, or pseudoaneurysm formation is identified.

Infections. Aortic graft infections are often catastrophic complications of aortic bypass surgery. Mortality is high, exceeding 30% in one series.[41] Often patients first develop groin infections (at the distal anastomoses). Diagnosis is frequently obvious. If undetected until 6 weeks or more after surgery, however, the groin infection usually has spread into the retroperitoneum. While a localized groin infection can be treated conservatively, once intraabdominal spread occurs, the entire graft must be resected.

Graft infection with extension into the retroperitoneum is suggested by CT when abnormal fluid collections and/or air are identified in the vicinity of the aortic graft. These collections are often irregular and septated[68,84,136] (Fig. 37-12). "Normal" perigraft fluid and hematomas may be confused with abscesses in the immediate postoperative period (within 6 weeks of surgery);[153] MRI may be helpful in differentiating subacute hematomas from other perigraft fluid, in these instances (a distinction that cannot always be made by CT). However, MRI is not capable of reliably differentiating sterile from infected (hemorrhagic or nonhemorrhagic) perigraft fluid.

Follow-up CT scans can be obtained in patients in whom infection is considered a likely diagnostic possibility and in whom retroperitoneal air visualized on CT may be secondary to recent surgery. Pathologic gas collections (often posterior and multilocular in relation to the graft) will increase in size over time, whereas post-

surgical collections (usually uniocular and anterior) and should diminish.[75] Ultimately, in problem cases and in symptomatic patients, a CT-guided needle aspiration may be required for diagnosis.[11,103,160]

CT or MRI evaluation of patients with suspected graft infections who are not in the immediate postoperative period (less than 3 months since surgery) is not nearly as difficult.[101] The presence of any perigraft soft tissue, fluid, or air in these patients should be viewed with extreme suspicion and considered a probable sign of infection.[128] CT scans on 33 of 35 infected patients evaluated by Low and colleagues[128] were correctly identified as abnormal because of the presence of perigraft soft tissue (32 scans), perigraft fluid (10 scans), disruption of the aortic wrap (in 9 of 16 patients who had endoaneurysmorrhaphy), increased soft tissue between graft and wrap such that the distance between graft and wrap exceeded 5 mm (in 8 of these 16 patients), ectopic gas (12 scans) pseudoaneurysm formation (7 scans), and focal wall thickening of adjacent bowel (13 scans) (Fig. 37-12).

Aufferman and associates correctly diagnosed aortic graft infection in 17 of 20 patients on MRI.[12] These 17 patients all had perigraft fluid more than 3 months after surgery; this was characterized by low to medium signal intensity of T1-weighted images and high signal intensity on T2-weighted images. The three missed infections were in patients who did not have perigraft fluid. Postoperative perigraft fluid resolved in 10 of 13 patients who did not have infections, and was replaced by a low signal (on *both* T1- and T2-weighted images) perigraft collar which likely represented fibrosis.[7]

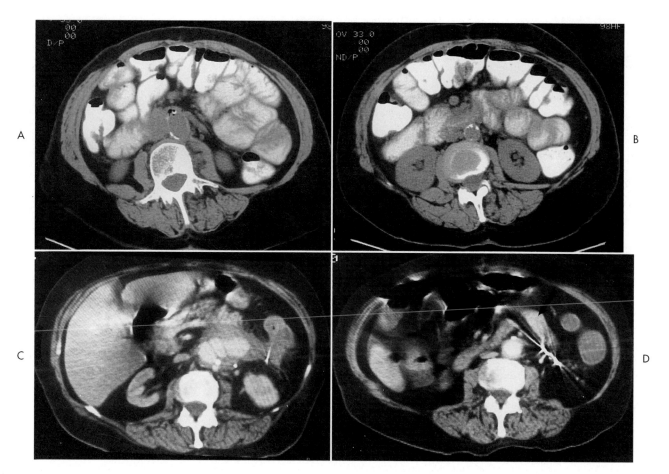

Fig. 37-13. Aortoenteric fistulae. **A,** A small amount of air is identified between the aortic graft and the adjacent duodenum. Distinction cannot be made between aortoenteric fistula and graft infection on the basis of this image. **B,** A slightly more cephalic scan on the same patient reveals mild thickening of the third portion of the duodenum. This finding, coupled with a history of gastrointestinal tract bleeding, suggested the correct diagnosis (unenhanced scans). **C,** Another patient was studied before oral (but after intravenous) contrast media administration. Note the extension of enhanced blood from the aorta (in a pseudoaneurysm) toward bowel in the left upper quadrant. **D,** A more cephalic scan demonstrates enhanced blood in the proximal jejunum *(arrow),* confirming the diagnosis of aortoenteric fistula.

Aortoenteric fistulae. Aortoenteric fistulae probably result from the persistent pulsatile pressure of the proximal graft anastomosis on the duodenum and/or from a low-grade infection that disrupts the suture line.[84] CT, the procedure of choice for detecting these fistulae, usually identifies indirect signs of their presence (including extraluminal air and bowel-wall thickening) (Figs. 37-13, *A,* 37-13, *B*). Visualization of high-attenuation extravasating blood in the duodenum in a patient given intravenous (but no oral) contrast is unlikely in a patient stable enough to undergo a CT examination, but can be seen in some instances (see Figs. 37-13, *C,* 37-13, *D*). For this reason CT examination to rule out aortoenteric fistulae is usually performed after oral contrast administration.

In the series by Low et al, only 10 and 12 of 23 cases of aortoenteric fistulae were specifically diagnosed by two observers; however, nonspecific findings (such as perigraft soft tissue) that suggested infection were identified in 19 and 20 cases.[128] Since symptoms are often (but not always) distinctive and treatment of aortoenteric fistulae and infected grafts is identical (graft resection), CT's failure to reliably distinguish between these two complications is probably not critical.

Pseudoaneurysms. Pseudoaneurysms occur most frequently in the femoral area,[84] and usually they are identified long after surgery. MRI usually can easily diagnose this complication because of the flow void seen on standard spin-echo sequences and the high-signal when limited flip-angle techniques are used. Dynamic enhanced CT is nearly as specific. On unenhanced CT, however, pseudoaneurysms must be distinguished from other perigraft masses and collections such as hematomas, abscesses, and lymphoceles.

VEINS

Normal anatomy

The inferior vena cava (IVC) is formed by the confluence of the two common iliac veins, usually at the level of the fourth or fifth lumbar vertebral bodies, just caudal to the aortic bifurcation. The IVC courses to the right of the aorta, becoming slightly more ventral in location just before it traverses the diaphragm.[107] The IVC is formed by the development and partial regression of the three paired venous systems in the embryo: the posteriorcardinal, subcardinal, and supracardinal veins. Normally, the right supracardinal vein becomes the infrarenal IVC, the subcardinal vein and its anastomoses become the perirenal and suprarenal IVC, and the confluence of hepatic veins forms the intrahepatic IVC. The upper portions of the right and left supracardinal veins form the azygos and hemiazygos systems.[37]

Failure of normal embryologic development may result in many possible venous anomalies, although only a relatively small number have actually been reported. Recognition of these variants on CT helps prevent confusion with enlarged retroperitoneal lymph nodes or other masses. Furthermore, knowledge of these abnormalities is very helpful before surgery, particularly in patients undergoing shunt surgery for portal hypertension, kidney donation, abdominal aortic aneurysm repair, or nephrectomy.[188] In one series,[16] 40% of retroaortic left renal veins were injured in a large group of patients undergoing abdominal aortic surgery.

Technique

Evaluation of the retroperitoneal venous anatomy is best performed using 1-cm-thick images at 1-cm intervals, after dynamic bolus intravenous contrast infusion. A rapid bolus of contrast can, in most instances, differentiate a blood vessel from a lymph node. Both the ability to follow a rounded structure on sequential images (indicating the vessel's tubular shape) and the higher attenuation of enhanced and flowing blood within the vessel lumen are useful in making this distinction.[185]

Transposition of the inferior vena cava (left-sided IVC)

A left-sided IVC, resulting from persistence of the infrarenal left supracardinal vein and regression of the right supracardinal vein, occurs in 0.2% to 0.5% of the population.[137] Commonly, a round tubular structure is detected to the left of the aorta and extending superiorly to the left renal vein. The suprarenal portion of the inferior vena cava continues cephalad in its normal right-sided location, because its subcardinal portion is not abnormally formed.[107]

Duplication of the IVC

Duplication of the IVC, occurring with an incidence of 0.2% to 3%,[93,137,190] results from the persistence of both the infrarenal right and left supracardinal veins. Usually the left-sided IVC drains into the right by emptying into the left renal vein. Only a right-sided IVC is seen cephalad to this level (since subcardinal development is again normal). It is not uncommon for one of the vessels to be dominant. Bolus CT examinations may not result in simultaneous and equal vessel enhancement, because contrast media may flow preferentially into the dominant vessel.[93]

In most cases CT demonstrates a rounded tubular structure on either side of the aorta, extending from just above the aortic bifurcation to the renal hila. A single normal prerenal IVC traverses the upper abdomen to the level of the diaphragm in its normal right paraaortic location (Fig. 37-14).

Circumaortic left renal vein

A renal venous collar around the aorta is thought to result from partial persistence of the posteriorly located left supracardinal vein and a midline left to right supracardinal anastomosis. This relatively common anomaly was reported in from 2.4% to 16% of patients. In a series of 433 patients, 4.4% were found on CT to have circumaortic left renal veins.[167]

The ventral portion of the left renal vein, usually normal in location, drains the inferior and ventral portions of the kidney. The dorsal vein, usually inserting several centimeters more caudally into an area of saclike dilatation of the IVC, drains the superior and dorsal aspects of the kidney.[188] The preaortic vein is always equal in size to or larger than the posterior vein.[167] The detection of a renal venous collar is usually incidental, although one case of hematuria and proteinuria ascribed solely to this variant has been reported.[177]

Both ventral and retroaortic components are frequently identified.[109] The presence of the retroaortic component can be suspected, however, even in the absence of its direct visualization, if a medially located triangular-shaped diverticulum off the IVC is identified at or below the level of the ventral left renal vein.

Retroaortic left renal vein

A retroaortic left renal vein forms when the ventral component of a circumaortic renal vein has involuted. This anomaly is less common than the renal venous collar, having been reported in 1% to 3.3% of patients.[167,188] In the previously cited review of 433 CT

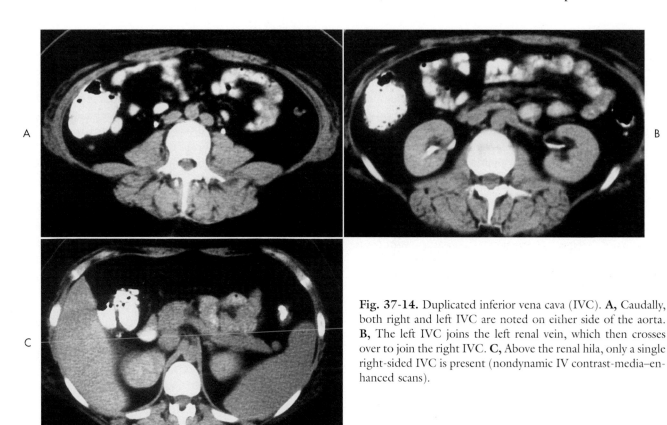

Fig. 37-14. Duplicated inferior vena cava (IVC). **A,** Caudally, both right and left IVC are noted on either side of the aorta. **B,** The left IVC joins the left renal vein, which then crosses over to join the right IVC. **C,** Above the renal hila, only a single right-sided IVC is present (nondynamic IV contrast-media–enhanced scans).

examinations, 1.8% of patients had retroaortic renal veins detected by CT. CT findings are notable for absence of a ventral left renal vein. The dorsally located renal vein is often visualized just caudal to the level of the renal hila (Fig. 37-15).

Periureteric venous ring or circumcaval ureter

Occasionally, the right ureter will be medially displaced by an abnormally positioned IVC or a periureteric venous ring at the level of the third or fourth lumbar vertebral bodies. This abnormality has been termed the *circumcaval ureter* and occurs with a frequency of 0.9 per 1,000 patients.[151] Most of the patients with this anomaly who were reviewed by Nielsen had a single right preureteric IVC, which was felt to represent persistence of the right posterior cardinal vein with failure of development of the infrarenal right supracardinal vein.[151,172] When present, symptoms (secondary to obstruction) usually appear late.

CT can diagnose circumcaval ureter, if the right ureter partially encircles the inferior cava, passing first posterior and then medial to the inferior vena cava.[116] Lateral positioning of the upper abdominal IVC in relation to the right ureter without an identifiable retroca-

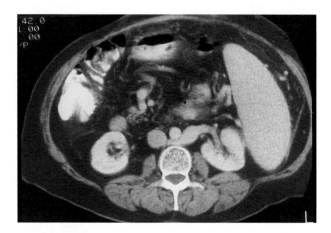

Fig. 37-15. Retroaortic left renal vein in a patient with splenomegaly (nondynamic enhanced scan).

val component of the ureter, although seen in all patients with circumcaval ureters, is most commonly a normal variant (visualized in 6% of the general population).[116]

Azygos continuation of the inferior vena cava

Azygos continuation of the IVC results from both the failure of the hepatic and right subcardinal veins to merge, and the persistence of a suprarenal right subcardinal to right supracardinal anastomosis, allowing venous drainage to continue up the azygos vein to the superior vena cava.[32] This anomaly was observed in 0.2% to 4.3% of patients undergoing cardiac catheterization for congenital heart disease. However, this is a heavily biased patient population, because 85% of patients with azygos continuation of the IVC have coexisting congenital heart disease. Associated abnormalities include asplenia, polysplenia, and abnormal abdominal and/or cardiac si-

tus. In another series of 1,055 noncardiac patients, none demonstrated this abnormality.[32,93,107]

CT may reveal enlarged azygos and hemiazygos systems in the upper abdomen and chest. These vessels may be confused with enlarged retrocrural lymph nodes, although their tubular nature and brisk enhancement after bolus injection of contrast material usually allow for their correct identification (Fig. 37-16). Cases of accessory azygos continuation of a left-sided cava also have been reported[37,48] (Fig. 37-17).

Other retroperitoneal venous abnormalities

Patients with inferior vena cava obstructions may develop dilated azygos and hemiazygos veins and other large retroperitoneal collaterals that can occasionally be confused with enlarged para-aortic lymph nodes.[48] Patients with portal venous hypertension may spontaneously decompress into their left renal vein or, more rarely, into lumbar veins (Fig. 37-18). Large vascular abdominal tumors may drain into retroperitoneal veins, with the increased blood flow frequently causing vessel enlargement. Normal retroaortic anastomoses between the azygos and hemiazygos veins may be prominent and confused with pathologic retrocrural nodes.[183]

The gonadal veins are usually seen just lateral to the ureter and anterior to the psoas muscles in the lower abdomen. They ascend parallel to and cross anteriorly over the ureters (approximately half way between the IVC bifurcation and the level of the renal hila) and then continue cephalad just medial to the ureters, usually emptying into the left renal vein (left gonadal vein) or the IVC (right gonadal vein). In one recent study the

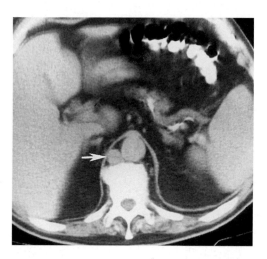

Fig. 37-16. Azygos continuation of the IVC. Note the marked enlargement of the azygos vein *(arrow)*. The subhepatic, suprarenal portion of the IVC was absent (nondynamic enhanced scan).

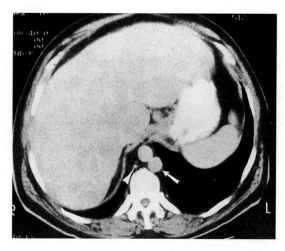

Fig. 37-17. Hemiazygos continuation of a left-sided IVC. The hemiazygos vein *(arrow)* is enlarged in this patient, while the azygos vein *(arrowhead)* is normal in size. The subhepatic, suprarenal portion of the IVC was absent. Note that the liver is enlarged and heterogeneous because of the presence of infiltrative metastatic disease (nondynamic enhanced scan).

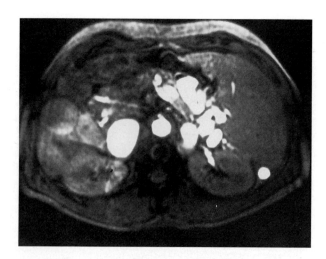

Fig. 37-18. Splenorenal shunt in a patient with portal hypertension. Limited flip-angle image readily identified the round high-intensity structures in the left upper quadrant as vessels. These could be confused with bowel or lymph nodes on a suboptimally enhanced CT scan.

right gonadal vein was visualized in 35 of 44 (80%) of normal patients.[166] The gonadal veins may enlarge in pregnant patients and in patients with portal hypertension.[166] On occasion they may appear prominent in patients in whom no etiology for dilatation can be identified (Fig. 37-19).

Distinction between dilated retroperitoneal veins and enlarged lymph nodes is usually easily accomplished with MRI, because in most instances the veins are characterized by signal void on spin-echo sequences and high signal on gradient-echo images (see Fig. 37-18).

Inferior vena cava thrombosis

Thrombus may be detected in the inferior vena cava or its branches.[63,97] Usually, on CT the involved vessel is enlarged. Prominent collateral vessels may be present. If intravenous contrast material has been administered, the thrombus itself is identified as a low-attenuation filling defect (in which case a definitive diagnosis can be made without any additional imaging being required). The wall of the thrombosed vessel enhances brightly (Fig. 37-20). IVC thrombus may be seen in patients as an extension of lower extremity or pelvic deep vein thrombosis. It may also form as a result of spread from either bland or tumor thrombus in the renal veins.

Septic thrombosis of the IVC is a rare finding, usually encountered in the critically ill. These patients must be managed aggressively with antibiotics and anticoagulants and, occasionally, even surgical ligation of the IVC. A specific diagnosis can be made by CT when air is identified within or adjacent to IVC clot (Fig. 37-21). Frequently, the infecting organism is not gas-producing,

however. Percutaneous aspiration can be performed in these cases to confirm the suspected diagnosis.[143]

Gonadal vein thrombosis

Gonadal vein thrombosis (GVT) is being diagnosed with increasing frequency, probably because it is so easy to identify on CT. GVT has been traditionally seen in postpartum females, in women with endometritis or pelvic inflammatory disease, or after gynecologic surgery.[91] It has more recently been detected in patients with malignancies (particularly those undergoing chemotherapy)[91] and in patients with a variety of gastrointestinal inflammatory diseases[92] (Fig. 37-22). Patients with

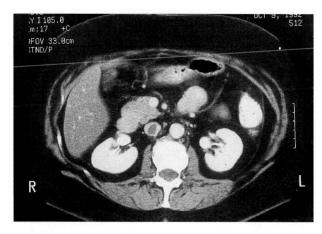

Fig. 37-20. IVC thrombus. Note that the margin between the clot and the surrounding blood is sharply defined. Delayed images would not reveal any significant change in this appearance (dynamic enhanced scan).

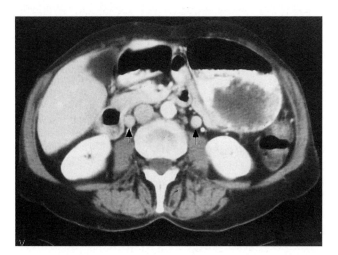

Fig. 37-19. Prominent gonadal veins, as demonstrated in this patient *(arrows)* should not be confused with enlarged retroperitoneal lymph nodes (dynamic enhanced scan).

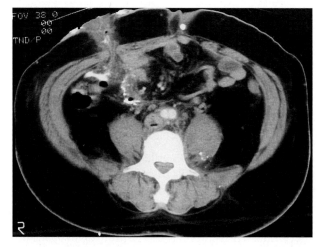

Fig. 37-21. Infected IVC thrombus. A punctate collection of air adjacent to the IVC thrombus indicates infection in this patient with a right lower quadrant ostomy (unenhanced scan).

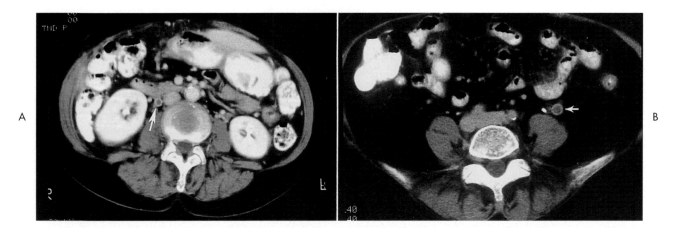

Fig. 37-22. Gonadal vein thrombosis. **A,** Low-attenuation clot is noted in the right gonadal vein *(arrow)* of this patient with breast carcinoma who was receiving high dose chemotherapy. **B,** Thrombus is easily visualized in the left gonadal vein *(arrow)* of another patient (enhanced scans).

typical postpartum or post-GYN surgery (GVT) have infected thrombus and must be treated with both antibiotics and anticoagulants. Appropriate treatment for patients with GVT related to malignancies or GI inflammation has not yet been determined with certainty; however, it appears that anticoagulation here is often unnecessary.[91,92]

MRI for evaluation of venous thrombosis

MRI offers several advantages over CT in the assessment of patients with abdominal venous thrombosis. Imaging can be performed in any plane. Intravenous contrast media is not required. Arrive and co-workers found that a combination of spin-echo (SE) and gradient-echo (GRE) imaging was more sensitive, increasing thrombus detection rate from 63% (SE alone) and 58% (GRE alone) to 82%.[10] Problems leading to false negative diagnoses included failure to visualize small partially occluding thrombi (on SE and GRE images) and misinterpreting low to intermediate signal thrombus as flow (on SE images). False positive diagnoses resulted from misinterpretation of slow flow as representing thrombus (on SE images) and from failing to detect high-intensity signal in small patent vessels (on GRE images).

Gadolinium-DTPA–enhanced MRI has been able to distinguish between bland and tumor thrombus in at least one case.[64] After contrast enhancement, tumor thrombus signal intensity was noted to increase significantly in a fashion similar to that of the patient's primary tumor. Such distinction can also be made on dynamic bolus CT, since again the vascularity of tumor thrombus can result in its brisk (and often heterogeneous) enhancement.

Other intraluminal or intramural lesions may be confused with clot, although these are exceedingly rare. Leiomyosarcomas of the IVC are the most common primary caval tumors. These occur most frequently in older women. Although they are slow-growing, they are associated with a poor prognosis.[201]

It is important not to confuse heterogeneous IVC enhancement ("pseudothrombus"—often seen on the early images of a dynamic enhanced CT) with thrombus.[54] Heterogeneous contrast enhancement is due to low attenuation of unenhanced centrally located blood (from the lower extremities and pelvis) surrounded by higher-attenuation enhanced blood (entering the IVC from the renal veins) on CT images obtained early in the course of a bolus injection of contrast media. Distinction can be made because unenhanced central blood is usually not nearly as well defined as is thrombus. Also, dynamic CT flow-artifact disappears as time passes. It will not be present if recuts are obtained (Fig. 37-23).[54]

Inferior vena cava filters

IVC filters are inserted in patients with lower extremity or pelvic venous thrombosis who have recurring pulmonary emboli despite anticoagulation or in whom a contraindication to anticoagulation exists. CT is at least as accurate as venography in determining whether the filter is positioned at the proper level (between the IVC bifurcation and the renal veins) and appropriately angulated.[142] CT can identify other complications that cannot be imaged by venography, such as filter perforation of the wall of the IVC and retroperitoneal hematomas (Fig. 37-24).[142]

MRI has been safely performed in patients with IVC filters, despite the fact that two of the more com-

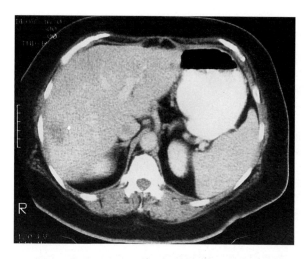

Fig. 37-23. IVC pseudothrombus. Early images on this dynamically enhanced CT demonstrate centrally not yet enhanced IVC blood from the pelvis and lower extremities surrounded by already enhanced blood from the renal veins. On delayed images, the IVC became homogeneous. Incidental note is made of low-attenuation lesions in the liver.

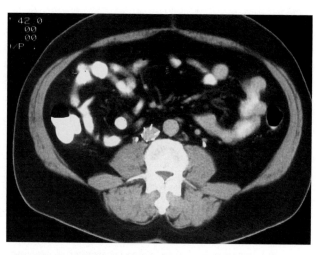

Fig. 37-24. Inferior vena cava filter. The metallic struts of this Kimray-Greenfield filter are easily demonstrated. Note that two of the anterior struts appear to extend through the wall of the IVC (nondynamic enhanced scan).

monly used types (Kimray-Greenfield and Bird's Nest filters) are ferromagnetic.[123,195] *In vitro* experiments have failed to detect any evidence that the small amount of magnetic torque that develops at a field strength of 1.5 T results in filter migration.[123,186] However, Liebman and colleagues caution that when filters are *angulated*, greater torque is exerted and the risk of filter movement increases.[123] Magnetic susceptibility artifacts caused by most filter types[186] degrade image quality to such an extent that abdominal MRI studies in these patients are of limited quality. MRI of the head, pelvis, spine, and extremities is usually artifact-free, however, and can be performed without complication.[195]

The small IVC

Flattening or significant decrease in the short axis diameter of the IVC (so that it appears "slit-like") has been described in severely hypovolemic patients.[94] Any patient in whom this finding is observed should have his or her venous pressures carefully monitored (see Fig. 37-5).

LYMPH NODES
Normal anatomy

Normal retroperitoneal lymph nodes commonly are seen by CT and appear as small soft-tissue masses adjacent to the great vessels. *Retrocrural nodes* are the most cephalad group of intra-abdominal nodes that can be identified. Normal retrocrural nodes do not exceed 6 mm in size.[47] Occasionally they may be confused with

other retrocrural structures, including azygos and hemiazygos veins and their anastomoses, and the thoracic duct.

Paraaortic and paracaval lymph nodes usually are well seen by CT because the great vessels are often surrounded by fat, allowing for sharp contrast between small lymph nodes and the surrounding retroperitoneum. Single paraaortic lymph nodes are considered normal on CT if they measure 11 mm or less in short axis diameter.[47]

Pelvic nodes are harder to identify than are retrocrural or paraaortic nodes. They follow the iliac vessels, dividing into internal and external iliac groups. The obturator nodes are particularly important, because they are the first site of lymph node spread of most pelvic tumors. These nodes (belonging to the external iliac chain) are best seen medial to the obturator internus muscle on CT images obtained just above the acetabulae. Pelvic nodes exceeding 15 mm in short axis diameter are considered abnormal,[50] whereas those under 10 to 12 mm are considered normal size.[107,145] Pelvic lymph nodes may be confused with unopacified loops of bowel, tortuous iliac vessels, or adnexal masses in women.

Technique

CT scanning for evaluation of patients with possible retroperitoneal lymphadenopathy must be performed after generous administration of oral contrast to maximally opacify any adjacent bowel. Intravenous contrast media is not mandatory but is helpful in distinguishing nodes from vessels, especially in the pelvis.[185] Contrast material injections should be performed as a dynamic bolus. Scans of 1-cm thickness at 1.0- or 1.5-cm intervals are obtained from the diaphragm to the pubic symphysis.

Evaluation of the retroperitoneum for lymph-node enlargement may be extremely difficult in pediatric patients, and in thin or cachectic adults as a result of a paucity of retroperitoneal fat.[107] Intravenous contrast material is particularly helpful in elucidating the anatomy of the retroperitoneum in these patients.

Lymphadenopathy

CT evaluation of retroperitoneal lymph nodes is most commonly performed on patients with known or suspected malignancies to rule out the presence of malignant lymphadenopathy. CT detects lymph-node abnormalities only by identifying enlargement. The majority of lymph nodes over 1.0 to 1.1 cm in short axis diameter will contain tumor cells in these patients. In some, however, enlargement may represent reactive hyperplasia, fatty replacement, reaction to chemotherapy or radiation therapy, or infection. Conversely, normal-size

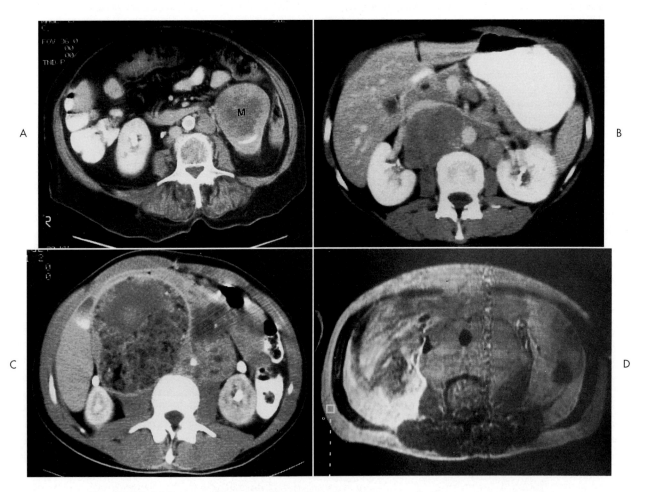

Fig. 37-25. Malignant retroperitoneal lymph-node enlargement. **A,** Para-aortic lymph node enlargement on a dynamically enhanced CT. Enlargement is due to metastases from a large left renal adenocarcinoma *(M).* **B,** Dynamically enhanced CT of non-Hodgkin lymphoma. Large nodal masses involve the para-aortic lymph node chains. The IVC is displaced anteriorly. **C,** Nondynamic enhanced CT of retroperitoneal lymph node metastases from testicular teratocarcinoma. Huge nodal masses with areas of fat, fluid, and calcification are characteristic. **D,** Intermediate spin-echo MRI scan in a patient with bulky lymph node metastases from prostate carcinoma. The flow void in the aorta and IVC makes the location of these vessels easy to determine in relation to the lymph node enlargement, even in the absence of a contrast media injection.

lymph nodes may contain microscopic metastases that will be missed by CT. This is particularly true in patients with Hodgkin lymphoma and primary pelvic malignancies.

Lymphography

Lymphography (LAG) is extremely valuable in patients with a wide variety of tumors, because LAG can identify alterations in the internal architecture of normal-size nodes, as well as lymph-node enlargement.[135] Another advantage of LAG is the low cost of follow-up examinations. After LAG, contrast material remains in lymph nodes for up to 1 year in 75% of patients, and up to 2 years in 35%.[95] An abdominal radiograph may therefore be obtained every 3 to 6 months to assess for any change. The cost of a plain radiograph is only a fraction of a follow-up CT.

CT has several important advantages over LAG. First, many more lymph node groups can be visualized. While LAG opacifies most lymph nodes in the external and common iliac, para-aortic, aortocaval, and paracaval chains,[95] paraaortic nodes not immediately contiguous to the aorta and IVC often are not visualized.[145] Internal iliac and presacral pelvic nodes are opacified only occasionally, and retrocrural, renal hilar, splenic, peripancreatic, periportal, and mesenteric nodes are never filled with contrast media.[95] All of these lymph node groups can be assessed by CT. CT can also evaluate other organs for possible tumor involvement (i.e., liver, spleen, and adrenal glands). Similarly, the extent of local spread of a primary tumor can be imaged. For these reasons CT has replaced LAG as the primary imaging modality in many cancer patients (Fig. 37-25). However, sensitivity in detecting malignant spread is greatest when both procedures are employed.[152,158,187]

Magnetic resonance imaging of lymph nodes

Normal lymph nodes have T1 values much longer than fat, but only slightly longer than that of muscle. T2 values are similar to those of fat, but longer than that of muscle. Dooms et al advocate using two pulse-sequences for best identification of lymph nodes, the first employing a short TR interval to maximize T1 weighting, and hence, differences between lymph nodes and fat; the second employing a long TR (and long TE) allowing increased T1 weighting and hence easy differentiation from muscle (such as the diaphragmatic crura).[45] Alternatively, Lee et al advocate a single compromise spin-echo sequence using an intermediate length TR (900 msec) and a short TE (30 msec), which they feel optimizes contrast between nodes and both fat and muscle.[118] A number of studies have suggested that MRI might be able to distinguish between residual tumor and fibrosis in patients who have been treated for a variety of retroperitoneal and pelvic neoplasms.[149,158] Mature fibrotic tissue usually has a low-signal intensity on T2-weighted images while malignant or acutely inflamed lymph nodes are of high signal intensity.

Many had hoped that tissue-specific differences in T1 and T2 values would also allow for the differentiation of nonfibrotic benign and malignant lymph nodes. This has not proved to be the case. Reliable differences in relaxation times between most enlarged benign and malignant retroperitoneal lymph nodes have not been discovered. Relaxation times of normal-size lymph nodes (those less than 10 mm in diameter) cannot be accurately measured because of variations caused by partial voluming.[46]

Several disadvantages of MRI must be stressed; these make CT the preferred screening examination in patients with possible lymphadenopathy. CT is still cheaper and often faster. Its superior resolution allows for identification of multiple small or borderline lymph nodes. MRI cannot identify calcification within lymph nodes, while CT can. Occasionally, bowel loops may be confused with nodes on MRI, although this problem may be eliminated with the use of paramagnetic oral contrast agents.

Non-Hodgkin lymphoma

Non-Hodgkin lymphomas (NHL) include a diverse group of lymphocytic neoplasms. The most common classification of NHL had been that of Rappaport,[167] although Bragg et al[15] and others advocate "the working formulation" as being more useful. Briefly, the working formulation classifies lymphomas as low, intermediate, or high grade. Rappaport's nodular lymphomas belong to low and intermediate grades, whereas histiocytic, lymphoblastic, and undifferentiated lymphomas (including Burkitt's) belong to the intermediate and high grades.

Low-grade lymphomas often are disseminated widely when first detected, yet they are slow-growing and patients may be followed for years. Chemotherapy or radiation therapy usually are used for palliation; although treatment may be initially deferred. These neoplasms may transform into higher-grade lymphomas.

Intermediate or high-grade lymphomas are less frequently widespread when discovered but are much more aggressive. Potent chemotherapy is required. Remission or even cure is the goal of therapy in these patients. Five-year survival statistics are much lower for most intermediate and high-grade lymphomas (23% to 45%) than for low-grade lymphomas (50% to 70%).

Lymphomas are staged, according to the Ann Arbor System, as follows:

- *Stage I disease:* Involvement of one nodal group
- *Stage II disease:* Involvement of more than one nodal group on the same side of the diaphragm
- *Stage III disease:* Malignant nodes on both sides of the diaphragm
- *Stage IV disease:* Extranodal spread

Certain populations are particularly susceptible to non-Hodgkin lymphoma. Patients who have had renal transplants, patients with AIDS, or patients who are immunocompromised for other reasons, are all at increased risk.

Imaging of non-Hodgkin lymphoma at presentation. CT has been the preferred imaging modality for evaluation of the retroperitoneum in patients presenting with NHL because involved nodes are usually enlarged. Most patients with NHL (as opposed to fewer than half with Hodgkin disease) will have abdominal involvement.[78] With NHL, bulky paraaortic lymphadenopathy is common. Mesenteric disease is seen in over half of patients (compared with less than 5% of those with Hodgkin disease).[145] Enlarged lymph nodes may appear as discrete masses or as confluent soft tissue obliterating the retroperitoneal fat, resulting in loss of definition of the fat planes between the aorta and IVC (see Fig. 37-25, *B*). Many other lymph node groups, such as retrocrural, gastrohepatic, paraceliac, periportal, peripancreatic, posterior iliac crest, and pelvic chains are frequently involved.[28,50] Lymph-node calcification at presentation is extremely unusual.[117]

CT-guided biopsy of patients presenting with potentially lymphomatous masses should be performed with core rather than aspiration biopsy needles, since pathologists often require histologic rather than cytologic specimens for accurate tumor characterization and grading.

LAG has a slightly superior sensitivity in detecting abnormal nodes in patients with non-Hodgkin lymphoma.[135] In the series reported by Pond et al, LAG was positive in 110 of 157 patients (70%) with NHL, while CT demonstrated enlarged lymph nodes in 88 of 139 patients (63%).[158] The small sacrifice in malignant node detection made by CT was partially compensated by CT's ability to examine adjacent organs for possible involvement.

Imaging of non-Hodgkin lymphoma at follow-up. CT is advocated for assistance in planning ports for radiation therapy,[15] as well as for following disease after treatment. Oliver, Bernardino, and Sones found several patterns on CT that indicated tumor response to therapy.[154] Reduction in overall abdominal lymphadenopathy correlated with clinical improvement in 48 of 56 of their patients, with five of the remaining eight patients having developed central nervous system disease accounting for their deterioration. Decreased lymph-node mass attenuation values with or *without* overall reduction in lymph node size, and/or increased mesenteric stranding, coincided with clinical improvement in all 26 patients. Post-treatment calcification of lymphomatous masses is rare but has been reported.[30]

Failure to completely eradicate retroperitoneal lymph node masses with chemotherapy does *not* necessarily indicate that viable tumor cells are present.[122] NHL patients with these residual fibrotic masses should be closely monitored with follow-up examinations to detect tumor recurrence; however, if these masses remain stable, treatment may be discontinued. MRI may be helpful in these instances, since, though there may be some overlap, tumor masses usually remain bright on T2-weighted images while chronic fibrosis or scar is dark.[58,118] Patients with MRI scans revealing high signal in residual masses should be more closely followed or even referred for biopsy.

Histiocytic lymphomas deserve special comment because these neoplasms have an extraordinarily high incidence of gastrointestinal tract involvement. In Burgener and Hamlin's series, patients presented with gastric involvement, peripancreatic masses, high paraaortic lymphadenopathy, mesenteric involvement, and ileocolic masses.[22] These locations should be examined carefully on CT scans of patients with this aggressive form of lymphoma.

AIDS-related lymphomas tend to be poorly differentiated and aggressive. Advanced disease is often present at the time of diagnosis, and prognosis is poor. AIDS-related NHL is often characterized on CT by lymph-node enlargement. Abdominal visceral organ involvement (resulting in hepatic, splenic, and gastrointestinal tract masses) and omental disease is more frequently seen in these patients.[192]

Hodgkin lymphoma

Hodgkin lymphoma is more common in adults in higher socioeconomic groups and peaks both in the third and fifth decades of life. The hallmark of Hodgkin lymphoma is the Reed-Sternberg cell. Unfortunately, this cell is relatively uncommon in pathologic specimens, and aspiration biopsies are often inadequate for establishing the diagnosis.[27,86]

Histologically, Hodgkin lymphoma is classified into several forms. The nodular sclerosing type is most frequent (50% to 80% of cases) and of intermediate aggressiveness. Lymphocytic predominant Hodgkin lymphoma, which carries the best prognosis, and lymphocytic depletion Hodgkin lymphoma, which carries the worst, are considerably less common (5% to 10% each). The mixed cellularity forms occur with somewhat higher frequencies (15% to 40%).[27] Staging of Hodgkin lymphoma is similar to that of non-Hodgkin's lymphoma.

Treatment of Hodgkin disease is based on accurate staging, because radiation therapy can be curative when all areas of tumor involvement are included in radiation ports.[25] In advanced disease, chemotherapy and radiation therapy often are used jointly, frequently with very favorable results. Ten-year survival has been reported at 85% in adults.[27] For this reason, careful follow-up of patients over many years is required.

In contrast to NHL, lymph-node involvement with Hodgkin disease less commonly results in bulky enlargement. Therefore, CT is less sensitive in detecting abdominal spread. Castellino et al[26] noted that CT identified abnormal para-aortic nodes in only 13 of 20 patients (65%) who were proved subsequently to have retroperitoneal disease at staging laparotomy, but LAG detected involvement of these nodes in 17 of 20 patients (85%). These authors (and others) recommend that LAG be performed for the evaluation of the retroperitoneal lymph nodes in all patients with Hodgkin lymphoma.[26,152]

Unlike LAG, CT can also evaluate the spleen for possible metastases. Unfortunately, correlation between spleen size and attenuation and splenic Hodgkin lymphoma is poor.[1] Single or multiple discrete low-attenuation masses detectable by CT are seen infrequently. The Southwest Oncology group recently found that CT was able to detect disease in only 10 of 68 spleens involved with Hodgkin lymphoma and in only 3 of 16 livers.[133] In addition, only about one third of patients with splenomegaly on CT have splenic involvement. Only massive splenomegaly correlates well with the spread of Hodgkin disease.

Currently, we recommend that LAG, as well as abdominal CT, be performed on patients presenting with Hodgkin disease. Follow-up plain radiographs are frequently sufficient to detect any changes within 12 to 18 months of LAG. A baseline CT may be obtained after completion of treatment[27] so that any residual fibrotic masses or stranding can be distinguished from recurrence.

MRI has not yet played a significant role in assessment of patients with Hodgkin lymphoma. A recent study found Hodgkin lymphomas to have a brighter signal on T2-weighted images than did other lymphomas. This was an unexpected finding because pathologically these lymph-node masses contained an increased amount of dense "active" fibrosis.[158] The clinical utility of this observation is not yet clear.

Testicular neoplasms

Testicular tumors, the most common cancers in men between 15 and 34 years of age,[51] are divided into germinal (95%) and nongerminal (5%) cell types. The most common germinal tumors (40%) are seminomas. Seminomas are extremely responsive to irradiation (with 10-year patient survival of 90%), and for this reason staging lymphadenectomy and chemotherapy are reserved only for patients with advanced disease. The lack of routine lymphadenectomy after orchiectomy in these patients explains why there is some difficulty acquiring data on the accuracy of CT and LAG in staging these patients. Surgical follow-up is rarely available.

The nonseminomatous germ cell tumors include teratocarcinoma, teratoma, choriocarcinoma, embryonal cell neoplasms, and yolk-sac tumors. Mixed cancers containing seminomatous and nonseminomatous elements may also be considered in this group, because the clinical course often follows that of the nonseminomatous cells.[51] These neoplasms do not respond as favorably to treatment. The percentage of patients who are disease-free at 3 years ranges from 26 (for patients with choriocarcinomas) to 62 (for patients with teratomatous neoplasms).

While some testicular tumors appear quite homogeneous on CT, others, particularly teratomatous neoplasms, often appear heterogeneous, containing areas of necrosis, fat and calcification (see Fig. 37-25, C). These neoplasms have been treated by orchiectomy followed by staging lymphadenectomy in many institutions.

Testicular neoplasms tend to metastasize via lymphatics rather than via the bloodstream. Lymphatics from the testicle drain into ipsilateral lymph nodes, which follow the course of the gonadal veins. Only occasionally do lymphatics drain into ipsilateral external iliac nodes. It is, therefore, more common that lymph node metastases involve para-aortic and paracaval rather than pelvic nodes. Typically, left-sided neoplasms can spread to involve lymph nodes in the left renal hilum (in the area where the left gonadal vein inserts into the left renal vein). Right-sided neoplasms can spread to paracaval lymph nodes (in the area where the right gonadal vein inserts into the IVC).

Imaging of testicular neoplasms at presentation. Testicular metastases tend to enlarge involved lymph nodes, thus facilitating their visualization by CT.[107] Low-attenuation lymph node metastases (less than 30 HU) have been reported in patients with testicular neoplasms. In one series, 10 of 57 patients evaluated by CT had such masses.[173] Although seven of these patients had previous therapy, the masses were found at presentation in three cases. Biopsies identified lipid-laden macrophages, cholesterol clefts, and necrosis in the post-treatment patients, and teratomatous elements and cystic spaces were identified in an untreated patient.

The sensitivity of CT in detecting metastatic nodes, ranging between 60% to 93% has not significantly exceeded that of LAG (56% to 93%).[49,95,145,187] Although the sensitivity for detecting lymph-node metastases increases when CT and LAG are used to gether,[124,187] reliance on both procedures for staging has shown decreased specificity. Tesoro-Tess et al report, for example, that LAG and CT together reduced false negative examinations from 27% to 10%; however, false positive results increased from 25% to 37% in the same patient population.[187] Nonetheless, these authors emphasize the importance of not overlooking subtle metastases. It is better to subject patients who do not need it to aggressive surgery or other therapy than to fail to appropriately treat those with lymph-node metastases.

Our recommendation for staging patients presenting with testicular neoplasms is to obtain a preliminary abdominal CT. If the CT is positive, LAG need not be performed. If the CT is negative, staging lymphadenectomy (with or without preceding LAG) should be considered.

Imaging of testicular neoplasms at follow-up. Residual fibrotic masses have been detected in patients after apparently successful treatment. As with patients with NHL, the persistence of these masses does not necessarily indicate that malignant or even benign teratomatous cells remain,[178] and this can sometimes be a problem. Patients with residual malignant tumor cells must receive additional therapy. Benign mature teratomas (which may differentiate from treated malignant nonseminomatous germ cell tumors) must be surgically removed, since they may undergo malignant transformation at any time.[182] Obviously, follow-up CT examinations must be scrutinized closely to exclude any possible changes in masses presumed to be fibrotic. In any given case there are no reliable CT features that permit distinction of recurrent or residual malignancy from benign teratoma, fibrotic scar, or necrosis.[182]

Our current recommendation is to follow patients with treated testicular neoplasms with serial CT examinations and serum tumor marker studies. LAG need not be performed. Percutaneous fine-needle aspiration biopsy of a residual mass can be performed if a patient has rising markers, or if the mass has changed in size or morphology. In equivocal cases, surgery will be required.

Other pelvic malignancies

The pelvic tumors that most commonly metastasize to pelvic and retroperitoneal lymph nodes are bladder, prostate, cervix, and, less frequently, ovarian carcinomas. The local manifestations of all these tumors are better assessed with MRI. All of these neoplasms frequently metastasize to nodes without enlarging them so that CT and even MRI identification of tumor spread to pelvic and retroperitoneal nodes is more difficult than with other tumors.[107] Reported sensitivities in detecting abdominal and pelvic lymph-node involvement range from 30% to 100% for bladder and prostate cancer and from 80% to 85% for cervical cancer. Specificities have also been less than optimal, ranging from 46% to 100%

for the three neoplasms.[70,95,114,196,197]

Studies on the value of lymphography in assessing retroperitoneal and pelvic nodes for metastases have also been characterized by significant differences and somewhat disappointing results. In a recent series by Chagnon et al, the rate of false positive results for LAG in 101 patients with bladder carcinoma was 40% (due to misinterpreting inflammatory changes as metastases), while the rate of false negative results was 48% (due to missing small microscopic tumor foci).[29] This suggests that LAG must be followed by percutaneous biopsy of any suspicious nodes.

We currently recommend initial local staging with MRI. LAG is only performed on patients with cervical carcinoma whose cross-sectional imaging studies fail to demonstrate metastatic disease. Any patients with bladder, prostate, or cervical cancer whose chemical or imaging studies do not suggest metastatic disease must go on to staging lymphadenectomy for most accurate determination of disease extent.

Benign causes of retroperitoneal lymphadenopathy

The presence of enlarged retroperitoneal lymph nodes is not diagnostic of malignancy. Many of the false positive CT scans and lymphograms in patients with lymphomas and pelvic neoplasms are caused by reactive lymphoid hyperplasia. Some nodes can undergo fatty replacement, occasionally visible with CT. Several inflammatory diseases have been specifically identified as causing, or being associated with, retroperitoneal lymphadenopathy.

HIV-infected patients. Enlarged lymph nodes or an increase in the number of normal-sized lymph nodes is frequently present in patients infected with the HIV virus. The most common etiologies for retroperitoneal lymphadenopathy in these patients are (1) lymph node or lymphadenopathy syndrome (LNS), (2) epidemic (disseminated) Kaposi sarcoma, (3) lymphoma, (4) *Mycobacterium tuberculosis* and *Mycobacterium avium-intracellulare* (MAI) infections, and (5) extrapulmonary *Pneumocystis carinii* (PC) infections. CT manifestations in patients with lymphoma and mycobacterial infections are described elsewhere.

Retroperitoneal lymphadenopathy was noted in 9 of 12 patients with LNS elsewhere in the series by Moon et al.[144] Although a variety of CT appearances was appreciated by these authors, most commonly they noted the presence of abnormally large numbers of normal-sized lymph nodes, rather than discrete bulky enlarged lymph nodes or confluent masses. Also, splenomegaly was identified frequently in these patients (Fig. 37-26, *A*).

When Kaposi sarcoma spreads systemically (epidemic form), CT studies performed after enhancement

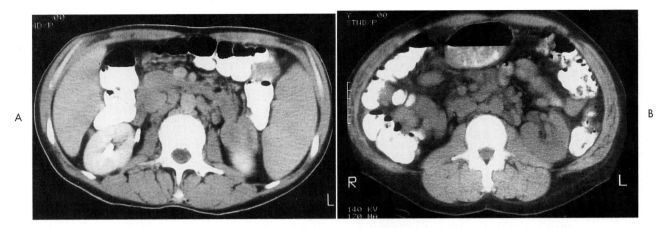

Fig. 37-26. A, Retroperitoneal lymph node enlargement and splenomegaly in an HIV-infected patient with no known malignancy (probable lymph node syndrome). **B,** Retroperitoneal lymph node enlargement and retroperitoneal lymph node enlargement in a patient with sarcoidosis (unenhanced scans).

with intravenous contrast media show involved retroperitoneal nodes to be more likely hyperattenuating (in comparison with the iliopsoas muscles) than are enlarged lymph nodes due to any of the other above described processes.[83] In the recent study by Herts and Associates, 80% of 33 patients with high-attenuation lymph nodes had disseminated Kaposi sarcoma.[93]

Extrapulmonary *Pneumocystis carinii* is rare, although it has been reported with increasing frequency over the past 5 years, perhaps because AIDS patients are living longer. Also, many patients now receive treatment (or prophylaxis) with aerosolized pentamidine, perhaps curbing the pulmonary but not the extrapulmonary manifestations of PC infections. Lymph nodes involved with PC infections tend to calcify over time, leading to a rather characteristic appearance. Other associated findings of extrapulmonary PC infection include multiple focal low-attenuation splenic and liver lesions, and pleural and peritoneal fluid.[129] Calcification has been noted to develop over time in all of these structures, as well as in the renal cortices and adrenal glands.

Myobacterium tuberculosis and *Mycobacterium avium-intracellulare* (MAI). Retroperitoneal lymphadenopathy has been detected by CT in many patients with abdominal mycobacterial infections. This was observed in 21 of 24 patients with lymph-node enlargement in a review by Hulnick et al.[89] Interestingly, mesenteric and peripancreatic adenopathy frequently overshadowed the adenopathy involving retroperitoneal nodes, perhaps reflecting the drainage routes of hematogeneously seeded organs in the gastrointestinal tract. Up to 83% of patients with *Mycobacterium tuberculosis,* in contrast to only 14% of patients with MAI infections, have enlarged lymph nodes with low-attenuation centers, a finding also described in some patients with malignancies, as well as in

patients with bacterial infections and Whipple disease.[83,89,161] The incidence of abdominal tuberculosis and MAI infections has increased dramatically over the past few years, because of the progression of the AIDS epidemic and the appearance of antibiotic-resistant strains.

Sarcoidosis. Retroperitoneal lymphadenopathy has been described in up to 69% to 75% of patients with sarcoidosis.[13,140] Recently, Britt and associates compared CT findings in patients with abdominal sarcoidosis with those in patients with non-Hodgkin lymphoma.[17] Although they found that retrocrural lymphadenopathy was much less frequent in patients with sarcoidosis and that sarcoid lymph nodes tended to be smaller, there was enough overlap to limit any ability to suggest a specific diagnosis in any given case (Fig. 37-26, *B*). Only rarely will abdominal lymph node enlargement be present without any mediastinal lymph-node involvement.

Other causes of benign lymph node enlargement. Patients with secondary amyloidosis and Castleman disease may occasionally develop enlarged retroperitoneal fibrotic masses or nodes.[66,100,184] Other infectious diseases also may be associated with intraabdominal lymphadenopathy. The CT appearance of these enlarged lymph nodes is often not specific, although briskly enhancing lymph nodes have been described in Castleman disease.[132]

Mimickers of lymphadenopathy

A variety of retroperitoneal structures can be confused with enlarged retroperitoneal lymph nodes, including unopacified loops of small bowel, collateral vessels, dilated lymphatics,[198] retroperitoneal hemorrhage, retroperitoneal fibrosis, and primary retroperitoneal tumors (Fig. 37-27). Usually distinctive features of each of these

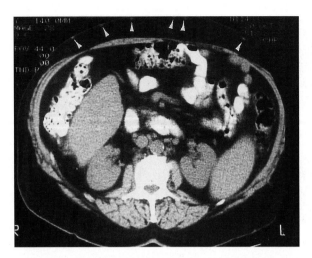

Fig. 37-27. Collateral vessels mimicking modest para-aortic lymphadenopathy in a patient with upper abdominal IVC occlusion. Note that subcutaneous collateral vessels are also present *(arrowheads)* (unenhanced scan).

abnormalities allows the radiologist to determine that these other findings do not represent pathologic lymph nodes.

PRIMARY RETROPERITONEAL NEOPLASMS

The vast majority of neoplasms in the retroperitoneum originate from viscera that have at least a partial retroperitoneal location, such as the colon, duodenum, pancreas, kidneys, adrenals, and ureters. Only 0.2% of retroperitoneal tumors are considered to be primary (i.e., not originating from a retroperitoneal organ).[79] Primary retroperitoneal masses are generally derived from mesenchymal or neurogenic cells or from embryonic rests.[24]

Primary retroperitoneal tumors usually do not present until they are quite large. This is apparently due to their capacity to grow unimpeded in the retroperitoneal space, before compromising adjacent organ function.[156] In a series by Lane and colleagues,[113] the range in average size of malignant tumors was 11 to 20 cm, and of benign tumors, 4 to 7 cm.

CT is the imaging study of choice for evaluation of patients with known or suspected retroperitoneal masses. If a mass is detected, a CT-guided biopsy can provide further characterization. Biopsies should be obtained using cutting or core needles because pathologic analysis often requires histologic samples, and distinction from lymphoma (often a diagnostic consideration) is more easily made.[156] Pathologists may also have difficulty distinguishing benign from malignant tumors (even when surgical specimens are obtained), and clinical behavior (such as the presence or absence of adjacent or-

gan invasion and distant metastases) may be used to classify a tumor as benign or malignant.

Most adult primary retroperitoneal neoplasms are treated surgically. While complete removal of the mass is preferred, in many instances only debulking is possible. Chemotherapy and external beam radiation of malignant tumors have limited effectiveness on most cell types (with the exception of rhabdomyosarcoma). Since malignant retroperitoneal neoplasms are relatively slow-growing, patients with unresectable tumors may live for years after initial surgery. Often, second and even third debulking procedures are performed. In a series we reported, median survival for patients with soft-tissue attenuation tumors (usually leiomyosarcomas) was 16 months. Median survival of patients with liposarcomas was 52 months.[34]

Malignant neoplasms

The majority of retroperitoneal tumors (66% to 90%) are malignant.[34,76,77,113] The frequency of various malignant retroperitoneal masses is somewhat dependent on the pathologist's classification system. Liposarcomas are considered by most to be the most frequent.[34,156] Leiomyosarcomas are slightly less common, with a variety of other malignancies also being encountered (malignant fibrous histiocytomas [MFH], fibrosarcomas, teratomas, rhabdomyosarcomas, and hemangiopericytomas). In the Mayo Clinic series reported by Lane et al, MFH was diagnosed most commonly, followed closely by liposarcomas and leiomyosarcomas.[113]

Liposarcomas can often be recognized on CT by the presence of low-attenuation fat (Fig. 37-28, *A*). This is nearly always seen in patients with well-differentiated (lipogenic) liposarcomas (which usually contain only a minimal amount of soft-tissue attenuation material and which are considered to be low-grade malignancies).[194] Myxoid liposarcomas (intermediate grade) and pleomorphic or poorly differentiated (high-grade) liposarcomas may contain recognizable fat on CT as well. Occasionally, tumors contain areas of homogeneously dispersed soft-tissue and fatty elements, which can volume average to water attenuation thereby making these regions look cystic[34] (Fig. 37-28, *B*). Rarely, there may be no recognizable fat, in which case liposarcomas cannot be distinguished from other retroperitoneal masses.

Although liposarcomas can be specifically diagnosed on MRI, there is no evidence that MRI is any more specific than CT. MRI has a theoretical advantage over CT in its ability to image in coronal and sagittal planes and thus better define the relationship of the tumor mass to the great vessels.

Leiomyosarcomas are large heterogeneous masses. They often have low-attenuation components that represent necrosis, and they do not contain fat or calcifica-

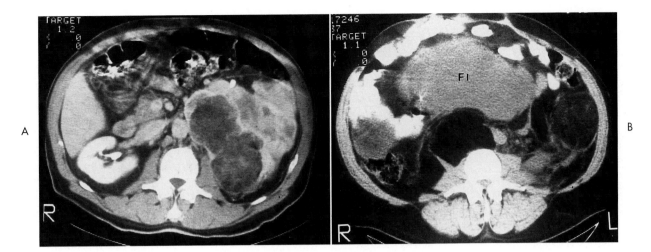

Fig. 37-28. Liposarcoma. **A,** A huge liposarcoma has heterogeneous attenuation ranging from fat to portions denser than muscle. **B,** In another patient with a liposarcoma, there is a large area of fluid attenuation *(Fl)* surrounded by fat (nondynamic enhanced scans).

tion.[138] Their appearance is never distinctive; however, their heterogeneity (as well as that of other retroperitoneal sarcomas of soft-tissue attenuation) can be contrasted with the homogeneity usually found in large lymphomatous masses. In our series, 11 of 12 large homogeneous retroperitoneal masses were lymphomas, while 20 of 26 heterogeneous soft-tissue attenuation masses were retroperitoneal sarcomas (nine of these being leiomyosarcomas).[34] Since lymphomas are often considered in the differential diagnosis of bulky retroperitoneal masses, this difference may be helpful in some instances.

Malignant fibrous histiocytomas are usually visualized on CT as heterogeneous soft-tissue attenuation masses containing areas of low attenuation, most likely representing necrosis.[168] Up to one fourth of MFHs contain dystrophic calcification, a finding that is extremely uncommon in other adult retroperitoneal masses.[113]

Neurofibrosarcomas are soft-tissue–density tumors on CT with attenuation values equal to or just below that of muscle. They are usually heterogeneous and therefore identical in appearance to leiomyosarcoma as well as some liposarcomas and malignant fibrous histiocytomas.[113] *Neuroblastomas* and *ganglioneuroblastomas* often contain calcification. They are usually seen in the pediatric population.[113]

Rhabdomyosarcomas are quite rare and are also seen in pediatric patients. They can be quite heterogeneous.[34]

Hemangiopericytomas tend to be hypervascular masses and therefore may demonstrate brisk enhancement on dynamic bolus CT,[69] a finding not seen in patients with most of the other primary retroperitoneal malignancies. One of 17 previously reported hemangiopericytomas also contained amorphous calcification.[69]

Benign neoplasms

The majority of benign lesions tend to originate from neural tissue or neural crest remnants. In a series by Lane et al, 22 of 31 benign neoplasms were paragangliomas, neurofibromas, neurilemomas, or ganglioneuromas.[113] The remaining tumors were hemangiomas, lymphangiomas, lipomas, teratomas, and a desmoid. Several other benign lesions have also been described, including retroperitoneal xanthogranuloma,[82] giant cell tumor,[77,76] sclerosing fibroma,[77,76] xanthofibroma,[77,76] and even lymphangiomyoma.[179]

About 10% of all pheochromocytomas are extra-adrenal, and most of these lie in the retroperitoneum. The most common site in which these *paragangliomas* lie is in the para-aortic region, from the level of the adrenals to the aortic bifurcation where the organ of Zuckerkandl is found. As with adrenal pheochromocytomas, paragangliomas may or may not be metabolically and clinically active. In their report of 31 tumors in 28 patients, Hayes et al found that 24 patients had hypertension (although 14 of these patients were asymptomatic).[80] However, catecholamine levels were elevated in all 18 patients who were studied.

A small minority (4 of 28 patients in the previous series) of paragangliomas are actually considered to be malignant. A diagnosis of malignancy is usually difficult for a pathologist to make. Instead, demonstration of local organ invasion or distant metastases is usually required. Paragangliomas are detected by CT as large smooth well-defined, soft-tissue masses in the immediate para-aortic region. A retroperitoneal mass not located adjacent to the aorta is unlikely to represent a paraganglioma.

Most small paragangliomas are homogeneous; however, larger lesions may undergo central necrosis and calcify. Paragangliomas are generally hypervascular and will enhance briskly on scans performed after intravenous contrast injection. As with adrenal pheochromocytomas, there is a risk of precipitating a hypertensive crisis by administering intravenous contrast media; for these reasons, unenhanced scans are preferred. Fortunately, paragangliomas are usually large enough that they are easily detected on unenhanced CT examinations.

Adrenal pheochromocytomas are identified easily with MRI by their extremely high signal intensity on T2-weighted images. Since metastatic deposits from pheochromocytomas also demonstrate this high signal intensity, it is reasonable to assume that paragangliomas would have similar characteristics.[58]

Neurogenic tumors include neurofibromas, neurilemomas (schwannomas), and ganglioneuromas. Neurofibromas contain Schwann cells and are commonly retroperitoneal in location; they are often seen in patients with neurofibromatosis.[113] Nerves generally course directly through these tumors and therefore cannot be dissected away from them. Neurilemomas are encapsulated tumors arising from peripheral nerve sheaths, usually in young to middle-aged adults.[106] They most often occur in the soft tissues of the head and neck and in the extremities. Less commonly, the retroperitoneum is involved. Nerve fibers do not traverse neurilemomas but instead are usually confined to the capsule of these tumors. Often, neurilemomas can be surgically dissected away from adjacent nerves and removed. Ganglioneuromas are essentially exclusively seen in children.

When imaged on CT, neurofibromas are seen as well-defined, sharply marginated homogeneous masses of near-water attenuation.[113] This low attenuation presumably reflects averaging of soft tissue and fat contained in neural sheath cells. These tumors are often located adjacent to the vertebral column, or deep to the psoas muscles (Fig. 37-29). Adjacent bone, particularly the neural foramena, may be smoothly eroded. Malignant degeneration may be suspected if the mass is or becomes increasingly heterogeneous, with large soft-tissue attenuation components. Neurilomomas are soft-tissue attenuation masses that usually contain prominent cystic areas (due to degeneration). They cannot be distinguished from other retroperitoneal tumors.

Lipomas are well-defined neoplasms composed of mature fat cells and bounded by a thin capsule. Except for fine septa, which may be seen traversing a lipoma, they are homogeneous and of fat density. Large lipomas may be difficult to distinguish from lipogenic liposarcomas (both for the radiologist and the pathologist).

Hemangiomas are unusual benign retroperitoneal tumors. On CT they are of soft-tissue density. Unlike many retroperitoneal masses, however, they enhance briskly when intravenous contrast material is administered. They may contain calcification.

Teratoma is one of the most radiographically characteristic tumors. These are congenital neoplasms that contain components of all three germ layers. Although the majority of patients are diagnosed before they are 6 months old, occasionally patients will not be recognized until they become adults.[42] CT often demonstrates cal-

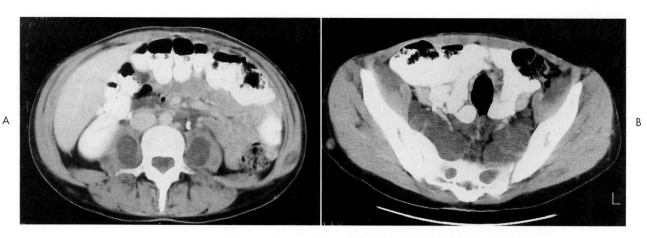

Fig. 37-29. Neurofibromas. **A,** Low-attenuation masses are identified within the psoas muscles and in the left posterolateral abdominal wall in this patient with neurofibromatosis. **B,** A more caudal scan reveals plexiform neurofibromas in the pelvis, adjacent to the sacrum, and in the subcutaneous tissues (nondynamic enhanced scans).

cification or even osseous elements. Fatty attenuation components may be visualized. A fat-fluid level, representing fat that floats on a denser layer of fluid and debris is occasionally present. A hairball may be recognized by CT as a rounded mass floating at the fat-fluid interface.[42,57] Occasionally a dermoid plug is seen as a soft-tissue mass projecting from the wall into the cyst cavity.[60] Although the incidence of malignancy is small (less than 1%), teratomas are usually removed because their continued growth can lead to complications such as rupture, infection, or torsion. Even benign teratomas may adhere to adjacent structures. Malignant degeneration is more common in postmenopausal women and usually occurs in the dermal plug. Although microscopic invasion cannot be excluded, the presence of an intact fat plane around the tumor indicates that the capsule has not been penetrated. Absence of a fat plane may be normal, particularly in an asthenic patients, or may represent local invasion or adherence.

Lymphangiomas are usually smooth, well-defined, near-water–attenuation masses discovered in young children. Retroperitoneal *xanthogranulomas* (representing either a local inflammatory reaction or a true benign neoplasm),[82] *lymphangiomyomas* (seen in a patient with lymphangioleiomyomatosis)[179] as well as other unusual benign masses have only been encountered in small numbers. No distinguishing characteristics of these masses have as yet been identified. On CT all of these lesions appear as inhomogeneous soft-tissue masses.

RETROPERITONEAL FIBROSIS

Retroperitoneal fibrosis (RPF) is a rare fibrotic process most frequently involving the caudal aspect of the retroperitoneum. On gross inspection RPF appears as a gray-white plaque of woody consistency that usually envelopes the aorta and inferior vena cava. On histologic examination, the disease is first characterized by proliferation of fibroblasts, acute inflammatory cells, and capillaries, all of which are surrounded by collagen fibers.[99] Usually, early RPF is characterized by a high fluid content. Over time, the cellular activity in the retroperitoneal plaque diminishes significantly. The collagen becomes hyalinized and much more tightly packed. Fluid content is minimal.[3] In 15% of patients, retroperitoneal fibrosis is associated with fibrotic processes elsewhere in the body (such as fibrosing mediastinitis, thyroiditis, sclerosing cholangitis, and orbital pseudotumors).[3]

In up to 70% of cases, no causative factor for retroperitoneal fibrosis can be identified. Recently, it has been postulated that the etiology of this idiopathic retroperitoneal fibrosis (most commonly seen in middle-aged to elderly men) may relate to an immune response to material that has leaked into the retroperitoneum from atherosclerotic plaques in the abdominal aorta.[20,21] The

substance suspected of eliciting such a response is an insoluble lipid called ceroid, which is frequently detected in macrophages in the aortic adventitia or in periaortic lymph nodes.

There are many known benign causes of retroperitoneal fibrosis, including medication ingestion (most commonly methysergide, but also beta blockers, methyldopa, hydralazine, antibiotics, and other analgesics), infections (particularly tuberculosis, syphilis, actinomycosis, brucellosis, and fungal infections such as histoplamosis), previous surgery or radiation treatment, abdominal aortic aneurysms, trauma, retroperitoneal hemorrhage, Marfan syndrome, and a variety of intra-abdominal inflammatory conditions (diverticulitis, appendicitis, extravasation from the urinary tract).[2,3,31,121]

In 8% to 10% of instances, malignant processes (primary neoplasms or metastatic disease) can provoke an extensive desmoplastic reaction in the retroperitoneum that cannot be distinguished from benign retroperitoneal fibrosis.

Patients often present with symptoms or signs related to compression of retroperitoneal structures. The ureters are most frequently involved. While ureteral obstruction may be clinically silent, some patients will have flank pain or tenderness. Others will develop oliguria or even anuria. Extrinsic narrowing of the inferior vena cava can cause lower extremity swelling with or without associated deep vein thrombophlebitis. Occasionally, the distal abdominal aorta can be so severely compressed that patients may develop vascular insufficiency (to the lower extremities, bowel, or kidneys).[3] In some instances symptoms and signs are vague, consisting of diffuse abdominal or back pain, fatigue, and weight loss.

Laboratory studies usually demonstrate significant elevation of the erythrocyte sedimentation rate. Nearly three fourths of all patients will have elevated blood urea nitrogen and creatinine levels.[3,121,180]

Diagnosis cannot be definitely made by any imaging study and is nearly always made at surgery. While CT-guided percutaneous biopsy is often technically feasible, a biopsy that does not detect malignant cells is not conclusive. Tumor cells in patients with the malignant form of RPF may be sparse in relation to the extensive surrounding inflammation and therefore may not be sampled when fine-needle aspiration or even core biopsies are performed.

Treatment for benign RPF consists of ureterolysis and/or steroids. Frequently, the ureters are wrapped in omentum and/or moved laterally over the psoas muscles or into the peritoneal cavity in the hope that, should response to steroids be limited or should the process recur, the ureters would be protected from further involvement.[43] In cases of perianeurysmal fibrosis, definitive treatment is aortic aneurysm repair. Treatment of the malignant type of RPF is palliative, consisting of urinary diversion for those patients with ureteral obstruction and appropriate chemotherapy or radiation therapy.

Prognosis in patients with benign RPF is excellent, while that for patients with malignant RPF is usually poor. Most patients with malignant RPF survive for only 3 to 6 months after diagnosis.[9,65,181]

Imaging of RPF

Since most patients with RPF have some degree of renal compromise, imaging evaluation is usually performed with unenhanced CT or MRI. In some patients with normal renal function, however, excretory urography (EU) will be obtained initially. It has been generally believed that RPF may be suspected on EU or retrograde pyelography when the mid to distal ureters are deviated medial to the lumbar vertebral pedicles. Unfortunately, medial deviation of the ureters can be seen in up to 18% of normal patients[171] and can also be caused by hypertrophy of the psoas muscles. Several studies have also failed to detect any difference in the position of the ureters in patients with RPF when compared with normal patients.[8,171] Most likely, RPF encases the ureters wherever they are located. The characteristic feature of RPF

on EU therefore tends to be its ability to grow in the retroperitoneum *without* displacing the ureters laterally.

The CT appearance of RPF ranges from minimal periureteral stranding to large lobulated masses obliterating the fat planes between the aorta and cava, indistinguishable from bulky lymphadenopathy (Fig. 37-30).[40,53,55,112] Often RPF also cannot be distinguished on CT from primary retroperitoneal neoplasms; however, several patterns have been identified to suggest RPF as the most likely diagnosis in some instances. RPF tends to be located at the level of the L4 vertebra[19] and also tends to be plaque-like and infiltrating rather than nodular.[55] The fibrotic mass of RPF may enhance with intravenous contrast.[39,40] RPF usually surrounds (rather than displaces) the anterior and lateral aspects of the great vessels (Fig. 37-31), although recently, two cases of benign RPF anteriorly displacing the aorta to a moderate extent have been reported.[18]

Other diseases that can have a CT appearance similar to that of RPF include lymphoma, or infection; primary retroperitoneal neoplasms; amyloidosis; and hemorrhage.[3,159] Occasionally, some of these processes will demonstrate features suggesting a specific diagnosis. Lymphadenopathy from lymphoma is often centered

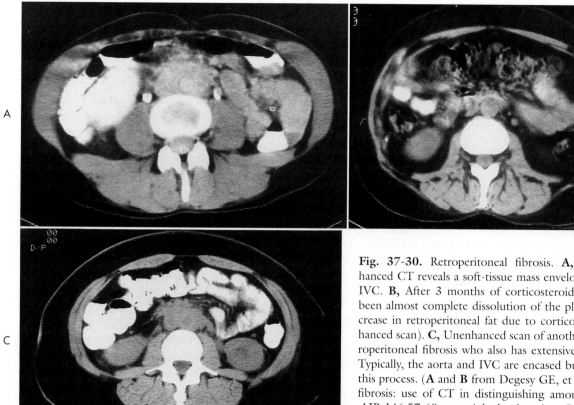

Fig. 37-30. Retroperitoneal fibrosis. **A,** Nondynamic enhanced CT reveals a soft-tissue mass enveloping the aorta and IVC. **B,** After 3 months of corticosteroid therapy there has been almost complete dissolution of the plaque. Note the increase in retroperitoneal fat due to corticosteroid use (unenhanced scan). **C,** Unenhanced scan of another patient with retroperitoneal fibrosis who also has extensive periaortic plaque. Typically, the aorta and IVC are encased but not displaced by this process. (**A** and **B** from Degesy GE, et al: Retroperitoneal fibrosis: use of CT in distinguishing among possible causes. *AJR* 146:57-60, copyright by American Roentgen Ray Society, 1986.)

more cephalad in the retroperitoneum and may be bulkiest at the level of the renal hila. Other primary and metastatic neoplasms usually displace the aorta and inferior vena cava as well as the ureters. Malignancies and infectious processes may invade and destroy adjacent bones or organs. Acute hemorrhage often has high attenuation on unenhanced scans; it also infiltrates between the fascial planes in a characteristic fashion.

CT can be used to follow patients after surgery and/or corticosteroid therapy. In one report, postsurgical steroids resulted in significant clinical improvement and in reduction in retroperitoneal masses on CT in two patients.[165] Figures 37-30, *A*, and 37-30, *B* illustrate a patient who experienced resolution of a large retroperitoneal inflammatory mass as a result of steroids.

MRI, offering several important advantages over CT, may represent the study of choice for evaluating patients with suspected RPF. First, the relationship of the mass to the great vessels is easily visualized on MRI. While mass and vessels can have identical attenuation values on unenhanced CT, flow-void in vessels on MRI allows for their identification on standard spin-echo sequences even when they are surrounded by extensive RPF. Second, MRI can image patients in coronal and saggital planes, again facilitating evaluation of the relationship of the RPF to the retroperitoneal vasculature. Also, at least in some instances, MRI may be able to identify patients with RPF by detecting low T2 signal intensity. Since mature fibrosis contains much collagen and little cellularity and fluid, it is not surprising that longstanding RPF is usually of low-signal intensity on T2-weighted images.* Acute benign RPF with its greater

*References 2, 3, 9, 120, 148, 202.

cellularity and fluid content will have intermediate or high signal intensities on T2-weighted sequences.[3,148]

Arrive and co-workers found that all cases of nonmalignant and malignant RPF could be differentiated on T2-weighted images, however, because the latter had heterogeneous signal intensities, while the former always had homogeneous intensities.[9] They also found that the T2-signal intensities were significantly higher in the malignant group, possibly at least partially because of their failure to include many (or even any) patients with "acute" nonmalignant RPF.

A specific diagnosis of benign RPF can probably be offered for any patient who has a retroperitoneal mass that is of low signal on both T1- and T2-weighted images. High or intermediate signal on either T1- or T2-weighted images is not specific.

MRI can be used to follow patients with RPF who are undergoing treatment. While in a few cases signal intensity has diminished over time (suggesting plaque maturation), in the majority of patients no intensity change has been detected.[202]

ILIOPSOAS

Anatomy

The psoas major muscles arise from the anterior and inferior surfaces of the transverse processes of T12 and L1 to L5, as well as from the adjacent vertebral bodies and intervertebral disks. They course inferiorly and fuse with the iliacus muscles before traversing under the inguinal ligament to insert onto the lesser trochanter of the femurs.[49,139] These bulky muscles are responsible for flexion of the thigh.

The psoas minor muscles, absent in 40% to 70% of individuals,[49,147] originate from the lateral aspects of T12 and L1 and travel caudad to insert onto the pecti-

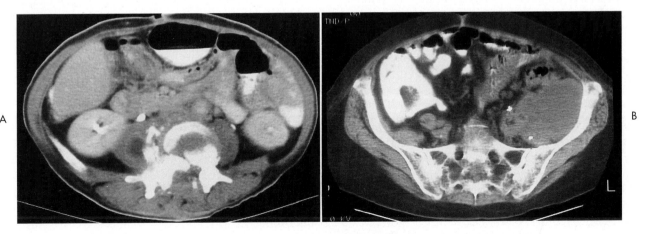

Fig. 37-31. Iliopsoas abscesses. **A,** Low-attenuation mass within the right psoas muscle represented purulent material at surgery (nondynamic enhanced scan). **B,** A large iliopsoas abscess on the left was successfully managed by percutaneous drainage (enhanced scan).

nal eminence of the ipsilateral iliac bone just anterior to the psoas major.

On CT and MRI, the psoas major muscles are visualized, lying immediately lateral to the lumber vertebra. Usually, the lateral aspect of the muscles is well defined by adjacent retroperitoneal fat; in children or cachectic adults, however, it may be obliterated by adjacent abdominal organs. The psoas major muscle reaches its largest cross-sectional size at the L3-L4 level. Subsequently, it thins as it fuses with the iliacus. The iliopsoas continues caudally into the thigh and is easily visualized throughout its course. The muscle is characterized by homogeneous attenuation, but a small linear zone of decreased density, representing fat surrounding branches of the lumbar plexus, may be identified within the lateral aspect of the muscle. The psoas minor muscles may occasionally be identified as small soft-tissue masses immediately anterior to the psoas major and, when observed, should not be confused with lymph nodes or retroperitoneal vessels. Often, the psoas minor muscles are contiguous with the anterior aspects of the psoas major and therefore are not distinguishable as discrete, separate structures.

Pathologic conditions

Abnormalities of the iliopsoas muscles usually result in asymmetric enlargement; however, some patients with neuromuscular disorders may demonstrate atrophy of the iliopsoas muscles on the affected side. Pathologic processes may diffusely infiltrate the iliopsoas and involve the entire length of the muscle from the diaphragm to the thigh. Common causes of iliopsoas pathologic disease include inflammation, neoplasm, and hematoma. Although clinical history, physical examination, laboratory tests, and CT or MRI findings often suggest the etiology of iliopsoas disease, in up to 20% of patients CT- or MRI-detected iliopsoas masses remained uncharacterized before percutaneous biopsy or surgery.[56] It is generally believed that in most instances MRI usually does not offer any significant advantage over CT in assessment of patients with iliopsoas disease.

Inflammatory processes

Inflammatory processes of the iliopsoas muscles account for 36% to 54% of CT or MRI detected psoas masses, according to two reports.[56,139] Patients frequently have abdominal or pelvic pain and fever, although symptoms may be absent. In the overwhelming majority of cases reported, abscesses developed from spread of adjacent infection of the kidneys, aortic bed, spine, pancreas, or bowel. Occasionally, iliopsoas abscesses are complications of abdominal surgery. Only rarely are these infections thought to originate in the iliopsoas muscles themselves (3 of 38 cases reported in the previously cited series).[56,139] Pyogenic infections are most frequent. The incidence of tuberculous spondylitis has dropped significantly over the past few decades.[44,56,162]

On CT, iliopsoas inflammatory masses display a variety of appearances, ranging from diffuse homogeneous enlargement of the psoas to discrete masses containing areas of low attenuation (Fig. 37-31). Punctate collections of gas are seen in a minority of patients and are thought to be specific indicators of infection; however, these have been observed also in a patient with a psoas metastasis.[56,98,162,199] Calcifications are detected occasionally on CT in inflammatory masses, particularly in patients with tuberculosis.[56] Adjacent destruction of lumbar vertebrae can be seen in patients whose iliopsoas disease represents spread from tuberculosis or pyogenic spondylitis. On MRI, inflammatory masses have increased signal on T2-weighted scans. Percutaneous aspiration of these masses yields grossly purulent fluid in some instances, but only solid tissue in others. Unfortunately, the CT and MRI appearance of iliopsoas phlegmon and iliopsoas abscess can be identical.[162,199]

CT or MRI evaluation of patients with iliopsoas infections must include thorough scrutiny of surrounding abdominal organs for possible associated inflammatory changes. Also, CT may be used to guide the percutaneous aspiration and placement of percutaneous abscess drainage catheters for definitive treatment of iliopsoas abscess, thus obviating the need for surgery.[147] It must be remembered, however, that the underlying cause of the infection (e.g., renal disease, pancreatitis) must be adequately treated to ensure successful management of the iliopsoas disease.

Neoplasms

Neoplasms involving the iliopsoas represent between one fourth and one third of CT-detected iliopsoas masses.[56,139] Metastatic lymph nodes in patients with non-Hodgkin's lymphomas, pelvic tumors, testicular cancer, renal malignancies, and malignant melanoma have all been noted to result in apparent iliopsoas enlargement and invasion. Similarly, primary retroperitoneal tumors, including liposarcomas, fibrosarcomas, and neurogenic neoplasms can involve the iliopsoas muscle also. Theoretically, neoplasms tend to invade rather than respect fascial planes; this results in large localized masses distorting only portions of the iliopsoas while spreading out to destroy adjacent bones and soft tissues. Yet, despite this apparent difference in growth pattern, specific identification of an iliopsoas mass as neoplastic remains impossible. As with abscesses, tumors may have enhancing rims and low-density centers[199] and occasionally may diffusely infiltrate large portions of the iliopsoas (Fig. 37-32). Only when fat is detected within a large iliopsoas

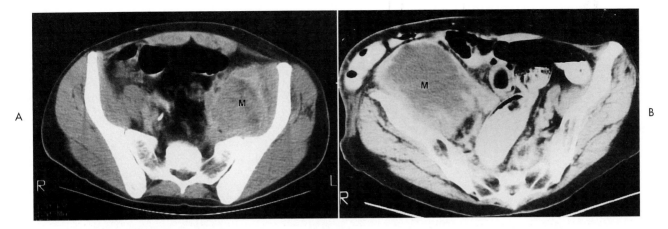

Fig. 37-32. Malignant masses involving the iliopsoas muscles. **A,** Primary retroperitoneal sarcoma results in a heterogeneous left iliopsoas mass *(M)*. **B,** Colon cancer metastasis *(M)* to right iliopsoas muscle. This mass would be difficult to distinguish from an abscess or hematoma (nondynamic enhanced scans).

mass can CT or MRI suggest the presence of a lipoma, liposarcoma, or teratoma. Otherwise, definitive diagnosis of an iliopsoas neoplasm can be made only by CT-guided needle biopsy or surgery.

Hemorrhage

Hemorrhage in and around the iliopsoas muscles is seen almost exclusively in patients with predisposing conditions. Iliopsoas hematomas have been described in patients with hemophilia, von Willebrand's disease, thrombocytopenia, leaking abdominal aortic aneurysms or grafts, traumatic injuries, and after femoral arteriography, as well as in patients receiving anticoagulants.[56,90,139] If the bleeding is relatively acute, CT can identify high-attenuation collections within enlarged iliopsoas muscles (Fig. 37-33). Fluid-fluid levels corresponding to layering of retracting high-attenuation clot under lower density blood components may be present. As in infectious processes, hematomas tend to spread between and not through fascial planes, and thus may expand along the entire length of the iliopsoas compartment. Bone destruction is not present. The hematoma will become progressively less dense with age, so that after several days it can have an identical appearance to an inflammatory or neoplastic mass. Old hematomas may undergo liquification and develop a central density near water. Superinfection is rarely a problem. Although percutaneous biopsy is sometimes helpful in excluding other diagnoses, clinical history and CT findings allow for appropriate identification of most patients with iliopsoas hematomas. In acute stages, hematomas may have a varied appearance on MRI; however, when subacute, iliopsoas hematomas will have high signal on T1-weighted images and lower signal on T2-weighted images.

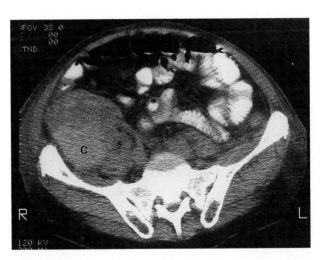

Fig. 37-33. Unenhanced CT of a spontaneous psoas hematoma in a patient receiving anticoagulants. Note the higher attenuation retracting clot *(C)* layering dependently.

Other iliopsoas masses

Cases of patients with incidentally discovered atherosclerotic aortic aneurysms and lumbar artery pseudoaneurysms masquerading as iliopsoas masses have been reported.[88,193] An atherosclerotic aneurysm might be expected in a patient with extensive atherosclerotic changes elsewhere in the abdomen. Pseudoaneurysms result from trauma or surgery, and many patients have a pulsatile mass and a bruit (Fig. 37-34). It is obviously important to identify the entire course of the aorta and iliac vessels in such patients. A bolus injection of contrast material, followed by dynamic sequential imaging, may demonstrate the abnormal vessel surrounded by

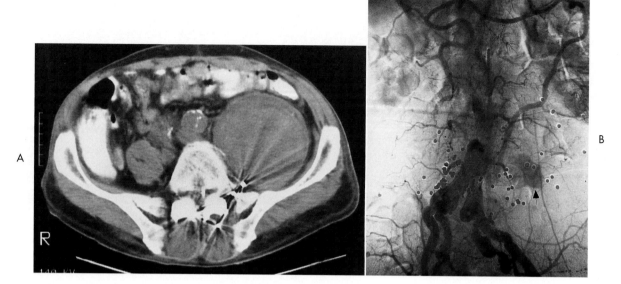

Fig. 37-34. Lumbar artery pseudoaneurysm. **A,** A large left iliopsoas mass is noted in this patient who had received a gunshot wound years previously (unenhanced scan). **B,** An arteriogram demonstrates contrast material pooling in the center of the pseudoaneurysm *(arrow).*

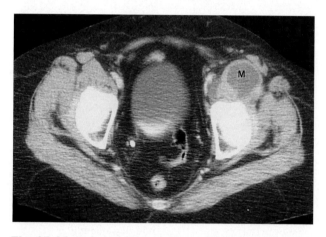

Fig. 37-35. Enlarged iliopsoas bursa. An asymptomatic low-attenuation groin mass *(M)* on this nondynamically enhanced CT of a patient with rheumatoid arthritis represents an unusually prominent iliopsoas bursa.

thrombus in the region of the psoas muscle. The presence of an aneurysm or pseudoaneurysm should be excluded before biopsy in patients with either a history or CT findings that suggest that these vascular abnormalities could be present.

Occasionally, the iliopsoas bursa may become distended with fluid, resulting in the appearance of a painless bulging mass, usually in the inguinal region. Enlarged iliopsoas bursae have been most commonly described in patients with rheumatoid arthritis or osteoar-

thritis. These small masses are of fluid attenuation on CT. While rounded or ovoid, they often contain a slight invagination toward the hip joint (Fig. 37-35). Communication with the hip-joint space, however, is only seen in some (15%) cases when arthrography is performed. Enlargement of the iliopsoas bursa should be included in the differential diagnosis of any groin mass.[38]

REFERENCES

1. Aisen AM, et al: Distribution of abdominal and pelvic Hodgkin disease: implications for CT scanning. *J Comput Assist Tomogr* 9(3):463-465, 1985.
2. Amis ES: Retroperitoneal fibrosis. *Urol Radiol* 12:135-137, 1990.
3. Amis ES: Retroperitoneal fibrosis. *AJR* 157:321-329, 1991.
4. Amparo EG et al: Magnetic resonance imaging of aortic disease: preliminary results. *AJR* 143:1203-1209, 1984.
5. Amparo EG et al: Aortic dissection: magnetic resonance imaging. *Radiology* 155:399-406, 1985.
6. Anagnostopolous CE, Prabhakar MJ, Kittle, CF: Aortic dissections and dissecting aneurysms. *Am J Cardiol* 30:263-273, 1972.
7. Anderson PE Jr, Lorntzen JE: Comparison of computed tomography and aortography in abdominal aortic aneurysms. *J Comput Assist Tomogr* 7(4):670-673, 1983.
8. Arger PH, Stolz JL, Miller WT: Retroperitoneal fibrosis: an analysis of the clinical spectrum and roentgenographic signs. *AJR* 119:812-821, 1973.
9. Arrive L, et al: Malignant versus nonmalignant retroperitoneal fibrosis: differentiation with MR imaging. *Radiology* 172:139-143, 1989.
10. Arrive L, et al: Diagnosis of abdominal venous thrombosis by means of spin-echo and gradient echo MR imaging: analysis with receiver operating characteristic curves. *Radiology* 181:661-668, 1991.

11. Auffermann W, et al: MR imaging of complications of aortic surgery. *J Comput Assist Tomogr* 11(6):982-989, 1987.

12. Aufferman W, et al: Incorporation versus infection of retroperitoneal aortic gradts: MR imaging features. *Radiology* 172:359-362, 1989.

13. Bach DB, Vellet AD: Retroperitoneal sarcoidosis. *AJR* 156:520-522, 1991.

14. Belville JS, et al: Spontaneous perinephric and subcapsular renal hemorrhage: evaluation with CT, US, and angiography. *Radiology* 172:733-738, 1989.

15. Bragg DG, Colby TV, Ward JH: New concepts in the non-Hodgkin lymphomas: radiology implications. *Radiology* 159:289-304, 1986.

16. Brener BJ, et al: Major venous anomalies complicating abdominal aortic surgery. *Arch Surg* 108:159-165, 1974.

17. Britt AR, et al: Sarcoidosis: abdominal manifestations at CT. *Radiology* 178:91-94, 1991.

18. Brooks AP, Reznek RH, Webb JAW: Aortic displacement on computed tomography of idiopathic retroperitoneal fibrosis. *Clin Radiol* 40:51-52, 1989.

19. Brun B, et al: CT in retroperitoneal fibrosis. *AJR* 137:535-538, 1981.

20. Buff DD, Bogin MB, Faltz LL: Retroperitoneal fibrosis: a report of selected cases and a review of the literature. *NY State J Med* 89:511-516, 1989.

21. Bullock N: Idiopathic retroperitoneal fibrosis. *Br Med J* 297:240-241, 1988.

22. Burgener FA, Hamlin DJ: Histiocytic lymphoma of the abdomen: radiographic spectrum. *AJR* 137:337-342, 1981.

23. Buss RW, et al: Emergency operation in patients with symptomatic abdominal aortic aneurysms. *Am J Surg* 156:470-473, 1988.

24. Cancer patient survival experience, Bethesda, Md., US Dept of Health and Human Services, NIH Publication No 80-2148, 1980.

25. Castellino RA, Marglin S, Blank N: Hodgkin disease, the non-Hodgkin lymphomas and the leukemias in the retroperitoneum. *Semin Roentgenol* 15:288-301, 1980.

26. Castellino RA, et al: Computed tomography, lymphography, and staging laparotomy: correlations in initial staging of Hodgkin disease. *AJR* 143:37-41, 1984.

27. Casatellino RA: Hodgkin disease: practical concepts for the diagnostic radiologist. *Radiology* 159:305-310, 1986.

28. Castellino RA: Lymph nodes of the posterior iliac crest: CT and lymphographic observations. *Radiology* 175:687-689, 1990.

29. Chagnon S, et al: Pelvic cancers: staging of 139 cases with lymphography and fine-needle aspiration biopsy. *Radiology* 173:103-106, 1989.

30. Cheng J, Castellino RA: Post-treatment calcification of mesenteric non-Hodgkin lymphoma: CT findings. *J Comput Assist Tomogr* 13(1):64-66, 1989.

31. Chong WK, Al-Kutoubi MA: Retroperitoneal fibrosis in Marfan's syndrome. *Clin Radiol* 44:386-388, 1991.

32. Churchill RJ, et al: Computed tomographic demonstration of anomalous inferior vena cava with azygos continuation. *J Comput Assist Tomogr* 4(3):398-402, 1980.

33. Cisternino SJ, Neiman HL, Malave SR, Jr: Diagnosis of retroperitoneal hemorrhage by serial computed tomography. *J Comput Assist Tomogr* 3(5):686-688, 1979.

34. Cohan RH, et al: Computed tomography of primary retroperitoneal malignancies. *J Comput Assist Tomogr* 12(5):804-810, 1988.

35. Cohan RH: Computed tomography of the abdominal aorta. *Contemp Diag Radiol* 13(19):1-6, 1990.

36. Cohen JM, Weinreb JC, Maravilla KR: Fluid collections in the intraperitoneal and extraperitoneal spaces: comparison of MR and CT. *Radiology* 155:705-708, 1985.

37. Cohen MI, et al: Accessory hemiazygos continuation of left inferior vena cava: CT demonstration. *J Comput Assist Tomogr* 8(4):777-779, 1984.

38. Constant O, Mitchell RA: Case of the monthe: an unusual inguinal swelling. *Br J Radiol* 60:1139-1140, 1987.

39. Cullenward MJ, et al: Inflammatory aortic aneurysms (periaortic fibrosis): radiologic imaging. *Radiology* 159:75-82, 1986.

40. Dalla-Palma L, et al: Computed tomography in the diagnosis of retroperitoneal fibrosis. *Urol Radiol* 3:77-83, 1981.

41. Daugherty SH, Simmons RL: Infection in bionic man. II. The pathobiology of infections in prosthetic devices. *Curr Prob Surg* 19:281-287, 1982.

42. Davidson AJ, Hartman DS, Goldman SM: Mature teratoma of the retroperitoneum: radiologic, pathologic, and clinical correlation. *Radiology* 172:421-425, 1989.

43. Degesys GE, et al: Retroperitoneal fibrosis: use of CT in distinguishing among possible causes. *AJR* 146:57-60, 1986.

44. Donovan PJ, Zerhourni EA, Siegelman SS: CT of the psoas compartment of the retroperitoneum. *Semin Roentgenol* 16(4):241-250, 1981.

45. Dooms GC, et al: Magnetic resonance imaging of the lymph nodes: comparison with CT. *Radiology* 153:719-728, 1984.

46. Dooms GC, et al: Characterization of lymphadenopathy by magnetic resonance relaxation times: preliminary results. *Radiology* 155:691-697, 1985.

47. Dorfman RE, et al: Upper abdominal lymph nodes: criteria for normal size determined by CT. *Radiology* 180:319-322, 1991.

48. Dudiak CM, Olson MC, Posniak HV: CT evaluation of congenital and acquired abnormalities of the azygos system. *Radiographics* 11:233-246, 1991.

49. Dunnick NR, Javadpour N: Value of CT and lymphography: distinguishing retroperitoneal metastases from nonseminomatous testicular tumors. *AJR* 136:1093-1099, 1981.

50. Einstein DM, et al: Abdominal lymphadenopathy: spectrum of CT findings. *Radiographics* 11:457-572, 1991.

51. Ellis JH, et al: Comparison of NMR and CT imaging in the evaluation of metastatic retroperitoneal lymphadenopathy from testicular carcinoma. *J Comput Assist Tomogr* 8(4):709-719, 1984.

52. Evancho AM, Osbakken M, Weidner W: Comparison of NMR imaging and aortography for preoperative evaluation of abdominal aortic aneurysm. *Magn Reson Med* 2:41-55, 1985.

53. Fagan CJ, Larrieu AJ, Amparo EG: Retroperitoneal fibrosis: ultrasound and CT features. *AJR* 133:239-243, 1979.

54. Fagelman D, et al: Inferior vena cava pseudothrombus in computed tomography using a contrast medium power injector: a potential pitfall. *J Comput Assist Tomogr* 11(6):1042-1043, 1987.

55. Feinstein RS, et al: Computed tomography in the diagnosis of retroperitoneal fibrosis. *J Urol* 126:255-259, 1981.

56. Feldberg MAM, Koehler PR, van Waes PFGM: Psoas compartment disease studied by computed tomography. *Radiology* 148:505-512, 1983.

57. Feldberg MAM, van Waes PFGM, Hendriks MJ: Direct multiplanar CT findings in cystic teratoma of the ovary. *J Comput Assist Tomogr* 8(6):1131-1135, 1984.

58. Fink IJ, et al: MR imaging of pheochromocytomas. *J Comput Assist Tomogr* 9(3):454-458, 1985.

59. Flak B, et al: Magnetic resonance imaging of aneurysms of the abdominal aorta. *AJR* 144:991-996, 1985.

60. Friedman AC, et al: Computed tomography of abdominal fatty masses. *Radiology* 139:415-429, 1981.

61. Friedman AC, et al: CT of benign cystic teratomas. *AJR* 138:659-665, 1982.

62. Garb M: The CT appearances of ruptured abdominal aortic aneurysms. *Australas Radiol* 33:154-156, 1989.

63. Gatewood OMB, et al: Renal vein thrombosis in patients with nephrotic syndrome: CT diagnosis. *Radiology* 159:117-122, 1986.

64. Gehl HB, Bohndorf K, Klose KC: Inferior vena cava tumor thrombus: demonstration by Gd-DTPA enhanced MR. *J Comput Assist Tomogr* 14(3):479-481, 1990.

65. Geller SA, Lin CS: Ureteral obstruction from metastatic breast carcinoma. *Arch Pathol* 99:476-478, 1975.

66. Glynn TP, Kreipke DL, Irons JM: Amyloidosis: diffuse involvement of the retroperitoneum. *Radiology* 170:726, 1989.

67. Godwin JD, Breiman RS, Speckman JM: Problems and pitfalls in the evaluation of thoracic dissection by computed tomography. *J Comput Assist Tomogr* 6(4):750-756, 1982.

68. Godwin JD, Korobkin M: Acute disease of the aorta: diagnosis by computed tomography and ultrasonography. *Radiol Clin North Am* 21(3):551-554, 1983.

69. Goldman SM, Davidson AJ, Neal J: Retroperitoneal and pelvic hemangiopericytomas: clinical, radiologic, and pathologic correlation. *Radiology* 168:13-17, 1988.

70. Golimbu M, et al: CAT scanning in staging of prostate cancer. *Urology* 28:305-308, 1981.

71. Gomes MN, Choyke PL: Improved identification of renal arteries in patients with aortic aneurysms by means of high resolution computed tomography. *J Vasc Surg* 6:262-268, 1987.

72. Gore I, Hirst AE, Jr: Atherosclerotic aneurysms of the abdominal aorta: a review. *Prog Cardiovasc Dis* 16:113-150, 1973.

73. Greatorex RA, et al: Limitations of computed tomography in leaking abdominal aortic aneurysms. *Br Med J* 297:284-285, 1988.

74. Guirguis EM, Barber GG: The natural history of abdominal aortic aneurysms. *Am J Surg* 162:481-483, 1991.

75. Haaga JR, et al: CT detection of infected synthetic grafts: preliminary report of a new sign. *AJR* 131:317-320, 1978.

76. Hadju SI, Hadju EO: *Cytopathology of sarcomas and other non-epithelial malignant tumors*, Philadelphia, 1976, WB Saunders Co.

77. Hadju SI: *Pathology of soft tissue tumors*, Philadelphia, 1979, Lea & Febiger.

78. Harell GS, et al: Computed tomography of the abdomen and the malignant lymphomas. *Radiol Clin North Am* 15:391-400, 1977.

79. Hartman DS: Retroperitoneal tumors and lymphadenopathy. *Urol Radiol* 12:131-134, 1990.

80. Hayes WS, et al: Extraadrenal retroperitoneal paraganglioma: clinical, pathologic, and CT findings. *AJR* 155:1247-1250, 1990.

81. Heiberg E, et al: CT characteristics of aortic atherosclerotic aneurysm versus aortic dissection. *J Comput Assist Tomogr* 9(1):78-83, 1985.

82. Hennessy OF, et al: Retroperitoneal xanthogranuloma: report of two cases with a review of the literature. *Australas Radiol* 34:347-349, 1990.

83. Herts BR, et al: High attenuation lymphadenopathy in AIDS patients: significance of findings at CT. *Radiology* 185:777-781, 1992.

84. Hilton S, et al: Computed tomography of the post-operative abdominal aorta. *Radiology* 145:403-407, 1982.

85. Hirst AE, Johns VJ, Kime SW, Jr: Dissection aneurysms of the aorta: a review of 505 cases. *Medicine* 37:217-219, 1958.

86. Hoppe RT: The contemporary management of Hodgkin disease. *Radiology* 169:297-304, 1988.

87. Hopper KD, Sherman JL, Ghaed N: Aortic rupture into the retroperitoneum. *AJR* 145:435-437, 1985.

88. Hulnick DH, et al: Lumbar artery pseudoaneurysm: CT demonstration. *J Comput Assist Tomogr* 8(3):570-572, 1984.

89. Hulnick DH, et al: Abdominal tuberculosis: CT evaluation. *Radiology* 157:199-204, 1985.

90. Illescas FF, et al: CT evaluation of retroperitoneal hemorrhage associated with femoral arteriography. *AJR* 146:1289-1292, 1986.

91. Jacoby WT, et al: Ovarian vein thrombosis in oncology patients: CT detection and clinical significance. *AJR* 155:291-294, 1990.

92. Jain KA, Jeffrey RB: Gonadal vein thrombosis in patients with acute gastrointestinal inflammation: diagnosis with CT. *Radiology* 180:111-113, 1991.

93. Jasinski RW, Yang CF, Rubin JM: Vena cava anomalies simulating adenopathy on computed tomography. *J Comput Assist Tomogr* 5(6):921-924, 1981.

94. Jeffrey RB, Federle MP: The collapsed inferior vena cava: CT evidence of hypovolemia. *AJR* 150:431-432, 1988.

95. Jing BS, Wallace S, Zornoza J: Metastases to retroperitoneal and pelvic lymph nodes: computed tomography and lymphangiography. *Radiol Clin North Am* 20(3):511-530, 1982.

96. Johansen K, et al: Ruptured abdominal aortic aneurysm: the Harborview experience. *J Vasc Surg* 13:240-247, 1991.

97. Johnson CD, et al: Renal adenocarcinoma: current generation CT staging. *AJR* 148:59-63, 1987.

98. Jones B, et al: Psoas abscess: fact and mimicry. *Urol Radiol* 2:73-79, 1980.

99. Jones JH, et al: Retroperitoneal fibrosis. *Am J Med* 48:203-208, 1970.

100. Joseph N, et al: Computed tomography of retroperitoneal Castleman disease (plasma cell type) with sonographic and angiographic correlation. *J Comput Assist Tomogr* 9(3):570-572, 1985.

101. Justich E, et al: Infected aortoiliofemoral grafts: magnetic resonance imaging. *Radiology* 154:133-136, 1985.

102. Kam J, Patel S, Ward RE: Computed tomography of aortic and aortoiliofemoral grafts. *J Comput Assist Tomogr* 6(2):298-302, 1982.

103. Katz BH, Black RA, Colley DP: CT-guided fine needle aspiration of a periaortic collection. *J Vasc Surg* 5:762-764, 1987.

104. Kazam E, Whalen J: Anatomy. In Margulis AR, Burhenne JH, editors: *Alimentary tract radiology*, vol 3, St. Louis, 1979, Mosby–Year Book.

105. Kazerooni EA, Bree RL, Williams DM: Penetrating atherosclerotic ulcers of the descending thoracic aorta: evaluation with CT and distinction from aortic dissection. *Radiology* 183:759-765, 1992.

106. Kim SH, et al: Retroperitoneal neurilemoma: CT and MR findings. *AJR* 159:1023-1026, 1992.

107. Korobkin M: Computed tomography of retroperitoneal vasculature and lymph nodes. *Semin Roentgenol* 16(4):251-267, 1981.

108. Korobkin M, et al: CT of the extraperitoneal space: normal anatomy and fluid collections. *AJR* 159:933-941, 1992.

109. Kumar D, Kumar S: Circumaortic left renal vein. *J Comput Assist Tomogr* 5(6):914-916, 1981.

110. Kunin M: Bridging septa of the perinephric space: anatomic, pathologic, and diagnostic considerations. *Radiology* 158:361-365, 1986.

111. Kvilekval KHV, et al: The value of computed tomography in the management of symptomatic abdominal aortic aneurysms. *J Vasc Surg* 12:28-33, 1990.

112. Lalli AF: Retroperitoneal fibrosis and inapparent obstructive uropathy. *Radiology* 122:339-342, 1977.

113. Lane RH, Stephens DH, Reiman HM: Primary retroperitoneal neoplasms: CT findings in 90 cases with clinical and pathologic correlation. *AJR* 152:83-89, 1989.

114. Lang EK: The use of imaging modalities in staging of carcinoma of the prostate and bladder. In Lang EK, editor: *Current concepts of uroradiology,* Baltimore, 1984, Williams & Wilkins.

115. LaRoy LL, et al: Imaging of abdominal aortic aneurysms. *AJR* 152:785-792, 1989.

116. Lautin EM, et al: CT diagnosis of cirumcaval ureter. *AJR* 150:591-594, 1988.

117. Lautin EM, et al: Calcification in non-Hodgkin lymphoma occurring before therapy: identification on plain films and CT. *AJR* 155:739-740, 1990.

118. Lee JKT, et al: Magnetic resonance imaging of abdominal and pelvic lymphadenopathy. *Radiology* 153:181-188, 1984.

119. Lee JKT, et al: Magnetic resonance imaging of abdominal aortic aneurysms. *AJR* 143:1197-1202, 1984.

120. Lee JKT, Glazer HS: Controversy in the MR imaging appearance of fibrosis. *Radiology* 177:21-22, 1990.

121. Lepor H, Walsh PC: Idiopathic retroperitoneal fibrosis. *J Urol* 122:1-6, 1979.

122. Lewis E, et al: Post-therapy CT-detected mass in lymphoma patients: is it viable tissue? *J Comput Assist Tomogr* 6(4):792-795, 1982.

123. Liebman CE, et al: MR imaging of inferior vena cava filters: safety and artifacts. *AJR* 150:1174-1176, 1988.

124. Lien HH, et al: Comparison of computed tomography, lymphography, and phlebography in 200 consecutive patients with regard to retroperitoneal metastases from testicular tumor. *Radiology* 146:129-132, 1983.

125. Limet R, Sakalihassan N, Adelin A: Determination of the expansion rate and incidence of ruptures or abdominal aortic aneurysms. *J Vasc Surg* 14:540-548, 1991.

126. Love L, Demos TC, Posniak H: CT of retrorenal fluid collections. *AJR* 145:87-91, 1985.

127. Love L: Radiolog anatomy of the retroperitoneum in general abdominal, pelvic, and genitourinary radiology. In Tavaras JM, Ferrucci JR, editors: *Radiology: diagnosis-imaging-intervention,* vol 4, Philadelphia, 1986, JB Lippincott Co.

128. Low RN, et al: Aortoenteric fistula with perigraft infection: evaluation with CT. *Radiology* 175:157-162, 1990.

129. Lubat E, et al: Extrapulmonary pneumocystis carinii infection in AIDS: CT findings. *Radiology* 174:157-160, 1990.

130. Lupetin AR, Beckman I, Daffner RH: CT diagnosis of traumatic abdominal aortic rupture. *J Comput Assist Tomogr* 14(2):313-314, 1990.

131. Machida K, Tasaka A: CT patterns of mural thrombus in aortic aneurysms. *J Comput Assist Tomogr* 4(6):840-842, 1980.

132. Magnusson A, et al: Contrast enhancement of pathologic lymph nodes demonstrated by computed tomography. *Acta Radiol* 30:307-310, 1989.

133. Mansfield CM, et al: Comparison of lymphangiography and computed tomography scanning in evaluating abdominal disease in stages III and IV Hodgkin's disease. *Radiology* 170:159-164, 1989.

134. Mantello MT, et al: Impending rupture of nonaneurysmal bacterial aortitis: CT diagnosis. *J Comput Assist Tomogr* 14(6):950-953, 1990.

135. Marglin SI, Castellino RA: Selection of an imaging modality for staging abdominal involvement in malignant lymphomas: lymphography or computed tomography. In Bennet JM, editor: *Controversies in the management of lymphomas,* Boston, 1983, Martinus Nijhoff.

136. Mark A, et al: CT evaluation of complications of abdominal aortic surgery. *Radiology* 145:409-414, 1982.

137. Mayo J, et al: Anomalies of the inferior vena cava. *AJR* 140:339-345, 1983.

138. McLeod AJ, Zornoza J, Shirkhoda A: Leiomyosarcoma: computed tomographic findings. *Radiology* 152:133-136, 1984.

139. Mendez G, Jr, Isikoff MB, Hill MC: Retroperitoneal processes involving the psoas demonstrated by computed tomography. *J Comput Assist Tomogr* 4(1):78-82, 1980.

140. Meranze S, et al: Retroperitoneal manifestations of sarcoidosis on computed tomography. *J Comput Assist Tomogr* 9(1):50-52, 1985.

141. Meyers MA: *Dynamic radiology of the abdomen: normal and pathologic anatomy,* Heidelberg, 1988, Springer-Verlag.

142. Miller CL, Wechsler RJ: CT evaluation of Kinray-Greenfield filter complications. *AJR* 147:45-50, 1986.

143. Miner DG, et al: CT-guided percutaneous aspiration of septic thrombosis of the inferior vena cava. *AJR* 148:1213-1214, 1987.

144. Moon KL, Jr, et al: Kaposi sarcoma and lymphadenopathy syndrome: limitations of abdominal CT in acquired immunodeficiency syndrome. *Radiology* 150:479-483, 1984.

145. Morehouse HT, Thornhill BA: Nodes or no nodes: CT of adenopathy. *CRC Critical Rev Diagn Imaging* 25(2):177-207, 1986.

146. Morettin LB, Kumar R: Small renal carcinoma with large retroperitoneal hemorrhage: diagnostic considerations. *Urol Radiol* 3:143-148, 1981.

147. Mueller PR, et al: Iliopsoas abscess: treatment by CT-guided percutaneous catheter drainage. *AJR* 142:359-362, 1984.

148. Mulligan SA, et al: CT and MR imaging in the evaluation of retroperitoneal fibrosis. *J Comput Assist Tomogr* 13(2):277-281, 1989.

149. Negendank WH, et al: Lymphomas: MR imaging contrast characteristics with clinical-pathologic correlations. *Radiology* 177:209-216, 1990.

150. Nevitt MP, Ballard DJ, Hallett JW, Jr: Prognosis of abdominal aortic aneurysms. *N Engl J Med* 321:1009-1014, 1989.

151. Nielsen PB: Retrocaval ureter: report of a case. *Acta Radiol (Stockh)* 51:179-188, 1959.

152. North LB, et al: Current use of lymphography for staging lymphomas and genital tumors. *AJR* 158:725-728, 1992.

153. O'Hara PJ, et al: Natural history of periprosthetic air on computerized axial tomographic examination of the abdomen following abdominal aortic aneurysm repair. *J Vasc Surg* 1(3):429-433, 1984.

154. Oliver TW, Jr, Bernardino ME, Sones PJ, Jr: Monitoring the response of lymphoma patients to therapy: correlation of abdominal CT findings with clinical course and histologic cell type. *Radiology* 149:219-224, 1983.

155. Oudkerk M, Overbosch E, Dee P: CT recognition of acute aortic dissection. *AJR* 141:671-676, 1983.

156. Papanicolaou N, Yoder IC, Lee MJ: Primary retroperitoneal neoplasms: how close can we come in making the correct diagnosis. *Urol Radiol* 14:221-228, 1992.

157. Parienty RA, et al: Computed tomography versus aortography in diagnosis of aortic dissection. *Cardiovasc Intervent Radiol* 5:285-291, 1982.

158. Pond GD, et al: Non-Hodgkin lymphoma: influence of lymphography, CT, and bone marrow biopsy on staging and management. *Radiology* 170:159-164, 1989.

159. Posner R, Saks AM, Leiman G: Diffuse retroperitoneal amyloidosis: further radiologic observations. *Br J Radiol* 64:469-471, 1991.

160. Rabinovici R, et al: CT guided periaortic fluid aspiration diagnosing aortic graft infection. *J Cardiovasc Surg* 29:318-319, 1988.

161. Radin DA: Intraabdominal mycobacterium tuberculosis vs mycobacterium avium-intracellulare infections in patients with

AIDS: distinction based on CT findings. *AJR* 156:487-491, 1991.

162. Ralls PW, et al: CT of inflammatory disease of the psoas muscle. *AJR* 134:767-770, 1980.

163. Rappaport H: Tumors of the hematopoetic system. In *Atlas of tumor pathology.* Section 2, fasicle no. 8, Washington, DC, 1966, Armed Forces Institute of Pathology.

164. Raptopolous V, et al: Renal fascial pathway: posterior extension of pancreatic effusions within the anterior pararenal space. *Radiology* 158:367-374, 1986.

165. Rauws EAJ, Mallens WMC, Bieger R: CT scanning for the follow-up of corticosteroid treatment of primary retroperitoneal fibrosis. *J Comput Assist Tomogr* 7(1):113-116, 1983.

166. Rebner M, et al: CT appearance of right gonadal vein. *J Comput Assist Tomogr* 13(3):460-462, 1989.

167. Reed MD, Friedman AC, Nealy P: Anomalies of the left renal vein: analysis of 433 CT scans. *J Comput Assist Tomogr* 6(6):1124-1126, 1982.

168. Ros PR, Viamonte M, Jr, Rywlin AM: Malignant fibrous histiocytoma: mesenchymal tumor of ubiquitous origin. *AJR* 142:753-759, 1984.

169. Rosen A, et al: CT diagnosis of ruptured abdominal aortic aneurysm. *AJR* 143:265-268, 1984.

170. Russell AJ, Ward AS: Prognosis of abdominal aortic aneurysm. *Br Med J* 301:446, 1990.

171. Saldino RM, Palubinskas AJ: Medial placement of the ureter: a normal variant which may simulated retroperitoneal fibrosis. *J Urol* 107:582-585, 1972.

172. Sasai K, et al: Right periureteric venous ring detected by computed tomography. *J Comput Assist Tomogr* 10(2):349-351, 1986.

173. Scatarige JC, et al: Low attenuation nodal metastases in testicular carcinoma. *J Comput Assist Tomogr* 7(4):682-687, 1983.

174. Scott RAP, Ashton HA, Kay DN: Abdominal aortic aneurysm in 4237 screened patients: prevalence, development, and management over 6 years. *Br J Surg* 78:1122-1125, 1991.

175. Seymour EQ: Aortoesophageal fistula as a complication of aortic prosthetic graft. *AJR* 131:160-161, 1978.

176. Shin MS, Berland LL, Ho KJ: Small aorta: detection and clinical significance. *J Comput Assist Tomogr* 14(1):102-103, 1990.

177. Simeone JF, Glickman MG, Itzchak Y: A complication of circumaortic renal vein obstruction in an obese patient. *J Urol* 117:784-785, 1977.

178. Soo CS, et al: Pitfalls of CT findings in post-therapy testicular carcinoma. *J Comput Assist Tomogr* 5(1):39-41, 1981.

179. Spencer JA, Smith MJ, Golding SJ: Lymphangioleiomyomatosis with unusual calcific retroperitoneal lymphangiomyoma: CT findings. *Eur J Radiol* 14:192-194, 1992.

180. Srinivas V, Dow D: Retroperitoneal fibrosis. *Can J Surg* 27:111-114, 1984.

181. Srinivas V, Dow D: Retroperitoneal fibrosis with azotemia secondary to metastaic breast cancer. *Br J Urol* 58:231, 1986.

182. Stomper, et al: CT and pathologic predictive features of residual mass histologic findings after chemotherapy for nonseminomatous germ cell tumors: can residual malignancy or teratoma be excluded? *Radiology* 180:711-714, 1991.

183. Takasugi JE, Godwin JD: CT appearance of the retroaortic anastomoses of the azygos system. *AJR* 154:41-44, 1990.

184. Takebayashi S, et al: Computed tomography of amyloidosis involving retroperitoneal lymph nodes mimicking lymphoma. *J Comput Assist Tomogr* 8(5):1025-1027, 1984.

185. Teefy SA, et al: Differentiating pelvic veins and enlarged lymph nodes: optimal CT techniques. *Radiology* 175:683-685, 1990.

186. Teitelbaum GP, Bradley WG, Klein BD: MR imaging artifacts, ferromagnetism, and magnetic torque of intravascular filters, stents, and coils, *Radiology* 166:657-664, 1988.

187. Tessoro-Tess JD, et al: Lymphangiography and computerized tomography in testicular carcinoma: how accurate in early stage disease? *J Urol* 133:967-970, 1985.

188. Thomas RV: Surgical implications of retroaortic left renal vein. *Arch Surg* 100:738-740, 1970.

189. Thorsen MK, et al: Dissecting aortic aneurysms: accuracy of computed tomographic diagnosis. *Radiology* 148:773-777, 1983.

190. Tisnado J, et al: Computed tomography of a double inferior vena cava: the "double cava" sign. *Comput Tomogr* 3:195-199, 1979.

191. Todd GJ, et al: The accuracy of CT scanning in the diagnosis of abdominal and thoracoabdominal aortic aneurysms. *J Vasc Surg* 13:302-310, 1991.

192. Townsend RR: CT of AIDS-related lymphoma. *AJR* 156:969-974, 1991.

193. Vibkakar SD, et al: Aortic aneurysm presenting as psoas enlargement. *J Comput Assist Tomogr* 5(6):925-928, 1981.

194. Wagliore MP, et al: Lipomatous tumors of the abdominal cavity: CT appearance and pathologic correlation. *AJR* 137:539-545, 1981.

195. Watanabe AT, et al: MR imaging of the bird's nest filter. *Radiology* 177:578-579, 1990.

196. Weinerman PM, et al: Pelvic adenopathy for bladder and prostate carcinoma: detection by rapid-sequence computed tomography. *AJR* 140:95-99, 1983.

197. Whitley NO, et al: Computed tomographic evaluation of carcinoma of the cervix. *Radiology* 142:439-446, 1982.

198. Williams MP, Olliff JFC: Case report: computed tomography and magnetic resonance imaging of dilated lumbar lymphatic trunks. *Clin Radiol* 40:321-322, 1989.

199. Williams MP: Non-tuberculous psoas abscess. *Clin Radiol* 37:253-256, 1986.

200. Yamaguchi T, et al: False lumens in type III aortic dissections: progress CT study. *Radiology* 156:757-760, 1985.

201. Young R, Friedman AC, Hartman DS: Computed tomography of leiomyosarcoma of the inferior vena cava. *Radiology* 145:99-103, 1982.

202. Yuh WT, et al: Magnetic resonance imaging in the diagnosis and follow-up of idiopathic retroperitoneal fibrosis. *J Urol* 141:602-605, 1989.

38

Computed Tomography of the Pelvis

JAMES W. WALSH

Computed tomography (CT) has been a premier pelvic imaging modality for the past 15 years. Its strengths and limitations in evaluating pelvic disease are well known, and indications for pelvic CT have been further refined by concomitant developments in ultrasound (US) and magnetic resonance imaging (MRI). This chapter discusses current indications for pelvic CT, especially in cancer staging and mass characterization.

ANATOMY

The pelvis is a bony ring that consists of four bones: the two innominate bones laterally and anteriorly

and the sacrum and coccyx posteriorly. The sacrum is inserted between the two innominate bones, and its alae support the psoas muscles and the lumbosacral nerve trunks (Fig. 38-1). Each innominate bone is composed of three fused parts: the ilium, ischium, and pubis. Within the innominate bone is the acetabulum, which is contained within the inverted Y formed by the anterior (iliopubic) and posterior (ilioischial) columns. The triangular-shaped anterior and posterior columns are connected by the quadrilateral plate, which forms the medial acetabular wall (Fig. 38-2).

The pelvis is divided into the greater (false) and the lesser (true) pelvis. The iliac wings bound the false pelvis and iliac fossae, which contain the ascending, descending, and sigmoid colon; small bowel loops; the psoas and iliacus muscles; and the major neurovascular

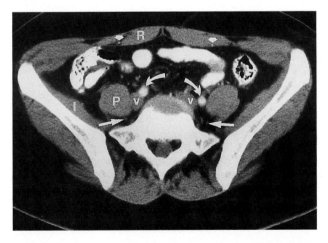

Fig. 38-1. CT scan through contrast-filled ascending and descending colon in the iliac fossae shows paired rectus abdominis *(R)*, psoas *(P)*, and iliacus *(I)* muscles. Common iliac arteries *(curved arrows)*, common iliac veins *(v)*, and lumbosacral trunks *(straight arrows)* are located anterior to the ala of the sacrum. The inferior epigastric arteries *(arrowheads)* are related to the posterior rectus muscles.

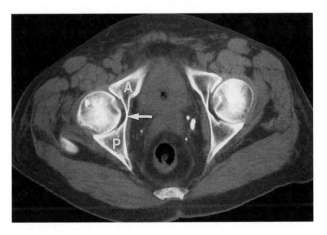

Fig. 38-2. CT scan through the femoral heads show the anterior column *(A)*, quadrilateral plate *(arrow)*, and posterior column *(P)* of the acetabulum.

bifurcations (see Fig. 38-1). The paired bellies of the rectus abdominis muscles form the anterior border of the false pelvis. The true pelvis lies below the sacral promontory, bounds the pelvic organs, and is separated inferiorly from the perineum by the pelvic diaphragm.

Muscles and nerves

The psoas major muscle passes caudad along the anterolateral border of the pelvis, tapers gradually, passes beneath the inguinal ligament anterior to the hip joint

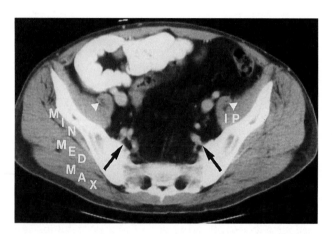

Fig. 38-3. CT scan at the inferior sacroiliac joints shows the external iliac arteries and veins medial to the iliopsoas muscles *(IP)*, which enclose the femoral nerves *(arrowheads)* and the posterior dividing branches of the internal iliac arteries and veins *(arrows)*. The gluteus minimus *(MIN)*, gluteus medius *(MED)*, and gluteus maximum *(MAX)* muscles compose the buttocks.

capsule, and ends in a tendon that inserts on the lesser trochanter of the femur (Figs. 38-1, 38-3, and 38-4). The iliacus is a fan-shaped muscle that fills the iliac fossa and narrows rapidly to insert on the lateral side of the psoas tendon and lesser trochanter (see Fig. 38-1). The femoral nerve lies in the fat plane between the psoas and iliacus muscles and passes caudally to lie under the inguinal ligament lateral to the femoral artery (Fig. 38-3). The gluteus minimus, gluteus medius, and gluteus maximus muscles lie posterior to the innominate bones (see Fig. 38-3).[123]

The muscles within the pelvis are divided into two groups: (1) the true pelvis muscles, the levator ani and coccygeus, and (2) the muscles that originate within the pelvis and form part of the pelvic wall, the obturator internus and the piriformis. The levator ani and coccygeus muscles compose the pelvic diaphragm, which is the floor of the pelvic cavity (see Fig. 38-4). The pelvic diaphragm is pierced by the urethra, vagina, and anus. The piriformis and obturator internus muscles form most of the lateral sidewall of the true pelvis (Fig. 38-5). The obturator internus muscle also extends into the perineum to form the lateral boundary of the ischiorectal fossa (see Fig. 38-4). The greater sciatic foramen lies between the ischial spine and sacrum, and the sciatic nerve passes through it on the anterolateral aspect of the piriformis muscle (see Fig. 38-5).[42,88]

The perineum is a diamond-shaped space below the pelvic diaphragm bounded anteriorly by pubic symphysis, laterally by the inferior pubic rami and ischial tuberosities, and posteriorly by the coccyx.[111] The triangular ischiorectal fossae are bordered laterally by the ischiopubic rami, medially by the pelvic diaphragm, and

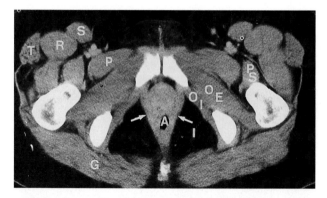

Fig. 38-4. CT scan through the symphysis pubis shows the obturator internus muscle *(OI)* and obturator externus *(OE)* on either side of the obturator foramen and the psoas muscle *(PS)* inserting on the lesser trochanter of the femur. Other muscles are the pectineus *(P)*, sartorius *(S)*, rectus femoris *(R)*, tensor fascia lata *(T)*, and gluteus maximum *(G)* muscles. The pelvic diaphragm *(arrows)* separates the anus *(A)* from the ischiorectal fossae *(I)* in the perineum.

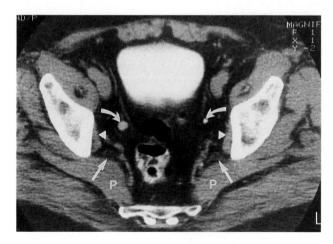

Fig. 38-5. CT scan through the sciatic notch shows the sciatic nerves *(straight arrows)* anterior to the piriformis muscles *(P)* and the obturator internus muscles *(arrowheads)* along the pelvic sidewalls. The pelvic ureters *(curved arrows)* are immediately posterolateral to the pelvic peritoneal reflections.

posteriorly by the gluteus maximus muscles (see Fig. 38-4).

Vessels, lymph nodes, and ureters

The abdominal aorta divides on the left side of the fourth lumbar vertebra into two common iliac arteries (see Fig. 38-1), which course laterally and caudad and divide opposite the L5-S1 disk space into the external and internal iliac arteries. Caudad to the aortic bifurcation, the inferior vena cava is formed by the confluence of the common iliac veins at the fifth lumbar vertebra. The external iliac arteries pass along the anteromedial border of the iliopsoas muscles. The internal iliac arteries lie posteriorly on the lumbosacral plexus, course toward the greater sciatic foramen, and divide into multiple branches at the level of the inferior sacroiliac joints (see Fig. 38-3). Only the superior and inferior gluteal arteries are consistently seen on CT as they exit the sciatic notch. The external and internal iliac veins lie medial and posterior to the corresponding arteries.

The pelvic lymph nodes are classified according to accompanying vessels. The common iliac lymph nodes are located lateral and posterior to the common iliac arteries. The hypogastric node is situated at the bifurcation of the external and internal iliac vessels (Fig. 38-6). The external iliac lymph nodes are arranged in three chains: (1) the lateral chain on the lateral aspect of the external iliac artery, (2) the middle chain anterior and medial to the external iliac vein, and (3) the medial chain posterior to the external iliac vein against the pelvic sidewall. The obturator node is considered one of the medial external iliac nodes.[121] The most common internal iliac nodes identified on CT are located anterior to the

piriformis muscle, around the inferior gluteal artery and vein (Fig. 38-7). The superficial inguinal lymph nodes lie distal to the inguinal ligament in the subcutaneous fat anterior to the femoral artery and vein. A report has identified an additional pelvic lymph node, the posterior iliac crest node, located in the iliac fossa between the psoas and iliacus muscles.[22]

The pelvic ureters cross anterior to the common iliac artery bifurcation and course posterior to the peritoneum (see Fig. 38-5). At the sciatic foramen, the ureters course medially toward the lateral angle of the bladder. In the male, they terminate anterior to the seminal vesicles (Fig. 38-8). In the female, the ureters lie lateral

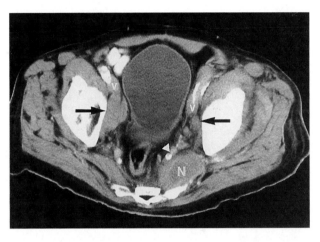

Fig. 38-7. Recurrent prostate cancer. CT scan through the sciatic notch shows bilateral obturator lymph node metastases *(arrows)* posterior to the external iliac veins *(v)* and a larger left internal iliac node metastasis *(N)* confluent with the piriformis muscle posterior to the inferior gluteal artery and vein *(arrowhead)*.

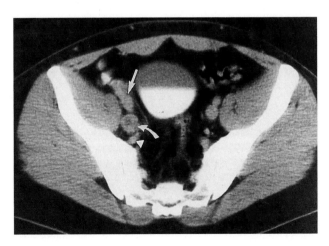

Fig. 38-6. CT scan through the bifurcation of the external iliac artery and vein anteriorly *(straight arrow)* and the internal iliac vessels posteriorly *(arrowhead)* shows a classic right hypogastric lymph node metastasis *(curved arrow)* from cancer of the prostate gland.

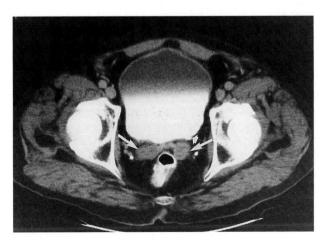

Fig. 38-8. CT scan shows seminal vesicles *(arrows)* between bladder and rectum and left pelvic ureter entering bladder *(arrowhead)*.

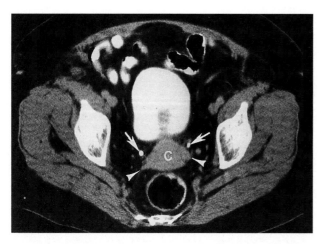

Fig. 38-9. CT scan through the cervix *(C)* shows triangular cardinal ligaments tapering laterally *(arrowheads)* and pelvic ureters *(arrows)* anteriorly.

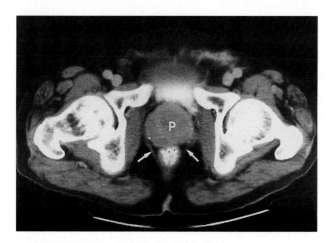

Fig. 38-10. CT scan shows normal prostate gland *(P)* between bladder and rectum and levator ani muscles *(arrows).*

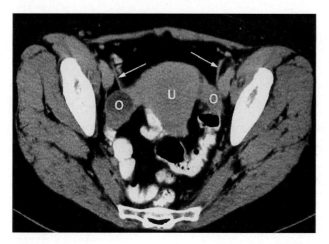

Fig. 38-11. CT scan through the uterus *(U)* and ovaries *(O)* shows round ligaments *(arrows)* tapering anterolaterally over the external iliac vessels.

or posterior to the ovaries and then course 1 to 2 cm from the lateral border of the cervix, where they pass through the cardinal ligaments to enter the bladder (Fig. 38-9).

Internal genital organs

The male internal genital organs are the prostate gland and the seminal vesicles. The seminal vesicles are two extraperitoneal lobulated pouches located superior to the prostate gland between the bladder and the rectum (see Fig. 38-8). They vary in size both in different patients and in the same individual. The prostate gland is a musculoglandular organ that lies posterior to the symphysis pubis between the bladder base above and the pelvic diaphragm below (Fig. 38-10).

The female internal genital organs are the ovaries, fallopian tubes, uterus, and vagina. The ovaries are usually located at the level of the uterine fundus and round ligaments (Fig. 38-11). They usually lie in a shallow depression, the ovarian fossa, which is bounded by the external iliac vessels laterally and the pelvic ureter posteriorly. The uterus is a pear-shaped organ between the bladder and rectum that is divided into a body (corpus) (Fig. 38-11) and cervix (see Fig. 38-9).

The broad ligaments are two fibrous sheets extending laterally from the uterus to the pelvic sidewall and covered on their anterior and posterior surfaces by peritoneum. They are not routinely seen on CT unless outlined by ascites. Between the leaves of the broad ligament are the parametrium, uterine artery (Fig. 38-12), fallopian tube, and round ligament. The round ligaments demarcate the superolateral border of the uterus and ascend anterolaterally over the external iliac vessels, pass

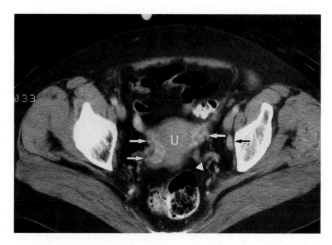

Fig. 38-12. CT scan through the uterus *(U)* shows a tortuous left uterine artery *(white arrowhead)* and prominent vascular plexus *(white arrows)* running within the broad ligament. A normal contrast-enhanced left obturator lymph node *(black arrow)* is present.

through the inguinal canal, and insert in the labia majora (see Fig. 38-11). The triangular cardinal ligaments are located at the base of the broad ligament and fan out from their attachments at the cervix to insert on fascia covering the pelvic diaphragm (see Fig. 38-9).[117] The uterosacral ligaments arise in continuity with the cardinal ligaments and pass posterolaterally around the rectum to insert on the sacrum.

Peritoneal and extraperitoneal spaces

The urinary bladder indents the parietal peritoneum reflecting over the dome, forming the intraperitoneal paravesical fossae laterally.[4] The proximal two thirds of the rectum is covered by peritoneum on its anterior and lateral sides, forming the pararectal fossae laterally. The distal one third of the rectum is covered only by anterior peritoneum, which reflects onto the seminal vesicles and bladder in the male to form the rectovesical pouch. In the female, the peritoneum covering the bladder and rectum is divided by the uterus and vagina into a shallow anterior vesicouterine recess and a large, deep, posterior rectouterine fossa (cul-de-sac or pouch of Douglas). The cul-de-sac is continuous with the pararectal and ovarian fossae.[4]

The extraperitoneal spaces of the pelvis are complex. Anterior to the peritoneum and posterior to the transversalis fascia, the umbilicovesical fascia spreads inferiorly from the umbilicus to surround the urachus, obliterated umbilical arteries, and urinary bladder.[5] This fascia divides the anterior extraperitoneal fat into a perivesical space and a prevesical space. The bladder, umbilical arteries, and urachus lie within the confines of the umbilicovesical fascia in the small perivesical space. The large potential prevesical space lies anterior to the umbilicovesical fascia and includes the retropubic space or

space of Retizius. The prevesical space has potential extensions into the anterior abdominal wall (rectus sheath), parametria (round ligaments), inguinal canal and scrotum, properitoneal fat, and retroperitoneum.[5]

EXAMINATION TECHNIQUE

Oral contrast opacification of small and large bowel is essential to perform a diagnostic pelvic CT study. Patients drink 450 ml of a 2% oral barium suspension the evening before the examination to opacify large bowel and 450 ml 45 minutes preceding the study to opacify pelvic small bowel. In patients with suspected ovarian cancer, pelvic inflammatory disease, endometriosis, diverticulitis, or rectal cancer, a 200 ml dilute water-soluble contrast enema may best delineate disease extent (Fig. 38-13). Intravenous contrast material is used to opacify the bladder and ureters; enhance solid tumor components of ovarian and bladder cancer (Fig. 38-14), endometrial sarcoma, and gestational trophoblastic disease; differentiate iliac vessels from lymph nodes (Fig. 38-15); delineate parametrial blood vessels (see Fig. 38-12); and enhance myometrium and visualize the endometrial cavity (see Fig. 38-15). With current high-resolution fast CT scanners, an optimum intravenous contrast enhancement technique uses a mechanical injector to give 150 ml of 60% contrast at the rate of 2 ml/second. Most of the contrast (100 ml) is used to image the pelvis, and the remaining 50 ml is given as a bolus for abdominal scans.

A standard pelvic CT scan consists of contiguous 8 to 10 mm sections from the level of the symphysis pubis cephalad to the iliac crest to optimize parenchymal enhancement as well as vascular opacification for lymph node metastasis detection. An optional technique on newer scanners is a dynamic screening study with con-

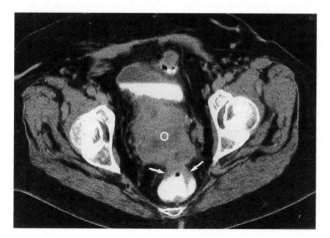

Fig. 38-13. Serous cystadenocarcinoma of the ovary. CT scan after water-soluble contrast enema shows solid ovarian cancer (*O*) invading the rectum (*arrows*) confirmed at surgery.

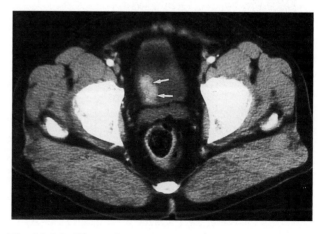

Fig. 38-14. CT scan during peak arterial contrast enhancement with a mechanical injector shows contrast-enhanced bladder cancer (*arrows*) confined to bladder wall.

tiguous 4 to 5 mm slices through the pelvis. In cancer staging or abdominopelvic mass evaluation, sections are then taken at 1 to 1.5 cm intervals from the iliac crest to the diaphragm to screen for hydronephrosis and metastatic disease. At the end of the abdominal study, additional 2 to 5 mm sections may be taken through pelvic tumor or small masses to define local extension better and eliminate the problem of volume averaging of mass and normal adjacent structures (Fig. 38-16). Delayed thin sections through the pelvis also show better the interface between mass and contrast-filled bladder and pelvic ureters.

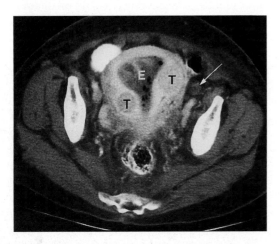

Fig. 38-15. Adenosquamous carcinoma of the endometrium. CT scan through an enlarged uterus during peak contrast enhancement shows hypodense tumor *(T)* invading the myometrium, gas bubbles in a dilated endometrial cavity *(E)*, and a left external iliac lymph node metastasis *(arrow)*.

BLADDER CANCER

Bladder cancer accounts for 4% of all malignant tumors. Ninety percent of these tumors are transitional cell carcinomas, with the majority occurring around the trigone and posterolateral walls of the bladder. Clinical staging methods include cystoscopy and biopsy for diagnosis, transurethral resection to assess depth of bladder invasion, and bimanual examination of the bladder under anesthesia to evaluate extravesical extension. The major limitation of clinical staging is the inaccuracy of bladder palpation to evaluate extraluminal tumor extension.

Over the past 15 years, CT has been the most commonly used imaging technique for staging bladder cancer.[24,59,66,82,85,92,102] CT is most useful for evaluating extravesical tumor extension, invasion of adjacent organs, and detection of lymph node metastases.[24,59,85] This information assists surgical decision making regarding candidates for radical cystectomy. The overall accuracy of CT staging varies from 64% to 81%.[66,102] The overall accuracy of lymph node assessment varies from 83% to 92%, with a false-negative rate of 25% to 40% due mainly to tumor in normal-size lymph nodes.[66,82] Although CT-MRI comparison studies have shown no significant difference in overall staging accuracy, MRI has advantages over CT in differentiating superficial from deep bladder muscle invasion, delineating tumors at the bladder base and dome with sagittal images, and detecting invasion of the prostate gland.[2,12,58] MRI is also useful when CT is equivocal for extraluminal extension or for invasion of adjacent organs.

In the United States, clinical staging criteria are based on the Jewett-Strong-Marshall classification (Table 38-1). Because CT cannot differentiate stages 0-A-B1-

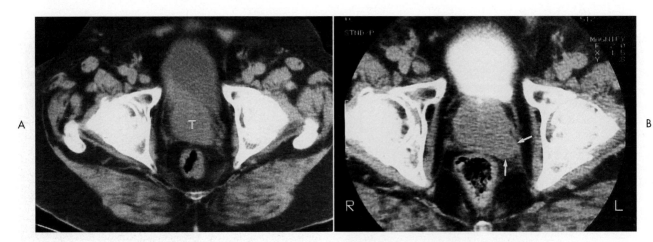

Fig. 38-16. Stage C prostate cancer. **A,** Ten millimeter section through prostate tumor *(T)* barely shows prominent left posterolateral margin. **B,** Five millimeter section shows focal mass *(arrows)* obliterating margins of left neurovascular bundle consistent with extracapsular tumor extension.

B2, CT stage criteria are stage B or less, tumor confined to bladder; stage C, irregular outer bladder wall or soft tissue infiltration into perivesical fat in region of tumor, or both; stage D1, loss of fat/fascial planes associated with mass between tumor and contiguous pelvic organs (prostate, seminal vesicles, uterus, vagina, obturator internus muscle, rectus abdominis muscle) or pelvic nodes larger than 1.5 to 2.0 cm in diameter; stage D2, enlarged lymph nodes above the aortic bifurcation or extrapelvic metastases.

The CT technique used to demonstrate intraluminal bladder tumor is a matter of individual preference and experience. The simplest method is to use urine (Figs. 38-14 and 38-17) or intravenous contrast medium (Fig. 38-18) to outline the borders of the tumor. Both the intraluminal and extraluminal components of bladder cancer may exhibit intravenous contrast enhancement (see Fig. 38-14).[58] Because the cystoscopist is best at evaluating stage 0-A-B1-B2 tumors, CT technique should focus on definition of gross extravesical tumor extension and detection of enlarged lymph nodes. Also, care must be taken to differentiate the bladder wall thickening and perivesical fat infiltration of bladder cancer from edema or fibrosis caused by previous biopsy, surgery, or radiation therapy.[92]

The CT findings of bladder cancer include irregular wall thickening, sessile polypoid mural lesions (see Figs. 38-14 and 38-17), and exophytic irregular masses filling the bladder lumen (see Fig. 38-18). Overdistention of the bladder lumen should be avoided. In such situations, postvoid sections through the tumor allow better scrutiny of peripelvic fat for extravesical tumor extension. Perivesical tumor (stage C) is characterized by soft tissue mass outside the bladder lumen associated with increased soft tissue density in perivesical fat (see Fig. 38-18). More advanced tumors (stage D1) may extend locally to invade surrounding organs or the peripheral borders of the true pelvis.

CT overstaging errors are due to either misinterpreting normal structures abutting the bladder as extravesical tumor extension or mistaking absence of fat planes between pelvic organs as evidence of local invasion. One study overstaged 27% of stage B or less tumors because of loss of fat planes between the seminal vesicles and posterior bladder wall.[66] Understaging CT errors are due to failure to demonstrate microscopic invasion of the perivesical fat[59,82] or to detect microscopic metastases to normal or slightly enlarged pelvic lymph nodes.[59,66]

CT is an excellent method to detect recurrent bladder cancer after cystectomy.[32,69,86] Although the most common site of tumor recurrence is the pelvis, the abdomen should also be scanned because isolated abdominal metastases occur in this disease.[32] Characteris-

Table 38-1. Jewett-Strong-Marshall staging system for classification of bladder cancer

Stage	Characteristics
0	Lesion limited to superficial mucosa
A	Submucosal invasion
B1	Superficial muscle invasion
B2	Deep muscle invasion
C	Perivesical invasion
D1	Spread to adjacent organs or pelvic lymph nodes
D2	Spread to extrapelvic lymph nodes or distant metastases

Data from Jewett HJ, Strong GH. *J Urol* 55:366-372, 1946; and Marshall VF: *J Urol* 68:714-723, 1952.

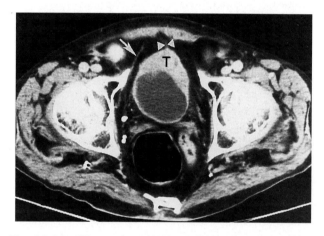

Fig. 38-17. CT scan through bladder tumor *(T),* outlined by urine, which is confined to the anterior wall. Median *(arrowheads)* and medial *(arrow)* umbilical ligaments are well seen.

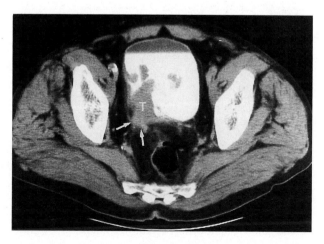

Fig. 38-18. Stage C bladder cancer. CT scan through bulky intraluminal tumor *(T)* outlined by opacified urine shows right posterolateral extension into perivesical fat *(arrows).*

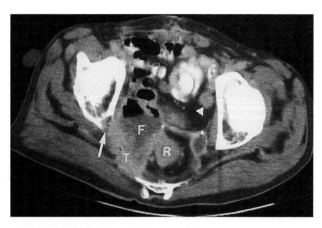

Fig. 38-19. Recurrent transitional cell bladder cancer after cystectomy. CT scan shows right posterior pelvic tumor recurrence *(T)* eroding ischial spine *(arrow)* and associated with a fluid collection *(F)* from a fistula to the rectum *(R)*. A metastatic left obturator lymph node *(arrowhead)* is also present.

Table 38-2. American Urological Association staging system for prostate cancer

Stage	Characteristics
A	Occult cancer
A1	Focal
A2	Diffuse
B	Cancer confined within prostatic capsule with no elevation of serum acid phosphatase
B1	Tumor <1.5 cm or 1 lobe
B2	Tumor >1.5 cm or >1 lobe
C	Cancer extending beyond prostatic capsule, including seminal vesicles, bladder, and urethra, or confined within capsule with elevated serum acid phosphatase
C1	No involvement of seminal vesicles
C2	Involvement of seminal vesicles
D	Metastatic disease
D1	Pelvic lymph node metastases
D2	Bone or distant lymph node or organ metastases

Data from Whitmore WF Jr. *Urol Clin North Am* 11:205-220, 1984.

tic CT findings, alone or in combination, are a mass in the cystectomy site, pelvic and retroperitoneal adenopathy, and liver metastases.[32,69,86] Bone erosion may be present adjacent to pelvic tumor masses (Fig. 38-19).

URACHAL CANCER—CYST

Urachal carcinoma is a rare malignancy, which accounts for less than 0.34% of all bladder carcinomas.[84] Eighty-five percent to 90% of these tumors are mucinous adenocarcinomas.[11] The cancer has a characteristic presentation as a mass anterosuperior to the bladder dome along the expected midline course of the urachus. CT findings in this tumor are usually diagnostic and consist of a vesical dome mass with a caudal intravesical part that occupies a portion of the bladder wall and a cephalad part that is primarily extravesical. This supravesical tumor component characteristically has a low attenuation owing to mucin produced by the tumor and contains peripheral or central calcification.[11]

CT has also been a useful technique to diagnose uninfected and infected urachal cysts.[95,105] Although CT can guide percutaneous catheter drainage of infected urachal cysts as short-term therapy, the high recurrence rate of infection usually requires total excision of the mass.[105]

PROSTATE CANCER

Prostate cancer is the most common male cancer in the United States and the second leading cause of cancer deaths in men. Diagnosis is usually established by prostate biopsy guided by digital examination or transrectal US or by positive prostate fragments after transurethral resection of the prostate. The standard staging workup includes digital rectal examination, serum acid

phosphatase and prostate-specific antigen levels, cell ploidy, and a bone scan. Cross-sectional imaging techniques are used to determine local extent of tumor and identify operative candidates. Methods of treatment include radical prostatectomy for stages A and B versus radiation therapy and hormones for advanced stages C and D disease. MRI with whole body and endorectal coils is now considered the most accurate preoperative staging technique for prostate cancer.[10,100,110]

Clinical staging is based on the American Urological Association staging system (Table 38-2). Because CT cannot differentiate stage A from stage B, CT stage criteria are stage B or less, tumor confined to prostate; stage C, extracapsular tumor extension to involve the periprostatic fat, seminal vesicles, bladder, rectum, obturator internus muscle; stage D1, pelvic nodes greater than 1.5 to 2.0 cm in diameter; stage D2, enlarged lymph nodes above the aortic bifurcation, bone metastases, or extrapelvic metastases.

CT is not an effective technique to differentiate stage B from stage C tumors and thus influence treatment decisions because of its low sensitivity in determining extracapsular tumor extension. CT has reported overall accuracies of only 58% in detecting seminal vesicle invasion and 64% in detecting periprostatic fat invasion (see Fig. 38-16, *B*).[89] Thus CT is most useful in evaluating advanced bulky disease (stages D1 to D2) with gross objective findings (Fig. 38-20).

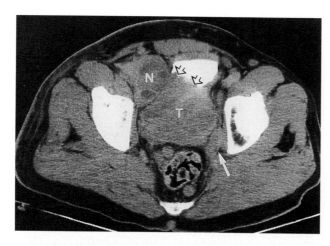

Fig. 38-20. Stage D2 prostate cancer. CT scan through a large prostate tumor *(T)* extending into the true pelvis to invade the bladder *(arrowheads)* and associated with right external iliac *(N)* and left internal iliac *(arrow)* lymph node metastases. Para-aortic lymph node metastases were present on abdominal sections.

The most common signs of advanced disease are extraprostatic soft tissue masses invading the posterior bladder base or seminal vesicles (stage C). These masses are commonly near the midline and cause asymmetrical thickening, irregularity, and nodularity of the posterior bladder wall and obliterate fat planes between the bladder and seminal vesicles. Associated pelvic (stage D1) and para-aortic (stage D2) lymph node metastases are usually easy to detect because they are large and multiple (see Fig. 38-20). Bone metastases should be evaluated on appropriate window and level settings.

The role of CT staging of prostate cancer has changed significantly because of its own inherent limitations as well as advances in transrectal US and MRI. Although the overall accuracy for CT staging is only 67% to 73%,[33,89] the overall accuracy for detection of lymph node metastases is 67% to 93%.[33,70,82,124] Thus CT retains a role in screening for advanced local disease and lymph node metastases. These images can be used for radiation therapy planning and assessing treatment response to therapy.

TESTICULAR CANCER

Cancer of the testis is an uncommon tumor, representing 2% of all cancers in men. It is the most common solid cancer in men aged 15 to 34 years. Malignant germ cell tumors of the testis are divided into seminomas and nonseminomas. The serum tumor markers human chorionic gonadotropin and alpha-fetoprotein for nonseminomas and lactic dehydrogenase for seminoma are important indicators of metastatic disease or disease response to treatment. The predominant metastatic route of testicular neoplasms is via the gonadal lymphatics to upper retroperitoneal, retrocrural, mediastinal, and supraclavicular lymph nodes.

CT has replaced lymphangiography for retroperitoneal lymph node screening because it is noninvasive and has an overall accuracy comparable to lymphangiography in testicular tumor staging.[56,106] If CT is negative or equivocal, a lymphangiogram can identify metastases in normal-sized nodes in a small proportion of cases.[56] The CT findings in metastatic testicular tumor are those of lymph node enlargement. Low attenuation areas in nodal metastases are common.[57,99] The most common sites of retroperitoneal lymph node metastases are para-aortic and paracaval nodes from T-11 to L-4 vertebral bodies. Pelvic lymphadenopathy is less common and is associated with tumor penetration of the testicular capsule, alteration of lymphatic drainage by previous inguinal surgery or transscrotal tumor biopsy, or caudal spread from upper retroperitoneal lymph nodes.

Follow-up CT scans are frequently used to assess treatment response or detect disease recurrence. Persistent but stable or resolving masses are common after chemotherapy for advanced seminoma. In contrast to nonseminomatous tumors, these masses most often represent fibrosis and do not warrant surgical excision.[107] In patients with treated nonseminomatous metastases, residual masses may represent residual malignancy, mature or immature teratoma, or necrosis and fibrosis.[108] In fact, enlarging retroperitoneal, mediastinal, or pulmonary masses in patients with negative serum tumor markers after chemotherapy for nonseminomatous tumor frequently represent mature teratoma.[72,87] These masses are predominately cystic and are cured by complete surgical excision. Because CT cannot reliably exclude malignancy in residual masses after treatment for nonseminomatous tumor, complete surgical excision of the mass may be required for optimal management of this disease.[108]

CERVICAL CANCER

Cervical cancer is the ninth most common cancer in women and is usually detected by an abnormal papanicolaou smear or discovery of a cervical mass associated with vaginal discharge or bleeding. Clinical staging of cervical cancer, as defined by the International Federation of Gynecology and Obstetrics (FIGO), consists of bimanual pelvic examination, chest radiography, excretory urography, barium enema, cystoscopy, and sigmoidoscopy (Table 38-3). Use of CT or MRI for staging often eliminates the need for urography or a barium enema. Because clinical staging has decreasing accuracy with more advanced disease, CT is an excellent complementary staging procedure because of its high accuracy

Table 38-3. International Federation of Gynecology and Obstetrics (FIGO) classification of cervical carcinoma

Stage	FIGO Classification
0	In situ
I	Confined to cervix
Ia	Microinvasive
Ib	All other cases of stage I
II	Extends beyond cervix but not to pelvic sidewall or lower third of vagina
IIa	No obvious parametrial involvement
IIb	Obvious parametrial involvement
III	Extends to pelvic sidewall or lower third of vagina or ureteral obstruction
IIIa	No extension to pelvic sidewall
IIIb	Extension to pelvic sidewall or ureteral obstruction
IV	Extends beyond the true pelvis or invades mucosa of bladder or rectum
IVa	Spread to adjacent organs
IVb	Spread to distant organs

Data from Beahrs OH, Henson DE, Hutter RVP, Myers MH, editors: *Manual for staging of cancer,* 3rd ed, pp 151-153, Philadelphia, 1988, JB Lippincott.

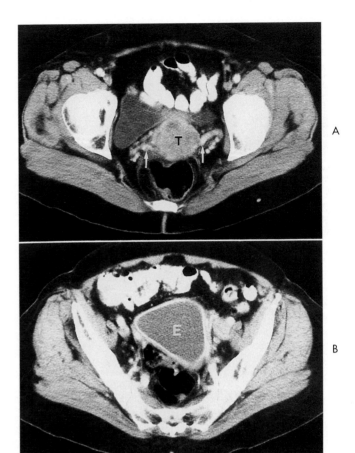

Fig. 38-21. Stage I cervical cancer. **A,** CT scan shows heterogeneous hypodense tumor *(T)* completely replacing the cervix and normal uterine arteries *(arrows)* and parametrial vessels without evidence of parametrial tumor extension. **B,** CT scan through an enlarged uterus with a dilated fluid-filled endometrial cavity *(E),* and thinned myometrium owing to tumor obstruction of the endocervical canal.

in advanced disease.[119] The overall accuracy of CT staging is 58% to 88%, but CT has an accuracy rate of only 30% to 58% in evaluating parametrial tumor extension.[48,64,118,119] MRI may become the procedure of choice to differentiate stage Ib from IIb cervical cancer because of its higher overall accuracy for evaluating parametrial tumor extension and higher predictive value for determining tumor confined to the cervix.[55,65,113]

CT is still an important imaging test for evaluating advanced cervical carcinoma. CT is indicated for any poorly differentiated lesion or a large bulky tumor, especially when detection of lymph node metastases is important.[7,19,45,118] In the detection of pelvic lymph node metastases, CT has an overall accuracy of 65% to 80%.[19,48,119] CT has a higher accuracy of 80% to 98% in detecting para-aortic lymph node metastases.[7,19,64,118]

CT staging criteria for cervical carcinoma are based on the FIGO staging classification (see Table 38-3). CT criteria for a stage I tumor are (1) intact peripheral cervix borders, (2) absence of parametrial soft tissue mass, and (3) intact periureteral fat planes (Fig. 38-21, *A*).[117] Normal structures, such as the cardinal and uterosacral ligaments, parametrial blood vessels (Fig. 38-21, *A*), or ovaries, should not be mistaken for parametrial tumor extension. The classic CT appearance of cervical cancer is a solid mass enlarging the cervix greater than 3.5 cm in diameter and containing hypodense ar-

eas from necrosis, ulceration, and diminished intravenous contrast enhancement (Fig. 38-21, *A*). Uterine enlargement with an endometrial fluid collection may be secondary to tumor obstruction of the endocervical canal (Fig. 38-21, *B*).[101]

CT criteria for parametrial tumor invasion (stage IIb) are (1) disruption of the peripheral cervix margins, (2) prominent parametrial soft tissue strands, (3) obliteration of periureteric fat planes, and (4) an eccentric parametrial soft tissue mass (Fig. 38-22).[117] The latter two findings are essential to make a definitive diagnosis of parametrial tumor extension. Pelvic sidewall extension (stage IIIb) is characterized by soft tissue mass extension to the obturator internus or piriformis muscles. CT detection of hydronephrosis or pelvic lymphadenopathy also indicates a stage IIIb tumor (Fig. 38-23). CT criteria for bladder or rectal involvement (stage IVa) are (1)

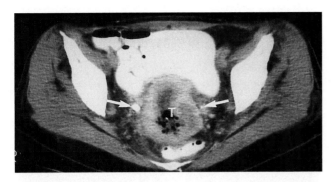

Fig. 38-22. Stage IIb cervical cancer. CT scan through a bulky cervical tumor *(T)* shows bilateral diffuse parametrial soft tissue mass surrounding the pelvic ureters *(arrows)*.

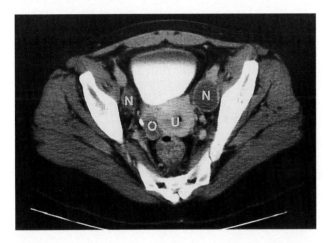

Fig. 38-23. Stage IIIb cervical cancer. CT scan through the uterus *(U)* and right ovary *(O)* shows bilateral hypodense obturator lymph node metastases *(N)* from known cervical cancer.

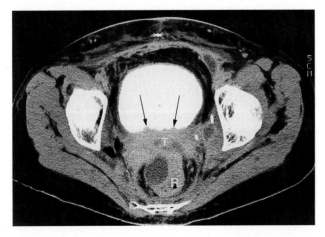

Fig. 38-24. Recurrent cervical cancer after hysterectomy. CT scan shows central pelvic tumor recurrence *(T)* involving the anterior rectum *(R)* and posterior bladder *(arrows)* and extending to both pelvic sidewalls.

focal loss of the perivesical/perirectal fat plane accompanied by focal wall thickening, (2) nodular indentations or serrations of the bladder/rectal wall, and (3) an intraluminal mass.[64,119]

CT is commonly used to screen patients with known or suspected recurrent cervical cancer.[7,45,64,122] Clinical examination and CT are complementary techniques to determine disease extent and assist decision making either to perform an exenterative procedure or alternative tumor resection for disease control or to document inoperable tumor with CT-guided biopsy. The classic CT findings of recurrent cervical cancer include central pelvic recurrence; parametrial, pelvic sidewall, and perineal tumor extension; bladder and rectal invasion; pelvic and para-aortic adenopathy; bone erosion from adjacent lymph node metastases; hydronephrosis; pelvic vein thrombosis; and liver metastases (Fig. 38-24). A major limitation of CT is the differentiation of recurrent tumor from radiation therapy or postsurgical fibrosis.[64,122] MRI may be a useful technique to distinguish recurrent tumor from posttreatment fibrosis.[30]

ENDOMETRIAL CANCER

Endometrial carcinoma is the most common female genital tract cancer, and most patients present with stage I to II disease owing to postmenopausal vaginal bleeding. Recommendations by FIGO have led to a new surgical staging system for endometrial carcinoma. The rationale for surgical management is that hysterectomy controls pelvic disease by removing gross tumor and permits pathological assessment of tumor grade, depth of myometrial invasion, and cervical extension. The surgeon also evaluates metastases to the adnexae, lymph nodes, omentum, and peritoneum. Thus the role of imaging tests in preoperative evaluation of this cancer is unclear. CT is not routinely used to evaluate clinical stage I to II tumors except for poorly differentiated carcinomas or endometrial sarcomas because of its low yield in demonstrating extrauterine cancer spread.[120] CT is used to screen patients with suspected advanced disease who are not surgical candidates.[6,120] The overall accuracy of CT staging is 84% to 92%.[6,29,120]

CT staging criteria for endometrial cancer are based on the FIGO staging classification (Table 38-4). Contrast-enhanced CT demonstrates endometrial tumor as a hypodense mass in the endometrial cavity (Fig. 38-25) or myometrium (Fig. 38-15), as an enlarged fluid-filled obstructed uterus,[101] or rarely as a contrast-enhancing myometrial lesion.[51] Endometrial tumor involvement of the cervix (stage IIA) is characterized on CT as cervical enlargement greater than 3.5 cm in diameter and heterogeneous cervical stroma.[6,53] Stage IIIA disease is characterized by transserosal tumor extension (Fig. 38-26) or metastatic disease to the ovary and

Table 38-4. FIGO surgical staging of endometrial cancer (1988)

Stage	Characteristics
IAG123	Tumor limited to endometrium
IBG123	Invasion <½ myometrium
ICG123	Invasion >½ myometrium
IIAG123	Cervical stromal invasion
IIIAG123	Tumor invades serosa or adnexae positive peritoneal cytology
IIIBG123	Vaginal metastases
IIICG123	Metastases to pelvic or para-aortic nodes
IVAG123	Tumor invasion bladder and/or bowel mucosa
IVB	Distant metastases including intra-abdominal and/or inguinal lymph node

Data from FIGO: Corpus cancer staging. *Int J Gynecol Obstet* 28:189-193, 1989.

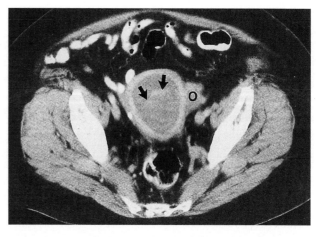

Fig. 38-25. Stage I uterine sarcoma. CT scan through the left ovary *(O)* and uterus shows polypoid tumor *(arrows)* in the fluid-filled endometrial cavity and intact myometrium.

fallopian tube. Limitations of CT staging are (1) difficulty in differentiating a leiomyoma from uterine cancer and (2) difficulty in determining the depth of myometrial invasion.

CT has been an important imaging modality in detecting persistent and recurrent endometrial carcinoma or sarcoma.[6,120] CT features include a central pelvic mass; pelvic and para-aortic lymphadenopathy; and mesenteric, peritoneal, omental, and liver metastases.[120]

GESTATIONAL TROPHOBLASTIC DISEASE

The serum human chorionic gonadotropin–beta subunit is the most accurate test to detect persistent gestational trophoblastic disease (GTD) and to monitor its treatment. CT is used for imaging persistent local pelvic and metastatic GTD because of its ability to screen the brain, chest, abdomen, and pelvis with one imaging test.[27,80,83,94] CT can detect persistent extrauterine GTD that has invaded the broad ligament, parametria, and pelvic fascia and muscles.[27,94] Also, chest CT can identify pulmonary metastases not detected by chest radiographs.[83]

The classic CT findings of uterine invasive mole or choriocarcinoma are eccentric hypodense foci in the myometrium or endometrial cavity associated with bilateral multilocular theca-lutein cysts.[27,80,94] Dynamic CT shows contrast-enhanced myometrial tumor components (Fig. 38-27, *A*), often in association with dilated uterine arteries in the parametria.[80] Dynamic CT also detects the classic hypervascular metastases of choriocarcinoma (Fig. 38-27, *B*).

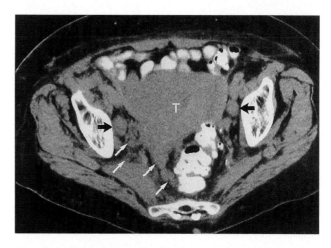

Fig. 38-26. Stage IIIc endometrial cancer. Five millimeters section through large uterine tumor *(T)* shows extensive right parametrial tumor extension *(arrows)* and bilateral obturator lymph node metastases *(arrows)*.

OVARIAN CANCER

Surgery is the staging procedure of choice in evaluating ovarian cancer. Surgery identifies the primary site of disease, determines the tumor spread pattern and stage, provides tumor excision for histologic diagnosis, and allows maximal tumor reduction. When preoperative evaluation of a suspected ovarian carcinoma is indicated, CT is currently considered the imaging modality of choice.[1,60,126] CT is often used to determine tumor extent and thus the amount of cytoreductive surgery that might be required. CT is not as accurate as surgical staging because it may not detect tiny peritoneal tumor implants or omental and mesenteric nodules. MRI has not

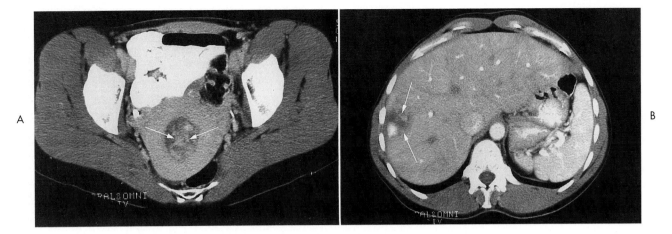

Fig. 38-27. Gestational trophoblastic disease. **A,** CT scan through uterus shows contrast-enhanced tumor *(arrows)* filling dilated endometrial cavity and intact myometrium. **B,** Dynamic CT scan through liver shows hypervascular metastasis *(arrows)*.

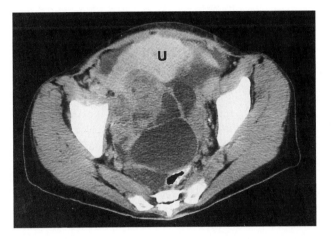

Fig. 38-28. Serous cystadenocarcinoma of the ovary. CT scan at sciatic notch shows huge cancer with multiple cystic loculi and solid components displacing the uterus *(U)* anteriorly.

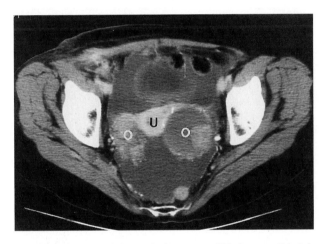

Fig. 38-29. CT scan through the uterus *(U)* shows solid right and cystic and solid left ovarian cancers *(O)* surrounded by ascites.

had a role in ovarian cancer staging because of its limitations in evaluating abdominal disease spread.

The CT features of ovarian cancer include a number of morphological tumor patterns: (1) a multiloculated cyst with thick septations and solid components (Fig. 38-28), (2) a thick-walled cyst, (3) a combined cystic and solid mass (Fig. 38-29), and (4) a uniformly solid mass (see Fig. 38-13). Calcifications and contrast enhancement may be present in the cyst wall or soft tissue tumor components. The CT appearance of ovarian metastases is indistinguishable from a primary ovarian cancer, and images of the stomach and colon should be carefully viewed as potential primary tumor sites.[23,77]

Ovarian cancers are most frequently found in the adnexae, cul-de-sac, or over the sacral promontory. CT is useful in detecting tumor involvement of small and large bowel; encasement of the pelvic ureter; hydronephrosis; metastases to the peritoneum, mesentery, greater omentum (Fig. 38-30), liver, spleen, and pelvic and para-aortic lymph nodes; ascites; and pseudomyxoma peritonei. CT detection of peritoneal tumor implants depends more on their location and surrounding ascites than on size (Fig. 38-31). The three sites where these implants are easiest to detect are the right subphrenic space, the greater omentum, and the cul-de-sac. Current CT scanners can detect 50% of peritoneal implants that are 5 mm in size.[15] CT can also detect psammomatous calcification in plaquelike tumor implants from serous cystadenocar-

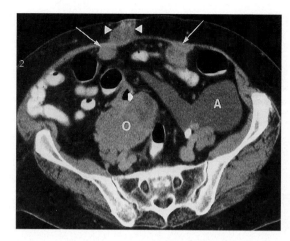

Fig. 38-30. CT scan through solid ovarian cancer *(O)* and ascites *(A)* shows nodular metastases in omental fat *(arrows)* and in the umbilicus *(arrowheads).*

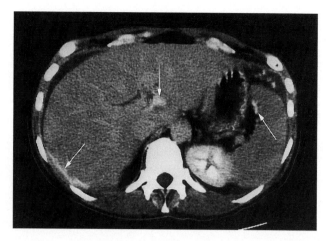

Fig. 38-32. CT scan shows calcified peritoneal tumor implants on the right posterior liver, in the superior recess of the lesser sac, and on the medial spleen *(arrows)* from psammomatous calcification associated with papillary serous cystadenocarcinoma of the ovary.

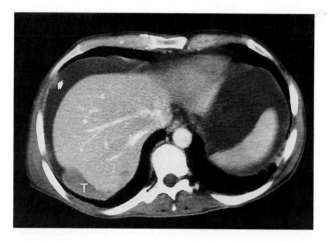

Fig. 38-31. CT scan shows ascites surrounding the liver and spleen, a large tumor implant on the right posterior diaphragm *(T)*, and a small peritoneal tumor implant *(arrowhead)* from metastatic ovarian cancer.

cinoma of the ovary, even in the absence of ascites (Fig. 38-32).[79] The major limitation of CT in staging ovarian cancer is the inability to detect peritoneal, mesenteric, and bowel surface tumor implants less than 5 mm in size.

CT is most commonly used to detect persistent or recurrent ovarian cancer and document tumor response to subsequent therapy.[78,103] CT detection of recurrent tumor, however, has been hampered by both a high false-negative rate owing to small volume tumor deposits and a high false-positive rate owing to misdiagnosis of adherent bowel loops as a tumor mass. These bowel "pseudotumors" may be due to adhesions or the effects of radiation therapy. A study shows that meticulous CT technique with thinner sections and better bowel con-

trast opacification has increased the overall accuracy of recurrent disease detection.[91]

FLUID COLLECTIONS

CT is an important imaging test for diagnosis and management of both intraperitoneal abscesses and extraperitoneal infections involving the iliopsoas muscle, buttock and hip, perirectal compartment, and perineum. CT-guided pelvic abscess drainage by various routes is also well established.[14,41] CT is indicated for evaluation of extraluminal abscesses related to diverticulitis, Crohn's disease (Fig. 38-33), or appendicitis; postoperative fluid collections; and large tubo-ovarian abscesses. Less common pelvic infections well suited for CT diagnosis are gas-forming abscess in diabetics, pyomyositis (Fig. 38-34),[50] supralevator versus infralevator abscess,[49] and a septic hip.[90]

The standard route for CT-guided pelvic abscess drainage is an anterolateral approach through the abdominal wall avoiding bowel, inferior epigastric vessels, and bladder (Fig. 38-35). When this approach is not possible, some pelvic abscesses can be drained through the greater sciatic foramen (Fig. 38-36, *A, B*).[14] A caudal approach through the sacrospinous ligament avoids the sacral plexus and the inferior gluteal vessels. The major disadvantage of this technique, however, is pain in 20% of patients.[14] Alternative routes for drainage of fluid collections in the cul-de-sac are a transrectal approach under CT guidance[41] or a transvaginal approach using US guidance.[116]

Lymphoceles are uncommon pelvic fluid collections that occur several weeks after pelvic lymphadenec-

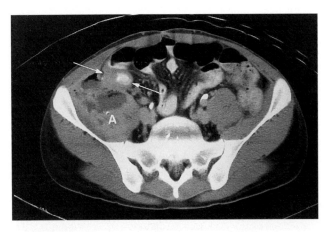

Fig. 38-33. CT scan shows right psoas muscle abscess *(A)* containing fluid and gas adjacent to thick-walled small bowel loop *(arrows)* owing to Crohn's disease.

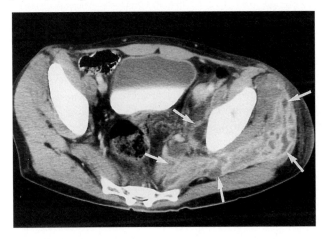

Fig. 38-34. Pyomyositis in a diabetic. CT scan shows extensive fluid collections surrounded by intravenous contrast enhancement involving the left obturator internus, piriformis, and gluteus medius muscles *(arrows)*. Blood cultures grew *Streptococcus pyogenes*.

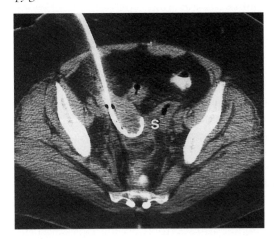

Fig. 38-35. CT scan through the sigmoid colon *(S)* shows a percutaneous catheter via an anterior approach draining a right paracolic abscess from diverticulitis.

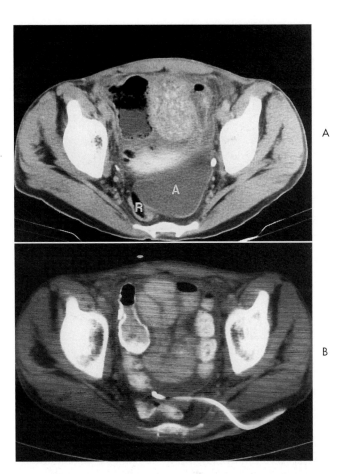

Fig. 38-36. Pelvic abscess. **A,** CT scan shows a pelvic fluid collection *(A)* anterolateral to the rectum *(R)*. **B,** CT scan shows successful catheter drainage through the left sciatic notch.

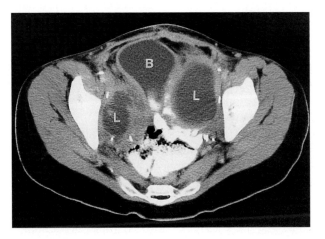

Fig. 38-37. CT scan through bladder *(B)* shows bilateral large lymphoceles *(L)* surrounded by surgical clips from pelvic lymph node dissection.

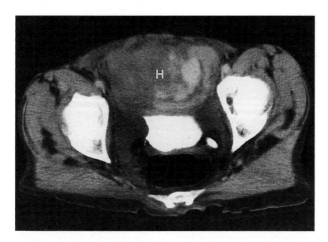

Fig. 38-38. Pubic fractures. CT scan shows large associated hematoma *(H)* in the prevesical space compressing the bladder posteriorly.

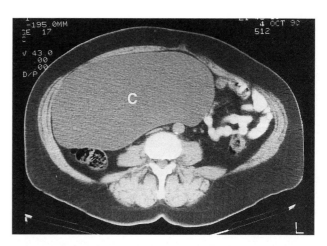

Fig. 38-39. Mucinous cystadenoma of the ovary. CT scan through purely cystic abdominal mass *(C)* in an asymptomatic 66-year-old woman with a palpable mass.

tomy (Fig. 38-37) or renal transplant surgery. These fluid collections characteristically can have a low CT attenuation value (e.g., 10 HU) owing to their fat content, and diagnostic needle aspiration may show characteristic lymphocytes and pathognomonic fat globules. Percutaneous management of lymphoceles requires long-term catheter drainage, and sclerosing agents may be beneficial in closing the lymphatic fistula.[115,125] CT is also a standard imaging test to identify high-density pelvic hemorrhage associated with trauma (Fig. 38-38), anticoagulants, groin catheterization, or a bleeding diathesis.

GYNECOLOGICAL MASSES

US is considered the screening modality of choice for a pelvic mass in women of childbearing age. Transabdominal and transvaginal US are commonly used to characterized ovarian cysts, endometriomas, dermoids, ectopic pregnancy, pelvic inflammatory disease, and uterine leiomyomas. One must be familiar, however, with the CT appearances of ovarian and uterine masses because these lesions may be discovered incidentally.[47,97] Also, middle-aged and older women with large palpable abdominopelvic masses are commonly referred for CT evaluation because the presumptive diagnosis is ovarian cancer. CT is considered superior to US for characterization of benign versus malignant ovarian epithelial tumors.[17] CT and MRI have an equivalent overall accuracy in the evaluation of epithelial tumors of the ovary.[44]

Ovarian masses

The CT features of an ovarian cyst are a homogeneous, unilocular water-density ovarian mass with smooth thin walls and no internal contents.[47,98] Ovarian cysts are frequently functional follicular or corpus lu-

teum cysts, which usually resolve in 1 to 3 months on follow-up US. The differential diagnosis of a cystic adnexal mass includes a cystic teratoma (dermoid), cystadenoma, endometrioma, paraovarian cyst, hydrosalpinx, large bladder diverticulum, mesenteric-duplication cyst, peritoneal inclusion cyst, and unopacified bowel loops. A purely cystic ovarian cancer is rare.[39] Cystadenomas may be unilateral or bilateral unilocular cysts, although they more frequently contain internal septations (Fig. 38-39). Paraovarian cysts arise in the broad ligament between the ovary and fallopian tube, are usually large and unilocular, and may occupy a midline position superior to the bladder. A hydrosalpinx is typically a tubular cystic adnexal mass associated with previous pelvic inflammatory disease or tubal ligation.[112] A peritoneal inclusion cyst is an adnexal collection of fluid between peritoneal adhesions and is associated with a history of multiple surgical procedures for trauma, pelvic inflammatory disease, or endometriosis.[54] Postmenopausal ovarian cysts are being increasingly detected and must be distinguished from ovarian cancer in this age group. Important criteria for diagnosis include a 5-cm maximum allowable diameter, unilocular cyst with no internal components, and no ascites.[46] They should be followed with serial US every 3 to 6 months.

CT criteria for complex adnexal masses include a thick wall, heterogeneous density, internal components, and contour irregularity. The differential diagnosis includes cysts complicated by hemorrhage, infection, or torsion; pelvic inflammatory disease or tubo-ovarian abscess; endometriosis; ectopic pregnancy; benign and malignant ovarian neoplasms; and pelvic abscess. Endometriomas and tubo-ovarian abscesses are usually evaluated with US, but they may be detected on CT done for

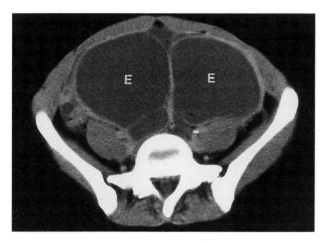

Fig. 38-40. CT scan through bilateral thick-walled giant ovarian endometriomas *(E)* in a 22-year-old woman with intermittent abdominal pain.

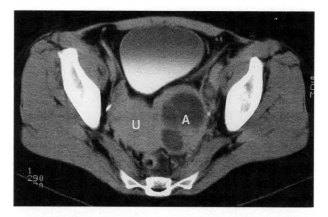

Fig. 38-41. CT scan through the displaced uterus *(U)* shows a thick-walled multilocular left tubo-ovarian abscess *(A)*.

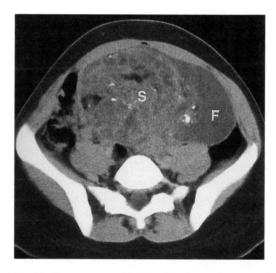

Fig. 38-42. Sixteen-year-old girl with elevated serum alpha-fetoprotein. CT scan through pelvic mass with smaller fluid component *(F)* and large solid component *(S)* containing small areas of fat and calcification indicating a malignant teratoma.

pelvic pain or fever. Older CT literature indicated no standard CT appearance for endometriosis,[35] but a more recent study reports small focal blood clots adjacent to the inner wall in 15% of endometriomas.[18] Bilateral endometriomas may have a characteristic CT pattern of bilateral thick-walled, multilocular cysts, which are indistinguishable from bilateral tubo-ovarian abscesses. (Fig. 38-40).

Tubo-ovarian abscess is a complication of pelvic inflammatory disease that occurs in as many as one third of women admitted for acute salpingitis. The CT spectrum of findings include a tubular fluid-density mass representing a hydrosalpinx or pyosalpinx, a septated thick-walled adnexal cyst representing an ovarian abscess (Fig. 38-41), poor fat planes between pelvic organs, anterior displacement of the mesosalpinx, thickened ureterosacral ligaments, rectosigmoid involvement, ureteractasis, para-aortic lymphadenopathy, and gonadal vein thrombosis.[31,128] In patients who fail antibiotic therapy, CT-guided abscess drainage has an 88% to 94% success rate, and surgery can be avoided in the majority of cases.[21,114]

Ovarian cystadenomas are common ovarian neoplasms, with serous and mucinous forms each composing 20% of all benign ovarian tumors. They may be purely cystic and unilocular (Fig. 38-39) but are more frequently multilocular with thin internal septations without wall thickening or internal solid papillary projections.[98] Mucinous cystadenomas, however, may contain high-density loculi of mucin, which simulates a solid tumor component, or prominent contrast-enhancing septations, which make the tumor indistinguishable from a borderline or malignant cystadenocarcinoma.[17,39] Mature cystic teratoma or dermoid is another common benign ovarian neoplasm. Although the diagnosis is commonly made with a pelvic pain film or US, CT can make a definitive diagnosis in the majority of cases.[16,38] The characteristic CT features include detection of fat, a dermoid plug, hair, teeth, and fat-fluid level. Although malignant teratomas are rare, CT detection of an irregular solid component greater than 5 cm should strongly suggest this diagnosis (Fig. 38-42).[16]

CT is an important imaging modality for differentiating benign from malignant ovarian neoplasms.[17,39,44] CT criteria for a malignant ovarian mass include thickening of the wall or internal septations, papillary projections, and solid tumor components.[39] When a solid component is detected in an ovarian mass, the mass should be considered malignant, although a few

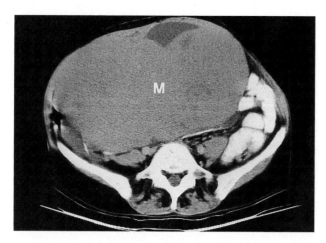

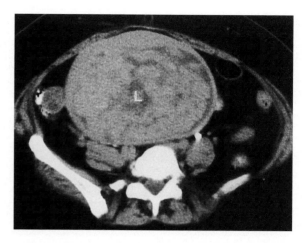

Fig. 38-43. Seventy-seven-year-old woman with large abdominopelvic mass. CT scan through huge, predominantly solid mass *(M)* simulating a giant leiomyoma. At surgery, a benign fibrothecoma of the ovary was removed.

Fig. 38-44. CT scan at iliac crest shows a typical heterogeneous enhancement pattern of a giant leiomyoma *(L)* of the uterus.

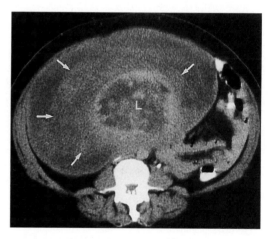

cases (5%) are benign solid tumors.[39] Some benign ovarian tumors, such as fibromas or Brenner's tumors, are uniformly solid and smoothly marginated (Fig. 38-43).[98] Both benign and malignant ovarian neoplasms may contain calcification. The differential diagnosis of a solid adnexal mass includes ovarian neoplasm, pedunculated uterine leiomyoma, metastasis, non-Hodgkin lymphoma, presacral tumor, and retroflexed uterus.

Ovarian (gonadal) vein thrombosis is associated with postpartum puerperal endometritis, obstetrical and gynecological surgery, and pelvic inflammatory disease. Eighty percent to 90% of the cases occur in the right ovarian vein. Both CT and MRI are diagnostic of this complication. The characteristic CT findings are an adnexal mass associated with a well-defined, tubular retroperitoneal mass extending from the pelvis to the infrarenal inferior vena cava.[96]

Uterine leiomyomas

Uterine leiomyomas are the most common solid uterine neoplasm, occurring in 20% to 40% of all women during the reproductive years. Leiomyomas are often found incidentally on CT, or they may present as a palpable mass (Fig. 38-44), sometimes associated with bleeding or pain, or cause symptoms owing to compression of the bladder or rectum. The characteristic CT features of uterine leiomyomas are lobulated uterine enlargement with a deformed outer contour; deformity and eccentricity of the endometrial cavity; mural thickening; a midline location and pear shape; and amorphous popcorn, whorllike, or rimlike calcification.[20,97,109] The presence of coarse dystrophic calcification is the most specific sign of leiomyoma.[20,62] Leiomyomas may be hy-

Fig. 38-45. CT scan through lower abdomen shows uterine leiomyoma *(L)* surrounded by swirls of high-density blood *(arrows)* owing to uterine hemorrhage.

podense, isodense, or hyperdense relative to normal myometrium and may be indistinguishable from endometrial cancer.[97] Leiomyomas may be complicated by necrosis or infection.[20] We have also noted symptomatic leiomyomas associated with infarction or internal hemorrhage (Fig. 38-45). Rare lipomatous uterine tumors caused by lipoleiomyoma or lipoma have also been reported.[28]

LYMPH NODES

CT is commonly used as a screening test for pelvic lymph node metastases from a wide variety of tumors. The overall CT accuracy is 73% to 77%, with a false-negative rate of 15% to 40% owing to tumor in normal-size lymph nodes.[67,121] Lymph node enlargement

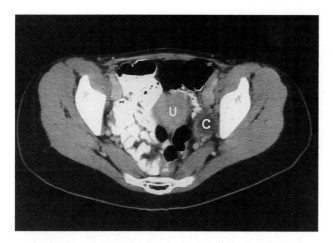

Fig. 38-46. CT scan through the uterus *(U)* shows an unusual lateral position for an ovarian cyst *(C)* simulating a hypodense obturator lymph node metastasis.

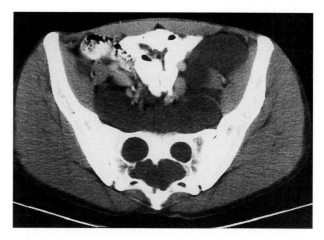

Fig. 38-47. Neurofibromatosis. CT scan shows classic multiple hypodense neurofibromas in the distribution of the femoral nerves and lumbosacral nerve trunks as well as widening of the sacral foramina by neurofibromas.

greater than 15 mm in diameter is the major criterion for diagnosis of metastatic lymphadenopathy, although lymph node enlargement may occasionally be due to chronic lymphadenitis, fatty replacement, or reactive hyperplasia. The differential diagnosis of lymph node metastases includes asymmetrical iliac veins, iliac artery aneurysm, venous thrombosis, a hydroureter, unopacified bowel loops, and the normal ovary (Fig. 38-46).

MUSCULOSKELETAL APPLICATIONS

Until the advent of MRI, CT was the imaging technique of choice in the evaluation of pelvic soft tissue and osseous tumors.[76] Now MRI is considered superior to CT for this application because of its multiplanar capability; superb soft tissue contrast; and ability to define interosseous tumor extent and tumor involvement of neurovascular bundles, specific muscle compartments, and joints.[26] When MRI is not available or contraindicated, CT is an excellent secondary imaging test for evaluating musculoskeletal tumors. Common pelvic soft tissue tumors assessed with CT are lipoma, neurofibroma (Fig. 38-47), ganglioneuroma, hemangiopericytoma, and various soft tissue sarcomas. Commonly evaluated pelvic osseous tumors are chondrosarcoma (Fig. 38-48), osteosarcoma, Ewing's sarcoma, multiple myeloma, lymphoma, metastases, and sacral chordoma.

In patients with sciatica, CT is used to distinguish a mass lesion involving the lumbosacral plexus from a nonstructural cause.[40,42,88] Key CT sections for mass detection are the sacral promontory where the lumbosacral trunk lies posterior to the common iliac vessels and the sciatic notch where the sciatic nerve exits. The types of CT-detected mass lesions causing lumbosacral plexopathy are recurrent pelvic cancers, lymphomas, soft tissue

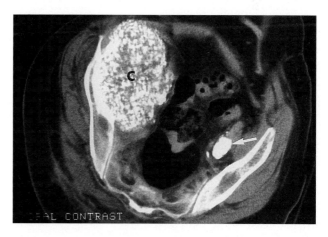

Fig. 38-48. CT scan shows classic right iliac wing chondrosarcoma *(C)* and contralateral hypogastric lymph node metastasis *(arrow)* containing calcified tumor matrix.

sarcomas, bone tumors, metastases, and internal iliac artery aneurysms.[40,42,88] A study suggests that MRI detects a greater percentage of mass lesions involving lumbosacral nerve roots than CT or bone scanning.[9]

Insufficiency stress fractures may occur in the sacrum after radiation therapy or secondary to osteoporosis. These vertical fractures typically occur in the sacral alae, parallel to the sacroiliac joints, and are easily mistaken for metastatic disease. CT is the most accurate means of displaying the fracture and excluding a destructive, neoplastic process.[25]

PELVIMETRY

Pelvimetry is performed to assess the feasibility of vaginal breech delivery. Over the past decade, digital CT pelvimetry has often replaced conventional radiographic pelvimetry because it reduces the absorbed radiation dose to the fetus.[34] The CT technique consists of an anteroposterior digital radiograph to measure the transverse pelvic inlet diameter, a lateral digital radiograph to measure the anteroposterior pelvic inlet diameter, and a single axial scan at the foveae of the femoral heads to measure the distance between the ischial spines.[34] The interspinous diameter is the most important measurement derived from pelvimetry because it is the narrowest midpelvis point where most cases of obstructed labor occur.[3] Careful positioning of the pelvis near the center of the gantry allows the most accurate CT cursor measurements.[34,127] Several problems with this technique, however, have been reported.[3,104,127] The ischial spines may be 0.9 to 1.2 cm below the foveae, and thus an axial scan through the foveae may overestimate the interspinous distance by an average of 1.0 cm.[3] Use of the lateral digital radiograph to localize the level of the ischial spines for an axial section often alleviates this problem. Newer measurement techniques to increase the accuracy of measuring the transverse diameter of the pelvic inlet have been reported.[104,127]

TRAUMA

Bladder injury in pelvic trauma can be classified into contusion, extraperitoneal rupture, intraperitoneal rupture, or combined space rupture. Bladder rupture is an uncommon injury, occurring in 10% of patients with pelvic fractures. Although cystography has been the gold standard for evaluation of bladder trauma, two studies suggest that CT cystography is as sensitive as cystography in detecting bladder injury.[61,71] The advantages of CT cystography are differentiation of extraperitoneal from intraperitoneal collections, visualization of associated pelvic fractures and hematomas, detection of other more life-threatening abdominal injuries, and minimization of patient movement.

The most crucial aspect of CT cystography is adequate bladder distention to detect contrast extravasation. This can be accomplished by instillation of 350 ml of 4% dilute contrast through an indwelling Foley catheter on the CT table[71] or by obtaining delayed CT images through the bladder after maximum antegrade filling with opacified urine.[61] Extraperitoneal bladder rupture is characterized by local extravasation of contrast medium and urine into perivesical fat, anterior thigh, and scrotum and is usually associated with pelvic fractures. Intraperitoneal rupture usually results from a direct blow to a distended bladder, with extravasation of opacified urine from the dome into the peritoneal spaces.

Numerous studies have shown the superiority of CT over plain films of the pelvis for characterizing acetabular and sacral fractures.[52,73,74,81] CT is complemen-

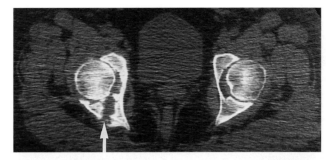

Fig. 38-49. CT scan shows a comminuted vertical fracture through the right posterior column *(arrow)* of the acetabulum.

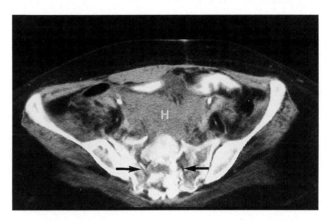

Fig. 38-50. Automobile accident. CT scan shows vertical fractures *(arrows)* through the body of the sacrum and a large anterior hematoma *(H)*.

tary to conventional radiography of the hip because of its axial display of both the anterior and posterior columns and the medial aspect of the acetabulum (quadrilateral surface). More recent development of surface[13] or volumetric[36] rendering CT techniques have enabled three-dimensional imaging of complex acetabular fractures. CT is especially useful for detecting fractures of the posterior acetabular lip (Fig. 38-49) and small intra-articular fracture fragments, mapping fracture fragment position and displacement, and assessing the integrity of the acetabular dome and quadrilateral surface.[52,73,74] Sagittal and coronal reconstructions improve appreciation of the superior hip joint and acetabular dome and allow the most accurate definition of the articular surface and weight-bearing support.[74]

Sacral injuries make up a major component of pelvic ring fractures, occurring in 4% to 74% of patients with pelvic fractures.[81] Sacral fractures are associated with an increased risk of neurological injury, vascular tear and hemorrhage, and pelvic instability. CT has a higher detection rate of sacral injuries than plain films and shows

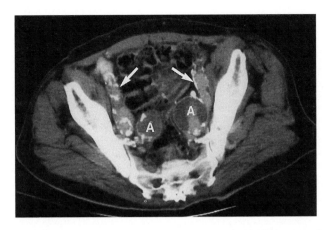

Fig. 38-51. CT scan shows tortuous vertical calcified external iliac arteries *(arrows)* and bilateral internal iliac artery aneurysms *(A)*.

the fracture configuration and extent better.[81] CT is useful for evaluation of sacroiliac diastasis, sacral or iliac lip fractures abutting the sacroiliac joint, vertical shear fractures, and comminuted fractures (Fig. 38-50).

INTERNAL ILIAC ARTERY ANEURYSM

Isolated internal iliac artery aneurysms are rare, but they represent potentially lethal lesions because of their insidious presentation; lack of symptoms until they are quite large; deep location in the pelvis; and difficulty in detection by palpation, radiography, or US. Patients with these aneurysms may present acutely with rupture, rectal bleeding, sacral erosion, and compression of the lumbosacral plexus. CT has been extremely successful in the diagnosis of this uncommon aneurysm and its complications (Fig. 38-51).[8,75,93]

PELVIC LIPOMATOSIS

Pelvic lipomatosis is a rare benign disorder characterized by overgrowth of unencapsulated fat within the pelvis. CT is a useful method to make the diagnosis, exclude a mass, and preclude the need for surgery.[43] The classic CT findings are excess pelvic fat causing a pear-shaped deformity of the bladder and straightening and elongation of the rectosigmoid. Less common findings are hydronephrosis and iliac vein compression.

UNDESCENDED TESTIS

The undescended testis is associated with increased risk of testicular cancer and infertility. Eighty percent of nonpalpable testes are located between the inguinal canal and the internal inguinal ring, and the remaining 20% occur between the internal inguinal ring and the lower pole of the kidney. US can be used to confirm a palpable undescended testis, but it has a low sensitivity in detecting impalpable testes.[37] CT is generally used for detection of impalpable testes in adults.[68,129] The classic CT findings are an oval soft tissue mass in the inguinal canal above the groin or in the internal inguinal ring medial to the external iliac vessels. CT detection of cryptorchid testes in children is difficulty because of their small size and the relative lack of body fat. MRI is probably the procedure of choice for localization of nonpalpable testes in young boys because of its superior sensitivity and lack of ionizing radiation.[63]

REFERENCES

1. Amendola MA, et al: Computed tomography in the evaluation of carcinoma of the ovary. *J Comput Assist Tomogr* 5:179-186, 1981.
2. Amendola MA, et al: Staging of bladder carcinoma: MRI-CT-surgical correlation. *AJR* 146:1179-1183, 1986.
3. Aronson D, Kier R: CT pelvimetry: the foveae are not an accurate landmark for the level of the ischial spines. *AJR* 156:527-530, 1991.
4. Auh YH, et al: Intraperitoneal paravesical spaces: CT delineation with US correlation. *Radiology* 159:311-317, 1986.
5. Auh YH, et al: Extraperitoneal paravesical spaces: CT delineation with US correlation. *Radiology* 159:319-328, 1986.
6. Balfe DM, et al: Computed tomography in malignant endometrial neoplasms. *J Comput Assist Tomogr* 7:677-681, 1983.
7. Bandy LC, et al: Computed tomography in evaluation of extrapelvic lymphadenopathy in carcinoma of the cervix. *Obstet Gynecol* 65:73-76, 1985.
8. Baron RL, Banner MP, Pollack HM: Isolated internal iliac artery aneurysms presenting as giant pelvic masses. *AJR* 140:784-786, 1983.
9. Beatrous TE, Choyke PL, Frank JA: Diagnostic evaluation of cancer patients with pelvic pain: comparison of scintigraphy, CT and MR imaging. *AJR* 155:85-88, 1990.
10. Bezzi M, et al: Prostatic carcinoma: staging with MR imaging at 1.5 T. *Radiology* 169:339-346, 1988.
11. Brick SH, et al: Urachal carcinoma: CT findings. *Radiology* 169:377-381, 1988.
12. Bryan PJ, et al: CT and MR imaging in staging bladder neoplasms. *J Comput Assist Tomogr* 11:96-101, 1987.
13. Burk L Jr, et al: Three-dimensional computed tomography of acetabular fractures. *Radiology* 155:183-186, 1985.
14. Butch RJ, et al: Drainage of pelvic abscesses through the greater sciatic foramen. *Radiology* 158:487-491, 1986.
15. Buy JN, et al: Peritoneal implants from ovarian tumors: CT findings. *Radiology* 169:691-694, 1988.
16. Buy JN, et al: Cystic teratoma of the ovary: CT detection. *Radiology* 171:697-701, 1989.
17. Buy JN, et al: Epithelial tumors of the ovary: CT findings and correlation with US. *Radiology* 178:811-818, 1991.
18. Buy JN, et al: Focal hyperdense areas in endometriomas: a characteristic finding on CT. *AJR* 159:769-771, 1992.
19. Camilien L, et al: Predictive value of computerized tomography in the presurgical evaluation of primary carcinoma of the cervix. *Gynecol Oncol* 30:209-215, 1988.
20. Casillas J, Joseph RC, Guerra JJ: CT appearance of uterine leiomyomas. *Radiographics* 10:999-1007, 1990.
21. Casola G, et al: Percutaneous drainage of tubo-ovarian abscesses. *Radiology* 182:399-402, 1992.
22. Castellino RA: Lymph nodes of the posterior iliac crest: CT and lymphographic observations. *Radiology* 175:687-689, 1990.

23. Cho KC, Gold BM: Computed tomography of Krukenberg tumors. *AJR* 145:285-288, 1985.

24. Colleen S, et al: Staging of bladder carcinoma with computed tomography. *Scand J Urol Nephrol* 15:109-113, 1981.

25. Cooper KL, Beabout JW, Swee RG: Insufficiency fractures of the sacrum. *Radiology* 156:15-20, 1985.

26. Dalinka MK, et al: The use of magnetic resonance imaging in the evaluation of bone and soft-tissue tumors. *Radiol Clin North Am* 28:461-470, 1990.

27. Davis WK, et al: Computed tomography of gestational trophoblastic disease. *J Comput Assist Tomogr* 8:1136-1139, 1984.

28. Dodd GD III, Budzik RF Jr: Lipomatous uterine tumors: diagnosis by ultrasound, CT, and MR. *J Comput Assist Tomogr* 14:629-632, 1990.

29. Dore R, et al: CT evaluation of myometrium invasion in endometrial carcinoma. *J Comput Assist Tomogr* 11:282-289, 1987.

30. Ebner F, et al: Tumor recurrence versus fibrosis in the female pelvis: differentiation with MR imaging at 1.5 T. *Radiology* 166:333-340, 1988.

31. Ellis JH, et al: CT findings in tuboovarian abscess. *J Comput Assist Tomogr* 15:589-592, 1991.

32. Ellis JH, et al: Transitional cell carcinoma of the bladder: patterns of recurrence after cystectomy as determined by CT. *AJR* 157:999-1002, 1991.

33. Emory TH, et al: Use of CT to reduce understaging in prostatic cancer: comparison with conventional staging techniques. *AJR* 141:351-354, 1983.

34. Federle MP, et al: Pelvimetry by digital radiography: a low-dose examination. *Radiology* 143:733-735, 1982.

35. Fishman EK, et al: Computed tomography of endometriosis. *J Comput Assist Tomogr* 7:257-264, 1983.

36. Fishman EK, et al: Volumetric rendering techniques: applications for three-dimensional imaging of the hip. *Radiology* 163:737-738, 1987.

37. Friedland GW, Chang P: The role of imaging in the management of the impalpable undescended testis. *AJR* 151:1107-1111, 1988.

38. Friedman AC, et al: CT of benign cystic teratomas. *AJR* 138:659-665, 1982.

39. Fukuda T, et al: Computed tomography of ovarian masses. *J Comput Assist Tomogr* 10:990-996, 1986.

40. Gaeta M, et al: Pelvic carcinomatous neuropathy: CT findings and implications for radiation treatment planning. *J Comput Assist Tomogr* 12:811-816, 1988.

41. Gazelle GS, et al: Pelvic abscesses: CT-guided transrectal drainage. *Radiology* 181:49-51, 1991.

42. Gebarski KS, et al: The lumbosacral plexus: anatomic-radiologic-pathologic correlation using CT. *Radiographics* 6:401-425, 1986.

43. Gerson ES, Gerzof SG, Robbins AH: CT confirmation of pelvic lipomatosis: two cases. *AJR* 129:338-340, 1977.

44. Ghossain MA, et al: Epithelial tumors of the ovary: comparison of MR and CT findings. *Radiology* 181:863-870, 1991.

45. Ginaldi S, et al: Carcinoma of the cervix: lymphangiography and computed tomography. *AJR* 136:1087-1091, 1981.

46. Goldstein SR, et al: The postmenopausal cystic adnexal mass: the potential role of ultrasound in conservative management. *Obstet Gynecol* 73:8-10, 1989.

47. Gross BH, et al: Computed tomography of gynecologic diseases. *AJR* 141:765-773, 1983.

48. Grumbine FC, et al: Abdominopelvic computed tomography in the preoperative evaluation of early cervical cancer. *Gynecol Oncol* 12:286-290, 1991.

49. Guillaumin E, et al: Perirectal inflammatory disease: CT findings. *Radiology* 161:153-157, 1986.

50. Hall RL, et al: Pyomyositis in a temperature climate. *J Bone Joint Surg* 72-A:1240-1244, 1990.

51. Hamlin DJ, Burgener FA, Beecham JB: CT of intramural endometrial carcinoma: contrast enhancement is essential. *AJR* 137:551-554, 1981.

52. Harley JD, Mack LA, Winquist RA: CT of acetabular fractures: comparison with conventional radiography. *AJR* 138:413-417, 1982.

53. Hasumi K, et al: Computed tomography in the evaluation and treatment of endometrial carcinoma. *Cancer* 50:904-908, 1982.

54. Hoffer FA, et al: Peritoneal inclusion cysts: ovarian fluid in peritoneal adhesions. *Radiology* 169:189-191, 1988.

55. Hricak H, et al: Invasive cervical carcinoma: comparison of MR imaging and surgical findings. *Radiology* 166:623-631, 1988.

56. Husband JE, Bellamy EA: Unusual thoracoabdominal sites of metastases in testicular tumors. *AJR* 145:1165-1171, 1985.

57. Husband JE, Hawkes DJ, Peckham MJ: CT estimations of mean attenuation values and volume in testicular tumors: a comparison with surgical and histologic findings. *Radiology* 144:553-558, 1982.

58. Husband JE, et al: Bladder cancer: staging with CT and MR imaging. *Radiology* 173:435-440, 1989.

59. Jeffrey RB, Palubinskas AJ, Federle MP: CT evaluation of invasive lesions of the bladder. *J Comput Assist Tomogr* 5:22-26, 1981.

60. Johnson RJ, et al: Abdomino-pelvic computed tomography in the management of ovarian carcinoma. *Radiology* 146:447-452, 1983.

61. Kane NM, Francis IR, Ellis JH: The value of CT in the detection of bladder and posterior urethral injuries. *AJR* 153:1243-1246, 1989.

62. Karasick S, Lev-Toaff AS, Toaff ME: Imaging of uterine leiomyomas. *AJR* 158:799-805, 1992.

63. Kier R, et al: Nonpalpable testes in young boys: evaluation with MR imaging. *Radiology* 169:429-433, 1988.

64. Kilcheski TS, et al: Role of computed tomography in the presurgical evaluation of carcinoma of the cervix. *J Comput Assist Tomogr* 5:378-383, 1981.

65. Kim SH, et al: Uterine cervical carcinoma: comparison of CT and MR findings. *Radiology* 175:45-51, 1990.

66. Koss JC, et al: CT staging of bladder carcinoma. *AJR* 137:359-362, 1981.

67. Lee JKT, et al: Accuracy of CT in detecting intraabdominal and pelvic lymph node metastases from pelvic cancers. *AJR* 131:675-679, 1978.

68. Lee JKT, et al: Utility of computed tomography in the localization of the undescended testis. *Radiology* 135:121-125, 1980.

69. Lee JKT, et al: Use of CT in evaluation of postcystectomy patients. *AJR* 136:483-487, 1981.

70. Levine MS, et al: Detecting lymphatic metastases from prostatic carcinoma: superiority of CT. *AJR* 137:207-211, 1981.

71. Lis LE, Cohen AJ: CT cystography in the evaluation of bladder trauma. *J Comput Assist Tomogr* 14:386-389, 1990.

72. Lorigan JG, et al: The growing teratoma syndrome: an unusual manifestation of treated, nonseminomatous germ cell tumors of the testis. *AJR* 151:325-329, 1988.

73. Mack LA, Harley JD, Winquist RA: CT of acetabular fractures: analysis of fracture patterns. *AJR* 138:407-412, 1982.

74. Magid D, Fishman EK: Computed tomography of acetabular fractures. *Semin US CT MR* 7:351-361, 1986.

75. Manaster BJ, Greenberg M, Rubin JM: Isolated internal iliac artery aneurysms. *J Comput Assist Tomogr* 6:845-846, 1982.

76. McLeod RA: Pelvic skeletal tumors. In Walsh JW, editor: *Computed tomography of the pelvis*, New York, 1985, Churchill Livingstone.

77. Megibow AJ, et al: Ovarian metastases: computed tomographic appeaances. *Radiology* 156:161-164, 1985.

78. Megibow AJ, et al: Accuracy of CT in detection of persistent or recurrent ovarian carcinoma: correlation with second-look laparotomy. *Radiology* 166:341-345, 1988.

79. Mitchell DG, et al: Serous carcinoma of the ovary: CT identification of metastatic calcified implants. *Radiology* 158:649-652, 1986.

80. Miyasaka Y, et al: CT evaluation of invasive trophoblastic disease. *J Comput Assist Tomogr* 9:459-462, 1985.

81. Montana MA, et al: CT of sacral injury. *Radiology* 161:499-503, 1986.

82. Morgan CL, et al: Computed tomography in the evaluation, staging, and therapy of carcinoma of the bladder and prostate. *Radiology* 140:751-761, 1981.

83. Mutch DG, et al: Role of computed axial tomography of the chest in staging patients with nonmetastatic gestational trophoblastic disease. *Obstet Gynecol* 68:348-352, 1986.

84. Narumi Y, et al: Vesical dome tumors: significance of extravesical extension on CT. *Radiology* 169:383-385, 1988.

85. Narumi Y, et al: Squamous cell carcinoma of the uroepithelium: CT evaluation. *Radiology* 173:853-856, 1989.

86. Oliva L, et al: CT evaluation of the pelvic cavity after cystectomy: observation in 40 cases. *J Comput Assist Tomogr* 8:734-738, 1984.

87. Panicek DM, et al: Nonseminomatous germ cell tumors: enlarging masses despite chemotherapy. *Radiology* 175:499-502, 1990.

88. Pech P, Haughton V: A correlative CT and anatomic study of the sciatic nerve. *AJR* 144:1037-1041, 1985.

89. Platt JF, Bree RL, Schwab RE: The accuracy of CT in the staging of carcinoma of the prostate. *AJR* 149:315-318, 1987.

90. Resnik CS, Ammann AM, Walsh JW: Chronic septic arthritis of the adult hip: computed tomographic features. *Skel Radiol* 16:513-516, 1987.

91. Reuter KL, Griffin T, Hunter RE: Comparison of abdominopelvic computed tomography results and findings at second-look laparotomy in ovarian carcinoma patients. *Cancer* 63:1123-1128, 1989.

92. Sager EM, et al: The role of CT in demonstrating perivesical tumor growth in the preoperative staging of carcinoma of the urinary bladder. *Radiology* 146:443-446, 1983.

93. Samuelsson L, Albrechtsson U: Ruptured aneurysm of the internal iliac artery. *J Comput Assist Tomogr* 6:842-844, 1982.

94. Sanders C, Rubin E: Malignant gestational trophoblastic disease: CT findings. *AJR* 148:165-168, 1987.

95. Sarno RC, Klauber G, Carter BL: Computer assisted tomography of urachal abnormalities. *J Comput Assist Tomogr* 7:674-676, 1983.

96. Savader SJ, Otero RR, Savader BL: Pureperal ovarian vein thrombosis: evaluation with CT, US, and MR imaging. *Radiology* 167:637-639, 1988.

97. Sawyer RW, Walsh JW: CT in gynecologic pelvic diseases. *Semin US CT MR* 9:122-142, 1988.

98. Sawyer RW, et al: Computed tomography of benign ovarian masses. *J Comput Assist Tomogr* 9:784-789, 1985.

99. Scatarige JC, et al: Low attenuation nodal metastases in testicular carcinoma. *J Comput Assist Tomogr* 7:682-687, 1983.

100. Schnall MD, et al: Prostate cancer: local staging with endorectal surface coil MR imaging. *Radiology* 178:797-802, 1991.

101. Scott WW Jr, et al: The obstructed uterus. *Radiology* 141:767-770, 1981.

102. Seidelmann FE, et al: Accuracy of CT staging of bladder neoplasms using the gas-filled method: report of 21 patients with surgical confirmation. *AJR* 130:735-739, 1978.

103. Silverman PM, et al: CT prior to second-look operation in ovarian cancer. *AJR* 150:829-832, 1988.

104. Smith RC, McCarthy S: Improving the accuracy of digital CT pelvimetry. *J Comput Assist Tomogr* 15:787-789, 1991.

105. Spataro RF, et al: Urachal abnormalities in the adult. *Radiology* 149:659-663, 1983.

106. Steinfeld AD: Testicular germ cell tumors: review of contemporary evaluation and management. *Radiology* 175:603-606, 1990.

107. Stomper PC, et al: CT evaluation of advanced seminoma treated with chemotherapy. *AJR* 146:745-748, 1986.

108. Stomper PC, et al: CT and pathologic predictive features of residual mass histologic findings after chemotherapy for nonseminomatous germ cell tumors: can residual malignancy or teratoma be excluded? *Radiology* 180:711-714, 1991.

109. Tada S, et al: Computed tomographic features of uterine myoma. *J Comput Assist Tomogr* 5:866-869, 1981.

110. Tempany CMC, et al: Invasion of the neurovascular bundle by prostate cancer: evaluation with MR imaging. *Radiology* 181:107-112, 1991.

111. Tisnado J, et al: Computed tomography of the perineum. *AJR* 136:475-481, 1981.

112. Togashi K, et al: Computed tomography of hydrosalpinx following tubal ligation. *J Comput Assist Tomogr* 10:78-80, 1986.

113. Togashi K, et al: Carcinoma of the cervix: staging with MR imaging. *Radiology* 171:245-251, 1989.

114. Tyrrel RT, Murphy FB, Bernardino ME: Tubo-ovarian abscesses: CT-guided percutaneous drainage. *Radiology* 175:87-89, 1990.

115. vanSonnenberg E, et al: Lymphoceles: imaging characteristics and percutaneous management. *Radiology* 161:593-596, 1986.

116. vanSonnenberg E, et al: US-guided transvaginal drainage of pelvic abscesses and fluid collections. *Radiology* 181:53-56, 1991.

117. Vick CW, et al: CT of the normal and abnormal parametria in cervical cancer. *AJR* 143:597-603, 1984.

118. Villasanta U, et al: Computed tomography in invasive carcinoma of the cervix: an appraisal. *Obstet Gynecol* 62:218-224, 1983.

119. Walsh JW, Goplerud DR: Prospective comparison between clinical and CT staging in primary cervical carcinoma. *AJR* 137:997-1003, 1981.

120. Walsh JW, Goplerud DR: Computed tomography of primary, persistent, and recurrent endometrial malignancy. *AJR* 139:1149-1154, 1982.

121. Walsh JW, et al: Computed tomographic detection of pelvic and inguinal lymph-node metastases from primary and recurrent pelvic malignant disease. *Radiology* 137:157-166, 1980.

122. Walsh JW, et al: Recurrent carcinoma of the cervix: CT diagnosis. *AJR* 136:117-122, 1981.

123. Wechsler RJ, Schilling JF: CT of the gluteal region. *AJR* 144:185-190, 1985.

124. Weinerman PM, et al: Pelvic adenopathy from bladder and prostate carcinoma: detection by rapid-sequence computed tomography. *AJR* 140:95-99, 1983.

125. White M, et al: Percutaneous drainage of postoperative abdominal and pelvic lymphoceles. *AJR* 145:1065-1069, 1985.

126. Whitley N, et al: Use of the computed tomographic whole body scanner to stage and follow patients with advanced ovarian carcinoma. *Invest Radiol* 16:479-486, 1981.

127. Wiesen EJ, et al: Improvement in CT pelvimetry. *Radiology* 178:259-262, 1991.

128. Wilbur AC, Aizenstein RI, Napp TE: CT findings in tuboovarian abscess. *AJR* 158:575-579, 1992.

129. Wolverson MK, et al: CT in localization of impalpable cryptorchid testes. *AJR* 134:725-729, 1980.

39

Magnetic Resonance Imaging of the Pelvis

ERIC K. OUTWATER

Since the first clinical reports of magnetic resonance (MR) imaging of the pelvis a decade ago,[23,32] both the technical quality and range of applications of pelvic MR imaging have steadily increased. High cost, slow spread of technical expertise in the community, as well as the absence of unequivocal clinical indications have delayed the widespread acceptance of MR as an important imaging technique in the pelvis. Nonetheless, MR imaging has some definite advantages over other techniques of pelvic imaging, and further technical advances will serve to expand the range of applications.

The great challenge in pelvic imaging is the search for a cross-sectional technique that combines very high resolution with high tissue contrast and tissue specificity, sufficient safety to apply to pregnant patients, and low-enough cost to apply in common clinical situations. Needless to say, no current technique currently fulfills all these criteria across a broad spectrum of applications. Ultrasonography is the current imaging procedure of choice for most pelvic disorders. Its safety is established, and it provides sufficient depiction of normal and pathologic anatomy for routine assessment of many gynecologic and almost all obstetric disorders. Endoluminal probes and color Doppler imaging further expand the applications of ultrasonography in the pelvis. Nonetheless, pelvic ultrasonography has serious limitations. It is not suitable for one of the largest potential clinical applications, tumor staging. Resolution and tissue contrast are not sufficient for accurate staging of any genitourinary malignancies, male or female. In addition, the accuracy of diagnosis of adnexal masses is not sufficient to obviate laparoscopy in many cases.

CT provides a more systematic examination of the pelvis, and it is better suited to defining bowel involvement in inflammatory and neoplastic disorders, compared with ultrasonography. CT is superior to ultrasound in depicting fat planes and adenopathy, which are important to staging of malignancies. Aside from adipose tissue, however, soft-tissue contrast is intrinsically poor on CT images in the pelvis. Zonal anatomy of the uterus or of the prostate is difficult to demonstrate by CT. This tissue contrast, as well as the potential radiation risk in women of childbearing age, limits the general applicability of CT in the pelvis.

Early investigators realized four potential advantages of MRI over conventional imaging techniques in the pelvis: (1) Direct multiplanar imaging, which is essential for clear depiction of organ anatomy and tissue planes in the pelvis, (2) Intrinsic soft tissue contrast of pelvic organs appeared to be high on MR images, because of the multiple parameters of tissue proton relaxation that contribute to the MR signal, (3) The unique characteristics of moving protons on MR images promised unequivocal identification of vessels without using intravascular contrast, and (4) MR imaging appeared to be safe in pregnant patients. These basic observations have provided the impetus for further research into potential clinical applications of MR imaging in the pelvis.

NEWER MR IMAGING TECHNIQUES IN THE PELVIS

The quality of MR images of the brain, spine, and musculoskeletal system exceeds that obtained in the chest, abdomen, and pelvis primarily because of motion effects (respiratory, bowel peristalsis, and cardiac) and the lack of local receiver coils in the latter applications. Pelvic MR images are the least susceptible to motion effects, but they still suffer from suboptimal resolution because of the relatively large fields of view necessary to sustain a satisfactory signal-to-noise ratio. In addition, long examination times are necessary to acquire the long TR/TE spin-echo images in multiple planes needed to portray the pelvic structures adequately. Helmholtz coil arrangements (e.g., paired 5-inch coils) increase signal to noise but they are essentially restricted to imaging a pre-identified single anatomic area and do not provide a systematic evaluation of the entire pelvis. Two technical innovations, multicoil and fast spin-echo sequences, can increase the signal-to-noise ratio in pelvic images and can shorten the acquisition time of long TR/TE pulse sequences. This time savings can be used for higher-resolution matrices, acquisitions in multiple planes, or thinner sections, all of which are important in imaging the uterine adnexae. These two innovations have general applicability in imaging the pelvic structures. In addition, improved methods of chemical shift imaging and vascular imaging allow for an added dimension to an overall examination of the pelvis.[191,253,254]

Surface coils

Two newer strategies have been developed for imaging the pelvis with surface coils. These are endoluminal surface coils and multiple arrays of external surface coils. Both of these take advantage of the higher signal-to-noise ratio achievable with small diameter receiver coils to achieve smaller fields of view and hence higher resolution than that obtainable with the whole-volume body coils in the bore of the magnet system. These techniques are more widely applicable to imaging the pelvis than are surface coil arrangements, (such as a single-loop anterior surface coil for imaging the scrotum) that have always been available.

Endoluminal surface coils increase the signal-to-noise ratio achievable with small (10 to 12 cm) fields of view. The sensitivity profile of these small diameter coils falls off steeply with distance away from the coil, so that they are suited only for perirectal structures and organs such as the prostate[235] and rectum.[45] Endorectal surface coils can also image the cervix with high resolution, and can show cervical carcinoma, as well as tumor invasion into the parametria.[176] Intravaginal coils for imaging the cervix have also been developed.[18] As a group, these coils are less suited for imaging very bulky cervical tumors or other gynecologic neoplasms.

Multicoil ("phased array") arrangements have been designed for imaging the spine, abdomen, chest, and pelvis. Multicoil technique uses multiple separate receiver coils, preamplifiers, receiver channels, digitizers, and memory.[102,224] The signal from each receiver is separately transformed and generates separate data sets that are then reconstructed into a single composite image using a sum of the squares algorithm. Each coil is designed with a smaller effective diameter than would otherwise be used for a given volume of interest. The result is a composite image that can adequately include a larger area, but with the same or higher signal-to-noise ratio

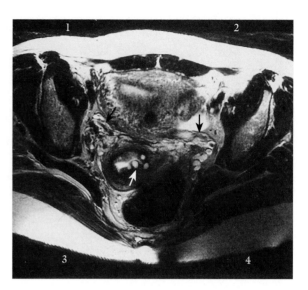

Fig. 39-1. Multicoil imaging of the pelvis. The white numbers (1 to 4) identify the transverse arrangement of the four coils. Coil number 4 is not receiving signal; this leads to a loss of signal intensity in the left posterior pelvis. Axial FSE image through the cervix and anteflexed uterine fundus shows dilated glands *(white arrow)* in the endocervical mucosa, an 8-mm uterine fibroid, and veins in the broad ligament *(black arrows)*. (TR/TE$_{eff}$ of 4000/140, 512 × 512 acquisition matrix, 28-cm FOV, 6-mm–slice thickness.)

of a smaller diameter coil.[102,224] The images in this chapter use a four-coil multicoil arrangement with two 5-inch coils anteriorly and two coils posteriorly. For imaging the true pelvis, coils can be arranged either cranio-caudad or transversely (Fig. 39-1).

Multicoil shares the disadvantages of all surface coils. The primary disadvantage is an intense signal near the coil, with a steep gradient of signal loss away from the coil.[168] This near-field effect renders the image very susceptible to ghosting artifacts that arise along the phase-encoding axis from motion of structures[168] (Fig. 39-2). These ghost artifacts may be ameliorated by judicious choice of phase-encoding direction, anterior saturation bands,[253] fat-suppression techniques, and physical restriction of the anterior pelvic wall. In addition, multicoil technology imposes additional burdens of increased memory demands and lengthened reconstruction times. Lastly, the signal-to-noise benefit of multicoil compared with the body coil may be lost in particularly large patients or in pregnant patients, because of the fall-off of sensitivity of the coils in the center of the imaging volume.[253]

Fast spin-echo imaging

The development of fast spin-echo sequences (variants called FSE, FAISE, Turbo spin echo) was con-

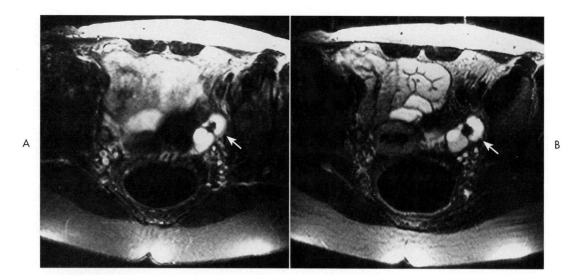

Fig. 39-2. Use of glucagon to suppress motion artifact. Axial FSE images before **(A)** and after **(B)** the intravenous administration of 0.1 mg glucagon. Glucagon significantly improves the definition of the ileal wall and also results in fewer ghosting artifacts in the phase-encoding (right-to-left) axis. In both images, the septated high signal intensity left ovarian mass *(arrow)* with a central low-signal–intensity mural nodule (cystadenofibroma) is well depicted. (TR/ TE$_{eff}$ of 4000/120, 256 × 256 acquisition matrix, 24-cm FOV, 6-mm–slice thickness.)

ceptually based on the RARE (rapid acquisition with re-laxation enhancement) pulse sequence first introduced by Hennig et al.[108] These sequences employ multiple closely spaced refocusing pulses, called an *echo train,* for every 90° pulse. Conventional spin-echo imaging uses a single refocusing pulse and acquires only one phase-encoded step per 90° pulse. Thus, a typical fast spin-echo sequence with an echo train length of 16 refocusing pulses reduces the acquisition time sixteenfold. This al-lows larger acquisition matrices, or a greater number of acquisitions. The drawback of FSE is that fewer sections can be obtained in multislice acquisitions because a greater portion of TR is devoted to the echo train. How-ever, interslice gaps can be avoided by performing two contiguous interleaved acquisitions.

Contrast in FSE may be manipulated by ordering of phase-encoding trajectories in k-space. The time be-tween the 90° pulse and the *n*th signal that is assigned to the lowest order phase-encoding step in k-space de-termines the effective TE (TE$_{eff}$). These low-order–phase encoding steps determine the relative contrast, or T2 weighting, of the sequence.[56,57] T2-weighted FSE im-ages generally show contrast similar to that of SE se-quences.[58,10] Compared with SE sequences, several mechanisms act, in most instances subtly, to alter tissue contrast. These include, among others, modulation of J-coupling effects in lipids, exaggeration of magnetiza-tion transfer effects, and T2-dependent alteration of the point-spread function.[56,57,90]

The most obvious difference in contrast between

FSE and SE image is the increased signal from fat on FSE images. In conventional SE sequences, lipid protons un-dergo phase dispersion as a result of the different chemi-cal shifts of these protons produced by spin-spin cou-plings (J-coupling) of hydrocarbon chain protons. This results in a relative loss in signal from lipids. In FSE im-ages this phase dispersion is reduced by frequent refo-cusing, resulting in a preservation of the lipid signal on FSE images. The exact clinical situation will determine whether the high signal fat on T-weighted sequences be-comes a help or a hindrance in interpreting the images. As a general rule, the use of a TE$_{eff}$, which is longer than the TE used in conventional T2-weighted spin-echo se-quences, is preferable. This achieves more heavily T2-weighted images with correspondingly less fat signal and relatively better conspicuity of edema, tumors, and so forth.

Almost all FSE and SE imaging is performed clini-cally with multislice sequences. In this mode, every slice receives irradiation from RF applied to the other slices at various frequencies off-resonance during application of the slice-select gradient.[173] This off-resonance irradia-tion has both direct saturation effects and magnetization transfer effects.[292] The effect of both of these is a reduc-tion in signal intensity, compared with an acquisition of a single slice only.[56,173] Direct saturation effects can be predicted by the Bloch equations; they are T1- and T2-dependent and will generally only occur in adjacent slices with a narrow gap because the effect is strongly depen-dent on the offset frequency.[292]

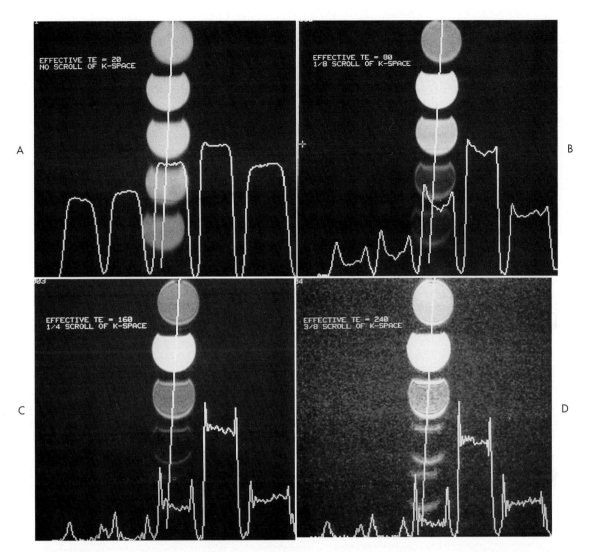

Fig. 39-3. Edge effects in fast spin-echo imaging. Shown are signal intensity histograms through the five phantoms which consist of *(from top to bottom)* vegetable oil, 0.1-mm, 0.2-mm, 0.3-mm, and 0.4-mm manganese chloride solution. The signal intensity plot of the line through the phantoms is shown at the bottom of each image. These FSE images were performed with an effective TE of 20 **(A)**, 80 **(B)**, 160 **(C)**, and 240 **(D)**. Note the enhancement of the edge in the phase encoding direction of the phantoms at the longer echo times, and edge blurring at the TE of 20, particularly in the phantoms with the shorter T2 values.

The magnetization transfer effect is less dependent on the offset frequency and can be demonstrated by observing the difference in contrast between a single-slice acquisition and a multislice acquisition performed with large interslice gaps to eliminate the direct saturation effect.[173] It results from irradiation of very broad spectrum (ultrashort T2) protons, which are associated with macromolecules. These protons transfer magnetization (saturation) to the surrounding water protons, which are the source of the observable MR signal. The result is signal loss in voxels containing a greater proportion of macromolecules. Seen in both SE[69] and FSE,[173]

it is more important in FSE because of the shorter time interval between successive 180° RF pulses that reduces the longitudinal relaxation of the saturated protons.[56,57,90]

The effect of magnetization transfer on MR signal in various normal tissues has been described in detail,[292,293] although the implications for pathologic tissue contrast in body applications in general, and pelvic applications in particular, have gone almost entirely unreported. For all practical purposes, the degree of this effect cannot be predicted for a given tissue, but must be empirically observed. In general, magnetization transfer reduces the signal of solid tissues, especially muscle, with lesser reductions of proteinaceous fluid and blood signal and virtually no effect on water or fat.[197,292,293] Tumors also demonstrate saturation transfer, whereas cysts do not.[197] In FSE imaging, magnetization transfer will lead to relatively lower signal in solid tissues, compared with cysts and other fluids, and will tend to add to the already high fat-tissue contrast.

Finally, the effects of the point-spread function can work to alter edge definition of some objects in FSE images.[56,57] FSE phase-encoded steps are acquired during the evolution of T2 decay. Just as contrast is determined by the position of the low spatial frequencies in k-space, the placement of high spatial frequencies determines the fidelity of edges. This can lead to an edge enhancement if the high spatial frequencies are collected at the early echoes (heavily T2-weighted), or it can result in edge blurring if the high spatial frequencies are collected at the late echoes (intermediate weighting).[56,57] Edge enhancement occurs with long T2 structures, whereas short T2 structures will tend to be blurred[90] (Fig. 39-3). In addition, small objects of relatively short T2 lose contrast on FSE images and may be obscured.[57] The practical result in pelvis imaging is a slight additional sharpness and conspicuity of cysts and other fluid collections in FSE images acquired with long TE_{eff} (>100 ms). This effect may combine with magnetization transfer effects to highlight small ovarian cysts and other small fluid collections.[191]

For the pelvis the fast spin-echo sequence is particularly well suited to heavily T2-weighted images with TE_{eff} of 80-140 and TR 3000-4000 ms.[254,253] A 256 × 256 acquisition matrix is used in conjunction with a 18 to 24 cm field of view when using the phased array coil, although finer matrices can be sustained in the pelvis. Four to five millimeter slices are obtained in an interleaved fashion. Respiratory gating and gradient-moment nulling are usually unnecessary because respiratory motion artifacts are not usually a significant problem in pelvic MRI. Artifacts related to bowel motion can be suppressed with the use of glucagon.

Chemical-shift imaging

Various forms of fat-suppression techniques have been developed and have widespread clinical utility in imaging the pelvis.[181,143] These include chemical-shift–sensitive methods (frequency-selective fat saturation[142]), phase-sensitive methods (Dixon technique[68,244] chopper-Dixon method,[261] and opposed-phase gradient-echo sequences[285]), and inversion recovery technique (STIR), which suppresses all tissues with a T1 approximating that of fat. The latter technique is not chemical-shift specific and therefore does not unequivocally identify fat-containing tissue.[181] It has generally limited applicability in evaluating the soft-tissue structures of the pelvis.

Frequency-selective fat saturation is the most widely available of the techniques. It can be applied to

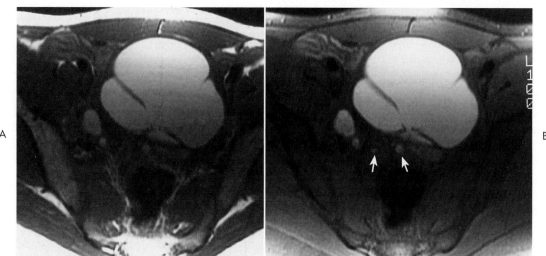

Fig. 39-4. Chemical shift imaging of endometriomas. **A,** Axial SE 800/11 image demonstrates bilateral adnexal masses with signal intensity approaching fat. The left adnexal mass is partially septated. **B,** Same pulse sequence performed with frequency selective presaturation of fat demonstrates that high signal intensity is not due to lipid. In addition, several small implants of endometriosis *(arrows)* are more easily seen. Note that the subcutaneous fat signal is also suppressed.

T1-weighted or T2-weighted images to suppress signal from all aliphatic lipid protons in the volume. It is most often used in T1-weighted sequences after injection of intravenous contrast to render enhancing structures more conspicuous relative to fat; it can also be used to differentiate hemorrhagic masses from fatty masses (Fig. 39-4). In T2-weighted images, it permits reduced bandwidth technique to increase the signal-to-noise of the images, and it highlights pathologic conditions that may have T2 times approaching that of fat.[184] Like the Dixon technique, frequency-selective saturation is very sensitive to magnetic-field inhomogeneities.[28,296]

Opposed-phase images can be generated using spin-echo (Dixon technique) or gradient-echo sequences. Gradient-echo sequences do not use a refocusing RF pulse to rephase fat and water protons, therefore lipid signal will cycle in and out of phase with the water signal during the period TE.[285] Voxels containing lipids and water will show higher signal intensity if the fat and water are in-phase and additive, rather than if they are out-of-phase and subtractive. At 1.5 T, these resonances will be in phase to yield maximum signal for voxels with lipid and fat at TEs that are a multiple of 4.4 ms, and out of phase at TEs that are a multiple of 2.2 ms. These opposed-phase gradient-echo images achieve exquisite sensitivity to lipid- and water-containing voxels, with complete loss of signal in those voxels having 50% of the signal a result of fat and 50% a result of water. Such opposed-phase images can be used to detect lipid in dermoids, since the sebaceous lipid is generally mixed with water protons. Boundary artifacts similar to those in inversion recovery images appear at fat-water interfaces in these images.[105]

Hybrid methods achieve maximal fat suppression by applying frequency-selective fat saturation to an opposed-phase image.[46,260] With frequency-selective fat saturation, some significant amount of residual signal remains in adipose tissue. This is due to the presence of olefinic lipids with resonances near that of water, and the steady-state effects of the fat-saturation pulse that produce residual longitudinal magnetization of lipid protons. With the addition of opposed-phase imaging, these residual longitudinal magnetizations will be out of phase at time TE, resulting in nearly complete loss of signal in adipose tissue.[46] Hybrid techniques are the most reliable for fat suppression. They aid in diagnosing masses that are mostly lipid, such as dermoids, and are also useful in contrast-enhanced images.

MR angiography in the pelvis

MR angiography can be used in the pelvis for an overall evaluation of veins or arteries. In general, two-dimensional time-of-flight (2DTOF) techniques are more serviceable than phase contrast because of the rapid time of acquisition and because the predominant direction of flow of most vessels in the pelvis is cephalocaudad, an ideal situation for axial 2DTOF acquisitions.

A sequence that can yield good results for the pelvic arteries and veins in the pelvis uses a minimum TE with gradient-moment nulling, TR of 33 to 45 ms, 30-cm field of view, 2.5-mm–slice thickness contiguously acquired, and a 128 × 256 acquisition matrix. A flip angle of 60° works well in most cases, although a lower flip angle may yield better results when prominent arterial pulsation artifact is present.[210,264] The use of multicoil will permit smaller fields of view for better resolution, although the very high signal in stationary tissue close to the coil will interfere with maximum intensity reconstruction algorithms.

MR angiography can provide gross evaluation of the major arteries of the pelvis to determine vessel or graft patency, vessel displacement or encasement by masses, or larger stenoses.[6] The resolution of MRA obtained with the body coil is far inferior to that obtained with contrast angiography. Therefore the assessment of stenoses by MRA is problematic, and other applications such as the identification of bleeding sites, small emboli, or sites of arterial wall injury cannot be reliably achieved.

MR venography can reliably demonstrate the common femoral veins, external and internal iliac veins, and the IVC[210,256] (Fig. 39-5). In addition, branches of the internal iliac veins are usually delineated. The demonstration of the iliac veins is, again, inferior to that of direct iliac or femoral-injection contrast venography but often superior to that of routine pedal injection for

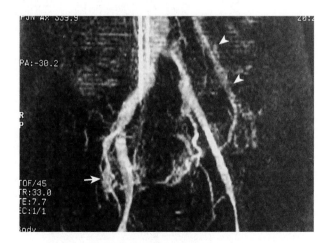

Fig. 39-5. Normal MR venography of the pelvis. Two-dimensional time-of-flight MR venography (TR/TE of 33/7.7 with flip angle of 45°, 2-mm–thick slices, 256 × 128 matrix) shows patency of the inferior IVC, common iliac veins, and external iliac veins. The uterine veins *(arrow)* and the prominent left gonadal vein *(arrowheads)* are somewhat more prominent that usual because this patient is postpartum.

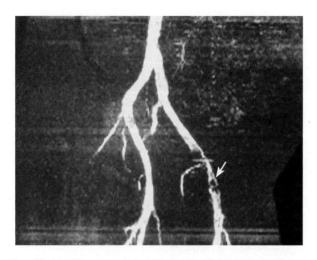

Fig. 39-6. MR venography diagnosis of thrombosis. Reconstruction from axial 2D time-of-flight gradient echo images (flip angle of 60°, 120 slices of 2.5-mm thickness, TR/TE of 7.7/45) shows filling defects in the left common femoral vein *(arrow)*. The presence of thrombosis was confirmed on venography.

lower-extremity venography. Venous occlusions due to thromboses or tumor encasement can be identified[6,256,264] (Fig. 39-6). Gadolinium enhancement may increase the conspicuity of thrombi.[83] The presence of an apparent flow defect on the MIP images must be compared with the axial gradient-echo or spin-echo images to verify the presence of thrombus (Fig. 39-7). Venous compression and magnetic-field inhomogeneity artifacts due to metal commonly cause an appearance similar to thrombus.

MRI ANATOMY OF THE PELVIS
Male genital system

Anatomic details of the male genital system are best appreciated with the highest possible resolution, which requires the use of surface coils to support smaller fields of view. For the scrotum, this is easily accomplished with a circular loop coil placed directly over the scro-

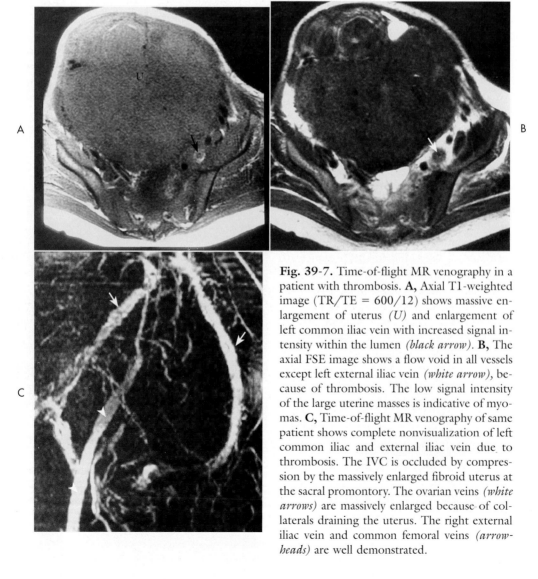

Fig. 39-7. Time-of-flight MR venography in a patient with thrombosis. **A,** Axial T1-weighted image (TR/TE = 600/12) shows massive enlargement of uterus *(U)* and enlargement of left common iliac vein with increased signal intensity within the lumen *(black arrow)*. **B,** The axial FSE image shows a flow void in all vessels except left external iliac vein *(white arrow)*, because of thrombosis. The low signal intensity of the large uterine masses is indicative of myomas. **C,** Time-of-flight MR venography of same patient shows complete nonvisualization of left common iliac and external iliac vein due to thrombosis. The IVC is occluded by compression by the massively enlarged fibroid uterus at the sacral promontory. The ovarian veins *(white arrows)* are massively enlarged because of collaterals draining the uterus. The right external iliac vein and common femoral veins *(arrowheads)* are well demonstrated.

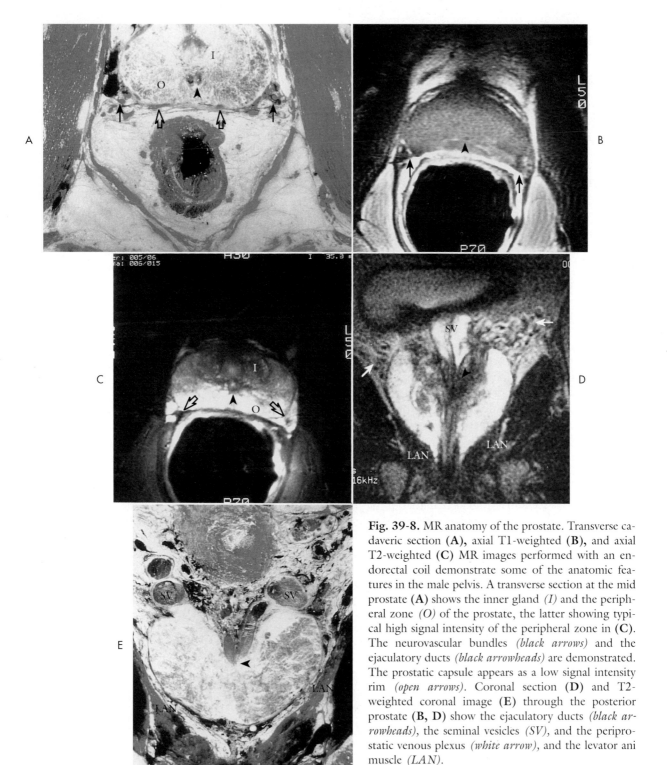

Fig. 39-8. MR anatomy of the prostate. Transverse cadaveric section **(A)**, axial T1-weighted **(B)**, and axial T2-weighted **(C)** MR images performed with an endorectal coil demonstrate some of the anatomic features in the male pelvis. A transverse section at the mid prostate **(A)** shows the inner gland *(I)* and the peripheral zone *(O)* of the prostate, the latter showing typical high signal intensity of the peripheral zone in **(C)**. The neurovascular bundles *(black arrows)* and the ejaculatory ducts *(black arrowheads)* are demonstrated. The prostatic capsule appears as a low signal intensity rim *(open arrows)*. Coronal section **(D)** and T2-weighted coronal image **(E)** through the posterior prostate **(B, D)** show the ejaculatory ducts *(black arrowheads)*, the seminal vesicles *(SV)*, and the periprostatic venous plexus *(white arrow)*, and the levator ani muscle *(LAN)*.

tum.[164,220,243] For the prostate, this is best achieved with a pelvic multicoil arrangement or the use of an endorectal coil. Body coil imaging with large fields will not permit the high resolution needed to identify important landmarks such as the prostatic capsule and the neurovascular bundles of the prostate.[121,203,233,265] T2-weighted images display the zonal anatomy of the prostate and the testicular adnexae to best advantage; acquisition in the axial and coronal or oblique coronal planes is usually the most desirable.[121,152,203,233,265] T1-weighted images are important for the assessment of the integrity of the periprostatic fat and neurovascular bundle, and for identification of sites of hemorrhage.

Prostate. The zonal anatomy of the prostate and its alteration due to benign prostatic hyperplasia is somewhat complex. For imaging purposes, whether by ultrasound or MRI, the prostate gland usually displays three main regions: *the central gland, the peripheral gland, and the anterior fibromuscular stroma*[121,154,209,234] (Fig. 39-8). The *central gland* in older men is usually involved to some degree by hyperplastic changes and displays generally lower signal intensity than does the surrounding *peripheral gland*.[139,204,231] The central gland, as it appears on MR images, includes the anatomic designations of the central and transition zones.[233,234] The central and transitional zones are histologically and anatomically distinct,[10,170] but the echogenicity on ultrasound and MR signal-intensity characteristics are similar. In addition, the distinction between these becomes distorted and obscured by the development of hyperplasia.[234] The peripheral gland, on the other hand, corresponds to the peripheral zone and displays higher signal on T2-weighted images because of the presence of generally larger and more numerous glandular lumens than that of the fibromuscular tissue of the central gland.[233] When the gland is affected with BPH, a thin low-signal intensity boundary usually appears between the central nodules and the peripheral gland. Finally, the *anterior fibromuscular stroma* is a low-signal–intensity structure occupying the anterior edge of the prostate[121,203] (Fig. 39-9).

The apex of the prostate, approximately the inferior 1.5 cm, is composed primarily of peripheral zone and urethra, unless considerable BPH is present. The apex is often best displayed in coronal T2-weighted images. The central zone of the prostate extends from the verumontanum to the base of the gland, becoming progressively wider superiorly. At the base, it occupies most of the transverse area of the prostate. The lower signal of this tissue, similar to that of prostate carcinomas, renders the base of the gland a difficult area in which to identify carcinomas or to judge the extent of carcinomas.

The prostatic capsule is not a true capsule but a thin fibromuscular band that blends with the prostatic stroma and, to a lesser extent, the periprostatic tissues.

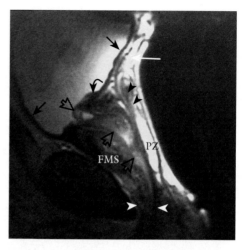

Fig. 39-9. Sagittal endorectal coil imaging of the prostate. Sagittal mid-line T2-weighted fast spin-echo image of the prostate demonstrates the seminal vesicles *(white arrow)*, ejaculatory ducts *(black arrowheads)*, bladder neck and prostatic urethra *(open arrows)*, membranous urethra *(white arrowheads)*, anterior fibromuscular stroma *(FMS)* and peripheral zone *(PZ)*, and bladder wall *(black arrows)*. Note small nodules of benign prostatic hypertrophy bulging the trigone of the bladder *(curved arrow)*.

This band is incomplete at the apex.[10,289] On T2-weighted images the prostatic "capsule" appears as a thin low-signal–intensity line marginating the prostate.[198,233,234] This band will tend to have similar signal intensity to tumors, rendering assessment of its integrity difficult when tumors abut the capsule. Posteriorly, the capsule blends with the rectovesical fascia of Denonvilliers.[10,289] Numerous nerves and vessels lie in the adjacent pericapsular fat. These are particularly prominent anterior to the apex, the anterior periprostatic plexus, and posterolateral to the peripheral zone, the neurovascular bundles. The latter are important structures to assess for nerve-sparing prostatectomy.[265]

The seminal vesicles are easily identified on MR images as convoluted tubular structures coursing posterior and superior to the base of the prostate (Fig. 39-10). The seminal fluid within the lumens results in high signal intensity on T2-weighted images; these lumens are surrounded by low signal intensity of the tubular walls.[198,233,234] The size of the seminal vesicles is highly variable. On occasion, the lumens may be nearly completely collapsed, with little fluid evident. Since spread of tumor to the seminal vesicles will usually occur directly from the base of the gland or via the ejaculatory ducts,[289] it is important to image the inferior aspect of the seminal vesicle separate from the (low-signal–intensity) base of the gland with coronal or sagittal images. Medially,

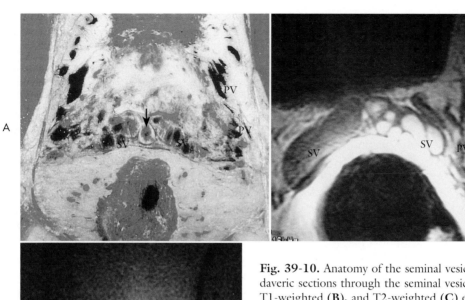

Fig. 39-10. Anatomy of the seminal vesicles. Cadaveric sections through the seminal vesicles **(A)**, T1-weighted **(B)**, and T2-weighted **(C)** endorectal coil images of the seminal vesicles show the slightly thick-walled vas deferens *(arrow)*, the seminal vesicles *(SV)* and the periprostatic venous plexus *(PV)*. Note that although there is T1 shortening throughout the left seminal vesicle and left vas deferens indicating the presence postbiopsy hemorrhage. This does not pose diagnostic difficulty because there is no low signal intensity on the T2-weighted FSE image to indicate the presence of tumor invasion.

the vesicles terminate just posterolateral to the ampullae of the *vas deferens,* which demonstrate a thicker low-signal–intensity wall (see Fig. 39-9). The course of the vas deferens can be traced from the spermatic cord in the inguinal canal laterally along the pelvic sidewall and then medially to the base of the prostate gland. The distal few centimeters of each vas widens to form the ampulla, which contains the tortuous lumen and a thicker muscular wall. This thickening should not be confused with seminal vesicle invasion by prostatic carcinoma (see Fig. 39-10).

Scrotum. Scrotal MR imaging is usually performed to evaluate testicular abnormalities. The testis, like the peripheral zone of the prostate, demonstrates a fairly long T2 and therefore has fairly high signal intensity on T2-weighted images.[14,164,220,243] The signal is homogeneous, except for faint, low-signal–intensity septae sometimes seen radiating from the low-signal mediastinum testis[164,243] (Fig. 39-11). The testis is invested in a thin low-signal intensity capsule that represents the tunica albuginea and tunica vaginalis.[14] The latter reflects over the bare area of the testis, thus serving to anchor the testis to the scrotal wall, and covers the interior of

the scrotum as the parietal tunica vaginalis.[14] The epididymus demonstrates somewhat inhomogeneous intermediate signal intensity on T2[243] (Fig. 39-12). High-signal venous vessels of the pampiniform plexus surround the vas deferens in the spermatic cord and frequently obscure it. Dilated vessels of varicoceles are easily recognized.

Female genital anatomy

Female genital anatomy is best displayed on T2-weighted images. The sagittal plane is ideal for demonstrating the uterine zonal anatomy and vaginal anatomy and for showing the relation of abnormalities of these organs to the bladder and rectum. Therefore, imaging in this plane and one other plane, usually axial, is considered important for adequately evaluating the female pelvis. T1-weighted images show poor soft-tissue contrast, containing information somewhat similar to that in CT scanning but important for definition of fat planes, adenopathy, and fat or hemorrhage in pathologic masses.

MR imaging can provide striking depiction of anatomy of the uterus, unavailable by other imaging techniques, together with corresponding characteriza-

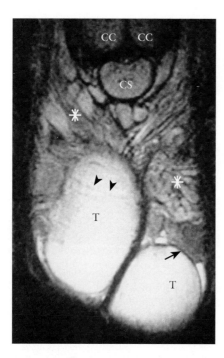

Fig. 39-11. Coronal anatomy of the scrotum. Coronal T2-weighted image performed with surface coil through the scrotum (FSE image with TR/TE effective of 4500/140) shows normal high signal intensity of the testes *(T)*. The head of the epididymis is seen with intermediate signal intensity *(arrow)*. The pampiniform plexus is demonstrated as tortuous venous vessels. *(asterisk)*. The faint septae radiating from the mediastinum testis *(arrowheads)* are seen in the right testis. Note the corpora cavernosum *(CC)* and corpora spongiosum *(CS)* at the base of the penis.

tion and diagnosis of uterine masses. The inner high-signal–intensity stripe represents the glandular tissue of the endometrium.[35,150,165] This is sharply demarcated from the very low-signal–intensity, deeper myometrium, the so-called junctional zone (Fig. 39-13). This represents a compact, more cellular smooth-muscle zone with a lesser water content, compared with the outer myometrium.[30,166,240] The bulk of the myometrium appears as intermediate-signal–intensity tissue with numerous small high-signal–intensity vessels running through it. To a variable degree, a thin, patchy subserosal low-signal–intensity layer may appear, also representing a smooth-muscle zone similar to the junctional zone.[150,165,240]

The signal intensity of the myometrium is variable; increased signal intensity on T2-weighted images occurs during the secretory phase.[167] The endometrium increases in thickness during the follicular phase of the cycle.[167] In oral contraceptive users, no such increase occurs; the endometrium is, in fact, thinner than normal throughout the cycle.[167] In addition, the signal intensity of myometrium on T2-weighted images is increased in users of oral contraceptives.[167] Blood products with variable signal intensity on T1- and T2-weighted images may appear in the uterine cavity during the menses and after D and C.[8,167] In postmenopausal women, the myometrium tends to lose signal so that the contrast between the junctional zone and the outer myometrium decreases or ceases. The atrophic endometrium in postmenopausal women may be difficult to identify by MR imaging.

The cervix demonstrates a very low-signal–intensity myometrium, continuous with the low signal

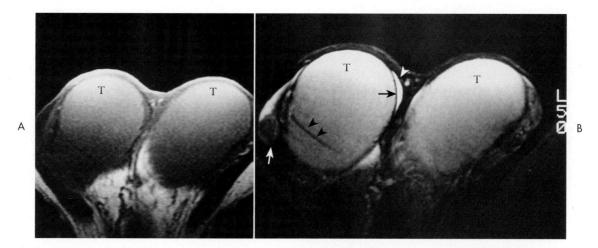

Fig. 39-12. Axial anatomy of the scrotum. **A,** Transverse T1 (500/15), and **B,** T2 FSE (TR/TE effective of 4000/115) shows the normal intermediate signal intensity of the testes *(T)* on T1-weighted image and high signal on the T2-weighted image. Radiating septae of the mediastinum testis on the right *(black arrowheads)* are seen. The epididymis on the right *(white arrow)* is seen. A small hydrocele on the right separates the tunica albuginea covering the testis *(black arrow)* from that covering the internal surface of the scrotum *(white arrowhead)*.

intensity of the junctional zone of the uterine corpus. This occupies a greater proportion of the cervical wall than it does of the uterine body, with a correspondingly thinner outer myometrium.[241] The cervical mucosa and submucosa can be distinguished from cervical canal glandular secretions.[165] Depending on the level, the cervix is bordered externally by lumen of the vaginal fornices (inferiorly, posteriorly, and laterally); vesicovaginal septum (anteriorly); parametrial tissues, including cardinal ligaments, uterosacral ligaments, and paracervical venous plexus (laterally); and peritoneum of the cul-de-sac (posteriorly) (Fig. 39-14). These adjacent structures serve as important sites of invasion of cervical carcinoma.

FSE and multicoil imaging with TE_{eff} of 80 ms or greater depicts the normal ovaries as having a low-signal–intensity central stroma with numerous high-signal–intensity follicular cysts (Fig. 39-15). These cysts may appear more numerous on high-resolution, long TR/TE FSE images than with conventional body-coil spin echo techniques, because of the higher resolution and contrast provided by heavily T2-weighted FSE sequences.[165,253] This appearance should not be confused with polycystic ovarian disease, which shows innumerable cysts peripherally situated with a fibrotic ovarian tunica (Fig. 39-16). The identification of ovarian follicular cysts on MR is critical in definitively identifying structures as ovaries. Small follicular cysts splayed around an adnexal mass can ascertain the ovarian origin of a mass (Fig. 39-17). Adnexal masses can be ascertained. Postmenopausal ovaries demonstrate fewer, smaller cysts or an absence of cysts.

Round ligaments are identified as low-signal–intensity structures coursing toward the inguinal canal (see Fig. 39-15). The peritoneal reflections of the broad ligament are not visualized except when bordered by ascites. However, the uterine arteries and veins of the inferior aspect of the broad ligaments can be seen serving as a

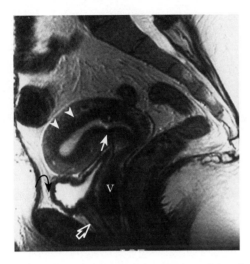

Fig. 39-13. T2-weighted sagittal imaging of female pelvic anatomy. Axial FSE image (TR/TE effective of 4000/126, with multicoil) demonstrates the uterus with a normal appearance of the junctional zone *(white arrowheads)*. Note the anterior indentation of the endometrium at the site of a prior C-section *(white arrow)*. Note the demonstration of the urethral wall *(open arrow)* and the normal bladder wall *(curved arrow)*. A tampon lies within the vagina *(V)*.

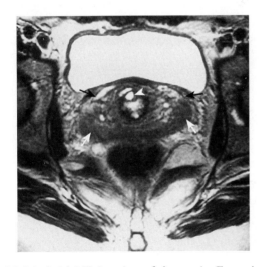

Fig. 39-14. Axial MR imaging of the cervix. Fast spin-echo T2-weighted image through the cervix and vaginal fornices *(white arrows)* shows the low signal intensity cervical myometrium. Several small nabothian cysts *(white arrowhead)* are also seen. Note the perivaginal and pericervical plexus veins appearing as high signal intensity structures in the perimetrium *(black arrows)*.

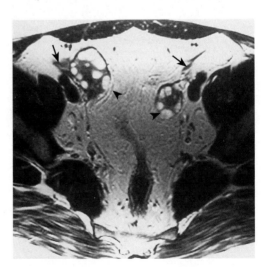

Fig. 39-15. Normal ovaries. Axial FSE image shows normal ovaries with several follicular cysts *(arrowheads)*. The round ligaments *(arrows)* are also seen. (TR/TE_{eff} of 4000/126, 256 × 256 acquisition matrix, 24-cm FOV, 5-mm–slice thickness.)

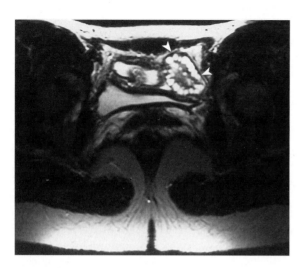

Fig. 39-16. Polycystic ovary. Axial 4000/126 FSE image through the bladder dome shows a left ovary with innumerable high signal intensity peripheral cysts surrounded by a slightly thickened low signal intensity tunica *(white arrowheads)*. (TR/TE$_{eff}$ of 4000/126, 256 × 256 matrix, 24-cm FOV, 5-mm–slice thickness.)

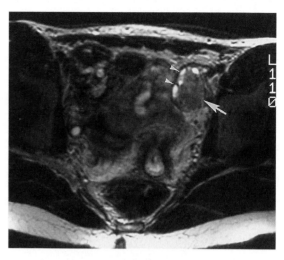

Fig. 39-17. Sertoli-Leydig cell tumor of the left ovary. FSE image through the cervix and left ovary depicts a solid mass arising within the left ovary *(arrow)*, displacing and deforming the small follicular cysts *(arrowheads)*. In this 17-year-old patient with virilization, the preoperative imaging diagnosis of ovarian stromal neoplasm was made. (TR/TE$_{eff}$ of 4000/140, 256 × 256 acquisition matrix, 18-cm FOV, 8-mm–slice thickness.)

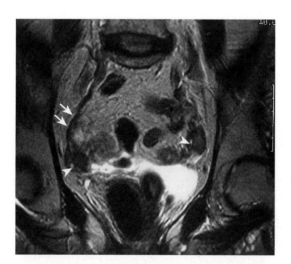

Fig. 39-18. Normal postmenopausal ovaries. The ovaries are small and low signal intensity on this coronal FSE image with TR/TE$_{eff}$ 4000/140. The ovarian vessels leading to the right ovary *(arrows)* and the presence of a tiny follicular cyst in each ovary *(arrowheads)* identify these structures as ovaries (Five-centimeter scale on left side of image). (TR/TE$_{eff}$ of 4000/140, 256 × 256 acquisition matrix, 24-cm FOV, 6-mm–slice thickness.)

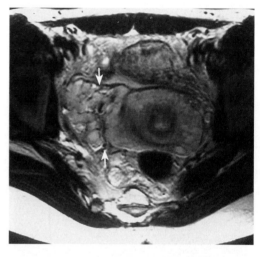

Fig. 39-19. Broad ligament pelvic arteriovenous malformation. The right broad ligament is significantly expanded by numerous venous channels *(arrows)*, which have intermediate to high signal intensity due to slowly flowing blood. Axial FSE 4000/120 image. (TR/TE$_{eff}$ of 4000/120, 256 × 256 acquisition matrix, 20-cm FOV, 5-mm–slice thickness.)

landmark for the broad ligament (Fig. 39-18). Normal fallopian tubes are usually not well depicted. Dilatation of the tubes by fluid or blood renders the tubes visible as serpentine high-signal–intensity structures with a discrete low-signal–intensity muscularis (Figs. 39-19 and 39-20).

Bladder and rectum

Four layers of the bladder wall are important for staging of bladder carcinoma: the mucosa, lamina propria, and two muscular layers. Depending on the pulse sequence used, the degree of bladder distension, and any pathologic processes affecting the bladder, usually one or two of these layers will be seen on MR images.[78] On T2-weighted images the hypointense muscularis of the wall can always be discerned; high-resolution studies may depict more than one muscular layer (see Fig. 39-14). Inflamed mucosa/lamina propria may exhibit high signal on T2-weighted images blending in with urine in the bladder.[110] Intermediate-weighted images may depict this abnormal layer as high-signal–intensity contrasting with low-signal–intensity urine.[78,79] Gadolinium enhanced T1-weighted images can depict the mucosa as a thin enhancing internal rim to the bladder wall.[189,262] In general, however, the mucosa will not be distinguished as a distinct layer by MR imaging.

The layered structure of the rectal wall is best depicted by high-resolution imaging with an endorectal coil (Fig. 39-21).[129] With this technique the muscularis can be discerned and the mucosa and submucosa can be seen, albeit intermittently even in the normal rectum.[45] High-resolution imaging of the rectal wall shows the low signal intensity of the mucosa and muscularis contrasted with the higher-signal–intensity submucosa on T2-weighted images.[129] No other technique can show the relationships of the rectum to important structures such as the puborectalis and levator ani with the multiplanar capability of MR.[281]

EVALUATION OF MALE PELVIS
Benign disorders

The value of MR imaging for benign disease affecting the male pelvis has not been well defined. Because of considerations of cost, availability, and the nature of the information needed, ultrasonography has proved most generally useful in imaging the scrotum and penis. Clinical evaluation alone serves to diagnose most infectious disease affecting the male genitalia, such as prostatitis and epidiymitis. Transrectal sonography can adequately visualize various developmental abnormalities affecting the prostate and seminal vesicles. MR imaging can in no way replace contrast radiography for evaluation of the urethra. Nonetheless, a number of applications for MR imaging have been described, and the technique may prove useful in selected cases in which conventional evaluation is inadequate.

MRI may be of value as an alternative to CT in localization of undescended testes. A testis is undescended in about 3% of infants, but the majority of these descend by the age of 1 year. Cryptorchidism affects ap-

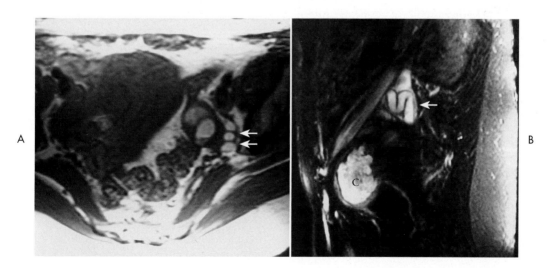

Fig. 39-20. Hematosalpinx. **A,** Axial SE 600/12 image shows hemorrhagic cysts in the left ovary with high signal intensity locules lying laterally outside the ovary *(white arrows)*. **B,** Sagittal FSE 3000/100 image demonstrates that this structure is a dilated fallopian tube *(arrows)*. *C* = chondrosarcoma in pubic ramus. (TR/TE$_{eff}$ of 3000/100, 256 × 256 acquisition matrix, 24-cm FOV, 4-mm–slice thickness.)

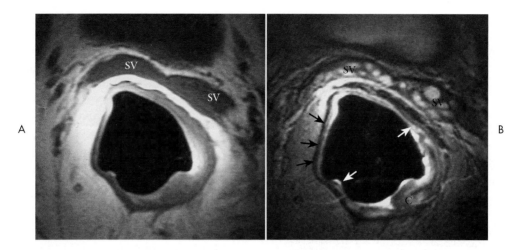

Fig. 39-21. Endorectal coil imaging of superficial rectal tumor. **A,** Axial T1-weighted spin-echo image (500/14) shows posterolateral rectal wall thickening. **B,** Axial fast spin-echo image (TR/TE$_{eff}$ of 3800/133) shows the mucosal tumor *(C)*. Note the low signal intensity rectal muscularis propria *(black arrows)*. Normal mucosa *(white arrows)* appears as a thin intermediate signal intensity stripe. (*SV* marks seminal vesicles.)

proximately 0.3% of the male population.[160] It may be bilateral in 25% of cases.[160] Histologic changes in the malpositioned testis begin as early as 2 years of age and include tubular atrophy, fibrosis, small size, and a paucity of germ cells.[59] The undescended testis is subject to a tenfold to fortyfold increased risk of malignancy and an increased incidence of infertility. Interestingly, there is an increased likelihood of both in the contralateral, normally descended testis as well.[59,160] Almost half of malignancies occurring in malpositioned testes occur in intra-abdominal testes.[160] The standard therapy for cryptorchidism is surgical, either orchiopexy for cases discovered early, or orchiectomy for patients beyond the age of 10.[159,160] Orchiopexy renders tumor surveillance easier and may decrease the incidence of malignancy.[159,160]

The vast majority of cases of cryptorchidism will not require radiologic evaluation, because the testis can be palpated in the inguinal canal. In approximately 4% of these cases, the testis cannot be palpated.[81] In these cases radiologic evaluation with CT or MR may be of benefit to localize the testis. CT has demonstrated utility in this regard,[151] but high sensitivity (94%) with MR imaging in a small series has also been reported.[81] The undescended testis may have lower signal intensity and smaller size on T2-weighted images than does the normal testis.[81] The importance of not confusing lymph nodes or the remnant pars intravaginalis gubernaculi has been stressed.[225] MR imaging has also been used to diagnose polyorchidism on the basis of typical signal intensity and testicular morphology of the supernumerary testis.[15]

Diagnostic imaging is not needed in most cases of epididymo-orchitis because the condition can be adequately evaluated on clinical grounds. Patients that do not respond to antimicrobial therapy, or for whom the clinical history and examination may be compatible with tumor, may require imaging to exclude an abscess or intratesticular mass.[278] The hallmark of intrascrotal infection is evidence of epididydmal inflammation: increased size, increased signal on T2-weighted images, sympathetic hydrocele, and increased vascularity.[13,278] The latter may manifest itself as increased numbers of vessels and signal voids seen in vessels usually displaying slower flow.[13,164,278] The testis often demonstrates evidence of orchitis as patchy areas of lower signal intensity, compared with normally high signal intensity of testicular parenchyma on T2-weighted images[13,164,278] (Fig. 39-22). The fluid usually evident in the scrotal sac may outline the bare area of the testis. Visualization of this structure will help to exclude testicular torsion, which may be in the clinical differential diagnosis of subacute scrotal pain.[164,278] If the fluid within the hydrocele is other than simple fluid (i.e., very long T1 and T2), then the presence of hemorrhage or infection of the fluid should be suspected. Because the testis itself has signal-intensity characteristics on T1- and T2-weighted images similar to that of fluid, identification of an intratesticular fluid collection such as an abscess may not be straightforward. Gadolinium-enhanced images may be of value in this regard to demonstrate necrotic or infarcted areas of the testis as nonenhancing areas.

Testicular torsion is related to abnormally diminutive attachments of the testis to the scrotal wall (the so-

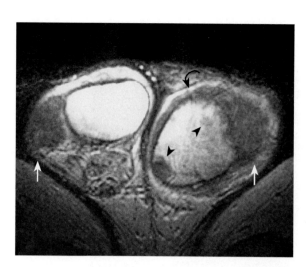

Fig. 39-22. Chronic epididymo-orchitis. Thirty-year-old male with pulmonary and scrotal sarcoidosis. The hallmarks of chronic epididymo-orchitis are present, including the marked enlargement at the epididymi *(arrows)*, patchy low signal in the testes *(black arrowheads)* as well as hydrocele *(curved arrow)*.

called bell-clapper deformity), resulting in the capacity of the testis to rotate and twist about the spermatic cord.[278] Depending on the degree and duration of twist, this causes congestion and interstitial hemorrhage in the testis, progressing to hemorrhagic venous infarction as a result of venous occlusion.[59] Arterial occlusion producing infarction occurs late and infrequently. Spermatic cord torsion typically occurs in the second and third decades. Testicular torsion is an acute surgical condition; if it is diagnosed within 24 hours, detorsion and orchiopexy may salvage the testis.

Dynamic testicular scintigraphy is the most common means of assessing for testicular torsion and has generally high accuracy rates.[112] Color Doppler ultrasonography has also been used, with 86% to 100% sensitivity and 100% specificity rates reported.[36,175] It is unlikely that MR imaging can improve on these results, since currently there is no way to definitively demonstrate flow or the absence of flow in the pampiniform plexus and testicular artery by MR. MR imaging reveals the parenchymal changes of torsion, with hemorrhage and edema within the epididymus and testis. This will produce lower-than-normal signal in the testicular parenchyma, often in a linear pattern radiating from the mediastinum.[270,278] The affected testicle tends to be smaller than normal. The epididymus will enlarge and demonstrate heterogeneous low-signal intensity, in a pattern very similar to that of epididymitis. A key finding, if it can be identified, is the twisted portion of the spermatic cord producing a vortex of helical low-signal structures

surrounded by high-signal–intensity edematous cord.[278] Because of the basic pattern of signal abnormality in the epididymus and testis, in the absence of this torsion knot it may be difficult to reliably distinguish torsion from inflammatory disorders of the testis. Torsion is typically not associated with the MR evidence of increased vascularity seen in epididymo-orchitis.[278]

MR imaging with an endorectal coil has also been used in men with ejaculatory dysfunction to identify developmental abnormalities of the prostate and seminal vesicles.[236] Prostatic cysts along the course of the ejaculatory ducts (Müllerian duct cysts),[98] seminal vesicle cysts associated with ipsilateral seminal vesicle and renal agenesis, seminal vesicle calculi, and some cases of chronic inflammatory disease of the prostate and seminal vesicles can be identified[236] (Fig. 39-23). Evidence of hemorrhage is frequently seen in the seminal vesicles (short T1 of fluid) in men with hemospermia. Acute or chronic prostatitis is a frequent histologic finding in the prostate and may mimic the MR findings of carcinoma in the peripheral zone.[203] Prostatitis usually manifests as patchy low-signal–intensity areas in the peripheral zone. Granulomatous prostatitis is indistinguishable from carcinoma by MR, with discrete low-signal–intensity nodular lesions (Fig. 39-24) or generalized low-signal intensity in the peripheral zone. Prostatic abscesses can easily be identified with MR imaging; and the multiplanar display may aid in the planning of surgical drainage (Fig. 39-25).

Malignancies of the male pelvis

Testicular carcinoma. Testicular malignancies are a leading cause of cancer in males in the 15- to 34-year age group, and they account for 8.8% of deaths in this group.[106] Approximately 10% are associated with undescended testes.[159,160] There are important genetic differences in incidence; the rate in Africans and African-Americans is very low. Testicular neoplasms are frequently misdiagnosed as epididymo-orchitis or other disorders on initial clinical examination.[199] Therefore, there may be a role for imaging to distinguish testicular masses from extratesticular processes (Fig. 39-26). Treatment, and to a certain extent MR imaging features, are dependent on the cell type and extent.[71,113,199]

Testicular neoplasms are broadly categorized into germ cell tumors (about 95%), lymphomas (5%), and sex cord-stromal tumors (2%). The latter are usually benign but capable of elaborating steroid hormones. Germ cell tumors are further subdivided into seminomatous and nonseminomatous tumors, an important distinction because of the different approaches to treatment of these two classes. In general, after orchiectomy and establishment of the histologic type of tumor, patients with seminomatous tumors receive radiation to the retroperitoneal lymph nodes, whereas patients with nonseminomatous

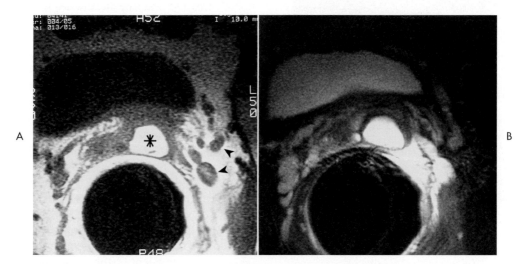

Fig. 39-23. MR evaluation of ejaculatory dysfunction. **A,** Axial spin echo T1-weighted image performed with the endorectal coil shows high signal intensity cystic mass in the left seminal vesicle *(asterisk)*. There are numerous periprostatic veins descending on the left *(black arrowheads)*, but there is a very atrophic seminal vesicle on the left. The T2-weighted fast spin echo image in **(B)** shows the cystic nature of the mass and again shows absence of seminal vesicle on the left. The right seminal vesicle is normal and better demonstrated on other images. These are typical findings of a Wolffian duct cyst with seminal vesicle aplasia. This was confirmed at pathology.

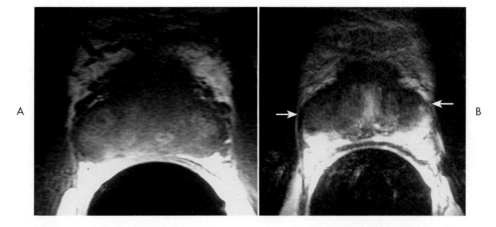

Fig. 39-24. Granulomatous prostatitis. **A,** Axial spin-echo T1-weighted image (TR/TE of 400/12) shows slightly hyperintense nodules within the prostate but a normal overall prostatic morphology. **B,** Axial fast spin echo (TR/TE_{eff} of 4000/140) shows hypoechoic nodules within the peripheral zone *(white arrows)*. Pathologic examination of the cystoprostatectomy specimen, in this patient who had been treated with BCG therapy for a bladder carcinoma, showed only granulomatous prostatitis. The appearance of the low-signal–intensity nodules in the peripheral zone, however, is quite compatible with carcinoma.

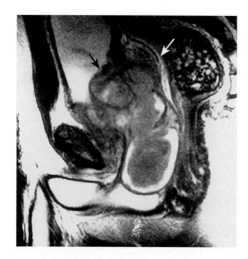

Fig. 39-25. Prostatic abscess. Sagittal FSE image in the midline of the pelvis, performed with multicoil, shows a huge mass involving the prostate extending up into the base of the bladder *(black arrow)*, seminal vesicle *(white arrow)*, and into the perineum. The heterogeneous material within this and the fluid characteristics of some of the mass are atypical for tumor. At surgery a large prostatic abscess with hemorrhagic material was drained transperineally.

tumors usually undergo retroperitoneal lymphadenectomy and chemotherapy.[71,113,199] However, only about 30% of germ cell tumors appear to be of one cell type when combined criteria of histology and tumor markers are used.[59]

Seminomas are the most common type of germ cell tumor. The peak age of incidence of these tumors is in the fourth and fifth decades, about one decade later than the peak for nonseminomatous tumors. Pathologically, these tumors appear as large solid masses without hemorrhage or necrosis, usually confined by the tunica albuginea. On MR images they appear as lobulated, more or less homogeneous intratesticular masses, with predominantly intermediate signal on T2-weighted images and contrasting with the high signal intensity of the remaining testicular tissue.[135] They are frequently large and can entirely replace the testicle (Fig. 39-27). Small associated hydroceles are common. As opposed to epididymo-orchitis, the testicular adnexa, particularly the epididymus, will appear normal, with testicular tumors that are confined by the tunica albuginea (Fig. 39-28). Of course, more advanced tumors extend into the epididymus and enlarge it.

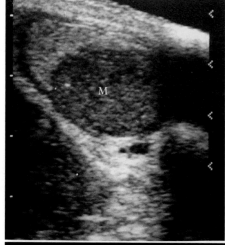

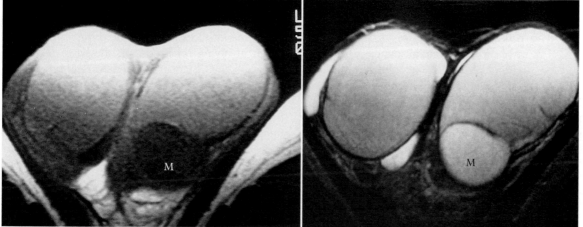

Fig. 39-26. MR differentiation of testicular mass. **A,** A 24-year-old man with palpable left sided testicular mass received an ultrasound examination, which demonstrated a left testicular mass *(M)* that has diffuse moderate echogenicity, believed to indicate a solid lesion. Increased through transmission, however, can be noted. **B,** T1-weighted (spin echo 500/15) and **C,** T2-weighted FSE images (TR/TE effective of 4000/115) shows a well-circumscribed left-sided mass *(M)*, which is very low signal on the T1-weighted images and very high signal intensity on the T2-weighted images, consistent with a cyst. Pathologic examination of this lesion showed an intratesticular left-sided epidermoid cyst. Note the small bilateral hydroceles in **(C).**

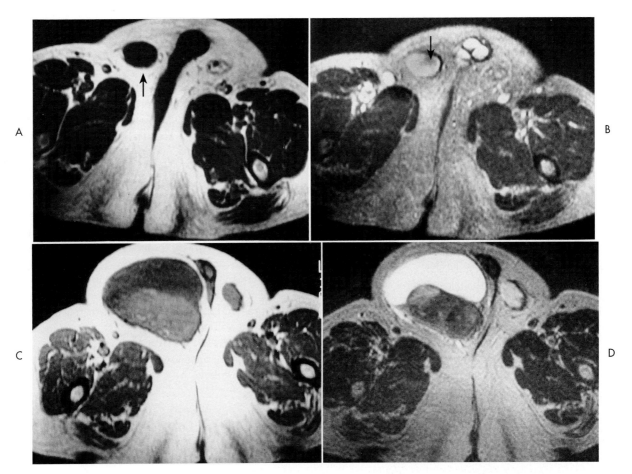

Fig. 39-27. Development of seminoma in a maldescended right testis. **A,** T1 500/20 spin echo image, and **B,** T2-weighted (2500/80 spin-echo image) demonstrates a malpositioned right testis *(arrow)* lying at the external orifice of the right inguinal canal. There is a abnormal low-signal intensity focus within this on the T2-weighted image *(arrow)*. The patient refused surgery. **C, D,** T1 (spin echo, 800/17) and FSE T2-weighted (TR/TE effective = 4000/ 140) images performed 10 months later show the large right scrotal and inguinal mass with solid components as well as a hydrocele. This proved to represent anaplastic seminoma. Note the left testis with predominantly normal signal intensity but small foci of low signal intensity *(black arrow)*, which proved to represent granulomatous orchitis.

Nonseminomatous tumors include embryonal cell carcinomas, yolk-sac tumors, teratomas, and choriocarcinomas; most, however, contain mixed elements. These tumors are much more likely to be locally advanced, and they have a higher likelihood of metastases, than do seminomas. MR images of these tumors demonstrate considerably more heterogeneity than do images of seminomas, with areas of high and low-signal on T2-weighted images.[135] They frequently demonstrate a thin low-signal–intensity capsule.[135]

MR imaging, like ultrasonography, cannot distinguish benign from malignant intratesticular masses, with the exception of simple lesions like cysts (see Fig. 39-26) or hematomas.[164,220,243,270] Therefore, orchiectomy is

indicated for any solid intratesticular mass. MR imaging may establish the presence of diffuse infiltrating neoplasm involving the testis, on the basis of diffusely decreased signal intensity, more accurately than can ultrasound.[270]

The role for pre-orchiectomy ultrasound or MR for local staging of testicular neoplasms has not been defined. Initial studies have indicated poor accuracies of both ultrasound and MR for this purpose.[270] Most attention has focused on cross-sectional imaging of the retroperitoneum for determination of lymphatic spread. Although MR imaging may be equally as sensitive as CT for the detection of enlarged lymph nodes,[72] it currently cannot distinguish carcinomatous lymphadenopathy

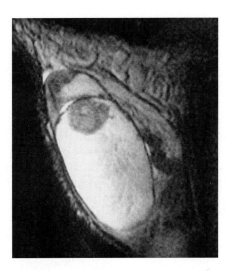

Fig. 39-28. MR evaluation of questionable clinical mass. Thirty-one-year-old male with question of a palpable abnormality in the testis. Sagittal FSE (TR/TE effective 4500/140) shows mass in the superior pole of the testis without involvement of the overlying epididymis. The mass is confined by the tunica albuginea. This proved to represent a Sartoli-Leydig cell tumor.

from benign lymphadenopathy. CT and MR have accuracy rates of 75% to 80% for staging the retroperitoneum of patients with testicular carcinoma.[106,207] Since lymphadenectomy obviously can improve on these rates and is often believed to be therapeutic, it is preferred for initial management of low-stage disease.[71,106,207]

Prostate carcinoma. Prostate carcinoma is the most common carcinoma discovered in men and is the third leading cause cause of cancer mortality, with an estimated 32,000 deaths per year.[26] Studies of autopsies and prostatectomy specimens have demonstrated that clinically inapparent prostate carcinomas have a very high general prevalence in older men, with over 80% incidence in men beyond the age of 80.[238,246] The majority of these incidental carcinomas are low-volume, well-differentiated carcinomas with a good prognosis without treatment.* Approximately nine tenths of these tumors will go undetected during the lifetime of the individual.[87] Relatively recent innovations such as PSA screening and ultrasound-guided biopsy, however, may considerably increase the numbers of carcinomas that are discovered.[44] In addition, there is suggestive evidence that now prostate carcinoma is discovered at an earlier stage than it was previously.[202]

Clinicopathologic studies of prostate carcinoma have revealed the major prognostic determinants of localized prostate carcinomas. Stage of disease, specifically

*References 87, 134, 170, 238, 246, 257, 290.

the presence of capsular penetration and seminal vesicle invasion, was one of the first variables to be identified.[40] These correlate with the presence of lymph node metastases, with poorer prognosis, and they are generally considered a relative contraindication to prostatectomy. The critical prognostic importance of cancer volume is also becoming realized. The incidence of lymph node metastases strongly correlates with the grade and volume of the tumor.[170,282] These important determinants of cancer volume, grade, and local stage have provided part of the impetus in the attempt to develop an imaging technique that could accurately image the extent and volume of prostate carcinoma.[188] MRI demonstrates a higher accuracy for measurement of prostate volume than does transrectal ultrasound.[216] This is especially important for calculations for PSA corrections to distinguish patients with PSA elevations due to BPH from those due to carcinoma.[44,194]

Most clinically significant prostate carcinomas arise in the peripheral zone of the prostate. Approximately 5% to 10% of carcinomas arise in the central zone of the prostate. The remainder occur within the transitional zone, from which most benign prostatic hyperplasia nodules also arise, or from the peripheral zone. These distinctions are important because cancers largely confined to the central zone, transitional zone, or within areas of BPH will generally not be apparent on either ultrasound or MR imaging. Fortunately most transitional zone tumors are low-volume, low-grade lesions that uncommonly extend outside the prostate or to the seminal vesicles.[93,170,290] This does not necessarily apply to all stage A lesions, however.[246,290] Incidental small foci of tumor discovered at TURP may require no treatment; however, many stage A2 lesions may represent high-volume disease and may benefit from prostatectomy.[149,299] Clinical staging of these patients is often inaccurate,[149,299] and although tumor grade and PSA level may help stratify these patients, an accurate staging modality would be of benefit in their management.[188,246]

Prostate tumors spread by invasion through the prostatic capsule, invasion of the seminal vesicles, invasion of the bladder base, and lymphatic spread to regional lymph nodes. Perineural invasion is a well-described feature of prostatic carcinoma, and although the presence of intraprostatic perineural spread is not in and of itself a significant finding,[40,170] the nerves serve as conduits to capsular transgression. Neural branches penetrate the capsule from the neurovascular bundle at the posterolateral edge of the prostate, at the superolateral margin, and at the apex.[170] These serves as the more common sites of capsular penetration (Fig. 39-29). At the apex, such capsular penetration frequently results in positive surgical margins because of the difficulty of obtaining tissue around the prostate deep within the surgi-

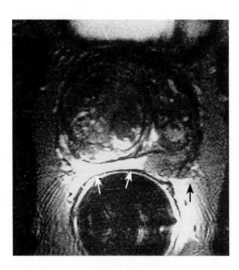

Fig. 39-29. Neurovascular bundle invasion by prostate carcinoma. Axial FSE (TR/TE effective 5000/140) image shows normal high signal intensity to the right peripheral zone *(white arrows)*. A low-signal intensity mass in the left posterolateral peripheral zone invades the left neurovascular bundle *(black arrow)* and destroys the capsule on the left side. Note the significant enlargement of the central gland with a typical appearance of benign prostatic hyperplasia.

cal field.[170,171] In prostatectomy specimens (i.e., clinically stage B carcinomas), capsular penetration is frequently very shallow, usually <3 mm.[171] This has important implications concerning the need for high-resolution imaging for its detection.

Seminal vesicle invasion has been categorized into three types, based on pathologic studies of prostatectomy specimens.[289] Type I, the most common (40% of specimens), involves extension along the ejaculatory ducts superiorly into the medial aspect of the seminal vesicles or ampullae of the vas deferens. Direct growth superiorly from the base of the prostate into the periprostatic tissue and then into the seminal vesicles represents Type II invasion (30%). Type III involvement (30%) indicates foci of tumor within the seminal vesicles without evident connection to tumor in the prostate. These foci may represent metastases. Capsular penetration is very frequent with Types I and II.[289]

Staging lymphadenectomy is generally performed before prostatectomy. The relative inaccuracy of lymphangiography and CT for determining spread to lymph nodes has led most urologists to sample nodes before attempting this surgery. Spread typically occurs first to the hypogastric, obturator lymph nodes and less commonly to the external iliac chains.[169] Evaluation of these nodes with CT or MRI can obviate lymphadenectomy if suspicious nodes can be proved by needle aspiration to contain metastasis. Lymphadenectomy has an associated complication rate of about 20% to 30%.[169]

The choice of treatment for prostatic carcinoma depends on many variables, including the clinical stage and grade of tumor, age of the patient, and concerns of the particular patient.[290] Options for treating early-stage disease range from no treatment[134,252,290] to hormonal manipulation, radiation, and prostatectomy. Stage A2 and B lesions show approximately equal survival rates with prostatectomy and radiation therapy.[87,290] However, rates of potency preservation above the approximately 50% level achievable with radiation therapy can only be attained with nerve-sparing prostatectomy, or possibly with radioisotope implants.[87,257]

The high levels of contrast between some carcinomas and the surrounding peripheral zone on MR images led to early enthusiasm for the technique for staging of prostate cancer.[115,120,204] Subsequent studies demonstrated fairly poor overall accuracy for MR staging of prostate carcinoma, at least with use of the standard body receiver coil (Table 39-1). Specifically, poor accuracy for staging results from inability to assess for capsular penetration, seminal vesicle invasion, and frequent inability to even identify the tumor nodule. There are several reasons why prostate tumors may not be identified on MR images: (1) Tumors may occur in the central gland where contrast with the surrounding tissue is nil, (2) Tumors may infiltrate into the stroma surrounding the peripheral zone so that, although possibly widespread, no MR signal intensity contrast is apparent, and (3) They may be imbedded in or surrounded by hemorrhage, prostatitis, or stromal fibrosis so as to be obscured. These factors may make judgment as to the extent of tumor difficult, and accurate determination of tumor volume impossible. These problems may apply equally to body coil and high-resolution endorectal coil imaging.

The hallmark of prostate carcinoma on T2-weighted images is a relatively low-signal–intensity nodule in the high-signal–intensity peripheral zone (Fig. 39-30).* The signal-intensity tissue within the prostate, whether fibrosis, tumor, or BPH, generally correlates with the number and size of glandular spaces versus the amount of fibromuscular stroma present.[214,231] Specifically, larger and more numerous glandular fluid-filled spaces results in higher signal intensity on T2-weighted images.[214] Therefore, benign prostatic hyperplasia tends to show signal intensity similar to that of carcinoma.[154,204] The conspicuity of tumor nodules in the peripheral zones depends to a large degree on the replacement of the normal glandular spaces of the peripheral zone with more cellular tumor.[214,231] If the tumor is infiltrative, however, it may not replace these glandular spaces. In addition, many other processes may mimic carcinoma by replacing these glandular spaces with other

*References 22, 24, 76, 120, 139, 154, 204, 223, 234.

Table 39-1. Staging accuracy of prostate carcinoma by MR imaging

N	% of tumors identified	Sensitivity	Specificity	Accuracy	Comments	Reference	Year
18		87	90	89	Clinical stage B patients	[24]	1987
46		75	88	83		[119]	1987
37	92	72	84	78		[22]	1988
20	71	38	100	82		[139]	1989
187	60	77	57	69	Multicenter prospective	[223]	1990
50		68	59	64	Neurovascular bundle invasion	[265]	1991
62		54	85	65	Capsular penetration	[76]	1991
22	95	93	84	84	Endorectal coil	[234]	1991
100		48	66	55	Capsular penetration	[232]	1992

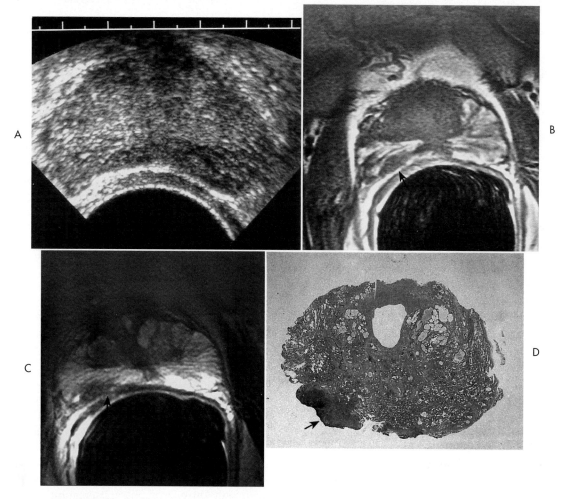

Fig. 39-30. Peripheral zone prostate carcinoma. **A,** Transrectal ultrasonography appears to suggest a left-sided area of hypoechogenicity. This was the site of suspected carcinoma in this patient. Biopsies of the left side were negative, whereas biopsy of the right mid-gland was positive. **B,** Axial T1-weighted endorectal coil image shows hemorrhage throughout the peripheral zone of the prostate. Hemorrhage does not enter a small focus in the right posterior peripheral zone *(arrow)*. **C,** T2-weighted fast spin-echo image shows the low signal intensity in the right peripheral zone *(arrow)* indicating the site of tumor. Note that signal intensity is similar to that in the central gland. **D,** Whole mount section of the prostate shows the right-sided cancer in the peripheral zone.

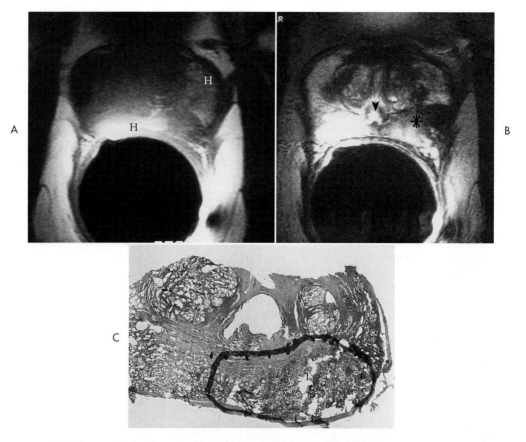

Fig. 39-31. MR evaluation of prostate carcinoma in the presence of hemorrhage. **A,** Axial T1-weighted image performed with the endorectal coil shows high signal intensity *(H),* indicating the presence of T1 shortening due to methemoglobin in the right posterior peripheral zone and left lateral peripheral zone. **B,** A T2-weighted image shows that some of the high signal intensity noted in **(A)** corresponds to low signal intensity in **(B).** There is, however, low signal intensity in the left posterior peripheral zone *(asterisk)* that does not correspond to high signal intensity in **(A),** thus indicating the presence of tumor. Note the urethra centrally *(black arrowhead).* **C,** Axial section through the prostate shows left-side tumor *(T)* corresponding to the low signal abnormality in **(B).** Note fibromuscular and glandular BPH with variable signal intensity in the central gland corresponding to the nodular changes seen in **(B).**

tissue.[43,289] Probably the most common benign process may be normal variation in the amount of stromal tissue in the peripheral zone, with areas of fibromuscular stroma causing low signal within the peripheral zone.[42,214] In some cases, prostate carcinoma may exhibit high signal intensity on T2-weighted images,[42,196] rendering differentiation from the peripheral zone difficult. Variants of prostate carcinoma, as well as other prostate neoplasms, often manifest high signal intensity on T2-weighted images.[17,67,196]

Since MR imaging is most often performed for staging purposes after biopsy, hemorrhage within the gland is a frequent finding. High signal intensity on T1-weighted images will persist for weeks or months after biopsy. It is difficult to locate tumor within an area of hemorrhage with certainty, since hemorrhage may cause some low signal on T2-weighted images (Fig. 39-31). Capsular penetration is most easily recognized on MR images when gross tumor is visualized outside of the confines of the capsule. Unfortunately, tumor penetration of the capsule often occurs on a smaller scale, frequently apparent only on microscopic examination. Indirect signs such as bulging of the capsule or slight irregularity may be of value in some cases (Fig. 39-32).[232,237,265] Particular attention must be paid to the prostate apex and base, not only because these are frequent sites of capsular penetration, but also because these may be particularly difficult areas to examine by MR imaging. Coronal images are important to evaluate tumor extension at the apex and base. Overall, MR imaging, at least using the body

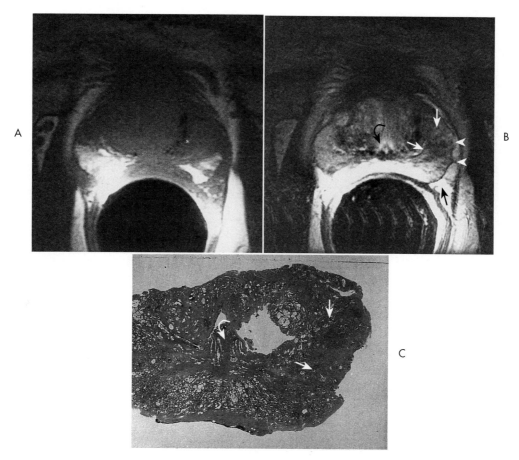

Fig. 39-32. MR evaluation of capsular penetration. **A,** Axial T1, **B,** T2-weighted FSE, and **C,** Whole-mount section of the prostate, showing a left-sided peripheral zone tumor *(white arrows)*. There is subtle capsular bulging *(arrowheads)* evident in **(B),** corresponding to capsular penetration in **(C).** Note signal voids in **(A)** and **(B)** from calcifications within the central gland; nodular changes indicative of benign prostatic hyperplasia are also seen. In **(A)** the T1-weighted images show evidence of methemoglobin in both the right and left sides of the peripheral zone, although this tends to be excluded from the more anterior tumor. The neurovascular bundle on the left *(black arrowheads)* is intact. Note the urethra *(curved arrow)* and utricle.

coil, has shown poor accuracies in recognizing capsular penetration.[232,265] Endorectal coil imaging may have value in evaluating patients after prostatectomy (Fig. 39-33).

The most reliable sign of seminal vesicle invasion by MRI is gross replacement of the fluid-filled lumens by low-signal–intensity tumor (Fig. 39-34). As in identification of the tumor nodule in the peripheral zone, care must be taken in interpreting areas of low signal intensity on the T2-weighted images that show high signal intensity on T1-weighted images, because these areas most likely represent hemorrhage.[179] Localized amyloid deposition in the seminal vesicles, an uncommon but not rare occurrence, will result in diffuse low signal throughout the seminal vesicles.[140] Carcinoma often in-

vades the seminal vesicles by invading through the walls, without replacement of the lumen with tumor; this form of spread is difficult if not impossible to recognize on MR images (Fig. 39-35).

In summary, the staging accuracies of MR for prostate carcinoma to date have been disappointing. This failure is particularly acute because, of all pelvic malignancies, prostate carcinoma has one of the strongest clinical rationales for accurate preoperative staging. Endorectal coil imaging offers high-resolution imaging of the prostate similar to intrarectal endosonography, but with better intraprostatic contrast. Although initial enthusiasm for endorectal coil imaging is high,[54,198,233] many of the problems discovered in body coil imaging may also pertain to endorectal coil imaging as well. These

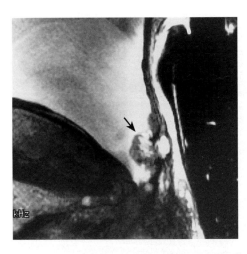

Fig. 39-33. Endorectal coil evaluation of the patient after prostatectomy. Sagittal midline FSE image, TR/TE effective of 4000/140 shows the bladder wall as a low-signal–intensity structure. Note the wide bladder neck down to the membranous urethra, representing the postprostatectomy appearance. In this patient with a rising PSA, a large nodule was found at the anastomotic site *(arrow)*. The appearance is suspicious for recurrent tumor; however, at surgery this proved to be recurrent benign prostatic hyperplasia.

include poor contrast of some tumors relative to the peripheral zone, infiltrative growth of some tumors into the seminal vesicles or across the capsule, and problems in evaluating central gland or anterior tumors.

BLADDER AND RECTUM
Bladder carcinoma

Bladder carcinoma is a very common tumor, the fourth most common tumor in men, and its incidence is rising.[26,215] Urothelial tumors demonstrate very different natural histories, depending on whether they are superficial or invasive. More than 70% of bladder cancer presents initially as a superficial (stage T1 or less) lesion.[215] Approximately 80% of these remain confined to the mucosa or submucosa through most of their natural history.[215,218] Tumors that have invaded the muscle of the bladder wall at presentation, however, have a much worse prognosis, with a much higher incidence of pelvic lymph node metastases and a high rate of recurrence after resection.[110,215,255]

The indicated treatment of bladder tumors varies according to whether the lesion is superficial or invasive (Table 39-2). Superficial tumors are candidates for intravesical therapy (TURB, cautery, photodynamic therapy) and intravesical chemotherapy or BCG.[215,255] Muscle-invasive tumors are generally treated with cystectomy, radiation therapy, or both. This distinction between T1 and T2 invasion is the most critical distinction that an imaging method must make to be useful as a stag-

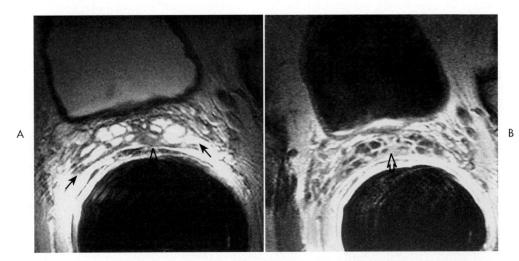

Fig. 39-34. Early seminal vesicle invasion. **A,** Axial T2-weighted fast spin-echo image of the seminal vesicles shows normal seminal vesicles laterally *(black arrows)*. Centrally, however, there is abnormal low signal intensity *(open arrow)* lying along the left seminal vesicle and surrounding the vas deferens. This represents early tumor invasion of the seminal vesicle. On the post gadolinium-enhanced T1-weighted image **(B)** it can be seen as an abnormal low-signal–intensity area enhances, proving that it is solid tissue. Note the normal enhancement of the walls of the seminal vesicles.

ing tool.[215,242] Staging by TURB is inaccurate, with approximately 30% of patients understaged by this method.[110,218,242] Bimanual examination under anesthesia improves the accuracy of clinical staging, and some advocate the use of this method to the exclusion of imaging for determination of T-stage.[96,110,255] The determination of depth of muscle invasion assumes less importance because the distinction is not supported by differences in survival.[242] The determination of spread of tumor into adjacent organs, in contrast, is very important because this may obviate cystectomy.

On T1-weighted images, little or no contrast is evident between bladder tumors and bladder wall[65,79,145] (Fig. 39-36). However, T1-weighted images provide sharp delineation of the external bladder wall and surrounding perivesical fat. T2-weighted images provide better demonstration of the bladder muscularis and show

Table 39-2. Local staging of bladder cancer

TNM system	Modified Jewett	Pathologic findings
TIS	CIS	Carcinoma in situ
Ta	O	Papillary tumor, noninvasive
T1	A	Invasion into lamina propria
T2	B1	Invasion into superficial muscle layer
T3a	B2	Invasion into deep muscle layer
T3b	C	Invasion into perivesical fat
T4a	D1	Invasion into prostate, uterus, vagina
T4b	D	Invasion into pelvic or abdominal wall

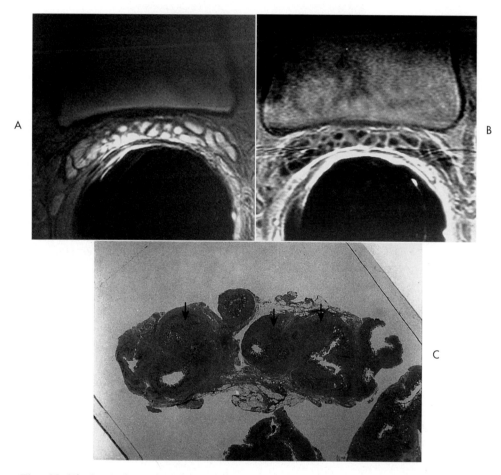

Fig. 39-35. Seminal vesicle invasion not apparent on MR. **A,** Axial FSE image, and **B,** gadolinium-enhanced T1-weighted spin-echo image through the seminal vesicles, performed with an endorectal coil in a patient with known prostate carcinoma shows normal-appearing seminal vesicles bilaterally. **C,** At surgery diffuse tumor infiltration of the walls of both seminal vesicles was discovered *(arrows).* This demonstrates the difficulty of detection of seminal vesicle invasion which does not fill the lumens of the seminal vesicles.

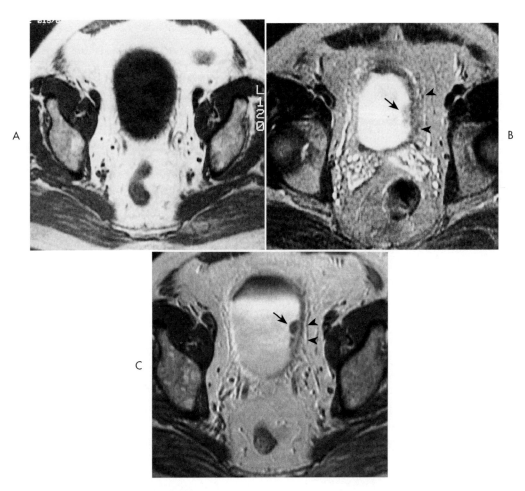

Fig. 39-36. MR evaluation of superficial of bladder carcinoma. **A,** Axial T1-weighted image (spin echo 600/18) shows no evidence of spread of tumor into the perivesical fat. The tumor itself, however, as well as the bladder wall are poorly seen because of poor contrast between the urine and the tumor or bladder wall. **B,** Spin-echo T2-weighted image (2500/80) demonstrates the tumor *(black arrow)* better than does the T1-weighted image. An intact low-signal–intensity bladder muscular *(black arrowheads)* is seen underneath the polypoid tumor indicating a superficial tumor. **C,** T1-weighted spin-echo axial image after the administration of gadolinium shows the gadolinium within the urinary bladder outlining the tumor. The bladder wall enhances slightly and forms a continuous band underneath the tumor, again verifying the superficial extent of tumor.

tumors as intermediate to high signal intensity. Depending on the TE and TR used, contrast between tumor and urine may be poor.[65,79,145] In addition, on T2-weighted images differentiation of tumor and perivesical fat may be suboptimal [145] (Figs. 39-37, 39-38). These considerations provide argument for the use of both T1- and T2-weighted images, in multiple planes, for judging the extent of bladder tumors.[65,79,145] These concerns have also contributed to the advocacy of gadolinium-enhanced imaging for the evaluation of bladder tumors (see Fig. 39-36). Bladder tumors show enhancement similar to that of bladder mucosa/submucosa, which becomes visible as a thin hyperintense lining to the bladder on contrast-enhanced T1-weighted images.[189,262] The additional contrast between muscularis and tumor evident on gadolinium-enhanced T1-weighted images has been claimed to facilitate staging in a number of studies.[190,262,263]

MR has achieved overall staging accuracies of the primary tumor of 60% to 85% (Table 39-3). The accuracies for separating tumors that have penetrated the bladder wall (T3b) from those that have not (T3a or less) range from 73% to 95%. This determination has been reported equivalent to[128,219] or superior to CT.[3,262,263] One report suggests that MR imaging is superior to transurethral ultrasound as well.[262]

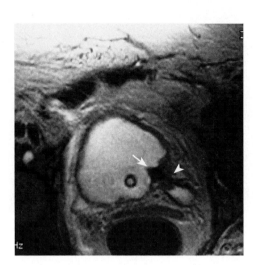

Fig. 39-37. MR evaluation of bladder carcinoma. FSE image (TR/TE effective of 4500/119 with multicoil) shows a left-sided tumor invading the bladder muscularis and ureteral orifice on the left *(arrow)*. Tumor growing into the perivesical fat and ureteral lumen can also be seen *(arrowhead)*. A Foley catheter is present in the bladder.

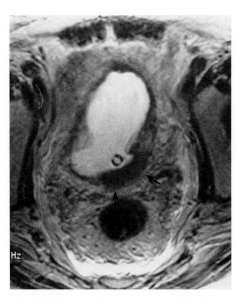

Fig. 39-38. MR imaging demonstration of bladder muscularis invasion. Fast spin-echo image (TR/TE effective of 5000/120, with multicoil) reveals low-signal–intensity tumor occupying most of the left posterolateral wall of the bladder. The tumor effaces the low-signal–intensity muscularis *(black arrows)* indicating deep invasion.

Table 39-3. Staging accuracy of bladder carcinoma by MR imaging

N	Staging criteria	Sensitivity (%)	Specificity (%)	Accuracy (%)	Comments	Reference
30	Extravesicle extension	82	62	73		128
23	Extravesicle extension			96		219
40	Overall TNM			60		39
	perivesical extension	67	100	85		ibid
	deep muscle invasion	95	95	95		ibid
68	Overall			69	Gadolinium-enhanced	190
	perivesical extension	93	95	95	Gadolinium-enhanced	ibid
11	Overall			64		3
79	Overall			85	Gadolinium-enhanced	263
57	Overall			74	Gadolinium-enhanced	262
	perivesical extension	96	83	89		ibid

Rectal carcinoma

Colorectal carcinoma is the most common cancer of the gastrointestinal tract and the second most common visceral cancer in the United States. It causes 11% to 13% of cancer deaths. Overall survival for rectal carcinoma with surgical therapy at 5 years is 40% to 60%. Ninety-five percent of rectal malignancies are adenocarcinomas.

Surgery is the major component of therapy for rectal carcinoma, and pathologic staging is the standard. The prognosis of rectal carcinoma is closely tied to the pathologic stage. The surgical approach is determined to some extent by preoperative estimation of the stage, but more importantly by the anatomic level of the rectal mass. The importance of accurate preoperative staging of rectal carcinoma is increasing because of evolutions in

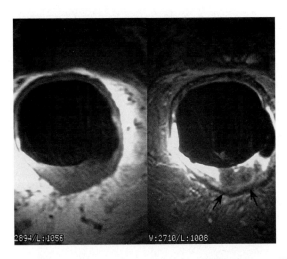

Fig. 39-39. Endorectal coil imaging of a rectal carcinoma. Endorectal coil images with T1-weighted *(left)* and T2-weighted FSE *(right)* images delineate the muscularis propria *(arrows)* underlying the tumor. Note that the low-signal–intensity muscularis on the FSE image is intact underneath the polypoid tumor, indicating that the muscularis at this level is not invaded. Note the seminal vesicles anteriorly.

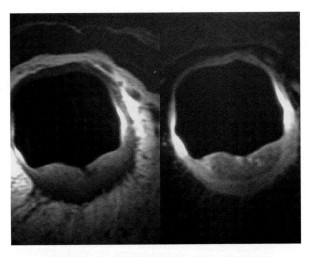

Fig. 39-40. Nonspecific stranding in perirectal fat. Image on the left represents the T1-weighted spin-echo image performed with an endorectal coil showing the tumor *(T)* with pronounced perirectal stranding in the perirectal fat (same patient as in Fig. 39-39). At pathology, the tumor was confined to the muscularis. This perirectal stranding is nonspecific and is due to small dilated vessels and lymphatics. The image on the right is performed with fat saturation and gadolinium enhancement showing a continuous enhancing muscularis beneath the polypoid, ulcerated, tumor.

the approach to treating these tumors. The use of preoperative radiation therapy has increased the need, at least on a research level, for assessment of the extent of these tumors and their response to radiation. Innovations in sphincter-sparing operations (as opposed to abdominoperineal resections) for very low lesions and local resections for superficial lesions has likewise increased the need for accurate determination of depth of invasion before surgery.

Locoregional recurrence is a much more significant problem in rectal carcinoma than in colon carcinoma.[66] Reported incidences of local recurrence after attempts at cure range from 10% to 40%.[66,157] The risk of recurrence depends partly on the tumor level; in comparison with higher rectal tumors, in distal rectal tumors the incidence of recurrence approximately doubles.[57] On T1-weighted imaging, rectal carcinoma appears as an intermediate signal intensity mass, similar in signal intensity to the rectal wall[37] (Fig. 39-39). An intrarectal contrast agent, either insufflated air or a short-T1 liquid, is helpful for identification of the intraluminal tumor,[62] although it is not clear that this is a helpful feature for actually gauging the transmural extent of tumor. T1-weighted images provide excellent definition of the perirectal fat surrounding the rectal wall. With high resolution, fine stranding in the perirectal fat radiating from the tumor can often be discerned (Fig. 39-40). This can occur in tumors confined by the wall and should not be interpreted as evidence of tumor spread. On T2-

weighted images, tumors have variable appearance, reflecting different histologic components of the tumor.[37] Most tumors are intermediate-signal intensity, but high-signal–intensity areas due to mucinous areas, and low-signal–intensity areas due to desmoplastic reaction, are common. Complete disruption of the very low signal intensity rectal muscularis propria is the key finding indicating early transmural penetration[45,129] (Fig. 39-41). Gadolinium-enhanced T1-weighted images, preferably performed with fat saturation, may also be useful. The muscularis enhances very little, providing some contrast between the enhancing tumor and muscularis.

Staging of rectal carcinoma by imaging methods is a complex issue that involves comparative assessment of imaging modalities for detection of hepatic metastases, lymphadenopathy, and depth of mural tumor invasion. Of the three modalities used for staging rectal carcinoma—transrectal ultrasound, CT, and MRI—only the latter two can provide a comprehensive evaluation of these areas. In a few published studies, MRI has achieved sensitivities of 75% to 100% and specifities of 66% to 100% for detection of transmural extension.[37,62,96] In one small study, endorectal coil imaging correctly staged 11 of 12 rectal cancers.[45] As with staging of most malignancies by imaging, the lack of sensitivity and specificity for the detection of metastases to lymph nodes is a

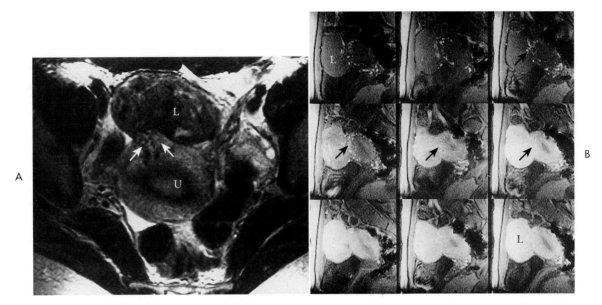

Fig. 39-43. MR characterization of pedunculated leiomyoma. **A,** Axial T2-weighted FSE image through the uterine fundus shows a large well-circumscribed low-signal–intensity mass *(L)* anterior to the uterine fundus *(U)*. The low signal intensity of this mass is suggestive of leiomyoma. In this case, vessels arising from the myometrium can be seen as supplying the mass *(white arrows)*, confirming its myometrial origin. **B,** Dynamic gadolinium enhancement of pedunculated leiomyoma shows a rapid enhancement of the leiomyoma *(L)* via vessels crossing from the myometrium *(arrow)*. Note the similar enhancement of the myometrium and the leiomyoma. There is less enhancement of the endometrium.

have also been described.[31,75,117] Synechiae may focally obscure the endometrial stripe.[75] Endometrial polyps exhibit equivalent or lower signal intensity than does normal endometrium.[31,117]

Leiomyomas. Leiomyomas (fibroids) of the uterus are the most common gynecologic disorder; relative to their frequency, however, few fibroids become symptomatic. In toto, fibroids demonstrate a highly variable signal on T2-weighted MR images, from homogenously hypointense to heterogenously hyperintense; however, the vast majority of leiomyomas display a characteristic appearance on MR, whether pedunculated or intramural, and will not be confused with other uterine tumors.[123,126,221,286] The vast majority of leiomyomas will show a predominantly *low signal* intensity on long TR/TE images.[126,156,277,286] They appear well defined and sharply marginated from surrounding myometrium. MR imaging can be used to differentiate pedunculated fibroids from other adnexal masses based on this typical signal intensity and morphology (Fig. 39-43).[9,221] Thin, hyperintense rims are sometimes seen,[185] as well as internal signal heterogeneity due to hyaline or myxoid degeneration.[123,126,277,286] These changes, however, are usually not extensive enough to mimic a malignant adnexal neoplasm. Subserosal tumors are particularly im-

portant to identify because of their propensity to cause uterine bleeding (Fig. 39-44). Only ovarian fibromas/ thecomas commonly have signal-intensity characteristics that match fibroids (Fig. 39-45). The gadolinium enhancement characteristics of fibroids are variable (Fig. 39-46). MR is more sensitive and specific than either ultrasound or hysterosalpingogram for the diagnosis of leiomyoma.[74]

Adenomyosis. Adenomyosis, first described in 1860 by Rokitansky, consists of the presence of endometrial glands and stroma deep within the myometrium.[11] Whorled hypertrophy of the myometrial smooth muscle occurs around the glands, accounting for the low-signal–intensity appearance of most of the lesion on MR imaging. High-signal–intensity foci appearing within the nodules on T2-weighted images represent the glandular epithelium[156,272] (Fig. 39-47). These are occasionally hemorrhagic.[11,272] Adenomyosis has a high prevalence in the female population, approximately 19% to 31%, although uncommonly is it symptomatic.[11] It is sometimes associated with menorrhagia and dysmenorrhea. The overall uterine size is enlarged in 60% to 80% of cases.[11,277]

Ovarian cysts. The morphology of functional ovarian cysts is as expected from the ultrasound appear-

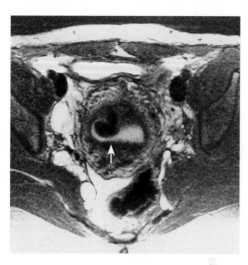

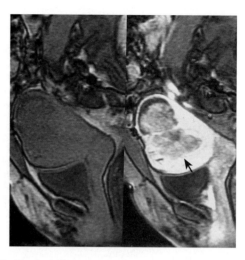

Fig. 39-44. Subserosal leiomyoma. In this patient with menorrhagia, this axial T2-weighted FSE image (TR/TE effective of 3500/80) demonstrates a submucosal leiomyoma *(white arrow)* protruding into the endometrium. Incidentally, note plexiform neurofibromas along the sciatic nerve in this patient with neurofibromatosis.

Fig. 39-45. Gadolinium enhancement of atypical leiomyoma. Dynamic sagittal images through the uterus performed before *(left)* and after *(right)* administration of intravenous gadolinium shows an extensively degenerated leiomyoma, which was proved at surgery. Note the somewhat bilobed nature of this mass with an extensive submucosal component *(black arrow)*.

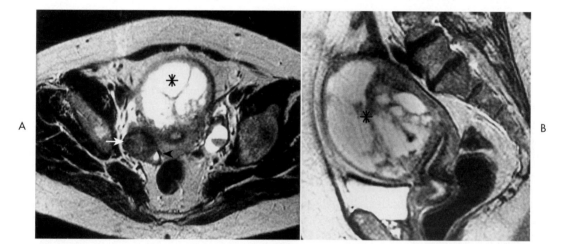

Fig. 39-46. MR evaluation of multiple pelvic masses. Axial **(A)** and sagittal **(B)** fast spin-echo images of the pelvis (TR/TE of 4000/108) show a low-signal–intensity well-defined mass in the right adnexa *(white arrow)*. The tiny follicular cysts *(arrowhead)* adjacent to this evident in **(A)** identify this as an ovarian mass. Although the signal intensity characteristics of this mass are similar to that of a typical leiomyoma, this bears no obvious relationship to the myometrium. The very large heterogeneous mass in the anterior myometrium *(asterisk)*, is nonspecific but consistent with a degenerated leiomyoma. The small left ovarian cyst with a hematocrit effect fluid level is a common finding in hemorrhagic corpus luteum cysts. Pathologic examination of these lesions showed a right ovarian fibroma, large degenerated uterine leiomyoma, and a small corpus luteum cyst in the left ovary.

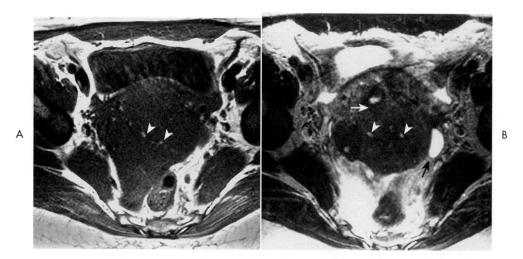

Fig. 39-47. MR appearance of focal adenomyosis. **A,** Axial spin echo T1-weighted image performed with multicoil demonstrates uterine enlargement with small punctate high signal intensity foci *(white arrowheads)*. **B,** Axial FSE T2-weighted image shows the typical appearance of adenomyosis with an ill-defined mass of low-signal–intensity tissue within the myometrium and several punctate high-signal–intensity foci *(white arrowheads)*. Note that the adenomyosis focally obscures the junctional zone posteriorly *(white arrow)*. Note the left peritubal cyst *(black arrow)*.

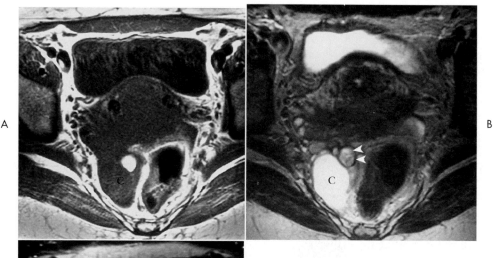

Fig. 39-48. MR appearance of an ovarian cyst. **A,** Axial T1-weighted spin-echo image performed with multicoil shows a larger cyst of the right ovary *(C)* adjacent to a small high signal intensity cystic lesion in the right ovary. The T2-weighted fast spin-echo image **(B)** shows the typical high-signal intensity of a simple ovarian cyst *(C)*. The high-signal–intensity small cyst identified in **(A)**, however, shows slightly lower signal on the T2-weighted image as well as a low-signal–intensity rim *(white arrowheads)*. This is a nonspecific appearance, however, it is compatible with the small endometrioma, which was indeed proven at surgery. **C,** Gadolinium-enhanced T1-weighted image performed with fat saturation shows a thick enhancing wall to the corpus luteum cyst *(white arrow)*.

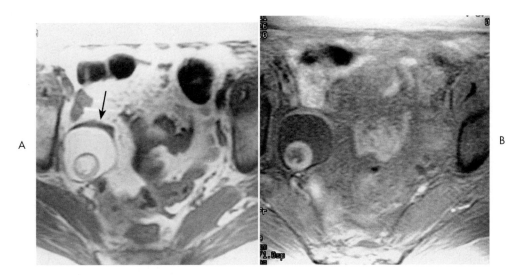

Fig. 39-49. Use of chemical shift image to diagnose ovarian dermoid. **A,** T1-weighted axial image performed with multicoil shows high-signal–intensity mass in the right adnexa *(black arrow).* Note the typical appearance of the dermoid plug within this mass. **B,** The same spin-echo T1-weighted sequence performed with frequency-selected fat saturation shows loss of signal within the fat within the pelvis as well as significant loss of signal within the mass in the right adnexa. This is diagnostic for a lipid-containing mass. By far the most common cause of a lipid-containing mass in the ovary would be a ovarian dermoid. Note that much of the dermoid plug does not show loss of signal with fat saturation.

ance. Small ovarian follicles normally stud the surface of ovaries of premenopausal women, and these are apparent on high-resolution MR images.[165,253] Follicular cysts show a thin smooth wall on MR images, and the cyst contents generally demonstrate the signal intensity of simple fluid, that is, low signal intensity on T1-weighted images and very high signal intensity on T2-weighted images. Corpus luteum cysts exhibit a thicker wall, which represents the luteinized lining (Fig. 39-48). This wall can demonstrate intense enhancement with gadolinium. MR imaging commonly reveals evidence of hemorrhage within corpus luteum cysts, with lower-signal–intensity blood or clot layering dependently in the cyst, and shortened T1 and T2 of the cyst contents relative to simple fluid.[193] Hemorrhagic cysts will rarely exhibit the significantly shortened T1 and T2 commonly seen with endometriomas.[275] On the other hand, some endometriomas will overlap in signal intensity with corpus luteum cysts.[195]

Dermoid cysts are a common cause of adnexal mass, accounting for approximately 20% of all ovarian neoplasms. Almost all of these lesions show some component that demonstrates lipid characteristics on MRI.[32,273] These areas will show signal intensity characteristics that approximates (but does not necessarily coincide with) the signal intensity of adipose tissue.[273] For definitive identification of these areas, a chemical-shift–selective technique should be employed to differentiate

these lesions from hemorrhagic lesions that may have similar signal intensity characteristics[143,180,181,273] (Fig. 39-49). Ovarian dermoid tumors may be diagnosed when lipid structures are demonstrable within the mass.[143,273] This is easily performed with frequency selective presaturation or chemical-shift–selective techniques.[143,180,181] Although not absolutely specific for dermoid, this finding in a uterine or ovarian mass virtually excludes a malignant tumor.[70]

Endometriomas. Endometriomas, or endometriotic cysts, are manifestations of advanced stage endometriosis.[288] They usually involve the ovaries and are bilateral in one third to one half of cases.[53,84] They are characterized by a wall that is usually thick and fibrotic but may be thin and attenuated. The cyst contains altered blood that varies from the usual semifluid or inspissated "chocolate" material to the much less common watery fluid.[53] Dense adhesions often fix the endometrioma to surrounding pelvic structures.

Studies of the MRI evaluation of endometriosis have demonstrated that endometriomas are reliably detected by MRI.[7,275,298] In contrast, MRI is insensitive compared with laparoscopy for the overall detection and staging of endometriosis, because it cannot reliably detect superficial implants and adhesions,[7] which are usually small and occur on peritoneal surfaces.

Endometriomas can reliably be distinguished from most other ovarian masses, including ovarian ma-

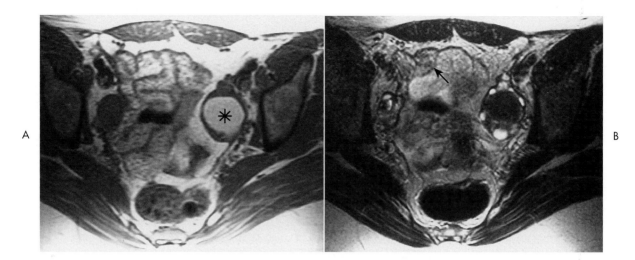

Fig. 39-50. Ovarian endometrioma. **A,** Axial SE TR/TE 600/12 image through the ovaries show a high-signal intensity–mass of the left adnexa *(asterisk).* **B,** FSE image shows significant low signal intensity *(shading)* within the mass, characteristic for an endometrioma. Several high-signal–intensity ovarian follicular cysts surround the mass, indicating its location within the ovary. (TR/TE$_{eff}$ of 4000/140, 256 × 256 acquisition matrix, 22-cm FOV, 5-mm–slice thickness.)

lignancies, by MRI criteria.[275] Endometriomas exhibit significantly variable appearances on T1- and T2-weighted spin-echo images, which differ nonetheless from simple (nonhemorrhagic) ovarian cysts.[298] Homogenously very hyperintense cysts on T1-weighted images that become hypointense on T2-weighted sequences, or multiple cysts that are entirely hyperintense on T1-weighted sequences, indicate endometriomas in the appropriate clinical setting[193,275] (Fig. 39-50). MR evidence of hemorrhage per se in a cystic mass is certainly not specific for a benign hemorrhagic cyst or endometrioma, since this feature is often seen in ovarian cystadenomas and carcinomas.[182,183,271] Togashi et al[275] reported several MRI criteria to be helpful in the diagnosis of endometriomas. These criteria include: (1) a cystic lesion that is hyperintense on short TR/TE images and shows "shading," or relative hypointensity, on long TR/TE images, and (2) multiple (>2) hyperintense lesions on short TR/TE images. Endometriomas may also be hyperintense on short TR/TE images and hyperintense without shading on long TR/TE images; however, this pattern of hyperintensity on T1- and T2-weighted sequences is nonspecific and is commonly seen in hemorrhagic cysts as well.[195] These criteria exclude lesions with solid nodules or obvious septations, or of very large size. Masses with signal intensity characteristic of hematomas are also excluded (Fig. 39-51). Using these criteria in a prospective study, endometrial cysts could be diagnosed with 90% sensitivity, 98% specificity, and 96% accuracy; no malignancies were erroneously diagnosed as

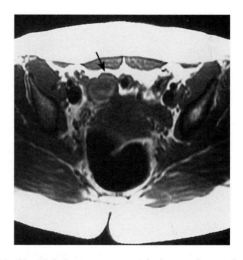

Fig. 39-51. Tubal pregnancy with hemorrhage. Axial SE 600/17 image shows a heterogenous mass in the right adnexa with peripheral high signal intensity *(arrow).* This appearance is characteristic of an subacute hematoma and is rarely seen in endometriomas. Surgery revealed an ectopic pregnancy. (TR/TE$_{eff}$ of 4000/90, 256 × 256 acquisition matrix, 24-cm FOV, 5-mm–slice thickness.)

endometriomas.[275] It should be noted that malignant transformation of endometriosis, though rare, can occur.[103] Ancillary findings that are commonly seen in endometriomas include low-signal–intensity rims that are due to the hemosiderin and fibrosis in the wall, and tethering to surrounding structures.[7]

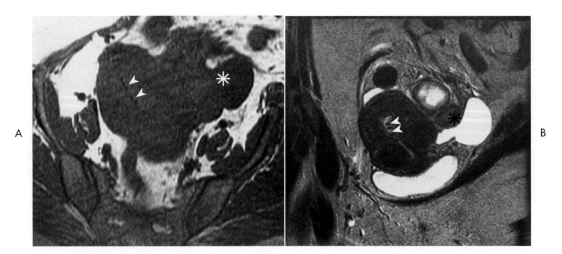

Fig. 39-52. Tubal ovarian abscess in association with IUD. **A,** T1-weighted spin-echo image shows large left adnexal mass *(asterisk)*. Punctate signal voids *(white arrowheads)* represent the IUD in the endometrial cavity. **B,** Coronal T2-weighted FSE image shows multilocular left adnexal mass with variable signal components, but mostly high signal intensity. Pathologic examination of tissue showed actinomyces.

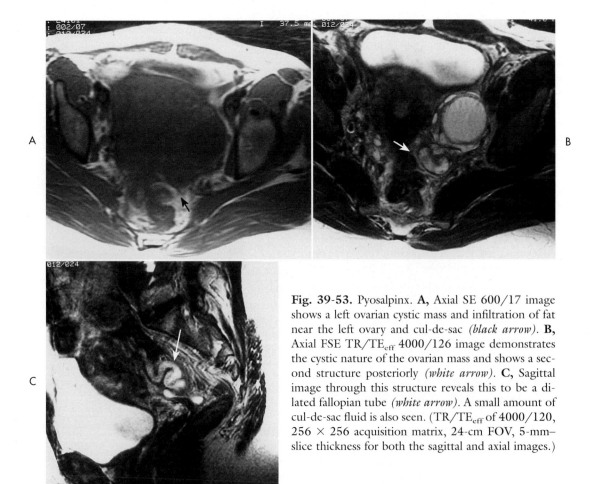

Fig. 39-53. Pyosalpinx. **A,** Axial SE 600/17 image shows a left ovarian cystic mass and infiltration of fat near the left ovary and cul-de-sac *(black arrow).* **B,** Axial FSE TR/TE$_{eff}$ 4000/126 image demonstrates the cystic nature of the ovarian mass and shows a second structure posteriorly *(white arrow).* **C,** Sagittal image through this structure reveals this to be a dilated fallopian tube *(white arrow).* A small amount of cul-de-sac fluid is also seen. (TR/TE$_{eff}$ of 4000/120, 256 × 256 acquisition matrix, 24-cm FOV, 5-mm–slice thickness for both the sagittal and axial images.)

Pelvic inflammatory disease. Tubo-ovarian abscess is a complication of pelvic inflammatory disease. In acute pyogenic salpingitis, pus emanating from the fallopian tube becomes confined by pelvic adhesions to form an abscess.[59] This abscess usually lies near or involves the ovary. Such abscesses appear on MR images as unilocular or multilocular cystic masses, usually with a thicker wall than that seen in functional ovarian cysts[117] (Fig. 39-52). The abscess fluid has variable signal but usually is very high signal intensity on T2-weighted images and low signal intensity on T1-weighted images.[117,183] Infiltration of pelvic fat surrounding the mass may be evident. Acute or chronic pelvic inflammatory disease is frequently accompanied by dilatation of the fallopian tube (Fig. 39-53). These pyosalpinges result from tubal obstruction with filling of the lumen with pus. Analysis of pyosalpinges or hydrosalpinges in more than one MR imaging plane may be necessary to recognize their tubal character.

Puerperal ovarian vein thrombophlebitis is an uncommon complication of postpartum endometritis. The disorder usually presents in the puerperium with prolonged fever after an initial trial of antibiotic therapy for endometritis. Approximately 80% of cases occur on the right side, and the thrombus may extend into the IVC. Once the diagnosis is made, anticoagulant therapy is often given. Either CT or MRI may be used for diagnosis.[230] Typically the thrombus will be slightly hyperintense on T1-weighted images and hyperintense on T2-weighted images.[158,230] Enlargement of the involved gonadal vein as well as surrounding stranding inflammatory changes are typical. Gradient-echo techniques easily demonstrate the absence of flow in the involved veins.

Obstetric applications. Ultrasonography is the primary modality for evaluation of obstetric complications. MRI may be useful in specific instances in which ultrasound is equivocal, such as in cases of extrauterine pregnancy or evaluation of placenta position.[4] Additional applications are limited by as yet unproven safety of MR imaging to the fetus and by the tendency of significant artifacts related to both fetal and maternal motion to degrade the MR images. These artifacts can be alleviated by administering intramuscular pancuronium to the fetus via an amniocentesis needle, although such an invasive procedure is rarely justified.

MRI is ideally suited to the evaluation of pelvic masses in pregnant patients when ultrasound in nondiagnostic.[4,87,287] MRI can reliably detect benign ovarian masses and diagnose dermoids and leiomyomas (Fig. 39-54), including those that may interfere with delivery.[4,87,287] Although adnexal masses are not uncommon in the pregnant patient, malignancies are rare; ovarian carcinoma occurs only in 1 of 17,000 to 38,000 pregnancies.[137] Ovarian tumors are one tenth as likely to be malignant in the pregnant patient, compared with those occurring without pregnancy.[19]

Malignancies of the female pelvis

MR imaging has not as yet achieved widespread use for staging of pelvic malignancies. In part, this is be-

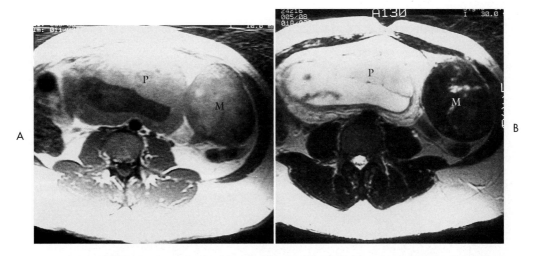

Fig. 39-54. MR evaluation of an adnexal mass in a pregnant patient. Ultrasound examination had a shown a large complex, partially solid mass. **A,** Axial spin-echo image (TR/TE of 700/12) and **(B)** axial T2-weighted fast spin-echo image (TR/TE effective of 3800/126) demonstrates the gravid uterus with the anterior placenta *(P)* as well as the left adnexal mass *(M)*. The signal intensity on the T2-weighted fast spin-echo image is very low for this mass, indicating a pedunculated leiomyoma. Small areas of hemorrhagic infarction are evident within the mass.

cause of lack of general availability of MR, but more importantly it is due to a lack of studies that demonstrate efficacy in well-defined clinical situations in which additional staging accuracy will affect patient outcome. Nonetheless, MRI can realize fairly high staging accuracies for some gynecologic malignancies, and persuasive arguments can be made for increased clinical use.[48,49,99,123,227]

Cervical carcinoma. Cervical epithelium can undergo a series of gradual histologic changes, from progressively severe dysplasia to carcinoma in situ (CIS) and invasive carcinoma. The detection of this progress with screening and biopsy has led to significant reduction in the mortality rate from this disease in the last 50 years.[26,59,206] The incidence of CIS surpasses invasive carcinoma by 4 to 1, with highest incidence around age 30, which is 10 to 15 years earlier than that of invasive carcinoma. Invasive carcinoma spreads by direct extension to adjacent organs, vagina, pelvic wall and bladder, and rectum. The failure to achieve control of this local disease is a major cause of treatment failures in advanced disease.[103,131,208,291] Metastatic lymphadenopathy occurs commonly in the pelvic lymph nodes, but it also involves the paraaortic chains in 17% to 29% of patients,[1,107,147,208,280] including 5% to 27% of stage IB and IIA lesions.[82,103,147,206] Locally advanced tumors may also disseminate along the peritoneum.[107,208]

The 5-year survival for invasive carcinoma is 80% to 90% for stage I, 75% for stage II, 35% for stage III, and 10% to 15% for stage IV.[109] The surgical approach for early-stage carcinoma includes total hysterectomy for stage IA, and radical hysterectomy for stage IB and II,

with radiation therapy reserved for bulky stage II, stage III and IV disease.[109,205,206] Anterior or posterior exenteration may be indicated for some stage IV disease with bladder or rectal involvement because of the risk of fistula formation after radiation treatment.[109]

The identification of cervical carcinoma on MR images is straightforward because of the normally very low signal intensity of the cervix on T2-weighted images, so that the high-signal–intensity lesion contrasts with the very low signal cervical stroma[23,144,294] (Fig. 39-55). Areas of coagulative necrosis may appear as small foci of lower signal.[249] The signal intensity of cervical carcinoma has a variable response to radiotherapy,[80,229] with a tendency to lose signal intensity on T2-weighted images in tumors responding to therapy. T1-weighted images fail to reveal smaller lesions because of a lack of contrast between cervix and tumor. Hematometra is not uncommon in cervical carcinoma, because of the occurrence of cervical obstruction or radiation-induced stenosis[29,239] (Fig. 39-56).

An important potential role for accurate noninvasive staging of cervical carcinoma exists, because clinical staging, based on clinical examination under anesthesia with cystoscopy and proctoscopy (Table 39-4), is inaccurate[103,107,147,208,280] when compared with pathologic findings. Surgical staging for clinical stage II-IV is not routinely performed and has significant morbidity.[107,147,227] Intraoperative findings of advanced-stage tumors will abort planned hysterectomy in up to 12% of patients with clinical stage I disease.[64,147] Patients treated with radiotherapy only may be under- or over-staged, causing adverse effects on mortality.[103] Therefore, if suf-

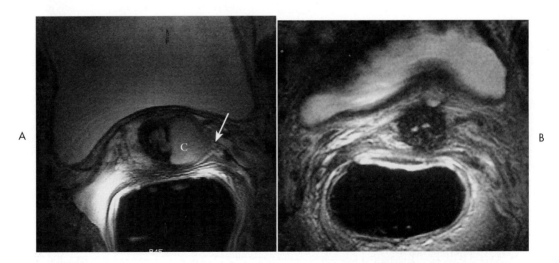

Fig. 39-55. Endorectal coil imaging of cervical carcinoma; stage IIB. **A,** Axial FSE (4000/140) image shows high-signal–intensity tumor (**C**) arising from the left cervical lip and growing into the left parametrium *(white arrow)*. **B,** Image after radiation therapy shows complete regression of the tumor and restoration of normal cervical signal intensity.

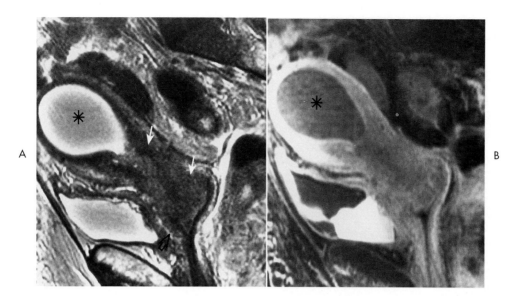

Fig. 39-56. Obstructed uterus due to endocervical adenocarcinoma. **A,** Sagittal FSE (TR/TE effective of 6000/119) shows a hematometra *(asterisk)* due to irregular intermediate-signal–intensity tumor *(white arrow)* obstructing the endocervical canal. Note that the normal low signal intensity of the cervical stroma is entirely disrupted because of infiltrating tumor and that the junctional zone in the low uterine segment is irregular and disrupted as a result of tumor infiltration. The anterior vaginal wall is irregularly thickened *(open arrow)* due to tumor involvement. Gadolinium-enhanced sagittal image **(B)** corresponding to the same level as in **(A)** demonstrates that the endocervical canal tumor enhances, though less than the normal myometrium and that the hematometra does not enhance. Notice the thickened enhancing tissue along the anterior vaginal wall indicating vaginal wall invasion.

Table 39-4. Staging accuracy of cervical carcinoma by MR imaging

Staging	N	Sensitivity (%)	Specificity (%)	Accuracy (%)	Ref
Overall	20			90	55
Overall	46			87	92
Overall	31			84	269
Overall	30			83	144
Overall	57			81	114
Overall	66			76	276
Overall	20			70	219
Vaginal involvement	57	100	89	93	114
Vaginal involvement	39	70	72	72	276
Parametrial involvement	57	89	87	93	114
Parametrial involvement	30	67	98	92	144
Parametrial involvement	19			90	249
Parametrial involvement	66	76	94	89	276
Parametrial involvement	25	100	80	88	248
Parametrial involvement	46	71	87	85	92
Parametrial involvement	20	0	83	79	283
Lymph node metastases	66	60	91	84	276
Lymph node metastases	30			78	144
Lymph node metastases	46	38	84	76	92
Pelvic sidewall involvement	57	86	96	95	114
Bladder involvement	57	100	96	96	114
Rectal involvement	57	100	100	100	114

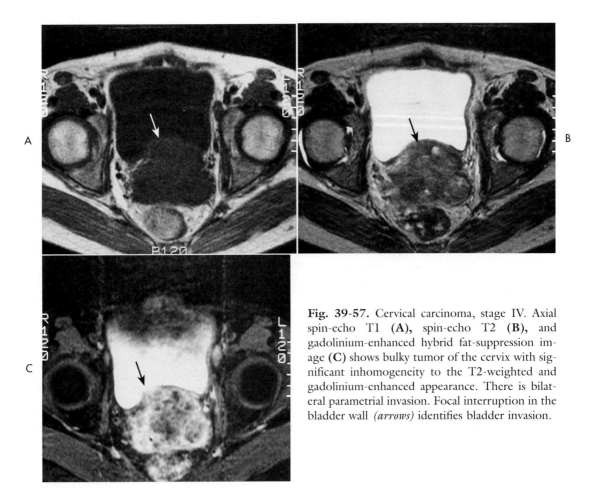

Fig. 39-57. Cervical carcinoma, stage IV. Axial spin-echo T1 **(A)**, spin-echo T2 **(B)**, and gadolinium-enhanced hybrid fat-suppression image **(C)** shows bulky tumor of the cervix with significant inhomogeneity to the T2-weighted and gadolinium-enhanced appearance. There is bilateral parametrial invasion. Focal interruption in the bladder wall *(arrows)* identifies bladder invasion.

ficient accuracy can be established, MR imaging may become a desirable substitute for clinical examination under anesthesia.[227]

Consistently high rates of accuracy for MR staging of cervical carcinoma (see Table 39-2) have been found in several studies. Overall accuracy rates of 76% to 83% are reported. Of course, MRI has no role in assessing most cases of cervical carcinoma, that is, carcinoma in situ, because these lesions are not visible on MR images. Stage IA lesions (microinvasive) are similarly difficult to detect by MR.[144,153,276] In one prospective study of 27 patients with stage 0 or IA lesions, no lesions were detected.[276] Larger lesions are easily appreciated, and accurate measurement of tumor volumes can be obtained.[35,101,153,249] Tumor volume is an important prognostic predictor of failure after radiation therapy, although it does not affect the FIGO clinical staging.[35,101,131,208,249]

The detection of parametrial spread relies on visualization of tumor invading the paracervical venous plexus. Invasion into the paracervical tissues can be excluded if a low-signal–intensity rim of cervical stroma surrounds the tumor (specificity 100%).[114,144,248,276] If this rim becomes effaced, parametrial spread is likely.* Bulky stage I tumors may displace the plexus laterally without invading it.† Tumors at the cervical lip that extend posterolaterally will protrude into the vaginal fornices; higher or anterior tumors will extend directly into the parametria[114] (see Fig. 39-55). Advanced tumors will grow along the sacrouterine ligaments and the cardinal ligaments to the pelvic side wall.[176,283,284] These features are best seen with side-by-side comparison of T1- and T2-weighted sequences for differentiation of tumor, paracervical venous plexus, and fat, since tumor and fat on T2-weighted sequences may exhibit little contrast.[248,283,284] Tumor invading the vaginal wall will interrupt the thin low-signal–intensity wall on T2-weighted sequences (see Fig. 39-56).‡ Similarly, if the low-signal–intensity muscularis of the bladder or rectum is focally disrupted, then spread into these organs is likely[55,92,114,144] (Fig. 39-57).

The role of gadolinium enhancement for staging

*References 114, 144, 219, 248, 274, 276.
†References 50, 114, 176, 226, 248, 276.
‡References 50, 55, 92, 114, 176, 274, 276.

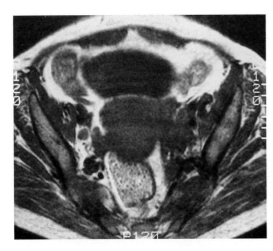

Fig. 39-58. Stage III cervical carcinoma. Spin-echo T1-weighted image demonstrates low-signal–intensity tumor extending to the left pelvic sidewall with extensive bilateral internal and external iliac adenopathy.

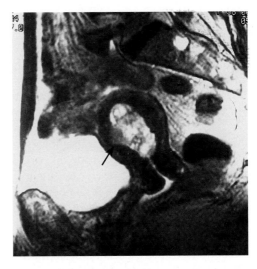

Fig. 39-59. MR imaging of endometrial carcinoma. Fast spin-echo image (FSE TR/TE 120/4000) shows a lobular tumor filling the entire endometrial cavity. This is a postmenopausal woman; the junctional zone is not well delineated. Polypoid tumor can be seen extending anteriorly into the myometrium *(arrow)* although it is clearly confined by myometrium. Pathology showed superficial myometrial invasion.

cervical carcinoma is not clear. Preliminary studies found similar information on enhanced T1-weighted images as on T2-weighted images, as well as an overall increase in staging accuracy with the enhanced images.[269] Hamm et al[97] and Thurner[267], however, reported that staging was not improved with Gd-DTPA administration. Intravenous contrast may be useful in specific problem-solving situations[122] or in combination with fat-suppression technique for excellent tumor-muscle differentiation on T1-weighted images (see Fig. 39-57).

A complete evaluation of patients with cervical carcinoma should include transverse T1-weighted images of the infrarenal paraaortic and iliac lymph node chains to detect enlarged lymph nodes (Fig. 39-58). Paraaortic metastatic adenopathy increases the stage of the disease and is a poor prognostic indicator.[1,101,103,208] The assessment of lymph nodes in cervical carcinoma is probably comparable to CT.[72] Experience with CT, however, indicates that size criteria alone are not sufficiently specific or sensitive for metastases[103,107,163] and must be supplemented by needle aspiration to provide diagnostic information.[16,99]

Endometrial carcinoma. Endometrial carcinoma is a disease of menopausal or postmenopausal women, with a peak incidence at age 55 to 65. Because of eradication of in situ cervical carcinoma detected by screening, endometrial carcinoma has become the more common invasive tumor in the United States.[60] Many endometrial carcinomas are surgically curable while confined to the uterus, however, so it has half the mortality of cervical carcinoma.[26] The risk factors include diabetes, hypertension, and those associated with prolonged unopposed estrogen stimulation: obesity, nulliparity, infertil-

ity, estrogen-secreting tumors, and exogenous estrogen administration.[59,60]

Endometrial carcinoma tends to proliferate within the endometrial cavity as a localized polypoid mass or as a diffuse tumor involving the entire endometrial surface.[59] Initially, invasion occurs through the myometrium or into the endocervical canal. Endometrial carcinoma commonly metastasizes to the adnexae or vagina, though frequently in microscopic deposits.[27,186] Pelvic or paraaortic lymph node metastases and positive peritoneal cytologies ensue with advanced tumors,[27,59,186] although these can occur with stage I disease.[27,59]

The most common finding on MR images in patients with small endometrial carcinomas is widening of the endometrial cavity as a result of the tumor or associated hematometra* (Fig. 39-59). Normal MRI scans occur in 15% to 19% of patients with endometrial carcinoma because small superficial lesions will blend in with the normal endometrium.[124,125] Masses of tumor within the endometrial cavity display variable signal intensity on T2-weighted images,[125,294] but they usually exhibit higher intensity than the uterine junction zone or myometrium.† Considerable signal heterogeneity due to necrosis, hemorrhage, and endocervical canal obstruction with hematometra is evident with larger tumors on T2-weighted images.[117,266,271] Gadolinium enhancement

---

*References 32, 117, 125, 211, 266, 294.
†References 91, 124, 125, 162, 211, 213, 295.

easily distinguishes vascularized tumor from areas of non-enhanced necrosis or fluid accumulation.[97,117,271] Usually, tumor enhances somewhat less than myometrial tissue, although the tumor-myometrial interface may often be obscured by gadolinium.[122]

The clinical utility of preoperative radiologic staging of endometrial carcinoma is not established.[162,187,227] Endometrial carcinoma is definitively staged using the surgical FIGO classification (see Table 39-3).[60] Treatment decisions are made, in part, on the basis of lymph node sampling or an assessment of relative risk for occult lymph node metastases.[187,186,27,34,161,60] The risk factors for paraaortic nodal metastases in Stage I/II disease include depth of myometrial invasion, presence of adnexal metastases, tumor grade, and grossly positive lymph nodes, all of which may be determined intraoperatively.* The role of preoperative radiation (e.g., intracavitary treatments) is unclear, although less toxicity to bowel may ensue, compared with postoperative radiotherapy.[34,155,192] MR imaging may be useful to plan radiation treatment portals.[227]

Staging of endometrial carcinoma by MRI requires demonstration of the tumor in relation to the myometrium and cervix, clear demonstration of the boundaries between uterus and bladder, rectum and vagina, and assessment of lymph nodes from the level of the kidneys through the pelvis. T2-weighted sagittal images display the uterine anatomy to best advantage, and these are considered most essential for showing intrauterine invasion. Transverse T1-weighted images are adequate for the evaluation of lymphadenopathy.

The depth of myometrial invasion is one of several pathologically defined risk factors that correlate with the surgical stage of disease, presence of lymph node metastases, and prognosis.† The most reliable sign of myometrial invasion on MR images is focal discontinuity in an otherwise intact junctional zone.‡ A distinct junctional zone, however, is not always visualized in postmenopausal women (see Fig. 39-59). A second sign in this case is focal thinning of the myometrium or irregularity of the tumor-myometrial interface (see Fig. 39-7).[125,211] Larger tumors and hematometra frequently thin the myometrium concentrically; therefore this is a nonspecific finding.[125,271] The prospective accuracy of determination of depth of invasion has been reported to be 74% to 94%.§ Invasion of the cervix can be diagnosed on MR images when high-signal–intensity tissue expands the endocervical canal or, more reliably, when tumor disrupts the low-signal–intensity cervical

stroma.[20,124,125,271] These findings are generally easily appreciated on MR[52,125,211]; reported accuracies for the detection of cervical invasion are 85% to 90%.[20,266]

Determination of stage III/IV disease requires assessment of the adnexae, uterine and cervical suspensory ligaments, pelvic lymph nodes, and bladder and rectal walls.[124,125,211,271] MR findings indicative of advanced disease include transmural interruption of the myometrium, serosal irregularity, and disruption of the low signal vaginal, bladder, or rectal muscularis.[52,124,125,271] Adnexal metastases, not uncommon, may be confused with normal high-signal ovaries or other ovarian pathologic condition.[52,73,211] In a prospective study, sensitivity for the detection of Stage III/IV disease by MRI was only 17%, and the positive predictive value for findings suggestive of advanced tumor was only 50%.[124]

The accuracy of MR staging of endometrial carcinoma has been reported to be 85% overall.[124,211,266] In one study[122] gadolinium-enhanced images were not shown to significantly improve accuracy, whereas other studies reported increased accuracy with contrast-enhanced imaging.[250]

Sarcomas of the uterus. Aside from malignancies arising from endometrium, uterine malignancies may originate from endometrial stroma (stromal sarcoma), pluripotential mesoderm (Müllerian mixed mesodermal tumors), and myometrial smooth-muscle origin (leiomyosarcomas).[59] In contrast to endometrial carcinoma, mesenchymal malignancies are often not detected with screening techniques and therefore are more likely to be in an advanced stage when diagnosed. Both lymphatic and hematogenous spread are more likely at presentation, compared with endometrial carcinoma.[12,47,51,245] Müllerian mixed mesodermal tumors are aggressive malignancies with a propensity for advanced stage at diagnosis.[12,25,59] Their biologic behavior and MR imaging characteristics are otherwise indistinguishable from endometrial carcinoma.[245,271,294] Tumors derived from endometrial stromal tissues include benign stromal nodules, low-grade stromal sarcoma (indistinguishable from benign nodules but with lymphatic invasion), and endometrial stromal sarcoma[12] (Fig. 39-60). The MR features of these tumors have not been reported.

Leiomyosarcomas arise from myometrial smooth muscle and usually occur in women between the ages of 40 and 60. Sarcomas are difficult to differentiate from leiomyomas histologically; typical criteria include greater than 10 mitoses per high-powered field, or more than 5 mitoses per high-powered field with nuclear atypia.[12,59] Given this subtle difference, it is unlikely that MR will prove useful in differentiating the two, although it serves to identify the myometrial origin of these tumors.[123,132] A large size at presentation and heterogeneously in-

---

*References 27, 34, 60, 138, 150, 161, 186, 192.
†References 27, 34, 138, 155, 161, 186.
‡References 124, 125, 211, 213, 271, 295.
§References 20, 52, 91, 124, 125, 211, 266, 295.

creased signal on T2-weighted images (see Fig. 39-10) distinguish sarcomas from the great majority of, but certainly not all, leiomyomas.[123,132] MR may prove useful in the unusual venoinvasive form of this sarcoma (intravenous leiomyomatosis) to demonstrate the extent of intravascular disease.[247]

Gestational trophoblastic disease. Gestational trophoblastic disease forms a spectrum of related condi-

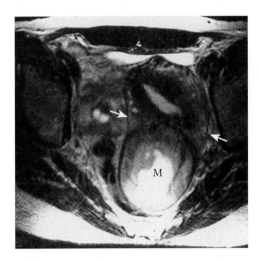

Fig. 39-60. Uterine sarcoma. Axial FSE image performed with multicoil demonstrates heterogenous intermediate signal intensity and mass *(M)* arising from the posterior uterine wall. Continuity of the mass with the myometrium can be seen *(white arrows)*. Note that the mass has internal necrosis, and that no part of the mass displays the usual low-signal–intensity areas of a uterine leiomyoma. Pathologic examination showed an endometrial stromal sarcoma.

tions that include molar pregnancy, invasive mole, and choriocarcinoma. After evacuation of a complete mole, 20% of patients develop persistent gestational trophoblastic disease, and 5% manifest metastases.[21] Chemotherapy achieves a high rate of cure, even when the tumor is widely metastasized.[21] The role of radiologic evaluation of patients with gestational trophoblastic disease lies primarily in the identification of metastases in the lung, brain, and liver.[21,127] MR imaging may be useful in demonstrating intrapelvic spread and tumor size. The signal intensity pattern of gestational trophoblastic disease is variable. Intratumoral hemorrhage frequently causes high-signal areas on T1-weighted sequences[119,271] (Fig. 39-61). Heterogeneity on T2-weighted sequences results from necrosis, hemorrhage, and cyst formation.[49,119,178] Large uterine vessels supplying the tumor appear as peritumoral signal voids (see Fig. 39-17).[119,178] Metastases to the vagina occur in 16% to 30% of cases.[21,127] Theca lutein cysts, which are frequently hemorrhagic,[49] occur in 30% to 50%[21,119] of cases.

Ovarian neoplasms. Ovarian carcinoma causes twice as many deaths as does any other gynecologic malignancy.[26] The incidence of epithelial ovarian carcinoma rises steadily between the ages of 30 and 70.[141]

Over 20 histologic types of tumors arise from the ovary. These are grouped into neoplasms of surface ovarian epithelium, germ cells, and sex cord-stromal origin.[59] The majority of malignant ovarian neoplasms in women are epithelial;[59,141,222] these include serous and mucinous cystadenocarcinomas, endometrioid carcinomas, and clear cell carcinomas.[59] These four neoplasms share similar clinical manifestations, frequency of bilaterality

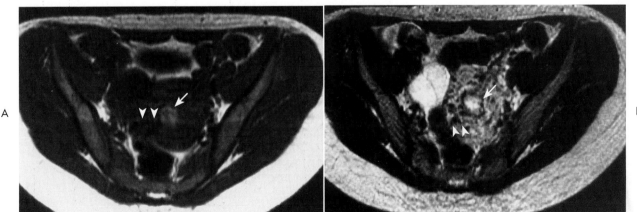

Fig. 39-61. Gestational trophoblastic disease. T1-weighted **(A)** and T2-weighted **(B)** images in a patient after evacuation of a complete mole shows high-signal–intensity mass embedded within the myometrium *(white arrows)*. Note on the T2-weighted spin-echo image in **(B)**, the punctate signal voids around the mass *(arrowheads)*. A right multiseptate theca lutein cyst is present.

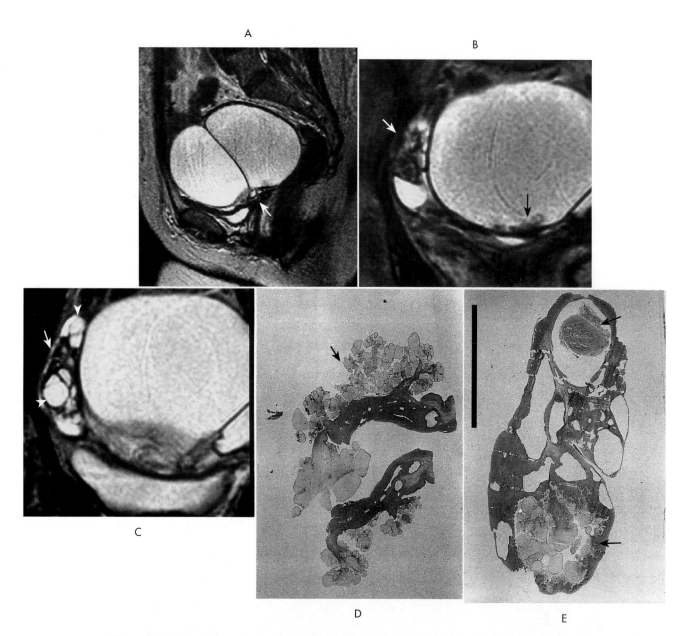

Fig. 39-62. Borderline ovarian carcinoma affecting both ovaries. **A,** Sagittal FSE image through the left adnexa shows a septated cystic mass arising from the left ovary. The identification of multiple small follicular cysts splayed out at the base of the mass *(white arrow)* identifies this as an ovarian origin. **B** and **C,** Two coronal images (fast spin-echo with TR/TE effective of 4000/120) demonstrate the cystic left adnexal mass compressing, but apparently not arising from, the right ovary *(white arrow)*. In **(B),** small papillary projections at the base of the mass *(black arrow)* identify this as a primary ovarian neoplasm. Although not giving rise to any mass, the right ovary is abnormal, displaying multiple irregular cysts with internal irregular projections consistent with papillary projections *(white arrowheads)*. **D,** Microscopic sections demonstrate the morphology of the papillary projections *(black arrow)* that were present in the multiseptate left ovarian mass shown in **(B)**. **E,** Whole mount section of the right ovary shows the irregular papillary projections *(arrows)* within the very small cysts of the right ovary even though no right ovarian mass was present (black bar >1.0 cm). Pathologic examination showed a serous cystadenocarcinoma of borderline malignancy affecting both ovaries.

(20% to 40% of cases), propensity for intraperitoneal metastasis, and a poor prognosis.[59,141,222] They have benign counterparts as well as low-grade forms, termed *borderline malignancies,* with significantly better prognosis (>90% 5-year survival) than higher grades.[59,222] Endometrioid and clear cell carcinoma resemble endometrial carcinoma histologically, frequently coexisting with endometriosis and synchronous endometrial carcinoma.[59] Clear cell carcinoma demonstrates a poorer prognosis and higher rates of lymphatic and hematogenous metastases.[133] Epithelial carcinomas indistinguishable from those of ovarian origin may arise in the peritoneum without ovarian involvement.[2]

In evaluating an adnexal mass by MR imaging, the first step is to establish that the mass is arising from the ovary (Fig. 39-62). High-resolution T2-weighted images are necessary to identify the ovaries and their relation to the mass. Heavily T2-weighted fast spin-echo images are helpful to identify small follicular cysts stretched around an ovarian mass. Gynecologic masses of other origin (e.g., peritubal cysts, pedunculated fibroids, some endometriomas, and hydrosalpinges) can be distinguished; these are almost always benign. In addition, criteria must

be applied to exclude benign causes of an ovarian mass: chemical-shift-specific behavior imaging for dermoids and previously described criteria for endometriomas and simple cysts.

Fairly high accuracy rates for distinguishing benign from malignant ovarian tumors by MR imaging have been reported, but whether this is sufficient for clinical management in difficult cases is unclear. Features on MR images that suggest malignancy in an adnexal mass include size greater than 4 cm; irregular or large solid components to a cystic mass; thick (>3-mm) septations; evidence of peritoneal, lymphatic, or hematogenous spread; or local invasion[38,251,258,267] (Figs. 39-63, and 39-64). Papillary projections within an ovarian mass establish that the mass is an ovarian neoplasm, although these can be seen in benign lesions (uncommonly), borderline lesions (commonly), and higher-grade malignant lesions (see Figs. 39-62, 39-65). Using these as well as other criteria described above, accuracy rates of 60% to 93% in determining benign from malignant masses by MRI have been reported,[251,258] with higher accuracy reported for Gd-DTPA–enhanced studies.[258,267] Accuracy of 86% in distinguishing benign from malignant epithe-

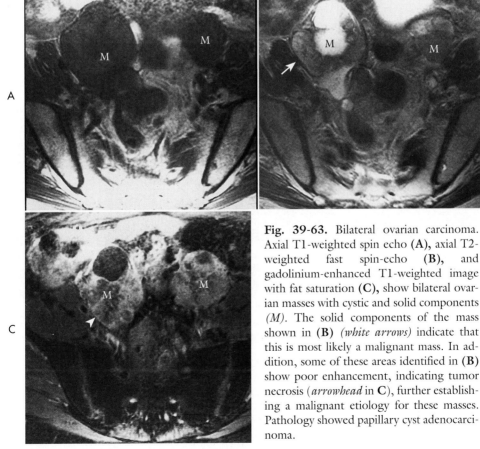

Fig. 39-63. Bilateral ovarian carcinoma. Axial T1-weighted spin echo **(A)**, axial T2-weighted fast spin-echo **(B)**, and gadolinium-enhanced T1-weighted image with fat saturation **(C)**, show bilateral ovarian masses with cystic and solid components *(M)*. The solid components of the mass shown in **(B)** *(white arrows)* indicate that this is most likely a malignant mass. In addition, some of these areas identified in **(B)** show poor enhancement, indicating tumor necrosis *(arrowhead* in **C)**, further establishing a malignant etiology for these masses. Pathology showed papillary cyst adenocarcinoma.

lial neoplasms has been described.[86] These results are comparable to those of 80% and 94% reported for US and CT, respectively.[38] One comparative study established a higher accuracy for the differentiation of benign and malignant ovarian masses for MRI, compared with transvaginal ultrasound and Doppler analysis.[238]

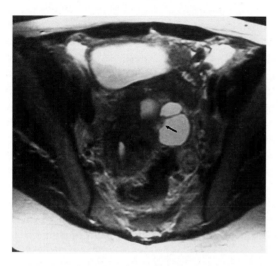

Fig. 39-64. Poorly differentiated epithelial ovarian carcinoma. Axial T2-weighted (FSE 2500/180, with multicoil) image shows cystic left adnexal mass with small mural nodule *(black arrow)* as well as a septation. Note small amount of ascites in the right and left paracolic gutter. Adenopathy in the left obturator chain is also present.

The signal intensity of cystic components of ovarian neoplasms varies, especially in mucinous tumors.[86,162,182,271] Specifically, signal may be hyperintense on T1-weighted images and intermediate on T2-weighted images as a result of hemorrhage, mucin content, or cell debris (see Fig. 39-14).[86,183,271,275] Gd-DTPA administration can assist in defining nodules, fluid loculi, and septa in complex adnexal masses.[86,97,258,268]

In contrast to endometrial and cervical carcinomas, ovarian carcinoma is usually diagnosed when it is not surgically curable. About 30% of ovarian carcinoma is surgically resectable by total hysterectomy and salpingo-oophorectomy (stage I and IIa disease).[222] The value of extensive debulking procedures for gross disease is controversial.[212]

Hysterectomy, salpingo-oopherectomy, omentectomy, and peritoneal inspection and washings comprise the definitive staging procedure for ovarian carcinoma.[33,141,222] Radiologic staging is inadequate primarily because of the high rates of microscopic peritoneal deposits throughout the abdomen.[33] Ascites is a nonspecific feature; as few as 40% of patients with ascitic fluid exhibit positive peritoneal cytologies.[33] In second-look restaging, even laparotomy may have a 20% false-negative rate.[85] These observations limit the application of CT as a substitute for surgical staging or restaging of ovarian carcinoma.[94,99,136,172] Similarly, MRI has no defined role in staging or second-look evaluations during therapy. Preliminary results, however, suggest that up to 75% accuracy rates may be achieved with contrast-enhanced

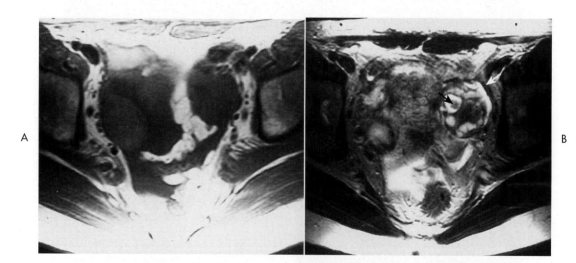

Fig. 39-65. Serous ovarian carcinoma of borderline malignancy in a 21-year-old woman. T1-weighted spin-echo images **(A)** and T2-weighted FSE (TR/TE$_{eff}$ of 4000/108) image **(B)** shows a small left ovarian cyst with internal papillary projections *(black arrowhead)*. The left fallopian tube *(white arrow)* is mildly dilated and adherent to the ovary (proved at laparotomy). At surgery, the left ovary was diffusely involved with tumor. (TR/TE$_{eff}$ of 4000/108, 256 × 256 acquisition matrix, 20-cm FOV, 5-mm–slice thickness.)

MRI staging of ovarian carcinoma,[258] and 83% accuracy can be achieved for detection of recurrent disease.[201]

In any case, the recognition of macroscopic intra-abdominal spread of ovarian carcinoma is crucial in using MRI to evaluate these patients. Solid or cystic peritoneal nodules can be diagnosed in many cases[86]; glucagon will help in this regard to suppress motion artifacts from bowel. The characteristic appearance of omental cake can be identified by its infiltrative margins and distinguished from bowel by Gd-DTPA enhancement if necessary.[117] Gadolinium-enhanced T1-weighted images with fat-suppression techniques may be particularly helpful for defining peritoneal spread.

COMPLICATIONS OF RADIATION AND SURGERY IN THE PELVIS

Common postoperative complications in the pelvis can be demonstrated by MR imaging. Hematomas, lymphoceles, abscesses, fistulas, and venous thromboses can be detected and characterized by MRI.[116] Fluid collections with peripheral hyperintense rims (the "ring sign") on T1-weighted images characterize hematomas.[117] Lymphoceles develop after lymphadenectomy, manifesting as sharply marginated cystic masses along the lymphatic chains and containing simple fluid.[116,291] Gadolinium enhancement of a mass with central fluid intensity and infiltrative borders characterizes most abscesses in the postoperative period.[116,123] Fistulas are common complications of radiotherapy of larger gynecologic neoplasms and surgery.[146] Enterovaginal and vesicovaginal fistulas are the most common types in this context.[146] MRI can demonstrate fistulous tracts on T2-weighted images as signal-intensity fluid tracts surrounded by lower-signal–intensity granulation tissue and fibrosis (Fig. 39-66).

External beam radiotherapy induces a number of changes in normal structures in the pelvis; these are evident on MR imaging. Some of these changes are summarized in Table 39-4. Radiation effects are dependent on the radiation dose and time elapsed since radiotherapy. Increased signal intensity on T2-weighted signal are usually acute or subacute changes and will not persist indefinitely.[5,77,259] Increased signal intensity should not be confused with tumor recurrence.[5,50] Bladder and rectal mucosal changes correlate, in part, with radiation cystitis and proctitis.[259]

The differentiation of recurrent pelvic carcinoma from postoperative fibrosis is a common clinical problem to which MR has been applied. Recurrent tumor in the pelvis usually appears as nodules or masses with higher signal intensity on T2-weighted images than occurs with fibrosis[77,88,89,130] (Fig. 39-67), although exceptions may occur.[63] Infiltrative recurrences without definable mass are not common.[77] Fibrotic scarring less than 6 months old shows slightly higher signal intensity than does late fibrosis (>1 year) and overlaps in signal intensity with tumor recurrences.[77,130] The surgical vaginal cuff and pelvic sidewall are common sites of recurrence of cervi-

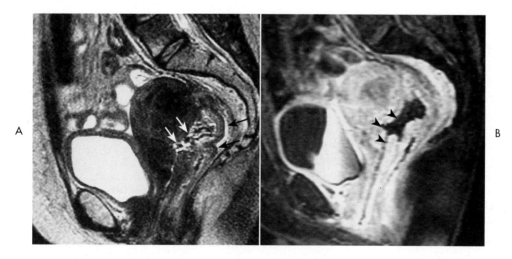

Fig. 39-66. Rectovaginal fistula on MR imaging. Sagittal T2-weighted FSE (**A**) and gadolinium-enhanced fat saturation image (**B**) in a patient after radiation for cervical carcinoma, in whom there was no clinical suspicion of fistula at the time of MR imaging, shows a high-signal–intensity tract *(white arrows)* on the FSE images extending from the rectum into the vaginal fornix. Note that although the posterior rectal wall is well delineated *(black arrows)*, there is a defect in the anterior rectal wall leading into the fistula. On the gadolinium-enhanced images, this appears as a nonenhancing tract *(black arrowheads)*. Incidentally noted are radiation changes in the spine and presacral space.

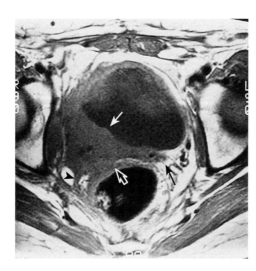

Fig. 39-67. MR evaluation of tumor recurrence. Axial T1-weighted image (spin echo 550/16) shows a right-sided tumor mass arising from the vaginal cuff. Note the normal appearance of the vaginal cuff on the left *(black arrow)*. The tumor invades anteriorly into the bladder *(white arrow)* and posteriorly into the rectal muscularis *(open arrow)*. Note also the right pelvic side wall and right uretero-sacral ligament invasion *(black arrowhead)*.

cal and endometrial carcinoma[82,131,291]; the incidence varies with the type of radiation given.[131,186,291] An accuracy of 80%, with a sensitivity of 82% and specificity of 78%, has been reported for the MR determination of recurrent cervical carcinoma.[291]

SUMMARY

MR imaging can delineate anatomy and pathologic conditions within the pelvis with higher intrinsic soft-tissue contrast than can ultrasound or CT, allowing for better characterization of lesions and their relation to surrounding organs. MR imaging demonstrated utility in diagnosing some of the more common gynecologic pelvic masses, although in both the male and female pelvis most attention has focused on the potential for MRI to stage, rather than diagnose, neoplasms. Currently, MR imaging has the greatest accuracy, as well as the potential for the greatest clinical utility, in the staging of cervical carcinoma. Endometrial carcinoma can also be staged by MRI with reasonable accuracy, although the clinical indications for preoperative endometrial carcinoma staging are less clear. Initial experience with bladder and rectal carcinomas is encouraging, although not clearly better than that of CT or clinical staging. On the other hand, MRI has proved to be somewhat disappointing in the staging of prostate cancer. Many of the problems inherent in staging tumors by MRI are common to all staging modalities. They arise from as yet suboptimal

tumor tissue contrast, low-image resolution, and the inability to distinguish benign from malignant lymphadenopathy. More recent techniques such as surface coil arrays, fast spin-echo sequences, endoluminal coils, and new contrast agents are contributing to the rapid pace of technologic advancement in the field of MRI of the pelvis.

REFERENCES

1. Alcock CJ, Toplis PJ: The influence of pelvic lymph node disease on survival for stage I and II carcinoma of the cervix. *Clin Radiol* 38:13, 1987.
2. Altaras MM, Aviram R, Cohen I, Cordoba M, et al: Primary peritoneal papillary serous adenocarcinoma: clinical and management aspects. *Gynecol Oncol* 40:230, 1991.
3. Amendola MA, Glazer GM, Grossman HB, et al: Staging of bladder carcinoma: MRI-CT-surgical correlation. *AJR* 146:1179, 1986.
4. Angtuaco TL, Shah HR, Mattison DR, et al: MR imaging in high-risk obstetric patients: a valuable complement to US. *Radiographics* 12:91, 1992.
5. Arrivé L, Change YCF, Hricak H, et al: Radiation-induced uterine changes: MR imaging. *Radiology* 70:55, 1989.
6. Arrivé L, Menu Y, Dessarts I, et al: Diagnosis of abdominal venous thrombosis by means of spin-echo and gradient-echo MR imaging: analysis with receiver operating characteristic curves. *Radiology* 181:661, 1991.
7. Arrivé L, Hricak H, Martin MC: Pelvic endometriosis: MR imaging. *Radiology* 171:687, 1989.
8. Ascher SM, Scoutt LM, McCarthy SM, et al: Uterine changes after dilation and curettage: MR imaging findings. *Radiology* 80:433, 1991.
9. Aubel S, Wozney P, Edwards RP: MRI of female uterine and juxta-uterine masses: clinical application in 25 patients. *Magn Reson Imaging* 9:485, 1991.
10. Ayala AG, Ro JY, Babaian R, et al: The prostatic capsule: does it exist? Its importance in the staging and treatment of prostatic carcinoma. *Am J Surg Pathol* 13(1):21, 1989.
11. Azziz R: Adenomyosis: current perspectives. *Obstet Gynecol Clinics North Am* 16:221, 1989.
12. Baggish MS: Mesenchymal tumors of the uterus. *Clin Obstet Gynecol* 17:51, 1974.
13. Baker LL, Hajek PC, Burkhard TK, et al: MR imaging of the scrotum: pathologic conditions. *Radiology* 163:93, 1987.
14. Baker LL, Hajek PC, Burkhard TK, et al: MR imaging of the scrotum: normal anatomy. *Radiology* 163:89, 1987.
15. Baker LL, Hajek PC, Burkhard TK, et al: Polyorchidism: evaluation by MR. *AJR* 148:305, 1987.
16. Bandy LC, Clarke-Pearson DL, Silverman PM, et al: Computed tomography in evaluation of extrapelvic lymphadenopathy in carcinoma of the cervix. *Obstet Gynecol* 65:73, 1985.
17. Bartolozzi C, Selli C, Olmastroni M, et al: Rhabdomyosarcoma of the prostate: MR findings. *AJR* 150:1333, 1988.
18. Baudouin CJ, Soutter WP, Gilderdale DJ, et al: Magnetic resonance imaging of the uterine cervix using and intravaginal coil. *Magn Reson Med* 24:196, 1992.
19. Beischer NA, Buttery BW, Fotune DW, et al: Growth and malignancy of ovarian tumours in pregnancy. *Aust NZ J Obstetr Gynaec* 11:208, 1971.
20. Belloni C, Vigano R, del Maschio A, et al: Magnetic resonance imaging in endometrial carcinoma staging. *Gynecol Oncol* 37:172, 1990.
21. Berkowitz RS, Goldstein DF: Gestational trophoblastic disease. *Semin Oncol* 16:410, 1989.

22. Bezzi M, Kressel HY, Allen KS, et al: Prostatic carcinoma: staging with MR imaging at 1.5T. *Radiology* 69:339, 1988.

23. Bies JR, Ellis JH, Kopecky KK, et al: Assessment of primary gynecologic malignanices: comparison of 0.15-T resistive MRI with CT. *AJR* 143:1249, 1984.

24. Biondetti PR, Lee JKT, Ling D, et al: Clinical stage B prostate carcinoma: staging with MR imaging. *Radiology* 162:325, 1987.

25. Bitterman P, Chun B, Kurman RJ: The significance of epithelial differentiation in mixed mesoderam tumors of the uterus: a clinicopathologic and immunohistochemical study. *Am J Surg Pathol* 14:317, 1990.

26. Boring CC, Squires TS, Tong T: Cancer statistics, 1991. *CA-A Cancer J Clin* 41:8, 1991.

27. Boronow RC, Morrow CP, Creasman WT, et al: Surgical staging in endometrial cancer: clinical-pathologic findings of a prospective study. *Obstet Gynecol* 63:825, 1984.

28. Borrello JA, Chenevert TL, Meyer CR, et al: Chemical shift-based true water and fat images: regional phase correction of modified spin-echo MR images. *Radiology* 164:531, 1987.

29. Breckenridge JW, Kurtz AB, Ritchie WGM, et al: Postmenopausal uterine fluid collection: indicator of carcinoma. *AJR* 139:529, 1982.

30. Brown HK, Stoll BS, Nicosia SV, et al: Uterine junctional zone: correlation between histologic findings and MR imaging. *Radiology* 179:409, 1991.

31. Brown JJ, Thurnher S, Hricak H: MR imaging of the uterus: low-signal-intensity abnormalities of the endometrium and endometrial cavity. *Magn Reson Imaging* 8:309, 1990.

32. Bryan PJ, Butler HE, LiPuma JP, et al: NMR scanning of the pelvis: inital experience with a 0.3 T system. *AJR* 141:1111, 1983.

33. Buchsbaum HJ, Brady MF, Delgado G, et al: Surgical staging of carcinoma of the ovaries. *Surg Gynecol Obstet* 169:226, 1989.

34. Bucy GS, Mendenhall WM, Morgan LS, et al: Clinical Stage I and II endometrial carcinoma treated with surgery and/or radiation therapy: analysis of prognostic and treatment-related factors. *Gynecol Oncol* 33:290, 1989.

35. Burghardt E, Hofmann HMH, Ebner F, et al: Magnetic resonance imaging in cervical cancer: a basis for objective classification. *Gynecol Oncol* 33:61, 1989.

36. Burks DD, Markey BJ, Burkhard TK, et al: Suspected testicular torsion and ischemia: evaluation with color Doppler sonography. *Radiology* 175:815, 1990.

37. Butch RJ, Stark DD, Wittenberg J, et al: Staging rectal cancer by MR and CT. *AJR* 146:1155, 1986.

38. Buy JN, Ghossain MA, Sciot C, et al: Epithelial tumors of the ovary: CT findings and correlation with US. *Radiology* 178:811, 1991.

39. Buy J-N, Moss AA, Guinet C, et al: MR staging of bladder carcinoma: correlation with pathologic findings. *Radiology* 69:695, 1988.

40. Byar DP, Mostofi FK, VA Cooperative Urol Research Group: Carcinoma of the prostate: prognostic evaluation of certain pathologic features in 208 radical prostatectomies. *Cancer* 30:5, 1972.

41. Carrington BM, Hricak H, Nuruddin RN, et al: Müllerian duct anomalies: MR imaging evaluation. *Radiology* 176:715, 1990.

42. Carrol CL, Sommer FG, McNeal JE, et al: The abnormal prostate: MR imaging at 1.5T with histopathologic correlation. *Radiology* 163:521, 1987.

43. Carter HB, Brem RF, Tempany CM, et al: Nonpalpable prostate cancer: detection with MR imaging. *Radiology* 178:523, 1991.

44. Carter HB, Pearson JD, Metter J, et al: Longitudinal evaluation of prostate-specific antigen levels in men with and without prostate disease. *JAMA* 267(16):2215, 1992.

45. Chan TW, Kressel HY, Saul SH, et al: Rectal carcinoma: staging at MR imaging with endorectal surface coil. *Radiology* 181:461, 1991.

46. Chan TW, Listerud J, Kressel HY: Combined chemical-shift and phase-selective imaging for fat suppression: theory and initial clinical experience. *Radiology* 181:41, 1991.

47. Chang KL, Crabtree GS, Lim-Tan SK, et al: Primary uterine endometrial stromal neoplasms: a clinicopathologic study of 117 cases. *Am J Surg Pathol* 14:415, 1990.

48. Chang YCF, Arrive L, Hricak H: Gynecologic tumor imaging. *Semin Ultrasound CT MR* 10:29, 1989.

49. Chang YCF, Hricak H: Current status of MR imaging of the female pelvis. *Crit Rev Diagn Imaging* 29:337, 1989.

50. Chang YCF, Hricak H, Thurnher S, et al: Vagina: evaluation with MR imaging. Part II. Neoplasms. *Radiology* 169:175, 1988.

51. Chen S: Propensity of retroperitoneal lymph node metastasis in patients with stage I sarcoma of the uterus. *Gynecol Oncol* 32:215, 1989.

52. Chen SS, Rumancik WM, Spiegel G: Magnetic resonance imaging in stage I endometrial carcinoma. *Obstet Gynecol* 75:274, 1990.

53. Clement PB: Pathology of endometriosis. In Rosen PP, Fechner RE, editors: *Pathology Annual,* Norwalk, 1990, Appleton and Lange, vol 25, p 245.

54. Clements R, Griffiths GJ, Peeling WB: Staging prostatic cancer. *Clin Radiol* 46:225, 1992.

55. Cobby M, Browning J, Jones A, et al: Magnetic resonance imaging, computed tomography, and endosonography in the local staging of carcinoma of the cervix. *Br J Radiol* 63:673, 1990.

56. Constable RT, Anderson AW, Zhong J, et al: Factors influencing contrast in fast spin-echo MR imaging. *Magn Reson Imaging* 10:497, 1992.

57. Constable RT, Gore JC: The loss of small objects in variable TE imaging: implications for FSE, RARE, and EPI. *Magn Reson Med* 28:9, 1992.

58. Constable RT, Smith RC, Gore JC: Signal-to-noise and contrast in fast spin echo (FSE) and inversion recovery FSE imaging. *J Comput Assist Tomogr* 6(1):41, 1992.

59. Cotran RS, Kumar V, Robbins SL: *Robbins pathologic basis of disease,* ed 4, Philadelphia, 1989, WB Saunders.

60. Creasman WT, Eddy GL: Recent advances in endometrial cancer. *Semin Surg Oncol* 6:339, 1990.

61. Crucitti F, Doglietto GB, Bellantone R, et al: Accurate specimen preparation and examination is mandatory to detect lymph nodes and avoid understaging in colorectal cancer. *J Surg Oncol* 51:153, 1992.

62. de Lange EE, Fechner RE, Edge SB, et al: Preoperative staging of rectal carcinoma with MR imaging: surgical and histopathologic correlation. *Radiology* 176:623, 1990.

63. de Lange EE, Fechner RE, Wanebo HJ: Suspected recurrent rectosigmoid carcinoma after abdominoperineal resection: MR imaging and histopathologic findings. *Radiology* 170:323, 1989.

64. Delgado G, Bundy BN, Fowler WC, et al: A prospective surgical pathology study of stage I squamous carcinoma of the cervix: a Gynecologic Oncology Group study. *Gynecol Oncol* 35:314, 1989.

65. Dershaw DD, Panicek DM: Imaging of invasive bladder cancer. *Semin Oncology* 17(5):544, 1990.

66. Devesa JM, Morales V, Enriquez JM, et al: Colorectal cancer: the bases for a comprehensive follow-up. *Dis Colon Rectum* 31:636, 1988.

67. Dhom G: Unusual prostatic carcinomas. *Pathol Res Pract* 186:28, 1990.

68. Dixon WT: Simple proton spectroscopic imaging. *Radiology* 153:189, 1984.

69. Dixon WT, Engels H, Castillo M, et al: Incidental magnetization transfer contrast in standard multislice imaging. *Magn Reson Imaging* 8:417, 1990.

70. Dodd GD, Budzik RF: Lipomatous tumors of the pelvis in women: spectrum of imaging findings. *AJR* 155:317, 1990.

71. Donohue JP, Perez JM, Einhorn LH: Improved management of non-seminomatous testis tumors. *J Urol* 121:425, 1979.

72. Dooms GC, Hricak H, Crooks LE, et al: Magnetic resonance imaging of the lymph nodes: comparison with CT. *Radiology* 153:719, 1984.

73. Dooms GC, Hricak H, Tscholakoff D: Adnexal structures: MR imaging. *Radiology* 158:639, 1986.

74. Dudiak CM, Turner DA, Patel SK, et al: Uterine leiomyomas in the infertile patient: preoperative localization with MR imaging versus US and hysterosalpingography. *Radiology* 167:627, 1988.

75. Dykes TA, Isler RJ, McLean AC: MR imaging of Asherman syndrome: total endometrial obliteration. *J Comput Assist Tomogr* 5(5):858, 1991.

76. Ebert T, Schmitz-Dräger B-J, Bürrig K-F, et al: Accuracy of imaging modalities in staging the local extent of prostate cancer. *Urol Clin North Am* 18(3):453, 1991.

77. Ebner F, Kressel HY, Mintz MC, et al: Tumor recurrence versus fibrosis in the female pelvis: differentiation with MR imaging at 1.5 T. *Radiology* 166:333, 1988.

78. Fisher MR, Hricak H, Crooks LE: Urinary bladder MR imaging. Part I. Normal and benign conditions. *Radiology* 157:467, 1985.

79. Fisher MR, Hricak H, Tanagho EA: Urinary bladder MR imaging. Part II. Neoplasm. *Radiology* 157:471, 1985.

80. Flueckiger F, Ebner F, Poschauko H, et al: Cervical cancer: serial MR imaging before and after primary radiation therapy—a 2-year follow-up study. *Radiology* 184:89, 1992.

81. Fritzsche PJ, Hricak H, Kogan BA, et al: Undescended testis: value of MR imaging. *Radiology* 164:169, 1987.

82. Fu YS, Reagan JW: *Pathology of the uterine cervix, vagina, and vulva,* Philadelphia, 1989, WB Saunders, p 225.

83. Gehl H-B, Bohndorf K, Klose K-C: Inferior vena cava tumor thrombus: demonstration by GD-DTPA enhanced MR. *J Comput Assist Tomogr* 14:479, 1990.

84. Gerbie AB, Merrill JA: Pathology of endometriosis. *Clin Obstet Gynecol* 31:779, 1988.

85. Ghatage P, Krepart GV, Lotocki R: Factor analysis of false-negative second-look laparotomy. *Gynecol Oncol* 36:172, 1990.

86. Ghossain MA, Buy J, Ligneres C, et al: Epithelial tumors of the ovary: comparison of MR and CT findings. *Radiology* 181:863, 1991.

87. Gittes RF: Carcinoma of the prostate. *New Engl J Med* 324:236, 1991.

88. Glazer HS, Lee JKT, Levitt RG, et al: Radiation fibrosis: differentiation from recurrent tumor by MR imaging. *Radiology* 156:721, 1985.

89. Gomberg JS, Friedman AC, Radecki PD, et al: MRI differentiation of recurrent colorectal carcinoma from postoperative fibrosis. *Gastrointest Radiol* 11:361, 1986.

90. Gomori JM, Schnall MD, Grossman RI: Mechanisms of altered T2 contrast in fast spin echo MR. *Radiology* (in press).

91. Gordon AN, Fleischer AC, Dudley BS, et al: Preoperative assessment of myometrial invasion of endometrial adenocarcinoma by sonography (US), and magnetic resonance imaging (MRI). *Gynecol Oncol* 34:175, 1989.

92. Greco A, Masson P, Leung AWL, et al: Staging of carcinoma of the uterine cervix: MRI-surgical correlation. *Clin Radiol* 40:401, 1989.

93. Greene DR, Wheeler TM, Egawa S, et al: A comparison of the morphological features of cancer arising in the transition zone and in the peripheral zone of the prostate. *J Urol* 146:1069, 1991.

94. Guidozzi F, Soonendecker EWW: Evaluation of preoperative investigations in patients admitted for ovarian primary cytoreductive surgery. *Gynecol Oncol* 40:244, 1991.

95. Guinet C, Buy JN, Sezeur A, et al: Preoperative assessment of the extension of rectal carcinoma: correlation of MR, surgical, and histopathologic findings. *J Comput Assist Tomogr* 12:209, 1988.

96. Hall RR, Prout GR: Staging of bladder cancer: is the tumor, node, metastasis system adequate? *Semin Oncology* 19(5):517, 1990.

97. Hamm B, Laniado M, Saini S: Contrast-enhanced magnetic resonance imaging of the abdomen and pelvis. *Magn Reson Q* 6:108, 1990.

98. Hamper UM, Epstein JI, Sheth S, et al: Cystic lesions of the prostate gland. A sonographic-pathologic correlation. *J Ultrasound Med* 9:395, 1990.

99. Hann LE, Crivello MS: Imaging techniques in the staging of gynecologic malignancy. *Clin Obstet Gynecol* 29:715, 1986.

100. Hata K, Hata T, Manabe A, et al: A critical evaluation of transvaginal doppler studies, transvaginal sonography, magnetic resonance imaging, and CA 125 in detecting ovarian cancer. *Obstet Gynecol* 80:922, 1992.

101. Hawnaur JM, Carrington BM, Johnson RJ, et al: Factors predicting clinical outcome on magnetic resonance imaging of carcinoma of the cervix treated by radiotherapy. Abstract No. 275 presented at the Society for Magnetic Resonance in Medicine, San Francisco, 1991.

102. Hayes CE, Hattes N, Roemer PB: Volume imaging with MR phased arrays. *Magn Reson Med* 18:309, 1991.

103. Heaps JM, Berek JS: Surgical staging of cervical cancer. *Clin Obstet Gynecol* 33:852, 1990.

104. Heaps JM, Nieberg RK, Berek JS: Malignant neoplasms arising in endometriosis. *Obstetr Gynecol* 75:1023, 1990.

105. Hearshen DO, Ellis JH, Carson PL, et al: Boundary effects from opposed magnetization artifact in IR images. *Radiology* 160:543, 1986.

106. Heiken JP, Balfe DM, McClennan BL: Testicular tumors: oncologic imaging and diagnosis. *Int J Radiat Oncol Biol Phys* 10:275, 1984.

107. Heller PB, Malfetano JH, Bundy BN, et al: Clinical-pathologic study of stage IIB, III, and IVA carcinoma of the cervix: extended diagnostic evaluation for paraaortic node metastasis—a Gynecologic Oncology Group study. *Gynecol Oncol* 38:425, 1990.

108. Hennig J, Nauerth A, Friedburg H: RARE imaging: a fast imaging method for clinical MR. *Magn Reson Med* 3:823, 1986.

109. Herbst A, Ulfedler H, Hatch R: Gynecology. In Schwartz SI, Shires GT, Spencer FC, Storer EH, eds.: *Principles of surgery,* ed 4, New York, 1984, McGraw-Hill.

110. Herr HW: Staging invasive bladder tumors. *J Surg Oncol* 51:217, 1992.

111. Herrera L, Villareal JR: Incidence of metastases from rectal adenocarcinoma in small lymph nodes detected by a clearing technique. *Dis Colon Rect* 35:783, 1992.

112. Holder LE, Martire JR, Holmes ER, et al: Testicular radionuclide angiography and static imaging: anatomy, scintigraphic interpretation, and clinical indications. *Radiology* 125:739, 1977.

113. Horwich A: Current controversies in the management of testicular cancer. *Eur J Cancer* 27(3):322, 1991.

114. Hricak H, Lacey CG, Sandles LG, et al: Invasive cervical carcinoma: comparison of MR imaging and surgical findings. *Radiology* 166:623, 1988.

115. Hricak H: Many facets of prostate carcinoma. *Semin Ultrasound CT MR* 9(5):327, 1988.

116. Hricak H: Postoperative and postradiation changes in the pelvis. *Magn Reson Q* 6:276, 1990.

117. Hricak H, Carrington BM: *MRI of the pelvis: a text atlas,* Norwalk, 1991, Appleton and Lange.

118. Hricak H, Chang YCF, Cann CE, et al: Cervical incompetence: preliminary evaluation with MR imaging. *Radiology* 174:821, 1990.

119. Hricak H, Demas BE, Braga CA, et al: Gestational trophoblastic neoplasm of the uterus: MR assessment. *Radiology* 161:11, 1986.

120. Hricak H, Dooms GC, Jeffrey RB, et al: Prostatic carcinoma: staging by clinical assessment, CT, and MR imaging. *Radiology-main* 162:331, 1987.

121. Hricak H, Dooms GC, McNeal JE, et al: MR imaging of the prostate gland: normal anatomy. *AJR* 148:51, 1987.

122. Hricak H, Hamm B, Semelka RC, et al: Carcinoma of the uterus: use of gadopenetate dimeglumine in MR imaging. *Radiology* 181:95, 1991.

123. Hricak H, Lacey C, Schriock E, et al: Gynecologic masses: value of magnetic resonance imaging. *Am J Obstet Gynecol* 153:31, 1985.

124. Hricak H, Rubinstein LV, Gherman GM, et al: MR imaging evaluation of endometrial carcinoma: results of an NCI cooperative study. *Radiology* 179:829, 1991.

125. Hricak H, Stern JL, Fisher MR, et al: Endometrial carcinoma staging by MR imaging. *Radiology* 162:297, 1987.

126. Hricak H, Tscholakoff D, Heinrichs L, et al: Uterine leiomyomas: correlation of MR, histopathologic findings, and symptoms. *Radiology* 158:385, 1986.

127. Hunter V, Raymond E, Christensen C, et al: Efficacy of the metastatic survey in the staging of gestational trophoblastic disease. *Cancer* 65:1647, 1990.

128. Husband JES, Olliff JFC, Williams MP, et al: Bladder cancer: staging with CT and MR imaging. *Radiology* 173:435, 1989.

129. Imai Y, Kressel HY, Saul SH, et al: Colorectal tumors: an in vitro study of high-resolution MR imaging. *Radiology* 177:695, 1990.

130. Ito K, Kato T, Tadokoro M, et al: Recurrent rectal cancer and scar: differentiation with PET and MR imaging. *Radiology* 182:549, 1992.

131. Jampolis S, Andras EJ, Fletcher GH: Analysis of sites and causes of failures of irradiation in invasive squamous cell carcinoma of the intact uterine cervix. *Radiology* 115:681, 1975.

132. Janus C, White M, Dottino P, et al: Uterine leiomyosarcoma: magnetic resonance imaging. *Gynecol Oncol* 32:79, 1989.

133. Jenison EL, Montag AG, Griffiths CT, et al: Clear cell adenocarcinoma of the ovary: a clinical analysis and comparison with serous carcinoma. *Gynecol Oncol* 32:65, 1989.

134. Johansson J-E, Adami H-O, Andersson SO, et al: High 10-year survival rate in patients with early, untreated prostatic cancer. *JAMA* 267:2191, 1992.

135. Johnson JO, Mattrey RF, Phillipson J: Differentiation of seminomatous from nonseminomatous testicular tumors with MR imaging. *AJR* 154:539, 1990.

136. Johnson RJ, Blackledge G, Eddleston B, et al: Abdomino-pelvic computed tomography in the management of ovarian carcinoma. *Radiology* 146:447, 1983.

137. Jolles CJ: Gynecologic cancer associated with pregnancy. *Semin Oncol* 6:417, 1989.

138. Kadar N, Malfetano JH, Homesley HD: Determinants of survival of surgically staged patients with endometrial carcinoma histologically confined to the uterus: implications for therapy. *Obstet Gynecol* 80:655, 1992.

139. Kahn T, Bürrig K, Schmitz-Dräger B, et al: Prostatic carcinoma and benign prostatic hyperplasia: MR imaging with histopathologic correlation. *Radiology* 173:847, 1989.

140. Kaji Y, Sugimura K, Nagoaka S, et al: Amyloid deposition in seminal vesicles mimicking tumor invasion from bladder cancer: MR findings. *J Comput Assist Tomogr* 16(6):989, 1992.

141. Katz ME, Schwartz PE, Kapp DS: Epithelial carcinoma of the ovary: current strategies. *Ann Intern Med* 95:98, 1981.

142. Keller PJ, Hunter WW, Schmalbrock P: Multisection fat-water imaging with chemical shift selective presaturation. *Radiology* 164:539, 1987.

143. Kier R, Smith RC, McCarthy SM: Value of lipid- and water-suppression MR images in distinguishing between blood and lipid within ovarian masses. *AJR* 158:321, 1992.

144. Kim SH, Choi BI, Lee HP, et al: Uterine cervical carcinoma: comparison of CT and MR findings. *Radiology* 175:45, 1990.

145. Koelbel G, Schmiedl U, Griebel J, et al: MR imaging of urinary bladder neoplasms. *J Comput Assist Tomogr* 12(1):98, 1988.

146. Kuhlman JE, Fishman EK: CT evaluation of enterovaginal and vesicovaginal fistulas. *J Comput Assist Tomogr* 14:390, 1990.

147. Lagasse LD, Creasman WT, Shingleton HM, et al: Results and complications of operative staging in cervical cancer: experience of the gynecologic oncology group. *Gynecol Oncol* 9:90, 1980.

148. Lanzer P, Gross GM, Keller FS, et al: Sequential 2D inflow venography: initial clinical observations. *Magn Reson Med* 19:470, 1991.

149. Larsen MP, Carter HB, Epstein JI: Can stage A1 tumor extent be predicted by transurethral resection tumor volume, per cent or grade? A study of 64 stage A1 radical prostatectomies with comparison to prostates removed for stages A2 and B disease. *J Urol* 146:1059, 1991.

150. Lee JKT, Gersell DJ, Balfe DM, et al: The uterus: in-vitro MR-anatomic correlation of normal and abnormal specimens. *Radiology* 157:175, 1985.

151. Lee JKT, McClennan BL, Stanley RJ, et al: Utility of computed tomography in the localization of the undescended testis. *Radiology* 135:121, 1980.

152. Lee JKT, Rholl KS: MRI of the bladder and prostate. *AJR* 147:732, 1986.

153. Lien HH, Blomlie V, Kjorstad K, et al: Clinical stage I carcinoma of the cervix: value of MR imaging in determining degree of invasiveness. *AJR* 156:1191, 1991.

154. Ling D, Lee JKT, Heiken JP, et al: Prostatic carcinoma and benign prostatic hyperplasia: inability of MR imaging to distinguish between the two diseases. *Radiology* 158:103, 1986.

155. Mannel RS, Berman ML, Walker JL, et al: Management of endometrial cancer with suspected cervical involvement. *Obstet Gynecol* 75:1061, 1990.

156. Mark AS, Hricak H, Heinrichs LW, et al: Adenomyosis and leiomyoma: differential diagnosis with MR imaging. *Radiology* 163:527, 1987.

157. Marks G, Mohiuddin M, Masoin L, et al: High-dose preoperative radiation therapy as the key to extending sphincter-preservation surgery for cancer of the distal rectum. *Surg Oncol Clin North Am* 1:71, 1992.

158. Martin B, Mulopulos GP, Bryan PJ: MRI of puerperal ovarian-vein thrombosis *AJR* 147:291, 1986 (case report).

159. Martin DC: Germinal cell tumors of the testis after orchiopexy. *J Urol* 121:422, 1979.

160. Martin DC: Malignancy in the cryptorchid testis. *Urol Clin North Am* 9(3):371, 1982.

161. Marziale P, Atlante G, Pozzi M, et al: 426 cases of stage I endometrial carcinoma: a clinicopathological analysis. *Gynecol Oncol* 32:278, 1989.

162. Masselot J, Buthiau D: Gynecology. In Vanel D, McNamara MT, editors: *MRI of the body,* Paris, 1989, Springer-Verlag, p 223.

163. Matsukuma K, Tsukamoto N, Matsuyama T, et al: Preoperative CT study of lymph nodes in cervical cancer—its correlation with histological findings. *Gynecol Oncol* 33:168, 1989.

164. Mattrey RF: Magnetic resonance imaging of the scrotum. *Semin Ultrasound, CT MR* 12(2):95, 1991.

165. McCarthy S: Magnetic resonance imaging of the normal female pelvis. *Radiol Clin North Am* 30:769, 1992.

166. McCarthy S, Scott G, Majumdar S, et al: Uterine junctional zone: MR study of water content and relaxation properties. *Radiology* 171:241, 1989.

167. McCarthy S, Tauber C, Gore J: Female pelvic anatomy: MR assessment of variations during the menstrual cycle and with use of oral contraceptives. *Radiology* 160:119, 1986.

168. McCauley TR, McCarthy S, Lange R: Pelvic phased array coil: image quality assessment for spin-echo MR imaging. *Magn Reson Imaging* 10:513, 1992.

169. McDowell GC II, Johnson JW, Tenney DM, et al: Pelvic lymphadenectomy for staging clinically localized prostate cancer. *Urology* 35(6):476.

170. McNeal JE: Cancer volume and site of origin and adenocarcinoma in the prostate: relationship to local and distant spread. *Hum Pathol* 23(3):258,.

171. McNeal JE, Villers AA, Redwine EA, et al: Capsular penetration in prostate cancer: significance for natural history and treatment. *Am J Surg Pathol* 14(3):240, 1990.

172. Megibow AJ, Bosniak MA, Ho AG, et al: Accuracy of CT in detection of persistent or recurrent ovarian carcinoma: correlation with second-look laparotomy. *Radiology* 166:341, 1988.

173. Melki PS, Mulkern RV: Magnetization transfer effects in multi-slice RARE sequences. *Magn Reson Med* 24:189, 1992.

174. Melki PS, Mulkern RV, Panych LP, et al: Comparing the FAISE method with conventional dual-echo sequences. *JMRI* 1:319, 1991.

175. Middleton WD, Siegel BA, Melson GL, et al: Acute scrotal disorders: prospective comparison of color Doppler US and testicular scintigraphy. *Radiology* 177:177, 1990.

176. Milestone BN, Schnall MD, Lenkinski RE, et al: Cervical carcinoma: MR imaging with an endorectal surface coil. *Radiology* 180:191, 1991.

177. Mintz MC, Thickman DI, Gussman D, et al: MR evaluation of uterine anomalies. *AJR* 148:287, 1987.

178. Mirich DR, Hall JT, Kraft WL, et al: Metastatic adnexal trophoblastic neoplasm: contribution of MR imaging. *J Comput Assist Tomogr* 12:1061, 1988.

179. Mirowitz SA: Seminal vesicles: biopsy-related hemorrhage simulating tumor invasion at endorectal MR imaging. *Radiology* 185:373, 1992.

180. Mitchell DG: Benign disease of the uterus and ovaries. *Radiol Clin North Am* 30:777, 1992.

181. Mitchell DG: Chemical shift magnetic resonance imaging: applications in the abdomen and pelvis. *Top Magn Reson Imaging* 4(3):46, 1992.

182. Mitchell DG: Magnetic resonance imaging of the adnexa. *Semin Ultrasound CT MR* 9:143, 1988.

183. Mitchell DG, Mintz MC, Spritzer CE, et al: Adnexal masses: MR imaging observations at 1.5 T, with US and CT correlation. *Radiology* 162:319, 1987.

184. Mitchell DG, Vinitski S, Rifkin MD, et al: Narrow sampling bandwidth and fat suppression: effects on long TR/TE MRI of the abdomen and pelvis at 1.5 T. *AJR* 153:419, 1989.

185. Mittl RL, Yeh IT, Kressel HY: High-signal-intensity rim surrounding uterine leiomyomas on MR images: pathologic correlation. *Radiology* 180:81, 1991.

186. Morrow CP, Bundy BN, Kurman RJ, et al: Relationship between surgical-pathologic risk factors and outcome in clinical stage I and II carcinoma of the endometrium: a Gynecologic Oncology Group study. *Gynecol Oncol* 40:55, 1991.

187. Morrow CP, Schlaerth JB: Surgical management of endometrial carcinoma. *Clin Obstet Gynecol* 25:81, 1982.

188. Mulholland SG: The impact of radiology on the management of prostatic disease: a clinician's perspective. *Semin US, CT, MR* 9(5):335, 1988.

189. Neurerburg JM, Bohndorf K, Sohn M, et al: Urinary bladder neoplasms: evaluation with contrast-enhanced MR imaging. *Radiology* 172:739, 1989.

190. Neuerburg J-M, Bohndorf K, Sohn M, et al: Staging of urinary bladder neoplasms with MR imaging: is Gd-DTPA helpful? *J Comput Assist Tomogr* 15(5):780, 1991.

191. Nghiem HV, Herfkens RJ, Francis IR, et al: The pelvis: T2-weighted fast spin-echo MR imaging. *Radiology* 185:213, 1992.

192. Noren H, Granberg S, Friberg LG: Endometrial cancer stage II: 190 cases with different preoperative irradiation. *Gynecol Oncol* 41:17, 1991.

193. Nyberg DA, Porter BA, Olds MO, et al: MR imaging of hemorrhagic adnexal masses. *J Comput Assist Tomogr* 11:664, 1987.

194. Oesterling JE: Prostate-specific antigen: improving its ability to diagnose early prostate cancer. *JAMA* 267(16):2236, 1992.

195. Outwater EK, Schiebler ML, Owen RS, et al: MRI characterization of hemorrhagic adnexal masses: a blinded reader study. *Radiology* 1993 (in press).

196. Outwater E, Schiebler ML, Tomaszewski JE, et al: Mucinous carcinomas involving the prostate: atypical findings at MR imaging. *JMRI* 2:597, 1992.

197. Outwater E, Schnall M, Braitman LE, et al: Magnetization transfer of hepatic lesions: evaluation of a novel contrast technique in the abdomen. *Radiology* 182:535, 1992.

198. Parivar F, Waluch V: Magnetic resonance imaging of prostate cancer. *Hum Pathol* 23:335, 1992.

199. Patton JF, Hewitt CB, Mallis N: Diagnosis and treatment of tumors of the testis. *JAMA* 71(16):2194, 1959.

200. Pellerito JS, McCarthy SM, Doyle MB, et al: Diagnosis of uterine anomalies: relative accuracy of MR imaging, endovaginal sonography, and hysterosalpingography. *Radiology* 183:795, 1992.

201. Perkins AC, Powell MC, Wastie ML, et al: A prospective evaluation of OC125 and magnetic resonance imaging in patients with ovarian carcinoma. *Eur J Nucl Med* 16:311, 1989.

202. Petros JA, Catalona WJ: Lower incidence of unsuspected lymph node metastases in 521 consecutive patients with clinically localized prostate cancer. *J Urol* 147:1574, 1992.

203. Phillips ME, Kressel HY, Spritzer CE, et al: Normal prostate and adjacent structures: MR imaging at 1.5 T. *Radiology* 164:381, 1987.

204. Phillips ME, Kressel HY, Spritzer CE, et al: Prostatic disorders: MR imaging at 1.5 T. *Radiology* 164:386, 1987.

205. Photopulos GJ: Surgery or radiation for early cervical cancer. *Clin Obstet Gynecol* 33:872, 1990.

206. Piver MS: Invasive cervical cancer in the 1990s. *Semin Surg Oncol* 6:359, 1990.

207. Pizzocaro G, Nicolai N, Salvioni R, et al: Comparison between clinical and pathological staging in low stage nonseminomatous germ cell testicular tumors. *J Urol* 148:76, 1992.

208. Podczaski ES, Palombo C, Manetta A, et al: Assessment of pretreatment laparotomy in patients with cervical carcinoma prior to radiotherapy. *Gynecol Oncol* 33:71, 1989.

209. Poon PY, McCallum RW, Henkelman MM, et al: Magnetic resonance imaging of the prostate. *Radiology* 154:143, 1985.

210. Pope CF, Dietz MJ, Ezekowitz MD, et al: Technical variables influencing the detection of acute deep vein thrombosis by magnetic resonance imaging. *Magn Reson Imaging* 9:379, 1991.

211. Posniak HV, Olson MC, Dudiak CM, et al: MR imaging of uterine carcinoma: correlation with clinical and pathologic findings. *Radiographics* 10:15, 1990.

212. Potter ME, Partridge EE, Hatch KD, et al: Primary surgical therapy of ovarian carcinoma: how much and when. *Gynecol Oncol* 40:195, 1991.

213. Powell MC, Womack C, Buckley J, et al: Preoperative magnetic resonance imaging of stage I endometrial adenocarcinoma. *Br J Obstet Gynaecol* 93:353, 1986.

214. Quint LE, Van Erp JS, Bland PH, et al: Prostate cancer: correlation of MR images with tissue optical density at pathologic examination. *Radiology* 179:837, 1991.

215. Raghavan D, Shipley WU, Garnick MB, et al: Biology and management of bladder cancer. *New Engl J Med* 332(16):1129, 1990.

216. Rahmouni A, Yang A, Tempany CMC, et al: Accuracy of in-vivo assessment of prostatic volume by MRI and transrectal ultrasonography. *J Comput Assist Tomogr* 116(6):935, 1992.

217. Reuter KL, Daly DC, Cohen SM: Septate versus bicornuate uteri: errors in imaging diagnosis. *Radiology* 172:749, 1989.

218. Reuter VE: Pathology of bladder cancer: assessment of prognostic variables and response to therapy. *Semin Oncology* 17(5):524, 1990.

219. Rholl KS, Lee JKT, Heiken JP, et al: Primary bladder carcinoma: evaluation with MR imaging. *Radiology* 163:117, 1987.

220. Rholl KS, Lee JKT, Ling D, et al: MR imaging of the scrotum with a high-resolution surface coil. *Radiology* 163:99, 1987.

221. Riccio TJ, Adams HG, Munzing, DE, et al: Magnetic resonance imaging as an adjunct to sonography in the evaluation of the female pelvis. *Magn Reson Imaging* 8:699, 1990.

222. Richardson GS, Scully RE, Nikrui N, et al: Common epithelial cancer of the ovary (part I). *New Eng J Med* 312:415, 1985.

223. Rifkin MD, Zerhouni EA, Gatsonis CA, et al: Comparison of magnetic resonance imaging and ultrasonography in staging early prostate cancer. *New Engl J Med* 323:621, 1990.

224. Roemer PB, Edelstein WA, Hayes CE, et al: The NMR phased array. *Magn Reson Med* 16:192, 1990.

225. Rosenfield AT, Blair DN, McCarthy S, et al: The pars infravaginalis gubernaculi: importance in the identification of the undescended testis. *AJR* 153:775, 1989.

226. Rubens D, Thornbury JR, Angel C, et al: Stage IB cervical carcinoma: comparison of clinical, MR, and pathologic staging. *AJR* 150:135, 1988.

227. Russel AH, Anderson M, Walter J, et al: The integration of computed tomography and magnetic resonance imaging in treatment planning for gynecologic cancer. *Clin Obstet Gynecol* 35:55, 1992.

228. Sager EM, Talle K, Rosså S, et al: The role of CT in demonstrating perivesical tumor growth in the preoperative staging of carcinoma of the urinary bladder. *Radiology* 146:443, 1983.

229. Santoni R, Bucciolini M, Cionini L, et al: Modifications of relaxation times induced by radiation therapy in cervical carcinom: preliminary results. *Clin Radiol* 38:569, 1987.

230. Savader SJ, Otero RR, Savader BL: Puerperal ovariation vein thrombosis: evaluation with CT, US, and MR imaging. *Radiology* 167:637, 1988.

231. Schiebler ML. Tomaszewski JE, Bezzi M, et al: Prostatic carcinoma and benign prostatic hyperplasia: correlation of high-resolution MR and histopathologic findings. *Radiology* 172:13, 1989.

232. Schiebler ML, Yankaskas BC, Tempany C, et al: MR imaging in adenocarcinoma of the prostate: interobserver variation and efficacy for determining stage C disease. *AJR* 158:559, 1992.

233. Schnall MD, Bezzi M, Pollack HM, et al: Magnetic resonance imaging of the prostate. *Magn Reson Q* 6(1):1, 1990.

234. Schnall MD, Imai Y, Tomaszewski J, et al: Prostate cancer: local staging with endorectal surface coil MR imaging. *Radiology* 178:797, 1991.

235. Schnall MD, Lenkinski RE, Pollack RE, et al: Prostate: MR imaging with an endorectal surface coil. *Radiology* 172:570, 1989.

236. Schnall MD, Pollack HM, Van Arsdalen K, et al: The seminal tract in patients with ejaculatory dysfunction: MR imaging with an endorectal surface coil. *AJR* 159:337.

237. Schnall MD, Tomaszewski J, Pollack HM, et al: The bulging prostate gland—a sign of capsular involvement. *Proceedings of the Society for Magn Resonance in Medicine*, p 279.

238. Scott R Jr, Mutchnik DL, Laskowski TZ, et al: Carcinoma of the prostate in elderly men: incidence, growth characteristics and clinical significance. *J Urol* 101:602.

239. Scott WW, Rosenshein NB, Siegelman SS, et al: The obstructed uterus. *Radiology* 141:767, 1981.

240. Scoutt LM, Flynn SD, Luthringer DJ, et al: Junctional zone of the uterus: correlation of MR imaging and histologic examination of hysterectomy specimens. *Radiology* 179:403, 1991.

241. Scoutt LM, McCauley TR, Flynn SD, et al: Zonal anatomy of the cervix: correlation of MR imaging and histologic examination of hysterectomy specimens. *Radiology* 186:159, 1993.

242. See WA, Fuller JR: Staging of advanced bladder cancer: current concepts and pitfalls. *Urol Clin North Am* 19(4):663, 1992.

243. Seidenwurm D, Smathers RL, Lo RK, et al: Testes and scrotum: MR imaging at 1.5 T. *Radiology* 164:393, 1987.

244. Sepponen RE, Sipponen JT, Tanttu JI: A method for chemical shift imaging: demonstration of bone marrow involvement with proton chemical shift imaging. *J Comput Assist Tomogr* 8(4):585, 1984.

245. Shapeero LG, Hricak H: Mixed mullerian sarcoma of the uterus: MR imaging findings. *AJR* 153:317, 1989.

246. Sheldon CA, Williams RD, Fraley EE: Incidental carcinoma of the prostate: a review of the literature and critical reappraisal of classification. *J Urol* 626, 1980.

247. Shida T, Yoshimura M, Chihara H, et al: Intravenous leiomyomatosis of the pelvis with reextension into the heart. *Ann Thorac Surg* 42:104, 1986.

248. Sironi S, Belloni C, Taccagni GL, et al: Carcinoma of the cervix: value of MR imaging in detecting parametrial involvement. *AJR* 156:753, 1991.

249. Sironi S, Belloni C, Taccagni G, et al: Invasive cervical carcinoma: MR imaging after preoperative chemotherapy. *Radiology* 180:719, 1991.

250. Sironi S, Colombo E, Villa G, et al: Myometrial invasion by endometrial carcinoma: assessment with plain and gadolinium-enhanced MR imaging. *Radiology* 185:207, 1992.

251. Smith FW, Cherryman GR, Baylis AP, et al: A comparative study of the accuracy of ultrasound imaging, x-ray computerized tomography, and low field MRI diagnosis of ovarian malignancy. *Magn Reson Imag* 6:225, 1988.

252. Smith PH: The case for no initial treatment of localized prostate cancer. *Urol Clin North Am* 17(4):827, 1990.

253. Smith RC, Reinhold C, Lange RC, et al: Fast spin-echo MR imaging of the female pelvis. Part I. Use of a whole-volume coil. *Radiology* 184:665, 1992.

254. Smith RC, Reinhold C, McCauley TR, et al: Multicoil high-resolution fast spin-echo MR imaging of the female pelvis. *Radiology* 184:671, 1992.

255. Soloway MS: Invasive bladder cancer: selection of primary treatment. *Semin Oncol* 17(5):551, 1990.

256. Spritzer CE, Sostman HD, Wilkes DC, et al: Deep venous thrombosis: experience with gradient-echo MR imaging in 66 patients. *Radiology* 177:235, 1990.

257. Steinfeld AD: Questions regarding the treatment of localized prostate cancer. *Radiology* 184:593, 1992.

258. Stevens SK, Hricak H, Stern JL: Ovarian lesions: detection and

characterization with gadolinium-enhanced MR imaging at 1.5 T. *Radiology* 181:481, 1991.

259. Sugimura K, Carrington BM, Quivey JM, et al: Postirradiation changes in the pelvis: assessment with MR imaging. *Radiology* 175:805, 1990.

260. Szumowski J, Eisen JK, Vinitski S, et al: Hybrid methods of chemical-shift imaging. *Magn Reson Med* 9:379, 1989.

261. Szumowski J, Plewes DB: Separation of lipid and water MR imaging signals by Chopper averaging in the time domain. *Radiology* 165:247, 1987.

262. Tachibana M, Baba S, Deguchi N, et al: Efficacy of gadolinium-diethylenetriaminepentaacetic acid-enhanced magnetic resonance imaging for differentiation between superficial and muscle-invasive tumor of the bladder: a comparative study with computerized tomography and transurethral ultrasonography. *J Urol* 145:1169, 1991.

263. Tanimoto A, Yuasa Y, Imai Y, et al: Bladder tumor staging: comparison of conventional and gadolinium-enhanced dynamic MR imaging and CT. *Radiology* 185:741, 1992.

264. Teitelbaum GP, Ortega HV, Vinitski S, et al: Optimization of gradient-echo imaging parameters for intracaval filters and trapped thromboemboli. *Radiology* 174:1013, 1990.

265. Tempany CMC, Rahmouni AD, Epstein JI, et al: Invasion of the neurovascular bundle by prostate cancer: evaluation with MR imaging. *Radiology* 181:107, 1991.

266. Thorvinger B, Gudmundson T, Horvath G, et al: Staging in local endometrial carcinoma: assessment of magnetic resonance and ultrasound examinations. *Acta Radiol* 30:525, 1989.

267. Thurnher SA: MR imaging of pelvic masses in women: contrast-enhanced vs. unenhanced images. *AJR* 159:1243, 1992.

268. Thurnher SA, Hodler J, Baer S, et al: Gadolinium-DOTA enhanced MR imaging of adnexal tumors. *J Comput Assist Tomogr* 14:939, 1990.

269. Thurnher SA, von Schulthess GK, Marincek B: Staging of cervical carcinoma with contrast-enhanced MR imaging. Abstract No. 276 presented at the Society for Magnetic Resonance in Medicine, San Francisco, 1991.

270. Thurnher S, Hricak H, Carroll PR, et al: Imaging the testis: comparison between MR imaging and US. *Radiology* 167:631, 1988.

271. Togashi K, Konishi J: Magnetic resonance imaging in the evaluation of gynecologic malignancy. *Magn Reson Q* 6:250, 1990.

272. Togashi K, Nishimura K, Itoh K, et al: Adenomyosis: Diagnosis with MR imaging. *Radiology* 166:111, 1988.

273. Togashi K, Nishimura K, Itoh K, et al: Ovarian cyst teratomas: MR imaging. *Radiology* 162:6697, 1987.

274. Togashi K, Nishimura K, Itoh K, et al: Uterine cervical cancer: assessment with high-field MR imaging. *Radiology* 160:431, 1986.

275. Togashi K, Nishimura K, Kimura I, et al: Endometrial cysts: diagnosis with MR imaging. *Radiology* 180:73, 1991.

276. Togashi K, Nishimura K, Sagoh T, et al: Carcinoma of the cervix: staging with MR imaging. *Radiology* 171:245, 1989.

277. Togashi K, Ozasa H, Konishi I, et al: Enlarged uterus: differentiation between adenomyosis and leiomyoma with MR imaging. *Radiology* 171:531, 1989.

278. Trambert MA, Mattrey RF, Levine D, et al: Subacute scrotal pain: evaluation of torsion versus epididymitis with MR imaging. *Radiology* 175:53, 1990.

279. van Gils APG, Tham RTO, Falke THM, et al: Abnormalities of the uterus and cervix after diethylstilbestrol exposure: correlation of findings on MR and hysterosalpingography. *AJR* 153:1235, 1989.

280. van Nagell JR, Roddick JW, Lowin DM: The staging of cervical cancer: inevitable discrepancies between clinical staging and pathologic findings. *Am J Obstet Gynecol* 110:973, 1971.

281. Vanneuville G, Lenck LCh, Garcier JM, et al: Contribution of imaging to the understanding of the female pelvic fasciae. *Surg Radiol Anat* 14:147, 1992.

282. Villers A, McNeal JE, Freiha FS, et al: Multiple cancers in the prostate. Morphologic features of clinically recognized versus incidental tumors. *Cancer* 70:2313, 1992.

283. Waggenspack GA, Amparo EG, Hannigna EV: MR imaging of uterine cervical carcinoma. *J Comput Assist Tomogr* 12:409, 1988.

284. Waggenspack GA, Amparo EG, Hannigan EV, et al: MRI of cervical carcinoma. *Semin Ultrasound CT MR* 9:158, 1988.

285. Wehrli FW, Perkins TG, Shimakawa A, et al: Chemical-shift-induced amplitude modulations in images obtained with gradient refocusing. *Magn Reson Imaging* 5:157, 1987.

286. Weinreb JC, Barkoff ND, Megibow A, et al: The value of MR imaging in distinguishing leiomyomas from other solid pelvic masses when sonography is indeterminate. *AJR* 154:295, 1990.

287. Weinreb JC, Brown CE, Lowe TW, et al: Pelvic masses in pregnant patients: MR and US imaging. *Radiology* 159:717, 1986.

288. Weitzman GA, Buttram VC: Classification of endometriosis. *Obstet Gynecol Clin North Am* 16:61, 1989.

289. Wheelr TM: Anatomic considerations in carcinoma of the prostate. *Adv Urol Ultrasound* 16(4):623, 1989.

290. Whitmore WF Jr: Clinical management of prostatic cancer: an overview. *Am J Clin Oncol* 11(2):S88, 1988.

291. Williams MP, Husband JE, Heron CW, et al: Magnetic resonance imaging in recurrent carcinoma of the cervix. *Br J Radiol* 62:544, 1989.

292. Wolff SD, Balaban RS: Magnetization transfer contrast (MTC) and tissue water proton relaxation in vivo. *Magn Reson Med* 10:135, 1989.

293. Wolff SD, Eng J, Balaban RS: Magnetization transfer contrast: method for improving contrast in gradient-recalled-echo images. *Radiology* 179:133, 1991.

294. Worthington JL, Balfe DM, Lee JKT, et al: Uterine neoplasms: MR imaging. *Radiology* 159:725, 1986.

295. Yazigi R, Cohen J, Munoz AK, et al: Magnetic resonance imaging determination of myometrial invasion in endometrial carcinoma. *Gynecol Oncol* 34:94, 1989.

296. Yeung HN, Kormos DW: Separation of true fat and water images by correcting magnetic field inhomogeneity in situ. *Radiology* 159:783, 1986.

297. Yoder IC: Diagnosis of uterine anomalies: relative accuracy of MR imaging, endovaginal sonography, and hysterosalpingography. *Radiology* 185:343, 1992.

298. Zawin M, McCarthy S, Scoutt L, et al: Endometriosis: appearance and detection at MR imaging. *Radiology* 171:693, 1989.

299. Zincke H, Blute ML, Fallen MJ, et al: Radical prostatectomy for stage A adenocarcinoma of the prostate: staging errors and their implications for treatment recommendations and disease outcome. *J Urol* 146:1053, 1991.

PART VII

IMAGING OF THE MUSCULOSKELETAL SYSTEM

40

Musculoskeletal Tumors

AMILCARE GENTILI
MICHAEL P. RECHT

SKELETAL TUMORS

Many imaging modalities are available for the evaluation of skeletal lesions. In most cases, standard radiographs are sufficient in the detection of skeletal tumors[87] and when evaluated together with clinical data, such as age, gender, anatomical location, and clinical presentation, are the best predictor of the histology of the lesion. When a lesion is in an area in which anatomy is complex, however, such as in the spine, scapula, pelvis, or in a periarticular location, magnetic resonance imaging (MRI) and computed tomography (CT) are often necessary to characterize the tumor fully. Bone scintigraphy remains the method of choice for screening for skeletal metastases. Although MRI has been shown to be more sensitive than scintigraphy in detecting metastases, it is not an efficient technique for evaluating the entire skeleton.[29]

Although plain radiographs are often sufficient for diagnosis,[87] MRI and CT are fundamental in staging skeletal tumors. Optimal treatment of primary skeletal neoplasms in the absence of distant metastases includes complete surgical resection of the tumor. In the past, amputation was the treatment of choice. With improvement of surgical technique and aggressive chemotherapy, limb-sparing operations now can be performed without affecting survival and improving functional results. In planning resection, accurate preoperative staging is essential. The initial CT or MRI scan should be performed before biopsy because after biopsy it is often difficult to distinguish tumor from edema, hemorrhage, and granulation tissue. Numerous studies have compared the usefulness of CT and MRI in the staging of musculoskeletal tumors.[1,5,9–12,33,69,86,87,96,100] MRI is superior in determining muscle compartment and vascular involvement because of the intrinsic contrast between tumor mass, muscle, and fat without the need for contrast enhancement. In addition, MRI has the ability to produce images in multiple planes, allowing easier assessment of in-

tramedullary extent of tumor and intra-articular extension.[23] CT is superior in detecting subtle cortical invasion and periosteal and endosteal reactions and depicting matrix calcification or ossification. Both MRI and CT are useful to evaluate response to chemotherapy and radiation therapy.[39,92] Signs of response to treatment are decrease in tumor size, better delineation of the mass, reappearance of fat planes between muscle groups, and calcification or ossification of the tumor.

TECHNIQUE
Magnetic resonance imaging

In evaluating musculoskeletal masses, it is necessary to image in multiple planes using a variety of pulse sequences. T1-weighted sequences best evaluate the intramedullary extent of tumor, whereas T2-weighted images are used to define soft tissue extension and cortical involvement. STIR (short tau inversion recovery) sequences have also been advocated for the evaluation of musculoskeletal neoplasms because of their increased sensitivity to abnormal tissue leading to increased conspicuity of lesions.[84] The value of the intravenous administration of gadolinium-DTPA in the evaluation of musculoskeletal neoplasms remains controversial.[27,74,85] The initial MRI sequence is typically a T1-weighted large field-of-view coronal sequence, which enables the assessment of the size and location of the lesion. This sequence also is used to evaluate for the presence of skip lesions. Depending on the size of the lesion, subsequent sequences are performed with smaller fields of view and slice thicknesses. If possible, surface coils are also used for the remainder of the examination to increase resolution and signal-to-noise ratio further. Transaxial T1- and T2-weighted images are the next sequences performed and allow for the evaluation of soft tissue extension, involvement of cortical bone, and the relationship of the mass to the neurovascular bundle. Additional T1-weighted or STIR images are then acquired in either the sagittal or the coronal plane depending on if the lesion is located primarily anterior or posterior (sagittal) or medial or lateral (coronal).

Computed tomography

Imaging should be perpendicular to the region of interest if possible. Following a scout view, transaxial images are acquired with a slice thickness ranging from 2 to 10 mm depending on the lesion being evaluated and the extent of the lesion. The slice interval also depends on the size and extent of the lesion. The administration of intravenous contrast material is useful for determining lesion vascularity and relationship of the mass to the neurovascular bundle. Once acquired, images should be filmed with both soft tissue and bone window settings.

Benign skeletal tumors

Enchondromas. Enchondromas are a common benign primary osseous tumor and follow in frequency only nonossifying fibromas and exostosis. They have no sexual preference. Approximately 50% of enchondromas are in the hands. They are asymptomatic unless fractured or undergoing malignant transformation. Enchondromas are often an incidental finding discovered on radiographs obtained for another reason. Enchondromas typically are round or oval lesions with well-defined, lobu-

lated borders. The unmineralized matrix has soft tissue attenuation on CT scan and on MRI has homogeneous high signal on T2-weighted images. Calcifications with ring and arc appearances are suggestive of chondroid matrix.[2,17] These are best identified on plain radiographs and CT scans, but calcifications are not consistently identified on MRI scans. On MRI, when seen, calcification has low signal intensity on all sequences.

Benign and malignant chondroid lesions can have a similar appearance, making differentiation of a enchondroma from a low-grade chondrosarcoma often difficult or impossible. The presence, however, of a soft tissue mass, cortical erosion, or pain in absence of fracture increases the suspicion of malignancy.

Chondroblastoma. Chondroblastoma is a benign rare tumor of cartilaginous origin composed of chondroblasts. Its peak is in individuals between 10 and 20 years of age. It is more common in males with a 2:1 male-to-female ratio. It involves the epiphysis or apophysis but may extend into the metaphysis after destroying the growth plate.[41] CT accurately demonstrates the extent of the lesion as well as matrix calcifications and subtle cortical infractions. Extension through the growth plate, however, is best detected on conventional tomography or MRI because the growth plate is usually best visualized in the sagittal or coronal plane. On MRI, both

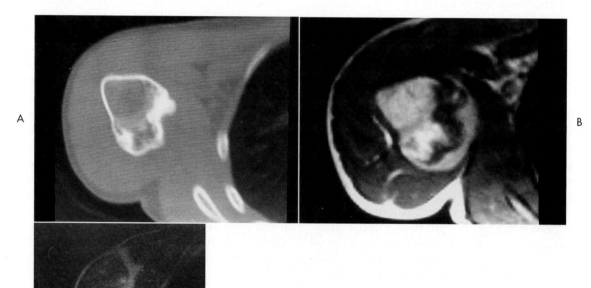

Fig. 40-1. Osteochondroma. A 9-year-old boy with a palpable mass. **A,** CT scan of the proximal humerus demonstrates continuity of the cortex and medullary cavity of the osteochondroma with that of the humerus, but the cartilage cup is not seen. Axial SE 2400/20 **(B),** and coronal SE 2100/90 **(C)** images of the humerus clearly demonstrate the cartilage cap as an area of high signal intensity.

T1- and T2-weighted images demonstrate a peripheral rim of signal void that corresponds to the sclerotic margin of the lesion. Abnormal signal intensity in large areas of bone marrow surrounding the lesion has been seen, probably representing bone marrow edema.[15,37]

Osteochondroma. Osteochondromas (exostosis) are the second most common benign tumor of bone after nonossifying fibromas. They predominate in males with a 1.5 to 2:1 male-to-female ratio. They are a congenital lesion but are usually discovered between 10 and 20 years of age. Multiple exostoses are uncommon, being only one tenth as frequent as a solitary exostosis, but they manifest themselves earlier, usually before 10 years of age. Ninety percent of osteochondromas originate from a long bone close to the metaphysis. The most common locations are around the knee (distal femur and proximal tibia) and proximal humerus. The morphology of an ostechondroma is more important than the signal intensity in making the diagnosis. The incidence of malignant transformation is approximately 1% for solitary osteochondromas and from 5% to 25% in cases of hereditary multiple exostoses. Both CT and MRI are useful in demonstrating the continuity of the cortex and medullary cavity of the osteochondroma with that of the parent bone (Fig. 40-1).[78] On MRI, the perichondrium is also well seen on T2-weighted images as an area of low signal surrounding the outer surface of the high signal of the cartilage cap.[54] MRI is also accurate in measuring the cartilage cap's thickness, whereas CT measurements of maximum cartilage thickness are often imprecise.[43] The thickness of the cartilage cap is important in distinguishing benign osteochondroma from an exostotic chondrosarcoma. According to most authors, the cartilage cap is usually thicker than 3 cm in chondrosarco-mas.[47] Other complications of osteochondromas include nerve injuries, vascular injury, and bursa formation.[70] The formation of a bursa over an osteochondroma is common and usually is asymptomatic, but if it becomes inflamed and distended, it can be painful. On T2-weighted images, bursal fluid has high signal intensity similar to that of the cartilage cap, and it can be difficult to differentiate between the two. On gradient echo sequences, cartilage has lower signal than fluid, and the diagnosis can be easily made. A more rare complication is the formation of an pseudoaneurysm adjacent to the exostosis.[72]

Chondromyxoid fibroma. Chondromyxoid fibroma is composed of three principal elements: chondroid, fibrous, and myxoid tissue. It is the least common of benign cartilaginous bone neoplasms. It has a male predominance with a 1.5 to 2:1 male-to-female ratio. It tends to occur around the knee joint but can involve any bone. The tumor is usually solid but may contain cystic or hemorrhagic areas. On MRI, the signal intensities of chondromyxoid fibroma vary with the proportion of chondroid, fibrous, and myxoid tissue present. CT may better delineate matrix calcification and sclerosis around the tumor than MRI.[97]

Osteoid osteoma. Osteoid osteomas are relatively frequent, following only osteochondromas and fibrous cortical defects in prevalence. They predominate in males with a 3:1 male-to-female ratio. They typically occur in teenagers and young adults and are rare before 5 and after 30 years of age. Osteoid osteomas are most frequent in the femur, tibia, and humerus and involve the diaphysis and less commonly the metaphysis. With spinal involvement, the posterior elements are typically affected. The main clinical symptom with osteoid osteo-

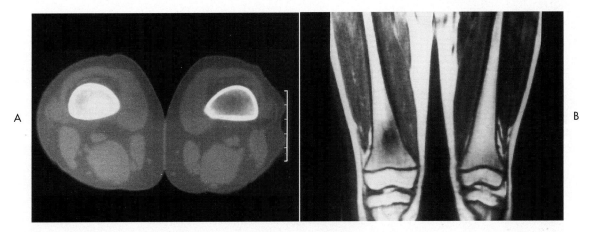

Fig. 40-2. Intramedullary osteoid osteoma. A 9-year-old girl with knee pain. **A,** CT scan demonstrates an area of sclerosis with a central lucency (nidus) in the medullary cavity. **B,** Coronal SE 650/20 image demonstrates an area of decreased signal intensity corresponding to sclerosis seen on CT; the nidus has intermediate signal intensity.

mas is pain relieved by aspirin. CT is accurate in detecting the nidus and is preferred to MRI for evaluating osteoid osteoma.[31,51,56] Occasionally an osteoid osteoma can be confused with a stress fracture on MRI owing to edema in the bone marrow. On CT, the typical appearance of an osteoid osteoma is an area of sclerosis surrounding a small, less than 1 cm radiolucent nidus (Fig. 40-2). Lesions larger than 1.5 cm are considered osteoblastomas. The nidus may contain calcifications, the amount of which can vary from none to almost complete calcification with only a thin peripheral rim of low density. To evaluate the nidus fully, thin-section CT with 2 mm slices is needed because the nidus is often less than 1 cm in diameter. The nidus enhances on dynamic CT scans. On MRI, the nidus has low signal intensity on T1-weighted images and variable intensity on T2-weighted images, depending on the degree of calcification of the

nidus. The surrounding bone marrow has low signal intensity on all pulse sequences if there is reactive sclerosis or high signal intensity on the T2-weighted images if there is edema (Fig. 40-3). When the osteoid osteoma is interarticular, an associated joint effusion may be detected.[79]

Osteoblastoma. Osteoblastoma is a rare benign tumor. It is at least four times less common than osteoid osteoma. It has a male predominance with a 2.5 : 1 male-to-female ratio. Its peak is in the second decade, and it is rare before 10 years of age and after 30 years of age. Its most common location is the spine, usually in the posterior elements. In the long bones, it is usually located in the metadiaphyseal region and rarely in adults can extend into the epiphyses. On CT, an osteoblastoma appears as an expansile lytic lesion, often with a mineralized matrix, surrounded by a thin bony shell. Dense scle-

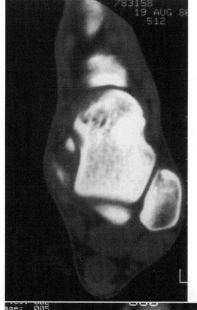

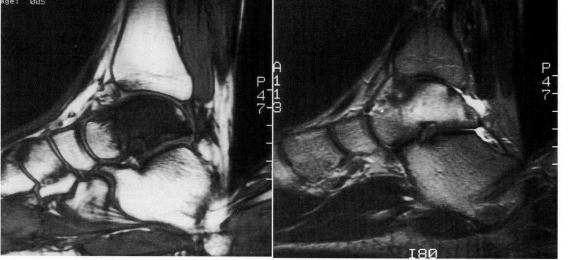

Fig. 40-3. Osteoid osteoma. **A,** CT scan demonstrates an area of sclerosis with a central lucency (nidus) in the talus. Calcifications are present in the center of the nidus. **B,** Sagittal T1-weighted image demonstrates decreased signal intensity in most of the talus owing to bone marrow edema. **C,** Sagittal T2-weighted image demonstrates high signal intensity in the bone marrow owing to edema. The nidus has also increased signal and is surrounded by a rim of low signal corresponding to sclerosis seen on CT.

rosis and periosteal reaction may occasionally be present. On MRI, it typically has low-to-intermediate signal intensity on T1-weighted images and high signal intensity on T2-weighted images. Edema in the surrounding soft tissues and in the bone marrow beyond the tumor margins is common.[5,20,53]

Nonossifying fibroma. Nonossifying fibroma and fibrous cortical defects have the same histology and differ only in size, with fibrous cortical defects being smaller. They are also called fibroxanthomas because they contain spindle-shaped fibroblasts and xanthoma (foam) cells. They are the most common benign lesion of bone and have been reported in 30% of normal children. They are a nonneoplastic developmental aberration. Most are asymptomatic and disappear spontaneously. There is a male predominance with a 1.5:1 male-to-female ratio. Their peak incidence is around 10 years of age. Nonossifying fibromas and fibrous cortical defects are usually localized to the metaphysis of a long bone and are most frequent about the knee (distal femur and proximal tibia). They are infrequent in the upper extremities.

Their radiographic appearance is often pathognomonic, and no additional studies are usually necessary. They are frequently seen as an incidental finding on MRI examinations of the knee and can have a varied MRI appearance (Fig. 40-4). In their early stages, when the lesion is completely lytic on plain radiographs, the lesion may have high signal on T1-weighted images owing to an abundance of xanthoma (foam) cells containing fat. Linear structures with low signal are often present and represent fibrous septa or osseous pseudosepta. When the lesion starts healing, it has low signal intensity on both T1- and T2-weighted images owing to increased fibrous collagen, mineralization, and possibly hemosiderin deposits.[75] The lesions are always well defined and are never surrounded by bone marrow edema.[49]

Simple bone cyst. Simple bone cyst is a benign cystic lesion of bone of unknown origin. It arises in the metaphysis of the bone but with growth tends to move away from the growth plate toward the diaphysis. It is a frequent bone lesion, following only nonossifying fibromas and exostosis in prevalence. It is more common in

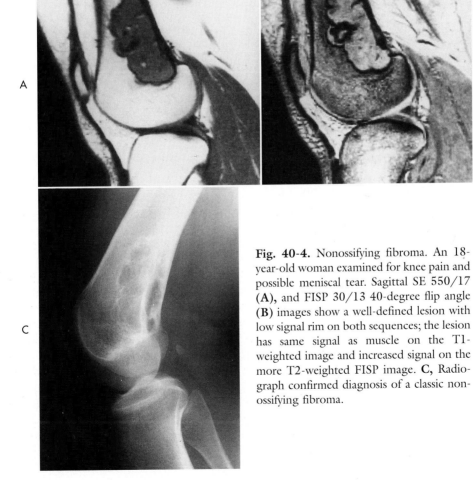

Fig. 40-4. Nonossifying fibroma. An 18-year-old woman examined for knee pain and possible meniscal tear. Sagittal SE 550/17 (**A**), and FISP 30/13 40-degree flip angle (**B**) images show a well-defined lesion with low signal rim on both sequences; the lesion has same signal as muscle on the T1-weighted image and increased signal on the more T2-weighted FISP image. **C,** Radiograph confirmed diagnosis of a classic nonossifying fibroma.

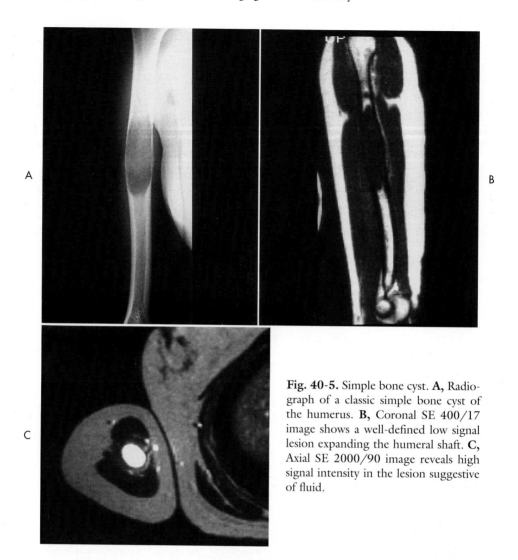

Fig. 40-5. Simple bone cyst. **A,** Radiograph of a classic simple bone cyst of the humerus. **B,** Coronal SE 400/17 image shows a well-defined low signal lesion expanding the humeral shaft. **C,** Axial SE 2000/90 image reveals high signal intensity in the lesion suggestive of fluid.

males with a 2.5:1 male-to-female ratio. It can be seen in any age group but is rare before 5 and after 20 years of age. The most common location of simple bone cysts is the proximal humerus followed by the proximal femur. All other locations are rare. Simple cysts are central, lytic, expansile lesions. Their radiographic appearance is usually diagnostic, and neither MRI nor CT is usually necessary. On MRI, they are well defined with low signal intensity on T1-weighted images and high signal intensity on T2-weighted images, owing to the fluid content of the cyst (Fig. 40-5). Typically, they are homogeneous on both T1- and T2-weighted images, unless hemorrhage has occurred. Peripheral low signal intensity borders represent reactive sclerosis. No edema is present in the surrounding bone marrow or muscle. CT is superior to MRI in detecting subtle infractions of the lesion.

Aneurysmal bone cyst. Aneurysmal bone cysts are expansile lytic lesions containing thin-walled cystic cavities of unknown origin. They can be seen in any age, but 75% are seen under 20 years of age, and they are rare after 30 years of age. They have a slight female predominance with a male-to-female ratio of 1:1.5. Aneurysmal bone cysts can occur in any bone but predominantly arise in the long bones and the spine. In the long bones, they are usually metaphyseal or metadiaphyseal. In the spine, they involve the posterior elements and may extend into the body, but involvement of the vertebral body alone is rare. On CT, an aneurysmal bone cyst appears as an expansile lesion with a thin cortical shell (Fig. 40-6). Fluid-fluid levels may be seen and are thought to represent sedimentation of degraded blood cell products within the cystic cavity.[42] Fluid levels are best seen if the patient is immobilized for some time before scanning. Fluid-fluid levels are a nonspecific finding and have also been described in giant cell tumors, chondroblastoma, and telangiectatic osteosarcomas.[90] On MRI, an aneurysmal bone cyst appears as a well-defined expansile mass with multiple internal septations surrounded by a well-

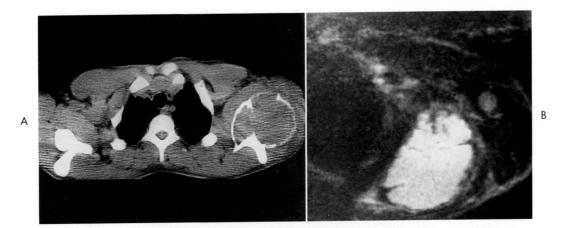

Fig. 40-6. Aneurysmal bone cyst. A 15-year-old boy with shoulder pain. **A,** CT scan shows a large lesion with marked expansion of the scapula. **B,** SE 2000/90 image shows a large scapular lesion with high signal intensity. Septations are present.

defined rim of low signal intensity of variable thickness on both T1- and T2-weighted images.[4,19,40,66,99] This low signal rim represents a bony shell. Fluid-fluid levels are often seen within well-defined cystic cavities.[40] On T1-weighted images, signal intensity in the cyst may be higher than in muscle owing to intracystic hemorrhage. One cavity may have markedly different signal characteristics than an adjacent cavity. The different signal characteristics probably reflect intracystic hemorrhage of different ages. Edema may be present in the surrounding muscles. Septations within the lesion enhance after administration of gadolinium-DTPA, but the cystic component does not enhance.

Giant cell tumor. Giant cell tumor is relatively frequent, but malignant transformation is rare, occurring in less than 10% of lesions. It has a slight female preponderance, with an age peak between 20 and 49 years of age. It is rare before closure of the growth plate or after 50 years of age. Ninety percent of cases involve long bones, where the lesion is localized to the metaepiphyseal region. In the rare cases, it develops before closure of the growth plate and is localized in the metaphysis. More than 50% of giant cell tumors involve the knee (distal femur and proximal tibia metaepiphyseal region). Other bones that can be affected include the distal radius, sacrum, distal tibia, proximal humerus, pelvis, and proximal femur, in order of frequency. Other locations are rare.[22] On CT, giant cell tumors appear as lytic lesions with thinning and erosion of the cortex (Fig. 40-7).[25] A sclerotic margin may be present between the tumor and the normal marrow cavity. On MRI, giant cell tumors are well defined with a low signal rim or halo surrounding the tumor. On T1-weighted images, they have intermediate signal intensity and are usually homoge-

neous, whereas on T2-weighted images, they have intermediate-to-high signal intensity and may be inhomogeneous.[14,38,64,99] Focal areas with increased signal intensity may be seen on both T1- and T2-weighted images and represent hemorrhage. Fluid-fluid levels, which are frequently seen in aneurysmal bone cysts and telangiectatic osteosarcomas, are only rarely present in giant cell tumors.[90] Both CT and MRI accurately demonstrate the intraosseous and soft tissue extension of the tumor, but CT is superior in showing cortical destruction, whereas MRI is better in demonstrating intra-articular involvement owing to its multiplanar capability.[88]

Malignant skeletal tumors

Multiple myeloma. Multiple myeloma is a multifocal malignant proliferation of plasma cells. It is the most frequent primary malignant tumor of the skeleton. It has a male predominance with a 1.5 : 1 male-to-female ratio. It is common after 50 years of age and is extremely rare before 30. Because this neoplasm derives from bone marrow elements, it involves bones containing red marrow: the skull, ribs, sternum, pelvis, proximal humeral metaphysis, and proximal femoral metaphysis. At the time of diagnosis, it is often disseminated throughout the red marrow of the axial skeleton. Infiltration of bone marrow has two forms: diffuse and focal. In the diffuse form, the myeloma cells are mixed with the hematopoietic cells. In the focal form, normal bone marrow is displaced by nodules composed entirely by myeloma cells. In the focal form, untreated myelomatous lesions have decreased signal intensity on T1-weighted images and increased signal intensity on T2-weighted images when compared with the surrounding bone marrow.[30,65] CT scan of these patients demonstrates purely osteolytic le-

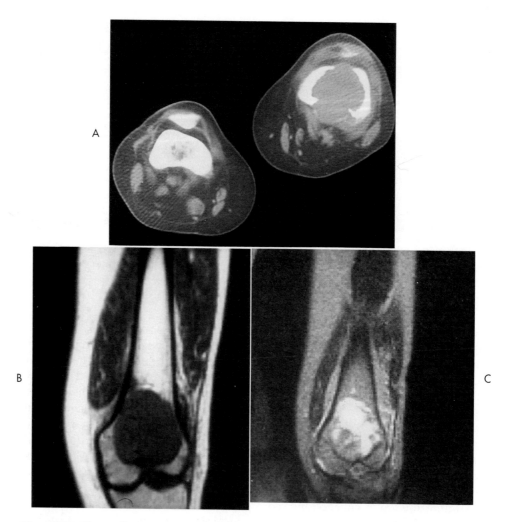

Fig. 40-7. Giant cell tumor. A 16-year-old girl with knee pain. **A,** CT scan demonstrates a lytic lesion of the distal femur with marked expansion and thinning of the cortex both anteriorly and posteriorly. On MRI a well-defined lesion is present. **(B)** The signal is same as muscle on coronal T1-weighted SE 600/17 image **(B)** and high on T2-weighted SE 2500/90 image **(C).**

sions in the trabecular bone, which occasionally extend to involve the cortex (Fig. 40-8).[80] After irradiation, these lesions have low signal intensity on both T1- and T2-weighted images and develop a sclerotic border on CT scan.

The diffuse form is difficult to image; the only manifestation on MRI scan is inhomogeneity of the bone marrow signal, which is difficult to quantitate and is subjective.[30,65] CT, plain radiographs, and scintigraphy may be negative.

Osteosarcoma. Osteosarcoma is a malignant neoplasm characterized by production of osteoid by the tumor cells. It is the second most common primary malignant tumor of bone after plasmacytoma. It is a rare tumor, representing only 0.2% of all malignant tumors. It

has a male predominance with a 2:1 male-to-female ratio. Its peak is in the second decade, and it is rare before 10 and after 30 years of age. Osteosarcoma can occur in any bone but has a strong preference for the distal femur, proximal tibia, and proximal humerus. Two thirds of osteosarcomas are localized to the knee or shoulder. Osteosarcomas can be divided into two categories: primary and secondary. Primary osteosarcomas arise de novo, whereas secondary osteosarcomas develop in abnormal bones. Underlying bone abnormalities include Paget's disease, radiation therapy, multiple enchondromas, multiple osteochondromas, chronic osteomyelitis, fibrous dysplasia, or infarct. Secondary osteosarcomas are usually in an older age group than primary osteosarcomas.

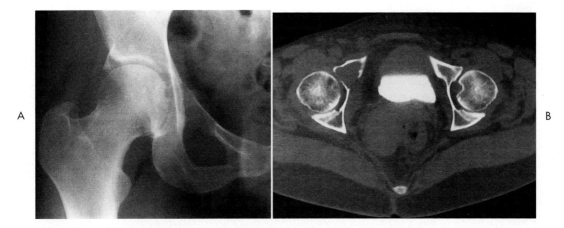

Fig. 40-8. Multiple myeloma. **A,** Radiograph of the right hip demonstrates a lytic lesion of the superior pubic ramus. **B,** CT confirms the presence of a lytic lesion with destruction of the cortex posteriorly; no sclerotic borders are present.

MRI is useful in staging the tumor and for follow-up after treatment.[13,28,32,67,73,82,81,100] The osteoblastic component of the tumor has low signal intensity on all sequences. The nonmineralized component has low signal on T1-weighted images and high signal on T2-weighted images. Bone marrow extension is best seen on T1-weighted images as loss of normal high bone marrow signal. Soft tissue extension is best seen on T2-weighted images because tumor and muscle may have the same signal intensity on T1-weighted images. CT is better than MRI in demonstrating matrix mineralization but is less accurate in detecting skip lesions and bone marrow and soft tissue extension (Fig. 40-9). Telangiectatic osteosarcomas contain large, cystic, blood-filled spaces with fluid-fluid levels that may mimic an aneurysmal bone cyst but usually are less well defined than aneurysmal bone cysts.[90]

In the last two decades, the development of aggressive chemotherapy has significantly improved the survival of patients with osteosarcoma, and imaging studies are being used to evaluate the tumor's response to treatment. CT findings of a positive response to treatment include marked decrease in size or complete disappearance of the soft tissue mass, increased calcification of the mass, improved delineation of the margins, and formation of a peripheral rim of calcification.[61,83] On MRI, decreased signal intensity of the nonmineralized mass on T2-weighted images is believed to represent fibrosis or sclerosis of the tumor. Persistent high signal may be due to either nonresponding tumor or necrotic tumor, reactive granulation tissue, or hemorrhage.[28,35,57] Administration of gadolinium cannot distinguish viable tumor from reactive inflammation because both enhance, but the lack of enhancement is indicative of tumor necrosis.[82]

Chondrosarcoma. Chondrosarcoma is a malignant chondroid tumor. It is the fourth most common primary malignant bone tumor after plasmacytoma, osteosarcoma, and Ewing's sarcoma. Its peak incidence is between 30 and 60 years of age. According to their intraosseous location, chondrosarcomas may be divided into central and peripheral. Most chondrosarcomas (approximately 75%) are primary and arise de novo, but the remaining 25% are secondary and develop from malignant transformation of a benign lesion, such as an enchondroma or an osteochondroma and rarely a chondroblastoma. Central chondrosarcomas occur both in tubular bones, such as the femur, proximal humerus, proximal tibia, and in flat bones, such as the pelvis. Peripheral chondrosarcomas most commonly arise in flat bones, such as the pelvis and ribs, and in the spine.

It is difficult to differentiate low-grade chondrosarcomas from benign chondroid lesions. The presence of pain in the absence of fracture, cortical destruction, and the presence of a soft tissue mass, however, are all signs suspicious for malignancy. On MRI, chondrosarcoma has a characteristic multilobular configuration. The lobules of hyaline cartilage have intermediate signal intensity, similar to that of muscle, on T1-weighted images (Fig. 40-10) and homogeneous high signal intensity on T2-weighted images.[17,35,57,93] The fibrous septa have low signal intensity on both T1- and T2-weighted images but enhance after gadolinium-DTPA administration.[2,32] Calcifications are common in low-grade chondrosarcoma and are best seen on conventional radiography and CT. Endosteal scalloping is also best depicted on CT and plain radiographs.

Ewing's sarcoma. Ewing's sarcoma is a malignant neoplasm probably of neuroectodermal origin. Among primary malignant neoplasms of bone, it follows

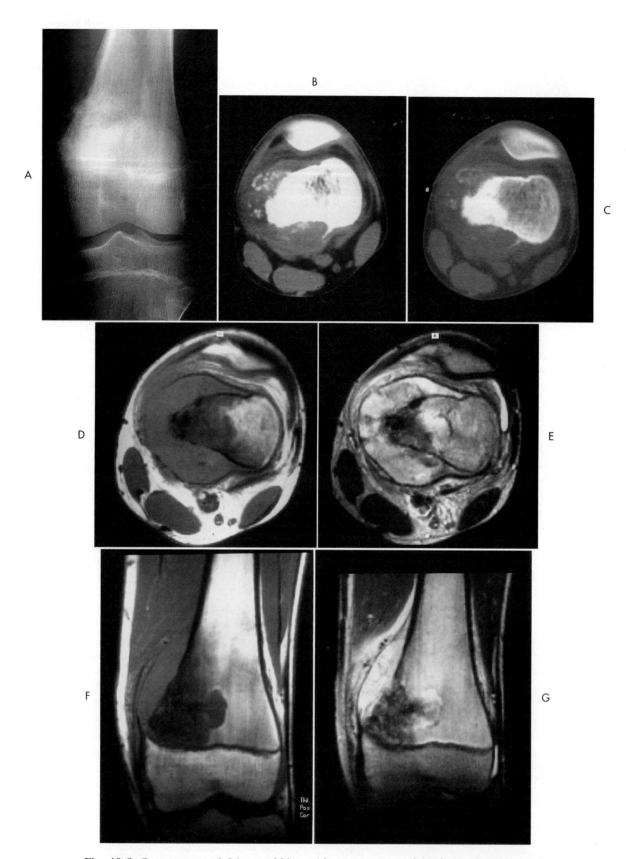

Fig. 40-9. Osteosarcoma. A 14-year-old boy with osteosarcoma of the femur. **A,** Radiograph demonstrates a sclerotic lesion in the metaphysis, with medial destruction of the cortex and periosteal reaction. Images from a CT scan with soft tissue **(B)** and bone windows **(C)** show a sclerotic lesion of the medial aspect of the femur with associated soft tissue mass and periosteal reaction. On MRI; axial SE 500/15 **(D),** SE 2000/70 **(E),** coronal SE 600/15 **(F),** and 2000/70 **(G)** images show the soft tissue component better than on CT, but periosteal reaction and soft tissue calcification are not as evident. An area of low signal is present on both T1- and T2-weighted images and corresponds to the area of sclerosis seen on CT.

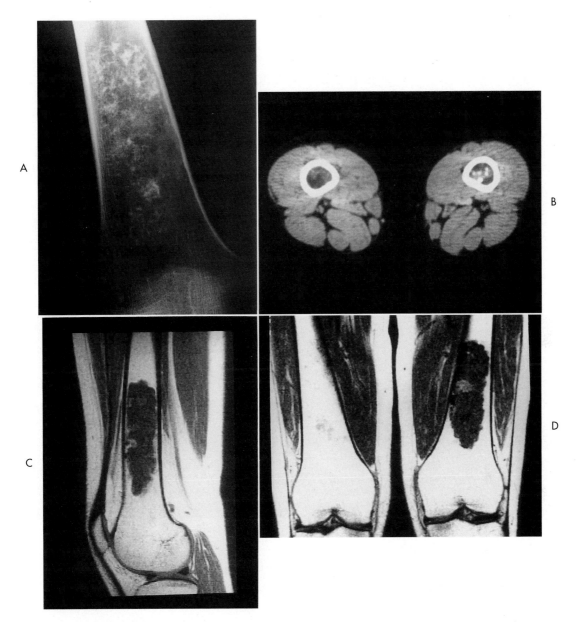

Fig. 40-10. Chondrosarcoma. Primary grade I chondrosarcoma in a 36-year-old woman. **A,** Radiograph of the knee demonstrates a lesion in the distal femur with cartilaginous matrix. **B,** CT scan also shows the calcifications in the matrix of the lesion. Sagittal **(C)** and coronal **(D)** SE 500/17 images demonstrate a lobulated lesion in the medullary cavity. The exact extension of the lesion is easily appreciated, but the matrix calcifications are poorly seen.

plasmacytoma, osteosarcoma, and chondrosarcoma in frequency. It has a male predominance with a 2:1 male-to-female ratio. Its peak is in the second decade, with 90% of cases between 5 and 25 years of age. It can involve any bone but has a predilection for the long bones and pelvis. In the long bones, it is localized to the diaphysis or metaphysis and until the growth plate is open does not extend to the epiphysis. MRI is useful in the

staging of Ewing's sarcoma and is better than CT in demonstrating bone marrow and soft tissue involvement.[34] MRI signal characteristics of Ewing's sarcoma are not specific and are similar to those of other malignant neoplasms.[13,28,36] The tumor has lower or equal intensity as muscle on T1-weighted images and high signal intensity on T2-weighted images (Fig. 40-11). MRI and CT are helpful in the evaluation of response to treat-

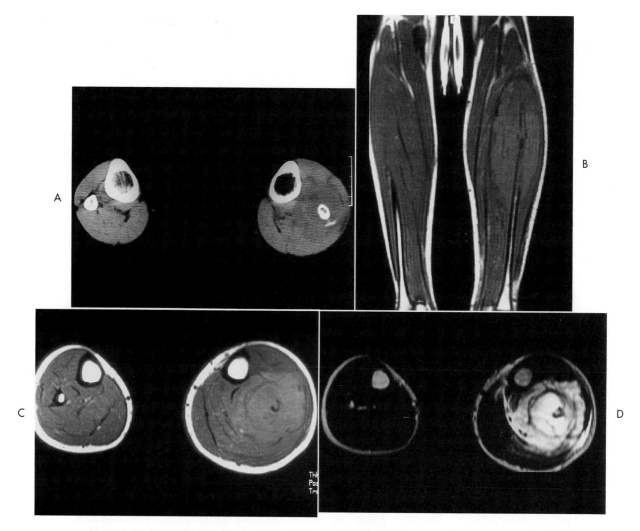

Fig. 40-11. Ewing's sarcoma. **A,** CT scan shows a large mass with density slightly lower than muscle surrounding the left tibia. Coronal SE 700/15 (**B**) and axial SE 800/15 (**C**) T1-weighted images demonstrate a large mass surrounding the fibula. This mass has similar signal intensity as muscle on T1-weighted images and high signal intensity on axial 2500/80 T2-weighted image (**D**).

ment. If the tumor is sensitive to treatment, it decreases in size, the periosteal reaction matures, and the bone becomes sclerotic.[28,39,55] High signal intensity on T2-weighted images after treatment does not always mean poor response because it may represent necrosis, reactive granulation tissue, or hemorrhage. Enhancement after gadolinium-DTPA cannot distinguish reactive changes from residual tumor, but the lack of enhancement indicates tumor necrosis.[28,39,55]

SOFT TISSUE TUMORS

CT has been widely used for the detection and staging of soft tissue tumors,[94] but MRI is now becoming the modality of choice for evaluation of soft tissue tumors owing to its intrinsic high soft tissue contrast.[23,24,68,87,95] MRI can accurately detect and stage soft tissue masses and is more sensitive for lesions than CT.

On MRI, benign lesions tend to have well-defined margins, have homogeneous signal intensity, do not encase neurovascular bundles, and are not surrounded by peritumoral edema.[6] Conversely, poorly defined margins, heterogeneous signal intensity, neurovascular bundle encasement, and peritumoral edema are typical of malignant lesions.[7,8] Unfortunately, there is a large overlap between benign and malignant lesions, and the ability of

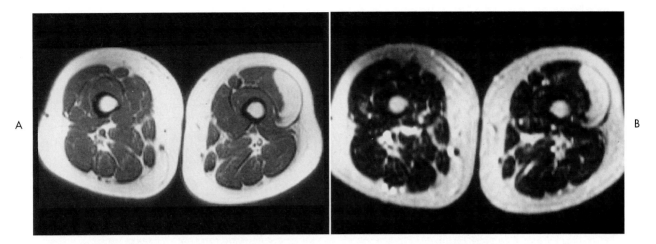

Fig. 40-12. Lipoma. Intramuscular lipoma in a 51-year-old woman. A lesion with the same signal intensity as subcutaneous fat is seen in the vastus medialis on both T1-weighted (**A**) and T2-weighted (**B**) images.

MRI to differentiate benign from malignant soft tissue masses remains controversial.[21,50]

Benign soft tissue tumors

Lipoma. Lipoma is a benign tumor composed by mature adipose tissue. It is the most frequent benign soft tissue tumor and is frequently asymptomatic. Superficial lipomas predominate in women, whereas deep lipomas are more common in men. The age peak for lipomas is between 40 and 60 years of age. Superficial lipomas are usually localized to the subcutaneous tissue of the trunk and proximal extremities. Deep lipomas are usually in the retroperitoneum, chest wall, and deep soft tissue of the hands and feet. On CT, lipomas have a low attenuation coefficient equal to subcutaneous fat and do not enhance after administration of contrast material. On MRI, they have the same signal characteristics as subcutaneous fat on all imaging sequences (Fig. 40-12). On both CT and MRI scans, lipomas have a homogeneous appearance, although occasional thin fibrous septa can be present.[16,52]

Vascular anomalies. Vascular anomalies include hemangiomas, venous malformations, arteriovenous malformations, arteriovenous fistulae, and mixed lesions. The term hemangioma has also been used generically to describe all of these vascular anomalies.[46] Vascular anomalies are more common in females. They are usually congenital except for posttraumatic arteriovenous fistulae.

On MRI, hemangiomas have the same signal intensity as muscle on T1-weighted images and high signal intensity on T2-weighted images. The signal is usually heterogeneous on T2-weighted images. On T1-weighted images, they may be either homogeneous or inhomogeneous.[98] Phleboliths are seen as focal areas of low signal intensity on all imaging sequences but are better identified on plain radiographs or CT (Fig. 40-13). Serpiginous areas of low signal intensity are occasionally seen and represent flow void in larger feeding arteries or draining veins. On MRI, arteriovenous malformations and arteriovenous fistulae have large tortuous vessels with flow void owing to rapidly flowing blood. Feeding and draining vessels can be identified as vascular structures, but differentiation of veins and arteries if not always possible.[18,62,71]

Desmoid tumor. Desmoid tumor is a tumor composed of fibroblasts. Histologically, it is benign and does not metastasize, but it is locally aggressive, infiltrates contiguous structures, and has a strong tendency to recur after resection. Desmoid tumor may occur at any age but most frequently is seen in the third and fourth decade. On cross-sectional imaging, desmoids have well-defined borders two thirds of the time, but in the remainder one third, there are infiltrative and poorly defined margins. CT scans obtained without contrast enhancement show variable attenuation relative to muscle. After intravenous contrast administration, desmoid tumors may or may not enhance. The majority are hyperdense or isodense with muscle on contrast-enhanced scans. On MRI, desmoid tumors have signal intensity lower than muscle on T1-weighted images, with variable signal intensity on T2-weighted images (Fig. 40-14). They may have an aggressive appearance and be confused with a malignant tumor.[7,20] The presence of areas of low signal intensity on both T1- and T2-weighted images, owing to fibrous tissue, is a clue to the correct diagnosis.

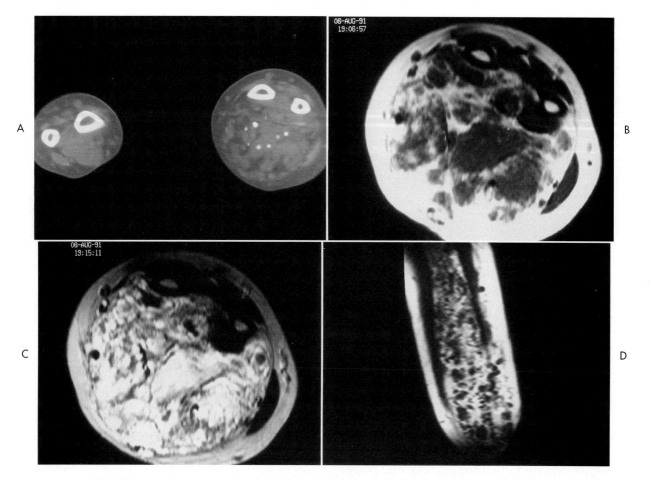

Fig. 40-13. Hemangioma. **A,** CT scan shows multiple phleboliths in the forearm within soft tissue mass. **B,** On T1-weighted images, the lesion is isointense with muscle, with areas of increased signal intensity corresponding to fat interposed between vascular elements. **C,** On T2-weighted images, the vascular elements have high signal intensity. **D,** Large tortuous vessels with flow void owing to rapidly flowing blood are seen on coronal T1-weighted image.

Intramuscular myxoma. Intramuscular myxoma is a rare benign tumor containing myxoid tissue. It occurs in older persons, between 40 and 70 years of age. Usually it is solitary and has a slow growth rate. Multiple myxomas have been seen in patients with fibrous dysplasias. The tumor is usually localized in a large muscle of the thigh, shoulder, or hip. On CT, it appears as a well-defined, homogeneous mass, with density lower than muscle. It typically does not enhance after administration of intravenous contrast material. On MRI, it has a low signal intensity on T1-weighted images and high signal intensity on T2-weighted images.[89]

Pigmented villonodular synovitis. Pigmented villonodular synovitis is a benign proliferative process of the synovial lining of a joint, bursa, or tendon sheath. The origin of this lesion is unknown. Repeat trauma, repeat intra-articular hemorrhage, and inflammation have

been suggested. A focal and a diffuse form exist. The focal form is more common and usually involves tendon sheaths of the hands; it is also called giant cell tumor of the tendon sheath. The diffuse form involves large joints, especially the knee. There is no sexual preference. The peak incidence is between 20 and 40 years of age. The MRI characteristics of pigmented villonodular synovitis are typical and often allow correct diagnosis. On MRI, the lesion has areas of low signal intensity on both T1- and T2-weighted images owing to deposition of hemosiderin within the tumor.[44,48] The presence of bone erosion on both sides of the joint also supports the diagnosis of pigmented villonodular synovitis. Joint effusion may be present. On CT, bone erosions have well-defined sclerotic borders. The soft tissue component may contain areas of high attenuation on nonenhanced scans, corresponding to deposits of hemosiderin.[77]

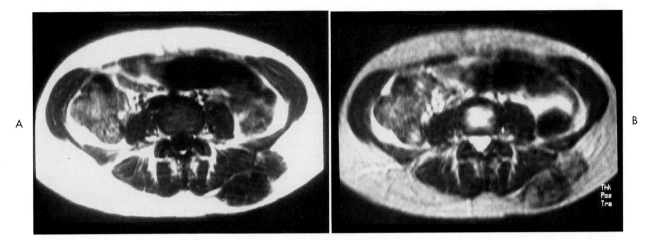

Fig. 40-14. Desmoid tumor. SE 540/15 **(A)** and SE 2000/80 **(B)** axial images demonstrate a lesion in the subcutaneous tissues of the back with low signal on the T1-weighted image and intermediate with area of low signal on the T2-weighted image. An area of low signal on both sequences is suggestive of the presence of fibrous tissue and helps in making the diagnosis of desmoid tumor.

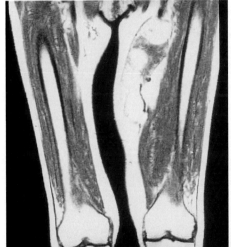

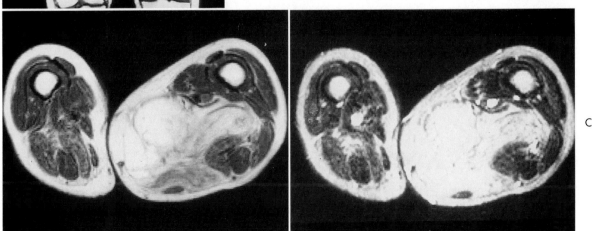

Fig. 40-15. Low-grade liposarcoma. Coronal SE 800/17 **(A)** and axial SE 800/17 **(B)** images demonstrate a large mass in the medial compartment of the thigh. A large part of the lesion has the same signal intensity as fat, but there are also areas with signal similar to muscle, making it possible to distinguish this lesion from a benign lipoma. **C,** On an axial SE 2500/90 T2-weighted image, the nonlipomatous portions of the tumor have signal intensity higher than fat.

Malignant soft tissue sarcoma

Liposarcoma. Liposarcoma is a malignant neoplasm of soft tissues containing cells with lipoblastic or lipocytic differentiation. It is the second most common malignant soft tissue tumor after malignant fibrous histiocytoma. Its peak incidence is between 50 and 60 years of age, and it is rare before 20 years of age. Liposarcomas are most common in the extremities, especially the thigh, and in the retroperitoneum. Liposarcomas can be divided into four groups based on their histologic characteristics: well differentiated, myxoid, round cell, and pleomorphic. The appearance of a liposarcoma on CT and MRI depends on its degree of differentiation.[45,52] Portions of the tumor containing fat have a low attenuation coefficient on CT scans and high signal intensity on T1-weighted MRI scans. The nonlipomatous portions of the tumor have a higher attenuation coefficient than fat on CT scans, and on MRI, they have a signal intensity similar to muscle on T1-weighted images (Fig. 40-15). and signal intensity higher than fat on T2-weighted images.[58] A well-differentiated liposarcoma can have the same characteristics of an atypical lipoma on both CT and MRI, and differentiation between these two entities can therefore be difficult.[16] More aggressive liposarcomas may contain no fat detectable on either CT or MRI (Fig. 40-16). In these cases, the appearance of the tumor is indistinguishable from other malignant soft tissue tumors.

Malignant fibrous histiocytoma. Malignant fibrous histiocytoma is a malignant tumor that develops from a primitive mesenchymal cell, with markers of histiocytoid differentiation. It is the most common malignant neoplasm of soft tissues. It is more common in men with an age peak between 50 and 70 years of age. Fifty percent are localized in the lower extremities, 20% in the upper extremities, and 20% in the abdominal cavity and retroperitoneum. Other locations are rare. On MRI, malignant fibrous histiocytoma has low signal intensity on T1-weighted images and heterogeneous high signal intensity on T2-weighted images (Fig. 40-17).[26,60] On CT, it has the same density as muscle and frequently contains areas of lower attenuation corresponding to areas

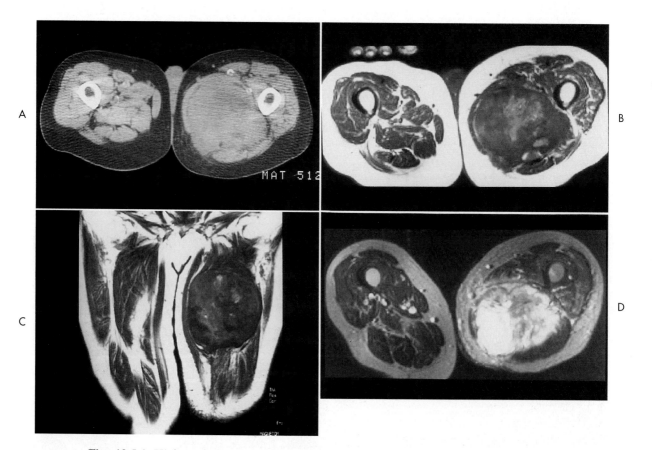

Fig. 40-16. High-grade liposaracoma. **A,** CT scan shows a large mass with heterogeneous density suggesting that portions of this mass are necrotic, but no fat density is identified. Axial **(B)** and coronal **(C)** SE 600/15 images show a large mass with heterogeneous signal; small foci with higher signal may represent hemorrhage or fat within the tumor **(D).**

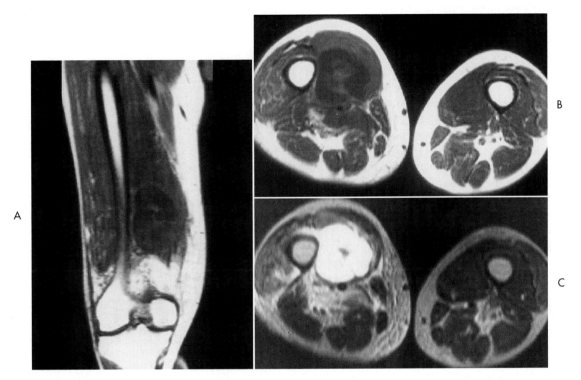

Fig. 40-17. Malignant fibrous histiocytoma. Coronal SE 600/15 (**A**) and axial 700/15 (**B**) T1-weighted images show a large mass of low signal intensity in the medial compartment of the thigh. **C,** On an axial SE 2500/80 T2-weighted image, this mass has heterogeneous high signal intensity.

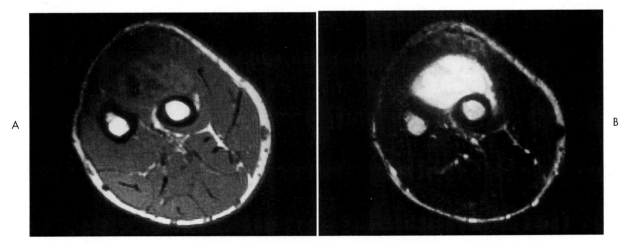

Fig. 40-18. Synovial sarcoma. Low-to-intermediate signal intensity is present on axial T1-weighted image (**A**), and heterogeneous high signal intensity is seen on axial T2-weighted image (**B**).

of necrosis.[76] MRI is better than CT in determining extension of tumor, but CT is superior in detecting bone involvement and calcifications within the tumor. Calcifications have been seen in up to 20% of malignant fibrous histiocytoma.[26]

Synovial sarcoma. Synovial sarcoma is a malignant tumor that develops from undifferentiated mesenchymal cells. It is a relatively frequent soft tissue tumor and follows malignant fibrous histiocytoma, liposarcoma, and rhabdomyosarcoma in prevalence. It has a slight male predominance and has an age peak between 15 and 35 years of age. Only 10% of synovial cell sarcomas are within a joint. Usually they are located adherent to a joint capsule, bursa, fascia, or tendon sheath. They are most common in the lower extremity. On MRI, synovial sarcoma has low-to-intermediate signal intensity on T1-weighted images and heterogeneous high signal intensity on T2-weighted images.[59,63] It is often multilocular with internal septation and occasionally fluid-fluid levels (Fig. 40-18).[90] Calcifications are present in 30% of the cases and are best seen on CT.[3] The presence of extensive calcifications indicates a better prognosis.[91]

REFERENCES

1. Aisen, et al: MRI and CT evaluation of primary bone and soft tissue tumors. *AJR* 146:749, 1986.
2. Aoki J, et al: MR of enchondroma and chondrosarcoma: ring and arcs of Gd-DTPA enhancement. *J Comput Assist Tomogr* 15:1011, 1991.
3. Azouz EM, Vickar DB, Brown KLB: Computed tomography of the foot. *J Canad Assoc Radiol* 34:85, 1984.
4. Beltran J, et al: Aneurysmal bone cysts: MR imaging at 1.5 T. *Radiology* 158:689, 1986.
5. Beltran J, et al: Tumors of the osseous spine: staging with MR imaging versus CT. *Radiology* 162:565, 1987.
6. Beltran J, et al: Increased MR signal intensity in skeletal muscle adjacent to malignant tumors: pathologic correlation and clinical relevance. *Radiology* 162:251, 1987.
7. Berquist TH, et al: Value of MR imaging in differentiating benign from malignant soft-tissue masses: study of 95 lesions. *AJR* 155:1251, 1990.
8. Berquist TH: Magnetic resonance imaging of musculoskeletal neoplasms. *Clin Orthop* 244:101, 1989.
9. Bloem JL, et al: Magnetic resonance imaging of primary malignant bone tumors. *Radiographics* 5:853, 1985.
10. Bloem JL, et al: Magnetic resonance imaging of primary malignant bone tumors. *Radiographics* 7:425, 1987.
11. Bloem JL, et al: Radiologic staging of primary bone sarcoma: MR imaging, scintigraphy, angiograph, and CT correlated with pathologic examination. *Radiology* 169:805, 1988.
12. Bohndorf K, et al: Magnetic resonance imaging of primary tumors and tumor like lesions of bone. *Skel Radiol* 15:511, 1986.
13. Boyko OB, et al: MR imaging of osteogenic and Ewing's sarcoma. *AJR* 148:317, 1987.
14. Brady TJ, et al: NMR imaging of forearms in healthy volunteers and patients with giant-cell tumor of bone. *Radiology* 144:549, 1982.
15. Brower AC, Moser RP, Kransdorf MJ: The frequency and diagnostic significance of periostitis, in chondroblastoma. *AJR* 154:309, 1990.
16. Bush CH, Spanier SS, Gillespy T: Imaging of atypical lipomas of the extremities: a report of three cases. *Skel Radiol* 17:472, 1988.
17. Cohen EK, et al: Hyaline cartilage—origin of bone and soft tissue neoplasms: MR appearance and histologic correlation. *Radiology* 167:477, 1988.
18. Cohen JM, Weinreb JC, Redman HC: Arteriovenous malformation of the extremities: MR imaging. *Radiology* 158:475, 1986.
19. Cory DA, et al: Aneurysmal bone cysts: imaging findings and embolotherapy. *AJR* 153:269, 1989.
20. Crim JR, et al: Widespread inflammatory response to osteoblastoma: the flare phenomenon. *Radiology* 177:835, 1990.
21. Crim JR, et al: Diagnosis of soft-tissue masses with MR imaging: can benign masses be differentiated from malignant ones? *Radiology* 185:581, 1992.
22. Dahlin DC: Giant cell tumor of bone: highlight of 407 cases. *AJR* 111:966, 1985.
23. Dalinka, et al: The use of magnetic resonance imaging in the evaluation of bone and soft-tissue tumors. *Radiol Clin North Am* 28:461, 1990.
24. Demas BE, et al: Soft-tissue sarcomas of the extremities: comparison of MR and CT in determining the extent of disease. *AJR* 150:615, 1988.
25. DeSantos LA, Murray JA: Evaluation of giant cell tumors by computerized tomography. *Skel Radiol* 2:205, 1978.
26. Dorfman MD, Bhagavan BS: Malignant fibrous histiocytoma of the soft tissue with metaplastic bone and cartilage formation: a new radiologic sign. *Skel Radiol* 8:145, 1982.
27. Erlemann, et al: Musculoskeletal neoplasms: static and dynamic Gd-DTPA-enhanced MR imaging. *Radiology* 171:767, 1989.
28. Fletcher BD: Response of osteosarcoma and Ewing sarcoma to chemotherapy: imaging evaluation. *AJR* 157:825, 1991.
29. Frank JA, et al: Detection of malignant bone tumors: MR imaging vs scintigraphy. *AJR* 155:1043, 1990.
30. Fruehwald FXJ, et al: Magnetic resonance imaging of the lower vertebral column in patients with multiple myeloma. *Invest Radiol* 23:193, 1988.
31. Gamba JL, et al: Computed tomography of axial skeletal osteoid osteomas. *AJR* 142:769, 1984.
32. Geirnaerdt MJA, et al: Cartilaginous tumors: correlation of gadolinium-enhanced MR imaging and histopathologic findings. *Radiology* 186:813, 1993.
33. Gillespy T, et al: Staging of intraosseous extent of osteosarcoma: correlation of preoperative CT and MR imaging with pathologic macroslides. *Radiology* 167:765, 1988.
34. Ginaldi S, deSantos LA: Computed tomography in the evaluation of small round cell tumors of bone. *Radiology* 134:441, 1980.
35. Golfieri R, et al: Primary bone tumors. MR morphologic appearance correlated with pathologic examinations. *Acta Radiol* 32:290, 1991.
36. Hall TR, Kangarloo H: Magnetic resonance imaging of the musculoskeletal system in children. *Clin Orthop* 244:119, 1989.
37. Hayes CW, Conway WF, Sundaram M: Misleading aggressive MR imaging appearance of some benign musculoskeletal lesions. *Radiographics* 12:1119, 1992.
38. Herman SD, et al: The role of magnetic resonance imaging in giant cell tumor of bone. *Skel Radiol* 16:635, 1987.
39. Holscher HC, et al: The value of MR imaging in monitoring the effect of chemotherapy on bone sarcomas. *AJR* 154:763, 1990.
40. Hudson TM, Hamlin DJ, Fitzsimmons JR: Magnetic resonance imaging of fluid levels in an aneurysmal bone cyst and in anticoagulated human blood. *Skel Radiol* 13:267, 1985.
41. Hudson TM, Hawkins IF: Radiologic evaluation of chondroblastoma. *Radiology* 139:1, 1981.

42. Hudson TM: Fluid levels in Aneurysmal bone cysts: a CT feature. *AJR* 141:1001, 1984.

43. Hudson TM, et al: Benign exostosis and exostotic chondrosarcomas: evaluation of cartilage thickness by CT. *Radiology* 152:595, 1984.

44. Jelinek JS, et al: Imaging of pigmented villonodular synovitis with emphasis on MR imaging. *AJR* 152:337, 1989.

45. Jelinek JS, et al: Liposarcoma of the extremities: MR and CT findings in the histologic subtypes. *Radiology* 186:455, 1993.

46. Kaplan PA, Williams SM: Mucocutaneous and peripheral soft-tissue hemangioma: MR imaging. *Radiology* 163:163, 1987.

47. Kenney PJ, Gilula LA, Murphy WA: The use of computed tomography to distinguish osteochondroma and chondrosarcoma. *Radiology* 139:129, 1981.

48. Kottal RA, et al: Pigmented villonodular synovitis: a report of MR imaging in two cases. *Radiology* 163:551, 1987.

49. Kransdorf MJ, et al: MR appearance of fibroxanthoma. *J Comput Assist Tomogr* 12:612, 1988.

50. Kransdorf MJ, et al: Soft-tissue masses: diagnosis using MR imaging. *AJR* 153:541, 1989.

51. Kransdorf MJ, et al: From the archives of AFIP. Osteoid osteoma. *Radiographics* 11:671, 1991.

52. Kransdorf MJ, et al: Fat-containing soft tissue masses of the extremities. *Radiographics* 11:81, 1991.

53. Kroon HM, Shurmans J: Osteoblastoma: clinical and radiologic finding in 98 new cases. *Radiology* 175:783, 1990.

54. Lee JK, Yao L, Wirth CR: MR imaging of solitary osteochondromas: report of eight cases. *AJR* 149:557, 1987.

55. Lemmi MA, et al: Use of MR imaging to assess results of chemotherapy for Ewing sarcoma. *AJR* 155:343, 1990.

56. Levine E, Neff JR: Dynamic computed tomography scanning of benign bone lesions: preliminary results. *Skel Radiol* 9:238, 1983.

57. Lodwick GS: The radiologist's role in managing chondrosarcoma. *Radiology* 150:275, 1984.

58. London J, et al: MR imaging of liposarcomas: correlation of MR features and histology. *J Comput Assist Tomogr* 15:832, 1989.

59. Mahajan H, Lorigan JG, Shirkhoda A: Synovial sarcoma: MR imaging. *Magn Reson Imaging* 7:211, 1989.

60. Mahajan H, et al: Magnetic resonance imaging of malignant fibrous histiocytoma. *Magn Reson Imaging* 7:283, 1989.

61. Mail JT, et al: Response of osteosarcoma to preoperative intravenous high-dose methotrexate chemotherapy: CT evaluation. *AJR* 144:89, 1985.

62. Meyer, et al: Biological classification of soft-tissue vascular anomalies: MR correlation. *AJR* 157:559, 1991.

63. Morton MJ, et al: MR imaging of synovial sarcoma. *AJR* 156:337, 1991.

64. Moser RP, et al: From the archives of the AFIP. Giant cell tumor of the upper extremity. *Radiographics* 10:83, 1990.

65. Moulopoulos LA, et al: Multiple myeloma: spinal MR imaging in patients with untreated newly diagnosed disease. *Radiology* 185:833, 1992.

66. Munk PL, et al: MR imaging of aneurysmal bone cyst. *AJR* 153:99, 1989.

67. Pan G, et al: Osteosarcoma: MR imaging after preoperative chemotherapy. *Radiology* 174:517, 1990.

68. Petasnick JP, et al: Soft-tissue masses of the locomotor system: comparison of MR imaging with CT. *Radiology* 160:125, 1986.

69. Pettersson H, et al: Primary musculoskeletal tumors: examination with MR imaging compared with conventional modalities. *Radiology* 164:237, 1987.

70. Prayer LM, et al: High-resolution real-time sonography and MR imaging in assessment of osteocartilaginous exostoses. *Acta Radiol* 32:393, 1991.

71. Rak KM, et al: MR imaging of symptomatic peripheral vascular malformations. *AJR* 159:107, 1992.

72. Recht MP, Sachs PB, LiPuma J, Clampitt M: Case report: a popliteal artery pseudoaneurysm in a patient with hereditary multiple exostoses diagnosed by MR and MR angiography. *J Comput Assist Tomogr* (in press).

73. Redmond OM, et al: Osteosarcoma: use of MR and MR spectroscopy in clinical decision making. *Radiology* 172:811, 1989.

74. Reuther G, Mutschler W: The value of CT and MRI in the diagnosis of cartilage-forming tumors [German]. *Rofo: Fortschritte Auf Dem Gebiete Der Rontgenstrahlen Und Der Nuklearmedizin* 151(6):647, 1989.

75. Ritshl, P, Hajeck PC, Pechmann U: Fibrous metaphyseal defects. Magnetic resonance imaging appearance. *Skel Radiol* 18:253, 1989.

76. Ros PR, Viamonte M, Rywlin AM: Malignant fibrous histiocytoma: mesenchymal tumor of ubiquitous origin. *AJR* 142:753, 1984.

77. Rosenthal D, Aronow S, Murray WT: Iron content of pigmented villonodular synovitis detected by computed tomography. *Radiology* 133:409, 1979.

78. Rosenthal RE, Wozney P: Diagnostic value of gadopentate dimeglumine for 1.5-T MR imaging of musculoskeletal masses: comparison with unenhanced T1- and T2-weighted imaging. *J Magn Reson Imag* 1:547, 1991.

79. Schlesinger AE, Hernandez RJ: Intracapsular osteoid osteoma of the proximal femur: findings on plain film and CT. *AJR* 154:1241, 1990.

80. Schreiman JS, McLeod R, Kyle RA, Beabout JW: Multiple myeloma: evaluation by CT. *Radiology* 154:483, 1985.

81. Seeger LL, Eckardt JJ, Bassett LW: Cross-sectional imaging in the evaluation of osteogenic sarcoma: MRI and CT. *Semin Roengenol* 24:174, 1989.

82. Seeger LL, et al: Preoperative evaluation of osteosarcoma: value of gadopentate dimeglumine-enhanced MR imaging. *AJR* 157:347, 1991.

83. Shirkhoda A, et al: Computed tomography of osteosarcoma after intraarterial chemotherapy. *AJR* 144:95, 1985.

84. Shuman WP, et al: Comparison of STIR and spin-echo MR imaging at 1.5 T in 45 suspected extremity tumors: lesion conspicuity and extent. *Radiology* 179:247, 1991.

85. Simon JH, Szumowski J: Chemical shift imaging with paramagnetic contrast material enhancement for improved lesion depiction. *Radiology* 171:539, 1989.

86. Sundaram M, McGuire MH: Computed tomography and magnetic resonance for evaluating the solitary tumor and tumor-like lesion of bone? *Skel Radiol* 17:393, 1988.

87. Sundaram M, McLeod RA: MR imaging of tumor and tumor like lesions of bone and soft tissue. *AJR* 155:817, 1990.

88. Tehranzadeh J, Murphy BJ, Mnaymneh W: Giant cell tumor of the proximal tibia: MR and CT appearance. *J Comput Assist Tomogr* 13:282, 1989.

89. Totty WG, Murphy WA, Lee JKT: Soft tissue tumors: MR imaging. *Radiology* 160:135, 1986.

90. Tsai JC, et al: Fluid-fluid level: a nonspecific finding in tumors of bone and soft tissue. *Radiology* 175:779, 1990.

91. Varila-Duran J, Enzinger FM: Calcifying synovial sarcoma. *Cancer* 50:345, 1982.

92. Vanel D, et al: Musculoskeletal tumors: follow-up with MR imaging after treatment with surgery and radiation therapy. *Radiology* 164:243, 1987.

93. Varma DGK, et al: Chondrosarcoma: MR imaging with pathologic correlation. *Radiographics* 12:687, 1992.

94. Weekes RG, et al: CT of soft-tissue neoplasms. *AJR* 144:355, 1985.

95. Weekes RG, et al: Magnetic resonance imaging of soft-tissue tumors: comparison with computed tomography. *Magn Reson Imaging* 3:345, 1985.

96. Wetzel LH, Levine E, Murphey MD: A comparison of MR imaging and CT in the evaluation of musculoskeletal masses. *Radiographics* 7:851, 1987.

97. Wilson AJ, Kyriakos M, Acckerman LV: Chondromyxoid fibroma: radiographic appearance in 38 cases and in review of the literature. *Radiology* 179:513, 1991.

98. Yuh WT, et al: Hemangioma of skeletal muscle: MR finding in five patients. *AJR* 149:765-768, 1987.

99. Zimmer WD, et al: Magnetic resonance imaging of aneurysmal bone cysts. *Mayo Clin Proc* 59:633, 1984.

100. Zimmer WD, et al: Magnetic resonance imaging of osteosarcoma. Comparison with computed tomography. *Clin Orthop Rel Res* 208:289, 1986.

41
The Foot

MARK SCHWEITZER

TRAUMATIC INJURIES

Ankle and foot fractures are common injuries most easily diagnosed and evaluated by routine radiography. Several of these injuries may, however, be radiographically occult or require more detailed evaluation provided by computed tomography (CT) or magnetic resonance imaging (MRI). These include bone bruises, occult fractures, fractures of the calcaneus talus, and navicular and triplane fractures of the tibia. It is in these injuries that CT and MRI play an important role. The mildest osseous injury is a bone bruise, contusion, or trabecular fracture. The latter is not an appropriate term since fractures by definition have cortical disruption. These purely intramedullary injuries were first described as incidental findings in the knee.[75,107] Similar injuries occur in the foot and ankle either secondary to indirect trauma, ligamentous injury, or as the result of direct compression.[74] On MRI they are poorly defined, inhomogeneous and reticulated. They are best seen on T1-weighted or STIR images, and when hyperacute to acute they demonstrate high signal on T2-weighted images[110] (Fig. 41-1). These injuries have not been described on CT. In the foot, in contradistinction to the knee, these injuries are painful and quite disabling. They are therefore treated more aggressively, similar to the treatment of a radiographically visible nondisplaced fracture. In addition, although nearly all knee bone bruises completely resolve by 3 months, similar-appearing injuries to the tarsal bones may be seen for up to between 6 and 12 months with continued symptoms. We therefore prefer the term *occult fracture* for this injury.

The next most serious injury is a stress response. These injuries occur with a milder force than is required to cause a true fracture. They are the result of repetitive activities. The activity is usually new or different. In response to a stress, according to Wolff's law, bone undergoes active remodeling. As an early stage of this remodeling, osteoclasts cause bone resorption, thus transiently weakening bone before new bone is formed. At the same time, muscle, in response to the new activity, is hypertrophying. This incongruity between muscle and bone

strength leads to stress response or stress fractures. The initial medullary injury is the stress response. As the bone further weakens, cortical breaks occur, leading to a stress fracture. A stress fracture is most likely the end result of a progression of injury and repair. First, bone resorbs as it remodels; added stress may then cause an MRI appearance of a marrow abnormality. Next a small cortical break occurs. This may act as a stress enhancer leading to a complete fracture.[28] When this injury occurs in normal bone (such as occurs in newly athletic individuals) it is termed a *fatigue fracture*. When the bone is diffusely abnormal, either secondary to osteoporosis, Paget's disease, or other conditions, it is termed an *insufficiency fracture*.

On MRI, foci of decreased intensity of T1-weighted images increasing in intensity on T2-weighted images are seen. Initially they are subtle, amorphous, and inhomogeneous. This is the stress response. After several days to weeks they appear globular and less subtle. Later linear fracture line, which remains low signal on T1-weighted images, may be seen[66,96,64.] The surrounding bone will appear inhomogeneously dark on T1-weighted images and bright on T2-weighted images. Occasionally, soft-tissue edema and, with juxta articular fracture, joint effusions will be seen.

Calcaneus

The calcaneus is the most commonly fractured tarsal bone. Its injury represents 60% of all tarsal fractures and 2% of all fractures.[47] The injuries are often disabling because of the slow healing time and symptomatic sequalae.[50] Three articular facets of the calcaneus articulate with the talus. The largest of these is the posterior facet, articulating with the talus at the true (posterior) subtalar joint. There is no anterior subtalar joint. The articulation of the anterior and middle facets with the talus is correctly termed the *talocalcaneal articulation of the talocalcaneal navicular joint*.[108] Most (75%) of calcaneal fractures are intra-articular, and these invariably involve the true subtalar joint.[47,50] Most cal-

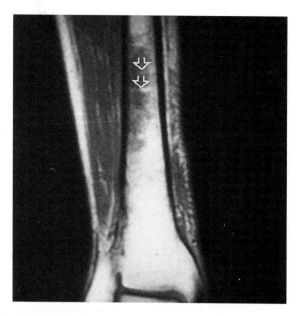

Fig. 41-1. Stress fractures characteristically only involve a portion of the medullary cavity, as seen in this coronal T1-weighted image; multiple horizontal lines are also seen *(arrows).*

caneal fractures are secondary to axial loading injuries. The primary fracture line is vertical and involves the sustentaculum tali and a variable portion of the posterior facet. The secondary fracture line determines the fracture type. In the more common joint-depression type this secondary line extends in a posterior direction horizontally just posterior to the posterior facet and exits superiorly to behind the posterior facet. In the tongue-type fractures, the secondary line extends horizontally posteriorly to exit at the tuberosity by the achilles. A third, less common type is comminuted.[47] Calcaneal stress fractures occur secondary to the antagonist actions of the achilles tendon and plantar ligament and aponeurosis. These may occur in military recruits or in patients with neurologic disorders or rheumatoid arthritis. MRI is the modality of choice in evaluating for the presence of stress fractures. These fractures occur posteriorly and have a vertical or oblique orientation. Since routine radiography visualizes complex calcaneal fractures in suboptimal detail, CT is the procedure of choice. Axial and coronal images should be performed at 3-mm intervals. Sagittal reconstructions are not usually necessary. From the CT, the type of fracture and number of fragments should be described. Of particular importance is the relative size of the sustentaculum tali fragment. Since the ligamentous attachments of the sustentaculum are strong, this is the most stable fragment. The remainder of the calcaneus tends

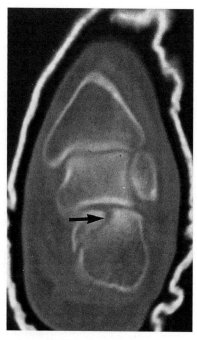

Fig. 41-2. A coronal CT image demonstrates a calcaneal fracture extending into the posterior facet even though there is only minimal articular depression *(arrow).*

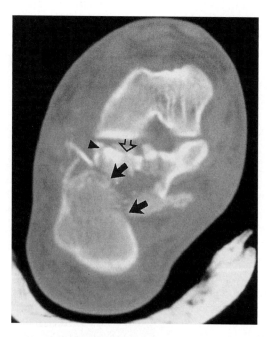

Fig. 41-3. Coronal CT image demonstrates a large (comminuted) *(arrow head)* sustentacular fragment involving nearly the entire posterior facet *(arrows).* There is approximately 3 mm of depression of the subtalar joint *(open arrow).* The entire medial fracture fragment is displaced inferiorly.

to displace laterally. The relative size of the sustentaculum fragment will determine the adequacy of its use as a buttress for fixation. Coronal images should be used to determine if the posterior facet is involved, and if involved the extent of depression, separation, and comminution of fragments (Fig. 41-2, 41-3). The presence of intra-articular bodies should also be assessed. The lateral fracture ligament is usually more depressed. Involvement of the middle facet should also be evaluated. Although involvement there has been considered rare, it was present in 75% of cases in one series. Since there are sparse trabculae in the calcaneus, interfragment gaps are frequent and CT images should be evaluated for the space between fragments. Widening in the coronal plane should also be evaluated. This may cause difficulty in wearing footwear. More importantly, the peroneal tendons are affected by this medial to lateral widening (Fig. 41-4). This may lead to peroneal tears, tendonitis, and subluxation or dislocation, and it may result in stenosing tenosynovitis. Although less frequently affected, the tendon of the flexor hallucis longus should also be assessed on CT or MRI examinations following calcaneal fractures. Lastly, axial images should be assessed for involvement of the calcaneal cuboid joint and degree of comminution of the lateral wall of calcaneus, which occurs with disruption of Gissane's angle (Fig. 41-5).

Following healing of calcaneal fractures in symptomatic patients images should be assessed for post-traumatic osteoarthritis, the most common sequelae of this injury. On CT this is demonstrated by joint space narrowing, irregularity, and the presence of a vacuum phenomenon in the subtalar joint. In 23% of patients intra-articular bodies will be seen. Nearly all fractures completely heal therefore non-union is an unusual complication. Involvement of the sural nerve of posterior tibial nerve may cause pain following fractures.[13] Fragments adjacent to, causing impression upon, or scarring in the known location of these nerves should be assessed. In particular, atrophy of the abductor digitii minimii is not rare following fractures occuring secondary to injury of the lateral plantar nerve.

Triplane fracture/epiphyseal injuries

The triplane fracture is an injury of the distal tibia that occurs in adolescents (average age 13.5 years) secondary to abnormal external rotation. This injury occurs in 6% to 10% of ankle fractures. There are three resultant fracture lines: sagittal, coronal, and axial. The axial

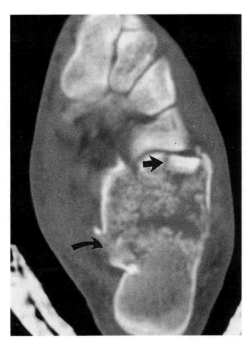

Fig. 41-4. On this axial CT image in a patient with a calcaneal fracture, involvement of the calcaneal cuboid joint is seen *(arrow)*. There is also extensive medial to lateral widening with fragment continuity with the peroneal tendons laterally and the flexor hallucis medially *(curved arrow)*. Extensive gaps between fracture fragments are seen as well.

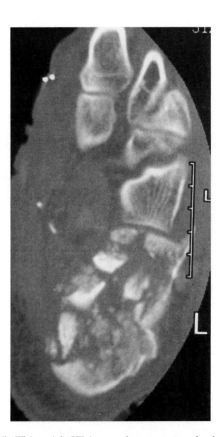

Fig. 41-5. This axial CT image demonstrates the least common calcaneal fracture comminuted. There is extensive disruption of the plantar calcaneus, with numerous fracture fragments.

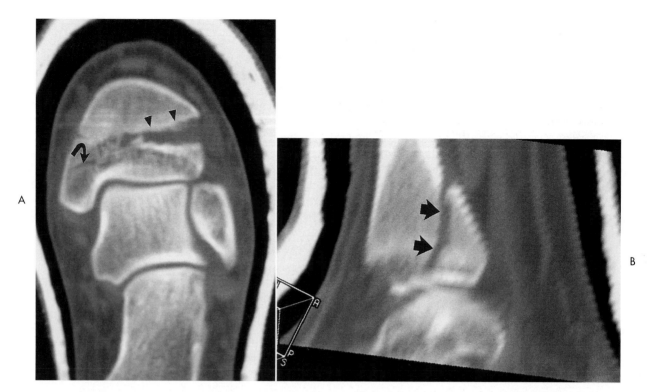

Fig. 41-6. Direct coronal CT image **(A)** demonstrates the axial fracture line extending through the partially open physis *(arrow heads)* and then coronally into the epiphysis more medially *(curved arrow)*. A sagittal CT reconstruction **(B)** demonstrates the posterior sagittal fracture *(arrows)* of the triplane fracture.

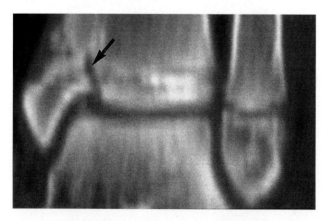

Fig. 41-7. A coronal reconstruction CT demonstrates a Salter IV fracture through the medial malleolus *(arrow)*.

fracture line occurs through the partially fused physis. It is important since asymmetric physeal closure resulting in growth disturbance, joint incongruity, and premature osteoarthritis are known complications. Classically, three fracture fragments are present: (1) the tibial shaft, (2) anterolateral epiphysis, and (3) posterior metaphysis with the remainder of the epiphysis. This classic three-fragment triplane has more complications than does the more common two-part triplane. This occurs because the third fragment prevents adequate closed reduction. The presence of a fibula fracture also increases the risk of an unsuccessful closed reduction.[36] The two-part triplane fracture consists of (1) the tibial shaft with the antero-medial epiphysis, and (2) the posterior metaphysis with the lateral epiphysis. CT may be used acutely or following reduction to evaluate the number and degree of displacement of fragments. (Fig. 41-6). CT may also be used to assess other Salter-type fractures (Fig. 41-7).

Talus

Fractures of the talus are an occasional indication for CT scanning. The talus is unusual since there are no muscle on tendon insertions. Most of the management problems involve fractures of the talus neck that make up 3% of all foot fractures. These fractures occur in a well-defined population, overwhelmingly male in the age range of mid-30s. Associated injuries are common. In fact, in only half of these patients is the talus fracture isolated. About 20% of these associated fractures involve the medial malleolus, with another 10% involving the calca-

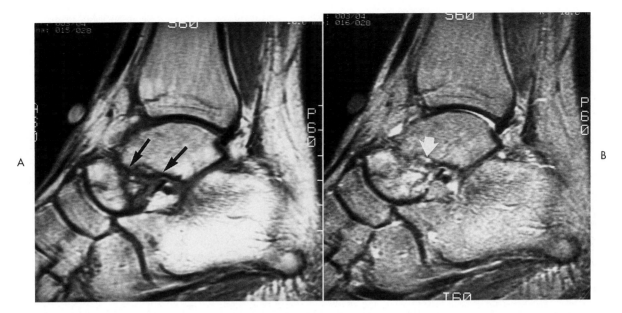

Fig. 41-8. In this patient with nonunion of a talus fracture, an intermediate signal intensity line is seen at the fracture *(arrow)* on a T1-weighted image **(A)**. The adjacent marrow is normal and there is therefore no evidence of avascular necrosis with T2-weighting **(B)** areas of fluid intensity *(arrows)* seen within the fracture lines consistent with nonunion. It should be noted that in acutely or subacutely imaged fractures this may represent normal healing.

neous.[52] The talus consists of a body, neck, and head. Since the neck is the only portion of the talus that is extraarticular, it acts as a bridge from the posterior facet to the anterior and middle facets and from the ankle and hindfoot articulations to the midfoot articulations. Most of the blood supply to the talus, similar to the navicular, extends distal to proximal. However, the talus blood supply is relatively complex; therefore increasing degrees of disruption progressively affect its blood supply.[1] Increased degrees of displacement will also affect the biomechanics of the subtalar articulations because a displaced talus acts like a man trying to keep opposite legs on floating logs that are progressively drifting apart. There are three proposed mechanisms for talus neck fractures: (1) a dorsal force on a braced foot and ankle as occurs in sudden braking; (2) the result of excessive supination, and (3) the result of a direct dorsal blow.[17]

The classifications of these fractures was first proposed by Hawkins and was later slightly modified. Class I is a nondisplaced fracture with congruent subtalar joints. When the subtalar joints are disrupted but the ankle joint remains intact, the fracture is termed a Class II. Complete dislocation of the talus body from the ankle joint is a Class III fracture. The rare Class IV fracture also has disruption of the talonavicular articulation.[49] Although as discussed the blood supply to the talus is complex, there are three main vessels that feed the talus. In Class I, one is disrupted, in Class II, two are disrupted,

and in Class III, all three are disrupted. AVN occurs in 13% to 16% of talus neck fractures. Therefore, the most frequent complication of these fractures, ischemic necrosis, is at least partially related to the Hawkins class. The incidence of AVN is decreased with aggressive surgical intervention, which is therefore indicated in Class II-IV fractures.[16] Two other complications of the injuries are malunion and osteoarthritis[16,72] (Fig. 41-8). Malunion occurs in up to 27% of cases and is usually dorsal or varus; typically in Type II fractures it is treated by conservative means. Osteoarthritis may affect either the tibiotalar as subtalar joints and is also related to the severity of the initial injury. Secondary osteoarthritis occurs in up to 97% of cases.[16] The usual indication for CT scanning involves evaluation of the congruity of the adjacent articulations, particularly after closed reduction. By evaluation of the degree of comminution and displacement, prognostication can also be performed. CT following healing may also allow precise evaluation of malunion and the extent of arthritic changes when surgical reconstruction is considered.

Lis-Franc fracture

Although initially described in horseback riders, currently these injuries occur as a complication of diabetes with neuroarthropathy, or less commonly as a result of motor-vehicle accidents, or falls. The mechanism is forced plantar flexion with rotation. Anatomically the transverse ligament connects the bases of the two second to fifth metatarsal. Therefore the lesser rays tend to move as a unit, a phenomenon that explains the typical pattern of Lis-Franc fracture. Since the second metatarsal is also recessed relative to the remaining metatarsals and has a tight attachment to the cuneiform, it provides stability of the Lis-Franc joint. Therefore all Lis-Franc injuries first involve the base of the second metatarsal. Two types of Lis-Franc fractures occur homolateral and divergent. In the former, either metatarsals 2-5 or 1-5 all displace laterally, and in the divergent the first metatarsal displaces medially. CT may be used to evaluate for presence of the not uncommon subtle Lis-Franc fractures or to assess for associated fractures (typically cuboid) and articular congruity following reduction.[43]

Navicular fractures

Navicular fractures are uncommon. The usual type is a stress fracture that is difficult to visualize using routine radiography.[104] These fractures occur in the middle third of the bone and are sagittally oriented. Typical patients are in their 20s and are involved in sports, usually basketball.[63] CT or MRI may be helpful in visualizing these lesions. Since patients typically have symptoms of vague plantar pain and have a 7-month delay before accurate diagnosis, these injuries are not infrequent "incidental findings." Approximately one third of these patients will go on to nonunion.[46]

Osteochondritis dissecans (OCD)

Osteochondritis dissecans (OCD) is a common disorder that may affect the femur, capitellum, or talus. It is more common in adolescents and young adults and usually affects males. Osteochondral lesion/injury is a better term for this disorder, with OCD best reserved for characteristic lesions in younger patients. Although fracture was initially thought to be the sequelae of bone necrosis, most authors now believe it to be the cause of this disorder, with necrosis the result. Talar OCD accounts for 1% of all talus fractures and 4% of all cases of OCD. OCD of talus, however, occurs in 6.5% of all ankle sprains.[92] OCD in locations in the foot and ankle other than the talus is exceedingly rare. The cause of this injury is a shear, rotatory, or even compressive (particularly medial talar OCD) force. When the injury occurs early in life, the cartilage is resilient as it transmits the vector to the underlying bone. Since the bone is less elastic than is cartilage, the bone may fracture without a chondral fracture. However, shear injuries may displace cartilage even in young patients. With aging cartilage, elasticity is decreased; this leads to transchondral and osseous fractures at the time of injury. Even when the cartilage is not fractured, it is still traumatized leading to premature degeneration. Healing of OCD resultsfrom ingrowth of

capillaries across a reduced immobile fragment. Any motion at the fracture site will shear off the capillary buds.[9] Healing of this lesion is therefore dependent on both the osseous stability of the fragment and the degree of intactness of the overlying cartilage, since both of these factors affect the degree of immobilization. The imaging stage of the lesion is therefore the main determinant of prognosis.[84] Osteoarthritis occurs in up to 20% of patients with OCD but as much as 75% of those with loose OCD. Loose fragments are surrounded by a high signal interface around the fragment on T2-weighted or STIR images. Any lesion with an underlying cyst is also invariably loose.[73] Irregular high signal or incompletely circumferential high signal is consistent with a partially loose fragment.[27] The fragment itself is of variable signal intensity. This fragment signal intensity is of no clinical significance. MR can also assess the intactness of the overlying cartilage with high-resolution techniques.[29] The cartilage may be initially fractured, may subsequently became fractured, or may

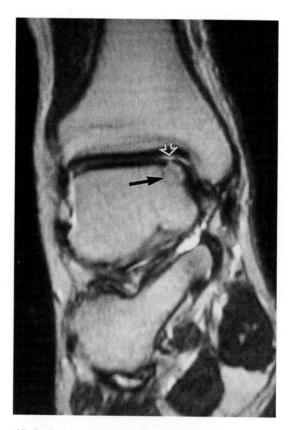

Fig. 41-9. On this T2-weighted coronal image an osteochondral defect is seen medially. The fragment is isointense to adjacent marrow, and no high signal rim is seen around it *(black arrow)*. There is therefore no definite evidence of loosening. Disruption of the articular cartilage *(open arrow)* is noted; the fragment is therefore considered loose in situ.

subsequently become degenerated. The subset of OCD with an overlying cartilage defect is termed *loose in situ* (Fig. 41-9).

Most osteochondral lesions are felt to be secondary to chronic stress rather than occurring as a single episode. The lateral talar OCD, however, is usually the sequelae of a specific injury and is less frequently stable than medial talar OCD. Medial OCD, which is slightly more common, most frequently has cup-in-a-hole appearance with lateral OCD more frequently seen as a horizontally oriented wafer. Medial talar OCD is also more commonly posterior than is lateral OCD. Anterior medial OCD-like lesions in the talus usually represent subchondral cysts (geodes) from osteoarthritis.

Ligament injuries

Inversion injuries are the most common ankle injury and among the most common musculoskeletal complaints that bring patients to the emergency room. Most ankle sprains occur in 15- to 35-year-old patients. It is estimated that on average an individual strains his ankle once every three decades. These sprains account for 25% to 50% of injuries that occur in volleyball, soccer, and football.[12] Since the medial (deltoid) ligament is so strong, avulsions occur medially. The lateral ligamentous complex is where ankle ligament sprains occur. The laterally supporting ligamentous structures can be divided into ankle and hindfoot ligaments.[7] The anterior group

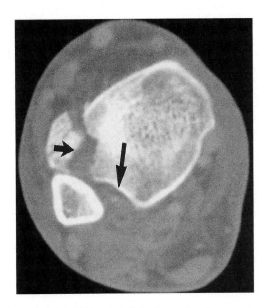

Fig. 41-10. Axial CT image of the lower leg demonstrates disruption of the distal tibia fibular articulation with the fibular subluxed anteriorly out of its sulcus *(large arrow)*. A large avulsion fragment is seen at the tibial insertion of the anterior tibiofibular ligament *(small arrow)*. This avulsion represents an adult talleux fracture.

consists of the anterior talo fibular ligament; and calcaneal fibular ligament (the lateral collateral ligament) the posterior talofibular is also part of the lateral collateral ligament, although it is only rarely injured.[12] Supporting the hindfoot are the medial fibers of the inferior extensor retinaculum, the cervical ligament, and the interosseous talocalcaneal ligament. Acute ankle injuries typically affect the anterior talofibular ligament; the calcaneal fibular ligament is next most frequently affected. Acute injuries can be divided by grade or strains. Grade I is the stretching and microscopic injury to the ligament. Grade II means a partial tear, and Grade III denotes complete tears. There is significant controversy as to whether to surgically or conservatively treat these acute injuries. However, 10% to 20% of patients with lateral ankle ligament injuries will suffer chronic symptoms, and the severity of initial injury does not correlate well with these long-term symptoms.[2] Most patients with chronic symptoms will eventually require surgical intervention.[38] The role of MRI, particularly in acute injuries, is currently unclear. Most MRI abnormalities are incidental or occur in patients with chronic, nonspecific symptoms. The anterior and posterior talofibular ligament are seen best on axial MRI images. The anterior ligament has an oblique course that is more anterior medially. The posterior talofibular ligament is horizontal.[34] The anterior ligament does not normally demonstrate internal signal; it is usually half the thickness of the posterior ligament. The posterior ligament on high-resolution images gives the appearance of internal signal secondary to the microanatomy of its fascicles.[82] The calcaneofibular ligament is best seen on coronal images. When the calcaneofibular ligament is injured, the anterior talofibular ligament is nearly always injured as well. The anterior tibiofibular is infrequently torn, but it may be avulsed off the tibia (Fig. 41-10). Injury to the anterior talofibular ligament may also demonstrate an osseous avulsion (Fig. 41-11) or more commonly joint fluid violating its anterior boundary. In acute ligament sprains, edema is seen in the adjacent subcutaneous fat. The ligament when injured may demonstrate internal signal on any imaging sequence. The ligament may also appear widened with irregular margins. With chronic instability, the ligament may scar and thicken and thus either demonstrate unusually low signal on T2-weighted images or become wavy.

The inferior extensor retinaculum inserts into the lateral-most aspect of sinus tarsi, where it is best seen on lateral sagittal images. The cervical ligament lies in the anterior sinus tarsi extending from a tubercle on the inferior lateral talar neck to the dorsal calcaneous. It may be seen on coronal or sagittal MR images. The interosseous talocalcaneal ligament, seen just posterior to the cervical ligament, is a thicker band. Injuries to the lateral-ligaments may therefore cause abnormally high signal in-

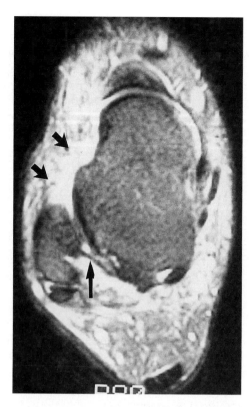

Fig. 41-11. On an axial T2-weighted image the posterior aspect of articular fluid is well marginated by the posterior talofibular ligament *(long arrow)*. The fluid extends too far anteriorly with an irregular margin secondary to a tear of the anterior talofibular *(short arrows)* ligament.

tensity within the sinus tarsi. The MRI differential diagnosis for this appearance is sinus tarsi syndrome, which may cause a similar appearance of high signal. In sinus tarsi syndrome, however, the morphologic integrity of the hindfoot ligaments is intact. Sinus tarsi syndrome may occur idiopathically or in patients with rheumatoid arthritis or gout. One additional complication, the anterior-lateral ankle impingement syndrome, may occur in patients as the sequelae of ankle sprains. In this syndrome there is development of hypertrophic synovium in the lateral talofibular sulcus.[5] On MRI the lateral aspect of the joint on axial image, particularly posterior to the anterior talofibular ligament, fills in with pannous displacing fluid posteriorly.

OSTEONECROSIS

Osteonecrosis (AVN) refers to the death of medullary bone. AVN may occur secondary to trauma, corticosteroid administration, marrow infiltrate processes, ethanol abuse, pancreatitis, collagen vascular diseases, or pregnancy, or it may be idiopathic. The most commonly affected tarsal bone is the talus, followed in frequency by the navicular and the metatarsal heads. AVN of the talus may follow fractures of the talus neck (Hawkins type) or occur in patients with systemic lupus erythematosus. Navicular AVN occurs idiopathically or in association with (possibly a result of) fractures, frequently of a stress type. Metatarsal-head AVN may occur either idiopathically, usually in adolescent females, or as a complication podiatric surgery. On MRI, AVN is characterized by marrow replacement with well-defined margins. On MR the region of necrosis has variable signal intensities. It may present as an edema-like pattern (decreased signal intensity on T1-weighted images and increased signal on T2-weighted images), or it may behave like acute blood, fatty marrow, or sclerotic bone.[76] Changes are best seen on T1-weighted or STIR images. The hallmark of bone necrosis on MR is the reactive interface between viable (reactive) and necrotic bone.[31] On T2-weighted images this appears as an inner rim of increased signal intensity and an outer rim of increased signal intensity. This double-line sign, when seen, is pathognomic. In the tarsal bones, however, this reactive interface may not always be discernable. The most frequent pattern of tarsal necrosis is decreased signal on T1-weighted images. In particular, collapse of articular surfaces is an important MR finding because of osteoarthritic sequelae. An MRI staging system has been proposed, and although this staging system appears to be temporarily accurate, we prefer to make use of traditional orthopedic classifications when describing these lesions. The major differential diagnostic considerations on MRI (when the double-line sign is absent) are osteomyelitis, traumatic disorders, osteochondral injury, and Sudek's atrophy (RSD). In osteomyelitis there is nearly always an associated soft-tissue mass that is absent in AVN. Traumatic disorders are the most difficult MRI differential. The margin of a fracture tend to be poorly defined and infiltrative, in contrast to the geographic margins of AVN. OCD of the talar dome may mimic AVN; in fact, historically many authorities believed that OCD was the sequelae of AVN. When AVN occurs in association with OCD, however, it is the sequelae and not the cause of the OCD. A high-signal regular interface with adjacent bone and the characteristic location in the medial on lateral talar dome distinguishes OCD from AVN. Sudek's atrophy, although traditionally thought of as a marrow edema process, rarely causes an MRI appearance of "marrow edema."[59] Infrequently in this disorder, muscle edema, and in the late stages muscle atrophy, may also be seen. Marrow edema does occur in transient osteoporosis of the hip as well as in a related disorder, regional migratory osteoporosis, which may be seen in the foot.[109] However, the latter disorder is usually associated with joint effusions and soft-tissue and muscle edema.

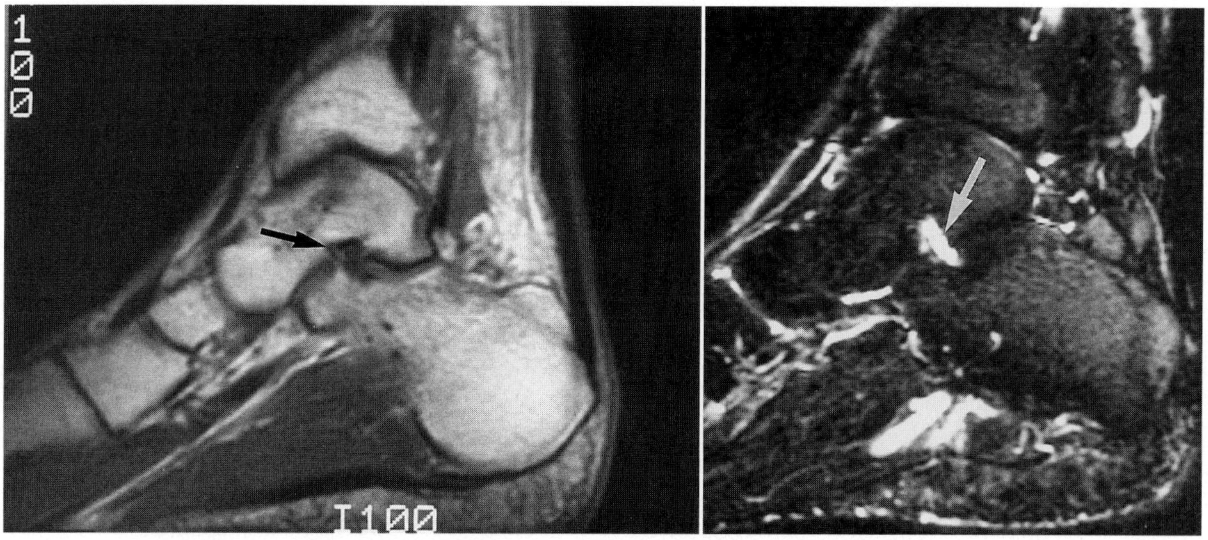

Fig. 41-12. Loss of marrow fat on a sagittal T1-weighted image **(A)** *(arrow)*. Increases in intensity on s STIR image **(B)** is seen consistent with chronic sinus tarsi syndrome.

SYNOVIAL FLUID

The evaluation of synovial fluid is both the blessing and the curse of MR imaging. It is a blessing because in vivo assessments of fluid can be made accurately for the first time. It is a curse because the determination of when fluid is abnormal is often difficult. Ankle fluid, when seen in large amounts, is abnormal; in particular, distention of the anterior joint recess in a supine, plantarflexed foot signifies an ankle joint effusion. Subtalar fluid frequently is seen distending the posterior recess, even in asymptomatic patients. However, the ankle and subtalar joints communicate in up to 15% of patients and even more commonly in patients with articular disease. Therefore, it may be difficult to determine the origin of articular fluid seen in either of these articulations. Articular fluid outside of the ankle and subtalar joints is abnormal. There are 13 tendons, 12 of which have sheaths, that cross the ankle. The presence of small amounts of fluid in most of these sheaths is frequent in a large percentage of asymptomatic patients. The particular exception to this is that normal patients rarely have fluid about the anterior tendons and the distal PTT. Fluid in these locations is abnormal. The presence of large amounts of fluid is particularly common about the tendon of the flexor hallucis longus but may be seen in many tendons. There is a strong relationship between fluid in various tendon sheaths as well as fluid in articulations. Therefore even when large amounts of fluid are seen it may be difficult to determine the precise origin.[91]

There are numerous bursae about the ankle and foot, some of these are normal and some are acquired.

Visible fluid in nearly all of these, however, is abnormal. The exception to this is the retrocalcaneal bursae. However, when large amounts of fluid are seen in this bursae, this may occur from mechanical causes (Hagland's syndrome), inflammatory causes (rheumatoid arthritis or Reiter's syndrome), or secondary to achilles tendon disorders.

HEEL PAIN

Heel pain is a frequent complaint. The clinical differential diagnosis includes calcaneal stress fractures, tarsal tunnel syndrome, sinus tarsi syndrome (Fig. 41-12), or plantar fascitis. Clinicians classify this pain based on location as achilles (posterior), PTT or tarsal tunnel (medial), peroneal (lateral), and plantar fascitis or plantar fibromatosis (plantar/posterior). Plantar heel pain typically occurs in overweight patients, often diabetic and elderly. The symptoms are frequently bilateral. Disorders of the plantar fascia are the typical cause of pain in these patients. This fascia is a multilayered aponeurotic complex consisting of central, medial, and lateral components. The aponeurosis originates from the plantar calcaneus, mostly from the medial tuberosity. During walking, running, and other activities, this fascia tightens with traction at its calcaneal origin.[51] Disorders of this complex therefore have a mechanical origin; they are either secondary to overpronation or a result of either cavus deformity (or most commonly) repetitive microtrauma. The latter usually affects the origin and proximal aponeurosis. This may result in enthesopathy either at the insertion of the plantar aponeurosis or, less frequently, at the long plantar ligament.[102] Plantar fascitis, advertial bursitis at the aponeurotic origin, and tear of the aponeurosis also occur. Plantar fascitis is the most frequent syndrome imaged, and the clinical diagnosis is usually straightforward. Plantar fascitis is usually a manifestation of chronic stress resulting in microtears with subsequent inflammation and repair. This disorder is common in the running athlete as well as in obese patients.

In MR of plantar fascitis, the plantar fascia may appear thickened, usually close to the calcaneal insertion. Frequently, subcutaneous edema or edema deep to the aponeurosis may be seen. The differential diagnosis on MR would be plantar fibromatosis, which is seen more distally in the subcutaneous fat. Plantar fibromatosis has different clinical presentation and will demonstrate low to isointense signal on T2-weighted images.[8] It will appear bright on STIR images. Patients with recalcitrant plantar fascitis symptoms often demonstrate areas of abnormal marrow within the adjacent calcaneus; this is believed to represent stress fractures.

Achilles tendon

The achilles tendon is the largest and strongest tendon in the body. After the plantaris, this tendon is also the longest. Since all normal tendons are exceedingly strong, when a stress is applied to a normal tendon, the tendon itself rarely fails. The point of failure will typically be the apophyseal growth plate in children or the enthesis in adults. A force more than double the strength of maximal physiologic forces is necessary before the mildest tendon injury occurs. Therefore for a tendon to tear, regardless of the force, it must be degenerated. Even in very young patients all torn tendons are presumed to be degenerated. The achilles tendon has a watershed area similar to that of the supraspinous 2 to 4 mm above the insertion leading to degeneration; this is where most true achilles disorders occur.[20] Most tendons in the body, with the particular exception of the peroneals, follow a recognized sequence of injury. Using the rotator cuff as a model, the first stage is tendonitis. Only for a fraction of time is the tendon with "tendonitis" inflamed; therefore, histologic evidence of inflammation is often absent. Without treatment and with continued activity these patients may go on to chronic tendonitis. Some of these patients will go on to the next stage, that of interstitial (partial) tears. Finally, some of these patients may progress to complete tears. Since the normal achilles tendon is so strong, nearly all patients with even early stages of disease will manifest tendon degeneration. Usually males are affected by achilles disorders more frequently than are females. This first stage begins in patients who are in their 30s and often progresses. Patients are often runners or "weekend athletes."

The achilles tendon is unusual in that of the 13 tendons that cross the ankle, it is the only one to lack a synovial sheath. Teliogically, this occurs because the achilles does not curve and therefore the lubrication value of the synovial sheath is not necessary. True synovitis of the achilles tendon therefore does not occur, the equivalent disorder being peritendonitis.[48] Peritendonitis is often clinically termed *acute achilles tendonitis*. On MR imaging with T2-weighted sequences, high signal around the tendon is seen. This high signal is not as rounded and well defined as is seen in true synovitis. This abnormal signal tends to predominate medially; this occurs because the tendon moves medially as a result of foot strike and overpromotion. Edema in Kagar's (the pre-achilles) fat pad may be seen, particularly with fat-suppressed techniques. When present, this implies a more painful and acute disorder. In friction-caused peritendonitis (resulting from ill fitting or uncomfortable shoes), abnormalities are seen posteriorly about 1 to 2 cm above the distal tendon. The normal tendon has no internal signal on any sequence except at its insertion. The tendon with tendonitis may or may not develop internal signal. When internal signal is present it is most sensitively seen on T1-weighted images. Any signal visible on T2-weighted images is invariably abnormal (Fig. 41-13). Differentiation between abnormal signal caused by tendonitis, as opposed to that caused by partial tears, is often difficult unless the area of signal is linear on longitudinal images.

In chronic achilles tendonitis the tendon enlarges.[86] On axial MR images the normal achilles tendon is kidney-shaped except at its insertion where it may be flat or oval.[69] The normal tendon is uniform in size from the soleus insertion to the calcaneus. With enlargement on sagittal images, focal thickening will be seen 2 to 4 cm above the insertion. On cross-sectional images the tendon loses its normal lenticular shape and becomes ovoid; with severe disease it becomes rounded. Internal signal is atypical with chronic tendonitis. When it occurs it is globular and parallels the long axis of the tendon. These longitudinal areas of abnormal signal are frequently resected since they may progress to interstitial and eventually complete tendon tears.[39] Complete achilles tears usually occur 2 to 4 cm from the insertion, in a degenerated tendon (tendonopathy). There frequently is a visible tendon gap.[56] This gap will be minimized or absent with plantar flexion. A treatment for achilles tears, in fact, casts the foot in plantar flexion. With complete tears the achilles may thicken secondary to retraction. Uncommonly these tears occur proximally, although these proximal tears are actually myotendonous junction tears of the medial head of the gastrocnemius. Least frequently, achilles tears occur at the insertion on the calcaneus or as an avulsion at the calcaneal insertion. On routine radiography occasionally an ossification is seen

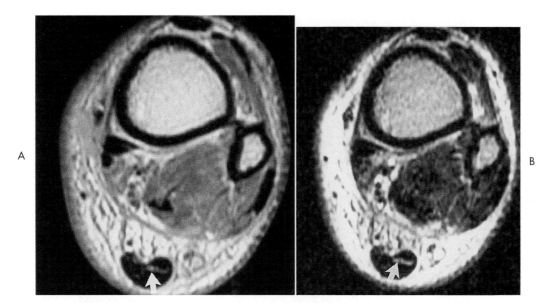

Fig. 41-13. Although normally shaped, the upper achilles tendon, demonstrates areas of internal signal on T1-weighted images *(arrow)* **(A)**. With T2-weighting **(B)** the interstitial tears become more obvious *(arrow)*. This represents a probable interstitial tear of the achilles tendon.

within the achilles tendon, giving the appearance of a fractured enthesophyte or an old avulsion. However, typically this appearance is caused by tendon degeneration with subsequent ossification.

Lastly, when evaluating patients with complete achilles tendon tears, one should assess the presence of atrophy in the muscle belly of the gastrocnemius and soleus. Irreversible atrophy is present when the muscle is fatty-infiltrated; it may be present if the muscle is small. If muscle atrophy is present, tendon repair may fail. Therefore, a tendon transfer will be the procedure of choice.

Posterior tibial tendon

The posterior tibial tendon (PTT) arises from the interosseous membrane, intermuscular septum, and proximal tibial and fibula. The myotendinous junction occurs in the distal third of the leg. As the tendon continues distally it becomes the most anterior of the medial ankle tendons passing just behind the medial malleolous. This tendon is enclosed in a synovial sheath beginning 6 cm above the ankle which ends 1 to 2 cm before its main (navicular) insertion. Distally the tendon divides into two major slips; the more clinically important one inserts on the tubercle at the medial navicular. The PTT inverts the hindfoot, maintains the plantar arch, and aids in plantar flexion. The antagonist muscle for the PTT is the peroneus brevis. PTT disorders are more common in females, especially those who are middle-aged to el-

derly and sedentary. Patients usually present with chronic pain exacerbated by weight bearing.[68] In younger patients this tendon is injured as a result of athletic activity. There is also an association with seronegative arthropathy (HLA Cw6), particularly in young males. Dysfunction of the PTT has a gradual onset following a progression of synovitis to tendonitis to a partial or interstitial and eventually complete tear. Since the symptoms are usually nonspecific, most patients see several physicians, with complaints of increasing severity, before a correct diagnosis is made.[55]

The typical location for injury is at or just below the medial malleolus, although distal (insertional) tears are not uncommon. Tears occur at the medial malleoulus because of a zone of relative hypovascularity[40] and because of friction stress of the PTT against the medial malleolus. A grading system for tears has been developed. Type I are partial ruptured tendons with longitudinal splits and tendon hypertrophy. Type II refers to partial tears with tendon attrition, and Type III injury describe complete tears.[87] Synovitis of the PTT is difficult to diagnose by MRI because fluid may be seen within its sheath in asymptomatic patients. However, when fluid is seen distally by its insertion this is nearly always abnormal. Since there is no tendon sheath in this location, this "fluid" typically has the appearance of adjacent edema or peritendonitis. Although the distal-most PTT may be heterogeneous on T1-weighted images and less frequently T2-weighted images, signal elsewhere within the

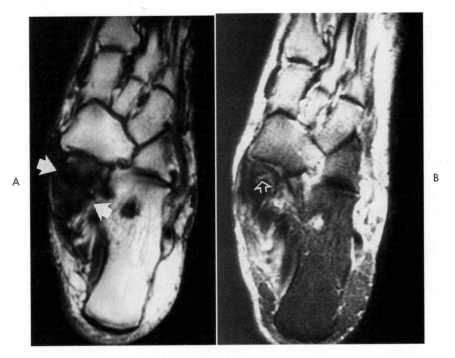

Fig. 41-14. T1 **(A)** axial image demonstrates a globular, thickened, and irregular distal PTT. On a T2-weighted image **(B)**, although the globular abnormal tendon remains predominantly dark, focal areas of high signal are seen *(arrow).* This is consistent with a navicular insertional avulsion of the PTT.

tendon is abnormal (Fig. 41-14). The PTT is typically twice the diameter of the adjacent flexor digitorum longus tendon. When this ratio is disturbed the tendon is also either atrophic from partial tears or more likely hypertrophic from chronic injury and inflammation. When completely torn a fluid-filled gap may be present, or the tendon may be retracted. Not infrequently, however, fibrosis and scarring may give the appearance of only a subtly abnormal tendon that is completely torn at surgery. The presence of either a cornuate (hypertrophied medial tubercle) or accessory navicular should raise the suspicion for a PTT tear because both these anomalies are associated with PTT disorders. In addition, the relationship of the talus to the navicular on sagittal images should be assessed. With PTT tears the talus will plantarflex and the navicular will be displaced.[90] Sagittal images where the first metatarsal is seen are the images best for evaluating this relationship. Evaluation of the muscle belly, particularly on large field-of-view sagittal images, are useful for the evaluation of muscle atrophy. Since the presence of muscle atrophy may preclude tendon repair, adjacent tendons may then be assessed by MR as possible routes of reconstruction. The subtalar joint should be evaluated for the presence of osteoarthritic change. If this is present most surgeons will perform a fusion rather than a tendon repair or reconstruction.

Peroneal tendons

The peroneus longus and brevis are the major lateral musculotendinous stabilizers of the ankle. These muscles act also as pronators and evert the foot. The peroneus longus (PL) arises from the lateral condyle of tibia, head of the fibula, and proximal intermuscular septum. The peroneus brevis (PB) arises from the lower two thirds of the fibula and proximal intermuscular septum and lies just anterior to the PL. The myotendonious junction of PL occurs at the level of the soleous insertion onto the achilles, while the myotendonious junction of the PB occurs quite distally often below the distal fibula. The PL tendon lies lateral and posterior to the PB tendon. The PB tendon continues anteriorly to insert on the base of the fifth metatarsal. The PL tendon crosses below the trochlear process of the calcaneus to the medial midfoot to insert on the first metatarsal.[18] The PB and PL share a common synovial sheath until the region of Chopart's joint with the sheath beginning 3.5 cm above the lateral malleolus and extending to 4 cm below the malleolus. To prevent bow-stringing, these tendons are held tightly in place by the superior and inferior peroneal retinacula.

Disorders of the peroneal tendons do not follow the sequence of disorders for the other tendons in the foot and ankle. Tenosynovitis, which is common in most

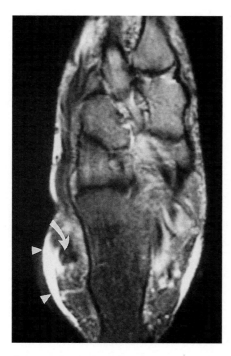

Fig. 41-15. Internal signal is seen within the peroneal tendons *(curved arrow)* on a T2-weighted (fat-suppressed) image consistent with peroneus brevis and longus tendonitis. The tendons are morphologically intact and not torn. A small amount of fluid is seen within the tendon sheath, and there is subcutaneous edema as well *(arrow heads)*.

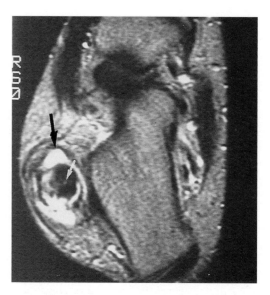

Fig. 41-16. On an axial T2-weighted image the peroneal tendons are enlarged with irregular margins. The peroneus brevis, anteriorly, also appears to demonstrate a focal area of internal signal *(white arrow)*. A large amount of synovial fluid is seen about these tendons *(black arrow)*, with areas of low signal representing synovial proliferation. Surgery confined a partial tear of the peroneus brevis with extensive proliferative synovitis.

foot tendons, is infrequent in the peroneals and when it occurs is secondary to mechanical abnormalities. In addition, patients may present initially with complete tears, which is an uncommon clinical situation for other foot tendons.[103] As seen on MRI, fluid about these tendons is nonspecific. Synovial fluid about the peroneals is frequent in asymptomatic patients. In addition, since the PL and PB share a common sheath, fluid related to one tendon will be seen to involve the other sheath. Tenosynovitis may be seen in patients with osteoarthritis and osteophyte formation, or as a sequelae of calcaneal fractures with broadening and compression of these tendons between the lateral aspect of the calcaneus and the fibula.[88] Internal signal in these tendons is uncommon but represents tendonitis/interstitial tears and is always abnormal. More frequently seen in peroneal disorders is enlargement of the PB (Fig. 41-15). What is also particular to the peroneal tendons is tendon subluxation/dislocation. Tendon dislocations are usually rare, with the exception of biceps tendon and infrequently the PTT, and may be the reason that patients with peroneal disorders often initially present with rupture. Peroneal subluxations typically affect male patients, often with relatively minor symptoms; they occur in skiers, skaters, and in soccer and basketball players.[18] In chronic subluxa-

tions the patient may complain of the ankle giving way with lateral instability. On MR images, particularly with inversion stress, the tendon will be seen lateral to the lateral aspect of the fibula. This displacement will be even more obvious in patients with peroneal dislocations. Both subluxations and dislocations may demonstrate absent or torn peroneal retinacula and a hypoplastic, absent (flat), or convex peroneal groove in the distal fibula. A sharp lateral margin of the fibula will cause accelerated tendon attrition in those patients leading to tear. Ruptures of the peroneal tendons are otherwise rare, invariably affect the PB, and usually occur at the region of the calcaneal cuboid joint. Stenosing tenosynovitis may occur where any sheathed tendon passes through an enclosed curved passageway. Stenosing tenosynovis occurs as sequelae of inflammation, with fibrosis and hypertrophy of the sheath limit passage.[45] The prototype for this disorder occurs in the upper extremity and is termed de Quervain's disease. In the foot this disorder typically affects the peroneal tendons, although the PTT or even Flexer Hallucis Longus may be involved. On MRI T1-weighted images demonstrated peritendon/sheath intermediate signal, which remains low signal and globular appearing on T2-weighted images. Some synovial fluid will also be seen (Fig. 41-16). The location for this disorder is typically underneath reticular or in the tarsal tunnel. Tendon splits are a final entity affecting the peroneus brevis. These splits result from mechanical attrition within the fibula groove as a sequelae of trauma. The trauma results in lateral ankle instability and an imcompetent superior peroneal retinaculum.[94] The resulting subluxation may result in peroneus brevis splits. On MRI the PB enlarges, becoming lentiform. With time the PL appears to act as a chisel bisecting the PB, which results in the appearance of "three" peroneal tendons.

Tibialis anterior tendon

Anterior tibial tendon tears are rare;[83] however, they may present as an anterior soft-tissue mass.

COALITIONS

Tarsal coalitions are an important cause of foot pain and deformity, with talocalcaneal and calcaneonavicular coalition being the two most common types. Whereas calcaneonavicular coalitions are usually well visualized on conventional radiographs, the nature, location, and extent of talocalcaneal radiographs and coalitions are best ascertained with computed tomography (CT). The true incidence of tarsal coalition in the general population is not known but is probably far less than 1%. Most patients with talocalcaneal coalition are symptomatic, often presenting during puberty. A few who are asymptomatic may develop symptoms following traumatic events. These symptoms include the painful peroneal, spastic flatfoot. Certain patients have unexplained talar or hindfoot pain with diminished subtalar motion.

Physical examination usually reveals a pes planus forefoot abduction and excessive calcaneal valgus standing. Like calcaneonavicular bars, talocalcaneal coalitions are often bilateral, with a prevalence of 50% in some series. Talocalcaneal coalition ossification occurs between 12 and 16 years of age, with an average of 18 years at clinical presentation. Men are more commonly affected than women. Talocalcaneal coalitions typically affect the middle medial facet. Osseous coalitions are clearly seen by CT, along with bridging medullary bone (Fig. 41-17). On MRI, low signal in the region of the osseous coalition is usually seen.[89] The appearance of bridging marrow may also be noted. Cartilaginous coalitions appear to have pseudoarticulation,[70] articular surfaces that are less curved, and congruent regular than normal joints (see Fig. 41-11). In addition, secondary signs are helpful in the CT diagnosis of both fibrous as well as cartilaginous coalitions. The best of these signs are subchondral sclerosis in the sustentaculum, the presence of productive charges about the middle facet, and a characteristic medial spur off the calcaneus adjacent to the distal PTT; the latter two best seen on axial images. The MR diagnosis of fibrous and cartilaginous coalitions is subtle, but many of these will be seen by MRI only and not by CT. Abnormal articular cartilage, joint anatomy, and productive change are the best signs of nonosseous coali-

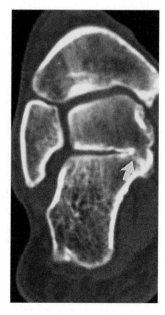

Fig. 41-17. Coronal CT images demonstrate an osseous coalition of the middle facet with bridging marrow *(arrow).*

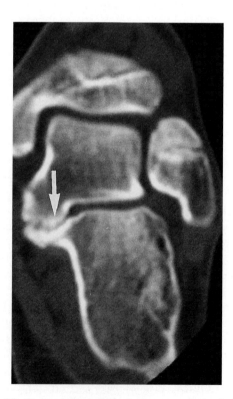

Fig. 41-18. Coronal CT images demonstrate irregularity, sclerosis, and hypertrophy of the middle facet consistent with a nonosseous coalition *(arrow).*

tions (Fig. 41-18). The only sign present may be decreased subchondral signal, a manifestation of subchondral sclerosis.

TARSAL TUNNEL

The medial ankle tendons pass through an enclosed anatomic boundary that is termed the *tarsal tunnel*. The roof of this tunnel is the flexor retinaculum, which prevents the tendons from bow-stringing while curving around the maleolus. The floor of the tunnel consists of the tibia proximally, the medial talus and systemtaculum tali, and the medial calcaneus distally. Septae emanate from the flexor retinaculum, dividing the tunnel into four "lanes" for the PTT, as well as for flexor digitorum longus tendon, the neurovascular bundle, and the flexor hallucis longus tendon.[112] These fibrous septae provide a relatively rigid fixation of these structures; therefore subtle traction from scarring or small space-occupying lesions may cause neurologic complaints.[19] Tarsal tunnel syndrome is diagnosed when there is compression or entrapment of the posterior tibial nerve. Symptoms include burning, pain, and paresthesia of the toes, sole of foot, and the medial heel. Symptoms, typically aggravated by weight bearing, may radiate proximally.[19] Neurologic symptoms are variable because of the inconstant level of nerve bifurcation.[25] Not infrequently patients with tarsal tunnel syndrome may present with symptoms of sinus tarsi syndrome because of overlap in

innervation. Tarsal tunnel syndrome is only partially analogous to the prototype of entrapment neuropathy, the carpal tunnel syndrome. EMG results, clinical evaluation, and even surgical results are much less consistent than with carpal tunnel syndrome. Patients may be imaged either for an evaluation of the cause of this syndrome or because of nonspecific symptoms that have led to a misdiagnosis. Because of this, and despite the fact that 50% of cases are idiopathic, MRI may play a more significant role in tarsal tunnel syndrome than it does in carpal tunnel syndrome. The MRI, however, is usually normal. Although tendon sheath fluid and "hypervascularity" have been described, these are nonspecific signs. MRI should be performed to exclude the possibility of a mass such as a neuroma, lipoma, ganglion, synovial cyst or varicosities.[53] MRI may also show edema, mass affect, or post-traumatic scarring within the tarsal tunnel[57] (Fig. 41-19).

INFECTION

Infection of the foot is common. Approximately half of all cases of cellulitis involve the lower extremity. Older patients are frequently affected because of such risk factors as venous disease, soft-tissue edema, and decreased lymphatic drainage. The rarer necrotizing infection that spares muscle is seen in younger patients. Soft-tissue infection, particularly in diabetes, may be indolent and lead to abscesses. These abscesses usually involve the

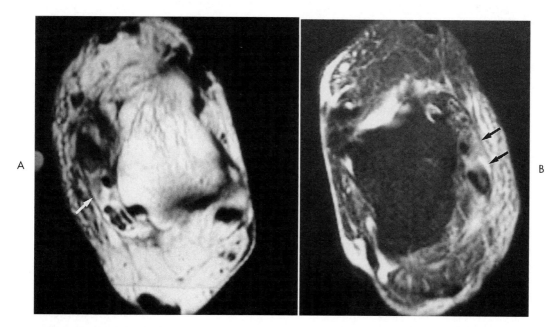

Fig. 41-19. In this patient with tarsal tunnel syndrome, a T1-weighted image **(A)** demonstrates low signal intensity replacing fat within the tunnel *(arrow)*. This area increases in intensity on T2-weighted images **(B)** representing edema within the tarsal tunnel. No mass was identified. Edema is also seen superficial to the flexor retinaculum *(arrows)*, a not uncommon finding in tarsal tunnel syndrome.

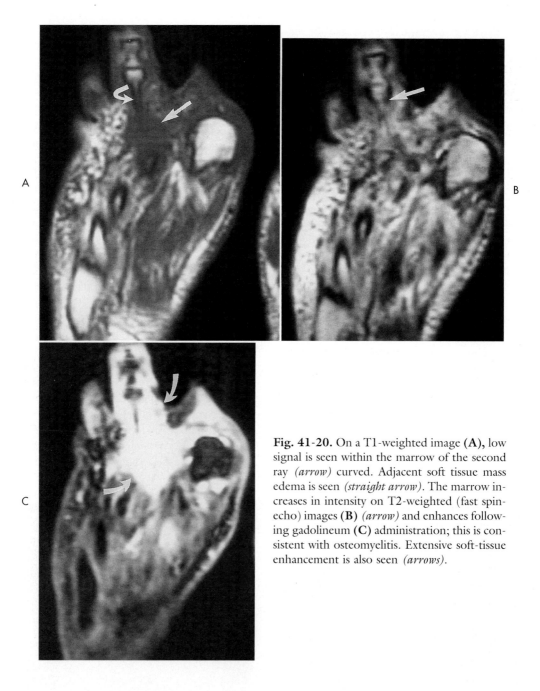

Fig. 41-20. On a T1-weighted image **(A),** low signal is seen within the marrow of the second ray *(arrow)* curved. Adjacent soft tissue mass edema is seen *(straight arrow)*. The marrow increases in intensity on T2-weighted (fast spinecho) images **(B)** *(arrow)* and enhances following gadolineum **(C)** administration; this is consistent with osteomyelitis. Extensive soft-tissue enhancement is also seen *(arrows)*.

central compartment of the foot spreading along the flexor tendon sheaths. When the soft-tissue infection spreads to bone it usually involves the calcaneus, metatarsals, or talus.[113] Hematogenously spread osteomyelitis is rare in the foot except in children. In the diabetic patient there is a complex interplay of infection, infarction, and sensory neuropathic condition resulting in a "neuropathic arthropathy."[4] The Lis-Franc joint is most commonly affected, followed by the metatarsphalageal and subtalar joints. Cellulitis as seen on MR is manifested by subcutaneous and less frequently by deep-muscle edema without mass effect. Diffuse high signal on T2-weighted image, common in diabetic patients, typically affects the plantar soft-tissue deep to the plantar aponeurosis. Soft-tissue fluid collections, with or without enhancement after gadolineum administration, is also common in diabetic patients.[6,78] These collections are typically but not necessarily seen near tissue ulcerations.

Osteomyelitis as seen on MR is usually manifested by low signal intensity within the marrow on T1-weighted sequences, frequently of significantly increased intensity on T2-weighted sequences, particularly with fat suppression[71,77,101,106] (Fig. 41-20). On STIR images the infection will also show high signal intensity, al-

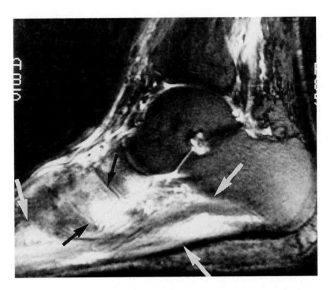

Fig. 41-21. Extensive subcutaneous edema with a distribution predominantly plantarly *(white arrows)* is seen in this patient with neuropathic disease. Sagittal STIR image demonstrates high signal in the navicular and medial cuneiform *(black arrows).*

though false positive STIR images may infrequently occur as a sympathetic response in cases of septic arthritis and in neuropathic disease[32] (Fig. 41-21). Intravenous gadolineum may be useful in complicated cases when marrow and soft-tissue enhancement may help to differentiate postoperative and neuropathic changes from infection.[79] Neuroarthropathy may produce collapse of the midfoot. Neuropathic disease usually demonstrates low signal on most imaging sequences. Occasionally increased signal is seen on T2-weighted images, even without infection.[45,94] Little enhancement with contrast, however, is usually seen. Fluid in tendon sheaths is quite common in diabetes and rarely of clinical significance; however, when tendon sheath enhancement is seen with gadolineum administration, soft-tissue infection is nearly always present.

MRI OF TUMORS

The evaluation of osseous and soft-tissue tumors is an important role of MRI. The incremental increase in diagnostic use is, however, more significant for soft tissue than it is for osseous tumors. This is because the evaluation of soft-tissue tumors was limited before the advent of MRI.

Soft-tissue tumors

Soft-tissue tumors of the feet and ankle are common. The most common are Kaposi's sarcoma, ganglions, and Morton's neuroma. Neural tumors, usually Morton's neuroma or schwannomas, make up two thirds

of resected lesions. Somewhat less common are tumors originating the skin or fatty/fibrous tissue. Of these latter tumors, plantar fibromas and giant cell tumors of tendon sheath are most common.[58] Also commonly seen are hemangioma, usually about the ankles. Location is helpful in evaluation of lesions of the foot. Dorsally, most will be ganglions or giant cell tumors of tendon sheath. In the nailbed, fibromas, glomus tumors, and pyogenic granulomas are most common. In the plantar aspect of the foot they are usually fibromas, giant cell tumors, lipomas or epidermal inclusion cysts. In the tarsal tunnel, neural tumors and ganglions are most frequent. The malignant counterparts to these lesions, such as malignant fibrous histiocytomas or liposarcoma, are rare.

On CT most tumors demonstrate soft-tissue attenuation similar to that of muscle.[26] The peritumoral edema is difficult to separate from tumor on CT; this limits detailed preoperative localization.[44] CT remains ideal for evaluation of soft-tissue calcifications. It is also useful for tumors with specific attenuation characteristics such as lipomas. MRI is a significant advance in imaging soft-tissue tumors; it is secondary to more precise anatomic localization and potentially improved preoperative diagnosis.[26,44] Most tumors, however, do not have specific signal characteristics.[60] These tumors are low signal on T1-weighted sequences and increase in signal on T2-weighted sequences. Lipomas, however, demonstrate high T1 and moderate T2 signal, similar to subcutaneous fat.[62] Other tumors that contain fat include liposarcomas and hemangiomas.[14,22] Other causes of high signal on a T1-weighted image include hemorrhage in aggressive necrotic tumors such as malignant fibrous histiocytomas (MFH), or protein (as in neural tumors, MFH, and synovial sarcoma). Fibrous tumors such as aggressive fibromatosis,[61,85] plantar fibromatosis, and some neurofibromas (only centrally)[97] demonstrate decreased signal on all sequences (except STIR in fibromatosis). Schwannomas are identified in the region of a peripheral, but not cutaneous, nerve. These tumors have high signal on T2-weighted sequences, often with a central area of lower signal.[97] Fibromas have variable signal characteristics but are seen within the plantar fat adjacent to the aponeurosis, usually close to the calcaneus.[61,85] Morton's neuromas are usually low signal on most imaging sequences.[33] Pigmented villonodular synovitis shows areas of decreased signal on both T1 and T2 images, secondary to hemosiderin deposition.[54,95] A similar appearance may be seen with giant cell tumor of tendon sheath, rheumatoid arthritis, and fibromatosis.[3,93] Synovial cysts and ganglion cysts demonstrate fluid characteristics[5,37,98] (Fig. 41-22). They are localized adjacent to joints, and ganglia are septated and will have a connection to the joint. Because of the proteinaceous fluid they contain they will be isointense to muscle on T1-

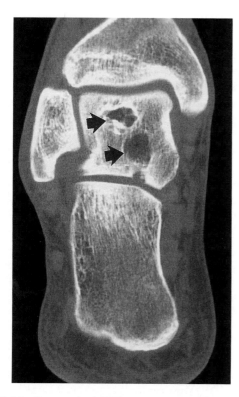

Fig. 41-22. On a sagittal FSE image a large, lobulated fluid-intensity ganglion is seen deep to the metatarsals.

weighted images. Synovial sarcomas may have appearance remarkably similar to a simple synovial cyst, although a portion of its margin will be slightly irregular. They tend to have more aggressive growth patterns, and they grow along a tendon sheath.[10] On T1-weighted images signal is typically slightly hyperintense to muscle. Hemangiomas will have increased signal on T1 and T2 sequences. This signal, however, will be less intense than fat on T1 sequences and greater than fat on T2 sequences. These appear septated or lobulated and have infiltrative margins routinely violating anatomic barriers. Calcifications in tumors will be visualized as regions of signal void. This may be difficult to distinguish from flow voids in highly vascular tumors (such as giant cell or aneurysmal bone cysts) or from hemosiderin in necrotic tumors. The differentiation of tumor from surrounding edema may be difficult. Typically the most prominent edema in soft-tissue tumors is seen with MFH, which typically tracts up and down as a single muscle.[67] Either on STIR images or immediately following contrast administration, the tumor and its pseudo-capsule can usually be distinguished from the edema.

The MR appearance is also helpful in evaluating the aggressiveness of a tumor. Benign tumors have smooth margins and homogeneous signal on all sequences, and they lack neurovascular or osseous involvement.[11,100] A low signal rim around a tumor is often seen with benign lesions. However, this is nonspecific and may occur in malignant lesions as well. These tumors are not necessarily encapsulated histologically. Malignant tumors frequently have a high T2-signal–intensity rim secondary to invasion of surrounding musculature. They will also be larger in size and will have more irregular margins and more heterogeneous signal characteristics, both on T2-weighted images as well as on contrast-enhanced images.

Bone tumors

Osseous tumors continue to be initially evaluated by plain radiography. MRI, however, is useful in localizing tumors and staging their extent. Most tumors have nonspecific signal characteristics. MRI is therefore unable to render a specific preoperative diagnosis. Signal characteristics may help narrow the differential diagnosis, however. The role of CT is limited to complex bones (tarsal), and the evaluation of the degree of cortical involvement (Fig. 41-23). CT, however, remains the modality of choice in evaluating osteoid osteoma.

Primary bone tumors of the feet are rare, accounting for only 4% of all bone tumors and only 3% of resected foot malignancies. The staging system is based on both histologic grade (I, low; II, high; III, metastasic) as well as whether the tumor is compartmental or extracompartmental.[35] In the foot, most bone neoplasms are primary. Benign bone neoplasms are more common than are malignant ones. The most common benign tumors are enchondromas and osteoid osteomas. The most common primary malignant tumors are chondrosarcomas and Paget's sarcoma. Metastatic tumors are rare and usually occur as a result of colorectal, renal, or bladder primaries. Certain bone tumors have a propensity for a specific anatomic location in the feet. Aneurysmal bone cysts and chondrosarcomas are most common in the calcaneus. In the anterior calcaneus, intraosseous lipomas and unicameral bone cysts are most common. Chondromyxoid fibroma and fibrous dysplasia occur frequently in metatarsals. The talus is the usual location for osteoid osteoma and osteoblastoma. Enchondromas occur in the proximal and middle phalanges and metatarsals.

Osteosarcomas demonstrate low signal on T1- and high signal on T2-weighted sequences.[41,99] Matrix calcifications may be seen as areas of signal void. Cortical breakthrough, adjacent soft-tissue extension, and peritumoral edema may be noted. The signal characteristics are variable and may be affected by the tumor subtype. For example, telangeclatic osteosarcomas may show areas of increased signal on both T1- and T2-weighted sequences. Fluid levels may also be noted in telangiectatic osteosarcomas, but this is a nonspecific finding.[105] Osteoid osteomas show high

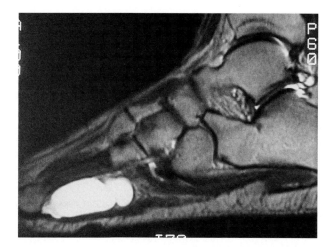

Fig. 41-23. Coronal CT images demonstrate well-defined cystic lesions in the talus *(arrows)* that apparently contain marrow fat. The upper cyst has sclerotic margins as well. Extensive osteoarthritic change is seen around the subtalar joint; these lesions may represent subchondral cysts.

signal intensity on T2-weighted sequences. The nidus may be visualized as an area of decreased signal.[42,111] Intravenous gadolineum may help in identifying the nidus since this will significantly enhance. Extensive edema surrounding this tumor is also seen both in marrow as well as in adjacent musculature.[24] This extensive edema maybe also seen in chondroblastomas and less frequently and intensely in osteoblastomas, eosinophilic granuloma, and aneurysmal bone cysts. Most frequently, fibrous dysplasia demonstrates decreased signal on T2-weighted sequences.[81] However, frequent islands of cartilage and cystic areas may be seen demonstrating increased T2 signal. Nonossifying fibromas will be cortically based lesions with decreased T2 signal. A low-signal rim will be seen with healing and will increase in thickness with time. Occasional nonossifying fibromas will demonstrate increased signal on T2-weighted images. Hyaline cartilage tumors such as enchondromas, osteochondromas, and chondrosarcomas will show a lobulated high signal on T2-weighted sequences.[21] Nonhyaline cartilage tumors such as chondroblastomas and synovial chondromatosis will show decreased T2 signal, although there is a significant amount of overlap.[65] Aneurysmal bone cysts demonstrate septations and fluid/fluid levels. The cystic areas may show varying signal intensity dependent on the stage of blood breakdown. Small diverticula-type outpouchings have been described. A well-defined low-signal rim is also frequently noted. High signal internally on T1-weighted images is characteristic, as is susceptibility artifact on gradient-echo images.[23,80] Intraosseous lipomas have signal characteristics similar to those of subcutaneous fat, will high T1 and moderate T2 signal.[30] A

central signal void corresponding to calcification/ossification noted on radiography may be seen. Although the previously described signal characteristics are useful in evaluating tumors, traditional criteria such as cortical breakthrough, soft-tissue mass, and periosteal reaction remain optimal for determining degree of aggressiveness. Marrow infiltrative tumors such as lymphomas, leukemia, metastatic disease, and multiple myeloma will show a decrease in the normal high-signal marrow on T1 sequences. On T2-weighted and STIR sequences the signal intensity will increase. Small adjacent soft-tissue masses or reaction will often be seen, most commonly in lymphoma and in aggressive subtypes of multiple myeloma.

REFERENCES

1. Adelaar RS: The treatment of complex fractures of the talus. *Orthop Clin North Am* 20(4):691-707, 1989.
2. Balduini FC, Vegso JJ, Torg JS, et al: Management and rehabilitation of ligamentous injuries to the ankle. *Sports Med* 4:364-380, 1987.
3. Balsara ZN, Stainken BF, Martinez AJ: Case report: MR image of localized giant cell tumor of the tendon sheath involving the knee. *J Comput Assist Tomogr* 13:159-162, 1989.
4. Bamberger DM, Daus GP, Gerding DN: Osteomyelitis in the feet of diabetic patients: long-term results, prognostic factors, and the role of antimicrobial and surgical therapy. *Am J Med* 86:653-666, 1987.
5. Bassett F, Gates H, Billys J, et al: Talor impingement by the anteroinferior tibio fibula ligament. *J Bone Joint Surg* 72A:55-59, 1990.
6. Beltran J, Campanni DS, Knight C, et al: The diabetic foot: magnetic resonance imaging evaluation. *Skeletal Radiol* 19:37-41, 1990.
7. Beltran J, Munchow AM, Khabini A, et al: Ligaments of the lateral aspect of the ankle and sinus tarsi: an MR imaging study. *Radiology* 177:455-458, 1990.
8. Berkowitz JF, Kier R, Rudiel S: Plantar fascitis: MR imaging. *Radiology* 179:665-667, 1991.
9. Berndt AL, Harty M: Tranchondral fractures (osteochondritis dissecans) of the talus. *J Bone Joint Surg* 41A:988-1020, 1959.
10. Bernreuter WK, Sartoris DJ, Resnick D: Magnetic resonance imaging of synovial sarcoma. *J Foot Surg* 29:94-100, 1990.
11. Bloem JL, Taminiau AHM, Eulderink F, et al: Radiographic staging of primary bone sarcoma: MR imaging, scintigraphy, angiography and CT correlated with pathologic examination. *Radiology* 169:805-810, 1988.
12. Boruta PM, Bishop JO, Braly WG, et al: Acute lateral ankle ligament injuries: a literature review. *Foot Ankle* 11:107-113, 1990.
13. Bradley SA, Davies AM: Computed tomographic assessment of old calcaneal fractures. *Br J Radiol* 63:926-933, 1990.
14. Buetow PC, Kransdorf MJ, Moser RPJ, et al: Radiologic appearance of intramuscular hemangioma with emphasis on MR imaging. *AJR* 154:563-567, 1990.
15. Burk DLJ, Dalinka MK, Kanal E, et al: Meniscal and ganglion cysts of the knee: MR evaluation. *AJR* 150:331-336, 1988.
16. Canale ST: Fractures of the neck of the talus. *Orthopaedics* 13(10):1105-1115, 1990.
17. Canale ST, Kelly FB: Fractures of the neck of the talus. *J Bone Joint Surg* 60A(2):143-156, 1978.
18. Church CC: Radiographic diagnosis of acute peroneal tendon dislocation. *AJR* 129:1065-1068, 1977.

19. Cimino WR: Tarsal tunnel syndrome: a review of the literature. *Foot Ankle* 11:47-52, 1990.

20. Clement P, Tauter J, Smart G: Achilles tendonitis and peritendonitis: etiology and treatment. *Am J Sports Med* 12:179-184, 1989.

21. Cohen EK, Kressel HY, Frank TS, et al: Hyaline cartilage-origin bone and soft tissue neoplasms: MR appearance and histologic correlation. *Radiology* 167:477-481, 1988.

22. Cohen EK, Kressel HY, Perosio T, et al: MR imaging of soft-tissue hemangiomas: correlation with pathologic findings. *AJR* 150:1079-1081, 1988.

23. Cory DA, Fritsch SA, Cohen MD, et al: Aneurysmal bone cysts: imaging findings and embolotherapy. *AJR* 153:369-373, 1989.

24. Crim JR, Mirra JM, Eckardt JJ, et al: Widespread inflammatory response to osteoblastoma: the flare phenomenon. *Radiology* 177:835-836, 1990.

25. Dellon AL, Mackinnon SE: Tibial nerve branching in the tarsal tunnel. *Arch Neurol* 41:645-646, 1984.

26. Demas BE, Heelan RT, Lane J, et al: Soft-tissue sarcomas of the extremities: comparison of MR and CT in determining the extent of disease. *AJR* 150:615-620, 1986.

27. DeSmet AA, Fisher DR, Burnstein MI, et al: Value of MR imaging in staging osteochondral lesions of the talus (osteochondritis dissecans). *AJR* 154:555-558, 1990.

28. Deutsch AL: Traumatic injury of bone and osteonecrosis. In Deutsch AL, Mink RH, Kern R, editors: *MRI of the foot and ankle.* New York, Raven Press, pp 75-109.

29. Dipaola D, Nelso DW, Colville MR: Characterizing osteochondral lesions by magnetic resonance imaging. *Arthroscopy* 7:101-104, 1991.

30. Dooms GC, Hricak H, Sollitto RA, et al: Lipomatous tumors and tumors with fatty component: MR imaging potential and comparison of MR and CT results. *Radiology* 157:479-483, 1985.

31. Ehman RL, Berquist TA, McLead RA: MR imaging of early avascular necrosis: reply. *Radiology* 168:282-283, 1988.

32. Erdman WA, Tamburro F, Hayson HT, et al: *Radiology* 180:533-539, 1991.

33. Erickson SJ, Corale PB, Carrera GF, et al: Interdigital (Morton) neuroma: high-resolution MR imaging with a soleroid coil. *Radiology* 181:833, 1991.

34. Erickson SJ, Smith JW, Ruiz ME, et al: MR imaging of the lateral collateral ligament of the ankle. *AJR* 156:131-136, 1991.

35. Enneking WF, Spanier SS, Goodman MA: A system for the surgical staging of musculoskeletal sarcoma. *Clin Orthop* 153:106-120, 1980.

36. Feldman F, Singson RD, Rosenberg FS, et al: Distal tibial triplane fractures: diagnosis with CT. *Radiology* 164:429-435, 1987.

37. Feldman F, Singson RD, Staron RB: Magnetic resonance imaging of para-articular and ectopic ganglia. *Skeletal Radiol* 18:353-358, 1989.

38. Freeman MAR, Dean MRE, Hanham IWF: The etiology and prevention of functional instability of the foot. *J Bone Joint Surg* 47B:678-685, 1965.

39. Frey C, Shereff M: Tendon injuries about the ankle in athletes. *Clin Sports Med* 7:103-117, 1988.

40. Frey C, Shereff M, Greenridge N: Vascularity of the posterior tibial tendon. *J Bone Joint Surg* 72A:884-888, 1990.

41. Gillespie TI, Manfrini M, Ruggieri P, et al: Staging of intraosseous extent of osteosarcoma: correlation of preoperative CT and MR imaging with pathologic macroslides. *Radiology* 167:765-767, 1988.

42. Glass RBJ, Poznanski AK, Fisher MR, et al: Case report: MR imaging of osteoid osteoma. *J Comput Assist Tomogr* 10:1065-1067, 1986.

43. Goiney RC, Connel DG, Nichols DM: CT evaluation of tarsonetatarsal fracture-dislocation injuries. *AJR* 144:985-990, 1985.

44. Golfieri R, Baddeley H, Pringle JS, et al: MRI in primary bone tumors: therapeutic implications. *Eur J Radiol* 12:201, 1991.

45. Gould N: Tenosynovitis of the flexor hallucis longus tendon at the great toe. *Foot Ankle* 2:46-48, 1981.

46. Greaney RB, Gerber FH, Laughlin RL: Distribution and natural history of stress fractures in U.S. Marines. *Radiology* 146:339-346, 1983.

47. Guyer BH, Levinsohn EM, Fredrickson BE, et al: Computed tomography of calcaneal fractures: anatomy, pathology, dosimetry, and clinical relevance. *AJR* 145:911, 1985.

48. Hamilton WG: Foot and ankle injuries in dancers. *Clin Sports Med* 7:143-173, 1988.

49. Hawkins LG: Fractures of the neck of the talus. *J Bone Joint Surg* 52A:991-1002, 1970.

50. Heger L, Wulff K, Seddigi MSA: Computed tomography of calcaneal fractures. *AJR* 145:131-137, 1985.

51. Hicks JH: The mechanics of the foot. II. The plantar aponeurosis and the arch. *J Anat* 88:25-30, 1954.

52. Hindman BW, Ross SDK, Sowerby MRR: Fractures of the talus and calcaneus: evaluation by computed tomography. *CT* 10:191, 1986.

53. Janecki CJ, Dovberg JL: Tarsal tunnel syndrome caused by neurilemoma of the medial plantar nerve. *J Bone Joint Surg* 59A:127-128, 1977.

54. Jelinek JS, Kransdorf MJ, Utz JA, et al: Imaging of pigmented villonodular synovitis with emphasis on MR imaging. *AJR* 152:337-342, 1989.

55. Johnson KA: Tibialis posterior tendon rupture. *Clin Orthop* 177:140-147, 1982.

56. Keene JS, Lash EG, Fisher DR, et al: Imaging of achilles tendon ruptures. *Am S Sports Med* 17:333-337, 1989.

57. Kerr R, Frey C: MR imaging in the evaluation of tarsal tunnel syndrome. *Foot Ankle* 14:159-164, 1993.

58. Kirby EJ, Shereff MJ, Lewis MM: Soft-tissue tumors and tumor-like lesions of the foot. *J Bone Joint Surg* 71A:621-626, 1989.

59. Koch E, Hofer HO, Sialer G, et al: Failure of MR imaging to detect reflex sympathetic dystrophy of the extremities. *AJR* 156:113-115, 1991.

60. Kransdorf MJ, Jelinek JS, Moser RPJ, et al: Soft-tissue masses: diagnosis using MR imaging. *AJR* 153:541-547, 1989.

61. Kransdorf MJ, Jelinek JS, Moser RPJ, et al: Magnetic resonance appearance of fibromatosis: a report of 14 cases and review of the literature. *Skeletal Radiol* 19:495-500, 1990.

62. Kransdorf MJ, Moser RPJ, Meis JM, et al: Fat-containing soft-tissue masses of the extremities. *RadioGraphics* 11:81-106, 1991.

63. Lee JK, Yao L: Occult introsseous fracture: detection with MR imaging. *Radiology* 168:749-750, 1988.

64. Lee JK, Yao L: Stress fractures: MR imaging. *Radiology* 169:217-220, 1988.

65. Lee JK, Yao L, Wirth CR: MR imaging of solitary osteochondromas: report of eight cases. *AJR* 149:557-560, 1987.

66. Lynch TCP, Crues JV, Morgan FW, et al: Bone abnormalities of the knee: prevalence and significance at MR imaging. *Radiology* 171:761-766, 1989.

67. Mahajan H, Kim EE, Wallace S, et al: Magnetic resonance imaging of malignant fibrous histiocytoma. *Magn Reson Imaging* 7:283-288, 1989.

68. Mann RA, Thompson FM: Rupture of the posterior tibial tendon causing flat foot. *J Bone Joint Surg* 67A:556-561, 1985.

69. Marcus DS, Reider MA, Kellerhouse LF: Achilles tendon injuries: the role of MR imaging. *JCAT* 13:480-486, 1989.

70. Mascioch C, D'Archivio C, Banile A, et al: Talocalcaneal coali-

tion: computed tomography and magnetic resonance imaging diagnosis. *Eur J Radiol* 15:22-28, 1992.
71. Mason MD, Zlatkin MB, Esterhai JL, et al: Chronic complicated osteomyelitis of the lower extremity: evaluation with MR imaging. *Radiology* 173:355-359, 1989.
72. McKeever FM: Treatment of complications of fractures and dislocations of the talus. *Clin Orthop* 30:45-52, 1963.
73. Mesgurzadeh M, Sapega AA, Bonakdarpour A, et al: Osteochondritis dissecans: analysis of mechanical stability with radiography, scintigraphy and MR imaging. *Radiology* 165:775-786, 1987.
74. Mink JH, Deutsch AL: MRI of the musculoskeletal system: a teaching file. In Mink JA, Deutsch AL, editors: New York 1990, Raven Press, pp 251-391.
75. Mink JH, Deutsch AL: Occult cartilage and bone injuries of the knee: detection, classification, and assessment with MR imaging. *Radiology* 170:823-829, 1989.
76. Mitchell DG, Kressel HY: MR imaging of early avascular recesses. *Radiology* 169:281-282, 1988.
77. Modic M, Feiglin D, Piraino D, et al: Vertebral osteomyelitis: assessment using MR. *Radiology* 157:157-166, 1985.
78. Moore TE, Yuh WTC, Kathol MH, et al: Pictorial essay abnormalities of the foot in patients with diabetes mellitus: findings on MR imaging. *AJR* 157:813-817, 1991.
79. Morrison W, Schweitzer ME, Mitchell DG, et al: The utility of gadolineum enhanced fat suppressed MRI in the diagnosis of osteomyelitis. *Radiology* (in press).
80. Munk PL, Helms CA, Holt RG, et al: MR imaging of aneurysmal bone cysts. *AJR* 153:99-101, 1989.
81. Norris MA, Kaplan PA, Pathria MN, et al: Fibrous dysplasia: magnetic resonance imaging. *Clin Imaging* 14:211, 1990.
82. Noto AM, Cheung Y, Rosenberg TS, et al: MR imaging of the ankle: normal variants. *Radiology* 170:121-124, 1989.
83. Pooley BJ, Kudelkap, Menelaus MB: Subcutaneous rupture of the tendon of tibialis anterior. *J Bone Joint Surg* 52A:1-20, 1970.
84. Pritsch M, Horoshouski H, Farine J: Arthroscopic treatment of osteochrondral lesions of the talus. *J Bone Joint Surg* 68A:862-865, 1986.
85. Quinn SF, Erickson SJ, Dee PM, et al: MR imaging in fibromatosis: results in 26 patients with pathologic correlation. *AJR* 156:539-542, 1991.
86. Quin SF, Murray WT, Clark RA, et al: Achilles tendon: MR imaging at 1.5 T. *Radiology* 164:767-776, 1987.
87. Rosenberg ZS, Cheung Y, Jahss MG, et al: Rupture of posterior tibial tendon: CT and MR imaging with surgical correlation. *Radiology* 169:229-235, 1988.
88. Rosenberg ZS, Feldman F, Singson RD: Peroneal tendon injuries: CT analysis. *Radiology* 161:743, 1986.
89. Sarno RC, Carter BL, Bankoff MS, et al: Computed tomography in tarsal coalition. *JCAT* 8:1155, 1984.
90. Schweitzer ME, Karasick D, Mitchell D, et al: Posterior tibial tendon tears: utility of secondary signs for MRI diagnosis. *Radiology* (in press).
91. Schweitzer ME, VanLeersum M, Wapner K, et al: Fluid in the ankle shown by MR imaging: amount and distribution in normal and abnormal ankles. *AJR* (in press).
92. Shea MP, Manoli A: Osteochondral lesions of the talar dome. *Foot Ankle* 14:48-55, 1993.
93. Sherry CS, Harmes SE: MR evaluation of giant cell tumors of the tendon sheath. *Magn Reson Imaging* 7:195-201, 1989.
94. Sobel M, Geppert MJ, Olsen EJ, et al: The dynamics of peroneus brevis tendon splits: a proposed mechanism, technique of diagnosis and clssification of injury. *Foot Ankle* 73:413-422, 1992.
95. Spritzer CE, Dalinka MK, Kressel HY: Magnetic resonance imaging of pigmented villonodular synovitis: a report of two cases. *Skeletal Radiol* 16:316-319, 1987.
96. Stafford SA: MRI in stress fracture. *AJR* 147:533-556, 1986.
97. Stull MA, Moser RPJ, Kransdorf MJ, et al: Magnetic resonance appearance of peripheral nerve sheath tumors. *Skeletal Radiol* 20:9-14, 1991.
98. Sundaram M, McGuire MH, Fletcher J, et al: Magnetic resonance imaging of lesions of synovial origin. *Skeletal Radiol* 15:110-116, 1986.
99. Sundaram M, McGuire MH, Herbold DR: Magnetic resonance imaging of osteosarcoma. *Skeletal Radiol* 16:23-29, 1987.
100. Sundaram M, McGuire MH, Herbold DR: Magnetic resonance imaging of soft tissue masses: an evaluation of fifty-three histologically proven tumors. *Magn Reson Imaging* 6:237-248, 1988.
101. Tang JS, Gold RH, Bassett LW, et al: Musculoskeletal infection of the extremities: evaluation with MR imaging. *Radiology* 166:205-209, 1988.
102. Tanz SS: Heel pain. *Clin Orthop* 28:169-177, 1963.
103. Thompson FM, Pattern AH: Rupture of the peroneus longus tendon. *J Bone Joint Surg* 71A:293-294, 1989.
104. Torg JS, Pavlov H, Cooley LH, et al: Stress fractures of the tarsal navicular: a retrospective review of twenty-one cases. *J Bone Joint Surg* 63A:700-712, 1982.
105. Tsai JC, Dalinka MK, Fallon MD, et al: Fluid-fluid level: a nonspecific finding in tumors of bone and soft tissue. *Radiology* 175:779-782, 1990.
106. Unger EC, Moldofsky PJ, Gatenby RA, et al: Diagnosis of osteomyelitis by MR imaging. *AJR* 150:605-610, 1988.
107. Vellet AD, Marks PH, Fowler PJ, et al: Occult posttraumatic osteochondral lesions of the knee: prevalence, classification and short-term sequelae evaluated with MR imaging. *Radiology* 178:271-276, 1991.
108. Wechsler RJ, Karasick D, Schweitzer ME: Computed tomography of talocalcaneal coalition: imaging techniques. *Skeletal Radiol* 21:353, 1992.
109. Wilson AS, Murphy WA, Hardy DC, et al: Transient osteoporosis: transient bone marrow edema. *Radiology* 167:757-760, 1988.
110. Yao L, Lee JK: Occult intraosseous fracture: detection with MR imaging. *Radiology* 167:749-751, 1988.
111. Yeager BA, Schiebler ML, Wertheim SB, et al: Case report: MR imaging of osteoid osteoma of the talus. *J Comput Assist Tomogr* 11:916-917, 1987.
112. Zeiss J, Fenton P, Ebraheim N, et al: Normal magnetic resonance anatomy of the tarsal tunnel. *Foot Ankle* 10:214-218, 1990.
113. Zlatkin MB, Pathria M, Sartoris DJ, et al: The diabetic foot. *Radiol Clin North Am* 25:1095-1105, 1987.

42
The Hip

MARK D. MURPHEY

The hip joint is a large and complex articulation that can be involved by numerous pathologic conditions. These include abnormalities resulting from trauma, infection, avascular necrosis, neoplastic involvement, and synovial-based processes. In addition, manifestations of congenital and developmental changes are not infrequently recognized in the hip. While conventional radiographs remain the initial imaging technique in most instances, computed tomography (CT) and/or magnetic resonance imaging (MRI) is often the next radiologic method of evaluation. The advantages of CT and MR imaging are that both eliminate overlying osseous structures that can limit assessment with radiographs. Also, the surrounding soft-tissue structures are well demonstrated as a result of improved contrast resolution. Unfortunately, clinical evaluation of, and distinction between, the various causes of hip pain usually yields nonspecific and ultimately unrewarding results. It is therefore important that we as radiologists are aware of the disease manifestations that commonly occur about the hip as seen on CT and MR images. The purpose of this chapter is to discuss and illustrate the application of CT and MR imaging to assessment of pathologic conditions involving the hip joint.

CONGENITAL AND DEVELOPMENTAL ABNORMALITIES

Developmental dysplasia of the hip (DDH), previously termed *congenital hip dysplasia* (CDH), is most often evaluated, radiologically, by ultrasonography and radiographs. MR imaging, however, can also be used to evaluate DDH; just as with sonography, MR does not expose these young patients to radiation. MR imaging can be particularly helpful in evaluating patients who fail initial treatment and in evaluating older children after ossification of the capital femoral epiphysis where sonography can be difficult to perform.[72,83,88] Axial and coronal MR images are most useful, and small surface coils with high spatial resolution are necessary to best evalu-

ate the changes of DDH.[72] Coronal images allow assessment of the shape of the acetabulum and femoral head coverage. MR images also improve evaluation of surrounding soft-tissue structures, including the labrum, iliopsoas tendon, capsular tissue, ligamentum teres, transverse acetabular ligament, and associated fibrofatty pulvinar (Fig. 42-1).[88] Ligamentous structures may invaginate into the joint, not allowing reduction of the articulation.[149] The acetabular labrum normally is a triangular area of fibrocartilage superolaterally. It can also insinuate into the joint and make nonoperative reduction impossible.[72] The ligaments and labrum are low intensity on all pulse sequences and are often accentuated by surrounding joint fluid on long TR images. Capsular tissue is intermediate intensity on all pulse sequences.

CT is most useful in evaluation of DDH after intraoperative reduction. Injection of contrast into the joint is also often performed at intraoperative reduction. The performance of CT as soon as possible after intraoperative arthrography allows contrast surrounding the nonossified femoral head to be identified to help access alignment and its relationship to the acetabulum.[27,117,149] The adequacy of reduction can then be well evaluated by CT.[68,86,88] The overlying cast, usually present, does not create artifact on CT and helps limit motion.

Conversion defects (herniation pits) result from an abrasive effect of the anterior hip capsule in an area of the anterosuperior subcapital region of the femoral neck. This phenomenon is common (4% to 5% of the adult population) and occurs in an area where there are often normal cortical defects.[5,114,118] The medullary canal is exposed to erosion from the overlying soft tissues and synovium, which creates a subcortical pit.[5] This developmental alteration, increasingly visualized on CT and MR images, is important to recognize as an incidental finding and not a cause of hip pain. In addition, conversion defects must be distinguished from other pathologic conditions (including osteoid osteoma, avascular necro-

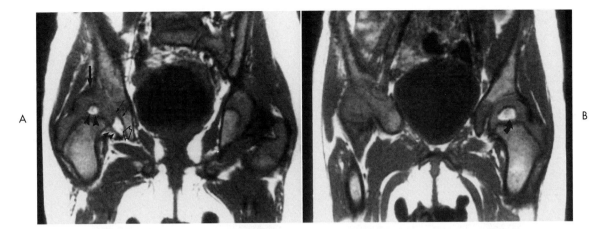

Fig. 42-1. A 22-month-old girl with developmental dysplasia of right hip. **A** and **B,** Coronal T1-weighted MR images show delayed ossification of right capital femoral epiphysis *(large arrowheads)* compared with left side *(curved arrow)*, and displacement superolaterally. There is thickening of the fibrofatty pulvinar *(open arrow)*, transverse acetabular ligament *(small arrowheads)*, and ligamentum teres *(small arrows)* on the right that limited reduction of the hip. However, the acetabular labrum is not infolded *(large arrow)* to block reduction. (Case courtesy of Edgar Colon, M.D.)

sis, chronic abscess, and intraosseous ganglion) with which they may be confused. CT and radiographs reveal a subchondral area of soft-tissue attenuation replacing the marrow or radiolucency, respectively, with surrounding sclerosis in the anterior subcortical region of the superolateral femoral neck (Fig. 42-2, A and B).[118] On MR imaging, herniation pits show marrow replacement in this subcapital region with a rim of low intensity on all pulse sequences corresponding to the area of sclerosis (Fig. 42-2, C). This appearance is seen best on axial and coronal MR images. Internally the lesions are primarily composed of fibrocollagenous tissue that largely remains low to intermediate signal intensity on all MR imaging pulse sequences. Small, focal, high-intensity regions on T2-weighted MR images may be apparent in a majority of patients; these regions represent fluid components creating heterogeneous signal intensity in combination with the fibrous tissue (Fig. 42-2, D).[114] The connection to the cortex can usually be detected on both CT and MR imaging (best seen in the axial plane) and may have a linear or channellike appearance. Herniation pits range in size from 5 mm to several centimeters and can enlarge over time.[118] The lesion location and imaging characteristics should allow distinction from other pathologic considerations.

Proximal femoral focal deficiency (PFFD) represents a congenital partial absence of the upper femur with resultant shortening.[126] The degree of deficiency of the proximal femur is extremely variable and can be difficult to assess on radiographs. There has been only limited use of CT and MR imaging to evaluate PFFD reported in the literature.[149] However, assessment is important in presurgical planning because of the wide variation in the degree of the gap between the femoral head and subtrochanteric femur. The gap between the femoral head and subtrochanteric femur may be small with pseudarthrosis, or it may be fibro-osseous or devoid of connecting tissue.[126] MR imaging or CT can be used to assess this osseous gap and the femoral head, which is delayed in ossification (Fig. 42-3). These structures and the resultant coxa varus deformity cannot be adequately evaluated with radiographs because the gap will be radiolucent whether it is filled with fibro-osseous tissue or absent. CT will show the nonossified areas as soft-tissue attenuation; however, this is difficult to distinguish from surrounding muscle. MR imaging is more valuable because of improved contrast resolution and multiplanar imaging capability. On MR images the femoral head, if present, shows intensity of yellow marrow, while fibrous tissue will be low intensity on all pulse sequences (Fig. 42-3, B). Pseudarthrosis may show high intensity fluid on long TR images.[126] Evaluation of PFFD is often best accomplished with coronal images. The presence of a femoral head and the connection between the upper femur and subtrochanteric femur is vital information to guide orthopedic reconstruction (Fig. 42-3, B and C).

Abnormalities of rotation and version (degree of hip anteversion) may be congenital, but it is more often a result of trauma. CT has been used to evaluate both types of abnormalities.[4,68,117] Axial images obtained through the femoral head and neck and additional images of the distal femoral condyles are needed. Measurements from these images are used to obtain both femoral anteversion and rotational abnormalities. These de-

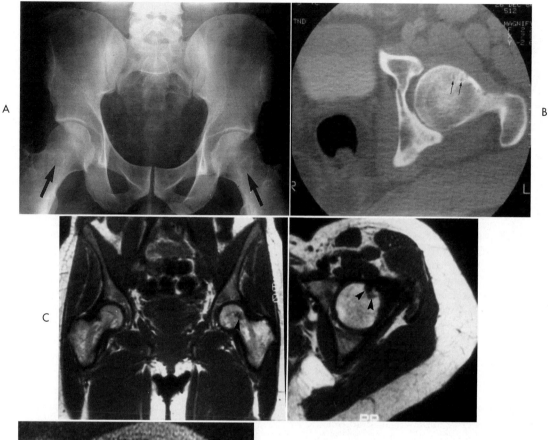

Fig. 42-2. Asymptomatic patients with conversion defects. **A,** Pelvis radiograph shows large conversion defects bilaterally seen as subcapital lucencies with surrounding sclerosis *(large arrows)*. **B,** CT shows a small herniation pit in the anterior subchondral region *(small arrows)* with vertical extension toward the cortex. **C,** T1-weighted MR images in the coronal *(left image)* and axial *(right image)* planes reveal herniation pits as focal areas of marrow replacement *(large arrowheads)*. This has a channel-like appearance extending towards the anterior cortex on the axial plane. **D,** Axial T2-weighted MR reveals heterogeneous signal in the conversion defect *(small arrowheads)* consistent with both fluid and fibrocollagenous tissue.

formities may require orthopedic correction with the use of osteotomies, and CT is necessary to direct surgical management. MR imaging could be used in a similar manner; however, there has been only limited experience in the literature.

SYNOVIAL ABNORMALITIES

Abnormalities primarily involving the cartilage and synovium of the hip are common. These include arthritis (both osteoarthritis and inflammatory arthropathy), and more infiltrative disorders such as pigmented villonodular synovitis (PVNS), synovial chondromatosis, and amyloidosis.

Conventional radiography remains the primary modality by which arthropathy of the hip is evaluated. However, CT and MR imaging can provide valuable information about the extent of disease, visualization of the surrounding soft tissue involvement, and a means of identifying other causes of hip pain. Detection of cartilage defects and thinning in osteoarthritis continues to challenge the contrast and spatial resolution capabilities of MR imaging. The clinical use of the CT and MR im-

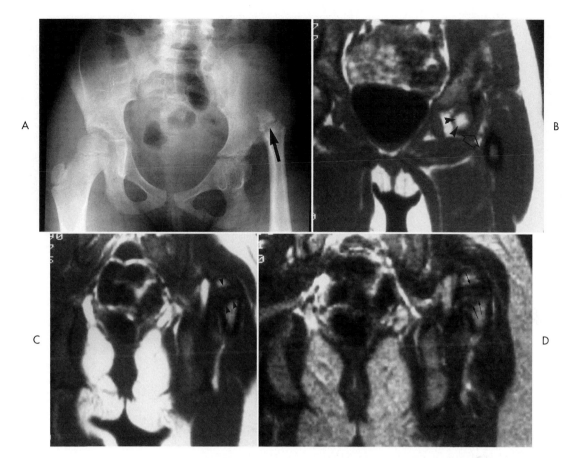

Fig. 42-3. A 6-year-old with proximal femoral focal deficiency. **A,** Pelvis radiograph shows deficiency of the proximal femur with lucent cleft in upper portion of remaining femur *(large arrow)*. **B,** Coronal T1-weighted MR image was performed to evaluate for possible surgical reconstruction. MR image shows that there is a capital femoral epiphysis seen as high signal (fatty marrow) not well recognized on radiograph *(large arrowheads)*. The femoral head, however, is not connected to the remainder of the femur where there is intervening tissue *(open arrow)* and thus cannot be used for reconstruction. More posteriorly, a coronal T1-weighted MR image **(C)** shows the upper remaining femur with low intensity gap at its upper extent *(small arrowheads)*. This area stays low intensity on T2-weighted coronal MR image **(D)** consistent with fibrous tissue *(small arrows)* rather than pseudoarthrosis, which may show high signal intensity.

aging in evaluation of osteoarthritis of the hip appears limited at this time.[26,93]

Involvement of the hip by inflammatory arthritis, both rheumatoid arthritis and the seronegative spondyloarthropathies, is not infrequent. Because the hip is a relatively noncapacious joint space, radiographs demonstrate erosions relatively early in the disease. MR imaging, and to a much lesser degree CT, can detect the extent of pannus formation that is common to all inflammatory arthritides but not evident on radiographs (Fig. 42-4).[137,169] Pannus generally shows low intensity on T1-weighted MR images and high intensity on T2-weighted MR images. Pannus can be difficult to differentiate from synovial fluid, also frequently present with involvement of the hip by inflammatory arthritis. Subtle differences between pannus and synovial fluid may be apparent on both T1- and T2-weighted MR images. Pannus may show slighter higher signal intensity on short TR images and have more heterogeneous signal intensity on long TR images (Fig. 42-4, *B*). Intravenous gadolinium injection can alleviate this difficulty.[137] Areas of synovitis and pannus formation have been shown to dramatically enhance after contrast injection in a linear and nodular pattern, respectively.[1,22,85] Imaging should be performed early after injection because on delayed images synovial fluid also shows enhancement.[78,124,125] Osseous erosions are better demonstrated by both CT and MR imaging, as compared with radiographs, because of improved delineation of exposed cortical surfaces.[137,169] In addition, MR imaging provides multiplanar imaging capabilities.

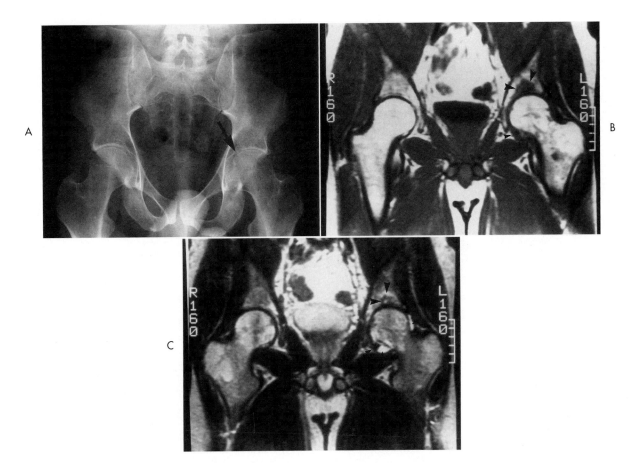

Fig. 42-4. A 29-year-old man with monarticular left hip pain for six months. **A,** Pelvis radiograph shows mild axial narrowing of the hip without erosions *(large arrow).* **B,** Coronal T1-weighted MR image shows soft tissue thickening (synovitis) about the hip of intermediate intensity *(small arrowheads).* There is a large area of marrow replacement in the superior acetabulum *(large arrowheads).* **C,** On the T2-weighted coronal MR image synovitis reveals increased intensity *(small arrowheads)* and there is heterogeneous signal in the acetabular erosion *(large arrowheads)* suggesting a fibrous component to the tissue. Erosion was not seen on CT (not shown), and low-grade infection could not be excluded. Patient had a history of psoriasis and subsequently developed polyarticular disease typical of psoriatic arthritis in other joints.

Bursal extensions from the hip joint (Fig. 42-5) can also be detected by CT and MR imaging and are not infrequently seen in patients with inflammatory arthritis, particularly rheumatoid arthritis.[120,158] Pannus may occasionally stay relatively low intensity on T2-weighted MR images (Fig. 42-4, *C*). This phenomenon may be the result of hemorrhage and deposition of hemosiderin (paramagnetic effect shortening T2 relaxation time) or fibrosis in more chronic areas of inflammation.[1,22] Fibrotic components within pannus are often more prominent in the seronegative spondyloarthropathies.

Overall, MR imaging of inflammatory arthritis of the hip can be very useful. It allows determination of the extent of synovial hypertrophy and pannus formation, as well as the degree of bone erosion and articular cartilage thinning. Knowledge of these factors is important in pa-

tient management. MR imaging can also be used to monitor the effects of therapy by quantitating the volume of pannus.[124,125]

PVNS represents a family of diseases of benign synovial hypertrophy. The degree of villous or nodular synovial hypertrophy as well as pigment deposition of hemosiderin is variable. PVNS occurs in 2 to 11 individuals per million, with relatively equal incidence in males and females.[40,54,60,126] PVNS is almost always a monoarticular disease and usually affects individuals in their second to fourth decades of life. The two basic forms of PVNS are diffuse and localized. The localized form of PVNS often involves the fingers and accounts for approximately 75% of cases.[12,74] It is also referred to as giant cell tumor of tendon sheath (GCTTS) and can involve tenosynovial tissues about the hip. The diffuse form of PVNS fre-

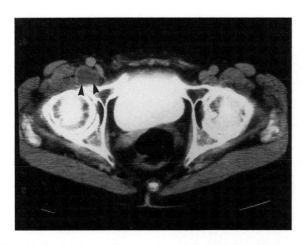

Fig. 42-5. CT shows iliopsoas bursal fluid collection *(arrowheads)* with higher attenuation fibrous wall *(arrows)* resulting from iliopsoas bursitis.

quently affects larger joints. The knee is most commonly involved; however, the hip joint is the second most frequently affected articulation. The pathogenesis of PVNS is unknown; possible etiologies include neoplasia, disorder of lipid metabolism, repetitive trauma, and the most commonly supported theory of an inflammatory process. Patients with PVNS often complain of longstanding pain and decreased range of motion.

Radiographic changes with PVNS of the hip are frequent as compared with involvement of the knee joint. This is a result of the relatively nondistensible hip joint with synovial thickening causing early extrinsic pressure erosions in the vast majority of cases.[60] These extrinsic erosions on both sides of the joint are well seen on both CT and MR imaging (Fig. 42-6). Coronal and sagittal MR images often demonstrate the erosive changes and their relationship to the hip joint to best advantage. CT and MR imaging reveal nodular synovial masses, and there is associated joint effusion in nearly 80% of cases.[126] This effusion when aspirated is a xanthochromic to brownish-stained bloody fluid. On CT there is soft-tissue thickening about the hip, and the synovial based masses often have higher attenuation than the surrounding muscle because of deposition of hemosiderin.[32,42] These areas of focal synovial masses are usually associated with localized pockets of joint effusion that may extend into the iliopsoas and obturator bursae. Injection of dilute contrast, followed by CT examination, will reveal nodular filling defects and synovial thickening identical to the findings at arthrography (Fig. 42-6, *B*).

MR imaging of the diffuse form of PVNS is usually very characteristic.[19,71,79,140] Synovial thickening with nodular excrescences arising from the joint surface are well shown on MR imaging. These areas are of heterogeneous signal intensity on all pulse sequences, although low signal intensity predominates (Fig. 42-6, *C* and *D*). The hypointensity is caused by hemosiderin deposition. Specifically, the unpaired electrons of iron in the ferric state (Fe^{+3}) interacts with adjacent water molecules, which results in shortening of the T2 relaxation time.[71,140] These effects are directly related to the square of the magnetic field and are thus accentuated with high–field-strength MR units.[140] Focal areas of synovial fluid, low intensity on T1-weighted images and high intensity on T2-weighted MR images, are also usually present within the hip joint involved by PVNS. Typically these fluid collections in PVNS are surrounded by a peripheral rind of low intensity hemosiderin-laden tissue on T2-weighted MR images. The areas of synovial proliferation are hypervascular and show significant enhancement after intravenous contrast injection with either CT or MR imaging.

The localized form of PVNS infrequently involves the tenosynovial tissues about the hip. GCTTS is more variable in the degree of hemosiderin deposition and CT or MR imaging may show similar characteristics as diffuse PVNS with low signal intensity on T1- and T2-weighted images.[12,70,74] MR imaging may, however, be less distinctive in cases of GCTTS by showing significant high signal intensity within a mass adjacent to the hip on long TR images.[12,74]

MR imaging and CT are important in follow-up of patients with PVNS to detect recurrences, which are frequent. Synovectomy is the usual initial treatment, however, because of the difficulty in removing all synovial tissue estimates of recurrence are as high as 40% to 50%.[54] External radiation therapy and injection of a beta-emitting agent into the joint tagged to radiocolloid, producing a nonsurgical synovectomy, may be used as adjuvant treatment methods.[126] Recurrent disease is identical in appearance to the initial characteristics previously described on both CT and MR imaging.

Synovial chondromatosis is caused by cartilage metaplasia occurring within the synovial membrane.[106,160] While many authors consider this a neoplastic disorder, inflammatory and traumatic etiologies have also been postulated.[69] The disease is usually seen between the ages of 20 and 50 and is twice as frequent in men. Typical clinical symptoms include joint pain of long duration and locking with limitation of range of motion.

Cartilage metaplasia within the hyperplastic synovium is seen pathologically in synovial chondromatosis.[106,160] These villous nodules often become detached from the synovium and are then free intraarticular bodies. These intraarticular fragments of cartilage may grow, deriving nourishment from synovial fluid, or reattach to the synovial lining where they may grow or be reabsorbed. The cartilage fragments may undergo endochondral ossification, at which point the term *synovial osteo-*

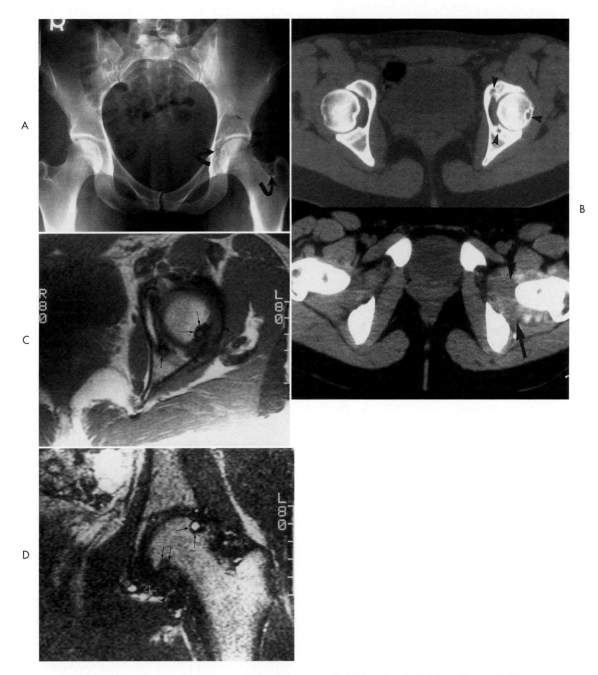

Fig. 42-6. A 27-year-old female with 5 year history of left hip pain. **A,** Pelvis radiograph shows extrinsic erosive changes *(curved arrows)* on both sides of the joint. **B,** CT scans before (**B,** *upper image*) and after intraarticular contrast injection (**B,** *lower image*) also reveal extrinsic erosions of acetabulum and femur *(large arrowheads)* and soft tissue thickening displacing the contrast *(large arrows)*. Axial T1-weighted (**C**) and coronal T2-weighted (**D**) MR images reveal extensive thickening about the hip *(small arrowheads)* causing extrinsic osseous erosions seen as areas of marrow replacement *(small arrows)*. The majority of this material stays low intensity on the long TR/TE image, although pockets of high intensity fluid are seen on the T2-weighted image *(open arrows)*. This appearance is due to hemosiderin in this patient with pigmented villonodular synovitis, confirmed at surgical synovectomy.

chondromatosis is appropriate. The synovial tissue of the tendons and bursa about the hip may also be involved by an identical process termed *tenosynovial chondromatosis.*

The cartilage fragments calcify in 70% to 95% of cases of synovial chondromatosis, and these areas often have a diagnostic ring-type appearance on radiographs (Fig. 42-7).[126] CT is often the optimal examination to detect, characterize, and localize these chondroid calcifications.[23,75] Smaller chondroid bodies are often solidly calcified on CT scans. Ossification of the cartilaginous bodies may be seen on CT scans, with a cortical rim and trabecular bone centrally containing yellow marrow. This may demonstrate a target appearance because at times there is a central dot of chondroid tissue with calcification. MR imaging of the mineralized intraarticular bodies is variable, depending on the degree of cartilage and ossification.[31] Noncalcified cartilaginous tissue will be low to intermediate intensity on T1-weighted images and very high intensity on T2-weighted images because hyaline cartilage is composed of 75% to 80% water.[82] Calcified intraarticular bodies will show low intensity on all MR imaging pulse sequences (Fig. 42-7, *C*); however, smaller fragments are better detected by CT or radiographs.[31] Ossification appears as low intensity on all pulse sequences if composed of cortical bone, and it appears as the intensity of fat (high intensity on T1-weighted image, intermediate intensity on T2-weighted image) if composed of trabecular bone on MR imaging. A target appearance corresponding to the osteochondral bodies on MR imaging may also be apparent. MR imaging and CT may detect as associated joint effusion. Soft-tissue thickening about the hip in the noncalcified areas of cartilage metaplasia will have attenuation similar or less than that of muscle on CT scans. On MR imaging, synovial chondromatosis may show low-signal–intensity areas (corresponding to calcified chondral bodies) on all pulse sequences surrounded by high intensity fluid or noncalcified cartilage metaplasia on T2-weighted images, an appearance exactly opposite of that in PVNS (Fig. 42-7). Low-intensity fibrous septation may be present within the synovial metaplasia on long TR images. CT and MR imaging may show extrinsic erosion and secondary osteoarthritis, a finding more frequent when synovial chondromatosis involves the hip as opposed to larger joints such as the knee, because of its relative lack of distensibility.[115,143] Synovial chondromatosis may rarely undergo malignant degeneration to chondrosarcoma.[126] Identification by CT or MR imaging of osseous invasion or destruction should suggest this complication. Multiple intraarticular osteochondral bodies may also be apparent after involvement of the hip joint by infection, trauma, or arthritis. This process, often termed *secondary synovial chondromatosis,* should be distinguished from the primary type by associated changes about the

hip joint. In addition, multiple rings of growth with calcification/ossification often create an appearance of lamination to the osteochondral intraarticular bodies. This multiple ring appearance is not usually seen in primary synovial chondromatosis.[106,160]

Amyloid deposition within the tenosynovial tissues and osseous structures about the hip occurs more commonly with secondary amyloidosis, as compared with primary amyloidosis. Secondary amyloidosis is associated with multiple myeloma (5% to 10% of patients) and chronic inflammatory diseases.[9,34,126] Patients with chronic renal failure who are receiving long-term hemodialysis are being increasingly reported to show a unique form of secondary amyloidosis with deposition of beta-2-microglobulin.[13,34,37,56] Camacho and co-workers reported an incidence of amyloidosis of 35% in a group of 88 patients receiving hemodialysis longer than 4 years.[33] All forms of amyloidosis appear to have some proclivity for deposition about the hip, both within bone and also within the tenosynovial tissue. The osseous lesions usually have a punched-out appearance, are eccentric or occur from extrinsic erosion, and reveal a thin sclerotic margin on radiographs and CT. MR images show marrow replacement on T1-weighting (Fig. 42-8, *A*). Femoral lesions often predispose to pathologic fracture. Both CT and MR images reveal diffuse thickening about the joint with intraarticular deposition of amyloid. This thickening is similar to muscle attenuation/signal intensity on CT and T1-weighted MR images, respectively. Interestingly T2-weighted MR images show that the signal intensity within the amyloid deposition remains low to intermediate, although high signal from focal fluid collections are also frequently present (Fig. 42-8, *B*).[96,130] Pathologically, this low intensity is most likely related to the fibrillar collagenlike composition of amyloid. Injection of intravenous contrast may reveal enhancement of the synovial thickening on CT or MR images (Fig. 42-8, *C*). The MR and CT appearance is similar to that of PVNS; however, amyloidosis is typically polyarticular with bilateral hip involvement, in contrast to monarticular disease in PVNS.[126]

Hemophilia, an X-linked recessive genetic disorder caused by a deficiency of clotting factor, is associated with repetitive intraarticular, intramuscular, and intraosseous episodes of bleeding.[126] Hemosiderin is progressively deposited within the synovial membrane with each bleeding episode, ultimately resulting in synovial hypertrophy and pannus formation. Hip involvement, though not frequent, may show progressive joint destruction and spontaneous dislocation. MR and CT reveal synovial thickening, and on long TR images the hemosiderin-laden synovial tissue stays low to intermediate signal intensity, similar to PVNS.[84,164,168] Synovectomy can be helpful in patient treatment; however, it

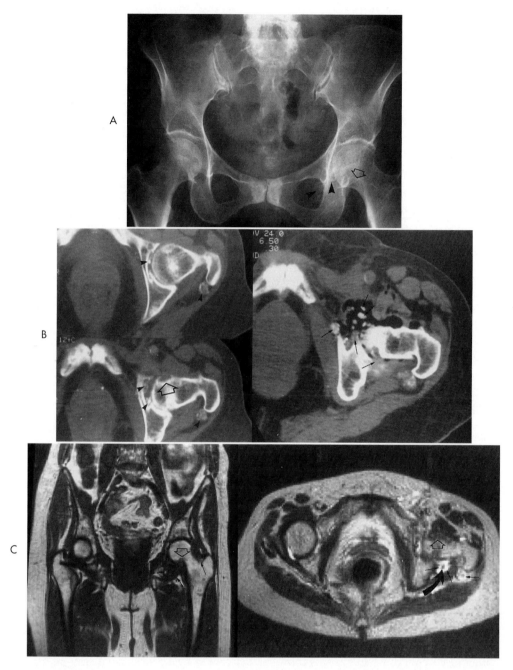

Fig. 42-7. A 67-year-old woman with 2 year history of left hip pain. **A,** Pelvis radiograph shows subtle multifocal areas of calcification about the hip *(large arrowheads)* with extrinsic erosion *(open arrow)*. CT scans before (**B,** *left image*) and after intraarticular air injection (**B,** *right image*) reveal calcification *(small arrowheads),* some of which have a typical ring-like appearance of chondroid and extrinsic erosion *(open arrow)*. After intraarticular injection, nodular soft tissue areas of synovial metaplasia and calcification *(small arrows)* are surrounded by air. Coronal T1-weighted (**C,** *left image*) and axial T2-weighted (**C,** *right image*) MR images show thickening about the hip *(small arrows)* and extrinsic erosion *(open arrow)*. High intensity on T2-weighted image represents fluid and synovial metaplasia *(small arrows)* with filling defect representing a calcified fragment *(curved arrow)*.

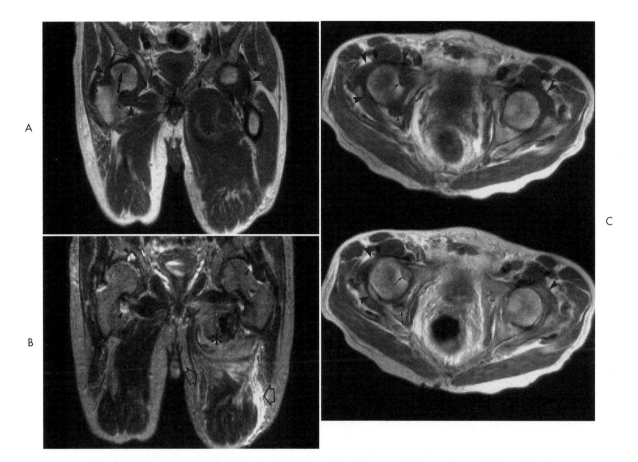

Fig. 42-8. A 43-year-old man on chronic hemodialysis for renal failure. Coronal T1-weighted (**A**) and T2-weighted (**B**) MR images show thickening of the tissues about both hips *(large arrowheads)* with marrow replacement from acetabular erosions *(small arrows)*. The T2-weighted image reveals that much of this tissue remains low in signal intensity, although there are pockets of high intensity fluid *(small arrowheads)*. There is a focus of decreased marrow signal from avascular necrosis on the right *(large arrow)*. Axial T1-weighted pre- (**C,** *upper image*) and post- (**C,** *lower image*) intravenous gadolinium injection also shows extrinsic erosions *(small arrows)* and thickening about the soft tissue of the hip that enhances with contrast *(large arrowheads)*. The changes about the hips are related to amyloid deposition. **A** and **B,** Large mass in the left medial thigh (*) on coronal images represents a spontaneous hemorrhage resulting from heparin administration during dialysis. The hematoma has areas of high signal intensity on T1- and T2-weighted images with heterogeneity. There is marked associated edema *(open arrows)* seen on the long TR images owing to hemorrhage dissecting throughout the surrounding tissues.

must be performed before cartilage destruction occurs. MR imaging can also be useful in this determination.[67] Areas of soft tissue or intraosseous hemorrhage also occur about the hips in hemophilia. Hermann and colleagues described soft-tissue hemorrhage on MR imaging, with acute hematoma (1 to 6 days) having similar appearance to muscle on T1 weighting and low signal on long TR images.[67] Beyond 1 week after hemorrhage, signal intensity increases on both T1- and T2-weighted images. These hematomas may subsequently ossify (myositis ossificans or heterotopic bone formation) with cortical bone peripherally and trabecular bone with yellow marrow centrally. This zonal pattern of ossification beginning peripherally is distinctive and is best detected by CT in its earliest phases.

INFECTION

Infection of the bone or soft tissue about the hip or septic arthritis is often very difficult to detect on initial radiographs. Osseous manifestations of osteomyelitis, such as bone destruction and periosteal reaction, are frequently not apparent on radiographs for 10 to 14 days after the onset of infection.[126] The metaphysis of the proximal femur is intraarticular because the hip capsule attaches in the intertrochanteric region. Infection localizing to this region, a frequent pattern in children because of vascular supply, may thus gain rapid access to the joint if the process extends through the osseous cortex.[58] Bacterial infection of the hip joint can then lead to rapid and irreparable cartilage damage and joint destruction. Early recognition of osteomyelitis, septic arthritis, and soft-tissue abscess about the hip is therefore imperative to prevent these dire sequelae and improve clinical outcome. CT and MR imaging provide excellent methods to identify and localize foci of infection at an early stage. In addition, both CT and MR imaging can help distinguish inflammation such as cellulitis from abscess formation.

Osteomyelitis about the hip is most commonly caused by hematogenous seeding; however, other routes of spread are caused by involvement from a contiguous soft-tissue infection, and direct implantation such as from a puncture wound or following surgery.[126] Although CT and MR imaging findings in osteomyelitis may be nonspecific, both are sensitive indicators of infection of the marrow space, in the appropriate clinical setting (Fig. 42-9). CT changes indicative of osteomyelitis are cortical destruction (particularly with osteomyelitis arising from contiguous spread), periosteal reaction, and increased attenuation within the marrow space.[10,58] Inflammation in the surrounding soft tissues is also often visualized on CT, seen as muscle and skin thickening, and soft-tissue stranding in the subcutaneous fat. MR imaging is superior to CT in identification of acute osteomyelitis, primarily because of improved contrast resolution.[14,18,58] Acute osteomyelitis reveals replacement of fatty marrow with low to intermediate signal intensity on T1-weighted images and high signal intensity on T2-weighted images.[51,111,144] These changes represent inflammatory and edematous tissue and usually demonstrate ill-defined margins and similar changes in the surrounding soft tissues. Sensitivity of MR imaging in detecting osteomyelitis has been reported by Erdman et al to be up to 98%; however, specificity was lower at 82%.[51] Both sensitivity and specificity of MR imaging are superior to that of CT and scintigraphy.[51,58]

The degree of activity in sites of chronic osteomyelitis often creates a clinical dilemma. Identification of new bone destruction, as well as the presence of irregular periosteal reaction and sequestra, are findings that suggest active osteomyelitis. CT can be very helpful to detect these findings, particularly sequestra, which are small sclerotic avascular bone fragments surrounded by granulation tissue (Fig. 42-9, A and B).[10,58] Though sequestra are not by definition infected, they provide an ideal milieu for organisms and must be considered foci of residual infection in the appropriate clinical setting. It is my belief that because of improved spatial resolution,

CT is better suited to detect sequestra; overall, however, MR imaging may be superior to all other methods (including indium WBC scanning) in identifying active areas of osteomyelitis. Marrow replacement is seen on T1-weighted MR images in chronic osteomyelitis because of fibrosis and osseous sclerosis, regardless of the activity of the infection. On T2-weighted MR images, however, active foci of infection will show high intensity.[38,103,153] Sequestra will be low intensity on T1 and T2 weighted images, but the surrounding inflammatory tissue shows a high intensity halo on long TR images. Subacute osteomyelitis, such as a Brodie's abscess, can be identified on CT and MR imaging as a focal intraosseous fluid collection, often elongated or channellike in shape with surrounding sclerosis (Fig. 42-9, B and C).[101] The fluid may be complex, having higher CT attenuation or intensity on T1-weighted MR images than does simple fluid. The surrounding sclerosis is low intensity on all MR images.

Soft-tissue infection about the hips can involve the joint or surrounding muscles. CT and MR imaging are helpful because of their ability to identify anatomically localized fluid collections. While infected and non-infected fluid collections have a similar appearance, in the appropriate clinical setting the detection of localized fluid is strong evidence of infection. In addition, a focal, infected fluid collection usually requires drainage for adequate treatment. CT and MR imaging changes suggesting an infected fluid collection are internal debris or septations and a thick wall (best seen on post-contrast images with enhancement).[41] MR imaging, again because of its superior contrast resolution, is better than CT in detection of fluid collections (Fig. 42-9, D). CT should be performed with intravenous contrast in cases in which an abscess is a consideration.[10,58] The absence of focal fluid collections by imaging essentially excludes localized soft-tissue infection.

The location of the fluid collection about the hip will determine the infected site: septic joint, bursitis, tenosynovitis, soft-tissue abscess, or sinus tract/fistula (Fig. 42-9, D). Septic bacterial arthritis involving the hip is a surgical emergency, as mentioned previously, because of the rapid cartilage destruction that can result. Hip joint infection is common in infancy and childhood. CT and MR imaging will show nonspecific joint fluid. MR imaging, in addition, can reveal early cartilage destruction indicative of infection. More indolent infections, including tuberculous and fungal, often result in a prominent synovitis and MR images may simulate a noninfectious inflammatory arthritis. Associated osteomyelitis is frequently associated with septic arthritis of the hip, because of both joint anatomy and cartilage loss, which expose underling bone to infection. Tendons involved by infection reveal fluid within the sheath. This fluid sur

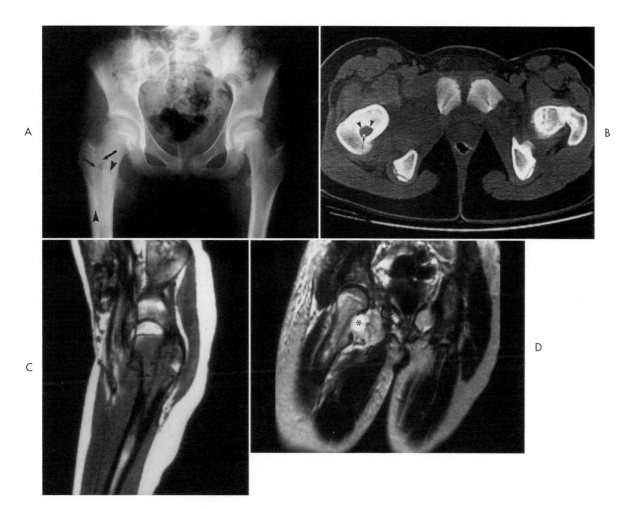

Fig. 42-9. A 13-year old girl with 1 year history of intermittent right hip pain now worsening with fever and clinical signs of sepsis. Patient had a history of bladder infection caused by staphylococcus aureus one year earlier. **A,** Pelvis radiograph shows channel-like lucency *(large arrows)* with associated sclerosis *(large arrowheads)* in the proximal femur. **B,** CT shows Brodie's abscess *(small arrowheads)* with sequestra *(small arrow)*. There is soft tissue thickening posteriorly although focal fluid collection is not seen. **C,** Sagittal T1-weighted MR image reveals marrow replacement in the proximal femur *(curved arrow)* with channel-like abscess *(small arrowheads)*. **D,** Coronal T2-weighted MR image shows soft tissue changes of focal abscess (*) and more diffuse edema *(open arrows)* posteromedially. The intraosseous abscess had extended into the soft tissues causing the patient's acute symptoms. Both soft tissue and intraosseous abscess were drained at surgery; culture revealed *Staphylococcus aureus* as the causative organism. Soft tissue abscess was larger on a more posterior coronal T2-weighted MR image (not shown).

rounds the tendon, which has high attenuation on CT and low intensity on all MR image pulse sequences. Soft-tissue abscess may be superficial or deep focal fluid collections. Cellulitis has an appearance of inflammation and edema, with muscle and skin thickening and soft tissue stranding in the subcutaneous tissue on CT as well as diffuse heterogeneous linear high intensity seen on T2-weighted MR images.[14,18,144] CT and MR imaging allow distinction of the nonlocalized changes of cellulitis from the focal fluid mass of a soft-tissue abscess (Fig. 42-9, *D*). This determination is vital to guide patient management because cellulitis is treated medically, whereas abscess requires drainage. Sinus or fistula tracts are more common in adults; they are seen as linear tracts on CT and MR images. On CT these tracts have high-attenuation walls, and on MR images there is often high intensity representing fluid within the tracts on long TR images. Sinus tracts are not unusual sequelae of osteomyelitis of the ischial tuberosities in paraplegic patients with chronic decubitus ulcers (Fig. 42-10). These sinus

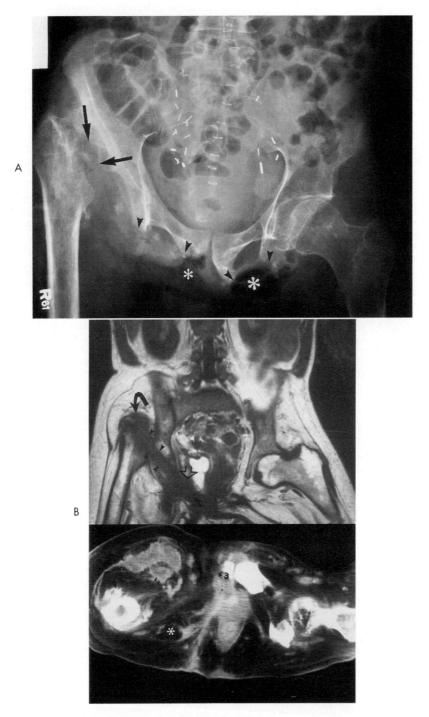

Fig. 42-10. Paraplegic 35-year-old man with chronic decubitus ulcers and fevers. **A,** Pelvis radiograph shows bone destruction and production about the ischial tuberosities *(large arrowheads)* from chronic osteomyelitis and subcutaneous air related to the decubitus ulcers (*). There is also chronic destruction of the right femoral head *(large arrows)*. Coronal T1-weighted MR (**B,** *upper image*) image reveals sinus tract *(small arrowheads)* extending from ischial area of osteomyelitis *(open arrow)* which seeded the right hip joint resulting in an additional site of pyarthrosis and osteomyelitis *(curved arrow)*. CT (**B,** *lower image*) shows bone destruction about the right hip *(curved arrows)* and large fluid collection anteriorly representing abscess *(small arrows)* and subcutaneous air (*).

tracts may seed the hip joints, causing septic arthritis, osteomyelitis, and joint destruction.

TRAUMA

Trauma about the hip is common. The two most frequent groups of fractures are those involving the acetabulum and proximal femoral neck. Acetabular fractures and fracture dislocations are usually due to motor vehicle accidents, and the complex anatomy and fracture patterns often require additional imaging beyond radiographs. Femoral neck fractures are usually easily diagnosed on radiographs and only infrequently require further radiologic evaluation.

Acetabular fractures constitute between 20% and 25% of all pelvic fractures in adults.[138] These fractures have a high association with concomitant injuries to the genitourinary system and vascular structures. Radiographs with oblique (Judet) views are often difficult to evaluate in determining the extent of involvement for presurgical planning.[73] CT is the modality of choice to evaluate these injuries.[62,64] Axial images should be performed with contiguous slices not thicker than 3 mm. Sagittal and coronal reconstructions and three-dimensional (3D) images are often helpful for the radiologist and more importantly for the orthopedic surgeon to conceptualize the fracture pattern before surgery.[53,102,136]

The normal acetabulum is formed by two columns, one anterior (iliopubic) and the other posterior (ilioischial); these unite superiorly in the shape of an inverted "Y." Medially, the bone between the anterior and posterior columns is the quadrilateral plate, and the acetabular socket is completed superiorly by the weight-bearing surface termed the *roof*.[132] Acetabular fractures have been divided into five basic or elementary patterns: posterior wall, transverse, posterior column, anterior column, and anterior wall. In addition complex fractures occur with various combinations of the elementary components.[73,91,116]

Fractures of the posterior column or wall account for nearly 30% of all acetabular fractures.[127] Fractures of the posterior wall are most common and are often a result of posterior hip dislocation (Fig. 42-11). The extent of posterior wall defect is well evaluated on CT and is important to determine both hip stability after reduction and the need for operative fixation. Posterior dislocation is the most common type of hip dislocation (85% to 90%).[127] CT allows identification of associated intraarticular fragments and impaction fracture or shearing osteochondral fractures of the femoral head, which are common sequelae of this injury.[127,146] The impaction fractures (seen in 13% to 61% of posterior hip dislocations) involve the anterior surface of the femoral head and are due to compression of the femur on the posterior

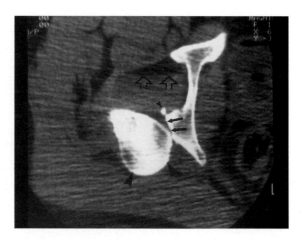

Fig. 42-11. Posterior column fracture with dislocation in a 30-year-old after motor vehicle accident. CT shows the femoral head posteriorly dislocated *(large arrowheads)* with small intraarticular fragment *(small arrowhead)*, fractured posterior column *(large arrows)*, and lipohemarthrosis in the joint *(open arrows)*.

acetabulum during dislocation. Large portions of the femoral head can be sheared (seen in 7% to 10% of posterior hip dislocations) from the remainder of the femur during dislocation (Fig. 42-12). These can be difficult to detect on radiographs, and CT is helpful to direct surgical fixation. Posterior column fractures are associated with central dislocations, and the fracture is directed obliquely across the posterior inferior acetabular fossa and inferior pubic ramus. This fracture separates the posterior column from the remainder of the iliac bone. Anterior column and wall fractures account for only 6% to 7% of acetabular fractures and may be associated with anterior hip dislocation.[138] Analogous to posterior column fractures, anterior column injuries divide this area from the remainder of the innominate bone. Anterior wall fractures only involve a portion of the anterior column. Anterior hip dislocations account for 10% to 15% of all hip dislocations.[62,64] Associated impaction fractures of the femoral head are not uncommon, and may be detected only on CT as a cortical indentation along the posterolateral femoral head. Transverse fractures (8% to 10% of acetabular fractures) are axially oriented injuries involving both columns (Fig. 42-13).[138] These fractures separate the innominate bone into superior and inferior fragments, usually at the level of the acetabular roof. They are often associated with central fracture dislocations.

Complex acetabular fractures combining two or more elementary fracture components are common. Frequently observed patterns include transverse and posterior wall (associated with posterior and central hip dislocation), fractures of both columns, and T-shaped fracture.[62,64,138] The T-shape injury combines a transverse fracture with a vertical component usually extending into

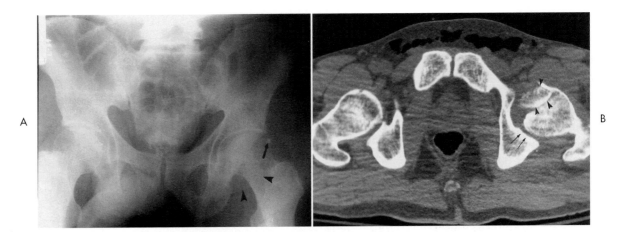

Fig. 42-12. Shearing femoral head osteochondral fracture resulting from posterior hip dislocation in a 39-year-old man sustained after motor vehicle accident. **A,** Pelvis radiograph following reduction shows small fragment superolateral to left hip *(large arrow);* however, large osteochondral femoral head fragment is only vaguely seen *(large arrowheads).* **B,** CT at lower extent of the acetabulum shows large osteochondral femoral head fragment *(small arrowheads)* that is rotated 180 degrees with its articular surface facing the remainder of the femur. Posterior column of the acetabulum is largely intact *(small arrows).* Subcutaneous air is seen anteriorly from associated soft tissue injury.

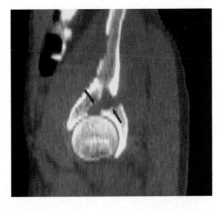

Fig. 42-13. Transverse acetabular fracture in a 25-year-old man sustained in an automobile accident. Sagittal CT reconstruction shows the axially oriented fracture *(arrows)* involving both columns at the level of the acetabular roof dividing the innominate bone into superior and inferior fragments.

and dividing the obturator ring. CT, in addition to initially evaluating acetabular fractures, can be used to assess both the adequacy of reduction after fixation and the position of metallic devices (particularly to exclude intraarticular location).[11] Some artifact is produced by the orthopedic fixation; however, these devices are relatively small in the acetabulum, and the use of bone windows and reconstructions will usually allow adequate evaluation on CT.

Femoral neck fractures are common, with over 250,000 subcapital fractures occurring annually in the U.S.[43] The vast majority of these fractures are well evaluated with radiographs. However, in a small per-

centage of patients the initial radiographs may be normal or equivocal, particularly in older patients. Scintigraphy may be falsely negative in these older osteoporotic patients for up to 4 or 5 days.[92] MR imaging can be quite helpful in those patients, and only coronal T1-weighted images are needed to detect an abnormality. If the marrow signal is normal, a fracture is immediately excluded. Fractures often have a linear or bandlike oblique or horizontal marrow replacement pattern seen on T1-weighted images (Fig. 42-14, *A*).[17,121] On T2-weighted MR images, areas around the fracture line will show increased intensity due to hemorrhage and edema; however, the fracture line often remains low intensity (Fig. 42-14, *B*).[128,167] This low intensity on long TR images may not be apparent in all cases, particularly before callus formation begins. Stress fractures have a similar appearance on MR images; these are frequent in the pubic rami and supraacetabular region in older patients (insufficiency fracture) and medial femoral neck in young patients (fatigue fracture).[89] Pubic rami and femoral neck insufficiency fractures (normal stress on bone of deficient elastic resistance) in elderly osteoporotic patients occasionally simulate pathologic fractures. This is caused by posttraumatic osteolysis simulating an osteolytic lesion or callus formation subacutely suggesting a chondroid or osteoid-producing neoplasm.[126] This appearance can be particularly confusing when previous radiographs, at the time of the acute fracture, are not available for review. In these cases, CT is often useful to define the linear fracture plane and surrounding callus and to confirm no evidence of a soft-tissue mass (although

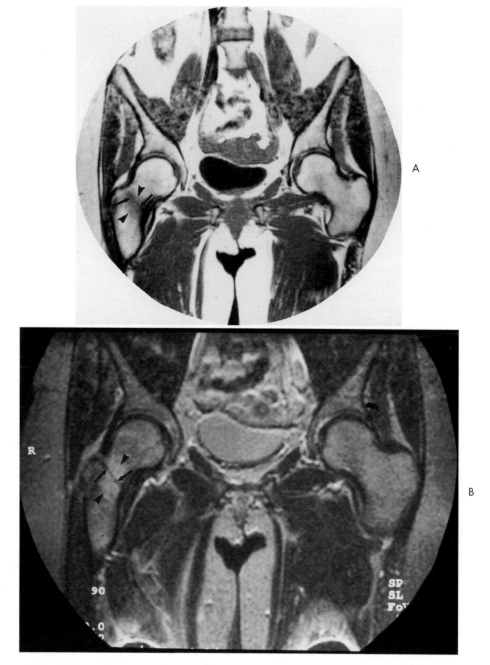

Fig. 42-14. Occult femoral neck fracture in a middle aged woman with hip pain. **A,** Coronal T1-weighted MR image shows a linear band of low intensity in the basicervical region of the right femoral neck *(arrows)* representing the fracture with surrounding marrow replacement from edema and hemorrhage *(arrowheads)*. **B,** Coronal T2-weighted MR image shows fracture line remaining low intensity *(arrows)* and marrow edema become high signal intensity *(arrowheads)*. Radiograph (not shown) revealed vague sclerosis in this area of the femoral neck, retrospectively. (Case courtesy of Harold Campbell, M.D.)

muscle thicken ing may be present) (Fig. 42-15). These factors exclude neoplastic involvement as a reasonable consideration.

MR imaging can also be used to evaluate muscle tears and hemorrhage about the hip;[45] these most fre-quently involve the rectus femoris muscle anteriorly and the hamstrings posteriorly. The appearance of intramus-cular hemorrhage is somewhat inconsistent; however, the most characteristic pattern is increased signal on both T1- and T2-weighted images with the area of involve

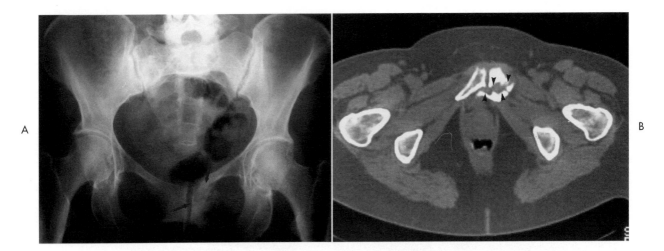

Fig. 42-15. Pubic insufficiency fracture in a 61-year-old woman simulating a neoplasm. **A,** Pelvis radiograph shows changes in the symphysis on the left with sclerosis suggesting a chondroid or osteoid producing lesion *(arrows)*. **B,** CT reveals linear fracture plane and surrounding callus *(arrowheads)* resulting from the healing fracture and no evidence of soft tissue mass.

ment being much larger on long TR images (Fig. 42-8, *A* and *B*).[45,131,154] Chronically, low intensity areas on all pulse sequence may be apparent because of hemosiderin and fibrosis. The area involved on MR images is frequently irregular and infiltrative, representing blood dissecting between muscle bundles. The multiplanar imaging capability of MR is also helpful to assess the degree of muscle disruption and to direct intervention when tears are complete.

NEOPLASM

Neoplastic involvement about the hip, both benign and malignant, can involve either the osseous structures or soft tissues. CT and MR imaging can provide localization and characterization of these neoplastic lesions, factors that are invaluable in staging and preoperative planning. Advantages of MR imaging include multiplanar imaging and superior contrast resolution as well as lack of ionizing radiation. While MR imaging has supplanted CT as the modality of choice in evaluation of many musculoskeletal masses, CT can still play an important role. Osseous neoplasms that produce mineralized matrix are often better evaluated by CT.[161,162] CT allows improved characterization of the matrix, particularly important when this is subtle, to determine if the lesion is of osteoid or chondroid derivation.

Numerous primary osseous neoplasms occur about the hip; however, commonly encountered lesions include osteoid osteoma, chondroblastoma, and chondrosarcoma. Patients' symptoms usually include nonspecific pain. Radiography should be the initial imaging in any case of suspected osseous neoplasms. The radiographs are of primary importance to identify the lesion,

characterize its margin and aggressiveness, detect any matrix formation, and provide a reasonable differential diagnosis. CT and/or MR imaging may then be performed to further characterize the lesion and delineate its extent.

Osteoid osteoma is common, accounting for 10% to 12% of primary benign skeletal neoplasms.[81] These lesions are seldom larger than 1.5 to 2.0 cm in diameter and are classified by their location as cortical, cancellous, or rarely subperiosteal. Cortical lesions are most frequent in long bones such as the tibia and femur and are usually easily identified as a small radiolucent nidus with extensive reactive sclerosis. The cancellous lesions are most common about the hip, with the proximal femur involved more frequently than the acetabulum. These lesions are often very difficult to detect on radiographs because of their small size and lack of prominent reactive sclerosis resulting from limited periosteal tissue in this region.[35] Patients' clinical findings suggest inflammatory synovitis, and the classic history of night pain relieved by aspirin may not be apparent. Patients are usually between 10 and 20 years of age, and males are affected about 2 to 3 times as frequently as females.[81] Radiographs of the hip may be nonspecific, showing disuse osteopenia. Periosteal reaction may only be seen inferior to the joint capsule attachment, in the subtrochanteric region.[76] Because of these difficulties, CT is often of great help in identifying these lesions and is usually preferable to MR imaging. On CT scans the nidus is a well-defined area of decreased attenuation with a variable degree of surrounding reactive sclerosis (Fig. 42-16, *A*). The nidus, which is composed of osteoid and woven bone, may show mineralization on CT in approximately

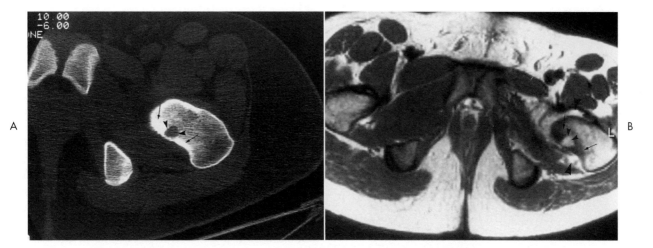

Fig. 42-16. Intraarticular osteoid osteoma in a 16-year-old boy with hip and knee pain. **A,** CT shows a focal low-attenuation nidus *(small arrowheads)* in the endosteal region of the femoral neck medially with mild associated reactive sclerosis *(arrows)*. **B,** Proton density axial MR image reveals osteoid osteoma nidus of intermediate intensity *(small arrowheads)* with reactive sclerosis showing low signal *(arrows)*. Reactive joint effusion resulting from lymphofollicular synovitis is also seen *(large arrowheads)*.

50% of cases.[61,81,134] This mineralization is usually a solitary central focus within the nidus but may be ringlike or multifocal; rarely, the entire nidus is ossified. MR imaging is usually not necessary to detect these lesions, and the appearance has reported to be quite variable, depending on the degree of mineralization. The nidus may be low to intermediate intensity on T1-weighted MR images. On T2-weighted MR images, the nidus may remain low to intermediate intensity if mineralized, or it may be of signal intensity similar to fat or higher if nonmineralized (Fig. 42-16, *B*).[61,81] This can create a target appearance, with the low intensity rim representing sclerosis. There may be extensive marrow edema surrounding the nidus that can obscure the lesion on long TR images. Both CT and MR images may show an associated joint effusion resulting from a lymphofollicular synovitis, as well as contrast enhancement of the vascular nidus (Fig. 42-16, *B*). A reactive soft-tissue mass has been reported on MR imaging, with osteoid osteoma.[20,166] However, this should not be surprising or confused with a more aggressive process. It represents another manifestation of associated inflammatory response seen with these lesions. CT is invaluable for localizing the nidus for the orthopedic surgeon before open resection and can also be used to direct needle placement before surgical removal.[77,141] In addition, CT can be used to treat osteoid osteoma by guiding core needle or electrode placement for percutaneous removal (Fig. 42-17) or ablation, respectively, while the patient is on the CT table.[8,47,105,129]

Chondroblastoma is a benign chondroid neoplasm involving primarily the epiphysis of young patients between 10 and 20 years of age. One of the most common sites is the proximal femur, which is involved in 16% of cases.[25] The lesion is usually seen on radiographs as a radiolucency within the epiphysis eccentrically (Fig. 42-18, *A*) that may extend into the metaphysis (55% of cases).[126] There is usually a rim of surrounding sclerosis. Thick periosteal reaction may be seen in 50% of patients with proximal femoral lesions.[29] The periosteal reaction is distal to the lesion about the femoral neck and subtrochanteric region (Fig 42-18). The differential diagnosis of epiphyseal lesions in the proximal femur includes eosinophilic granuloma and infection. CT can be helpful to detect distinctive chondroid calcification (ring and arc appearance) that is present in up to 60% of cases of chondroblastoma and which can be difficult to identify on radiographs (Fig. 42-18, *B*).[25] MR imaging shows marrow replacement within the lesion (seen on T1-weighted images) that may stay low intensity on long TR images or may become high intensity. Persistent low intensity in chondroblastoma on long TR images is unusual for most osseous neoplasms. This appearance is seen in chondroblastomas with high cellularity and less mature chondroid (Fig. 42-18, *C*). Areas of chondroid mineralization will also stay low intensity on all MR pulse sequences. As with osteoid osteomas, MR imaging may show extensive surrounding marrow edema with chondroblastoma. In addition, both CT and MR images may show hip joint effusion with chondroblastoma (Fig. 42-18).

Numerous differing primary and metastatic osseous malignancies can occur about the hip. Multiple myeloma and metastatic foci are well evaluated by MR imaging and typically show marrow replacement on T1-weighted images and high signal intensity on long TR

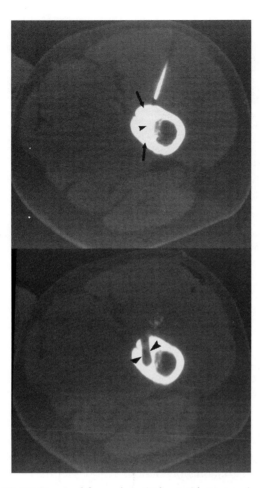

Fig. 42-17. Proximal femoral cortical osteoid osteoma in a 22-year-old man with percutaneous removal under general anesthesia on CT scanner. CT scans show initial localizing needle placement *(upper image)* directed toward the low attenuation nidus *(small arrowhead)*. Marked reactive cortical thickening is present *(arrows)*. Craig needle apparatus was then used to remove a core of bone including the nidus. The core tract is seen *(lower image, large arrowheads)* with removal of the low attenuation nidus. Patient was discharged from hospital within 1 day of this procedure.

images (Fig. 42-19). Myelomatous areas of involvement, diffuse or focal, occasionally stay low intensity on T2-weighted MR images (Fig. 42-19).[45,112,122,123] Osteoblastic metastases often show significant areas of low intensity on T2-weighted MR images corresponding to the sclerosis, and high attenuation on CT. The size, extent, and presence of associated soft-tissue mass are well evaluated on MR imaging; this information can be important in patient management.

CT shows myeloma and lytic metastatic lesions as areas of higher attenuation in the marrow space, and the degree of cortical involvement is easily assessed. CT and MR imaging are helpful in evaluating metastatic and myelomatous lesions to determine impending

pathologic fracture of the proximal femur (high-risk if lesion is larger than 2 to 3 cm in size or greater than 50% of the cortex is involved) and to guide the need for prophylactic fixation and radiation therapy (Fig. 42-19).[59,148]

Chondrosarcoma is one of the more frequent primary bone malignancies to involve the osseous structures about the hip. Approximately 25% of all chondrosarcomas involve the pelvis, with many occurring about the proximal femur (particularly the clear-cell variety) and acetabulum in the region of the triradiate cartilage (Fig. 42-20).[119,126] CT can be very helpful in identifying and characterizing the chondroid matrix, appearing as rings and arcs of calcification, in cases in which radiographs are not adequate because of both lack of contrast resolution and complex pelvic anatomy (Fig. 42-20, *B*).[6,40] CT also allows identification of any associated soft-tissue mass, which is frequent in higher grade chondrosarcomas (up to 50% of cases).[126,159] MR imaging is superior to CT in demonstrating the extent of marrow and soft-tissue involvement in chondrosarcoma or other osseous neoplasms about the hip. Marrow replacement is seen on T1-weighted images, and relative high intensity is seen on T2-weighted images. Mineralization is of low intensity on all pulse sequences; however, it is less well characterized than on CT.[159] The multiplanar imaging capability of MR is important in assessing osseous neoplasms about the hip for surgical planning. Detection of hip joint invasion is particularly important because resection of structures on both sides of the joint is then required. Involvement of the joint is usually best shown on coronal and sagittal images with soft-tissue mass within the articulation, and associated effusion (Fig. 42-20, *C*). The absence of a joint effusion in cases of osseous malignancy about the hip essentially excludes joint involvement, in my experience.

Soft-tissue masses about the hip, both benign and malignant, are not infrequent.[50,77] MR imaging has largely supplanted CT as the modality of choice in evaluation of these masses.[145,161,162] A specific histologic diagnosis by MR imaging is apparent in a relative minority of cases (lipoma, hemangioma); however, the contrast resolution of MR imaging allows exquisite distinction of tumor from surrounding soft tissue and osseous structures.[80,82] Staging of soft-tissue neoplasm for presurgical planning is also aided by the multiplanar imaging capability of MRI.[139,142]

MR imaging is also important to assess the effects of chemotherapy and radiation therapy on tumor size and extent, for both osseous and soft-tissue components of musculoskeletal neoplasms.[52,155,156] In general, a decreased intensity on T1-weighted images and an increased intensity on long TR images suggest a

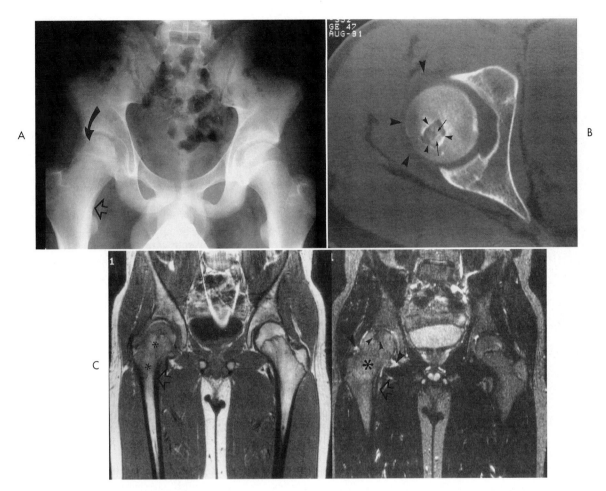

Fig. 42-18. Chondroblastoma of the right femoral head in a 14-year-old boy with several months of hip pain. **A,** Pelvis radiograph shows deformity of right femoral head with periosteal reaction in the medial femoral neck *(open arrow)*. Lytic lesion *(curved arrow)* is difficult to detect. **B,** CT reveals the lytic lesion *(small arrowheads)* with surrounding sclerosis and chondroid matrix within the chondroblastoma *(arrows)*. Joint effusion is also identified *(large arrowheads)*. Coronal T1-weighted MR image (**C,** *left image*) reveals diffuse marrow replacement in the right proximal femur (*) with the chondroblastoma difficult to distinguish as focal lesion. Periosteal reaction is seen as increased intensity within the medial femoral neck cortex *(open arrow)*. Coronal T2-weighted MR image (**C,** *right image*) shows diffuse mild increased marrow signal intensity in the right femur from edema (*). The chondroblastoma shows low intensity *(small arrowheads)* because of chondroid matrix and high cellularity (proven at pathology). Associated high signal intensity joint effusion *(large arrowheads)* and periosteal reaction *(open arrow)* are also seen.

response to therapy with necrosis and edema. MR imaging is also vital in postoperative evaluation to detect early soft-tissue recurrence. Edema resulting from surgery and radiation results in irregular, nonlocalized, often linear areas of high intensity on long TR images that does not disrupt the muscle texture pattern on T1-weighted images.[21,155,156] However, any nodular regions not characteristic of fluid (seroma or lymphocele) that disrupt the muscle textural pattern on T1-weighted images should be considered residual or recurrent tumor.[21] Recurrent osseous neoplasm will be

seen as new areas of marrow replacement. MR images after the intravenous injection of gadolinium is useful to distinguish vascular tissue (neoplasm, granulation tissue, inflammation) from nonvascular components (hemorrhage, necrosis, seroma, lymphocele, abscess) following surgery.[52,155] Vanel and co-workers have suggested that tumor recurrence can be distinguished from other tissues using dynamic contrast-enhanced subtraction MR imaging.[156] Neoplastic tissue shows enhancement in the early stages (first 2 minutes), in contrast to nonneoplastic tissue, which enhances at a later time.[156]

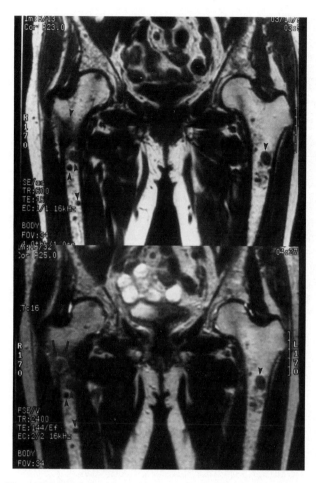

Fig. 42-19. Multiple myeloma involvement of the proximal femora in a 65-year-old woman. Coronal T1-weighted *(upper image)* and T2-weighted *(lower image)* MR images reveal multiple focal areas of marrow replacement *(arrowheads)* resulting from myelomatous involvement. The majority of these lesions remain low intensity on the T2-weighted image, although in the right femur the largest lesion shows mild increased intensity *(arrows)*. The size of this lesion suggests impending pathologic fracture, and the right femur was prophylactically internally fixed with an intramedullary rod.

AVASCULAR NECROSIS AND TRANSIENT OSTEOPOROSIS

Osteonecrosis of the hip is caused by insufficient vascular supply to the femoral head. Avascular necrosis (AVN) of the femoral head results from numerous abnormalities including trauma, steroids, collagen vascular disease, alcoholism, pancreatitis, hemoglobinopathies, and Gaucher's disease.[30,49,126] AVN may also be idiopathic both in adults and children (Legg-Calvé-Perthes disease). Traumatic osteonecrosis is the most frequent cause of AVN, usually related to femoral neck fracture or hip dislocation, with increasing incidence associated with the degree of displacement and delay in reduction.[49] AVN related to trauma is usually unilateral,

whereas nontraumatic osteonecrosis is commonly bilateral in up to 70% of patients.[49] The frequent sequelae of AVN, collapse and joint deformity with subsequent osteoarthritis and pain often leads to orthopedic intervention. Numerous treatment modalities are available, including a variety of joint replacements, joint fusion, or joint-preserving surgery such as core decompression or osteotomy. The use and success of core decompression, which reduces the intramedullary pressure that many authors believe is the underlying cause of AVN, is controversial in reports in the orthopedic literature.[16,36] However, there is general agreement that this procedure, if used, must be performed at the earliest stages of AVN to be of significant benefit.

Various staging systems have been used to assess femoral head AVN, with the most frequent classification being that developed by Ficat and Arlet.[7] This system is based on conventional radiographs. In stage 0 disease, patients are asymptomatic as shown by normal radiographs and bone scan; only biopsy reveals changes of AVN. Stage 1 disease corresponds to patients with pain, decreased range of motion, abnormal bone scan, and normal radiographs. In stage 2, radiographs show femoral head osteoporosis with areas of cystic lucency and sclerosis that progress to the subchondral collapse (crescent sign) in stage 3 disease. Stage 4 disease corresponds to progressive femoral head collapse with normal hip joint space. Finally, in stage 5, there are secondary osteoarthritic changes on both the femoral and acetabular sides of the joint, with narrowing.

MR imaging is clearly the most sensitive and specific radiologic modality currently available to detect the early changes of AVN of the femoral head.[28,39,55] The sensitivity of MR in detecting AVN in symptomatic patients has ranged from 88% to 100% in studies of Markisz et al and Beltran and co-workers; sensitivity was 10% to 20% more than with bone scan.[15,100] However, there is some delay between the histologic changes and development of MR imaging abnormalities of AVN; the extent of this gap remains unclear.[55,57,147]

The typical marrow pattern seen on MR imaging with AVN is variably sized areas of decreased intensity on T1-weighted images, usually in the anterosuperior subchondral aspect of the femoral head (Figs. 42-21, 22). This area may be homogeneous or heterogeneous with band, ring, wedge or crescentic configuration, often with regions of higher signal intensity centrally.[151] In the study by Mitchell and co-workers, this defect was present in 96% of patients, with the rim remaining low intensity on both T1-weighted images (94% of cases) and on long TR/TE sequences (86% of cases) (Fig. 42-21).[108-110] The appearance of AVN on long TR/TE MR images is more variable but often adds specificity. A high-signal intensity line within the low-intensity rim ("double

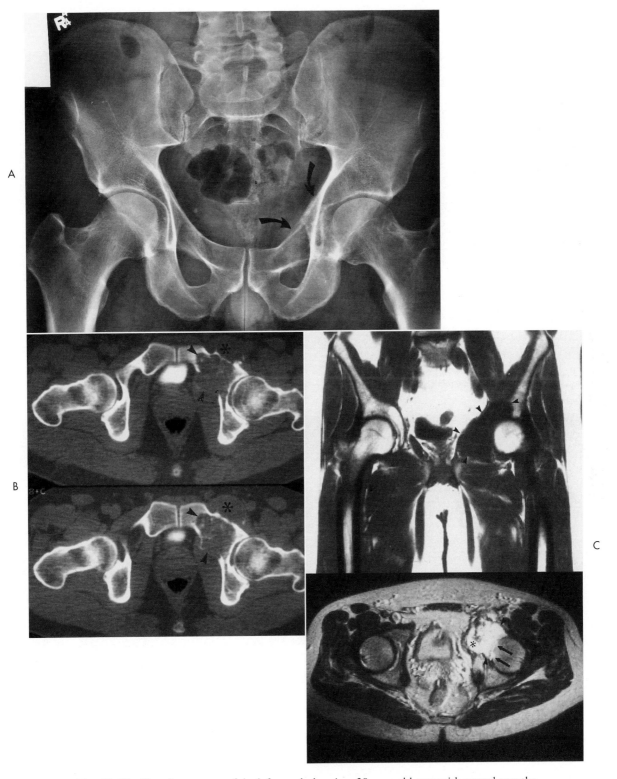

Fig. 42-20. Chondrosarcoma of the left acetabulum in a 30-year-old man with several months history of vague hip pain. **A,** Pelvis radiograph shows subtle aggressive bone destruction of the medial left acetabulum with permeation of the iliopectineal line *(curved arrows)*. **B,** CT scans show bone destruction with chondroid matrix formation *(large arrowheads)* and associated soft tissue mass (*). Coronal T1-weighted image (**C,** *upper image*) and axial T2-weighted image (**C,** *lower image*) reveal marrow replacement *(small arrowheads)* and soft tissue mass (*) which becomes high signal intensity on the long TR/TE image. The soft tissue mass has invaded the hip joint as evidenced by the fact that the soft mass abuts the femoral head *(arrows)*.

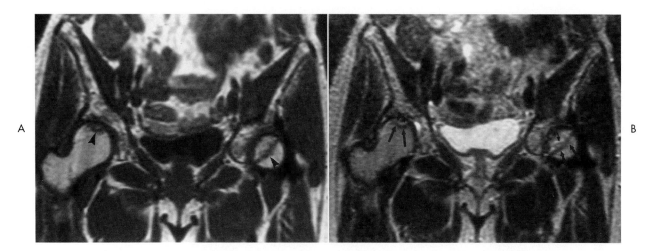

Fig. 42-21. Avascular necrosis (AVN) of both femoral heads in a 41-year-old woman on steroids for longstanding SLE. **A,** Coronal T1-weighted MR image shows focal crescentic areas of decreased marrow signal typical of AVN in both femoral heads *(arrowheads)*. **B,** Coronal T2-weighted MR image shows linear high signal *(small arrows)* with persistent low signal rim *(large arrows)* consistent with the "double outline sign" characteristic of AVN. The area of AVN has fatlike signal on the left typical of class A changes and predominantly low signal intensity on the right (fibrous tissue) typical of class D changes.

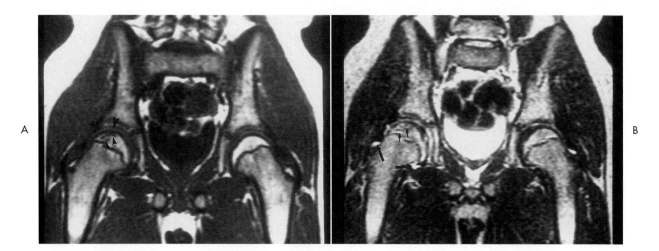

Fig. 42-22. Legg-Calve-Perthes disease in a 7-year-old boy with recent onset of right hip pain. Pelvic radiographs (not shown) were normal. **A,** Coronal T1-weighted MR image shows band-like areas of marrow replacement in the superolateral aspect of the right femoral head *(small arrowheads)*. Overlying cartilage *(large arrowheads)* appears intact, and femoral head is well covered by the acetabulum. **B,** Coronal T2-weighted image reveals the areas of AVN to be largely high signal intensity *(small arrows)* consistent with class C changes (fluid-like). Small associated joint effusion is also present *(large arrows)*.

outline" sign) has been described in 80% of patients with AVN in one series (Fig. 42-21, *B*).[108-110] Mitchell and co-workers have developed an MR imaging classification scheme based on the appearance of the central zone.[108-110] This area may simulate fat (Class A: high signal on short TR/TE images, intermediate on T2-weighting [Fig. 42-21]), blood (Class B: high signal on short and long TR/TE images), fluid (Class C: low signal on short TR/TE images and high intensity on long TR/TE images [fig. 42-22]), or fibrous tissue (Class D: low signal on all images [Fig. 42-21]). Class A and B changes appear to correspond to early stages 1 and 2 of AVN, while Class C and D correlate with the later stages 3 and 4.[108-110] In addition, clinical symptoms are usually most severe with class D changes and least prominent with class A findings. The MR imaging findings correspond to the histologic changes seen with AVN. Areas of low intensity on all sequences correspond to fibrosis or sclerosis, whereas regions of low intensity on short TR/TE images that become high intensity on long TR/TE images represent granulation tissue attempting to repair avascular regions. Marrow with residual high signal intensity on short TR/TE images represents necrotic tissue that is not invaded by granulation tissue. The manifestations of AVN are usually best evaluated on coronal MR images; however, sagittal and axial sequences can be helpful in assessing regions of collapse.[87] MR imaging may also be useful in the assessment of patients with AVN after core decompression, to evaluate for revascularization, further collapse, and any change in the volume of tissue involved.[113,150]

MR imaging of AVN may occasionally be nonspecific and show only diffuse marrow edema without focal defects as described in six patients by Turner and colleagues.[152] This pattern can also be seen with transient osteoporosis of the hip. Use of intravenous contrast medium may help in this distinction and in earlier recognition of AVN. Areas of contrast enhancement are seen in regions of viable marrow and granulation tissue, whereas avascular regions will be nonenhancing.[94,151] Additional associated MR findings with AVN are small hip joint effusion and premature conversion of hematopoietic to fatty marrow. This premature conversion was seen in over 60% of patients with AVN in the study by Mitchell et al and may be caused by ischemia.[107]

MR imaging in Legg-Calvé-Perthe disease shows identical changes as in other causes of AVN (Fig. 42-22). The capital femoral epiphysis often reveals necrosis centrally, with peripheral portions of viable epiphysis.[48,49] Peripheral portions of viable epiphysis may also develop or increase in size with revascularization and healing.[48,135] This is important for treatment because viability of the lateral aspect of the epiphysis corresponds to a reduced risk of further deformity or to an extension of AVN.[135] In these patients, bracing can be discontinued and the patient can begin weight bearing. MR imaging can also assess the shape of the cartilaginous portions of the femoral head and the degree of containment by the acetabulum. This determination is vital in identifying those children who require treatment by an osteotomy (25% of patients). This information previously required arthrography.[48]

CT is less sensitive than MR imaging in detecting AVN. The earliest sign on CT of AVN is alteration of the asterisk, which is a starlike condensation of trabeculae within the femoral head.[44] Changes in the asterisk in early AVN have been described as central or peripheral clumping or sclerosis (Fig. 42-23). CT is probably superior to MR imaging in longstanding AVN to delin-

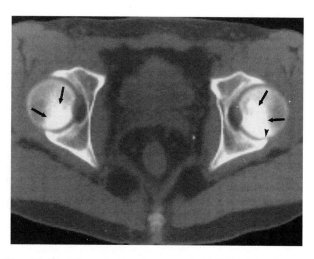

Fig. 42-23. Bilateral avascular necrosis (AVN) of the femoral heads in a 22-year-old man on steroids for Crohn's disease. CT shows focal sclerosis in both femoral heads posteriorly (*arrows*) typical of AVN with minimal cortical collapse (*arrowhead*) on the left.

eate structural deformity of the femoral head such as subchondral fracture, collapse, and calcified intraarticular fragments. In cases in which osteotomy is planned as a temporizing procedure, CT is often useful in determining which femoral surface is best preserved.[98,133] This information guides the surgeon in determining the feasibility and type of osteotomy to perform.

Transient osteoporosis of the hip, as originally described in women, almost exclusively involved the left hip in the third trimester of pregnancy.[49,126] It is now recognized as being actually more common in middle-aged men in either hip. Patients' symptoms are severe hip pain and decreased range of motion that resolves spontaneously in 6 to 12 months.[163] The etiology is poorly understood, and the disease has been associated with a type of reflex sympathetic dystrophy syndrome. It may be migratory, with subsequent involvement of the opposite hip or an adjacent joint. Radiologic changes may simulate indolent infection, osteonecrosis, or infiltrative neoplasm. The underlying pathologic condition appears to be bone marrow edema.[66] Current terminology may refer to this entity as transient bone marrow edema syndrome.

Radiographs usually show osteopenia, and bone scan reveals intense activity focally within the femoral head (unlike AVN, which often has central photopenia). MR imaging demonstrates diffuse marrow abnormalities that usually extend from the subchondral femoral head to the intertrochanteric and subtrochanteric regions. There is low signal intensity on T1-weighted MR images and high signal intensity on T2-weighted sequences (Fig. 42-24).[2,24,63] These MR imaging changes reflect the

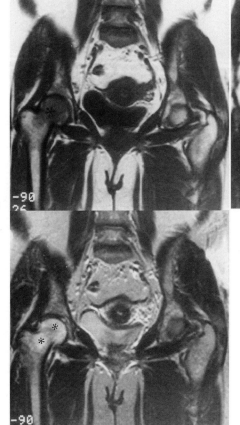
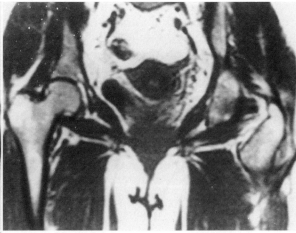

Fig. 42-24. Transient osteoporosis of the hip in a 47-year-old woman with several months history of right hip pain. Pelvis radiograph and bone scan (not shown) revealed osteopenia of the right proximal femur and diffuse marked increased activity about the right femoral head, respectively. Coronal T1-weighted (**A,** *upper image*) and T2-weighted (**A,** *lower image*) MR images show marrow replacement in the right femoral head and neck that becomes high intensity on the long TR image (*) consistent with marrow edema. Three months later symptoms had resolved and T1-weighted coronal MR image (**B**) has largely returned to normal. No focal subchondral areas of marrow replacement are seen on any image to suggest avascular necrosis.

nonspecific marrow edema that is present. Focal marrow defects in the subchondral region should be searched for diligently on MR imaging, because in contrast to AVN these are usually absent in transient osteoporosis. Intravenous gadolinium injection may also be useful in these patients to help distinguish AVN from transient osteoporosis.[65,66,157] In transient osteoporosis there will be mild diffuse homogeneous enhancement of the marrow space and edema seen on postinjection T1-weighted images, greater than that seen in contralateral normal femoral marrow (Fig. 42-25). This is in contradistinction to AVN, in which contrast enhancement is heterogeneous with avascular foci showing persistent low intensity signal resulting from lack of enhancement. According to Bloem and colleagues, MR imaging changes will gradually improve in transient osteoporosis of the hip without residual defects in a 6- to 10-month time frame, and return to normal marrow signal (Fig. 42-24, *B*).[24,90] These MR imaging findings will lag behind clinical improvement.

The relationship between transient osteoporosis of the hip and AVN is unclear. However, some researchers now believe that both entities are related, with marrow edema being the important common pathologic fea-

ture.[66] Transient osteoporosis of the hip could thus represent a forme fruste of AVN, with ischemia and resultant edema that for some reason does not progress to focal necrosis. Turner and colleagues recently reported six patients with a bone marrow edema pattern seen on MR imaging without focal defects that showed AVN at biopsy.[152] Studies with larger numbers of patients are required to further investigate the relationship between these two conditions.

CONCLUSION

Joint pain is a frequent presenting clinical symptom for a variety of pathologic conditions that can involve the hip. Radiographs should be the initial radiologic study performed to assess these patients. Although radiographs may provide diagnostic information in some cases, in many instances further imaging is necessary. CT, and more recently MR imaging, are the radiologic modalities of choice to provide this additional assessment. In this chapter I have attempted to describe and illustrate the CT and MR imaging appearances of commonly encountered pathologic conditions involving the hip. Recognition of these characteristics as seen on CT and MR imaging is important to provide our clinical col-

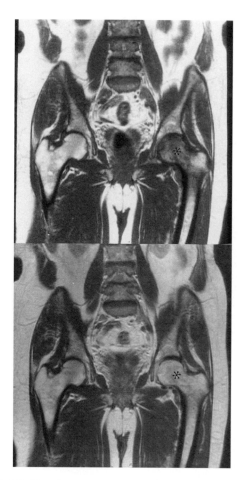

Fig. 42-25. Transient osteoporosis of the hip in a 77-year-old man with a 3 month history of left hip pain. Coronal T1-weighted MR images before *(upper image)* and after intravenous gadolinium injection *(lower image)* show marrow replacement diffusely in the left femoral head and neck (*) that enhances with contrast to become isointense to normal marrow (*), respectively. No focal nonenhancing areas are seen as would be expected with avascular necrosis. Long TR MR image (not shown) revealed increased intensity in the left femoral head and neck consistent with edema and small joint effusion. Patient symptoms and MR imaging changes resolved over the next three months without treatment.

leagues with specific information that often allows diagnosis and directs patient management.

REFERENCES

1. Adam B, et al: Rheumatoid arthritis of the knee: value of gado-pentetate dimeglumine-enhanced MR imaging. *AJR* 156:125, 1991.
2. Alarcon GS, Sanders C, Daniel WW: Transient osteoporosis of the hip: magnetic resonance imaging. *J Rheumatol* 14:1184, 1987.
3. Anda S, Terjesen T, Kvistad KA: Computed tomography measurements of the acetabulum in adult dysplastic hips: which level is appropriate? *Skeletal Radiol* 20:267, 1991.
4. Anda S, et al: Acetabular angles and femoral anteversion in dysplastic hips in adults. *J Comput Assist Tomogr* 15:115, 1991.
5. Angel JL: The reaction area of the femoral neck. *Clin Orthop* 32:130, 1964.
6. Aoki J, et al: MR of enchondroma and chondrosarcoma: rings and arcs of Gd-DTPA enhancement. *J Comput Assist Tomogr* 15:1011, 1991.
7. Arlet J, Ficat RP: Diagnostic de l'osteo-necrose femoro-capitale primitive au stade. *I Rev Chir Orthop* 54:637, 1968.
8. Assoun J, et al: Osteoid osteoma: percutaneous resection with CT guidance. *Radiology* 188:541, 1993.
9. Athanasou NA, et al: Joint and systemic distribution of dialysis amyloid. *Radiology* 181:616, 1991 (abstract).
10. Azouz EM: Computed tomography in bone and joint infections. *J Can Assoc Radiol* 32:102, 1981.
11. Baird RA, et al: Radiographic identification of loose bodies in the traumatized hip joint. *Radiology* 145:661, 1982.
12. Balsara AN, Stainken BF, Martinez AJ: MR image of localized giant cell tumor of the tendon sheath involving the knee. *J Comput Assist Tomogr* 13:159, 1989.
13. Bardin T, et al: Synovial amyloidosis in patients undergoing long-term hemodialysis. *Arthritis Rheum* 28:1052, 1985.
14. Beltran J, et al: Infections of the musculoskeletal system: high-field-strength MR imaging. *Radiology* 164:449, 1987.
15. Beltran J, et al: Femoral head avascular necrosis: MR imaging with clinical-pathologic and radionuclide correlations. *Radiology* 166:215, 1988.
16. Beltran J, et al: Core decompression for avascular necrosis of the femoral head: correlation between long-term results and preoperative MR staging. *Radiology* 175:533, 1990.
17. Berger PE, et al: MRI demonstration of radiographically occult fractures: what have we been missing? *RadioGraphics* 9:407, 1989.
18. Berquist TH, et al: Magnetic resonance imaging: application in musculoskeletal infection. *Magn Reson Imaging* 3:219, 1985.
19. Bessette PR, et al: Gadolinium-enhanced MRI of pigmented villonodular synovitis of the knee. *J Comput Assist Tomogr* 16:992, 1992.
20. Biebuyck J-C, Katz LD, McCauley TR: Soft tissue edema in osteoid osteoma. *Skeletal Radiol* 22:37, 1993.
21. Biondetti PR, Ehman RL: Soft-tissue sarcomas: use of textural patterns in skeletal muscle as a diagnostic feature in postoperative MR imaging. *Radiology* 183:845, 1992.
22. Bjorkengren AG, et al: MR imaging of the knee in acute rheumatoid arthritis: synovial uptake of gadolinium-DOTA. *AJR* 155:329, 1990.
23. Blacksin MF, et al: Synovial chondromatosis of the hip: evaluation with air computed arthrotomography. *Clin Imaging* 14:315, 1990.
24. Bloem JL: Transient osteoporosis of the hip: MR imaging. *Radiology* 167:753, 1988.
25. Bloom JL, Mulder JD: Chondroblastoma: clinical and radiological study of 104 cases. *Radiology* 157:851, 1985 (abstract).
26. Bongartz GE, et al: Degenerative cartilage lesions of the hip—magnetic resonance evaluation. *Magn Reson Imaging* 7:179, 1989.
27. Brody AS, Ball WS Jr, Towbin RB: Computed arthrotomography as an adjunct to pediatric arthrography. *Radiology* 170:99, 1989.
28. Brody AS, et al: Avascular necrosis: early MR imaging and histologic findings in a canine model. *AJR* 157:341, 1991.
29. Brower AC, Kransdorf MJ, Moser RP: Frequency and diagnostic significance of periostitis in chondroblastoma. *AJR* 154:309, 1990.
30. Brower AC, Kransdorf MJ: Imaging of hip disorders. *Radiol Clin North Am* 28:955, 1990.

31. Burnstein MI, et al: Case Report 502, *Skeletal Radiol* 17:458, 1988.

32. Butt YP, Hardy G, Ostlere SJ: Pigmented villonodular synovitis of the knee: computed tomographic appearances. *Skeletal Radiol* 19:191, 1990.

33. Camacho CR, et al: Radiological findings of amyloid arthropathy in long-term hemodialysis. *Eur Radiol* 2-4:305, 1992.

34. Casey TT, et al: Tumoral amyloidosis of bone of beta-2-microglobulin origin in association with long term hemodialysis: a new type of amyloid disease. *Hum Pathol* 17:731, 1986.

35. Cassar-Pullicino VN, McCall IW, Wan S: Intra-articular osteoid osteoma. *Clin Radiol* 45:153, 1992.

36. Chan T, et al: Aseptic necrosis of the femoral head: progression of MRI appearance following core decompression and grafting. *Skeletal Radiol* 20:103, 1991.

37. Cobby MJ, et al: Dialysis-related amyloid arthropathy: MR findings in four patients. *AJR* 157:1023, 1991.

38. Cohen MD, et al: Magnetic resonance differentiation of acute and chronic osteomyelitis in children. *Clin Radiol* 41:53, 1990.

39. Coleman BG, et al: Radiographically negative avascular necrosis: detection with MR imaging. *Radiology* 168:525, 1988.

40. Crim JR Seeger LL: Diagnosis of low-grade chondrosarcoma. *Radiology* 189:504, 1993.

41. Dangman BC, et al: Osteomyelitis in children: gadolinium-enhanced MR imaging. *Radiology* 182:743, 1992.

42. Darrason R, et al: Role of arteriography and x-ray computed tomography in the current evaluation of pigmented villonodular synovitis. *J Radiol* 69:645, 1988.

43. Deutsch AL, Mink JH, Waxman AD: Occult fractures of the proximal femur: MR imaging. *Radiology* 170:113, 1989.

44. Dihlmann W: CT analysis of the upper end of the femur: the asterisk sign and ischemic bone necrosis of the femoral head. *Skeletal Radiol* 8:251, 1982.

45. Dooms GC, et al: MR imaging of intramuscular hemorrhage. *J Comput Assist Tomogr* 9:908, 1986.

46. Dorwart RH, et al: Pigmented villonodular synovitis of synovial joints: clinical, pathologic and radiologic features. *AJR* 143:877, 1984.

47. Doyle T, King K: Percutaneous removal of osteoid osteomas using CT control. *Clin Radiol* 40:514, 1989.

48. Egund N, Wingstrand H: Legg-Calve-Perthes disease: imaging with MR. *Radiology* 179:89, 1991.

49. Ensign MF: Magnetic resonance imaging of hip disorders. *Semin Ultrasound, CT MR* 11:288, 1990.

50. Enzinger FM, Weiss SW: *Soft tissue tumors,* ed 2, St. Louis, 1988, Mosby.

51. Erdman WA, et al: Osteomyelitis characteristics and pitfalls of diagnosis with MR imaging. *Radiology* 180:533, 1991.

52. Erlemann R, et al: Musculoskeletal neoplasms: static and dynamic Gd-DTPA-enhanced MR imaging. *Radiology* 171:767, 1989.

53. Fishman EK, et al: Advanced three-dimensional evaluation of acetabular trauma: volumetric image processing. *J Trauma* 29(2):214, 1989.

54. Flandry F, Hughston JC: Current concepts review pigmented villonodular synovitis. *J Bone Joint Surg* 69A(6):942, 1987.

55. Genez BM, et al: Early osteonecrosis of the femoral head: detection in high-risk patients with MR imaging. *Radiology* 168:521, 1988.

56. Gielen JL, et al: Growing bone cysts in long-term hemodialysis. *Skeletal Radiol* 19:43, 1990.

57. Glickstein MF, et al: Avascular necrosis versus other diseases of the hip: sensitivity of MR imaging. *Radiology* 169:213, 1988.

58. Gold RH, Hawkins RA, Katz RD: Bacterial osteomyelitis: findings on plain radiography, CT, MR, and scintigraphy. *AJR* 157:365, 1991.

59. Gold RI, et al: An integrated approach to the evaluation of metastatic bone disease. *Radiol Clin North Am* 28(2):471, 1990.

60. Goldman AB, DiCarlo EF: Pigmented villonodular synovitis: diagnosis and differential diagnosis. *Radiol Clin North Am* 26:1327, 1988.

61. Goldman AB, Schneider R, Pavlov H: Osteoid osteomas of the femoral neck: report of four cases evaluated with isotopic bone scanning, CT and MR imaging. *Radiology* 186:227, 1993.

62. Griffiths HJ, et al: Computed tomography in the management of acetabular fractures. *Skeletal Radiol* 11:22, 1984.

63. Grimm J, et al: MRI of transient osteoporosis of the hip. *Arch Orthop Trauma Surg* 110:98, 1991.

64. Harley JD, Mack LA, Winquist RA: CT of acetabular fractures: comparison with conventional radiography. *AJR* 138:413, 1982.

65. Hauzeur JP, et al: Study of magnetic resonance imaging in transient osteoporosis of the hip. *J Rheumatol* 18:1211, 1991.

66. Hayes CW, Conway WF, Daniel WW: MR imaging of bone marrow edema pattern: transient osteoporosis, transient bone marrow edema syndrome, or osteonecrosis. *RadioGraphics* 13:1001, 1993.

67. Hermann G, Gilbert MS, Abdelwahab IF: Hemophilia: evaluation of musculoskeletal involvement with CT, sonography, and MR imaging. *AJR* 158:119, 1992.

68. Hernandez RJ: Evaluation of congenital hip dysplasia and tibial torsion by computed tomography. *J Comput Tomogr* 7:101, 1983.

69. Jaffe HL: *Synovial chondromatosis and other articular tumors.* In *Tumors and tumorous conditions of the bones and joints,* Philadelphia, 1958, Lea & Febiger.

70. Jelinek JS, et al: Giant cell tumor of the tendon sheath: MR findings in nine cases. *AJR* 162:919, 1994.

71. Jelinek JS, et al: Imaging of pigmented villonodular synovitis with emphasis on MR imaging. *AJR* 152:337, 1989.

72. Johnson ND, et al: MR imaging anatomy of the infant hip. *AJR* 153:127, 1989.

73. Judet R, Judet J, Letournel E: Fractures of the acetabulum: classification and surgical approaches for open reduction. *J Bone Joint Surg* 46A:1615, 1964.

74. Karasick D, Karasick S: Giant cell tumor of tendon sheath: spectrum of radiologic findings. *Skeletal Radiol* 21:219, 1992.

75. Karlin CA: The variable manifestations of extraarticular synovial chondromatosis. *AJR* 137:731, 1981.

76. Klein MH, Shankman S: Osteoid osteoma: radiologic and pathologic correlation. *Skeletal Radiol* 21:23, 1992.

77. Kneisl JS, Simon MA: Medical management compared with operative treatment for osteoid-osteoma. *Radiology* 185:294, 1992 (abstract).

78. Konig H, Sieper J, Wolf K: Rheumatoid arthritis: evaluation of hypervascular and fibrous pannus with dynamic MR imaging enhanced with Gd-DTPA. *Radiology* 176:473, 1990.

79. Kottal RA, et al: Pigmented villonodular synovitis: a report of MR imaging in two cases. *Radiology* 163:551, 1987.

80. Kransdorf MJ, et al: Soft-tissue masses: diagnosis using MR imaging. *AJR* 153:541, 1989.

81. Kransdorf MJ, et al: From the archives of the AFIP: osteoid osteoma. *RadioGraphics* 11:671, 1991.

82. Kransdorf MJ, Meis JM: From the archives of the AFIP: extraskeletal osseous and cartilaginous tumors of the extremities. *RadioGraphics* 13:853, 1993.

83. Krasny R, et al: MR anatomy of infants hip: comparison to anatomical preparations. *Pediatr Radiol* 21:211, 1991.

84. Kulkarni MV, et al: MR imaging of hemophiliac arthropathy. *J Comput Assist Tomogr* 10:445, 1986.

85. Kursunoglu-Brahme ST, et al: Rheumatoid knee: role of gadopentetate-enhanced MR imaging. *Radiology* 176:831, 1990.

86. Lafferty CM, et al: Acetabular alterations in untreated congenital dysplasia of the hip: computed tomography with multiplanar reformation and three-dimensional analysis. *J Comput Assist Tomogr* 10(1):84, 1986.

87. Lafforgue P, et al: Early-stage avascular necrosis of the femoral head: MR imaging for prognosis in 31 cases with at least 2 years of follow-up. *Radiology* 187:199, 1993.

88. Lang P, et al: Three-dimensional CT and MR imaging in congenital dislocation of the hip: clinical and technical considerations. *J Comput Assist Tomogr* 12:459, 1988.

89. Lee JK, Yao L: Stress fractures: MR imaging. *Radiology* 169:217, 1988.

90. Leonidas JC: MR imaging of transient osteoporosis. *Radiology* 170:281, 1989.

91. Letournel E: Acetabulum fractures: classification and management. *Clin Orthop* 151:81, 1980.

92. Lewis SL, et al: Pitfalls of bone scintigraphy in suspected hip fractures. *Br J Radiol* 64:403, 1991.

93. Li KC, et al: MRI in osteoarthritis of the hip: gradations of severity. *Magn Reson Imaging* 6:229, 1988.

94. Li KCP, Hiette P: Contrast-enhanced fat saturation magnetic resonance imaging for studying the pathophysiology of osteonecrosis of the hips. *Skeletal Radiol* 21:375, 1992.

95. Libshitz HI, et al: Multiple myeloma: appearance at MR imaging. *Radiology* 182:833, 1992.

96. Liu S-K, Moroff S: Case Report 733. *Skeletal Radiol* 22:50, 1993.

97. Madewell JE, Sweet DE: *Tumors and tumor-like lesions in or about joints.* In Resnick D, Niwayama G, editors: *Diagnosis of bone and joint disorders,* ed 2, Philadelphia, 1988, WB Saunders, pp 3889-3943.

98. Magid D, et al: Femoral head avascular necrosis: CT assessment with multiplanar reconstruction. *Radiology* 157:751, 1985.

99. Maistrelli G, et al: Osteonecrosis of the hip treated by intertrochanteric osteotomy: a 4- to 15-year follow-up. *Radiology* 172:294, 1989 (abstract).

100. Markisz JA, et al: Segmental patterns of avascular necrosis of the femoral heads: early detection with MR imaging. *Radiology* 162:717, 1987.

101. Marti-Bonmati L, et al: Brodie abscess: MR imaging appearance in 10 patients. *J Magn Reson Imaging* 3:543, 1993.

102. Martinez CR, et al: Evaluation of acetabular fractures with two- and three-dimensional CT. *RadioGraphics* 12:227, 1992.

103. Mason MD, et al: Chronic complicated osteomyelitis of the lower extremity: evaluation with MR imaging. *Radiology* 173:355, 1989.

104. Matsuno T, Hasegawa I, Masuda T: Chondroblastoma arising in the triradiate cartilage: report of two cases with review of the literature. *Skeletal Radiol* 16:216, 1987.

105. Mazoyer J-F, Kohler R, Bossard D: Osteoid osteoma: CT-guided percutaneous treatment. *Radiology* 181:269, 1991.

106. Milgram JW: Synovial osteochondromatosis: a histopathological study of thirty cases. *J Bone Joint Surg* 59:792, 1977.

107. Mitchell DG, et al: Hematopoietic and fatty bone marrow distribution in the normal and ischemic hip: new observations with 1.5T MR imaging. *Radiology* 161:199, 1986.

108. Mitchell DG, et al: Avascular necrosis of the hip: comparison of MR, CT, and scintigraphy. *AJR* 147:67, 1986.

109. Mitchell DG, et al: Femoral head avascular necrosis: correlation with MR imaging, radiographic staging, radionuclide imaging, and clinical findings. *Radiology* 162:709, 1987.

110. Mitchell DG, et al: Avascular necrosis of the femoral head: morphologic assessment of MR imaging with CT correlation. *Radiology* 161:739, 1986.

111. Modic MT, et al: Magnetic resonance imaging of musculoskeletal infections. *Radiol Clin North Am* 24:247, 1986.

112. Moulopoulos LA, et al: Multiple myeloma: spinal MR imaging in patients with untreated newly diagnosed disease. *Radiology* 185:833, 1992.

113. Neuhold A, et al: Bone marrow edema of the hip: MR findings after core decompression. *J Comput Assist Tomogr* 16:951, 1992.

114. Nokes SR, et al: Herniation pits of the femoral neck: appearance at MR imaging. *Radiology* 172:231, 1989.

115. Norman A, Steiner GC: Bone erosion in synovial chondromatosis. *Radiology* 161:749, 1986.

116. Pennal GF, et al: Pelvis disruption: assessment and classification. *Clin Orthop* 151:12, 1980.

117. Peterson HA, et al: The use of computerized tomography in dislocation of the hip and femoral neck anteversion in children. *J Bone Joint Surg* 63B:198, 1981.

118. Pitt MJ, et al: Herniation pit of the femoral neck. *AJR* 138:1115, 1982.

119. Present D, et al: Clear cell chondrosarcoma of bone: a report of 8 cases. *Skeletal Radiol* 20:187, 1991.

120. Pritchard RS, et al: MR and CT appearance of iliopsoas bursal distention secondary to diseased hips. *J Comput Assist Tomogr* 14:797, 1990.

121. Quinn SF, McCarthy JL: Prospective evaluation of patients with suspected hip fracture and indeterminate radiographs: use of T1-weighted MR images. *Radiology* 187:469, 1993.

122. Rahmouni A, et al: MR appearance of multiple myeloma of the spine before and after treatment. *AJR* 160:1053, 1993.

123. Reinus WR, et al: Plasma cell tumors with calcified amyloid deposition mistaken for chondrosarcoma. *Radiology* 189:505, 1993.

124. Reiser MF, Naegele M: Inflammatory joint disease: static and dynamic gadolinium-enhanced MR imaging. *J Magn Reson Imaging* 3:307, 1993.

125. Reiser MF, et al: Gadolinium-DTPA in rheumatoid arthritis and related diseases: first results with dynamic magnetic resonance imaging. *Skeletal Radiol* 18:591, 1989.

126. Resnick D, Niwayama G: *Diagnosis of bone and joint disorders,* ed 2, Philadelphia, 1988, WB Saunders.

127. Richardson P, Young JWR, Porter D: CT detection of cortical fracture of the femoral head associated with posterior hip dislocation. *AJR* 155:93, 1990.

128. Rizzo PF, et al: Diagnosis of occult fractures about the hip: magnetic resonance imaging compared with bone-scanning. *Radiology* 189:295, 1993 (abstract).

129. Rosenthal D, et al: Ablation of osteoid osteomas with a percutaneously placed electrode: a new procedure. *Radiology* 183:29, 1992.

130. Ross LV, et al: Hemodialysis-related amyloidomas of bone. *Radiology* 178:263, 1991.

131. Rubin JI, et al: High-field MR imaging of extracranial hematomas. *AJR* 148:813, 1987.

132. Saks BJ: Normal acetabular anatomy for acetabular fracture assessment: CT and plain film correlation. *Radiology* 159:139, 1986.

133. Sartoris DJ, et al: Computed tomography with multiplanar reformation and 3-dimensional image analysis in the preoperative evaluation of ischemic necrosis of the femoral head. *J Rheumatol* 13:153, 1986.

134. Schlesinger AE, Hernandez RJ: Intracapsular osteoid osteoma of the proximal femur: findings on plain film and CT. *AJR* 154:1241, 1990.

135. Scoles PV, et al: Nuclear magnetic resonance imaging in Legg-Calve-Perthes disease. *J Bone Joint Surg* 66A:1357, 1984.

136. Scott WW Jr, Fishman EK, Magid D: Acetabular fractures: optimal imaging. *Radiology* 165:537, 1987.

137. Senac MO Jr, et al: MR imaging in juvenile rheumatoid arthritis. *AJR* 150:873, 1988.

138. Shirkoda A, Brashear R, Staab EV: Computed tomography of acetabular fractures, *Radiology* 134:683, 1980.

139. Shuman WP, et al: Comparison of STIR and spin-echo MR imaging at 1.5 T in 45 suspected extremity tumors: lesion conspicuity and extent. *Radiology* 179:247, 1991.

140. Spritzer CE, Dalinka MK, Kressel HY: Magnetic resonance imaging of pigmented villonodular synovitis: a report of two cases. *Skeletal Radiol* 16:316, 1987.

141. Steinberg GG, Coumas JM, Breen T: Preoperative localization of osteoid osteoma: a new technique that uses CT. *AJR* 155:883, 1990.

142. Sundaram M, McGuire MH, Herbold DR: Magnetic resonance imaging of soft tissue masses: an evaluation of fifty-three histologically proven tumors. *Magn Reson Imaging* 6:237, 1988.

143. Szypryt P, et al: Synovial chondromatosis of the hip joint presenting as a pathological fracture. *Br J Radiol* 59:399, 1986.

144. Tang JSH, et al: Musculoskeletal infection of the extremities: evaluation with MR imaging. *Radiology* 166:205, 1988.

145. Tehranzadeh J, et al: Comparison of CT and MR imaging in musculoskeletal neoplasms. *J Comput Assist Tomogr* 13:466, 1989.

146. Tehranzadeh J, Vanarthos W, Pais MJ: Osteochondral impaction of the femoral head associated with hip dislocation: CT study in 35 patients. *AJR* 155:1049, 1990.

147. Tervonen O, et al: Clinically occult avascular necrosis of the hip prevalence in an asymptomatic population at risk. *Radiology* 182:845, 1992.

148. Thrall JH, Ellis BI: Skeletal metastases. *Radiol Clin North Am* 25(6):1155, 1987.

149. Toby EB, Koman LA, Bechtold RE: Magnetic resonance imaging of pediatric hip disease. *J Pediatr Orthop* 5:665, 1985.

150. Tooke SM, et al: Results of core decompression for femoral head osteonecrosis. *Clin Orthop* 226:99, 1986.

151. Totty WG, et al: Magnetic resonance imaging of the normal and ischemic femoral head. *AJR* 143:1273, 1984.

152. Turner DA, et al: Femoral capital osteonecrosis: MR findings of diffuse marrow abnormalities without focal lesions. *Radiology* 171:135, 1989.

153. Unger EC, et al: Diagnosis of osteomyelitis by MR imaging. *AJR* 150:605, 1988.

154. Unger EC, et al: MRI of extracranial hematomas: preliminary observations. *AJR* 146:403, 1986.

155. Vanel D, et al: Musculoskeletal tumors: follow-up with MR imaging after treatment with surgery and radiation therapy. *Radiology* 164:243, 1987.

156. Vanel D, et al: Dynamic contrast-enhanced subtraction MR imaging in follow-up of aggressive soft-tissue tumors: a prospective study of 74 patients. *Radiology* 189(P):205, 1993.

157. Vande Berg BE, et al: Avascular necrosis of the hip: comparison of contrast-enhanced and nonenhanced MR imaging with histologic correlation. *Radiology* 182:445, 1992.

158. Varma DGK, et al: MR appearance of the distended iliopsoas bursa. *AJR* 156:1025, 1991.

159. Varma DGK, et al: Chondrosarcoma: MR imaging with pathologic correlation. *RadioGraphics* 12:687, 1992.

160. Villacin AB, Brigham LN, Bullough PG: Primary and secondary synovial chondrometaplasia: histopathologic and clinicoradiologic differences. *Hum Pathol* 10:439, 1979.

161. Weekes RG, et al: CT of soft-tissue neoplasms. *AJR* 144:355, 1985.

162. Wetzel LH, Levine E, Murphey MD: A comparison of MR imaging and CT in the evaluation of musculoskeletal masses. *RadioGraphics* 7:851, 1987.

163. Wilson AJ, et al: Transient osteoporosis: transient bone marrow edema? *Radiology* 167:757, 1988.

164. Wilson DA, Prince JR: Imaging of hemophilic pseudotumors. *AJR* 150:349, 1988.

165. Wing VW, et al: Chronic osteomyelitis examined by CT. *Radiology* 154:171, 1985.

166. Woods ER, et al: Reactive soft-tissue mass associated with osteoid osteoma: correlation of MR imaging features with pathologic findings. *Radiology* 186:221, 1993.

167. Yao L, Lee JK: Occult intraosseous fracture: detection with MR imaging, *Radiology* 167:749, 1988.

168. Yulish BS, et al: Hemophilic arthropathy: assessment with MR imaging. *Radiology* 164:759, 1987.

169. Yulish BS, et al: Juvenile rheumatoid arthritis: assessment with MR imaging. *Radiology* 165:149, 1987.

43

The Knee

STEVEN SHANKMAN
JAVIER BELTRAN

Magnetic resonance imaging (MRI) has revolutionized our ability to picture the soft tissue structures of the musculoskeletal system. Increased soft tissue contrast coupled with multiplanar slice capability allows us to visualize the muscles, tendons, ligaments, cartilage, and bone marrow in a way that is unprecedented. Although the knee is a common site for all disorders occurring in and about joints, the large majority of cases requiring MRI are traumatic in nature. The role of computed tomography (CT) in the evaluation of internal derangement of the knee has always been limited owing to its inability to depict normal and abnormal soft tissue anatomy accurately. It remains the modality of choice, however, in certain situations, such as tibial plateau fracture. The following emphasizes standard spin echo MRI of the traumatized knee. Normal anatomy is discussed and other disorders affecting the knee joint are included.

TECHNICAL CONSIDERATIONS

MRI of the knee is performed using a transmit receive general purpose extremity surface coil manufactured by most companies. The knee is placed in full extension and about 15 degrees external rotation to visualize the anterior cruciate ligament (ACL). In general, small field of view (FOV) of 14 to 16 cm and 3 mm slice thickness is recommended.

Different institutions use different pulse sequences for knee imaging. When using spin echo two-dimensional Fourier transform (2DFT) techniques, three planes of section (axial, sagittal, and coronal) are obtained. It is convenient to obtain a proton density (PD)–weighted and T2-weighted set of images in one plane (e.g., 2000/20 to 80 TR/TE), frequently the sagittal. The axial plane can be imaged using T1-weighted pulse sequences (e.g., 500/20 TR/TE) or alternatively T2*-weighted, gradient echo techniques, which allow good visualization of the articular cartilage (e.g., 400/

9/75, TR/TE/flip angle). The same T2* sequence can be used in the coronal plane. Another alternative for articular cartilage imaging is the use of fat-suppressed spoiled gradient echo technique. Software developments allow fast spin echo techniques, which produce similar contrast with a fraction of the time it takes to obtain classic spin echo sequences (e.g., 3600/20-80).

Alternatively, one can use radial imaging, with multiple oblique planes oriented in a radial fashion centered over each side of the tibial plateau, with extra sections oriented along the axis of the ACL. This technique can be used also with 2DFT gradient echo pulse sequences and provides images similar to those obtained with conventional arthrography.

Three-dimensional Fourier transform (3DFT) volume acquisition techniques are becoming more popular owing to software improvements and availability of workstations. These techniques are obtained using gradient echo pulse sequences with short TR/TE (e.g., 18/9/30, TR/TE/flip angle). The advantages of 3DFT data acquisition include improved signal-to-noise ratio and reconstruction of true contiguous slices of about 1 mm in infinite planes of section, with minimal distortion.

Finally, for kinematic studies of the femoropatellar joint for patellar tracking abnormalities, multiple images can be obtained with ultra-fast gradient echo techniques in the axial plane during active flexion and extension of the knee within the gantry.

MENISCI

Anatomy

The menisci of the knee are two semilunar, C-shaped fibrocartilaginous disks that sit on the peripheral margins of the essentially flat tibial plateau. The upper surfaces of both menisci are concave and articulate with the convex femoral condyles. Both menisci measure approximately 4 to 7 mm in height at the periphery and 1 mm or less at the free edge. The peripheral one third

1477

contain neurovascular structures, whereas the remaining two thirds are strictly fibrocartilaginous.

The lateral meniscus has the same width throughout, approximately 7 to 10 mm. It is shaped like a three quarter circle with its anterior and posterior horns attached to the tibia immediately in front of and behind the intercondylar eminence. The central attachment sites are narrower in width. The peripheral margin of the lateral meniscus is attached to the capsule except posterolaterally, where the popliteus tendon crosses it, and more posteriorly and centrally near the central attachment site, where the capsule does not extend anteriorly into the joint.

The medial meniscus is shaped more like a half circle. Although its posterior horn is attached to the tibia just posterior to the posterior lateral meniscal attachment, its anterior horn attaches far anteriorly, approximately 10 to 14 mm anterior to the anterior horn of the lateral meniscus. The width of the medial meniscus gradually tapers from posterior to anterior in contrast to the lateral meniscus. The peripheral margin of the medial meniscus is more firmly attached to the joint capsule and to the tibial plateau itself, the latter via the coronary ligament. As with the lateral side, the capsule does not extend anteriorly into the joint near the posterior central attachment site.

The transverse ligament connects the anterior horns of both menisci. Its thickness varies from 1 to 4

mm. It arises at the most anterior-superior portion of the lateral meniscus and crosses in front of the ACL tibial attachment merging with the superior portion of the posterior aspect of the anterior horn of the medial meniscus.

The meniscofemoral ligaments are inconstant, 3 to 4 mm fibrous bands arising from the posterior horn of the lateral meniscus, attaching to the lateral aspect of the medial femoral condyle. The ligaments of Humphrey and Wrisberg arise together, the former coursing anterior to the posterior cruciate ligament (PCL) and the latter posterior to the PCL (Figs. 43-1 and 43-2).

MRI appearance

In general, sagittal images best show the anterior and posterior horns of the medial and lateral menisci. Coronal images best show the meniscal bodies (Figs. 43-3 and 43-4).

Sagittal cross sections show the posterior horn of the medial meniscus as an isosceles triangle, the sides nearly twice as long as the base. The neurovascular portion of the posterior horn of the medial meniscus is extensive, sometimes measuring 4 to 6 mm in width (Fig. 43-5).

The anterior horn of the medial meniscus is about one half the width of the posterior horn, appearing more as an equilateral triangle. It may vary in its appearance, sometimes appearing almost rounded. It sits on the extreme edge of the anterior tibia, the transverse ligament joining it more superiorly and somewhat posteriorly. This

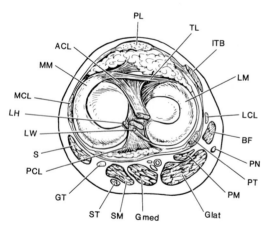

Fig. 43-1. Normal anatomy. *AC,* articular cartilage; *ACL,* anterior cruciate ligament; *BF,* biceps femoris; *Glat,* gastrocnemius lateral head; *Gmed,* gastrocnemius medial head; *GT,* gracilis tendon; *ITB,* iliotibial band; *LCL,* lateral collateral ligament; *LH,* ligament of Humphrey; *LM,* lateral meniscus; *LW,* ligament of Wrisberg; *MCL,* medial collateral ligament; *MM,* medial meniscus; *PCL,* posterior cruciate ligament; *PL,* patellar ligament; *PM,* plantaris muscle; *PN,* peroneal nerve; *Prox TFJ,* proximal tibia-fibula joint; *PT,* popliteus tendon; *S,* sartorius; *SM,* semimembranosus; *ST,* semitendinosus; *TL,* transverse ligament.

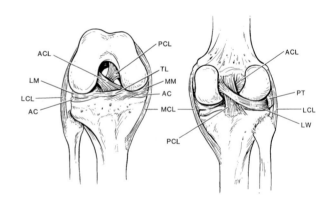

Fig. 43-2. Normal anatomy. *AC,* articular cartilage; *ACL,* anterior cruciate ligament; *BF,* biceps femoris; *Glat,* gastrocnemius lateral head; *Gmed,* gastrocnemius medial head; *GT,* gracilis tendon; *ITB,* iliotibial band; *LCL,* lateral collateral ligament; *LH,* ligament of Humphrey; *LM,* lateral meniscus; *LW,* ligament of Wrisberg; *MCL,* medial collateral ligament; *MM,* medial meniscus; *PCL,* posterior cruciate ligament; *PL,* patellar ligament; *PM,* plantaris muscle; *PN,* peroneal nerve; *Prox TFJ,* proximal tibia-fibula joint; *PT,* popliteus tendon; *S,* sartorius; *SM,* semimembranosus; *ST,* semitendinosus; *TL,* transverse ligament.

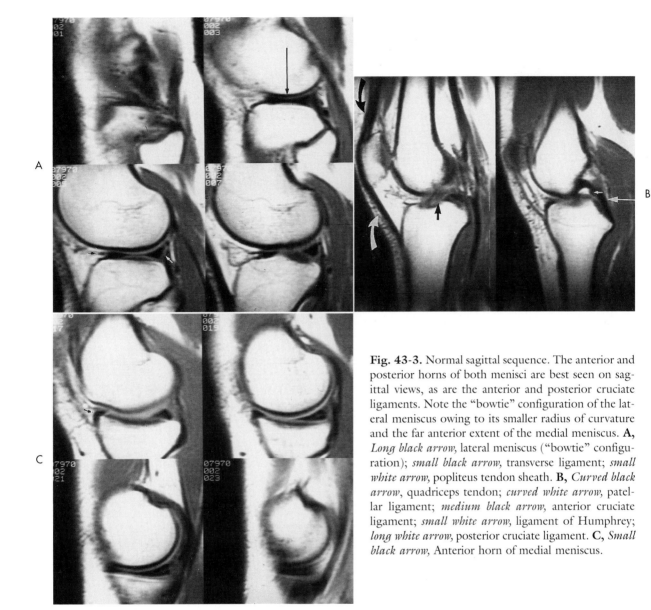

Fig. 43-3. Normal sagittal sequence. The anterior and posterior horns of both menisci are best seen on sagittal views, as are the anterior and posterior cruciate ligaments. Note the "bowtie" configuration of the lateral meniscus owing to its smaller radius of curvature and the far anterior extent of the medial meniscus. **A,** *Long black arrow,* lateral meniscus ("bowtie" configuration); *small black arrow,* transverse ligament; *small white arrow,* popliteus tendon sheath. **B,** *Curved black arrow,* quadriceps tendon; *curved white arrow,* patellar ligament; *medium black arrow,* anterior cruciate ligament; *small white arrow,* ligament of Humphrey; *long white arrow,* posterior cruciate ligament. **C,** *Small black arrow,* Anterior horn of medial meniscus.

junction may create an "arrowhead" appearance, pointing posteriorly. The lower portion represents the anterior horn attachment site, and the upper portion represents the transverse ligament junction (Fig. 43-6).

On the lateral side, the transverse ligament attaches to the most anterior-superior aspect of the anterior horn and may appear as a round dot anterior to the meniscus and should not be confused with a tear (Figs. 43-7, 43-8, and 43-9).[14] The anterior horn of the lateral meniscus is in fact the most uncommon site for a meniscal tear. The anterior and posterior horns of the lateral meniscus are of about equal size, the anterior being slightly smaller, both appearing as isosceles triangles.

The posterior horn of the lateral meniscus differs from the medial in that its attachment to the capsule is interrupted by the popliteus tendon, and this should not be mistaken for a tear (Fig. 43-10).[14] The ligament of Wrisberg is usually seen at its origin at the superior margin of the posterior horn. It may appear as a round dot adjacent to the superior aspect of the posterior horn and should not be confused with a tear (Fig. 43-11).[37]

The more peripheral sagittal images show the bodies of the medial and lateral menisci, although not optimally. On both sides, the menisci appear as flat bands. On the lateral side, owing to its smaller radius of curvature, more central slices show a "bowtie" configuration. Volume averaging of the capsule and menisci on extreme peripheral slices may be confused with a tear of the meniscal body (Fig. 43-12).[14] This normal increased signal may also represent truncation artifact. Parallel signal lines are produced in the phase encoding direction

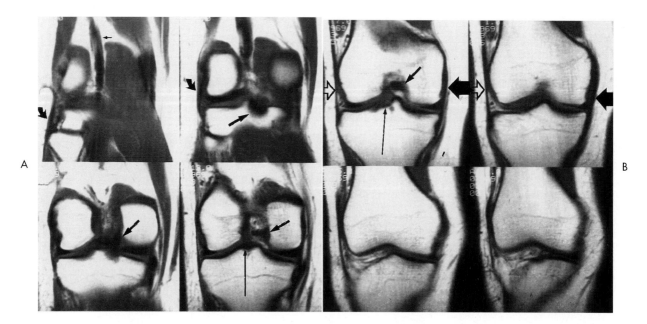

Fig. 43-4. Normal coronal sequence. The bodies of both menisci are seen best on coronal views, as are the medial and lateral collateral ligaments. Note the decreasing width of the medial meniscus as it courses anteriorly where it attaches at the anterior margin of the tibial plateau. *Smallest arrow,* Popliteal artery; *curved arrow,* lateral collateral ligament; *short arrow,* posterior cruciate ligament; *long arrow,* anterior cruciate ligament; *hollow arrow,* iliotibial band; *thick arrow,* medial collateral ligament.

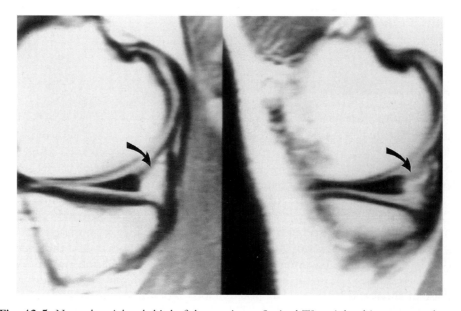

Fig. 43-5. Normal peripheral third of the meniscus. Sagittal T1-weighted images reveal normal increased signal intensity at the periphery of the posterior horn of the medial meniscus where neurovascular structures and fatty tissue are present *(arrow)*. This may be quite prominent, sometimes measuring 4 to 6 mm in width.

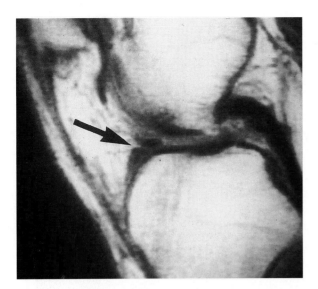

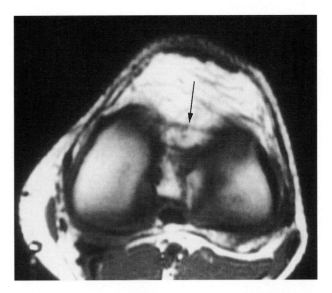

Fig. 43-6. Normal anterior horn of the medial meniscus. Sagittal T1-weighted image shows the "arrowhead" configuration of the anterior horn of the medial meniscus. The "arrowhead" points posteriorly with the lowermost anterior portion representing the anterior horn of the medial meniscus and the higher portion representing the transverse ligament attachment. The cleft in between should not be confused with a tear *(arrow)*.

Fig. 43-8. Transverse ligament. Axial T1-weighted image shows the transverse ligament extending from the medial to the lateral joint compartments *(arrow)*.

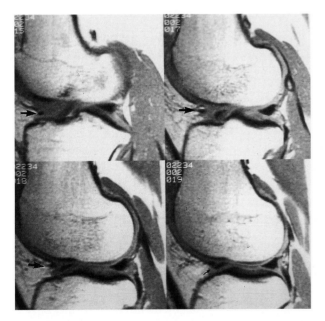

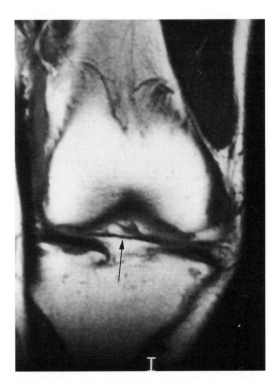

Fig. 43-7. Transverse ligament. Sagittal T1-weighted images show the transverse ligament *(arrow)* joining the anterior horn lateral meniscus. The junction *(small arrow)* should not be confused with a tear.

Fig. 43-9. Transverse ligament. Coronal T1-weighted image, far anteriorly, shows the transverse ligament extending from the medial to the lateral compartments of the knee *(arrow)*.

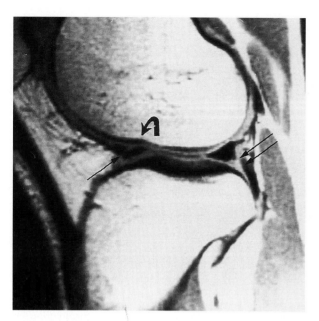

Fig. 43-10. Popliteus tendon sagittal view. Sagittal T1-weighted image shows the normal high signal intensity of the popliteus tendon sheath at the posterior horn of the lateral meniscus *(double arrow)*. Also, note the transverse ligament attachment to the anterior horn of lateral meniscus. The plane between them should not be mistaken for a tear *(arrow)*. The normal indentation of the lateral condylar surface representing the junction of its tibial and patellar articular surfaces should not be confused with an osteochondral fracture. The cartilage and subchondral cortex are intact *(curved arrow)*.

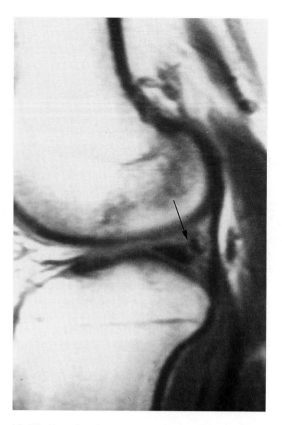

Fig. 43-11. Pseudo tear posterior horn of the lateral meniscus. Sagittal T1-weighted image shows the takeoff of the ligament of Wrisberg at the posterior horn of the lateral meniscus. The signal between the ligament of Wrisberg and the lateral meniscus itself *(arrow)* should not be confused with a tear.

at edges where there is a large, abrupt transition in tissue signal intensity.

Coronal cross sections at the midportion of the knee best show the bodies of both menisci. They appear triangular in shape, the lateral slightly larger than the medial. The capsular attachment on the medial side is incorporated into the tibial or medial collateral ligament. A small amount of fat may be interposed between the body of the medial meniscus and the capsule.

Posteriorly, coronal cross sections show the posterior horns as flat bands. On the lateral side, the popliteus tendon courses upward and laterally at 45 degrees (Figs. 43-13 and 43-14). Synovium extends superior and inferiorly about the tendon through the opening in the capsule and appears as increased signal intensity, linear in nature. This is seen on both the sagittal and the coronal images as medium signal intensity on T1-weighted and spin density images and high signal intensity on T2-weighted images.

More anteriorly, coronal images show the anterior horn of the lateral meniscus as bandlike. The anterior horn of the medial meniscus is quite small and extends more anteriorly than the lateral.

The avascular portions of the normal menisci and the transverse and meniscofemoral ligaments appear dark, without signal on all pulse sequences. The peripheral vascular zones are of low-to-medium signal intensity on T1-weighted and spin density images and of medium-to-high signal intensity on T2-weighted images. This is most prominent at the posterior horn of the medial meniscus seen best on sagittal cross section. With age, degeneration leads to indistinct focal areas of medium-to-high signal intensity in the avascular portion of the menisci.[15]

Meniscal trauma

Traumatic meniscal tears are usually longitudinal, produced when the femoral condyle compresses the meniscus, usually superiorly to inferiorly, posteriorly to anteriorly, and from without inward. These tears may extend along the radius of the meniscus or be localized to one segment, usually the posterior horn. An extensive tear with central displacement of the free edge is referred to as a bucket-handle tear, the handle representing the displaced free margin. Incomplete partial-thickness tears

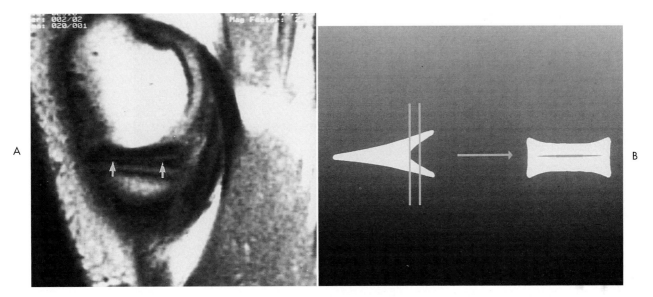

Fig. 43-12. Far peripheral sagittal pseudo tear. Far sagittal T1-weighted image of the medial joint compartment shows normal linear high signal intensity representing volume averaging of the joint capsule, concave surface of the meniscus periphery, and normal fat in between *(arrows)*. This may represent truncation artifact as well.

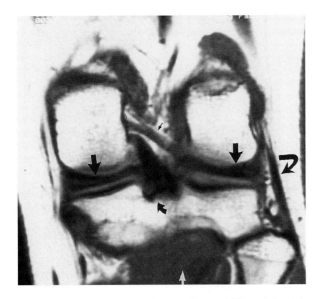

Fig. 43-13. Posterior coronal view. Coronal T1-weighted image shows the posterior horns of both menisci as rather large flat bands that should not be confused with discoid menisci *(large black arrows)*. Of note are the posterior cruciate ligament *(small curved arrow)*, ligament of Wrisberg *(small black arrow)*, fibular collateral ligament *(large curved arrow)*, and the popliteus muscle belly *(white arrow)*.

are usually seen at the posterior horn and extend to an articular surface, usually the inferior one.

Meniscal tears may result in abnormal signal within the meniscus, abnormal size and shape of the meniscus, and abnormal position of meniscal fragments.

Increased signal intensity representing a torn meniscus is best seen on T1-weighted and spin density images and may not be seen on T2-weighted images. These are more helpful when synovial fluid insinuates itself within the tear. Such signal changes represent a torn meniscus only when it extends to the superior or inferior articular surface (Figs. 43-15 and 43-16). The periphery of the meniscus does not represent such a surface. Such findings may be seen only on one image or in one plane but are still diagnostic. Also, altering the gray scale of an image should be done cautiously in that false-positive images result by exaggerating intrameniscal signal. When one is not sure whether or not signal extends to the articular surface, a true tear is probably not present. Controversy still exists as to whether or not intrameniscal signal, globular or linear, represents degeneration in that many such cases have resolved with follow-up examination. Of note, however, is the "meniscus-within-a-meniscus" appearance, in which increased signal is seen throughout the meniscus cross section. This represents a meniscal tear approximately 50% of the time (Fig. 43-17).

Nondisplaced peripheral separations may be difficult to detect. The most specific finding is irregular, jagged increased signal intensity at the periphery that brightens on T2-weighted images (Fig. 43-18).

More extensive tears may alter the size, shape, and position of the meniscus. When a portion of the free margin of the meniscus is detached, a bucket-handle tear, the remaining peripheral portion appears small and often truncated. The displaced portion usually lies in the intercondylar notch beneath the ACL or PCL (Fig. 43-

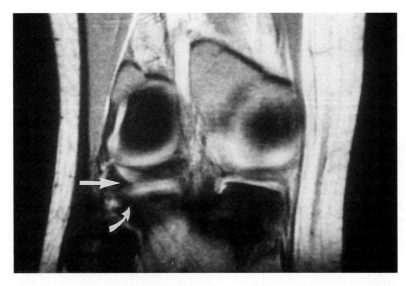

Fig. 43-14. Popliteus tendon coronal view. Coronal T1-weighted image, far posteriorly, shows the popliteus muscle belly extending laterally *(curved arrow)* and popliteus tendon itself *(straight arrow)* crossing through the posterior horn of the lateral meniscus.

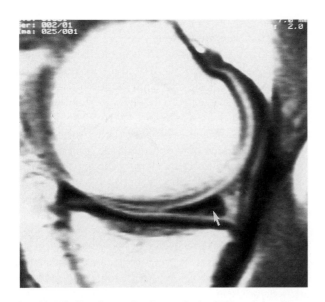

Fig. 43-15. Simple meniscal tear. Sagittal T1-weighted image shows linear high signal intensity at the posterior horn of the medial meniscus extending to the inferior articular surface *(arrow).*

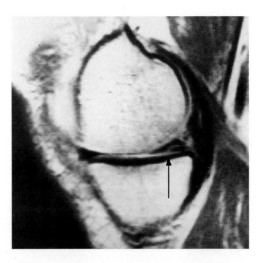

Fig. 43-16. Nondisplaced meniscal tears. Sagittal T1-weighted image shows high signal intensity at the posterior horn of the medial meniscus extending to the inferior articular surface *(arrow).*

19). Occasionally, it may flip anteriorly above the anterior horn (Fig. 43-20). Coronal views are helpful in further identifying such displaced fragments. These should not be confused with the central attachment sites of posterior meniscal horns.

Small radial tears of the free edge, almost always seen laterally, are referred to as parrot beak tears. They are best seen on coronal images. On sagittal views, the "bowtie" configuration of the lateral meniscus may be disrupted centrally (Fig. 43-21).[2,10,26,27,36]

Thin section CT of the menisci after air-contrast arthrography has been used for evaluation of tears. This technique has met with limited acceptance, conventional arthrography being favored until the advent of MRI.

Postoperative meniscus

The MRI appearance of the postsurgical meniscus depends on the nature of the surgical intervention-

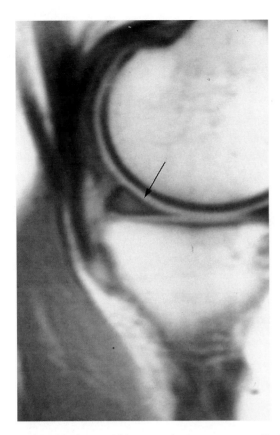

Fig. 43-17. Meniscus within a meniscus appearance. Sagittal T1-weighted image shows increased signal intensity throughout the confines of the posterior horn of the medial meniscus. Although signal does not extend to the articular surface, a true tear is seen at arthroscopy 50% of the time.

After partial meniscectomy, it can be quite difficult to evaluate tearing of the meniscal remnant. The arthroscopically normal meniscal stump varies in its MRI appearance. It may demonstrate a smooth contour with homogeneous signal intensity. Standard MRI criteria for meniscal tears are useful only in this situation. Other such "normal" stumps may demonstrate an irregular surface contour with inhomogeneous signal intensity. In fact, such a postoperative appearance represents a normal meniscal remnant most of the time. In such a setting, however, it is nearly impossible to delineate true pathology (Fig. 43-22).[35]

Peripheral meniscal tears are often treated conservatively or with arthroscopic repair. In either situation, it has been shown that persistent increased signal intensity at the periphery of the meniscus remains unchanged from that seen on preoperative studies in patients who have become asymptomatic and presumably healed. The presence of such signal therefore should not be misinterpreted as meniscal retear. In this regard, some cases of false-positive MRI examinations may in fact represent

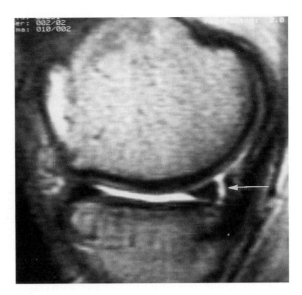

Fig. 43-18. Peripheral tear. Sagittal T2-weighted images show high signal intensity at the periphery of the posterior horn of the medial meniscus *(arrow)*. A joint effusion is present.

older injuries that have healed by the time arthroscopic examination is performed.[8]

Discoid meniscus

A discoid meniscus refers to a meniscus, almost always the lateral one, that is not C-shaped but rather like a disk and covers most of the tibial plateau to varying degrees rather than just its periphery. It is prone to tearing and is usually seen in children and adolescents. They may be asymptomatic and incidentally noted. Although seen in youngsters, it is believed that they are more developmental than congenital in that the fetal meniscus never assumes such a shape. MRI shows the signal void of the meniscus extending toward the intercondylar notch. Although much has been said about the increased number of routine sagittal images on which the discoid meniscal body should be seen (Fig. 43-23), it is simpler to judge such an enlarged meniscus on the coronal view (Fig. 43-24).[34]

ANTERIOR CRUCIATE LIGAMENT
Anatomy

The ACL extends from its semicircular attachment at the posterior aspect of the medial surface of the lateral femoral condyle to the anterior intercondylar region of the tibia, just medial to the midline, just lateral and anterior to the anterior tibial spine. This attachment is therefore several millimeters posterior to the anterior tibial margin. It is just posterior to the transverse ligament and just anterior to the central attachment of the anterior horn of the lateral meniscus. The tibial attachment is larger than the femoral and fanlike in shape. The

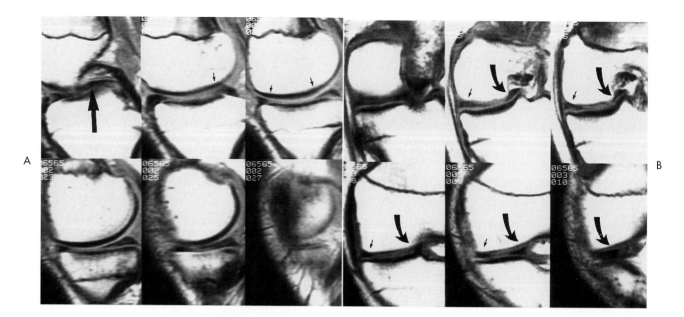

Fig. 43-19. Bucket-handle tear. **A,** Sagittal T1-weighted images show a bucket-handle tear of the medial meniscus. The central portion is displaced into the intercondylar notch *(large arrow)*. Note the distorted size and shape of the peripheral portion *(small arrow)*. **B,** Coronal T1-weighted images show the irregular periphery *(small arrows)* and the displaced central portion *(curved arrow)*.

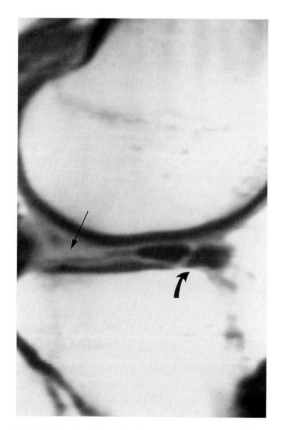

Fig. 43-20. Displaced meniscal tear. Sagittal T1-weighted image shows virtual absence of the posterior horn of the lateral meniscus *(straight arrow)*. The displaced fragment *(curved arrow)* has flipped anterior to the anterior horn of the lateral meniscus.

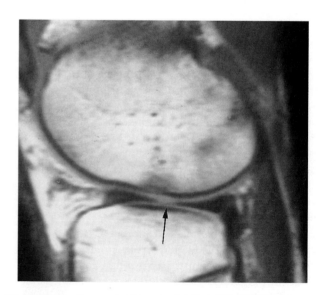

Fig. 43-21. Parrot beak tear. Sagittal T1-weighted image shows increased signal intensity interrupting the "bowtie" configuration of the lateral meniscus *(arrow)* indicative of a parrot beak tear.

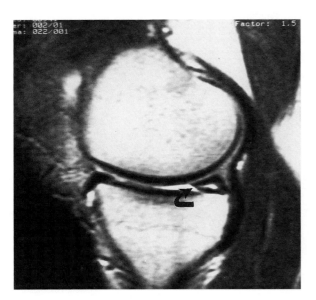

Fig. 43-22. Partial resection of the meniscus. Sagittal T1-weighted image shows partial resection of the posterior horn of the medial meniscus. Note the marked increase in signal within a clinically "normal" stump *(arrow)*.

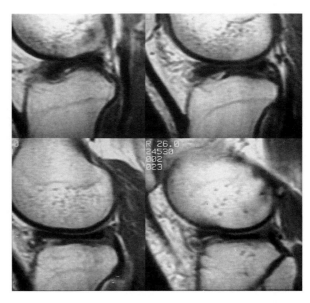

Fig. 43-23. Discoid meniscus sagittal views. Sagittal T2-weighted images show the lateral meniscus extending too far centrally consistent with a discoid meniscus.

ligament measures approximately 4 × 1 cm (Figs. 43-1, 43-2, 43-25, and 43-26). It may consist of two or more distinct bundles separated by loose connective tissue and fat more prominent at the mid and distal portions. Two distinct bands, the smaller anteromedial and larger posterolateral, have been identified. The former is taut in flexion, and the latter is taut in extension. Synovium covers all of the anterior surface of the ACL.

MRI appearance

The ACL is best seen on sagittal oblique images achieved by externally rotating the lower extremity about 10 to 15 degrees. The knee is usually extended during the examination, and the ligament therefore should appear taut, angled about 60 degrees to the tibial plateau. If the knee is flexed more than 5 degrees, it may appear lax. Occasionally, oblique coronal images may be necessary to define the ligament. In general, the ACL may appear as a solid low signal intensity band or three to four separate low signal intensity bundles. The tibial attachment is usually better seen than the femoral attachment site because of partial volume averaging of the proximal ligament with the lateral femoral condyle. Normally, increased signal intensity on T1-weighted and spin density images at the tibial insertion may be seen presumably due to the decreased density of the ligament itself and or interposed fat (Fig. 43-27).

Coronal and axial images are also useful in evaluating the ACL. Posterior coronal images show the ACL as a curvilinear low signal intensity band adjacent to the horizontal segment of the PCL, near the medial surface of the lateral femoral condyle. More anteriorly, the ACL courses obliquely in the intercondylar area to the tibial plateau (Fig. 43-28). Proximally the signal intensity is uniformly low, whereas distally it may be slightly increased.

Axial images proximally show the ACL as a low signal intensity band flattened against the medial surface of the lateral femoral condyle. Distally the ligament is not as well seen (Figs. 43-29 and 43-30).

Of note on all imaging sequences is the presence of fat at the intercondylar notch, adjacent to the ACL origin.

ACL trauma

Tears of the ACL occur more commonly at its proximal portion. Complete or partial avulsions occur more commonly at the femoral origin, whereas avulsion fractures are more common at the tibial insertion.

Acute tears result in edema and hemorrhage, which is seen as low-to-medium signal intensity (more than the normal ligament) on T1-weighted and spin density images. Markedly high signal intensity is seen on T2-weighted images. Smaller tears may cause no contour abnormalities but may lead to unsharpness of the fasciculi within the ligament. Larger tears may alter both the shape and the course of the ligament.

Larger incomplete tears and complete tears may produce a mass of edema and hemorrhage usually at the proximal portion. This appearance should not be con-

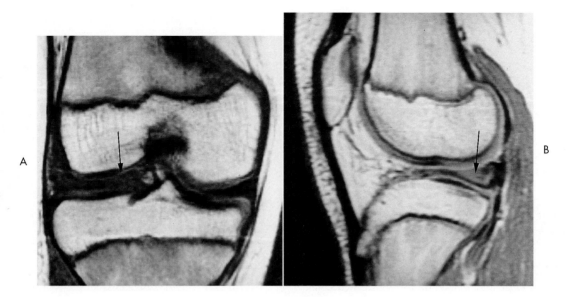

Fig. 43-24. Discoid meniscus. **A,** Coronal T1-weighted image shows a large, discoid lateral meniscus extending to the intercondylar notch with internal high signal areas *(arrow).* **B,** Sagittal proton density–weighted image better shows the tear present *(arrow).*

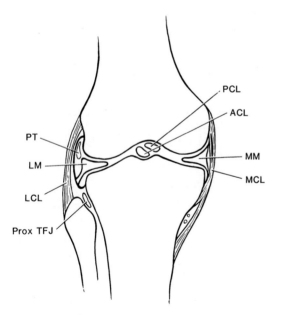

Fig. 43-25. Normal anatomy. *ACL,* Anterior cruciate ligament; *deep PB,* deep patellar bursa; *LH,* ligament of Humphrey; *LM,* lateral meniscus; *LW,* ligament of Wrisberg; *MCL,* medial collateral ligament; *MM,* medial meniscus; *PCL,* posterior cruciate ligament; *PL,* patellar ligament; *Pre PB,* prepatellar bursa; *Prox TFJ,* proximal tibia-fibula joint; *PT,* popliteus tendon; *SPB,* suprapatellar bursa; *Sup PB,* superficial patellar bursa.

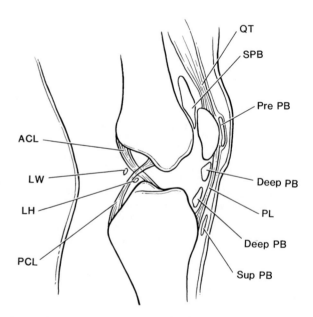

Fig. 43-26. *ACL,* Anterior cruciate ligament; *deep PB,* deep patellar bursa; *LH,* ligament of Humphrey; *LM,* lateral meniscus; *LW,* ligament of Wrisberg; *MCL,* medial collateral ligament; *MM,* medial meniscus; *PCL,* posterior cruciate ligament; *PL,* patellar ligament; *Pre PB,* prepatellar bursa; *Prox TFJ,* proximal tibia-fibula joint; *PT,* popliteus tendon; *SPB,* suprapatellar bursa; *Sup PB,* superficial patellar bursa.

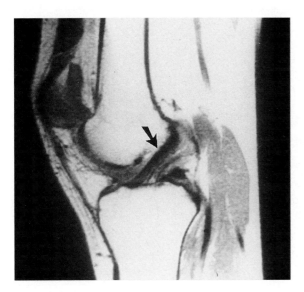

Fig. 43-27. Normal anterior cruciate ligament. Sagittal T1-weighted image shows a normal low signal intensity ACL *(arrow)*. Slight increased signal intensity at the tibial attachment site is normal.

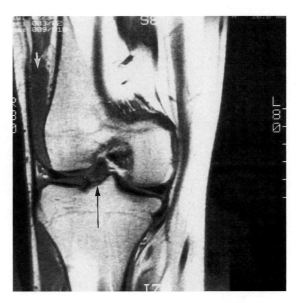

Fig. 43-28. Anterior cruciate ligament coronal view. Coronal T1-weighted image shows the fanlike ACL insertion *(black arrow)*. Joint fluid is evident at the suprapatellar gutters *(white arrow)*.

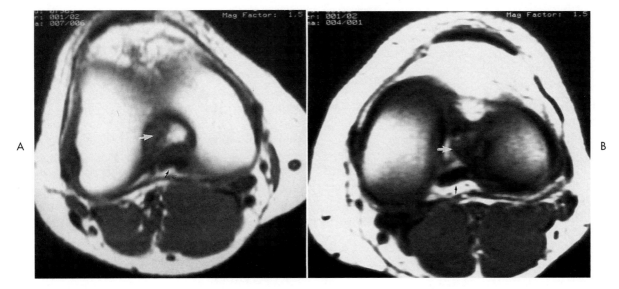

Fig. 43-29. Anterior cruciate ligament/posterior cruciate ligament on the axial view. Axial T1-weighted images show the normal ACL flattened against the lateral femoral condyle *(white arrows)*. The PCL is always better seen as a low signal intensity structure coursing posteriorly and laterally *(black arrows)*.

fused with normal volume averaging of the medial portion of the lateral femoral condyle (Fig. 43-31). These larger tears may alter the position of the ligament, producing sagging or posterior bowing (Fig. 43-32). A complete disruption may allow the ligament to lie horizontal in the intercondylar notch (Fig. 43-33). A complete tear, however, may be present with a normally po-

sitioned ligament and is seen as complete interruption of the fibers with high signal intensity edema and hemorrhage at the interrupted site.

Indirect signs of ACL tear include buckling of the PCL, anterior translation of the tibia relative to the femur (Fig. 43-34), posterior displacement of the lateral meniscus from the tibial plateau, indentation of the an-

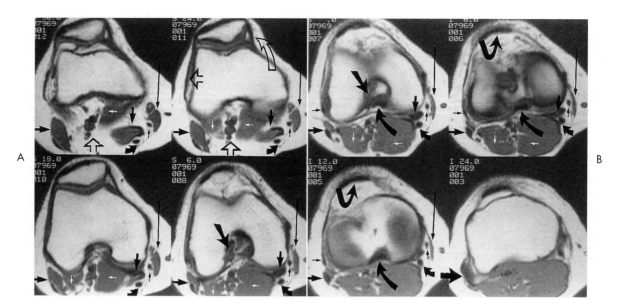

Fig. 43-30. Normal axial images. *Horizontal medium black arrow,* Biceps femoris muscle and tendon. *Horizontal small black arrow,* Fibular collateral ligament. *Horizontal large black arrow,* Conjoined tendon. *Vertical long black arrow,* Sartorius muscle and tendon. *Vertical small black arrows,* Gracilis tendon. *Vertical medium black arrow,* Semimembranosus muscle and tendon. *Small curved black arrow,* Semitendinosus tendon. *Large curved black arrow,* Posterior cruciate ligament. *Looped black arrow,* Patellar ligament. *Vertical white arrow,* Gastrocnemius muscle, lateral head. *Horizontal white arrow,* Gastrocnemius muscle, medial head. *Horizontal hollow arrow,* Lateral patellar retinaculum. *Vertical hollow arrow,* Popliteal artery and vein. *Curved hollow arrow,* Medial patellar retinaculum. *Oblique black arrow,* Anterior cruciate ligament.

terior margin of the medial femoral condyle, and fairly specific combinations of bone contusions to be described subsequently.

Chronic incomplete tears of the ACL may cause laxity. Diffuse nonhomogeneous, moderately increased signal intensity may be present on the T1-weighted and spin density images. The ligament itself may have an indistinct margin or may not be seen at all. Occasionally a chronic tear may demonstrate a normal MRI appearance owing to scar formation.

It should be stressed that the normal ACL may not be seen well on routine sagittal oblique images, and this is a commonly encountered problem. Repositioning of the oblique sagittal plane may be necessary. Oblique coronal views and axial and standard coronal views may also be necessary (Fig. 43-35). If the ACL is not seen on at least one image after attempts to picture it, it must be assumed to be torn.[16,26,31,38]

ACL repair

Most ACL repairs are intra-articular in nature and consist of arthroscopic ACL reconstruction with patellar bone–central third patellar tendon–tibial bone autografts. It has been shown that MRI demonstrates a well-defined intact low signal intensity autograft in clinically stable postoperative knees. Revascularization, which takes place 4 to 9 months postoperatively, may increase the signal intensity of the graft leading to isointensity with the intra-articular space. This may account for discrepancies in graft size. In this regard, focal and diffuse signal changes may be physiological. Therefore, postoperative evaluation seeks continuity of the graft itself rather than contour deformities or abnormal signal patterns (Fig. 43-36).[30]

POSTERIOR CRUCIATE LIGAMENT
Anatomy

The PCL arises at the lateral surface of the medial femoral condyle and extends to the posterior surface of the intercondylar region, below the level of the articular tibial plateau. It is wider and thicker than the ACL. It is arcuate in shape when the knee is extended or slightly flexed. It becomes taut with increasing flexion (see Figs. 43-1, 43-2, 43-25, and 43-26).

MRI appearance

Sagittal images best show the ligament as a uniformly low signal intensity structure with a near horizontal takeoff at the femoral origin and then an abrupt descent at about 45 degrees to the tibia. This angled por-

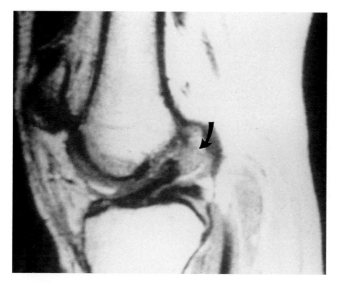

Fig. 43-31. Pseudo tear of the anterior cruciate ligament. Sagittal T1-weighted image of an obliquely positioned knee shows volume averaging at the proximal aspect of the ACL with the medial aspect of the lateral femoral condyle *(arrow)*.

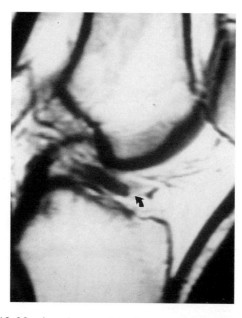

Fig. 43-33. Anterior cruciate ligament tear. Sagittal T1-weighted image shows a complete tear of the ACL, which is lying nearly horizontal within the intercondylar notch *(arrow)*.

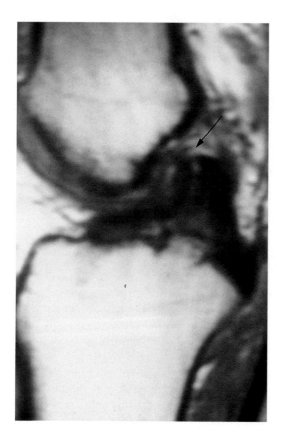

Fig. 43-32. Anterior cruciate ligament tear. Sagittal T1-weighted image shows buckling of the ACL with increased signal intensity at its proximal portion consistent with a tear *(arrow)*.

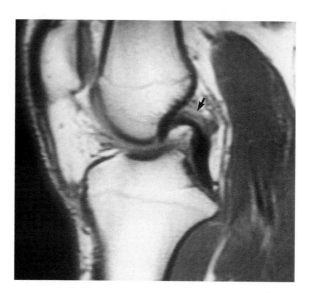

Fig. 43-34. Buckling of the posterior cruciate ligament. Sagittal T1-weighted image shows buckling of the PCL *(arrow)*. This is an indirect sign of the ACL tear present in this patient. Also note anterior subluxation of the tibia.

tion of the PCL is normally directed toward the femur and not posterior to it, unless the knee is hyperextended. In 20% to 25% of cases, the meniscofemoral ligaments of Humphrey and Wrisberg are seen as low signal intensity dots anterior and posterior to the PCL and should not be mistaken for displaced meniscal fragments (Fig. 43-37).

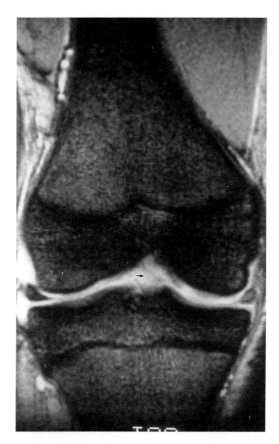

Fig. 43-35. Anterior cruciate ligament tear on the coronal view. Coronal gradient echo image shows no identifiable ACL at the intercondylar notch (*small arrow*) indicative of a tear.

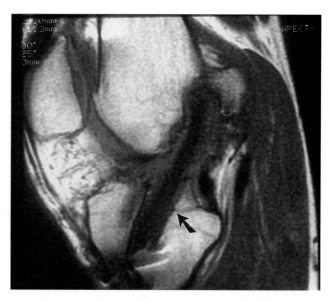

Fig. 43-36. Anterior cruciate ligament reconstruction. Sagittal T2-weighted image shows a normal-appearing ACL repair with patella tendon autograph (*arrow*). (Photograph courtesy of Dr. Padron of Madrid, Spain.)

PCL trauma

Tears of the PCL are uncommon. Perhaps 50 ACL tears are imaged for every 1 PCL tear. Most are incomplete and occur in the midportion of the ligament. Others involve the tibial insertion, where avulsion fracture may be present.

Tears of the PCL are best seen on sagittal images. Acute intrasubstance tears produce zones of increased signal intensity secondary to edema and hemorrhage (Fig. 43-38). With disruption or detachment of the ligament, similar signal changes are seen, and the ligament itself may appear redundant.[11] Trauma to the PCL can be seen on axial and coronal images as well (Fig. 43-39).

MEDIAL COLLATERAL LIGAMENT
Anatomy

The tibial or medial collateral ligament (MCL) is a broad, flat band, 2 cm in width and 2 to 4 mm in thickness. The superficial fibers extend from the medial epicondyle of the femur to the tibia, attaching about 2 cm below the joint line and then extending 3 to 4 cm more distally across the medial concavity of the proximal tibia,

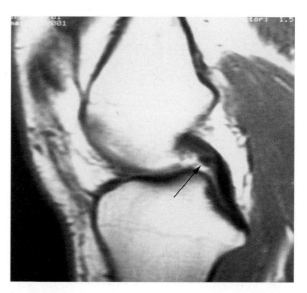

Fig. 43-37. Normal posterior cruciate ligament with the ligament of Humphrey. Sagittal T1-weighted image shows the normal course of the PCL. The anterior low signal intensity "dot" represents the ligament of Humphrey in cross section (*arrow*).

where fat and blood vessels are normally present. The deep fibers, which are really part of the joint capsule, attach loosely to the periphery of the body of the medial meniscus, where a small bursa or small amount of fat may intervene. A more firm attachment is to the tibia just below the joint line, in effect forming the coronary ligament. A small amount of fat may be present between the superficial and deep fibers of the MCL. In addition, nu-

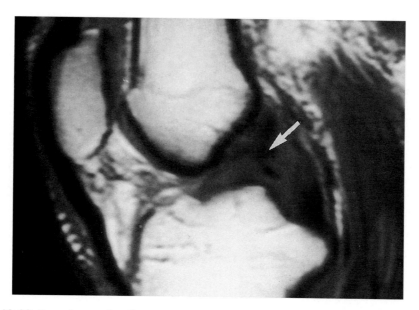

Fig. 43-38. Posterior cruciate ligament tear. Sagittal T1-weighted image shows no identifiable PCL configuration. Hemorrhage and edema replace the region of a complete tear *(arrow)*.

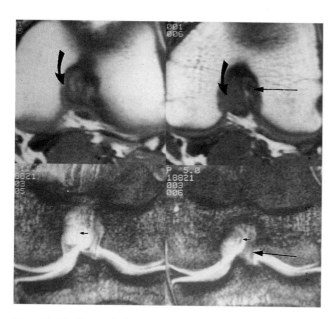

Fig. 43-39. Tear of the posterior cruciate ligament on axial and coronal views. Axial T1-weighted images show no identifiable PCL at its origin *(curved arrows)*. Gradient echo coronal images show no identifiable PCL at the intercondylar notch *(small arrows)*. The normal ACL is well defined *(large arrow)*.

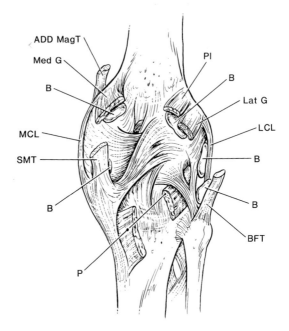

Fig. 43-40. Normal anatomy. *ADD Mag T,* Adductor magnus tendon; *B,* bursa; *BFT,* biceps femoris tendon; *G,* gastrocnemius; *Gr,* gracilis; *ITB,* iliotibial band; *Lat G,* lateral head gastrocnemius; *LCL,* lateral collateral ligament; *MCL,* medial collateral ligament; *Med G,* medial head gastrocnemius; *P,* popliteus; *Per L,* peroneus longus; *PL,* patellar ligament; *S,* sartorius; *SM,* semimembranosus; *SMT,* semimembranosus tendon; *Sol,* soleus, *ST,* semitendonosus; *VM,* vastus medialis; *VL,* vastus lateralis.

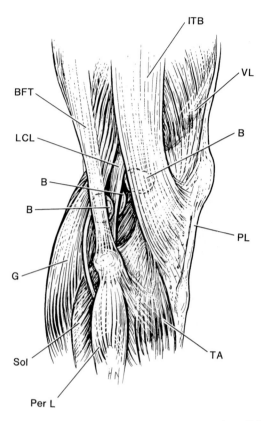

Fig. 43-41. *ADD Mag T,* Adductor magnus tendon; *B,* bursa; *BFT,* biceps femoris tendon; *G,* gastrocnemius; *Gr,* gracilis; *ITB,* iliotibial band; *Lat G,* lateral head gastrocnemius; *LCL,* lateral collateral ligament; *MCL,* medial collateral ligament; *Med G,* medial head gastrocnemius; *P,* popliteus; *Per L,* peroneus longus; *Pl,* plantaris; *PL,* patellar ligament; *S,* sartorius; *SM,* semimembranosus; *SMT,* semimembranosus tendon; *Sol,* soleus, *ST,* semitendonosus; *VM,* vastus medialis; *VL,* vastus lateralis.

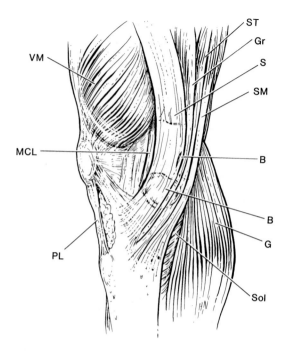

Fig. 43-42. *ADD Mag T,* Adductor magnus tendon; *B,* bursa; *BFT,* biceps femoris tendon; *G,* gastrocnemius; *Gr,* gracilis; *ITB,* iliotibial band; *Lat G,* lateral head gastrocnemius; *LCL,* lateral collateral ligament; *MCL,* medial collateral ligament; *Med G,* medial head gastrocnemius; *P,* popliteus; *Per L,* peroneus longus; *Pl,* plantaris; *PL,* patella ligament; *S,* sartorius; *SM,* semimembranosus; *SMT,* semimembranosus tendon; *Sol,* soleus; *ST,* semitendonosus; *VM,* vastus medialis; *VL,* vastus lateralis.

merous bursa may be present between the MCL and bone, between the deep and superficial fibers, and between the MCL and pes anserinus (Figs. 43-1, 43-2, 43-25, 43-40, 43-41, and 43-42).

MRI appearance

The MCL is best seen on coronal images as a homogeneously low signal intensity structure on all pulse sequences. Moderately increased signal may be seen between the superficial and deep fibers and below the superficial fibers at the distal tibial attachment site, where fat is normally interposed (see Fig. 43-4).

MCL trauma

Traumatic injuries of the MCL are common and range from intrasubstance tears (grade 1 sprain) to incomplete tears (grade 2 sprain) to complete disruption (grade 3 sprain). These are best seen on coronal images. A grade 1 sprain appears as increased signal within the ligament secondary to intrasubstance edema. Fluid may

be seen on both sides of the ligament as well. All of these changes are best noted on spin density and T2-weighted images. When internal signal extends to the superficial or deep surface, a grade 2 sprain is diagnosed (Fig. 43-43). A grade 3 sprain is seen as complete disruption of the low signal intensity band with redundancy of its proximal and distal portions. The ligament may be stripped from its femoral and tibial attachments, in which case hemorrhage and edema are seen as increased signal medial to the ligament (Figs. 43-44 and 43-45). This should be distinguished from fluid in the gutters of the suprapatellar bursa.[2,10,27]

LATERAL COLLATERAL LIGAMENT
Anatomy

The lateral or fibular collateral ligament is a tubular cord arising at the lateral epicondyle of the femur above the popliteus groove extending inferiorly and posteriorly to the fibular head, where it is joined with the biceps femoris insertion, the conjoined tendon. In contrast to the MCL, the lateral collateral ligament is separate and apart from the lateral joint capsule, with the lateral geniculate veins and arteries interposed (see Figs. 43-1, 43-2, 43-25, 43-40 through 43-42).

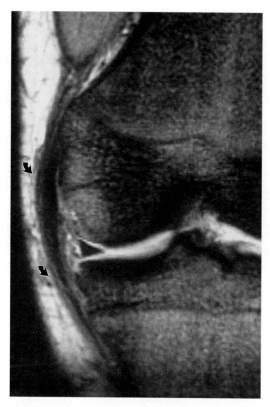

Fig. 43-43. Medial collateral ligament tear. Coronal gradient echo image shows thickening of the medial collateral ligament with increased signal intensity within *(curved arrow)*. This represents a grade 2 sprain with signal extending to the superficial and deep surfaces.

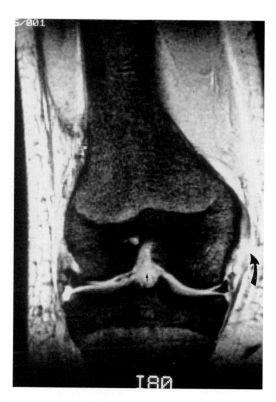

Fig. 43-44. Medial collateral ligament tear grade 3. Coronal gradient echo image shows complete disruption of the medial collateral ligament *(curved arrow)*. In addition, a normal ACL is not seen at the intercondylar region and is therefore torn *(small arrow)*.

MRI appearance

The lateral collateral ligament is best seen on coronal images as a uniformly low signal intensity cord on all pulse sequences (Figs. 43-4 and 43-46).

Lateral collateral ligament trauma

Injuries to the fibular collateral ligament are usually due to severe trauma involving varus force. Hemorrhage and edema with or without disruption of the ligament may be present. Signal intensity changes, as expected, reflect the edema present (Figs. 43-47, 43-48).[2,10,27] Avulsion of the lateral capsule at its tibial insertion is often associated and referred to as a Segond fracture, the lateral capsular sign.[40]

CT of the cruciate and collateral ligaments was never routinely performed.

PITFALLS IN THE EVALUATION OF INTERNAL DERANGEMENT OF THE KNEE

Transverse ligament

The attachment sites of the transverse ligament to the anterior horns of the medial and lateral menisci may mimic a tear on sagittal views (see Figs. 43-3 and 43-7).

Meniscofemoral ligaments

The takeoff of the ligament of Wrisberg at the posterior horn of the lateral meniscus may mimic a meniscal tear on sagittal views. When seen on end at its midportion, it may mimic a joint body posterior to the PCL. Similarly, a thick or low-lying ligament of Humphrey may appear as a displaced meniscal fragment (see Fig. 43-11).

Popliteus tendon

The popliteus tendon and synovium crosses the posterolateral aspect of the posterior horn of the lateral meniscus, causing an oblique region of increased signal intensity, and should not be confused with a meniscal tear (see Figs. 43-3, 43-4, 43-10, and 43-14).

Posterior menisci central attachment sites

The posterior horns of both menisci at the central attachment sites are not attached to the joint capsule and therefore may appear irregular on sagittal views. The posterior horns are seen on coronal views as flat bands that should not be confused with discoid menisci (see Fig. 43-13).

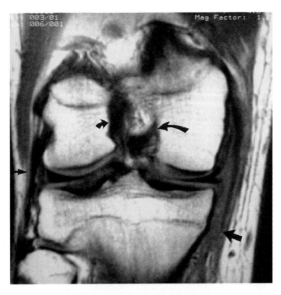

Fig. 43-45. Medial collateral ligament tear grade 3. Coronal T1-weighted image shows complete disruption of the medial collateral ligament *(large arrow)*. Edema and hemorrhage surround the ligament. Also, note the origins of the ACL *(small curved arrow)* and PCL *(large curved arrow)*. Portions of the FCL are seen *(small arrow)*.

Meniscocapsular junction

Far peripheral sagittal sections may show increased signal at the bodies of both menisci owing to volume averaging of the normal concavity of the meniscal body periphery with the joint capsule. Coronal images are normal (see Fig. 43-12).

Peripheral meniscus

Increased signal at the periphery of the meniscus represents the normal neurovascular portion, which can be quite prominent especially at the posterior horn of the medial meniscus (see Fig. 43-5).

ACL origin

Sagittal images may volume average the ACL and its origin at the lateral femoral condyle. This may mimick a proximal tear. Brightening on T2-weighted images, however, is not seen (see Fig. 43-31).

BONE AND BONE MARROW

The cortical bone of the distal femur, proximal tibia, and patella is of low signal intensity on all pulse sequences.

The signal intensity of the medullary canal is reflective of the changing amounts of hematopoietic and fatty bone marrow with age, the latter increasing with time. Older patients may have residual islands of hematopoietic marrow, which should not be confused with infiltrative disease. The epiphyseal portion of the distal fe-

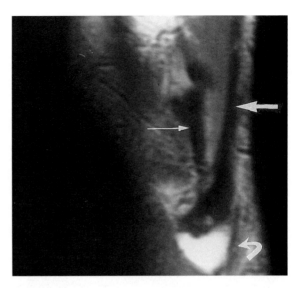

Fig. 43-46. Conjoined tendon. Sagittal T1-weighted image, far lateral, shows the tendon of the biceps femoris *(thick arrow)* inserting with the fibular collateral ligament *(thin arrow)* as the conjoined tendon at the fibular head *(curved arrow)*.

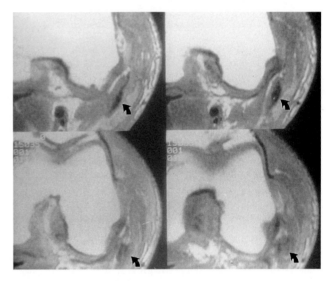

Fig. 43-47. Tear of the lateral collateral ligament complex. Axial T1-weighted images show no identifiable fibular collateral ligament. The biceps femoris tendon is irregular proximally and completely torn distally *(curved arrows)*. In addition, no identifiable ACL or PCL is seen at the intercondylar notch.

mur and proximal tibia and the epiphysioid patella always contain predominantly fatty marrow. The sensitivity of MRI to bone marrow alterations makes it ideal for detecting traumatic injuries.

Essentially four types of bone injury occur about the knee: bone bruise or contusion; osteochondral fracture; stress fracture; and obvious fractures of the femoral

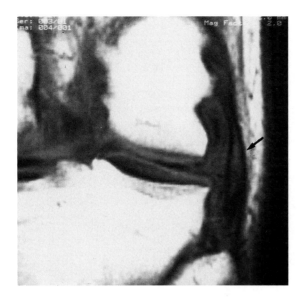

Fig. 43-48. Lateral collateral ligament tear. Coronal T1-weighted image shows intermediate signal intensity replacement of the lateral collateral ligament, which is split, redundant, and discontinuous *(arrow)*.

shaft, tibial plateau, and patella. Some of these are occult in nature; others are not.

A bone bruise represents an acute, occult microfracture of subchondral trabecular bone with subsequent hemorrhage and edema. The cortex and articular cartilage are infarct. They may be secondary to direct trauma or associated with twisting injuries and internal derangement of the knee. They resolve in 6 to 8 weeks. These injuries were not apparent before MRI. They appear as ill-defined subchondral reticulated or stellate regions of low signal intensity on T1-weighted images and high signal intensity on T2-weighted images (Fig. 43-49).[23,25,41]

An acute osteochondral fracture may be impacted or displaced. Displaced osteochondral fragments are best seen on T2-weighted images, especially if a joint effusion is present. These are often seen at the medial patellar facet and anterior-lateral femoral condyle secondary to patellar femoral dislocation (Fig. 43-50). Impacted osteochondral lesions are commonly seen at the anterior-lateral femoral condyle. Decreased signal intensity is seen on T1-weighted images at the impaction site, with increased signal seen about the impaction site on T2-weighted images secondary to edema. The overlying cartilage may be intact (Fig. 43-51).[23,25,39]

Chronic osteochondral fractures (osteochondritis dissecans) are well seen with MRI. Some believe that increased signal intensity at the base of the osteochondral fracture on T2-weighted images represents a loose or unstable fragment.[7] The ability to evaluate the overlying cartilage, however, remains less reliable (Figs. 43-52 and 43-53).[23,39]

CT arthrography may delineate acute and chronic osteochondral defects but is unreliable.

Stress fractures may be occult in nature. They appear as linear, low signal intensity bands, away from the joint on T1- and T2-weighted images. Increased signal may be seen about the impacted fracture site on T2-weighted images, reflecting the associated edema (Fig. 43-54).[21]

CT may detect stress fractures, especially those that are longitudinal in nature (Fig. 43-55).[1]

Tibial plateau fractures result from extreme valgus force at the knee and represent a common type of knee injury. Both CT and MRI can define the fracture and degree of depression. Because osseous detail is better seen with CT, tibial plateau fractures are often best studied in this manner complimented with two- and three-dimensional reconstructions. Fracture fragmentation and displacement and depression may be seen more clearly (Fig. 43-56).[29] MRI, of course, allows visualization of the cruciate and collateral ligaments and menisci.

PATTERNS OF INJURY

Although the structures of the knee and their respective injuries have been discussed separately, most trauma to the knee results in patterns of injury involving multiple structures.

The ACL principally resists anterior translation of the tibia and secondarily resists internal tibial rotation. This explains why twisting injuries of the ACL occur without direct trauma. Such injuries usually involve valgus stress as well. As a result, tearing of the ACL may be associated with distractive forces at the medial joint compartment and compressive forces at the lateral joint compartment. The former may produce injuries to the peripheral medial meniscus and MCL. The latter may produce lateral meniscus tears, bone contusion, or osteochondral fracture at the lateral femoral condyle and posterior lateral tibia. These two articular surfaces are in contact only following ACL tear and internal rotation of the tibia. Bony injury at the posterolateral tibia always occurs in these situations, whereas the lateral femoral condyle may be spared. Therefore the pattern of posterior lateral tibial injury with or without lateral femoral injury predicts ACL tear.

A less common mechanism of ACL tear involves hyperextension without rotation. This would allow impaction at the anterior femoral condyle and anterior tibia without injury to the menisci or collateral ligaments. Hence, this pattern of "kissing" contusions predicts isolated ACL tear.

The least common mechanism of ACL injury involves varus stress and external rotation of the tibia. As expected, distractive forces result at the lateral joint compartment with compressive forces seen medially. Typi-

Text continued on p. 1503.

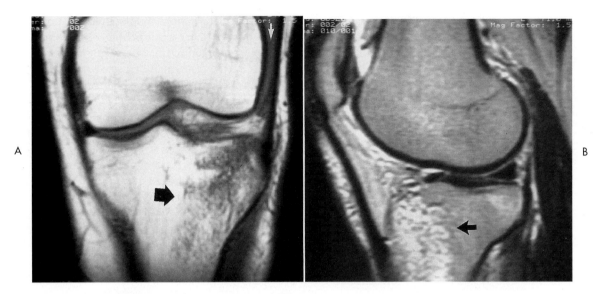

Fig. 43-49. Bone bruise. **A,** Coronal T1-weighted image shows an ill-defined, subchondral reticulated or stellate region of low signal intensity beneath the lateral tibial plateau *(black arrow)*. Fluid is seen at the suprapatellar bursae, at the lateral gutter *(white arrow)*. **B,** Sagittal T2-weighted image shows increased signal intensity indicative of edema/hemorrhage.

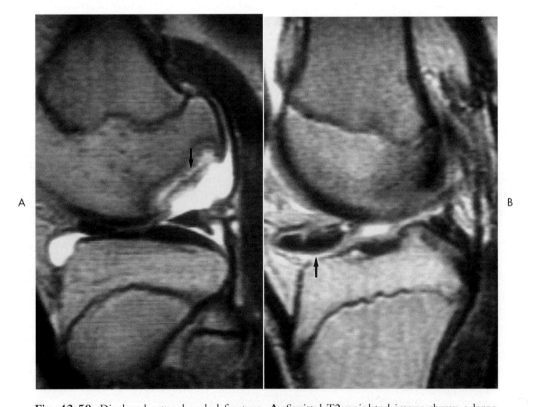

Fig. 43-50. Displaced osteochondral fracture. **A,** Sagittal T2-weighted image shows a large osteochondral defect at the posterior aspect of the lateral femoral condyle *(arrow)*. A large joint effusion is present. **B,** Sagittal T2-weighted image more centrally shows the detached bony fragment anteriorly *(arrow)*. The low signal intensity of the fragment is suggestive of secondary osteonecrosis.

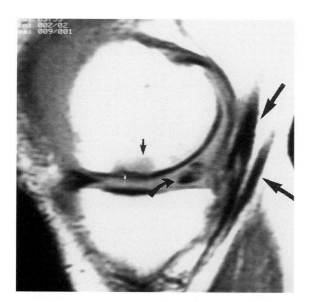

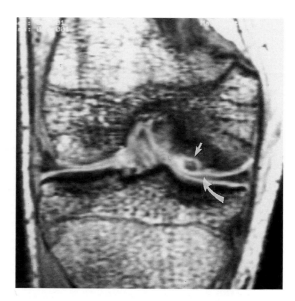

Fig. 43-51. Impacted osteochondral fracture. Sagittal T1-weighted image shows a small, impacted osteochondral fracture at the medial femoral condyle. Edema *(small black arrow)* surrounds the impacted cortex *(white arrow)*. Of note is the torn posterior horn of the medial meniscus *(curved arrow)*. The tendons of the pes anserinus are seen posteriorly *(large black arrows)*. Joint effusion is present at the suprapatellar bursa.

Fig. 43-52. Osteochondritis dissecans. Coronal gradient echo image shows an osteochondral defect at the notch aspect of the medial femoral condyle *(arrow)*. A defect is seen at the adjacent articular cartilage *(curved arrow)*. High signal intensity surrounds the osteochondral fragment. There is controversy as to whether or not this represents a loose fragment or a healing one. Of note is the fanlike insertion of the ACL. Also, note the medial collateral ligament and iliotibial band.

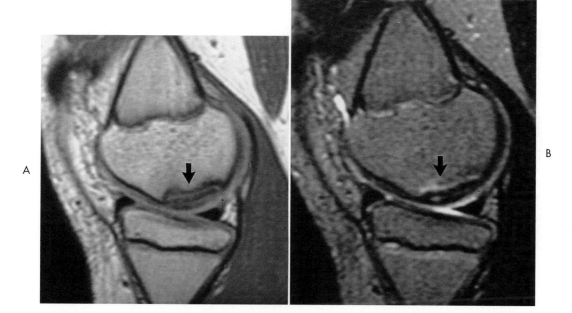

Fig. 43-53. Osteochondritis dissecans. Sagittal proton density–weighted and T2-weighted images shows an osteochondral defect *(arrow)* at the notch aspect of the medial femoral condyle. The overlying cortex appears intact. High signal intensity at the base of the defect may represent granulation tissue or be indicative of loosening.

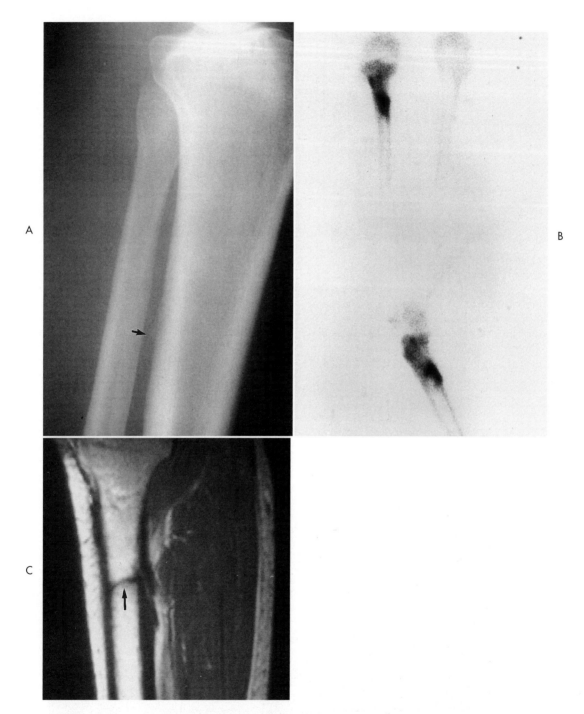

Fig. 43-54. Stress fracture. **A,** Lateral view of the proximal right leg shows faint periosteal reaction at the posterior aspect of the proximal tibia *(arrow)*. **B,** A bone scan shows increased uptake at the posterior aspect of the proximal right tibia. **C,** Sagittal T1-weighted image shows linear signal loss at the proximal tibia indicative of stress fracture *(arrow)*.

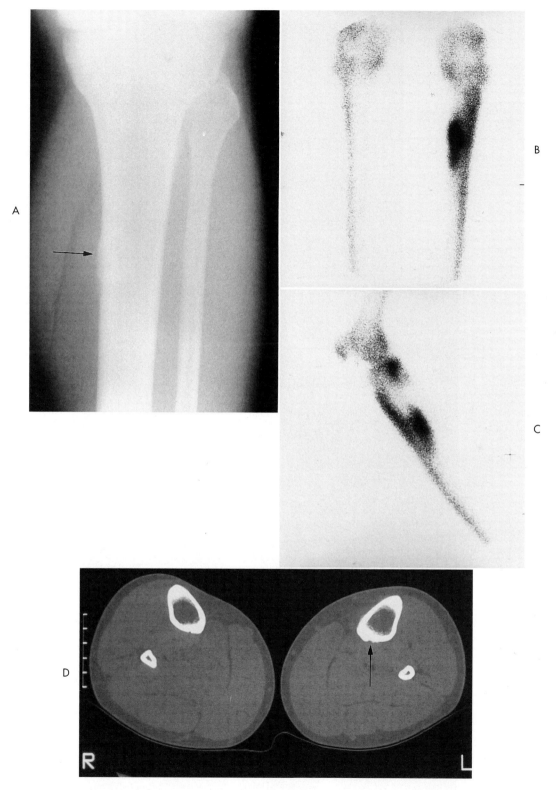

Fig. 43-55. CT of stress fracture **A,** An anteroposterior radiograph of the proximal left leg shows faint periosteal reaction at the medial proximal tibia *(arrow).* **B** and **C,** Frontal and lateral bone scan shows uptake at the posteromedial proximal tibia. **D,** CT scan shows a linear cleft at the posteromedial cortex of the left tibia indicative of a fatigue fracture in this marathon runner *(arrow).*

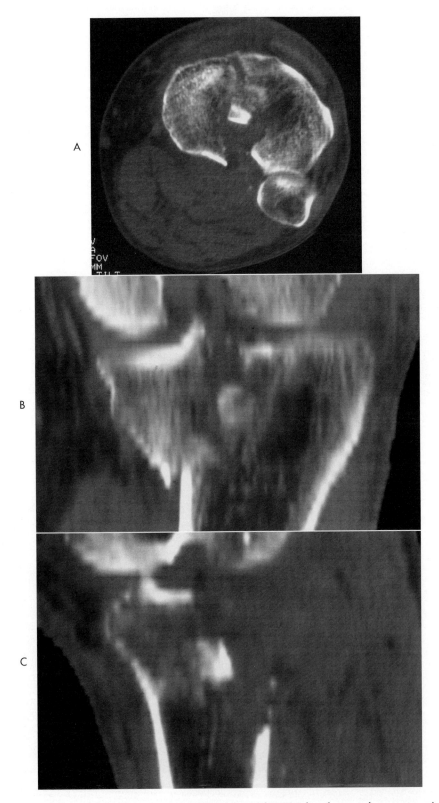

Fig. 43-56. Tibial plateau fracture. Axial CT image with sagittal and coronal reconstructions shows the degree of comminution of the tibial plateau fracture. The central depressed fracture is well seen and appears rotated.

cally, there is disruption of the lateral collateral ligament complex. Avulsion fracture of the lateral capsule at the tibia is referred to as a Segond fracture. Such a finding is associated with ACL tear more than 90% of the time. MRI may not show the fracture fragment itself, but edematous changes at the lateral tibial rim are always present and again suggest the presence of an ACL tear.[18,28,31]

MUSCLES AND TENDONS

Ten muscles and their respective tendons cross the knee joint. The anterior quadriceps represents the rectus femoris, vastus medialis, vastus intermedius, and vastus lateralis, which insert on the proximal pole of the patella. The anterolateral tensor fascia lata and its ilio-tibial band insert at Gerdy's tubercle at the anterolateral tibia. The posterolateral biceps femoris inserts with the fibular collateral ligament as the conjoined tendon at the fibula head. The posteromedial sartorius, gracilis, and semitendinosus insert at the posteromedial tibia, proximally at the pes anserinus. The posteromedial semimembraneous inserts separately, slightly more posteriorly. The medial and lateral heads of the gastrocnemius arise respectively at the posterior supracondylar region of the femur. The popliteus muscle belly rests at the posterior proximal tibia, its tendon coursing intraarticularly through the posterior horn of the lateral meniscus, toward the popliteus groove of the femur. The plantaris muscle originates at the posterolateral supracondylar femur, and its tendon, the longest in the body, courses toward the ankle (Figs. 43-1, 43-26, 43-40 through 43-42, and 43-57).

EXTENSOR MECHANISM

The extensor mechanism of the knee includes the quadriceps muscle and tendon, the patella ligament, and the components of the patella-femoral joint.

QUADRICEPS TENDON

The rectus femoris, vastus intermedius, vastus medialis, and vastus lateralis muscles converge to insert as the quadriceps tendon at the superior pole of the patella. The fascia of these four individual muscles combine to varying degrees to form a multilayered structure. The overall thickness of the quadriceps tendon is 8 ± 2 mm. The transverse width of the tendon averages 35 ± 7 mm. Usually the vastus medialis and vastus lateralis merge producing a three-layered quadriceps tendon, with the fascia from the rectus femoris seen anteriorly and the fascia from the vastus intermedius seen posteriorly. It is also common for the fascia of the vastus medialis and lateralis muscles to combine with each other and either the fascia of the rectus femoris or vastus intermedius muscles producing a two-layered tendon. This laminar structure can easily be

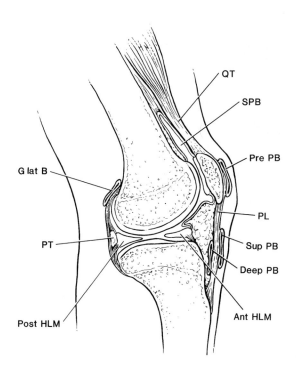

Fig. 43-57. Normal anatomy. *Ant HLM,* Anterior horn lateral meniscus; *deep PB,* deep patellar bursa; *G lat B,* gastrocnemius lateral head bursa; *PL,* patellar ligament; *post HLM,* posterior horn lateral meniscus; *pre PB,* prepatellar bursa; *PT,* popliteus tendon ; *QT,* quadriceps tendon; *SpB,* suprapatellar bursa; *sup PB,* superficial patella bursa.

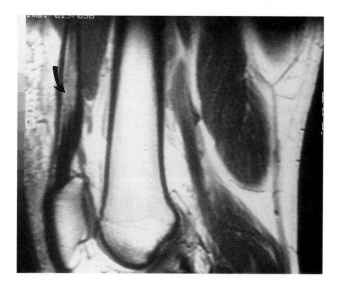

Fig. 43-58. Partial tear of the quadriceps tendon. Sagittal T1-weighted image shows increased signal intensity at the proximal portion of the quadriceps tendon indicative of partial tearing *(arrow).* The fascia from the vastus medialis and vastus lateralis are involved with sparing of the fascia from the rectus femoris and vastus intermedius muscle.

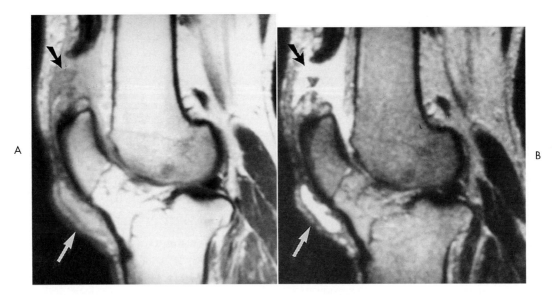

Fig. 43-59. Quadriceps tendon rupture. Sagittal proton density–weighted and T2-weighted images show complete disruption of the quadriceps tendon *(black arrow)*. Incidentally noted is a prepatellar bursitis *(white arrow)*.

seen with axial and sagittal MRI. Attention to these layers is paramount in that partial ruptures of the quadriceps tendon tend to involve one of these fascial groups. This may be difficult to detect clinically (Fig. 43-58). Full-thickness tears are more obvious (Fig. 43-59).[42]

PATELLAR LIGAMENT

The patellar ligament extends from the distal pole of the patellar to the anterior tibial tubercle. Its sagittal dimension is 3.7 ± 1.2 mm proximally, 4.3 ± 1.1 mm at the midportion, and 5.6 ± 1.1 mm distally. It is a fairly uniform low signal intensity structure seen best on sagittal images. The syndrome of patellar tendinitis really represents partial tearing and degeneration, usually of the proximal portion with secondary inflammation. Increased thickness of the proximal part, more than 7 mm, is the greatest indication of disease in symptomatic patients (Fig. 43-60). Other findings include indistinct margin with increased signal changes.[9] Others have shown, however, that these same changes can be seen in asymptomatic individuals.[32] Complete rupture leads to discontinuity, redundancy, and retraction of the ligament.

Damage to the quadriceps tendon and patellar ligament may be due to trauma or chronic overuse or be secondary to underlying systemic illnesses, such as hyperparathyroidism, gout, and rheumatic diseases. Damage to the patella-femoral articulation may be secondary to malalignment and tracking problems.

PATELLA-FEMORAL JOINT

Patella tracking abnormalities can be imaged with axial CT or MRI of the patella-femoral joints performed

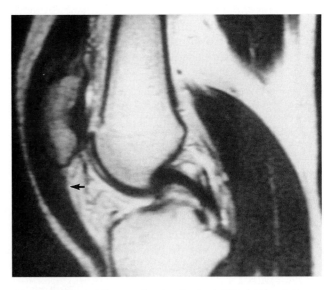

Fig. 43-60. Patellar tendinitis. Sagittal T1-weighted image shows thickening of the patellar ligament proximally *(arrow)*.

during incremental knee flexion. Both show the relationship of the patella to the femoral trochlea sulcus during the initial 30 degrees of flexion when most pathology is evident. MRI better defines the medial and lateral retinacula, although CT may image these structures as well. The patellar cartilage itself is better seen with MRI. CT arthrography may evaluate gross cartilage defects.

At 0 degrees of flexion, the patella-femoral joint is not congruent with the patella laterally displaced. With increasing flexion, the medial and lateral retinacula tighten, and the patella descends toward the midline. Eventually, congruence of the patella and trochlea is reached. In a normal knee, this state of patella-femoral

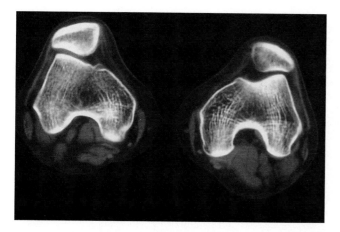

Fig. 43-61. Patellofemoral instability. Axial CT images of the patellar femoral joints show bilateral patellofemoral subluxation. Note the medial and lateral retinacula, neither of which appear taut.

congruence is reached with a lesser degree of flexion than in an abnormal knee. There remains then a wide range of what is normal and abnormal. Additional factors contributing to patella-femoral malalignment include structural abnormalities, such as misshapen patella and hypoplastic femoral trochlea sulcus and abnormally high position of the patella itself (Figs. 43-61, 43-62; and 43-63).[33]

ARTICULAR CARTILAGE

Because degeneration of the patella cartilage is such a common problem in young and older individuals, it has been extensively studied. The term "chondromalacia patella" has been used synonymously with both actual cartilage softening and the clinical syndrome of patella-femoral pain in adolescents and young adults.

The degree to which standard spin echo sequences predict the stages of patella cartilage degeneration, however, remains controversial. Based on these routine protocols for evaluating internal derangement of the knee, certain conclusions can be drawn. The articular cartilage is of uniformly low-to-intermediate signal intensity on T1-, spin density–, and T2-weighted images. Focal signal intensity changes appear to represent localized cartilaginous defects, especially when multiple pulse sequences are used. Spin density images alone are relatively insensitive to cartilage abnormalities. Normal-appearing cartilage may underestimate the degree of pathology present. These conclusions can apparently be applied to evaluation of the femoral and tibial cartilage as well. Although the consensus is that MRI is best suited for the evaluation of articular cartilage, different pulse sequences may be required.[6,12,13,17,24]

Inversion recovery sequences, chemical shift selective techniques, and numerous gradient echo sequences have been proposed. Magnetic resonance arthrography using a dilute gadolinium solution has been investigated. A less invasive technique involving intravenous gadolinium injection followed by diffusion of the agent across the synovium into pre-existing joint effusion appears to produce an arthrographic effect within 15 minutes.

Known pitfalls in the evaluation of articular cartilage include the chemical shift and volume averaging artifacts. The spatial misrepresentation of the interface of predominantly water- and fat-containing tissues occurs in the frequency encoding direction. Therefore, cartilage whose surface is perpendicular to the frequency encoding axis appears thicker or thinner than it actually is. This artifact may be reduced by decreasing the field of view or by repeating the imaging sequence after rotating the frequency and phase encoding gradients.

Volume averaging occurs whenever the imaged interface is not perpendicular to the imaging plane. The curved surfaces of the patella and femoral condylar cartilage are therefore prone to such artifacts. Imaging in at least two planes may be necessary. Also, the femoral and tibial cartilage is thinner than the patellar cartilage and hence more susceptible to volume averaging in this regard.

BURSAE

Numerous bursae are present about the knee joint. Anteriorly, two superficial bursae sit anterior to the extensor mechanism, the prepatellar bursa at the level of the patella itself, and a second bursa anterior to the patellar ligament. One or two deep patellar bursae sit posterior to the patellar ligament (see Figs. 43-26 and 43-57).

Posteriorly, bursa reside beneath the medial and lateral heads of the gastrocnemius. The former is adjacent to and usually connected with the semimembraneosus bursa. This gastrocnemius-semimembranosus bursa commonly communicates with the joint itself and represents the so-called "popliteal cyst" (Figs. 43-40 and 43-64).

Numerous bursae are present at the lateral and medial aspects of the knee joint. Laterally, bursae reside between the fibula collateral ligament and the joint capsule, the biceps femoris and fibula collateral ligament, and a third beneath the iliotibial tract. Medially, bursae reside beneath the tibial collateral ligament and the pes anserinus. A bursa may be present between the superficial and deep fibers of the tibial collateral ligament as well (see Figs. 43-41 and 43-42).

JOINT CAPSULE

The knee is the largest, most complex joint in the body. Its fibrous capsule is just as complex. Anteriorly the aponeurosis of the vastus medialis and lateralis extends from the medial and lateral margins of the quadriceps tendon, patella, and patellar ligament, poste-

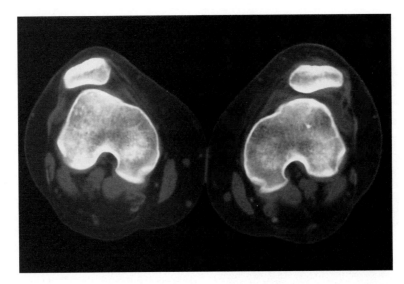

Fig. 43-62. Patellofemoral instability. Axial CT scan shows bilateral patellar femoral subluxation. The femoral trochlea grooves are shallow. A joint effusion is noted on the left.

riorly to the respective tibial and fibular collateral ligaments and tibial plateau. This anterior portion of the capsule is referred to as the medial and lateral patella retinacula.

Medially the fibrous capsule attaches at the femoral condyle just above the articular cartilage and at the tibia just below the plateau. The medial meniscus attaches to the capsule and the tibial collateral ligament complex. The coronary ligament refers to that portion of the capsule that attaches the inferior margin of the peripheral medial meniscus to the tibia.

Laterally the fibrous capsule attaches at the femoral condyle just above the popliteus tendon groove and at the tibia just below the plateau. The lateral meniscus attaches to the lateral capsule, more loosely than the medial, along its periphery except posteriorly, where the popliteus muscle and tendon interpose. The synovial membrane extends through an opening in the capsule posterolaterally between the popliteus tendon and the meniscus and more inferiorly between the tendon and the tibial cortex, often referred to as the subpopliteal recess.

NONTRAUMATIC DISORDERS

Nontraumatic conditions affecting the knee joint include the development of cystic masses, proliferative disorders of the synovium, osteonecrosis, inflammatory arthritis, osteoarthritis, and hematopoietic and neoplastic diseases.

Cystic masses about the knee

Synovial cysts about the knee represent distended bursa, which may or may not be inflamed. The most

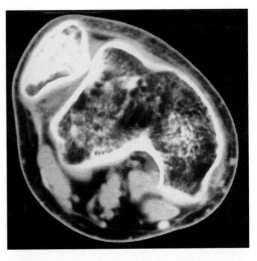

Fig. 43-63. Patellofemoral dislocation. Axial CT scan of the right knee in this patient with cerebral palsy shows chronic patellofemoral dislocation. The femoral trochlear sulcus is hypoplastic.

commonly encountered is the popliteal cyst, which usually communicates with the joint (Fig. 43-64). Isolated bursitis is also seen, pes anserinus bursitis representing such an entity. Other cystic masses about the knee include ganglion cysts and meniscal cysts.

Meniscal cysts occur at the joint line and are invariably associated with a degenerative, horizontal cleavage tear of the meniscus. Ganglion cysts may or may not have a definable communication with the joint and may occur in atypical locations, attached to tendon sheaths, within muscles, or near the proximal tibiofibula joint.

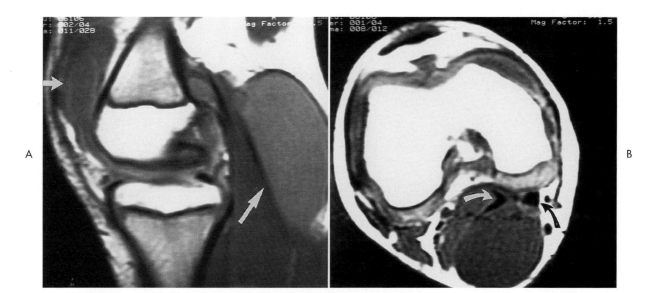

Fig. 43-64. Popliteal cyst. Sagittal and coronal T1-weighted images show fluid in the knee joint and popliteal cyst, the latter representing a distended, communicating semimembranosus-medial gastrocnemius bursa. **A,** The sagittal image shows low signal intensity fluid at the "cyst" and suprapatellar bursa *(small arrow)*. Normal high signal intensity fatty marrow is seen at the epiphyses. **B,** The axial images show the fluid-filled bursa and its relationship to the semimembranosus tendon *(curved black arrow)* and the medial gastrocnemius tendon *(curved white arrow)*.

Before any resection, the cystic nature of such a knee mass must be ascertained. The relationship to the joint must be evaluated, and associated intra-articular disease must be sought. MRI is most suited to study these issues. Generally speaking, cystic lesions on MRI have increased signal intensity on T2-weighted images and are well circumscribed with smooth walls. Because ganglion and meniscal cysts may contain a gelatinous substance high in protein content, short TR/TE images may not show lower signal intensity.

Mensical cysts are probably secondary to degenerative tears of the menisci. Synovial fluid is forced through the tear and accumulates at the meniscal-capsular junction. The larger cysts are seen posteromedially, where they may enlarge without restraint if they are posterior to the tibial collateral ligament (Fig. 43-65). These may be mistaken for popliteal cysts. Laterally, cysts appear to be more contained by the fibula collateral ligament and the iliotibial band and therefore are usually smaller (Fig. 43-66). The detection of the meniscal tear is essential in that treatment of only the cyst itself results in recurrence.

Ganglion cysts are not associated with meniscal tears but may or may not show communication with the joint capsule. Multiple components may be present. More common locations include the proximal tibiofibular joint and adjacent to the suprapatellar pouch (Fig. 43-67).[5]

Although CT may show fluid-containing structures about the knee, communication with the joint and meniscal tears is not demonstrated.[22]

Pigmented villonodular synovitis

Pigmented villonodular synovitis (PVNS) is a rare monarticular proliferative disorder of the synovium occurring in adults. The most common site of involvement is the knee. Although conventional radiographs may show associated pressure erosions of the underlying bone, most cases involving the knee demonstrate normal osseous structures at the time of clinical presentation. Soft tissue masses within the knee joint may be appreciated on plain films. MRI reveals the proliferative synovial mass throughout the confines of the joint capsule. The signal intensity characteristics may vary owing to the presence of abundant hemosiderin, inflamed synovium, and joint effusion. Certainly the presence of multiple areas of low signal intensity on all pulse sequences is a clue to the abundant hemorrhage present (Fig. 43-68). The differential diagnosis, however, includes other disorders that may be accompanied by hemarthrosis, such as hemophilia, synovial hemangioma, and inflammatory arthritis.

CT arthrography shows nonspecific nodular proliferation of the synovium. Osseous erosions are demonstrated.

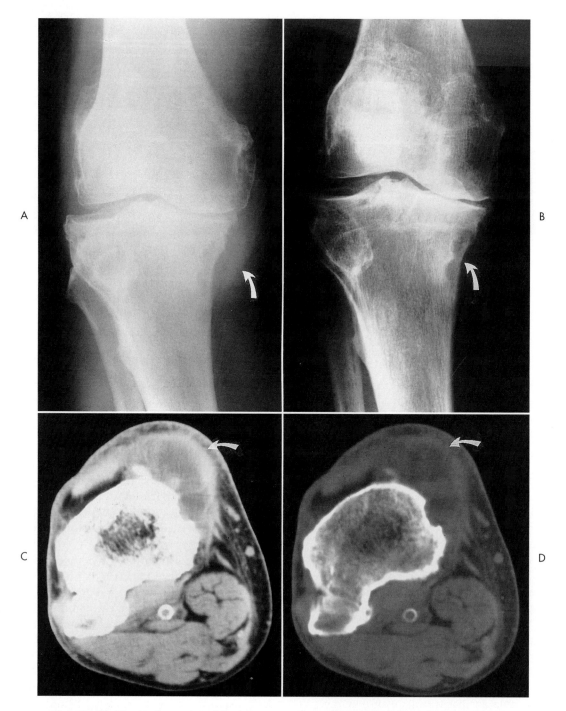

Fig. 43-65. Meniscal cyst. **A** and **B**, Anteroposterior radiographs of the right knee show osteoarthritis with a soft tissue mass medially causing pressure erosion of the proximal medial tibia *(arrow)*. **C** and **D**, CT scan shows a fluid-filled mass eroding the adjacent tibia *(arrow)*.

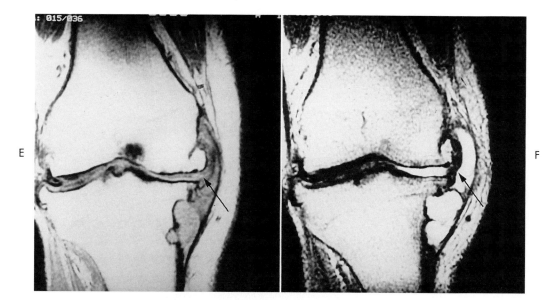

Fig. 43-65, cont'd. E and **F,** Coronal proton density–weighted and T2-weighted images show the cystic structure communicating with the osteoarthritic joint. The lateral meniscus is degenerated, and what remains of the medial meniscus has been displaced beyond the joint margins *(arrow)*. A meniscal cyst was found at surgery.

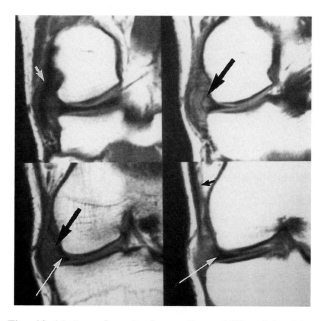

Fig. 43-66. Lateral meniscal cyst. Coronal T1-weighted images show a small lateral meniscal cyst *(large black arrow)* and an associated meniscal tear *(large white arrow)*. Note the relative containment by the fibular collateral ligament *(small white arrow)* and the iliotibial band *(small black arrow)*.

Synovial chondromatosis

Synovial chondromatosis represents the other major proliferative disorder of the synovium. As with PVNS, it is a rare monarticular disease that is seen principally in adults. Cartilaginous metaplasia of the synovium leads to the production of multiple cartilage bodies within the confines of the joint. The knee is most commonly involved. As with PVNS, osseous erosions may be present. Although PVNS virtually never calcifies, cartilaginous bodies are prone to such calcification and ossification. The x-ray appearance of multiple calcified and ossified bodies of similar size distributed throughout the confines of the joint capsule is diagnostic of the disorder. When these bodies are not calcified, MRI detects them and is diagnostic.

CT arthrography shows multiple bodies in the joint as well. Plain CT may detect calcification not apparent on x-ray and in this regard may differentiate this entity from PVNS.

Osteonecrosis

Spontaneous osteonecrosis of the knee is an idiopathic disorder of middle-aged and elderly adults usually affecting the weight-bearing portion of the medial femoral condyle less frequently affecting the medial tibial plateau, lateral femoral condyle, and lateral tibial plateau. Its onset is heralded by acute pain. X-ray films are normal for approximately 4 to 6 weeks. MRI, however, usually demonstrates a poorly defined zone of decreased signal intensity on T1-weighted images at the subchondral bone. On T2-weighted images, a poorly defined ring of moderately high signal intensity may be noted about the lesion. Associated osteoarthritis and degenerative tearing of the medial meniscus may be present. It has been demonstrated that such meniscal tears precede the necrotic event.[4] Of course, degenerative cleavage tears are com-

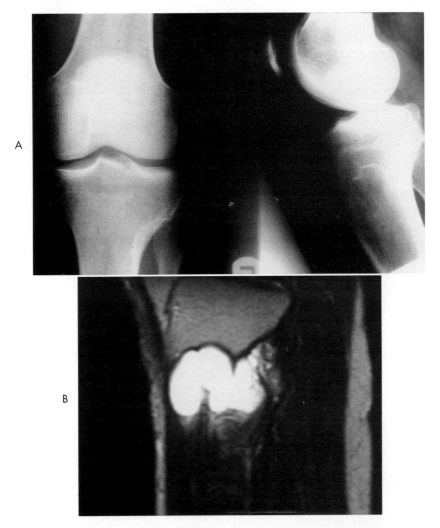

Fig. 43-67. Ganglion cyst. **A,** Anteroposterior and lateral radiographs of the left knee reveal osseous erosion at the lateral aspect of the proximal left tibia. **B,** Sagittal T2-weighted image shows a high signal intensity mass at the lateral aspect of the proximal left tibia near the proximal tibia-fibula joint. A ganglion cyst was removed surgically.

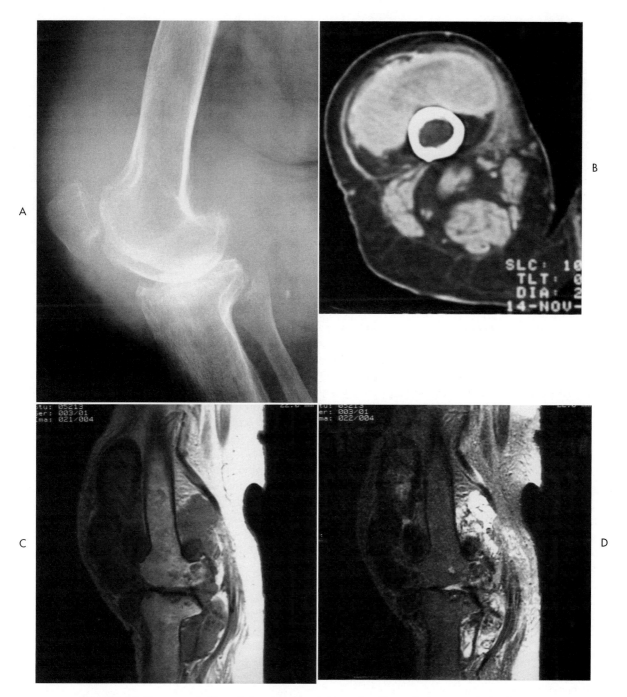

Fig. 43-68. Pigmented villonodular synovitis. **A,** Lateral radiograph shows marked soft tissue prominence within the joint capsule associated with osseus erosions. **B,** Axial CT scan shows mixed attenuation fullness at the suprapatellar bursa. **C** and **D,** Sagittal proton density–weighted images and T2-weighted images show the extent of the mixed signal mass within the joint. Persistent low signal areas on both sequences, especially those at the capsular margins, indicate extensive hemosiderin deposition and a probable diagnosis of PVNS.

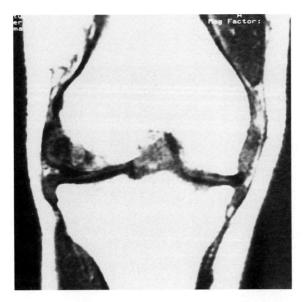

Fig. 43-69. Rheumatoid arthritis. Coronal T1-weighted image shows mixed signal intensity pannus within the joint capsule leading to osseous erosions.

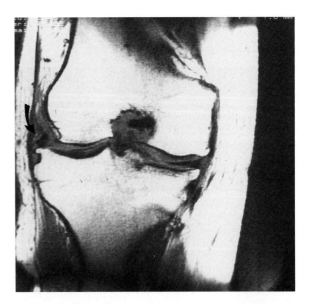

Fig. 43-70. Osteoarthritis. Coronal T1-weighted image shows marked lateral compartment narrowing, osteophyte formation, and lateral subluxation of the tibia. The lateral meniscus is degenerated, and what remains rests beyond the margin of the joint (*curved arrow*).

mon in the population susceptible to osteonecrosis of the knee.

Eventually, bone necrosis progresses to fracture and collapse of the subchondral bone with fragmentation of the articular cartilage. Osteoarthritis then may be secondary to the necrosis or exist coincidentally before the necrotic event.[3]

Inflammatory arthritis

The role of MRI in the care of patients with inflammatory arthritis is controversal. Certainly, MRI can show early erosions. It can also differentiate among joint effusion, active pannus formation, and chronic pannus and fibrosis with the aid of gadolinium. Both joint fluid and active pannus brighten on T2-weighted images, but only active pannus significantly enhances after gadolinium administration on T1-weighted images. Fibrotic pannus does not enhance with gadolinium on T1-weighted images and does not brighten on T2-weighted images. These distinctions are important to patient management in some but not all centers at this time (Fig. 43-69).[20]

Osteoarthritis

Osteoarthritis may be coincidentally present when other disorders are sought. Osteophyte formation, subchondral sclerosis, subchondral cyst formation, and cartilage loss can all be appreciated.

Degeneration of the menisci is independent of degeneration of the femorotibial compartments. It usually precedes the development of osteoarthritis, although it may accelerate the process. Therefore, associated degen-

erative horizontal cleavage tears of the menisci may be seen. These represent the extension of internal meniscal disruption to the free edge. Inferior articular surface, or capsular margin. The development of meniscal cysts has already been discussed.

With advancing osteoarthritis, what remains of the menisci may become adherent to the marginal osteophytes and eventually extruded beyond the margins of the joint. As the femorotibial compartments narrow, the meniscus may be forced between the joint capsule and underlying bone often to a point above or below the level of the joint itself (Fig. 43-70).

Hematopoietic and neoplastic diseases

As mentioned, MRI is exquisitely sensitive to changes in bone marrow, and hence myeloproliferative disorders, neoplasms, marrow reconversion and marrow failure are all well seen. One can imagine that processes affecting the marrow itself can be imaged long before trabecular bony changes are seen (Fig. 43-71). Such changes are necessary before CT can be of value.

It becomes clear that MRI has become the primary imaging modality of the knee. CT, however, remains helpful in evaluating any lesion characterized by calcification or ossification. As discussed earlier, both CT and MRI are also useful in evaluation of patellar-femoral instability and tibial plateau fractures.

Osteoid osteoma remains one bone lesion that is best diagnosed with thin section CT scanning often fol-

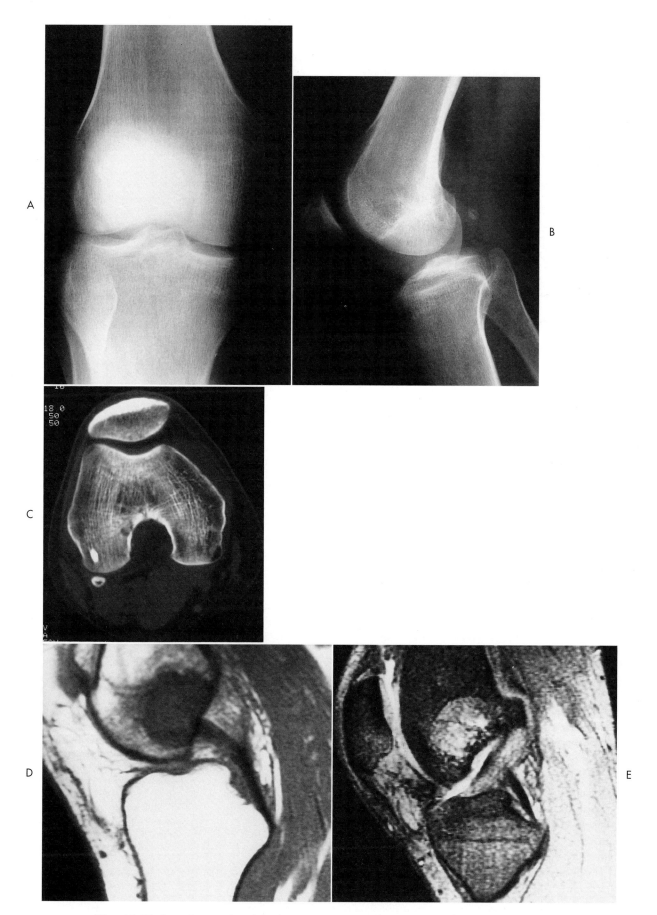

Fig. 43-71. Lymphoma. **A** and **B,** Anteroposterior and lateral radiographs of the right knee are normal. **C,** CT scan of the condylar region show vague rarefaction. **D** and **E,** Sagittal T1-weighted and gradient echo images show a focal abnormality at the condylar region, which represented non-Hodgkin lymphoma before gross trabecular destruction.

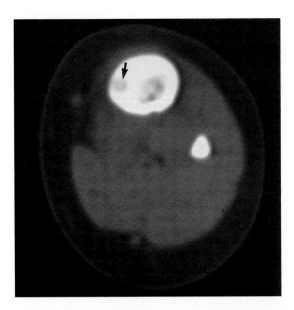

Fig. 43-72. Osteoid osteoma. CT scan of the proximal left leg shows the nidus with central mineralization *(arrow)*.

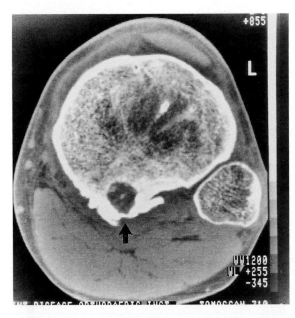

Fig. 43-73. Osteoid osteoma. CT scan of the proximal left leg shows a well-defined nidus with central mineralization and associated periosteal reaction at the posterior aspect of the proximal left tibia *(arrow)*.

lowing localization with bone scan (Figs. 43-72 and 43-73).[19] It more clearly defines the tiny nidus, whereas MRI may reveal a more vague region of bone marrow edema. Detection of tumor calcification or ossification is also more clearly seen with CT scanning and may be missed altogether with MRI. This is particularly useful in the evaluation of other bone-forming tumors and cartilage tumors.

ACKNOWLEDGMENT

The authors gratefully acknowledge Celena Cinetti for her valuable assistance in preparing this chapter.

REFERENCES

1. Allen GJ: Longitudinal stress fractures of the tibia: diagnosis with CT. *Radiology* 167:799-801, 1988.
2. Beltran J: *MRI musculoskeletal system,* ed 1, New York, 1990, Gower Medical Publishing.
3. Bjorkengren AG, Al Rowaih A, Lindstrand A, et al: Spontaneous osteonecrosis of the knee: value of MR imaging in determining prognosis. *AJR* 154:331-336, 1990.
4. Brahme SK, Fox JM, Ferkel RD, et al: Osteonecrosis of the knee after arthroscopic surgery: diagnosis with MR imaging. *Radiology* 178:851-853, 1991.
5. Burk DL Jr, Dalinka MK, Kanal E, et al: Meniscal and ganglion cysts of the knee: MR evaluation. *AJR* 150:331-336, 1988.
6. Chandnani VP, Ho C, Chu P, et al: Knee hyaline cartilage evaluated with MR imaging: a cadaveric study involving multiple imaging sequences and intraarticular injection of gadolinium and saline solution. *Radiology* 178:557-561, 1991.
7. DeSmet AA, Fisher DR, Graf BK, Lange RH: Osteochondritis dissecans of the knee: value of MR imaging in determining lesion stability and the presence of articular cartilage defects. *AJR* 155:549-553, 1990.
8. Deutsch AL, Mink JH, Fox JM, et al: Peripheral meniscal tears: MR findings after conservative treatment or arthroscopic repair. *Radiology* 176:485-488, 1990.
9. El-Khoury GY, Wira RL, Berbaum KS, et al: MR imaging of patellar tendinitis. *Radiology* 184:849-854, 1992.
10. Firooznia HF, Golimbu C, Rafii N, et al: *MRI and CT of the musculoskeletal system.* St. Louis, 1992, Mosby-Year Book.
11. Grover JS, Bassett LW, Gross ML, et al: Posterior cruciate ligament: MR imaging. *Radiology* 174:527-530, 1990.
12. Hayes CW, Conway WF: Evaluation of articular cartilage: radiographic and cross-sectional imaging techniques. *Radiographics* 12:409-428, 1992.
13. Hayes CW, Sawyer RW, Conway WF: Patellar cartilage lesions: in vitro detection and staging with MR imaging and pathologic correlation. *Radiology* 176:479-483, 1990.
14. Herman LJ, Beltran J: Pitfalls in MR imaging of the knee. *Radiology* 167:775-781, 1988.
15. Hodler J, Haghighi P, Pathria MN, et al: Meniscal changes in the elderly: correlation of MR imaging and histologic findings. *Radiology* 184:221-225, 1992.
16. Hodler J, Haghighi P, Trudell D, Resnick D: The cruciate ligaments of the knee: correlation between MR appearance and gross and histologic findings in cadaveric specimens. *AJR* 159:357-360, 1992.
17. Hodler J, Resnick D: Chondromalacia patellae. *AJR* 158:106-107, 1992.
18. Kaplan PA, Walker CW, Kilcoyne RF, et al: Occult fracture patterns of the knee associated with anterior cruciate ligament tears: assessment with MR imaging. *Radiology* 183:835-838, 1992.
19. Klein MH, Shankman S: Osteoid osteoma: radiologic and pathologic correlation. *Skel Radiol* 21:23-31, 1992.
20. Konig H, Sieper J, Wolf KJ: Rheumatoid arthritis: evaluation of hypervascular and fibrous pannus with dynamic MR imaging enhanced with Gd-DTPA. *Radiology* 176:473-477, 1990.
21. Lee JK, Yao L: Stress fractures: MR imaging. *Radiology* 169:217-220, 1988.
22. Lee R, Cox G, Neff J, et al: Cystic masses of the knee: arthrographic and CT evaluation. *AJR* 148:329-335, 1987.
23. Lynch TCP, Crues JV III, Morgan FW, et al: Bone abnormalities

of the knee: prevalence and significance at MR imaging. *Radiology* 171:761-766, 1989.

24. McCauley TR, Kier R, Lynch KJ, Okl P: Chondromalacia patellae: diagnosis with MR imaging. *AJR* 158:101-105, 1992.
25. Mink JH, Deutsch AL: Occult cartilage and bone injuries of the knee: detection, classification, and assessment with MR imaging. *Radiology* 170:823-829, 1989.
26. Mink JH, Levy T, Crues JV III: Tears of the anterior cruciate ligament and menisci of the knee: MR imaging evaluation. *Radiology* 167:769-774, 1988.
27. Mink JH, Reicher MA, Crues JV III: *Magnetic resonance imaging of the knee*, ed 1, New York; 1987, Raven Press.
28. Murphy BJ, Smith RL, Uribe JW, et al: Bone signal abnormalities in the posterolateral tibia and lateral femoral condyle in complete tears of the anterior cruciate ligament: a specific sign? *Radiology* 182:221-224, 1992.
29. Rafii M, Firooznia H, Golimbu C, et al: Computed tomography of tibial plateau fractures. *AJR* 142:1181-1185, 1984.
30. Rak KM, Gillogly SD, Schaefer RA, et al: Anterior cruciate ligament reconstruction: evaluation with MR imaging. *Radiology* 178:553-556, 1991.
31. Remer EM, Fitzgerald SW, Friedman H, et al: Anterior cruciate ligament injury: MR imaging diagnosis and patterns of injury. *Radiographics* 12:901-915, 1992.
32. Schweitzer ME, Mitchell DG: MR imaging of the patella tendon: buckling and other normal variants. Abstract *RSNA*, 1992.
33. Shellock FG, Mink JH, Deutsch AL, Fox JM: Patellar tracking ab-normalities: clinical experience with kinematic MR imaging in 130 patients. *Radiology* 172:799-804, 1989.
34. Silverman JM, Mink JH, Deutsch AL: Discoid menisci of the knee: MR imaging appearance. *Radiology* 173:351-354, 1989.
35. Smith DK, Totty WG: The knee after partial meniscectomy: MR imaging features. *Radiology* 176:141-144, 1990.
36. Stoller DW, Martin C, Crues JV III, et al: Meniscal tears: pathologic correlation with MR imaging. *Radiology* 163:731-735, 1987.
37. Vahey TN, Bennett HT, Arrington LE, et al: MR imaging of the knee: pseudotear of the lateral meniscus caused by the meniscofemoral ligament. *AJR* 154:1237-1239, 1990.
38. Vahey TN, Broome DR, Kayes KJ, Shelbourne KD: Acute and chronic tears of the anterior cruciate ligament: differential features at MR imaging. *Radiology* 181:251-253, 1991.
39. Vellet AD, Marks PH, Fowler PJ, Munro TG: Occult posttraumatic osteochondral lesions of the knee: prevalence, classification, and short-term sequelae evaluated with MR imaging. *Radiology* 178:271-276, 1991.
40. Weber WN, Neuman CH, Barakos JA, et al: Lateral tibial rim (Segond) fractures: MR imaging characteristics. *Radiology* 180:731-734, 1991.
41. Yao L, Lee JK: Occult intraosseous fracture: detection with MR imaging. *Radiology* 167:749-751, 1988.
42. Zeiss J, Saddemi SR, Ebraheim NA: MR imaging of the quadriceps tendon: normal layered configuration and its importance in cases of tendon rupture. *AJR* 159:1031-1034, 1992.

44
The Shoulder

TAMARA MINER HAYGOOD
KATHLEEN GALLAGHER OXNER
J. BRUCE KNEELAND
MURRAY K. DALINKA

When organizing this chapter about shoulder imaging, a subject to which hundreds of articles and one complete book[124] have already been devoted, we faced some thorny decisions about what topics to include and how much attention to devote to each. The desire to be comprehensive weighed against the need to restrict ourselves to a discussion of reasonable length. We chose to emphasize disorders that are unique to the shoulder at the expense of those that occur elsewhere as well. Thus, for example, we strove for a more detailed discussion of rotator cuff disease than of neoplasms, all of which occur at other sites and none of which claim the shoulder as a favorite location. No scheme will please everyone, but we hope this arrangement will be satisfactory to the majority of our readers.

ANATOMY

For purposes of this chapter, the shoulder will be considered to include the glenohumeral joint, the acromioclavicular joint, and related soft tissues. The glenohumeral joint is relatively shallow, with the humeral head large in comparison to the glenoid fossa. This configuration grants mobility at the expense of stability. The labrum is a meniscus-like fibrous or fibrocartilaginous structure that runs about the edge of the glenoid. It is firmly attached inferiorly but may be loosely attached or even unattached superiorly. It serves to increase the depth of the glenoid, providing more contact area and thus more stability for the glenohumeral joint.[15,78,99]

Surrounding the glenohumeral joint is the joint capsule, which attaches to both the anatomic neck of the humerus and the scapula. Its scapular attachment is variable, with three different types being generally recognized based on its attachment at the midpoint of the glenoid. The Type I capsule attaches to the anterior labrum.

Type II capsules attach to the glenoid just medial to the labrum. Type I and II are both stable configurations and may be difficult to tell apart at imaging. Type III capsules are relatively loose and attach farther medially along the glenoid. Although Type III capsules may be a normal variant, they are associated with anterior instability.[78,85]

Compared with the capsules of other joints, the glenohumeral joint capsule is relatively loose and allows maximal movement of the joint. There are three normal extensions of the joint capsule where joint fluid may be seen at imaging in patients with an effusion. The first is a communication with the sheath of the long head of the biceps as it runs through the intertubercular groove. The second reaches under the coracoid process to communicate with the subscapular bursa. The third is the axillary recess or axillary pouch, a loose fold of thickened capsule at the inferior extent of the capsule that tightens when the arm is abducted.[76]

Three glenohumeral ligaments represent thickened areas of the joint capsule. The superior glenohumeral ligament runs from the superior glenoid tubercle and nearby labrum to the fovea capitis of the humerus. It is the most consistent of the three in its course and is often identified at cross-sectional imaging. The middle glenohumeral ligament is the most variable of the three in its course and thickness. It is located anterior to the joint and generally runs in an inferolateral direction from the glenoid just below the glenoid tubercle to the lesser tuberosity of the humerus.[16,29]

The inferior glenohumeral ligament complex consists of distinct anterior and posterior bands separated by the axillary pouch. This ligament complex is the most important of the three glenohumeral ligaments as a stabilizer. It is also the one that stands out least from the joint

1516

capsule. It is the least often visualized in axial imaging, though the axillary pouch may be seen in coronal projection. The complex runs from the inferior labrum to the humeral neck. It stabilizes the joint against both anterior and posterior dislocation.[91]

A number of other ligaments also help stabilize the shoulder. The coracoacromial ligament passes beneath the deltoid and above the subacromial-subdeltoid bursa. It supports the shoulder against upward pressure. The coracohumeral ligament runs from the lateral aspect of the base of the coracoid to insert on the humerus adjacent to the greater tuberosity, where its fibers blend at its insertion site with those of the joint capsule. It passively supports the humerus when it hangs at the side. It is also a major stabilizer of the biceps tendon in its groove. The coracoclavicular ligament is made up of two parts, the trapezoid ligament and the conoid ligament. The former runs from the coracoid process to the undersurface of the distal clavicle, and the latter runs from the coracoid to the conoid tubercle of the clavicle. The acromioclavicular ligament strengthens the superior portion of the tight-fitting acromioclavicular joint capsule. Both it and the coracoclavicular ligament stabilize the acromioclavicular joint.[76,105]

Four muscles, the supraspinatus, the infraspinatus, the teres minor, and the subscapularis, together with their tendons, form the rotator cuff. All originate on the scapula and insert on the humerus. They are responsible for abduction and internal and external rotation of the glenohumeral joint. The supraspinatus is the most often injured of these muscles. It arches superiorly over the humerus to insert superolaterally on the greater tuberosity. The infraspinatus and teres minor also insert on the greater tuberosity, each a little more inferiorly and posteriorly. The subscapularis has a broad origin on the anterior scapula and inserts with multiple tendon slips onto the lesser tuberosity.

The large deltoid muscle extends from a very broad origin on the distal clavicle and acromion to insert into the deltoid tubercle of the lateral aspect of the proximal humeral diaphysis. Occasionally a proximal tendon slip of the deltoid arises from the undersurface of the clavicle or acromion, where it may mimic a spur. The deltoid is external to the rotator cuff and separated from it by the subacromial-subdeltoid bursa and its associated extrasynovial fat pad. The subacromial-subdeltoid bursa does not normally communicate with the glenohumeral joint. The peribursal fat pad has a rather variable appearance. Obliteration of a portion of this fat pad may occur in normal shoulders at MRI and in shoulders with rotator cuff pathology.[21,47,75,86]

Between the greater and lesser tuberosity lies the bicipital groove, also called the intertubercular sulcus. This depression cradles the tendon of the long head of the biceps brachii, which originates from the superior glenoid tubercle and superior labrum. Its proximal tendon passes anteriorly over the humeral head through the rotator interval, which separates the supraspinatus and subscapularis muscles. It then passes through the bicipital groove to the muscle belly. The tendon is secured in its groove superiorly by the coracohumeral ligament, its most important stabilizer, and by the transverse humeral ligament, to which the subscapularis tendon may lend some fibers. More inferiorly, the tendon of the pectoralis major also contributes to stabilization of the biceps tendon in its groove.[24]

The coracoacromial ligament forms part of the coracoacromial arch, which consists of the coracoacromial ligament and the structures it connects—the coracoid process of the scapula and the anterior acromion. This relatively immobile complex not only provides support to the shoulder but may also impinge on the tendon of the supraspinatus muscle, causing tendinitis and contributing to an eventual tear. Three different configurations of the acromion have been described. Type I is flat inferiorly. Type II curves smoothly. In Type III the most anterior portion of the acromion has a hooked shape. Type II and III are believed to be associated with increasing risk of rotator cuff disease.[5] The inferior margins of the acromion and distal clavicle usually lie at approximately the same level in the coronal plane. A low-lying acromion, which is positioned somewhat inferior to the distal end of the clavicle, may also lead to rotator cuff pathology, though there are no definitive criteria to separate a normally positioned acromion from a low-lying acromion or to differentiate a low-lying acromion from a high-riding clavicle, as may occur following an acromioclavicular joint separation.[48]

Three neurovascular structures are important to the imaging anatomy of the shoulder. Running on the posterior aspect of the scapula are the suprascapular nerve and artery. The nerve arises from the upper trunk of the brachial plexus and passes through the suprascapular notch. It then runs deep to the supraspinatus muscle. When it emerges from beneath the supraspinatus, it passes through the spinoglenoid notch. It carries both sensory and motor fibers and supplies motor innervation to the supraspinatus and infraspinatus muscles.[33,76]

Another vascular structure of imaging importance is the anterolateral branch of the anterior circumflex humeral artery. This small vessel runs for a short distance next to the tendon of the long head of the biceps within the intertubercular groove. It can be mistaken for a bicipital tendon disorder, particularly on gradient-echo sequences in which arterial flow appears bright.[76]

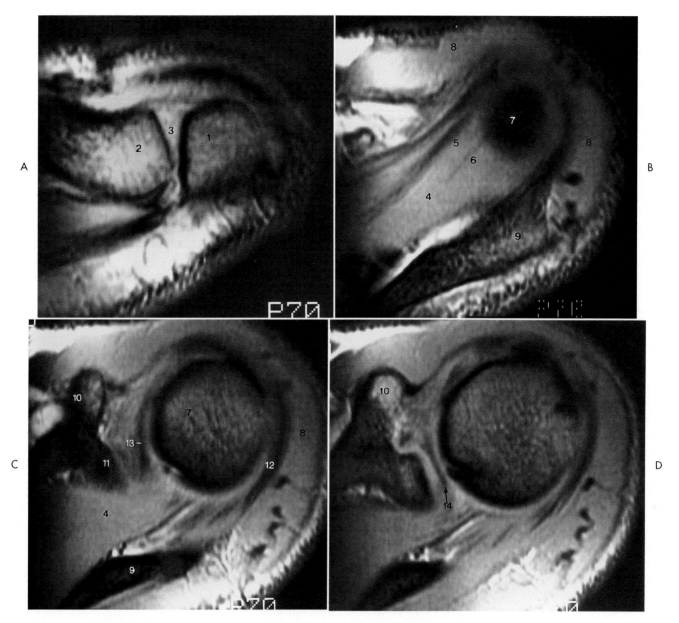

Fig. 44-1. MRI axial views of the shoulder (see text for details). *1*, Acromion. *2*, Clavicle. *3*, Acromioclavicular joint. *4*, Supraspinatus muscle. *5*, Anterior main tendon. *6*, Posterior tendon slip. *7*, Humeral head. *8*, Deltoid muscle. *9*, Scapular spine. *10*, Coracoid process. *11*, Glenoid. *12*, Infraspinatus muscle/tendon. *13*, Superior glenohumeral ligament. *14*, Superior labrum. *15*, Coracohumeral ligament. *16*, Anterior labrum. *17*, Posterior labrum. *18*, Glenoid articular cartilage. *19*, Greater tuberosity. *20*, Lesser tuberosity. *21*, Bicipital groove. *22*, Middle glenohumeral ligament. *23*, Bicipital tendon. *24*, Subscapularis muscle and tendon.

Continued.

CROSS-SECTIONAL ANATOMY

The following section describes the anatomy of the shoulder from the viewpoint of cross-sectional imaging in the three planes often obtained in MRI: axial, coronal oblique, and sagittal oblique. It is illustrated in Figs. 44-1 (*A-E*), 44-2 (*A-E*), and 44-3 (*A-E*).

Axial projection (Fig. 44-1)

A, At the level of the acromioclavicular joint, the acromion curves in on the lateral side of the shoulder to meet the distal end of the clavicle. It is not unusual for the ends of the bones to be oriented at slightly different angles. **B,** At the level of the top of the humeral head,

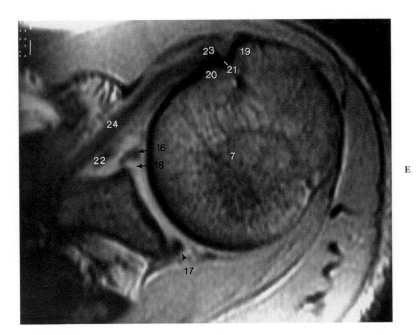

Fig. 44-1, cont'd.

the supraspinatus muscle will be seen arching across the humerus from posteromedial to anterolateral and may appear to surround the humeral head. A large, principal tendon arises from the anterior, fusiform portion of the muscle. Small individual tendon slips arise from the posterior supraspinatus, which morphologically resembles a strap muscle. Note that the course of the main tendon is angled slightly differently than the muscle.[118] The deltoid forms a thick semicircle of muscle external to the supraspinatus. The scapular spine can be noted posteriorly as it runs laterally and superiorly to form the acromion. **C,** At the level of the top of the coracoid process of the scapula, the humeral head normally has a round shape. The top of the glenoid is usually seen here, but it is not uncommon for the labrum to be inapparent. The supraspinatus muscle projects between the glenoid and inferior extension of the scapular spine. The infraspinatus tendon emerges anteriorly to attach to the greater tuberosity. Running from posterior to anterior between the glenoid and humeral head at this level is a black structure that may represent the superior glenohumeral ligament. Because of the variation in the course of the glenohumeral ligaments, their identification at imaging is sometimes more art than science. A Hill-Sachs deformity, if present, will be identified at this level or higher. **D,** Closer to the base of the coracoid, the superior labrum may become identifiable. **E,** The level where the humeral head is the largest in cross-sectional area is the best place to see the labrum in axial imaging. The normal posterior labrum has a relatively constant blunt triangular shape. The anterior labrum may vary considerably in

shape. It may appear either round or pointed and may exhibit longitudinal or transverse clefts.[41,67,72,85] Both anteriorly and posteriorly the articular cartilage comes to the edge of the glenoid, and this forms an area of increased signal that burrows beneath the internal edge of the labrum and must not be mistaken for a tear.[59] At this level the humeral head will have an oblong shape with two identations. Anteriorly, the greater and lesser tuberosities surround the bicipital groove, in which rests the tendon of the long head of the biceps. Posteriorly is a small concavity or flattening of the humerus that may be mistaken for a Hill-Sachs deformity.[107] Other structures routinely visualized here include the anterior joint capsule, middle glenohumeral ligament, and subscapularis muscle and tendon.

Coronal oblique projection (Fig. 44-2)

A, The subscapularis muscle runs anterior to the scapular blade and just beneath the base of the coracoid to attach to the lesser tuberosity. Inferior to this are the flow voids of axillary vessels within the quadrilateral space. Superiorly the anterior-most extent of the clavicle gives origin to a portion of the deltoid. **B,** More posteriorly the anterior humeral head may be seen with the greater and lesser tuberosities and the dark bicipital tendon within its groove. The coracohumeral ligament runs at an angle with respect to this plane of imaging, but portions of it may be seen. **C,** At the midglenoid, the glenohumeral articulation is well seen. It is best visualized in the coronal projection at the point at which the glenoid is most prominent. Also well seen at this level is the

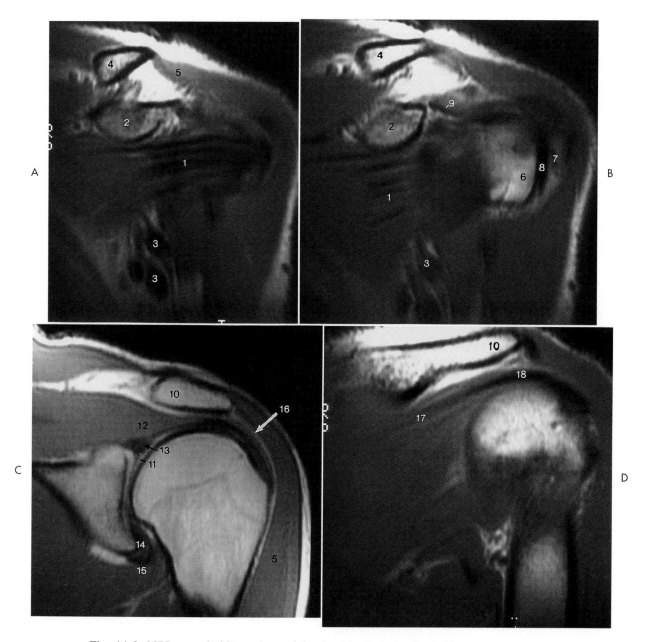

Fig. 44-2. MRI coronal oblique views of the shoulder (see text for details). *1,* Subscapularis muscle. *2,* Coracoid process. *3,* Axillary vessels. *4,* Clavicle. *5,* Deltoid. *6,* Lesser tuberosity. *7,* Greater tubersity. *8,* Bicipital tendon. *9,* Coracohumeral ligament. *10,* Acromion. *11,* Humeral articular cartilage. *12,* Supraspinatus muscle and tendon. *13,* Superior labrum. *14,* Inferior labrum. *15,* Inferior glenohumeral ligament/axillary recess. *16,* Fat stripe. *17,* Infraspinatus muscle. *18,* Infraspinatus tendon.

tendon of the supraspinatus and the peribursal fat stripe. A portion of the inferior glenohumeral ligament is seen below the inferior labrum. **D,** Far posterior in the shoulder the infraspinatus muscle and tendon pass under the acromion to insert on the greater tuberosity. Depending on the degree of internal or external rotation, this attachment site may not always be visualized in the same plane as the muscle. It may be quite difficult in an individual

patient to decide where the supraspinatus muscle ends and the infraspinatus begins.

Sagittal oblique projection (Fig. 44-3)

A, The four rotator cuff tendons blend at their insertion sites into a fibrous band that appears on MRI as a solid arc of dark signal draped across the humeral head. The deltoid muscle projects external to the rota-

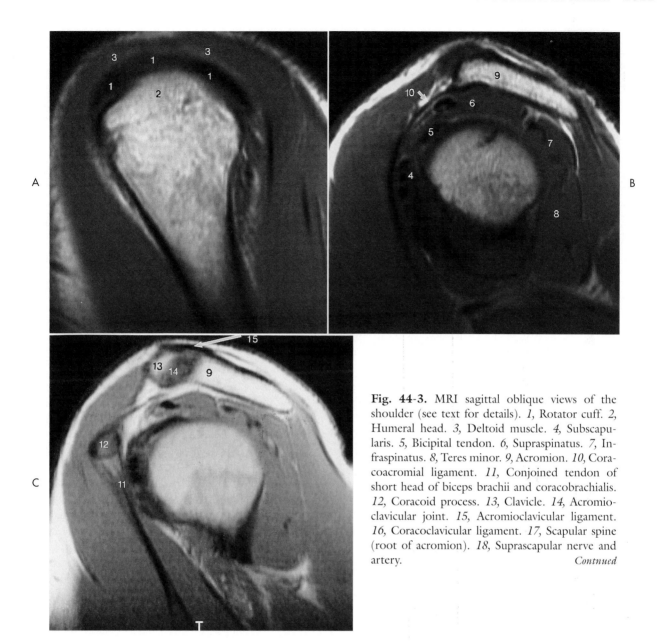

Fig. 44-3. MRI sagittal oblique views of the shoulder (see text for details). *1*, Rotator cuff. *2*, Humeral head. *3*, Deltoid muscle. *4*, Subscapularis. *5*, Bicipital tendon. *6*, Supraspinatus. *7*, Infraspinatus. *8*, Teres minor. *9*, Acromion. *10*, Coracoacromial ligament. *11*, Conjoined tendon of short head of biceps brachii and coracobrachialis. *12*, Coracoid process. *13*, Clavicle. *14*, Acromioclavicular joint. *15*, Acromioclavicular ligament. *16*, Coracoclavicular ligament. *17*, Scapular spine (root of acromion). *18*, Suprascapular nerve and artery. *Continued*

tor cuff. The physeal scar is often visible in adults. To distinguish anterior from posterior in the sagittal projection, note that a supine patient's arm will usually tilt backwards a bit from the shoulder, so as a first approximation the direction the distal humerus points may be taken as posterior. **B,** At the level of the medial humeral head the rotator cuff muscles are separate from one another. (The infraspinatus and teres minor may, however, be inseparable both anatomically and tomographically.) The biceps tendon is seen close to the humeral head in the rotator interval between the subscapularis and supraspinatus. The coracoacromial ligament is the dark structure arching anteriorly and inferiorly from the inferior margin of this slightly hooked acromion. **C,** Slightly more medially the lateral aspect of the coracoid process

becomes visible. The coracoid is a reliable marker for anterior. **D,** Farther medially the coracoid process arises from its base on the scapula. One of the coracoclavicular ligaments projects between the coracoid and the clavicle. **E,** At the level of the scapular "Y" the suprascapular artery and nerve are seen running beneath the body of the supraspinatus muscle and through the spinoglenoid notch.

TECHNIQUE

In evaluation of bony trauma, noncontrast CT of the shoulder is often useful. Contiguous 5-mm slices in the axial plane beginning at the acromioclavicular joint are sufficient to find or exclude fractures. The scan should extend a few centimeters below the most inferior

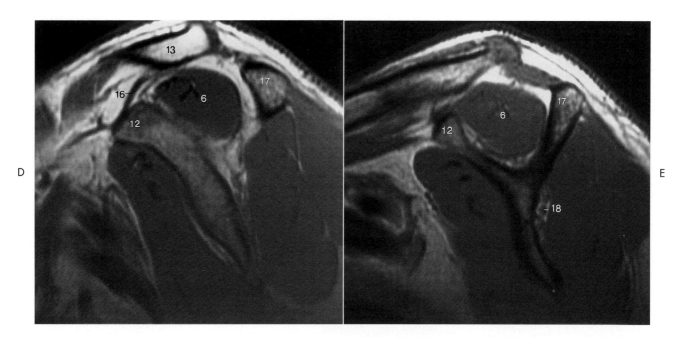

Fig. 44-3, cont'd.

fracture line. If coronal, sagittal, or three-dimensional reconstruction is desired, thinner cuts will provide smoother reconstructed images. A bone algorithm should be employed.[19]

CT arthrography is useful for evaluation of the joint capsule and intracapsular structures and for finding loose bodies within the joint. It may be the most accurate technique for studying the labrum. Fluoroscopy is used to guide a needle into the glenohumeral joint. One half to 3.0 ml of contrast material and approximately 10 ml of room air are introduced into the glenohumeral joint, and the needle is withdrawn. Contiguous slices are obtained at 3- to 4-mm intervals from a level just above the coracoid to below the glenoid fossa.[19,22,100,110-112,122]

CT arthrography has been overtaken in many imaging centers by MRI as the preferred technique for evaluation of intracapsular structures. MRI allows better concurrent evaluation of extracapsular structures such as the rotator cuff, is noninvasive, and does not require coordination with the fluoroscopy schedule. It does, however, have disadvantages. MRI is contraindicated in patients with intraorbital metal, pacemakers, and intracranial surgical clips. Ferromagnetic metallic surgical devices in the region being scanned may ruin the images. (This, of course, may also be a problem for CT.) Many claustrophobic patients can tolerate the confinement of a cylindrical superconducting magnet only with difficulty or not at all.

Depiction of intracapsular structures, the capsule itself, and the undersurface of the rotator cuff by MRI are greatly enhanced by a joint effusion, which is often conveniently present concomitantly with disease, particularly in young persons. When an effusion is not present, however, these structures become more difficult to interpret. To obtain the affect of an effusion, several investigators advocate the use of intraarticular Gd-DTPA in evaluation of both the rotator cuff and the glenoid labrum.[31] The procedure involves the fluoroscopically guided placement of the needle confirmed by a small injection of iodinated contrast followed by the injection of Gd-DTPA diluted approximately 1:250 with normal saline. The FDA has not granted approval for intraarticular injection of Gd-DTPA, so approval of an institutional review board must be obtained prior to performing these studies. An alternative procedure that does not require review board approval is the intraarticular injection of normal saline with acquisition of T2-weighted sequences (Fig. 44-4). These techniques have not been evaluated sufficiently to define their precise role, as compared with plain MRI. Disadvantages are that they turn a noninvasive technique into an invasive one and may create scheduling difficulties, particularly if fluoroscopy suites and magnetic imaging facilities are located at a substantial distance from one another.

Diagnostic MRI images of the shoulder depend on a number of technical considerations. Small field-of-view images with thin sections are essential to obtain sufficient spatial resolution. We use a 14- to 16-cm field of view (FOV) and a 3- to 4-mm–section thickness with a 0.5- to 1-mm intersection gap in all projections and for all pulse sequences. The larger FOV, section thickness, and intersection gap are used for larger patients. Local or surface radiofrequency coils provide a sufficient signal-

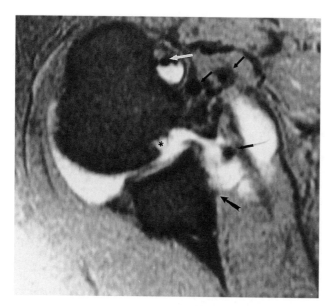

Fig. 44-4. Saline arthrogram. T2-weighted saline arthrogram, axial image. Distention of the glenohumeral joint with saline displays to advantage the anterior capsular stripping *(arrow)* and misshapen anterior labrum seen in this patient with multiple prior dislocations. Rounded areas of signal dropout anteriorly *(small arrows)* represent metallic artifact due to prior surgery. A small reverse Hill-Sachs defect is also present. (*) The biceps sheath is distended because of communication with the intraarticular fluid (tendon, *white arrow*). (Case courtesy of Timothy Greenan, M.D.)

to-noise ratio to support the necessary resolution. One final technical point that is often overlooked is the importance of stabilizing the shoulder to reduce motion artifact. Motion arises from a combination of respiratory and small voluntary movements by the subject. This small amount of motion can usually be effectively suppressed by placing a sandbag on the shoulder.

There is some disagreement among investigators concerning the ideal pulse sequences for imaging of the shoulder. For evaluation of the rotator cuff, most radiologists use a long TR, double echo sequence (e.g., 2500/20/80) obtained in an oblique coronal plane chosen to be parallel to the supraspinatus muscle or perpendicular to the glenoid fossa. We also obtain a second set of images in an oblique sagittal plane perpendicular to the coronal set using the same pulse sequence. Some radiologists prefer a short TR/TE sequence for the sagittal oblique plane, which has the advantage of shorter acquisition time but the disadvantage of lesser sensitivity to rotator cuff disease. For long TR/TE sequences we also recommend to those working on G.E. Signa systems use of the "classic" option with frequency centered on the water peak. This provides some fat suppression on the second echo. We do not routinely use other fat-suppression techniques. Recently some investigators have

advocated replacement of standard spin-echo sequences with fast spin-echo (FSE) sequences for evaluation of rotator cuff disease. It is not known at this time whether FSE sequences are as accurate as routine spin-echo sequences.

For evaluation of glenohumeral instability and the glenoid labrum we image in the axial plane and use either the long TR, double-echo sequences previously described or a 2D gradient echo sequence obtained with a TR/TE = 400-600/10 and flip angle of 20^0. One group of investigators advocates use of gradient-echo sequences with the shoulder in both neutral and externally rotated positions. (James Coumas, personal communication.) The relative accuracies of the various sequences is unknown.

ROTATOR CUFF DISEASE AND RELATED DISORDERS

Rotator cuff disease is a common cause of shoulder pain and disability. It is linked with impingement, glenohumeral instability and bicipital tendon disorders in a complex web of associations. It is impossible to speak or write comprehensively of one without bringing up the others, for whatever one may believe of the causal relationship of these disorders, patients with any one of them have an increased incidence of the others as compared with individuals not so affected.[46,79,87]

Fu has drawn from the work of many authors to propose a unifying theory linking rotator cuff disease to impingement and glenohumeral instability.[34] Intrinsic and extrinsic factors, acting together or separately, result in a common endpoint. Intrinsic factors, considered most important in the past by Codman and now by Ozaki, Ogata, and others, are those leading to degenerative changes within the substance of the rotator cuff with increasing age.[14,92,95] This degeneration may result from relative ischemia, believed by many investigators to exist within the distal portion of the supraspinatus tendon near its insertion site on the greater tuberosity. This zone of relative ischemia has been called the "critical zone" and corresponds to the most common site of rotator cuff disease, though its exact location and size varies from one subject to another.[60,77,102] Rotator cuff degeneration may incite secondary proliferative bony changes on the undersurface of the acromion. This in turn may lead to further cuff degeneration and ultimately to a cuff tear.[95] Overuse also exacerbates intrinsic degeneration.[34]

Extrinsic causes of rotator cuff disease relate to mechanical impingement by surrounding structures. The impingement can lead to inflammatory and degenerative change in the underlying tendons. The causes of impingement can be further divided into primary and secondary types.[34] Fu follows Neer[79] and Bigliani, Morrison, and April[5] in attributing primary impingement to contact between the coracoacromial arch or acromioclavicular joint and the underlying tendons. The anatomic relationship between the coracoacromial arch (consisting of the coracoid process, the coracoacromial ligament, and the undersurface of the anterior one third of the acromion), the acromioclavicular joint, and both the rotator cuff tendons and the tendon of the long head of the biceps, is very close. The supraspinatus tendon passes between the coracoacromial arch superiorly and the humeral head inferiorly to reach its insertion site on the greater tuberosity. The bicipital tendon passes through the same area, coming only slightly more anteriorly. Impingement on these tendons is particularly likely when the shoulder is flexed and internally rotated as during a tennis serve. Overuse in sports or work accelerates tendon degeneration resulting from either impingement or intrinsic degeneration.[5,34,79,81,87]

Neer divides the impingement syndrome into three stages. Stage I is characterized by edema and hemorrhage within the distal supraspinatus tendon and is usually reversible with conservative treatment. In Stage II impingement syndrome there is thickening and fibrosis of the subacromial-subdeltoid bursa, and tendinitis. The bursal changes compound the problem by decreasing the subacromial space available to the tendons. In Stage III disease a partial or full-thickness tear of the rotator cuff (or biceps tendon) occurs, along with osseous changes including anterior acromial osteophyte formation and degenerative changes in the greater tuberosity. Stage III lesions usually occur in patients over 40 years of age, while Stage I and II lesions are found in younger adults. Longstanding rotator cuff tears may lead, furthermore, to erosions of the humerus and glenohumeral destruction, termed rotator cuff arthropathy.[81,82,84]

Whereas primary impingement syndrome is caused by the effects of the coracoacromial arch and acromioclavicular joint on the rotator cuff in a normally positioned and functioning glenohumeral joint, secondary impingement syndrome is related to glenohumeral instability. Secondary impingement usually occurs in young athletic individuals involved in sports that demand overhead arm movement. Repetitive external rotation in abduction, as during the cocking phase of a baseball pitch, may lead to laxity of the capsule and mild instability. This is initially compensated for by an increase in the tone of the rotator cuff, which pulls the humeral head into the glenoid and enhances stability. With continued vigorous activity, however, the rotator cuff loses its ability to compensate, and the humeral head subluxes anteriorly. This subluxation is thought to result in secondary impingement.[34,45]

Patients with impingement syndrome present with a "painful arc" consisting of pain over the antero-lateral humeral head exacerbated by flexion and abduction, particularly in the 70° to 120° portion of the arc. Orthopedic surgeons test for impingement by injecting 10 cc of lidocaine into the subacromial region. If the condition is present, this will temporarily relieve the pain, hence a positive impingement test. Although the clinical presentation of primary and secondary impingement syndromes are sometimes similar, MRI may help differentiate between them. This is important because treatment differs significantly. Patients with primary impingement are usually treated with an anterior acromioplasty, with appropriate attention to the rotator cuff and biceps tendon. In patients with secondary impingement, treatment is aimed at the instability.*

Following are discussions of the role of imaging in diagnosis and evaluation of rotator cuff disease and related abnormalities. As Fu considered rotator cuff disease to be the final path to which impingement and intrinsic degeneration lead, it will be discussed first. We will then consider in turn primary impingement, glenohumeral instability and secondary impingement, and bicipital lesions.

Imaging of rotator cuff disease

Retrospective studies of Kneeland et al in 1986[55] and 1987[54] and a prospective study by Evancho et al in 1988[27] indicated that MR had potential for diagnosing rotator cuff pathologic conditions. Zlatkin et al[125] and Burk et al[7] in 1989 showed MR to be equal to or better than arthrography in the diagnosis of rotator cuff tears. Iannotti et al[43] in 1991 reported a 100% sensitivity and 95% specificity in the detection of full-thickness tears. In both Zlatkin and Iannotti's studies, MR accurately predicted the size of the full-thickness tears.[43,125] Iannotti also related the size of the tear to the degree of atrophy of the muscular portion of the rotator cuff, and this relationship has been confirmed by others.[28]

With increasing understanding of the signal patterns associated with rotator cuff abnormalities, MR has become highly accurate in diagnosing rotator cuff disorders.† Magnetic resonance imaging can depict the continuum between rotator cuff degeneration or tendinopathy and partial or full-thickness rotator cuff tears. Intrinsic cuff degeneration or tendinopathy is seen as increased signal within the distal tendon on proton-density images; this persists but does not intensify on T2-weighted images (Fig. 44-5). With more severe tendinopathy the tendon becomes thin or frayed. In these cases, minimally increased amounts of fluid may be present within the glenohumeral joint or subacromial-subdeltoid bursa.

Partial tear of the tendon may be intratendinous

---

*References 45, 46, 64, 65, 79, 81.
†References 7, 28, 43, 52, 101, 125.

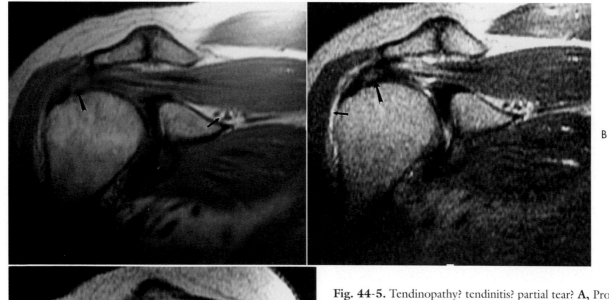

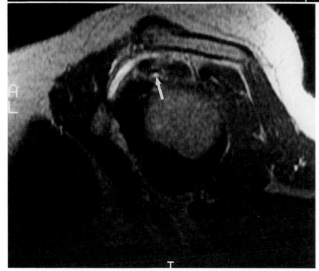

Fig. 44-5. Tendinopathy? tendinitis? partial tear? **A,** Proton-density–weighted (2500/14) coronal oblique image. The central tendon of the supraspinatus muscle is interrupted by an ill-defined area of increased signal in the "critical zone" near its attachment site *(arrow)*. Note the suprascapular neurovascular structures in the suprascapular notch *(small arrow)*. **B,** T2-weighted (2500/70) sagittal oblique image. The small area of increased signal in the supraspinatus tendon *(arrow)* has become relatively brighter with T2 weighting, and it is quite focal. Because of its focality, we believe this most likely represents a partial, intrasubstance tear of the supraspinatus tendon. There is fluid in the subdeltoid bursa *(small arrow)*. **C,** T2-weighted (2500/70) sagittal oblique image. This section is farther medial than the partial tear, yet a tiny bright spot is present near the anterior edge of the supraspinatus muscle *(white arrow)*. This most likely is joint fluid in the biceps interval that can be mistaken for a rotator cuff tear. Fluid in the subacromial-subdeltoid bursa is also seen to advantage.

in location or may occur on either the bursal or articular side of the tendon (Fig. 44-6). On MR, partial tears are depicted as focal areas of increased signal on short TE images; these areas increase in relative signal on long TE images but need not approach the signal intensity of joint fluid. The abnormal focus does not extend through the entire thickness of the tendon. There may be increased fluid within the glenohumeral joint, particularly if the partial tear is on the articular side. Alternatively, one may see fluid within the subacromial-subdeltoid bursa if the partial tear lies on the bursal side of the tendon. To distinguish partial instrasubstance tears from tendinitis can be a difficult but often a purely academic exercise because although some surgeons elect to operate for partial tears, both conditions are often treated conservatively, and even arthroscopic inspection may not yield the answer. In a patient who has had surgery for rotator cuff tear or intrinsic impingement, the situation is further compli-

cated by the presence of increased signal within the tendon secondary to the surgery.[94]

In a complete or full-thickness rotator cuff tear, the tendon is interrupted by an abnormal focus of bright signal extending across its complete superior to inferior extent on at least one section. The signal within the tendon gap is usually notably bright on T2-weighted images, presumably as a result of fluid. The tear is almost always associated with increased fluid in the glenohumeral joint, which may communicate through the defect directly with the subacromial-subdeltoid bursa (Figs. 44-7 to 44-9).

Large and usually longstanding cuff tears may demonstrate a full-thickness defect in the cuff, tendon retraction, atrophy of the involved muscles with associated fatty infiltration, and upward shift of the humeral head. Occasionally in such tears, little or no fluid will be visualized within the tendon, glenohumeral joint, or

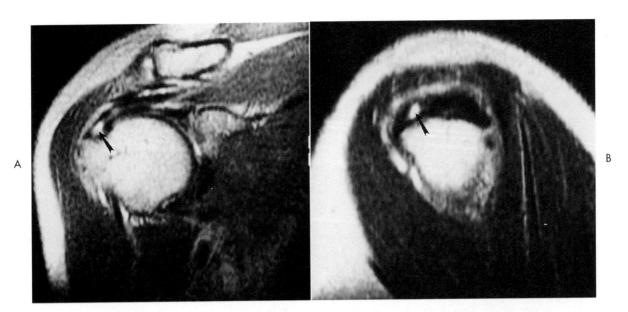

Fig. 44-6. Articular side partial tear. **A,** T2-weighted (2500/70) coronal oblique image. **B,** T2-weighted (2500/70) sagittal oblique image. On the articular side of the supraspinatus tendon is a bright gap *(arrow)* covered on the bursal side with a thin layer of remaining tendon. Increased joint fluid is present, and some fluid is present in the subdeltoid bursa.

subacromial-subdeltoid bursa (Figs. 44-10 and 44-11). In these cases, diagnosis will depend on the recognition of the other signs described above. Another occasional accompanying sign is irregularity of the bony elements of the glenohumeral joint due to rotator cuff arthropathy (Fig. 44-12). In large tears it is common for the injury to extend completely across the anterior to posterior dimension of the supraspinatus muscle and tendon, to involve parts or all of the infraspinatus and subscapularis. It is highly unusual, however, for a tear to involve those tendons without involving the supraspinatus.

Occasionally, in patients with a longstanding rotator cuff tear, there may be erosion of the undersurface of the acromioclavicular joint capsule, allowing fluid in the glenohumeral joint to communicate directly with the acromioclavicular joint. In arthrography this produces the "geyser" sign in which contrast injected into the glenohumeral joint is seen entering the acromioclavicular joint (Fig. 44-13). Fluid within the acromioclavicular joint on MR may also be associated with a rotator cuff tear but is often due to intrinsic disease of the acromioclavicular joint. In the same fashion fluid within the subacromial-subdeltoid bursa may be due either to an associated rotator cuff tear or to a subacromial-subdeltoid bursitis.

To avoid overcalling rotator cuff pathologic findings, one must be aware of a normal area of increased signal intensity in the distal supraspinatus tendon. It is located approximately 1 cm proximal to the insertion site of the tendon. It has been described by some authors as isointense with muscle.[47,74] Others refer to it merely as increased in signal without providing a point of reference. While most authors have noted it on short TE technique, Kaplan et al[47] found it to be most apparent on gradient-echo images, and Mirowitz also noted it in some T2-weighted image studies.[74] It has been identified in asymptomatic individuals and does not necessarily represent a pathologic finding. Several theories have been proposed to explain this area of increased signal. It may represent subclinical degenerative change within the tendon.[74,101,125] Conversely, Erickson et al[25] noted increased signal on T1-weighted images that they attributed to the "magic angle phenomenon," in which an artifactual focus of increased signal may occur on short TE images of a tendon oriented 55° to the constant magnetic field. They postulated that such increased signal may also be expected on intermediate-weighted images but not on long TE images.

A second possible pitfall concerns positioning of the shoulder. If the arm is internally rotated, the distal supraspinatus and infraspinatus tendons move anteriorly. This carries the distal infraspinatus tendon and small posterior supraspinatus tendon slips forward into the plane of the main supraspinatus tendon on oblique coronal images. The infraspinatus muscle routinely has multiple tendon slips with muscle interposed between them. The supraspinatus tendon may be divided into two structures—the anterior main tendon and smaller posterior slips. In addition, there are bits of fatty connective tissue between the supraspinatus and infraspinatus muscles.

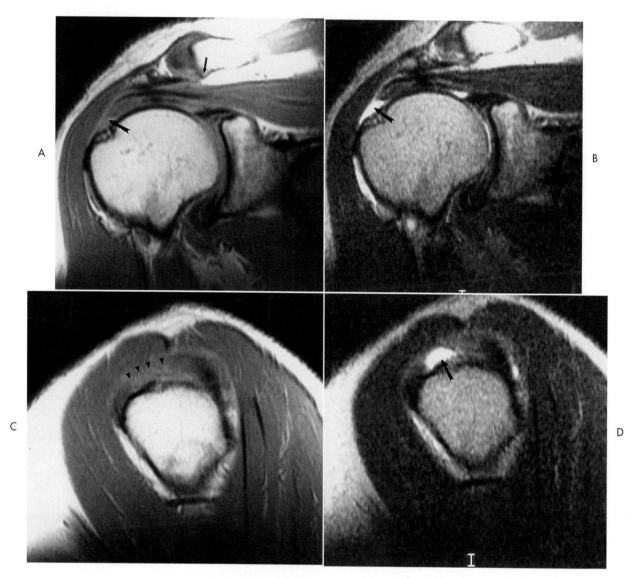

Fig. 44-7. Full-thickness tear. **A,** Proton-density–weighted (2500/14) coronal oblique image. A gap is present in the supraspinatus tendon near its insertion site *(arrow)*. Some proliferative changes affect the acromioclavicular joint, including a small, downward pointing spur *(small arrow)*. **B,** T2-weighted (2500/70) coronal oblique image. The tendon gap is very bright *(arrow)* and is most likely filled with fluid. There is no intact tendon above or below the abnormal area. **C,** Proton-density–weighted (2500/14) sagittal oblique image. Anterosuperiorly the normal dark band of the rotator cuff is interrupted by a fuzzy area of relatively increased signal *(arrowheads)*. **D,** T2-weighted (2500/70) sagittal oblique image. The anterior part of this area becomes very bright *(arrow)*. The remainder brightens only slightly. Often a tear will be adjacent to or surrounded by an area of tendinopathy.

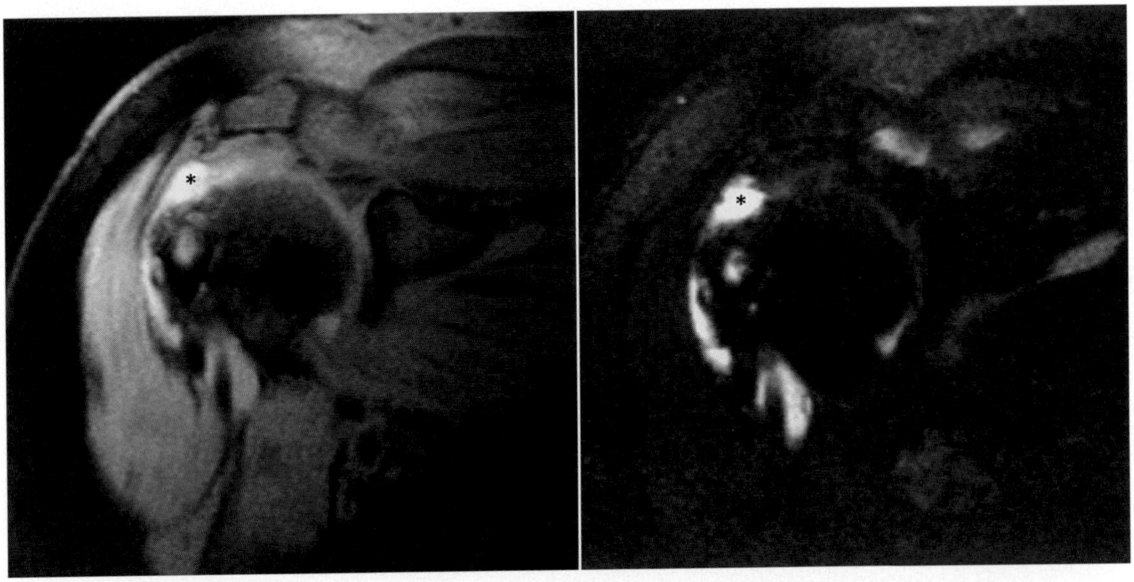

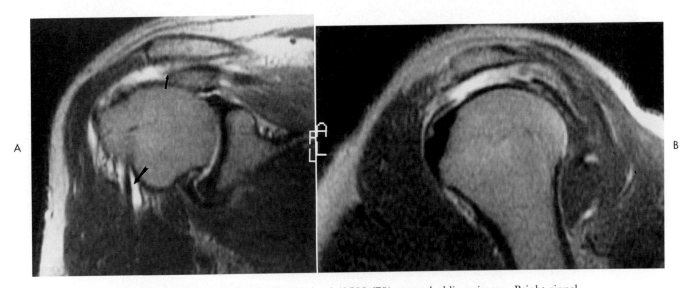

Fig. 44-8. Fat-suppression technique. **A,** Proton-density weighted (2000/15) coronal oblique image. **B,** T2-weighted (2000/90) coronal oblique image. Fat-suppression techniques may increase the conspicuity of a rotator cuff tear (*), as well as that of a small cystlike defect in the humeral head, but less detail may be discernible elsewhere. (Case courtesy of Thomas Hedrick, M.D., Houston, Texas.)

Fig. 44-9. Large cuff tear. **A,** T2-weighted (2500/70) coronal oblique image. Bright signal fluid spills from the glenohumeral joint through a large rent in the rotator cuff into the subacromial-subdeltoid bursa. Joint fluid also tracks down the sheath of the long head of the biceps brachii muscle *(arrow)*. The supraspinatus tendon is retracted *(small arrow)*. **B,** T2-weighted (2500/70) sagittal oblique image. The large size of this tear may be best appreciated on this sagittal image. At surgery it included all of the supraspinatus, most of the infraspinatus, and the superior part of the subscapularis.

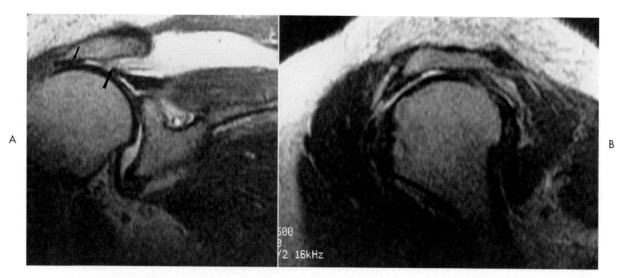

Fig. 44-10. Large chronic cuff tear. **A,** T2-weighted (2500/70) coronal oblique image. Relatively little joint fluid is present. The supraspinatus tendon is retracted nearly to the glenoid *(arrow)*, and the humeral head has translated superiorly and contacts the acromion. There is reactive modeling of the undersurface of the acromion and thickening of the cortex *(small arrow)*. **B,** T2-weighted (2500/70) sagittal oblique image. The acromion has a hooked shape.

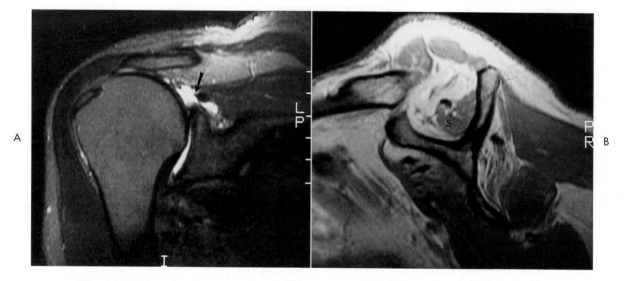

Fig. 44-11. Atrophy. **A,** T2-weighted (2500/70) coronal oblique image. The supraspinatus muscle and tendon are retracted to the glenoid *(arrow)*, and the humeral head is contacting the acromion. **B,** Proton-density–weighted (2500/14) sagittal oblique image. The supraspinatus *(S)* and infraspinatus *(I)* muscles are markedly atrophied.

This fatty tissue, along with the muscle interdigitated between slips of infraspinatus tendon or between the principal anterior supraspinatus tendon and the smaller posterior tendon slips, may result in an apparent area of increased signal on short TE images that fades on T2-weighted images. The correct conclusion may be reached by following the intact tendons on oblique sagittal images.[20,59,86,118]

Imaging of primary impingement

MR can be quite useful in the assessment of patients who have either primary or secondary mechanical impingement. Secondary impingement is caused by instability and will be considered below. This section will discuss primary impingement. Patients with impingement symptoms frequently have narrowing of the space between the acromion and the superior surface of the hu-

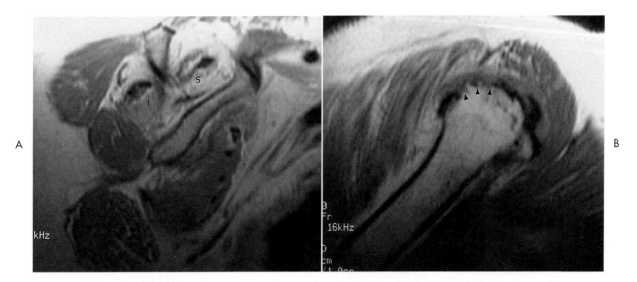

Fig. 44-12. Cuff arthropathy. **A,** Proton-density–weighted (2500/14) sagittal oblique image. Atrophy of the supraspinatus *(S)* and infraspinatus *(I)* muscles attests to longstanding rotator cuff tear. **B,** Proton-density–weighted (2500-14) sagittal oblique image. Jagged, irregular humeral cortex *(arrowheads)* is typical of cuff arthropathy. As this examination is filmed, anterior is to the right.

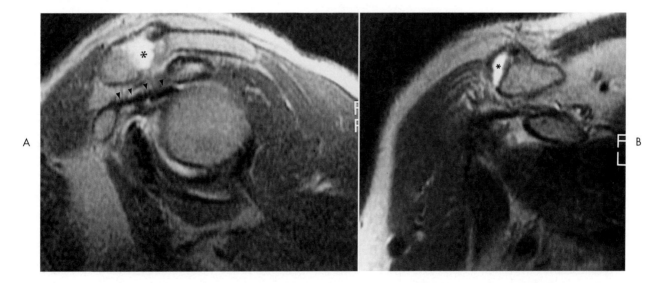

Fig. 44-13. Geyser sign. **A,** T2-weighted (2500/70) sagittal oblique image. Fluid fills the acromioclavicular joint (*) in this patient with a large rotator cuff tear (same individual as in Fig. 44-9). Note coracohumeral ligament *(arrowheads)*. **B,** T2-weighted (2500/70) coronal oblique image. This image, located at the most anterior extent of the acromioclavicular joint, also demonstrates fluid within the acromioclavicular joint (*). Such a finding may be due to intrinsic acromioclavicular disease and may be unrelated to rotator cuff disease, but in this case, no evidence of acromioclavicular disease was found at surgery.

meral head that is well delineated on MR in either the sagittal oblique or coronal oblique projections.[50,108] This narrowing may be related to the configuration of the anterior acromion or acromioclavicular joint. Bigliani and Morrison[5] describe an association between the shape of the undersurface of the anterior acromion and

the likelihood of rotator cuff tear. They establish three categories of acromial shape. Type I is flat (Fig. 44-14), Type II is curved, and Type III is hooked anteriorly. They find an increasing incidence of rotator cuff tears with type II and particularly with type III acromions. The association of hooked acromions and rotator cuff

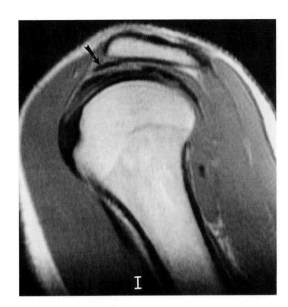

Fig. 44-14. Flat acromion. Proton-density–weighted (2500/14) sagittal oblique image. The undersurface of the acromion has a perfectly straight, flat shape. Note the coracoacromial ligament (*arrow*).

tears has been confirmed by others.[92] However, the practical application of Bigliani and Morrison's work to interpretation of shoulder MR is somewhat problematic. They performed their investigation using conventional radiography of the shoulder; in this the eye perceives a summation shadow composed of the entire acromion. MR, of course, demonstrates acromial shape tomographically. In MRI it is not unusual for the shape of the acromion to change from section to section. Thus, for example, an acromion with a flat configuration in one oblique sagittal section may have a curved shape in another (Fig. 44-15).

A low-lying acromion has also been implicated as a cause of impingement. The acromion is considered to be low if its inferior border is lower than that of the clavicle at the acromioclavicular joint. Unfortunately, there are no criteria for distinguishing a low-lying acromion from a high-riding clavicle (such as may result from a previous acromioclavicular joint separation).[48]

Degenerative changes at the acromioclavicular joint are variously considered either a cause or a result of impingement and rotator cuff disease. These include hypertrophic changes of soft tissue within the joint capsule as well as osteophytes that may project inferiorly from the acromion or clavicle. Spurs may visibly distort the supraspinatus muscle as it passes below them. At times it may be difficult to distinguish a spur from a tendinous or ligamentous attachment site, particularly because spurs may develop at such sites (Figs. 44-16, 44-17). Some authors[47] believe that spurs always contain marrow and thus will match other marrow-containing

bones in signal intensity. Our experience suggests that it is generally but not invariably true that spurs contain marrow.

Though there is an association between these configurations of the acromion and the acromioclavicular joint (described above) and impingement syndrome, these findings are common as well in asymptomatic individuals. One may, in fact, have visible indentation of the tendon by a portion of the coracoacromial arch and at the same time have no symptoms, much like an asymptomatic person may have a herniated lumbar disc. Therefore, impingement syndrome remains a clinical diagnosis. These findings may, however, reasonably be taken as support of clinically suspected impingement or may form a basis for suggestion of the diagnosis.

GLENOHUMERAL INSTABILITY

Glenohumeral joint stability depends on the supporting and restraining effect of the glenoid labrum, the joint capsule including the glenohumeral ligaments, and the rotator cuff. With failure of these structures, the glenohumeral joint becomes unstable. Instability may present clinically and anatomically as either subluxation or frank dislocation and may manifest chronically, recurrently, or as an isolated episode. Shoulder dislocations, which most commonly occur in an anterior and subcoracoid location, are usually secondary to acute trauma. During an initial episode of dislocation, the glenoid labrum and anterior capsule may become damaged, and an impaction fracture of the posterolateral humeral head, or Hill-Sachs deformity, may occur. These lesions predispose to recurrent dislocation, often after minimal or no trauma. Recurrent dislocations are common in young patients but become progressively less common with advancing age; they are relatively rare after age 40.[3,21,65,96,116]

Three types of instability have been described: traumatic, atraumatic, and voluntary. Traumatic instability is the most common, and its characteristics are outlined in the acronym TUBS[65]: Traumatic, Unilateral, Bankart, Surgery. The great majority of these patients have a history of shoulder TRAUMA, the instability is UNILATERAL, there is frequently an associated stripping of the labrum or joint capsule, the BANKART lesion, and SURGERY is often successful. It is far more common for traumatic instability to occur in an anterior direction than in a posterior direction.[3,65,96]

Atraumatic instability is considerably less common than traumatic instability. The acronym AMBRI is helpful.[65] Atraumatic, Multidirectional, Bilateral, Rehabilitation, Inferior capsular shift. A history of trauma is not characteristic (ATRAUMATIC). The instability is often MULTIDIRECTIONAL and may be BILATERAL. REHABILITATION with strengthening of the deltoid

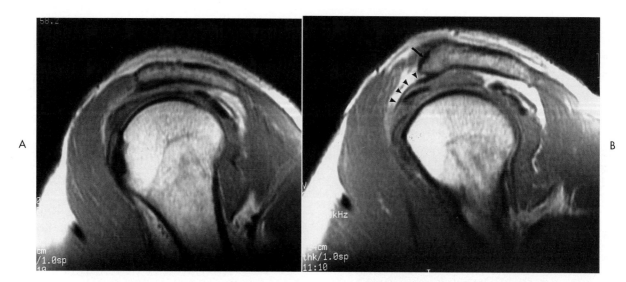

Fig. 44-15. A, Acromial variation. **A,** Proton-density–weighted (2500/14) sagittal oblique image. This relatively laterally placed section demonstrates an acromion with a smoothly curved undersurface. **B,** Proton-density–weighted (2500/14) sagittal oblique image. More medially, the same patient's acromion has a hooked shape *(arrow* at hook). Coracoacromial ligament *(arrowheads).*

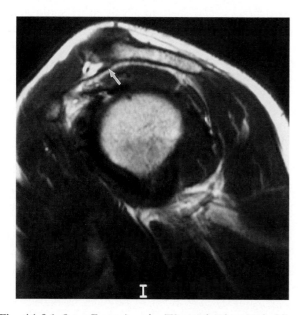

Fig. 44-16. Spur. Fast spin-echo T2-weighted sagittal oblique image. A spur containing marrow projects from the undersurface of the otherwise flat acromion at the attachment site of the coracoacromial ligament *(arrow).* The conjoined tendons of the short head of the biceps brachii muscle and the coracobrachialis are seen originating from the coracoid process.

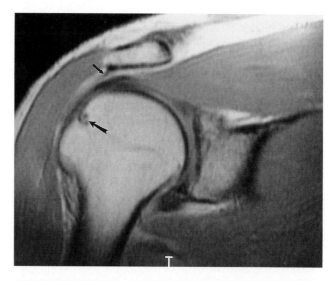

Fig. 44-17. Spurious spur. Proton-density–weighted (2500/14) coronal oblique image. A slender, black structure projects from the undersurface of the lateral acromion *(small arrow).* It represents a slip of deltoid tendon or a portion of the coracoacromial ligament (or both, as their fibers may fuse), but it may be mistaken for a spur. A small area of decreased signal *(arrow)* in the greater tuberosity or, in other cases, a small cyst, is a common finding and may be associated with rotator cuff disease.

and rotator cuff musculature is usually successful. If conservative therapy fails and surgery is indicated, however, an INFERIOR CAPSULAR SHIFT procedure is preferred. This is a reconstruction procedure in which the inferior capsule, particularly the inferior capsular recess,

is partially resected and then double-breasted to reinforce the capsule.[65,83]

Voluntary instability is the third category. The patient who voluntarily produces glenohumeral instability by muscle contraction alone may have a psychiatric or emotional disorder. In such patients physical therapy may be attempted but is frequently unsuccessful, and surgical stabilization is contraindicated. Patients who cease dislocating their shoulder and are without psychiatric problems may benefit from physical therapy or, if that fails, from surgery.[65,104]

Imaging of glenohumeral instability

MR or CT arthrography can often identify the anatomic residua of prior episodes of instability. Identification of the stigmata of instability does not, however, indicate whether the problem is ongoing, because anatomic changes may occur at a single episode of dislocation, and because it is rare to identify actual displacement of the humeral head at the time of imaging. The imaging signs of instability include labral and glenoid rim abnormalities, capsular stripping, and deformities of the humeral head.

Tears of the anterior inferior glenoid labrum are frequent in patients with recurrent anterior dislocation. Glenoid labral tears are identified by either complete absence of a portion of the labrum, displacement of the labrum from the glenoid rim, or abnormal linear areas of increased signal within the labrum. Similar criteria are used at CT arthrography (Fig. 44-18). CT arthrography is highly accurate in the diagnosis of tears of the glenoid labrum.[22,100,110-112,122] MRI's performance in the assessment of labral tears has been variable but generally good.[35,49,58,106,126] Anterior labral tears are the most easily diagnosed by both imaging modalities. Accuracy decreases with tears of the superior labrum and is poor with posterior or inferior labral tears. Isolated tears of the posterior or inferior labrum are relatively uncommon, however.[58]

To avoid overcalling labral tears, one must be aware of the many normal variations in appearance of the labrum. The posterior labrum has been described as rounded in its configuration by CT arthrography and as usually triangular in appearance by MRI. The configuration of the anterior labrum may vary considerably from one individual to another, and in the same person labral shape changes with rotation of the humerus.[78,106] With internal rotation, the anterior labrum assumes a large, globular configuration, but with external rotation it is attenuated and pointed (Fig. 44-19). The anterior aspect of the labrum may exhibit horizontal clefts or vertical notches. If this pattern is seen posteriorly, however, it suggests a tear. With gradient-echo imaging, an area of smooth, linear high signal within the anterior labrum may occasionally be seen. This finding alone does not indicate a tear; however, its etiology has not been ascertained.[41,67,72,85]

One must also be aware of normal structures that may be misinterpreted as labral tears. The hyaline articu-

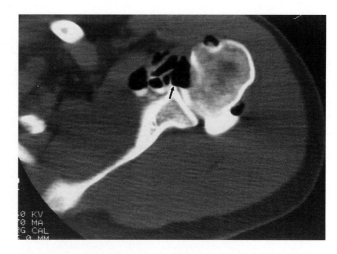

Fig. 44-18. CT arthrogram of labral damage. Gas within the joint capsule projects immediately adjacent to the glenoid cortex *(arrow)*. The anterior labrum is missing.

lar cartilage of the glenoid extends under the base of the labrum.[59,107] This produces a line of signal brighter than the dark, fibrous labrum; this may resemble a tear. At the level of the subscapularis tendon, the middle glenohumeral ligament runs parallel to the anterior labrum and is also of low signal. It may mimic a tear along the outer border of the labrum, but its true nature will usually be revealed by following it along its normal course on sequential images (Fig. 44-20).

Interpretation of labral images may be particularly difficult in the elderly because there is considerable overlap between pathologic labral changes and those associated with normal aging. Intrasubstance degenerative changes are noted in individuals after the age of 30 and increase in prominence with advancing age.[21,99] On proton-density or gradient-echo images, these may produce globular increased signal within the labrum.[67,85] The labrum may also appear small in the elderly.

The anterior joint capsule and glenohumeral ligaments are also important in maintaining shoulder stability.[116] In abduction and external rotation, the glenohumeral ligaments restrain the humeral head and prevent anterior instability. The configuration of the anterior capsule can be assessed with either MR or CT arthrography[100,110,111,122,126] and is best evaluated in the axial plane at the level of the mid glenoid. There is considerable variability in the medial attachment site of the anterior capsule.[22,78] Type III capsules, which attach medial to the labrum, may be congenital or secondary to traumatic stripping of the capsule from the anterior glenoid rim as a result of a previous episode of anterior instability. Whether as cause or effect, the more medially the anterior capsule inserts on the glenoid, the higher the likelihood of recurrent anterior instability. Laxity of the posterior capsule and stripping of the posterior capsule from

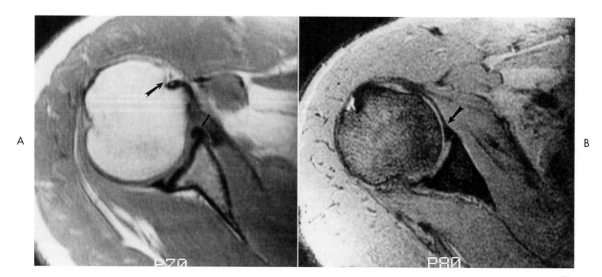

Fig. 44-19. Effect of rotation. **A,** Proton-density–weighted (2500/14) axial image. With the humeral head in internal rotation (note position of the bicipital groove, *arrow*), the anterior labrum has a rounded configuration *(small arrow).* **B,** Gradient-echo axial image. With external rotation, the same patient's anterior labrum assumes a pointed, triangular configuration *(arrow).* The attachment of the joint capsule to the tip of the labrum can be appreciated.

the glenoid rim have also been described on imaging studies in patients with posterior instability.[16]

The rotator cuff muscles also contribute to the stability of the glenohumeral joint. When the cuff is intact it counterbalances the upward pull of the deltoid muscle by pulling the humeral head snugly against the glenoid fossa. With anterior instability the work required of the cuff muscles increases, and if they fail, this allows unrestrained elevation of the humeral head by the deltoid, theoretically resulting in secondary impingement and further deterioration of the rotator cuff. In addition, rotator cuff tendinopathy or tear from other causes may also weaken the cuff and allow superior humeral translocation. In addition to the rotator cuff's role in counterbalancing the deltoid, the subscapularis muscle and tendon reinforce the anterior joint capsule. Weakness or laxity in these structures, both of which make up the anterior rotator cuff, predisposes to anterior subluxation of the humeral head. Rotator cuff disease associated with instability can be evaluated by MR with the same criteria used in assessing rotator cuff abnormalities alone.[63,65]

Glenohumeral dislocation can result in bony abnormalities that are sometimes visible on plain films but are clearly identified on either CT or MR. As the humeral head dislocates anteriorly, it impacts on the anterior glenoid rim, producing a bony Bankart lesion (anterior glenoid rim fracture) or a Hill-Sachs deformity. On axial images, Hill-Sachs lesions are visualized in the posterolateral border of the humeral head at or superior to the base of the coracoid process. They must not be con-

fused with the normal flattening of the humeral head, which is usually visualized more posteriorly and inferiorly but which may be found at the level of the coracoid in a patient with a large rotator cuff defect and superior translation of the humerus (Figs. 44-21 to 44-23).[49,107,123] In patients who have had a posterior dislocation, a "reverse" Hill-Sachs or trough lesion may be identified on the anteromedial margin of the head of the humerus in association with a posterior scapular or labral abnormality.

ABNORMALITIES OF THE BICEPS TENDON
Superior labral and associated biceps tears

Andrews et al.[2] first noted an increased incidence of a particular labral tear in athletes involved in throwing activities (e.g., baseball pitchers). These tears are found on the anterior superior glenoid labrum where the tendon of the long head of the biceps originates. The biceps tendon is subject to large forces during overhead throwing. It has been postulated, therefore, that forceful contraction of the biceps can result in fraying or tearing of the labrum. These tears may extend into the posterior portion of the labrum; they are then termed SLAP lesions (superior labrum, anterior and posterior).[113] Despite the labral tear, these patients usually have no anatomic instability of the glenohumeral joint. Although originally described in throwing athletes, SLAP lesions are also found in people who have been injured while catching a falling object or falling on an outstretched hand. In all cases there has been sudden contraction of

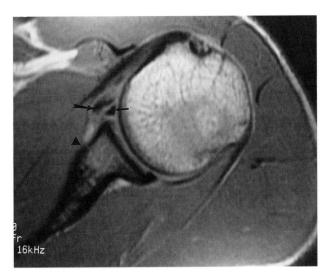

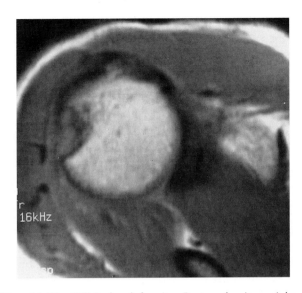

Fig. 44-20. Labral avulsion? Proton-density–weighted (2500/14) image. This patient suffered from recurrent anterior dislocation. A Hill-Sachs lesion was present on a higher section (Fig. 44-21). As we originally interpreted this image, the anterior labrum *(small arrow)* was displaced anteriorly and rotated counterclockwise from its anatomic position. The middle glenohumeral ligament projected anterior to the labrum *(arrow)*, and the capsule inserted far down the scapular neck *(arrowhead)*. At surgery 6 weeks later there was neither disruption of the labrum nor capsular stripping. The capsule could have reattached in the interval. Most likely the labral appearance was due to unusually prominent articular cartilage between the labrum and glenoid. This case illustrates the difficulty that may at times be encountered in interpretation of labral anatomy.

Fig. 44-22. Hill-Sachs deformity. Proton-density–weighted (2500/14) axial image. This Hill-Sachs deformity projects more laterally than the one in Fig. 44-21. The actual position may be slightly different from patient to patient, and the apparent position varies with the degree of internal or external rotation of the humerus at the time of imaging.

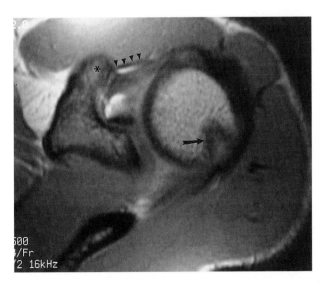

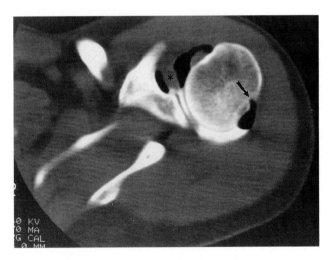

Fig. 44-21. Hill-Sachs deformity. Proton-density–weighted (2500/14) axial image. At the level of the coracoid process (*), a notch-shaped defect in the posterolateral humeral head *(arrow)* is typical of a Hill-Sachs defect in this patient with a history of recurrent anterior dislocation (same patient as in Fig. 44-20). Coracohumeral ligament *(arrowheads)*.

Fig. 44-23. CT arthrogram of Hill-Sachs deformity. A tiny but distinct Hill-Sachs deformity is present on the posterolateral humeral head *(arrow)*. Superior glenohumeral ligament (*).

the biceps muscle. There may be an associated injury to the long head of the biceps as well as the labral tear. SLAP lesions may be divided into four types, depending on the nature of the labral injury and whether there is associated biceps tendon damage. In Type I lesions the labrum is frayed, but it and the biceps tendon remain firmly attached to the glenoid. In Type II lesions the labrum is not only frayed but also stripped from the glenoid with the biceps tendon. If a "bucket-handle" type of tear occurs but does not extend to the region of the biceps origin, the injury is a Type III lesion. If the bucket-handle tear extends into the biceps tendon, then a Type IV lesion is present. These categories were established at arthroscopy. Precise criteria permitting diagnosis by MRI have not been firmly established.[9,40,113] At CT arthrography, the fraying of the labrum in a Type I tear and detachment of the labrum in a Type II lesion may be identified. In Type III and IV lesions a characteristic rounded area of attenuation less than labral tissue but greater than gas may be found; it is termed the "cheerio sign" and represents the bucket-handle tear.[42]

Bicipital tendinitis

Most cases of bicipital tendinitis are the result of mechanical impingement, occurring with rotator cuff disease in middle-aged or older patients. With flexion of the shoulder, the tendon of the long head of the biceps may become closely approximated to the coracoacromial ligament and the anterior acromion, particularly in the presence of a rotator cuff defect, and may be compressed between these structures and the humeral head.[21,87,97] This impingement will eventually result in tendinitis, inflammatory changes with flattening and thinning of the tendon that may lead to complete rupture.[84] Bicipital tendinitis can also occur in patients who have glenohumeral instability, particularly in the presence of pathologic conditions involving the superior labrum.

Early bicipital tendinitis is often undetected on imaging studies. Increased signal intensity within the abnormal tendon is rarely visualized on MRI (Fig. 44-24).

Morphologic abnormalities such as fraying, flattening, or absence of the tendon may sometimes be identified, particularly within the bicipital groove. Fluid within the bicipital tendon sheath will help delineate tendon morphology. The presence of fluid does not necessarily indicate bicipital tendon disease, however, because any fluid present often comes from the glenohumeral joint. In the rare instance when there is a disproportionately large amount of fluid within the biceps sheath in comparison with fluid within the joint, this should suggest bicipital abnormality.

Bicipital tendon dislocation

Bicipital tendon dislocation usually occurs in conjunction with large, longstanding tears of the rotator cuff that have extended to include the subscapularis tendon (Fig. 44-25). The tendon dislocation may be overlooked clinically because the symptoms are masked by the associated cuff tear. Other lesions necessary for bicipital tendon dislocation to occur include disruption of both the strong coracohumeral ligament, an important stabilizer of the biceps tendon,[63] and the weak transverse humeral ligament. In this setting the tendon of the long head of the biceps dislocates medially, moving posterior to the subscapularis tendon and muscle and into the glenohumeral joint, where it may be mistaken for a detached anterior labrum. Rarely, when the subscapularis tendon remains intact yet the coracohumeral and transverse humeral ligaments are disrupted, the biceps tendon will dis-

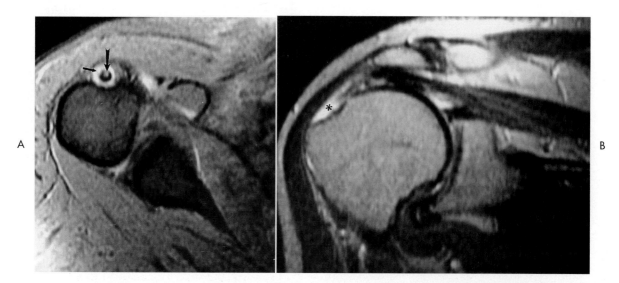

Fig. 44-24. Bicipital tendinitis. **A,** T2-weighted axial image. Fluid surrounds the bicipital tendon within the groove. In addition, an abnormal focus of high signal is present within the tendon *(arrow)*. The anterolateral branch of the anterior circumflex humeral artery may be identified *(small arrow)*. **B,** T2-weighted coronal oblique image. In this patient, as is commonly the case, biceps tendinitis is associated with rotator cuff disease. A large tendon gap (*) marks the location of a full-thickness tear of the supraspinatus muscle and tendon. (Case courtesy of Timothy Greenan, M.D., Washington, D.C.)

place extraarticularly and anterior to the subscapularis muscle. Occasionally, the biceps tendon lodges within the fibers of the distal subscapularis tendon.[11,12,98]

Besides allowing identification of the displaced biceps tendon, both CT arthrography and MR will show an empty bicipital groove. On axial MR images, particularly those using gradient-echo sequences, tiny bony spicules projecting into the bicipital groove may mimic the biceps tendon. They may be distinguished from it, however, because they will probably not be present on all the axial images where the biceps tendon would be expected to be seen. In addition, the far anterior coronal images will also show an empty bicipital groove.

Surgery is usually performed in the young and middle-aged patient with dislocation of the biceps tendon. The tendon is replaced in the bicipital groove, and the fibrous roof is reconstructed. Tenodesis is not necessary unless the tendon is severely attenuated. An acromioplasty is performed, as well as rotator cuff arthroplasty. In older patients, the treatment is usually directed to the rotator cuff disorder; the biceps tendon dislocation is considered secondary.

CALCIUM DEPOSITION DISEASES

Hydroxy apatite deposition disease, including its manifestations as calcific tendinitis or bursitis, idiopathic destructive arthritis (Milwaukee shoulder syndrome), and tumoral calcinosis, may all occur in the shoulder.

Calcific tendinitis can involve most tendons, but it most commonly involves the supraspinatus tendon. Patients are typically in middle age, though the disease has been reported in a child as young as 3 years of age. Women are affected more commonly then men. There is a predilection for the dominant shoulder. The etiology is unknown, but it is believed by some to be due to calcification of metaplastic cartilage in the relatively ischemic distal supraspinatus tendon. The deposits may also extrude from the tendon into a bursa, usually the subacromial-subdeltoid bursa, producing calcific bursitis. The deposits may erode bone. Pain is the presenting complaint and seems to be correlated with fluffy, ill-defined deposits occurring with resorption rather than with the well-defined deposits more commonly seen in asymptomatic patients. There is no association with other rotator cuff pathology.[70,90,117,119]

Plain films are generally sufficient for the diagnosis of calcific tendinitis. The calcium deposits are also readily apparent by CT. If an MRI study is obtained, a small calcium deposit may be missed. Larger ones may appear dark because of immobile protons in calcium. There may be obliteration of the peribursal fat pad, though that is quite nonspecific. If ossification has occurred and marrow is present in the deposit, the signal will match that of other marrow. Bursal deposits will have the same appearance as those in the tendons but are often accompanied by bursal fluid (Fig. 44-26).

Idiopathic destructive arthritis of the shoulder, or Milwaukee shoulder syndrome (for the city where it was first described), is another calcium crystal-related abnormality. It is most often seen in elderly women. It is characterized by large, blood-tinged effusions containing calcium hydroxyapatite and by extensive destruction of car-

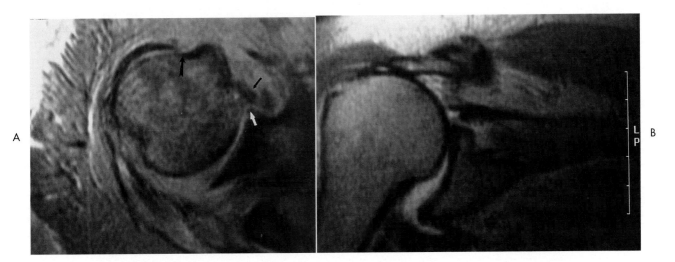

Fig. 44-25. Bicipital tendon dislocation. **A,** Gradient-echo axial image. The bicipital groove *(arrow)* is empty. The tendon of the long head of the biceps brachii muscle *(small arrow)* is displaced medially and posterior to the subscapularis tendon. It could be mistaken for an avulsed labrum, particularly since the anterior labrum of this elderly woman is diminutive *(white arrow)*. **B,** T2-weighted (2500/70) coronal oblique image. Like most biceps dislocations, this one accompanies an extensive tear of the rotator cuff.

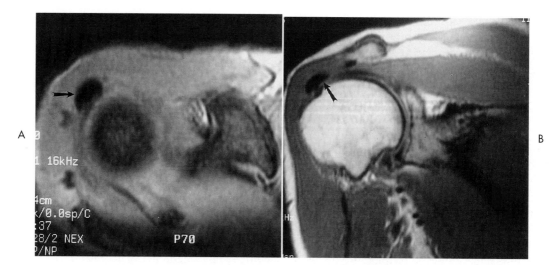

Fig. 44-26. Calcific tendinitis. **A,** Gradient-echo axial image. A large area of signal void *(arrow)* is present near the attachment site of the supraspinatus tendon. **B,** Proton-density–weighted (2500/14) coronal oblique image. Signal void is present in the relatively avascular area of the supraspinatus tendon *(arrow)*. This area was also dark on T2 weighting. Calcium was also apparent by plain films (not shown).

tilage and bone. It is often accompanied by derangement of the rotator cuff and/or proximal tendon of the long head of the biceps brachii. The calcium containing effusions distinguish it from simple rotator cuff arthropathy as does a tendency towards bilateral involvement and involvement of other joints, particularly the hips and knees. Milwaukee shoulder syndrome is generally diagnosed clinically. CT and MRI studies, if obtained, will demonstrate the effusions and destruction of articular surfaces. CT may also demonstrate calcium deposition on synovial surfaces.[36,37,66,88,120]

In *tumoral calcinosis,* amorphous, often liquid, deposits of calcium form near the joints, particularly the shoulder, hip, and elbow. The idiopathic form of the disease usually occurs in young persons who are otherwise healthy. There is a genetic component to this disease that has been reported concurrently in siblings and has a predilection for blacks. The same term is often used for similar chalky deposits occurring in conjunction with systemic disease, usually chronic renal failure. The diagnosis may be made by plain radiography, along with history, physical examination, and laboratory studies. Neither CT nor MRI are usually necessary. Occasionally, however, the plain film appearance of such masses may be confusing, and CT may help distinguish them from other calcified masses such as chondrosarcoma or osteosarcoma.[6,13,61,73,89]

INFLAMMATORY ARTHRITIS
RHEUMATOID ARTHRITIS

Rheumatoid arthritis is a common disease with a predilection for women of middle age. Either the gleno-

humeral joint, the acromioclavicular joint, or both may be involved, but it is unusual for the disease to present in the shoulder before it has manifested elsewhere. Indeed, the patient with shoulder involvement usually has progressive multiarticular disease before complaining of the shoulder.[18,71]

In the glenohumeral joint, as elsewhere, rheumatoid arthritis is characterized by osteopenia, effusions, progressive loss of joint space, and osseous erosions. The effusions may cause outpouchings of the synovium; when very large they are termed *giant synovial cysts.* Acromioclavicular involvement has a similar appearance, except that the scapula and clavicle are held in their respective locations by surrounding structures and do not migrate closer to one another with destruction of the joint surfaces. Thus, the acromioclavicular joint space will widen rather than narrow with rheumatic involvement.[18,71]

Inflammatory arthritides, especially rheumatoid arthritis, predispose the patient to tendon and ligament ruptures. In the shoulder, they may lead to rotator cuff tears. These may be diagnosed by arthrography, ultrasound, or MRI with the same criteria as for rotator cuff tears of other etiology.

Rheumatoid arthritis may be diagnosed by clinical and serologic means. Radiographic techniques are less useful in diagnosis than in plotting progression of disease and response to therapy. MRI is more sensitive than plain films to the presence of effusions and small erosions. Use of intravenous gadolinium helps distinguish pannus from effusions, because both may appear low in signal on unenhanced T1-weighted images and high in signal on T2-weighted images. Therefore, MRI may have

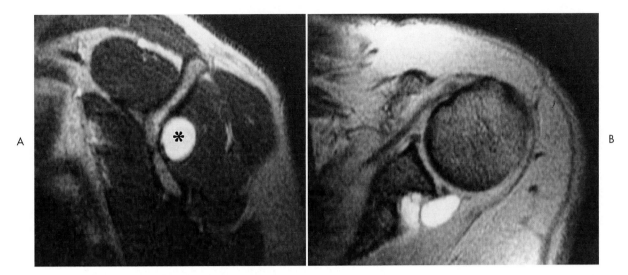

Fig. 44-27. Spinoglenoid notch ganglion. **A,** T2-weighted (2500/70) sagittal oblique image. A single rounded hyperintense mass (*) is present in the spinoglenoid notch of this young man who presented with shoulder pain. **B,** Gradient-echo axial image. At this level the lesion is composed of multiple smaller masses. On proton-density images, this mass was intermediate in signal, approximately isointense with muscle. This is the typical location and appearance of a spinoglenoid notch ganglion.

a role to play in evaluating therapeutic response. Most likely, however, the hands and wrists will be a more fruitful site of evaluation than will the shoulder.[4,32,103,121]

PIGMENTED VILLONODULAR SYNOVITIS

Pigmented villonodular synovitis is an uncommon disorder of unknown etiology. It usually affects young adults and is typically monoarticular, with most frequent involvement of the knee. It is rare in the shoulder.[23,30,109] Histologically PVNS demonstrates fatty areas together with hemosiderin deposition. This causes it to have a heterogenous appearance at both CT and MR imaging. The hemosiderin creates areas of decreased signal on intermediate weighting. The signal decrease becomes more prominent on T2 weighting. On gradient-echo imaging the paramagnetic affect of hemosidin causes even more dramatic signal loss. Effusions may be present.* One case that involved the shoulder is reported to have had very little hemosiderin at histology, demonstrating on MRI none of the signal dropout usually ascribed to hemosiderin.[109]

SUPRASCAPULAR NERVE ENTRAPMENT

Pressure on the suprascapular nerve as it courses across the posterior scapula is an uncommon cause of shoulder pain. Any mass that arises in the appropriate lo-

*References 8, 44, 53, 56, 62, 114.

cation can produce suprascapular nerve entrapment; reported causes include neoplasms and hematoma. The commonest cause, however, is a ganglion cyst. These cysts usually occur in young men. They most often arise at the spinoglenoid notch, from which they may extend superiorly into the supraspinatus fossa or inferiorly into the infraspinatus fossa. They may produce muscle paralysis and atrophy as well as pain. The infraspinatus muscle is most often affected, but the supraspinatus muscle may be involved as well.

Ganglia may be detected as a water-density mass by CT. On MRI they are approximately isointense with muscle on short TE images and very bright on T2-weighted images. If intravenous Gd-DTPA is administered, the cysts may enhance about their rim. They often appear septated. If muscle atrophy has ensued, this may also be apparent by MRI. There are three cases reported in which CT guided aspiration yielded relief. Other patients have successfully undergone surgery, and occasionally such cysts resolve spontaneously (Fig. 44-27).[33,93]

TRAUMA

Most fractures about the shoulder are adequately evaluated with plain radiography. In cases of complex fractures of the proximal humerus, CT may be helpful for pretreatment planning. Treatment of these fractures varies considerably, depending on their position in the widely used classification scheme of Neer that is based on the degree of separation or rotation of the four possible major fracture fragments (shaft, head, greater tuberosity, and lesser tuberosity). A fragment is considered displaced if it is distracted 1 cm or more from its neighbors or if it is angulated 45° or more from its proper location. Fractures without displacement are commonly treated with early mobilization, while those involving displacement of one of the tuberosities often require open reduction. It is important, therefore, to determine accurately the position of all fragments before definitive treatment is carried out. This may be difficult with plain radiographs alone. Castagno et al found that in 12 cases of acute fractures and five cases of persistent limitation of motion after treatment of fracture, CT provided useful information that was not evident on plain film. Even when the information is available on the plain films, evaluation of fragment location may be difficult, as evidenced by reports of high interobserver variability in classifying humeral fractures according to Neer's scheme.

CT may again be useful because it can provide a much more graphic depiction of fragments, particularly when 3D reconstruction is available. In addition to localizing major fracture fragments, CT can locate smaller ones; this is particularly useful for intraarticular fragments. Loose bodies of nontraumatic origin may, of course, also be located with CT (Fig. 44-28).[10,39,51,57,80]

CT may also be useful in detection of complex scapular fractures. These are rare injuries, usually seen in patients who have sustained multiple injuries due to direct, blunt trauma, often an automobile accident. They may be missed on initial plain radiography, particularly on the portable chest film often obtained on patients who have sustained severe trauma. When a suspected scapular fracture has not been revealed on such a film, it may be easier as well as more rewarding to obtain a CT study rather than plain films of the shoulder.[1,38,68,115]

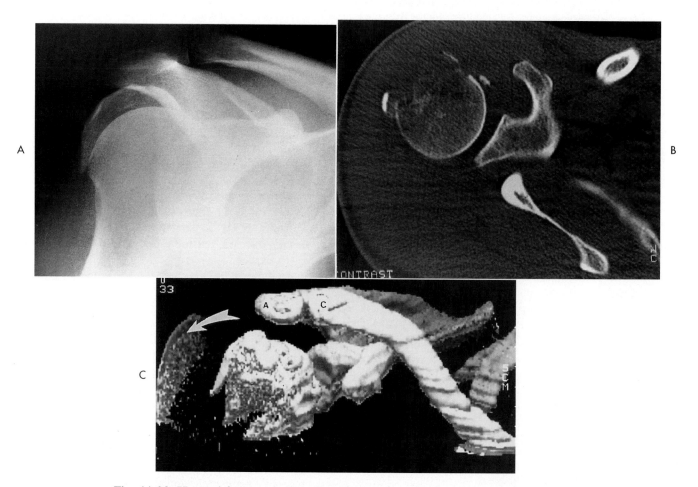

Fig. 44-28. Humeral fracture. **A,** Plain film. The humerus has been fractured. A crescent of bone typical of a detached greater tuberosity projects superolateral to the humeral head. **B,** Axial computed tomography. CT demonstrates more graphically than does the plain film the amount of damage that has occurred to the region of the greater and lesser tuberosities. **C,** Three-dimensional reconstruction; this shows the relationship of the detached greater tuberosity *(white arrow)* to the remainder of the humerus. Acromion *(A)*, clavicle *(C)*. (Case courtesy of Stein Rafto, M.D., Honolulu, Hawaii.)

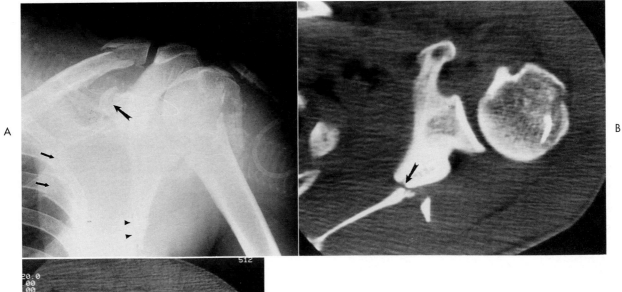

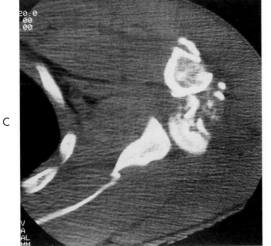

Fig. 44-29. Fractures. **A,** Plain film. Multiple fractures are present, including the proximal humerus, clavicle, coracoid process *(arrow)*, and at least two ribs *(small arrows)*. Fracture of the blade of the scapula is also present *(arrowheads)* but is somewhat difficult to see and could be missed. It is difficult to evaluate the glenoid. **B,** Axial CT, midglenoid level. The CT reveals the scapular blade fracture *(arrow)* as well as a relatively normal relationship between the humeral head and an unfractured glenoid. **C,** Axial CT, lower glenoid level. This section again confirms that the glenoid has not been fractured and demonstrates the relationship of humeral fracture fragments.

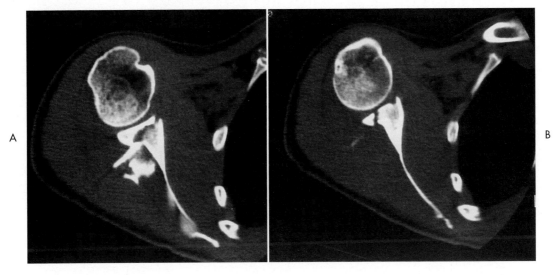

Fig. 44-30. Glenoid fracture. **A** and **B,** Axial CT. This fracture does extend to the articular surface of the glenoid.

Besides its use in fracture detection, CT may also be useful in evaluation of scapular fractures. Treatment of scapular fractures is less well established than is treatment of humeral fractures. Some surgeons believe that displaced fractures of the glenoid and spine should receive internal fixation, while others believe that these injuries, like other scapular fractures, may be satisfactorily

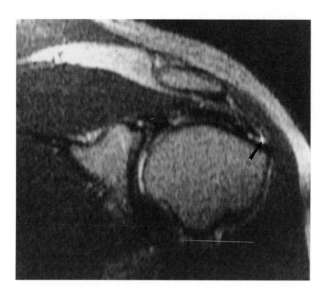

Fig. 44-31. Acute traumatic rotator cuff tear. T2-weighted (2500/70) coronal oblique image. This surgically proved full-thickness tear of the supraspinatus tendon *(arrow)* occurred as a result of trauma. The appearance is no different from that of other cuff tears.

treated by immobilization soon followed by range-of-motion exercises. In addition, the patient's other injuries may preclude surgical intervention. When treatment hinges on site of fracture and degree of displacement, however, CT may be more easily obtained and more revealing than plain films (Figs. 44-29 and 44-30).[1,69]

MRI has limited use in shoulder trauma. As in other areas of the body, it may reveal occult fractures. Acute trauma may cause a rotator cuff tear, particularly when superimposed on preexisting degeneration. The tear may be evaluated on MRI using the same criteria discussed above for tears not related to trauma (Fig. 44-31).

Avascular necrosis in the shoulder is seldom related to trauma. It may be well portrayed with MRI. Its appearance is similar in the shoulder to its appearance in other parts of the body.

TUMORS

In the region of the shoulder, as elsewhere in the musculoskeletal system, diagnosis of bone tumors may be most efficiently and accurately accomplished by plain film radiography. CT and MRI may occasionally add information useful to the characterization of a bone tumor. CT, for example, is more sensitive to the presence of calcium than are plain films and may therefore reveal matrix or periosteal calcification too faint to be seen on conventional radiographs. Either modality may demonstrate fluid-fluid levels. They are nonspecific, but they are commonest in aneurysmal bone cysts. Both CT and MRI are

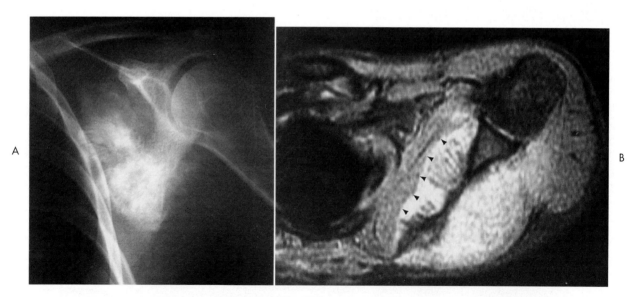

Fig. 44-32. Osteosarcoma. **A,** Plain film. Exuberant tumor new bone formation and sunburst periosteal reaction mark this scapular tumor as an osteosarcoma. **B,** Gradient-echo axial image. MRI delineated the extent of the tumor and demonstrated that the tumor edge *(arrowheads)* was free of the chest wall. Periosteal reaction can be seen as spiculated areas of low signal.

most useful, however, in staging local disease. The presence of soft tissue extension may be difficult to judge by plain films but is easily assessed by either CT or MRI. It is particularly important to determine whether the tumor involves a joint space, the axillary vascular structures, the brachial plexus, or the thoracic cage. MRI may at times overestimate the extent of soft-tissue involvement with tumor because perilesional edema may have an appearance similar to that of tumor. Both will often appear of decreased signal intensity on T1 weighting and of increased signal on T2 weighting. Dynamic intravenous gadolinium administration may be helpful in differentiation because edematous areas generally enhance more slowly than do tumor [26] (Fig. 44-32).

Soft-tissue tumors may be undetectable by plain films. Even very large ones may be noticeable as a nonspecific mass only. Several such tumors, however, have relatively characteristic appearances by MRI.[17] Lipomas have the same signal characteristics that fat has on all pulse sequences, including fat-suppression techniques. They will also demonstrate the CT attenuation of fat. They may be subcutaneous, intramuscular, or intermuscular in location. Ganglia are frequently septated and are of low signal intensity on T1 weighting and bright on T2 weighting. The spinoglenoid notch and infraspinatus fossa are the most common location about the shoulder. For many other soft-tissue masses, CT and MRI will not yield a specific diagnosis but will define the extent of local disease.

CONCLUSION

A great variety of diseases affect the shoulder. When CT or MRI evaluation is called for, in the majority of cases it will be in connection with trauma or a disorder in the spectrum of instability, intrinsic impingement, rotator cuff disease, and bicipital tendon disease. A solid understanding of these diseases will serve most radiologists well. For the future, work is needed on further definition of normal anatomy, particularly regarding the labrum, anterior capsule, and glenohumeral ligaments. In addition, more understanding is needed about the role that CT, CT arthrography, and MRI can play in the management of patients and about how the use of these studies affects clinical decision making and final outcome.

ACKNOWLEDGEMENTS

We would like to thank Mary Armstrong for her patient and precise word processing.

REFERENCES

1. Ada JR, Miller ME: Scapular fractures. *Clin Orthop* 269:174-180, Aug 1991.
2. Andrews JR, Carson WG Jr, McLeod WD: Glenoid labrum tears related to the long head of the biceps. *Am J Sports Med* 13(5):337-341, 1985.
3. Bankart ASB: The pathology and treatment of recurrent dislocation of the shoulder-joint. *Br J Surg* 26:23-29, 1938.
4. Beltran J, et al: Rheumatoid arthritis: MR imaging manifestations. *Radiology* 165:153-157, 1987.
5. Bigliani LU, Morrison DS, April EW: The morphology of the acromion and its relationship to rotator cuff tears. American Shoulder and Elbow Surgeons. *Orthop Trans* 10:228, 1986.
6. Bishop AF, et al: Tumoral calcinosis: case report and review. *Skeletal Radiol* 8:269-274, 1982.
7. Burk DL, et al: Rotator cuff tears: prospective comparison of MR imaging with arthrography, sonography, and surgery. *AJR* 153:87-92, July 1989.
8. Butt WP, Hardy G, Ostlere SJ: Pigmented villonodular synovitis of the knee: computed tomographic appearances. *Skeletal Radiol* 19:191-196, 1990.
9. Cartland JP, et al: MR imaging in the evaluation of SLAP injuries of the shoulder: findings in 10 patients. *AJR* 159:787-792, Oct 1992.
10. Castagno AA, et al: Complex fractures of the proximal humerus: role of CT in treatment. *Radiology* 165:759-762, 1987.
11. Cervilla V, et al: Medial dislocation of the biceps brachii tendon: appearance at MR imaging. *Radiology* 180:523-526, 1991.
12. Chan TW, et al: Biceps tendon dislocation: evaluation with MR imaging. *Radiology* 179:649-652, 1991.
13. Chew FS, Crenshaw WB: Idiopathic tumoral calcinosis. *AJR* 158:330, Feb 1992.
14. Codman EA: The classic rupture of the supraspinatus tendon. *Clin Orthop* 254:3-26, 1990.
15. Cooper DE, et al: Anatomy, histology, and vascularity of the glenoid labrum. *J Bone Joint Surg* 74A(1):46-52, Jan 1992.
16. Coumas JM, et al: CT and MR evaluation of the labral capsular ligamentous complex of the shoulder. *AJR* 158:591-597, March 1992.
17. Crim JR, et al: Diagnosis of soft-tissue masses with MR imaging: can benign masses be differentiated from malignant ones? *Radiology* 185:581-586, 1992.
18. Cruess RL: Rheumatoid arthritis of the shoulder. *Orthop Clin North Am* 11(2):333-342, 1980.
19. Dalinka MK, Boorstein JM, Zlatkin MB: Computed tomography of musculoskeletal trauma. *Radiol Clin North Am* 27(5):933-944, 1989.
20. Davis SJ, et al: Effect of arm rotation on MR imaging of the rotator cuff. *Radiology* 181:265-268, 1991.
21. DePalma AF: *Surgery of the shoulder.* Philadelphia, 1950, JB Lippincott.
22. Deutsch AL, et al: Computed and conventional arthrotomography of the glenohumeral joint: normal anatomy and clinical experience. *Radiology* 153:603-609, 1984.
23. Dorwart RH, et al: Pigmented villonodular synovitis of the shoulder: radiologic-pathologic assessment. *AJR* 143:886-888, 1984.
24. Erickson SJ, et al: Effect of tendon orientation on MR imaging signal intensity: a manifestation of the "magic angle" phenomenon. *Radiology* 181:389-392, 1991.
25. Erickson SJ: Long bicipital tendon of the shoulder: normal anatomy and pathologic findings on MR imaging. *AJR* 158:1091-1096, May 1992.
26. Erlemann R, et al: Musculoskeletal neoplasms: static and dynamic Gd-DTPA-enhanced MR imaging. *Radiology* 171:767-773, 1989.
27. Evancho AM, et al: MR imaging diagnosis of rotator cuff tears. *AJR* 151:751-754, Oct 1988.
28. Farley TE, et al: Full-thickness tears of the rotator cuff of the

shoulder: diagnosis with MR imaging. *AJR* 158:347-351, Feb 1992.

29. Ferrari DA: Capsular ligaments of the shoulder. *Am J Sports Med* 18(1):20-24, 1990.

30. Flandry F, Norwood LA: Pigmented villonodular synovitis of the shoulder. *Orthopedics* 12(5):715-718, 1989.

31. Flannigan B, Kursunoglu-Brahme S, Snyder S, et al: MR arthrography of the shoulder: comparison with conventional MR imaging. *AJR* 155:829-832, 1990.

32. Foley-Nolan D, et al: Magnetic resonance imaging in the assessment of rheumatoid arthritis—a comparison with plain film radiographs. *Br J Rheum* 30:101-106, 1991.

33. Fritz RC, et al: Suprascapular nerve entrapment: evaluation with MR imaging. *Radiology* 182:437-444, 1992.

34. Fu FH, Harner CD, Klein AH: Shoulder impingement syndrome. *Clin Orthop* 269:162-173, Aug 1991.

35. Garneau RA, et al: Glenoid labrum: evaluation with MR imaging. *Radiology* 179:519-522, 1991.

36. Halverson PB, et al: Milwaukee shoulder syndrome: eleven additional cases with involvement of the knee in seven (basic calcium phosphate crystal deposition disease). *Semin Arthritis Rheum* 14(1):36-44, August 1984.

37. Halverson PB, et al: Milwaukee shoulder syndrome: fifteen additional cases and a description of contributing factors. *Arch Intern Med* 150:677-682, March 1990.

38. Harris RD, Harris JH Jr: The prevalence and significance of missed scapular fractures in blunt chest trauma. *AJR* 151:747-750, Oct 1988.

39. Heppenstall RB: Fractures of the proximal humerus. *Orthop Clin North Am* 6(2):467-475, April 1975.

40. Hodler J, et al: Injuries of the superior portion of the glenoid labrum involving the insertion of the biceps tendon: MR imaging findings in nine cases. *AJR* 159:565-568, Sept 1992.

41. Holt RG, et al: Magnetic resonance imaging of the shoulder: rationale and current applications. *Skeletal Radiol* 19:5-14, 1990.

42. Hunter JC, Blatz DJ, Escobedo EM: SLAP lesions of the glenoid labrum: CT arthrographic and arthroscopic correlation. *Radiology* 184:513-518, 1992.

43. Iannotti JP, et al: Magnetic resonance imaging of the shoulder. *J Bone Joint Surg* 73A(1):17-29, Jan 1991.

44. Jelinek JS, et al: Imaging of pigmented villonodular synovitis with emphasis on MR imaging. *AJR* 152:337-342, 1989.

45. Jobe FW, et al: Anterior capsulolabral reconstruction of the shoulder in athletes in overhand sports. *Am J Sports Med* 19(5):428-434, 1991.

46. Jobe FW, Bradley JP: Rotator cuff injuries in baseball. *Sports Med* 6:378-387, 1988.

47. Kaplan PA, et al: MR imaging of the normal shoulder: variants and pitfalls. *Radiology* 184:519-524, 1992.

48. Keats TE, Pope TL: The acromioclavicular joint: normal variation and the diagnosis of dislocation. *Skeletal Radiol* 17:159-162, 1988.

49. Kieft GJ, et al: MR imaging of recurrent anterior dislocation of the shoulder: comparison with CT arthrography. *AJR* 150:1083-1087, May 1988.

50. Kieft GJ, et al: Rotator cuff impingement syndrome: MR imaging. *Radiology* 166:211-214, 1988.

51. Kilcoyne RF, et al: The Neer classification of displaced proximal humeral fractures: spectrum of findings on plain radiographs and CT scans. *AJR* 154:1029-1033, May 1990.

52. Kjellin I, et al: Alterations in the supraspinatus tendon at MR imaging: correlation with histopathologic findings in cadavers. *Radiology* 181:837-841, 1991.

53. Klompmaker J, et al: Pigmented villonodular synovitis. *Arch Orthop Trauma Surg* 109:205-210, 1990.

54. Kneeland JB, et al: MR imaging of the shoulder: diagnosis of rotator cuff tears. *AJR* 149:333-337, Aug 1987.

55. Kneeland JB, et al: Rotator cuff tears: preliminary application of high-resolution MR imaging with counter rotating current loop-gap resonators. *Radiology* 160:695-699, 1986.

56. Kottal RA, et al: Pigmented villonodular synovitis: a report of MR imaging in two cases. *Radiology* 163:551-553, 1987.

57. Kristiansen B, et al: The Neer classification of fractures of the proximal humerus: an assessment of interobserver variation. *Skeletal Radiol* 17:420-422, 1988.

58. Legan JM, et al: Tears of the glenoid labrum: MR imaging of 88 arthroscopically confirmed cases. *Radiology* 179:241-246, 1991.

59. Liou JTS, et al: The normal shoulder: common variations that simulate pathologic conditions at MR imaging. *Radiology* 186:435-441, 1993.

60. Lohr JF, Uhthoff HK: The microvascular pattern of the supraspinatus tendon. *Clin Orthop* 254:35-38, May 1990.

61. Longacre AM, Sheer AL: Tumoral calcinosis: case presentation and review of 55 cases in the literature. *J Fla Med Assoc* 61(3):221-225, March 1974.

62. Mandelbaum BR, et al: The use of MRI to assist in diagnosis of pigmented villonodular synovitis of the knee joint. *Clin Orthop* 231:135-139, 1988.

63. Matsen FA III, Arntz CT: Rotator cuff tendon failure. In Rockwood CA Jr, Matsen FA III, editors: *The shoulder,* Philadelphia, 1990, WB Saunders.

64. Matsen FA III, Arntz CT: Subacromial impingement. In Rockwood CA Jr, Matsen FA III, editors: *The shoulder,* Philadelphia, 1990, WB Saunders.

65. Matsen FA III, Thomas SC, Rockwood CA Jr: Glenohumeral instability. In Rockwood CA Jr, Matsen FA III, editors: *The shoulder,* Philadelphia, 1990, WB Saunders.

66. McCarty DJ, et al: "Milwaukee shoulder"—association of microspheroids containing hydroxapatite crystals, active collagenase, and neutral protease with rotator cuff defects. *Arthritis Rheum* 24(3):464-473, March 1981.

67. McCauley TR, Pope CF, Jokl P: Normal and abnormal glenoid labrum: assessment with multiplanar gradient-echo MR imaging. *Radiology* 183:35-37, 1992.

68. McGahan JP, Rab GT, Dublin A: Fractures of the scapula. *J Trauma* 20(10):880-883, Oct 1980.

69. McGinnis M, Denton JR: Fractures of the scapula: a retrospective study of 40 fractured scapulae. *J Trauma* 29(11):1488-1493, Nov 1989.

70. McKendry RJR, et al: Calcifying Tendinitis of the shoulder: prognostic value of clinical, histologic, and radiologic features in 57 surgically treated cases. *J Rheumatol* 9:75-80, 1982.

71. McNair MM, et al: A clinical and radiological study of rheumatoid arthritis with a note on the findings in osteoarthrosis. I. The shoulder joint. *Clin Radiol* 20:269-277, 1969.

72. McNiesh LM, Callaghan JJ: CT arthrography of the shoulder: variations of the glenoid labrum. *AJR* 149:963-966, Nov 1987.

73. Metzker A, et al: Tumoral calcinosis revisited—common and uncommon features. *Eur J Pediatr* 147:128-132, 1988.

74. Mirowitz SA: Normal rotator cuff: MR imaging with conventional and fat-suppression techniques. *Radiology* 180:735-740, 1991.

75. Mitchell MJ, et al: Peribursal fat plane of the shoulder: anatomic study and clinical experience. *Radiology* 168:699-704, 1988.

76. Moore KL: *Clinically oriented anatomy,* Baltimore, 1980, Williams & Wilkins.

77. Moseley HF, Goldie I: The arterial pattern of the rotator cuff of the shoulder. *J Bone Joint Surg* 45B(4):780-789, Nov 1963.

78. Moseley HF, Övergaard B: The anterior capsular mechanism in

recurrent anterior dislocation of the shoulder. *J Bone Joint Surg* 44B(4):913-927, Nov 1962.

79. Neer CS, Craig EV, Fukuda H: Cuff-tear arthropathy. *J Bone Joint Surg* 65A(9):1232-1244, Dec 1983.

80. Neer CS, Foster CR: Inferior capsular shift for involuntary inferior and multidirectional instability of the shoulder. *J Bone Joint Surg* 62A(6):897-908, Sept 1980.

81. Neer CS, Welsh RP: The shoulder in sports. *Orthop Clin North Am* 8(3):583-591, July 1977.

82. Neer CS: Anterior acromioplasty for the chronic impingement syndrome in the shoulder. *J Bone Joint Surg* 54A(1):41-50, Jan 1972.

83. Neer CS: Displaced proximal humeral fractures. *J Bone Joint Surg* 52A(6):1077-1089, Sept 1970.

84. Neer CS: Impingement lesions. *Clin Orthop* 173:70-77, March 1983.

85. Neumann CH, et al: MR imaging of the shoulder: appearance of the supraspinatus tendon in asymptomatic volunteers. *AJR* 158:1281-1287, June 1992.

86. Neumann CH, Petersen SA, Jahnke AH: MR imaging of the labral-capsular complex: normal variations. *AJR* 157:1015-1021, Nov 1991.

87. Neviaser TJ, et al: The four-in-one arthroplasty for the painful arc syndrome. *Clin Orthop* 163:107-112, March 1982.

88. Nguyen VD, Nguyen KD, Kamath V: Unusual feature of soft-tissue calcification in chronic renal failure: tumoral calcification. *Comput Med Imaging Graphics* 15(6):397-402, 1991.

89. Nguyen VD, Nguyen KD: "Idiopathic destructive arthritis" of the shoulder: a still fascinating enigma. *Comput Med Imaging Graphics* 14(4):249-255, July-Aug 1990.

90. Nutton RW, Stothard J: Acute calcific supraspinatus tendinitis in a three-year-old child. *J Bone Joint Surg* 69B(1):148, Jan 1987.

91. O'Brien SJ, et al: The anatomy and histology of the inferior glenohumeral ligament complex of the shoulder. *Am J Sports Med* 18(5):449-456, 1990.

92. Ogata S, Uhthoff HK: Acromial enthesopathy and rotator cuff tear. *Clin Orthop* 254:39-48, 1990.

93. Ogino T, et al: Entrapment neuropathy of the suprascapular nerve by a ganglion. *J Bone Joint Surg* 73A(1):141-147, Jan 1991.

94. Owen RS, et al: Shoulder after surgery: MR imaging with surgical validation. *Radiology* 186:443-447, 1993.

95. Ozaki J, et al: Tears of the rotator cuff of the shoulder associated with pathological changes in the acromion. *J Bone Joint Surg* 70A(8):1224-1230, Sept 1988.

96. Pappas AM, Goss TP, Kleinman PK: Symptomatic shoulder instability due to lesions of the glenoid labrum. *Am J Sports Med* 11(5):279-288, 1983.

97. Penny JN, Welsh RP: Shoulder impingement syndromes in athletes and their surgical management. *Am J Sports Med* 9(1):11-15, 1981.

98. Petersson CJ: Spontaneous medial dislocation of the tendon of the long biceps brachii. *Clin Orthop* 211:224-227, Oct 1986.

99. Prodromos CC, et al: Histological studies of the glenoid labrum from fetal life to old age. *J Bone Joint Surg* 74A(9):1344-1348, Oct 1990.

100. Rafii M, et al: CT arthrography of capsular structures of the shoulder. *AJR* 146:361-367, Feb 1986.

101. Rafii M, et al: Rotator cuff lesions: signal patterns at MR imaging. *Radiology* 177:817-823, 1990.

102. Rathbun JB, Macnab I: The microvascular pattern of the rotator cuff. *J Bone Joint Surg* 52B(3):540-553, Aug 1970.

103. Rominger MB, et al: MR imaging of the hands in early rheumatoid arthritis: preliminary results. *RadioGraphics* 13:37-46, 1993.

104. Rowe CR, Pierce DS, Clarke JG: Voluntary dislocation of the shoulder. *J Bone Joint Surg* 55A(3):445-460, April 1973.

105. Salter EG, Nasca RJ, Shelley BS: Anatomical observations on the acromioclavicular joint and supporting ligaments. *Am J Sports Med* 15(3):199-206, 1987.

106. Seeger LL, et al: MR imaging of the normal shoulder: anatomic correlation. *AJR* 148:83-91, Jan 1987.

107. Seeger LL, et al: Shoulder impingement syndrome: MR findings in 53 shoulders. *AJR* 150:343-347, Feb 1988.

108. Seeger LL, Gold RH, Bassett LW: Shoulder instability: evaluation with MR imaging. *Radiology* 168:695-697, 1988.

109. Sher M, et al: Case report 578. *Skeletal Radiol* 19:131-133, 1990.

110. Shuman WP, et al: Double-contrast computed tomography of the glenoid labrum. *AJR* 141:581-584, Sept 1983.

111. Singson RD, Feldman F, Bigliani L: CT arthrographic patterns in recurrent glenohumeral instability. *AJR* 149:749-753, Oct 1987.

112. Singson RD, et al: Recurrent shoulder dislocation after surgical repair: double-contrast CT arthrography. *Radiology* 164:425-428, 1987.

113. Snyder SJ, et al: SLAP lesions of the shoulder. *Arthroscopy* 6(4):274-279, 1990.

114. Steinbach LS, et al: MRI of the knee in diffuse pigmented villonodular synovitis. *Clin Imaging* 13:305-316, 1989.

115. Thompson DA, et al: The significance of scapular fractures. *J Trauma* 25(10):974-977, 1985.

116. Townley CO: The capsular mechanism in recurrent dislocation of the shoulder. *J Bone Joint Surg* 32A:370-380, 1950.

117. Uhthoff HK, Sarkar K: Calcifying tendinitis: its pathogenetic mechanism and a rationale for its treatment. *Int Orthop* 2:187-193, 1978.

118. Vahlensieck M, et al: Two segments of the supraspinous muscle: cause of high signal intensity at MR imaging? *Radiology* 186:449-454, 1993.

119. Vebostad A: Calcific tendinitis in the shoulder region. *Acta Orthop Scand* 46:205-210, 1975.

120. Weiss JJ, Good A, Schumacher HR: Four cases of "Milwaukee shoulder," with a description of clinical presentation and long-term treatment. *J Am Geriatrics Soc* 33(3): 202-205, March 1985.

121. Whitten CG, et al: The use of intravenous gadopentetate dimeglumine in magnetic resonance imaging of synovial lesions. *Skeletal Radiol* 21:215-218, 1992.

122. Wilson AJ, et al: Shoulder joint: arthrographic CT and long-term follow-up, with surgical correlation. *Radiology* 173:329-333, 1989.

123. Workman TL, et al: Hill-Sachs lesion: comparison of detection with MR imaging, radiography, and arthroscopy. *Radiology* 185:847-852, 1992.

124. Zlatkin MB, et al: Rotator cuff tears: diagnostic performance of MR imaging. *Radiology* 172:223-229, 1989.

125. Zlatkin MB, et al: The painful shoulder: MR imaging of the glenohumeral joint. *J Comput Assist Tomogr* 12(6):995-1001, 1988.

126. Zlatkin MB: *MRI of the shoulder*, New York, 1991, Raven Press.

PART VIII

SPECIAL CONSIDERATIONS

SPECIAL CONSIDERATIONS

45
Pediatric Imaging

STUART C. MORRISON

The use of computed tomography (CT) and magnetic resonance imaging (MRI) in the pediatric age group has continued to increase, and the indications for each study change. Ultrasound remains the modality of choice for the initial evaluation of the abdominal mass and retroperitoneum. CT remains the initial modality of choice for abdominal trauma and as the subsequent modality for many oncology patients (after initial diagnosis with either chest x-ray film or ultrasound). The indications for MRI are still evolving. The lack of ionizing radiation makes this modality especially attractive for children. In this chapter, the optimal scanning techniques and important clinical problems that occur in the pediatric age group are discussed. Rather than repeat general information about the different organs as noted in other chapters, information unique to this age-group is emphasized.

SCANNING RADIOGRAPHIC CT TECHNIQUE

Radiation doses for children are always of more concern because children have not reached their reproduction stage of life. In a review of radiation doses from CT scanning in children, Brasch and Cann[17] were able to show that the dosage, compared with an earlier study in 1977, had actually decreased 31%. Another major improvement was the reduction in scanning time that occurred in this period—less than 5 seconds a scan. The calculated mean dose for an abdominal CT scan was 1.5 rad. In another study, the absorbed entrance skin dose for chest and abdominal examinations was 1.1 to 2.4 rad.[48]

Several technical factors are important to note and adjust if optimal CT scans are to be obtained on children. These factors, which enhance spatial resolution and produce radiation savings, include proper choice of slice thickness, scan diameter, and milliamperage settings (Fig. 45-1, A and B).

Considering that the number of pixels is fixed,

one can improve the spatial resolution by using the smallest scan diameter possible. By decreasing the scan diameter, there are more pixels per area, thereby increasing the spatial resolution (assuming all other factors of slice thickness and milliamperes are constant). As noted by Hounsfield, the greater the number of pixels, the greater the spatial resolution. Thus the use of a 25 cm scan diameter rather than a 40 cm scan diameter significantly improves the spatial resolution (Fig. 45-1, C and D).

The slice thickness also has an impact on resolution seen on the scan image. The improvement of resolution can be best understood by remembering that each pixel on the scan image is really a voxel, or a rectangular volume measuring the width of the pixel size on the end and having a length corresponding to the slice thickness. If one uses a more narrow slice, the "averaging" within the slice is reduced, and resolution is improved (Fig. 45-1, E and F).

Furthermore, one should remember the relationship between the radiation dose and the contrast resolution. The amount of dosage required for good-quality scans depends on the body size being examined; large bodies remove more photons, and small bodies remove fewer photons. This means that one can use almost one half of the adult dose in an infant or child and see no difference in subjective or objective (phantom measurements) contrast or spatial resolution.[63] Current CT devices do not allow alterations with milliamperes, but in theory a CT machine could be manufactured that varied the milliamperes similar to a phototimer, and this could produce considerable decrease in dosage. The radiologists can make a subjective decision concerning acceptable noise; there is no question that beyond a certain level, additional milliamperes does not improve resolution.

Sedation

Children under 1 month of age rarely need sedation and can be satisfactorily immobilized after a normal

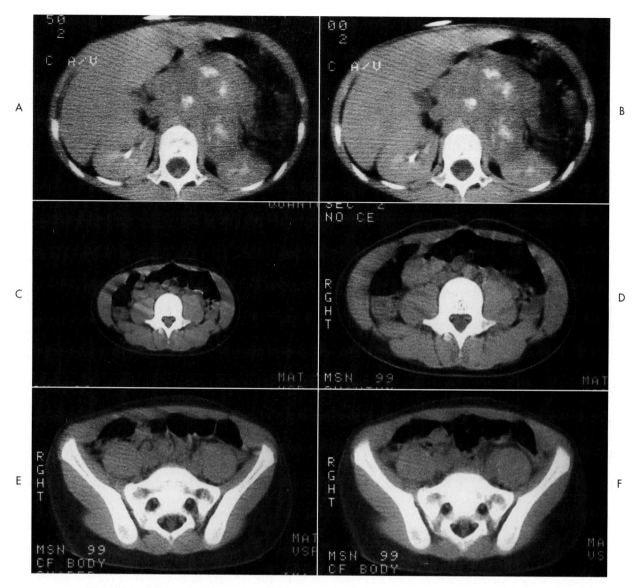

Fig. 45-1. Effect of milliamperage. **A,** Axial scan at 50 mA at the level of the kidneys in a child with neuroblastoma. **B,** Scan taken at an identical level with 100 mA. The 50 mA scan, half the dose of the 100 mA scan, shows similar resolution. Effect of scan diameter. **C,** Scan obtained with a 40 cm diameter. **D,** Scan of 25 cm scan diameter at an identical level shows increased spatial resolution. Effect of slice thickness. **E,** Scan obtained at 5 mm collimation through the pelvis clearly shows the right iliac vessel *(arrowhead)*. **F,** Scan taken with a 10 mm slice thickness shows a lack of resolution, with the iliac vessel on the right side poorly defined.

feeding. Oral chloral hydrate offers a wide safety margin for sedation. Given 30 minutes before the scan, this is the least depressant of all sedatives. It is useful in children up to approximately 2 years of age. For CT scans, a dose of 50 to 70 mg/kg is given orally. For MRI, the longer scan times require 75 to 100 mg/kg for satisfactory sedation. The maxumum dose is 2 g.

Children over 2 years of age can be sedated with intravenous sodium pentobarbital (Nembutal) at a dos-

age of 2 to 3 mg/kg. The maximum dose is 8 mg/kg. The advantage of this form of sedation is that the dosage can be titrated, and the response is fast and controlled.[129] The addition of fentanyl citrate (Sublimase) at a dosage of 1 µg/kg provides additive pain relief to the sedative effect of the barbiturate.

Continuous monitoring of the child is performed with pulse rate, electrocardiogram, and pulse oximetry together with visual inspection of the child, including chest wall motion. Appropriate pediatric resuscitative equipment and staff must be available.

Technique

To visualize fresh blood or calcification, images are obtained before the injection of contrast material. Feeding is withheld for approximately 3 to 4 hours before the study. Oral contrast material (diluted Hypaque or Gastrografin) is given 20 to 30 minutes before scanning starts. Children too young or too ill to cooperate are given this contrast material by a nasogastric tube, which is withdrawn into the distal esophagus before scanning.[75] Dynamic scanning, using 2 ml/kg of iodinated contrast material, is performed. From 40% to 50% of the total dose is rapidly injected, scanning is begun, and the remaining contrast material is injected during the first five or six slices.

UPPER AIRWAY

Choanal atresia is seen in newborns as severe difficulty in breathing because the neonate is an obligate nasal breather. Inability to pass a nasogastric tube is still the easiest and simplest way to confirm this diagnosis. Precise anatomy before surgery can be outlined by CT scanning, which can also discriminate the majority of cases, which are bony (90%), from membranous choanal atresia.[111] Unilateral choanal atresia is not often diagnosed until the second decade of life, and again CT scanning would be an excellent method for diagnosis.

Nasal obstruction may also be caused by nasal stenosis. Difficulty with passing a nasogastric tube, apneic spells during feeding, and chronic rhinorrhea were the usual symptoms in a large series of cases of nasal obstruction assessed by CT.[23] Scans are performed at a 10- to 15-degree angle to the hard palate in the axial plane, with 3 to 5 mm slices.

Paranasal sinus disease is common in young children. The value of plain films and CT scans remains controversial. Limited slice CT scans can provide superior anatomical detail than plain films with a fourfold to fivefold reduction in radiation exposure compared with a complete CT examination of the paranasal sinuses.[62] Complications of sinus disease, such as orbital cellulitis, subperiosteal abscess, and mucocele formation,[115] are well shown by CT scanning (Fig. 45-2).

AIRWAY

Ultrafast CT scanning or cine-CT provides more physiological data as well as anatomical information about the airway. Scans can be performed during quiet breathing in the supine position without sedation. Multiple axial views of the airway can be obtained followed by repeated scans at each level throughout the respira-

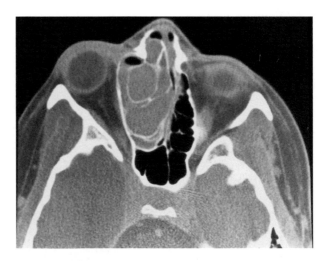

Fig. 45-2. Mucocele of ethmoid sinuses. Opacification with overexpansion of the anterior and middle ethmoid sinuses has occurred secondary to a mucocele related to previous ethmoid sinusitis.

tory cycle. With this sequence of scanning, many causes of chronic stridor in a child can be identified without the need for more invasive endoscopy, which also requires a sedative or general anesthetic.[57]

Laryngomalacia is the symptomatic obstruction caused by infolding of the aryepiglottic folds into the glottis during inspiration. Tracheomalacia is a dynamic narrowing of the trachea during expiration.

Vocal cord paralysis is demonstrated by failure of the vocal cords to abduct throughout the respiratory cycle with consequent persistent narrowing of the glottis. Tracheomalacia can be distinguished from a fixed focal stenosis of the trachea. For optimal results, both ultrafast CT scans (50 msec) and high-resolution images (100 msec) are necessary.[21] Ultrafast CT can also be helpful in symptomatic infants after repair of esophageal atresia and tracheoesophageal fistula.[74]

TRACHEA

Normal dimensions of length, anteroposterior diameter, transverse diameter, cross-sectional area, and volume of the normal growing trachea are reported by Griscom and Wohl.[61] A more complicated method for tracheal cross-sectional area has also been described.[46] Cross-sectional area may be useful in quantitating tracheal compromise by intrinsic or extrinsic masses. Plain films, even with high kilovolt peak and fluoroscopy, may still underestimate the degree of tracheal compression and appear normal.[78] This is especially important in infants with mediastinal masses, who are possibly going to be intubated and are at risk for respiratory compromise both during and after anesthesia.

Foreign bodies

Foreign bodies in the trachea are extraordinarily difficult to diagnose by plain films, which often show only overinflation of both lungs. CT scanning offers an excellent method for their localization.[10] The density discrimination of CT is so sensitive that foreign bodies that are not typically radiopaque, such as an albuminum tab or plastic material, can be seen.

Thymus

The thymus, a normal anterior mediastinal structure, can produce problems in interpretation on both chest x-ray films and CT scans. The normal thymus is a bilobed, arrowhead-shaped structure best seen at the level of the aortic arch. Rarely the normal thymus extends above the level of the left brachiocephalic vein and must not be mistaken for a pathological process.[31] The lateral border of the thymus is convex, smooth, and undulating in the extremely young; it may be concave in older children.[66] Occasionally a sharp, angular, lateral edge is identified. The normal thymus is molded by the heart and great vessels posteriorly and by the chest wall anteriorly.

In children under 10 years of age, the shape of the thymus is variable and may be difficult on CT to differentiate from other structures without contrast material.[7] Up to puberty, the thymus increases in size as a function of age. After puberty, the shape is more triangular, and fatty infiltration occurs, producing inhomogenicity in the density of the thymus. Before puberty, the CT numbers of the thymus are similar to chest wall muscle. Normal CT size measurements are available.[55] The normal thymus is never multilobar. Shape is the most important feature of the normal thymus, distinguishing it from the abnormal.

The shape of normal thymus varies slightly with age when images with MRI.[116] In children under age 5, the normal thymus is quadrilateral with biconvex lateral borders. In children older than 5 years, it is bilobed or triangular with straight lateral margins. On T1-weighted images, the intensity of the normal thymus is slightly greater than muscle and close to fat with T2-weighted images. The normal thymus is homogeneous in all sequences.

MRI measurements of the normal thymus[40] are greater than the CT measurements and correspond more closely to anatomical studies.

Rarely a normal thymus may occupy the posterior mediastinum. CT or MRI scanning can confirm that this represents a continuation of the normal thymus between the superior vena cava and trachea rather than a posterior mediastinal mass. The absence of a tissue plane between the posterior mediastinal mass and the normal

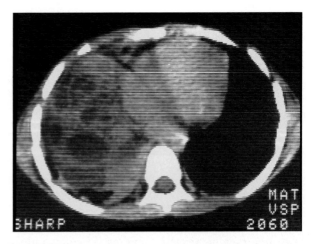

Fig. 45-3. Mediastinal lymphangioma (cystic hygroma). Mixed density mass is identified in the right mediastinum, almost completely filling the right hemithorax. This could be identified extending down from the neck.

thymus, which continues to have a smooth continuous lateral margin,[29] is an important imaging feature.

The thymus may change shape and size rapidly with stress, starvation, burns, fever, and exogenous steroids. The thymus atrophies during chemotherapy regardless of whether steroids are part of the chemotherapy regime.[25] "Rebound" enlargement of the thymus after chemotherapy for malignant tumors is seen in approximately 25% of children and should never be mistaken for infiltration of the thymus by malignant tissue.[26] Infiltration of the thymus with leukemia or lymphoma gives an inhomogeneous signal with MRI. Rarely, tumors[98] and cysts of the thymus occur and can be identified.

Mediastinal tumors

Mediastinal extension of lymphangiomas or cystic hygromas from the neck can be well documented by CT scan (Fig. 45-3) or MRI scans (Fig. 45-4). Although lymphadenopathies secondary to lymphoma (Fig. 45-5) and leukemia are clearly shown with either CT scanning or MRI, exact differentiation of the margins of the lymphomatous nodes from adjacent mediastinal structures can be difficult. Neither gallium imaging nor CT can reliably distinguish lymphoma from rebound thymic hyperplasia.[45] A rare form of leukemia occurring particularly in adolescent boys (T cell leukemia) primarily infiltrates the thymus. Other mediastinal tumors include teratoma (Fig. 45-6) and duplication cysts associated with the esophagus. Thyroid tumors are rare in childhood.

Comparison of imaging systems. CT scanning has shown superiority to plain film radiography in mediastinal lesions, adding additional information in 82% of cases, and in 65% it changed clinical management.[114] In

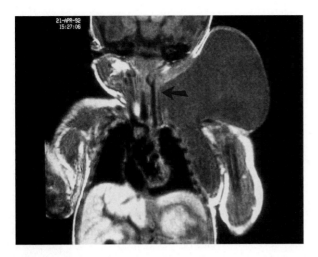

Fig. 45-4. Coronal MRI scan of the thorax and neck in a newborn. T1-weighted image shows a cystic hygroma (lymphangioma) on the left side of the neck extending into the left axilla and left lateral chest wall. There is no extension into the mediastinum. *Arrow* shows the left common carotid artery and bifurcation.

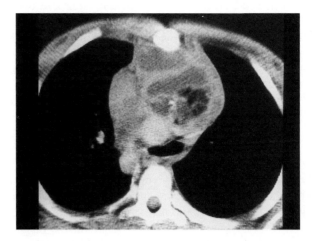

Fig. 45-6. Mediastinal teratoma. Anterior mediastinal mass is identified at the level of the carina and produces slight compression on the airway anteriorly. The variable densities (including fat and calcification) in the anterior mediastinal mass suggest teratoma.

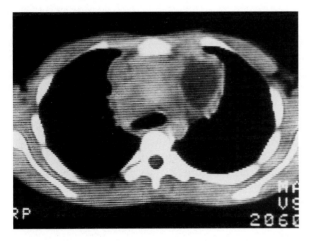

Fig. 45-5. Hodgkin's lymphadenopathy. Enlarged lymph node is identified in the mediastinum at the level of the carina. Low density of the enlarged node should not be mistaken for a cystic lesion. Contrast enhancement faintly shows the ascending and descending aorta adjacent to the lymphadenopathy.

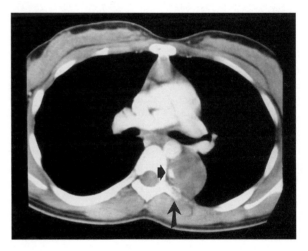

Fig. 45-7. Thoracic neuroblastoma. Axial CT of the thorax with bolus contrast enhancement shows a posterior mediastinal mass just posterior to the descending aorta and left main bronchus. *Arrow* shows bone destruction of the transverse process. *Arrowhead* shows calcification in the thoracic neuroblastoma.

this series, CT scanning was particularly helpful in assessing the full extent of malignant tumors and also in documenting that mediastinal masses were benign. In a comparison with MRI, the CT scan was better for identifying calcification (Fig. 45-7) and bronchial abnormalities.[119] Intraspinal extension of posterior mediastinal masses (such as neuroblastoma), however, and the distinction of masses and nodes from vascular structures were better seen on MRI. Therefore, CT scanning is thought to be the best choice for a mediastinal mass except for posterior mediastinal masses, in which the possibility of intraspinal spread (Fig. 45-8) is better documented with MRI.

MRI is now the imaging modality of choice for vascular anomalies in the mediastinum. Vascular rings[60] and other congenital anomalies[103] can be well seen without the need for contrast material or intervention with angiography. MRI can also assess the airway[54] and image adjacent mediastinal structures.

The mediastinum in children differs from the

adult in other ways than the relatively large size of the thymus. A normal finding is calcification in 13% of children in the ligamentum arteriosum.[13] In children, the azygoesophageal recess is not always concave as would be expected in normal adults. Almost all children under 2 years of age have a nonconcave azygoesophageal recess.[53] The incidence of a concave azygoesophageal recess increases with age throughout childhood.

LUNG

Congenital anomalies

Congenital anomalies of the lung are well seen on chest x-ray films; in the vast majority of cases, no other study is needed. Occasionally, when the diagnosis is in doubt, CT scanning has been described for the diagno-

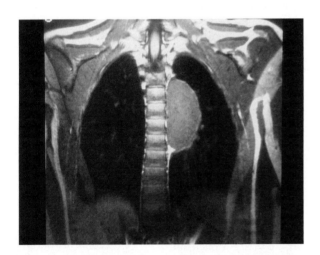

Fig. 45-8. Ganglioneuroma. Coronal T1-weighted image of the posterior mediastinum. Well-encapsulated posterior mediastinal mass was surgically removed and represents a ganglioneuroma. Coronal and axial MRI scans showed that the mass did not extend into the neural foramina or spinal canal.

sis of *congenital lobar emphysema,*[99] *tracheal bronchus,*[95] and *congenital cystic adenomatoid* malformation of the lung.[14] Congenital cystic adenomatoid malformation of the lung may appear in older children and even adults.[70] CT can best demonstrate the cystic and solid components and rule out other abnormalities, such as bronchiectasis. Diagnosis of a *pulmonary sequestration* can be specifically made after visualization of the feeding artery from the systemic circulation[49] by CT or MRI.

Infection

CT scans are helpful to define further anatomical information already demonstrated on the chest x-ray film (Fig. 45-9). Cavitation is better appreciated by CT scanning, and biopsy can be performed with CT guidance.[5]

Immunocompromised patients with pulmonary infiltrates constitute a diagnostic dilemma that occasionally can be helped by CT scanning. The demonstration of an air crescent or mural nodule by CT (Fig. 45-10) can suggest a diagnosis of invasive pulmonary aspergillosis in patients with leukemia who are granulocytopenic.[80] Unfortunately, this sign does not occur early in the course of the disease and usually is identified when the bone marrow is recovering. An earlier sign of a masslike infiltrate with a surrounding halo of low attenuation in the correct clinical setting suggests invasive pulmonary aspergillosis.

Bronchiectasis

Bronchiectasis can be diagnosed and separated into a cylindrical, cystic, or varicose type by CT scanning.[97] The lobes and segments involved can be identified, and this anatomical information has replaced the need for bronchography. Cystic fibrosis is the most common cause of bronchiectasis in children, and an objective scoring system using thin section CT[12] has been de-

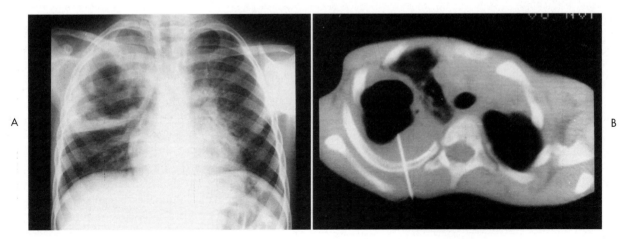

Fig. 45-9. A, Lung abscess. Cavitary infiltrate is identified in the right upper lobe of this infant. Sputum and blood cultures were negative. **B,** CT-guided biopsy of the abscess cavity; the culture grew anaerobic streptococci.

vised. This is particularly helpful for the preoperative evaluation of patients (Fig. 45-11) for lung transplant or lobectomy.

Tumors

Although thoracic masses are uncommon in children, their exact origin can be difficult to distinguish (Fig. 45-12). CT should be the next study after a chest x-ray film. It can help distinguish lung parenchymal masses from mediastinal masses[112] and thus avoid possible thoracotomy. CT scanning is the single best method for detection of metastatic disease. In children, hematogenous metastatic disease is most common from osteogenic sarcoma, Wilms' tumor, hepatoblastoma, hepatoma, germ cell tumors, and rhabdomyosarcoma.[28] A chest x-ray film, however, still is recommended as the initial study for metastatic disease. If multiple metastases are identified on the film, a CT scan is not necessary. If the plain film is negative, a CT scan should be performed. In fact, one problem with CT scanning is that it is too sensitive and not specific. In one study,[27] a third of all nodules identified on CT scanning of children with malignant tumors were shown not to be metastases. A nodule in a child with a known malignancy cannot therefore be assumed to represent a metastasis. Another problem is that malignant nodules that persist during chemotherapy do not necessarily indicate an inadequate response to the chemotherapy.[68] Surgical resection or percutaneous biopsy is the only way to confirm or exclude a diagnosis of metastasis.

Small cell tumor. A malignant small cell tumor of the thoracopulmonary region (Askin tumor) is a rare primary tumor that occurs typically in adolescents. The chest film shows a large mass, and it is often difficult to distinguish whether the involvement is primarily in the pleural space or lung parenchyma. CT scanning can define the anatomy of involvement of this tumor, which often infiltrates the chest wall, pleural space, and lung parenchyma.[96] The prognosis of patients with these tumors is grim because most tumors recur and the median survival after diagnosis is only 8 months.

LIVER

Common indications for imaging of the liver in children are the evaluation of primary liver tumors and metastic disease, abdominal trauma, infections, and abscess formation. Ultrasound examination is usually performed before the CT study, although no difference in sensitivity and specificity has been observed in a retrospective study of abdominal disease in children.[19] In comparison to MRI of the liver, CT scan is able to identify fatty infiltration and calcifications and to visualize the bile ducts, particularly when they are dilated.[132]

MRI demonstrates normal intrahepatic venous anatomy far better than CT scanning. This is true in normal and abnormal livers and can be helpful in assessment for transplantation to assess the size and patency of the portal vein.[39] Regardless of pathology on MRI, lesions are hypointense or isointense on T1-weighted images and hyperintense with T2-weighted images.

Diffuse disease and increased liver density

Low attenuation around the portal vein has a variety of causes in children.[113] These include tracking of blood from trauma, obstructive lymphedema following hepatic transplantation, and tumor infiltration. Other causes are perivascular inflammation from acute hepati-

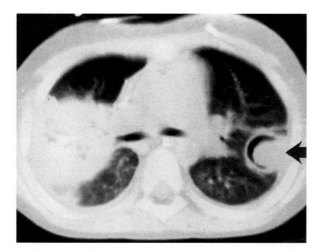

Fig. 45-10. Invasive aspergillosis. Axial CT scan at the level of the left and right main bronchi. Mural nodule or air crescent is well shown in the left lung peripherally *(arrow)*. Invasive aspergillosis in a child with acute lymphatic leukemia.

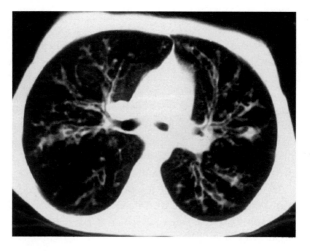

Fig. 45-11. Bronchiectasis. Axial 8 mm slice thickness scan of the chest in a patient with cystic fibrosis. Bronchiectasis is well shown bilaterally even with these thick slices.

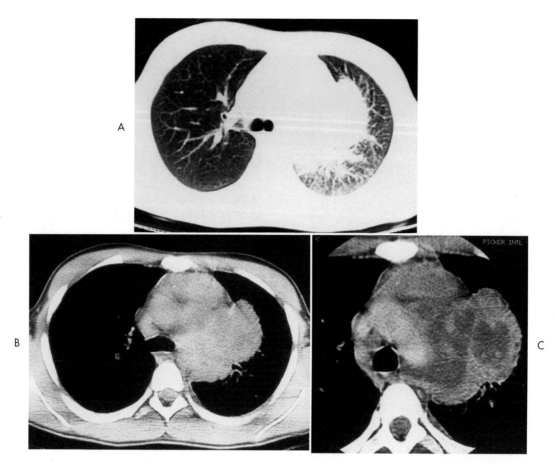

Fig. 45-12. Mediastinal lymphoma with interstitial lung pattern. **A,** CT scan taken just beneath the level of the carina with a wide window shows the interstitial lung disease on the left side together with a left-sided mass. **B,** With a narrower window, the mediastinal mass is clearly shown. Note that the interstitial lung pattern is not now appreciated. **C,** With contrast material injected, the aortic arch and superior vena cava are identified. The mediastinal mass shows mixed density and displaces the trachea slightly to the right but does not compress it. Biopsy showed this to represent a Hodgkin's lymphoma.

tis and bile duct proliferation with congenital hepatic fibrosis.

Increased density of the liver can be secondary to the deposition of iron or glycogen within the hepatic reticuloendothelial system or hepatic parenchyma. Transfusion hemosiderosis is the most common reason for this appearance in children (Fig. 45-13). In beta-thalassemia, iron is also deposited in the spleen, pancreas, bowel, and lymph nodes. The densely ferritinized lymph nodes may even be mistaken for calcifications.[93] In this group of patients, the density of the liver actually correlated with the degree of cirrhosis and hepatic fibrosis rather than with the amount of iron. On MRI scans, the paramagnetic effect of the ferric state of iron gives increased relaxation times resulting in low signal intensity of T1-weighted images and especially T2-weighted images.

Glycogen storage disease. In vitro experiments have shown that an increase of 1% in hepatic glycogen will produce a 2.8 HU increase in liver attenuation. Glycogen deposition in the liver in such glycogen storage diseases as von Gierke's disease (type I or glucose-6-phosphatase deficiency) may therefore show increased liver density ranging up to 20 HU greater than normal.[44] Glycogen is also deposited in the renal cortex; the CT scan can demonstrate this increase in cortical density secondary to glycogen deposition (Fig. 45-14).

Fatty infiltration of the liver may produce a 1.5 HU decrease in attenuation for every 1% increase in hepatic fat.[69] Fatty infiltration of the liver also occurs in glycogen storage disease. The resultant density of the liver depends on the balance of fatty infiltration and glycogen deposition. In glycogen storage disease, the liver may be of decreased, normal, or increased density, depending on the relative amounts of glycogen or fatty deposition. Older children with glycogen storage disease tend to have normal or reduced density livers. This is important

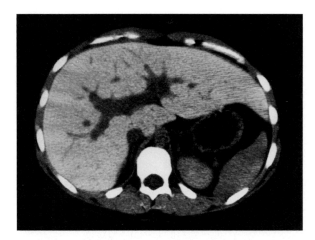

Fig. 45-13. Transfusion hemosiderosis. Unenhanced scan through the liver at the level of the portal vein shows increased density in the liver as well as enlargement of the liver. This child received multiple blood transfusions for aplastic anemia.

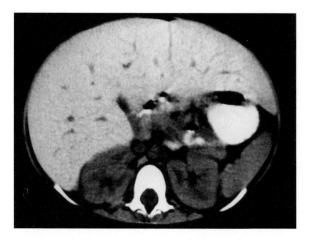

Fig. 45-14. Glycogen storage disease (Von Gierke's disease). Unenhanced study shows a large liver of increased density. The spleen is of normal size and density. Note the clear distinction between renal cortex and medulla secondary to glycogen being deposited in the renal cortex. (Courtesy Dr. N. Glazer, Akron Children's Hospital.)

because these children may develop adenomas and hepatomas, which appear as multiple or single well-defined round masses of slightly increased attenuation.

Other causes. Other causes of increased liver density include medications, such as amiodarone and cisplatinum,[2] which can both cause a diffuse increase in the density of the liver.

Fatty changes. Accumulation of fat in the liver produces decreased density. The CT density is directly related to the total content of fat, but CT is unreliable for accurate assessment of each major constituent (i.e., triglyceride and cholesterol).[69] The accumulation of fat in children, as in adults, can result from a number of causes:

1. Metabolic disorders, such as diabetes, malnutrition and cystic fibrosis.
2. Chemical exposures, such as toxins or chemotherapeutic agents.
3. Trauma.
4. Vascular injury.

As in adults, fatty metamorphosis in children can be focal in nature and simulate a mass lesion. The visualization of normal hepatic vessels crossing the lesion is helpful in differentiating focal fatty proliferation from other lesions.

Congenital anomalies

Choledochal cyst is best imaged with a combination of ultrasound and technetium-99m IDA scans.[64] Caroli's disease (a nonobstructive dilatation of intrahepatic bile ducts) can be specifically identified on CT when the "central dot" sign is demonstrated.[24] The "central dot" corresponds to intraluminal portal veins within the dilated bile ducts and was initially described with high-frequency ultrasound.[86] Caroli's disease may be associated with hepatic fibrosis and portal hypertension. Congenital hepatic fibrosis is associated with the infantile and juvenile forms of polycystic kidney disease and may be identified on the CT scan.

Infection

Abscesses in the liver are rare in children and may be pyogenic, fungal, or amebic. Whatever their cause, these abscesses are seen as areas of decreased attenuation, usually with an inhomogeneous pattern. Occasional nonuniform rim enhancement occurs after injection of contrast material. The presence of gas, although rare, usually means that pyogenic bacterial infection is the primary cause (Fig. 45-15). Such gas can also be caused by a fistula or rarely after trauma.[1] Fungal infections caused by *Candida* are usually seen in immunocompromised patients secondary to leukemia, aplastic anemia, or chronic granulomatous disease of children.[88] An amebic abscess cannot be distinguished by CT from other liver abscesses.[87] This serious, possibly life-threatening complication of amebic infection is rarely considered in young children. This may lead to an increased morbidity and mortality from this potentially curable infection.

Abscesses in the liver, kidney, or retroperitoneal spaces (Fig. 45-16) can be ideally visualized on CT examination. Aspiration for diagnosis and treatment can also be performed.

Reye's syndrome and other viral illness. Reye's syndrome is a fatty infiltration of the liver that occurs after a prodromal influenza illness or after varicella. Although this fatty infiltration is not specific in the correct clinical setting, it may be a helpful confirmatory finding.

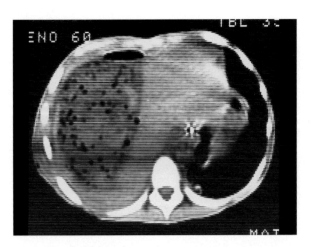

Fig. 45-15. Liver abscess with multiple gas collections. This liver abscess was secondary to portal pyemia and appendicitis.

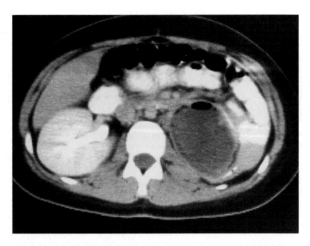

Fig. 45-16. Abscess in left nephrectomy space. Surgery for removal of a left multicystic dysplastic kidney. An abscess that developed in the left nephrectomy space was drained under CT guidance.

Liver tumors (benign)

Ultrasound examination is recommended for the initial evaluation of a child thought to have a hepatic tumor. Depending on the clinical suspicion, a CT scan or a radionuclide study is the second study of choice.[91] This integrated approach offers the greatest likelihood of a correct diagnosis in separating those lesions that need surgical exploration or biopsy from those for which this is unnecessary.

Infantile hemangioendothelioma. Infantile hemangioendothelioma is the most common vascular liver tumor of infancy and appears in the first 6 months of life as a rapidly enlarging upper abdominal mass. This mass gradually decreases in size over the next several months if the child can be supported without surgical intervention.[33] Heart failure is a less common complication than previously thought. Both CT and MRI scanning may offer a specific diagnosis of this liver tumor (Fig. 45-17). CT shows well-defined masses of slightly low density identified in the liver before contrast injection. With bolus injection of contrast material in dynamic scanning, a peripheral enhancement is identified that is extremely specific.[84] Enhancement continues centripetally, and on delayed scans the lesions can become isodense. A similar pattern of enhancement is seen in adults with cavernous hemangiomas, although these are rare in infants. This specific CT appearance may obviate the need for arteriography, unless embolization is being performed (Fig. 45-18). Approximately 40% of these lesions show calcification. A decreased caliber of the aorta distal to the origin of the hepatic artery is also occasionally seen.

MRI shows a low signal intensity on T1-weighted images and progressively higher signal intensity on T2-weighted images. This is a specific MRI appearance of these vascular hamartomas (see Fig. 45-17).

Focal nodular hyperplasia. Focal nodular hyperplasia, a rare benign "tumor," occurs occasionally in children. Often asymptomatic, this lesion is composed histologically of hepatocytes, Kupffer's cells, bile duct elements, and fibrous connective tissue.[4] The gross pathological appearance may be characteristic, with a central stellate scan and radiating septae of collagen. This appearance is occasionally identified on CT scans. More commonly, it is seen as a mass of decreased attenuation with well-defined margins that do not enhance. Uptake by technetium-sulphur colloid radionuclide scan occurs in approximately 55% of cases and is virtually diagnostic.

Mesenchymal hamartoma. Mesenchymal hamartoma is a rare liver tumor and is a developmental anomaly rather than a true neoplasm.[106] It consists of an admixture of bile ducts and mesenchymal tissue. Usually this tumor occurs within the first 2 years of life. A characteristic CT and ultrasound appearance has been described and consists of a predominantly cystic mass with internal septae.[126] There are variations in the size of the cysts and septae, but apart from the rare cystic hepatoblastoma, this appearance in a young child is almost diagnostic. The cystic component does not enhance with contrast material. The solid components may enhance. Following surgical removal of this hamartoma, the prognosis is excellent.

Malignant liver tumors

Primary liver cancer is the third most common form of abdominal malignancy in childhood, accounting for approximately 5% of all pediatric abdominal neoplasms. An integrated approach—starting with ultra-

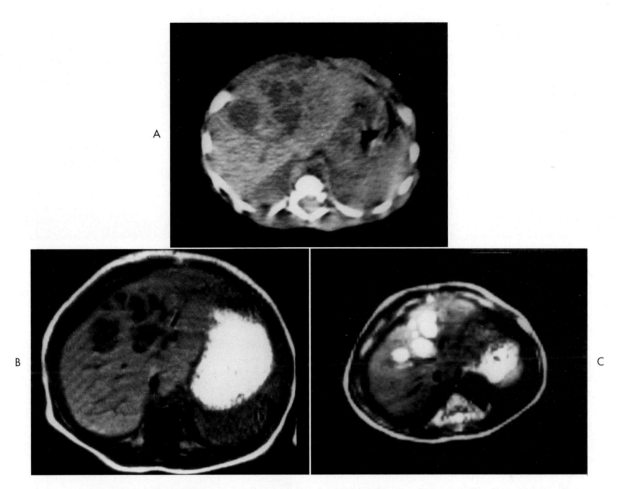

Fig. 45-17. Infantile hepatic hemangioendothelioma. **A,** Unenhanced axial CT scan of the liver demonstrates several low attenuation areas in the liver in this neonate with an upper abdominal mass. **B,** Axial T1-weighted MRI scan through the liver demonstrates low signal intensity in the areas in the liver. **C,** Axial T2-weighted MRI scan through the liver shows increased signal intensity in the hemangioendothelioma that increased even more with increased T2-weighted images.

sound examination of hepatomegaly—is recommended,[90] but once malignancy is suspected, CT scanning before and after contrast enhancement is advised. A similar pathway is recommended also for suspected metastatic disease to the liver. Metastases may occur to the liver from direct extension or hematogenous origin and is secondary to the common childhood tumors—neuroblastoma, Wilms' tumor (Fig. 45-19), and rhabdomyosarcoma. Lymphoma and leukemia also may produce focal or diffuse infiltration of the liver.

MRI has been shown to be accurate for the diagnosis of primary liver tumors.[16] Tumor resectability depends on accurate anatomical information of the liver and in particular the hepatic blood vessels. This can be better demonstrated by the multiple planes of imaging possible with MRI, whereas CT is limited to an axial plane. MRI is as good as CT in distinguishing benign from malignant liver tumors. Neither imaging modality can distinguish hepatoblastomas from hepatomas or even lymphoma of the liver.[16] MRI is more sensitive in the postoperative patient but cannot distinguish tumor recurrence from fibrosis and inflammation.

Hepatoblastoma. Hepatoblastoma is the most common primary malignancy of the liver in childhood. It is usually found in the first 3 years of life and is almost always associated with a raised serum alpha-fetoprotein level. Metastases occur to the lung and lymph nodes, and surgical resection together with chemotherapy is the only chance of a cure. This tumor presents on CT as a hypodense mass that is often inhomogeneous owing to hemorrhage or necrosis.[34] Hepatoblastoma shows enhancement with contrast material, which may accentuate the internal lobulation and nodularity (Fig. 45-20). Calcifications are identified on CT in approximately 50% of cases. Rarely, this tumor may appear completely cystic.[89] Because surgery offers the only hope of long-term cure

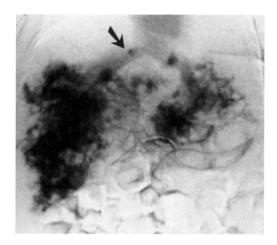

Fig. 45-18. Intra-arterial digital subtraction angiogram of infantile hemangioendothelioma. Note the multiple sites of hemangioendothelioma in both lobes of the liver and the rapid flow of contrast material into the enlarged hepatic veins *(arrow)* and right atrium.

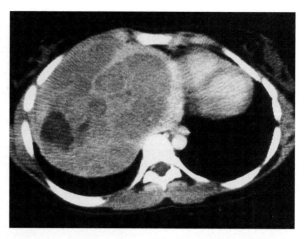

Fig. 45-19. Metastatic Wilms' tumor. The right lobe of the liver is almost totally replaced by a metastatic Wilms' tumor that recurred 7 years after initial treatment. The area of low density is thought to represent an area of necrosis or hemorrhage.

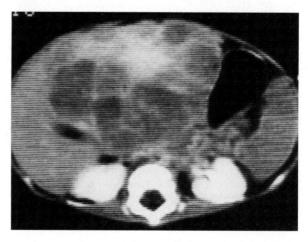

Fig. 45-20. Hepatoblastoma. Large mass identified throughout the entire left lobe of the liver shows contrast enhancement on this axial CT scan.

in patients with hepatoblastoma, accurate preoperative anatomical information of exactly which lobes are involved is essential for surgical resection. MRI shows the anatomical relationships (Fig. 45-21, *A*), and enhancement with gadolinium (Fig. 45-21, *B*) demonstrates the nodularity.

Hepatoma (hepatocellular carcinoma). The CT and MRI appearance of a hepatoma is identical to that of a hepatoblastoma. The peak incidence of this tumor is at 4 years, with a second peak in adolescence, and it is rare to find this tumor under the age of 2 years. Hepatoma is associated with hepatitis B infection (Fig. 45-22), biliary atresia and several metabolic diseases, such as cystinosis, type I glycogen storage disease and tyrosinemia. Children with tyrosinemia may develop regenerating nodules from cirrhosis. These are of high attenuation and may be difficult to distinguish by CT from multifocal hepatoma.[38]

Undifferentiated sarcoma of the liver. Undifferentiated sarcoma of the liver is an uncommon malignant tumor of mesenchymal origin.[107] It is composed of primitive mesenchymal cells without differential features. This tumor has several synonyms, which include mesenchymal sarcoma, embryonal sarcoma, and malignant mesenchymoma. The gross appearance, and therefore CT and ultrasound appearance, may be misleading because it can contain large cystic areas of degeneration that may be mistaken for a cystic benign tumor. Solid tumors also occur (Fig. 45-23). This lesion is seen in older children, adolescents, and young adults. Prognosis is poor, with a median survival of less than 1 year. The CT appearance shows a lesion with well-defined margins and internal septations. A pseudocapsule that enhances is of-

ten identified. The cystic areas correspond to cystic and myxoid degeneration of this tumor.

PANCREAS

Cystic fibrosis

In children with cystic fibrosis,[36] the pancreas is commonly replaced with fat and often maintains its shape in this manner. Other changes in the pancreas include calcification, small cysts, and occasionally extremely large cysts (see Fig. 32-87).[67] Children with cystic fibrosis are also at an increased risk of developing pancreatitis. Adjacent organs are commonly involved. Changes in the liver, ranging from fatty infiltration to cirrhosis; evidence of portal hypertension with splenomegaly; and gallstones can all be seen on CT scans.[32]

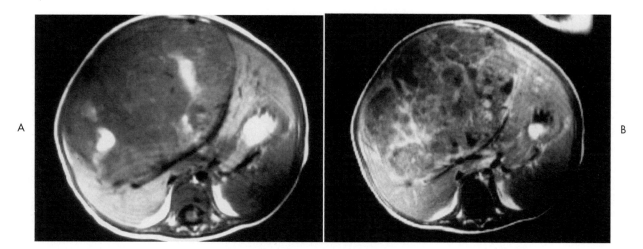

Fig. 45-21. Hepatoblastoma. **A,** MRI axial T1-weighted image of the upper abdomen shows a large liver tumor involving left and right lobes displacing the portal vein posteriorly. **B,** After gadolinium enhancement, the nodularity of this hepatoblastoma is better appreciated.

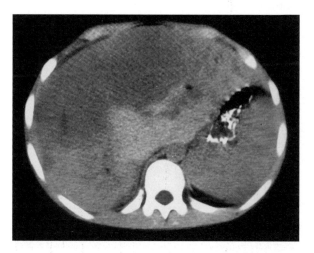

Fig. 45-22. Hepatoma. Axial CT scan of the liver without contrast material demonstrates multiple low-density areas in the left and right lobes of the liver. Multifocal hepatoma associated with hepatitis B infection.

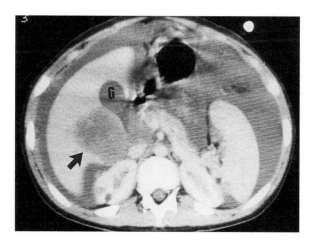

Fig. 45-23. Undifferentiated sarcoma of the liver. Low-density mass is identified in the right lobe of the liver *(arrow)* posterior to gallbladder *(G)*. Ascites is present with two low-density areas in the right kidney posteriorly. These represent simple cysts, which are unusual in children.

Pancreatitis

Acute pancreatitis in children is not as rare as was once thought. The CT pattern is similar to adults, with diffuse swelling and thickening of the renal fascia. Hereditary pancreatitis is the most common cause of recurrent pancreatitis in children. Extensive calcification and stone formation in the dilated main pancreatic duct as well as complications such as pseudocyst formation[56] are particularly well seen by CT scanning. Pseudocysts can be drained percutaneously under CT guidance.[72]

KIDNEY AND RETROPERITONEUM

In the neonate, the most common cause of an abdominal mass is hydronephrosis or a multicystic dysplas-

tic kidney, and ultrasound is the preferred initial imaging choice. After this period, CT scanning is the initial and best imaging modality for trauma and tumors of the kidney and retroperitoneum.[11] Children with urinary tract infections are best imaged with a combination of ultrasound and radionuclide scans. CT is helpful when a localized abscess or nephronia is suspected.

Neither the excretory urogram nor ultrasound is considered the optimal study for imaging the retroperitoneum.[117] Both CT and MRI scanning provide excellent visualization of the retroperitoneum, including the major vessels. Large masses in the retroperitoneum, especially on the right side (Fig. 45-24, *A*), can be embarrassingly difficult to localize with the axial images from

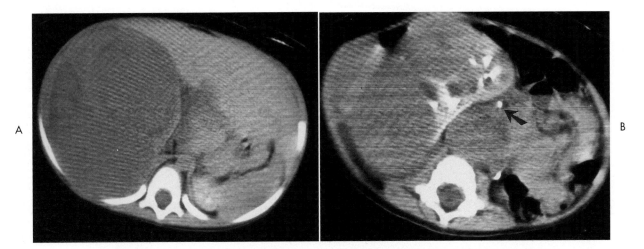

Fig. 45-24. A, Axial CT scan of the right upper quadrant demonstrates a large mass. It is difficult to tell if this mass originates from the adrenal, right kidney, or liver. **B,** Axial CT scan at a lower level of the abdomen demonstrates the Wilms' tumor that has displaced the right kidney inferiorly. Lymphadenopathy has displaced the right ureter *(arrow)* anteriorly.

a CT scan.[58] This is often even harder in children because of the relative lack of retroperitoneal fat planes. Lesions that appear to be intrahepatic on axial scans may in fact be extrahepatic (Fig. 45-24, *B*). MRI with its multiplanar capabilities is especially helpful in these cases.

The role of MRI in imaging the retroperitoneum and kidneys is not yet defined. Coronal T1-weighted images are best for anatomical information, including renal size and location.[41] The lower signal intensity of the renal pyramids can be clearly distinguished from the renal cortex on T1-weighted images (see Fig. 45-33).

Infection

In complicated cases of upper urinary tract infection, CT scanning can provide important information for diagnosis and therapy. Acute pyelonephritis demonstrates multiple low density, radially oriented areas extending from the central collecting system to the renal capsule (Fig. 45-25). Lobar nephronia is an acute nonsuppurative infection that appears on a CT scan as a low-density mass with a poorly marginated border (Fig. 45-26). Following contrast administration, the nephronia shows patchy enhancement that is still at a lower density than the surrounding normal renal parenchyma.[82] Renal abscesses are far better delineated, with a wall and a central low-density area that does not usually enhance. This distinction between a nephronia and abscess is important because the nephronia is treated with antibiotics,[104] and the abscess usually requires drainage (see Fig. 45-16).

Renal tumors

Mesoblastic nephroma (fetal renal hamartoma). Presentation is with a large abdominal mass in

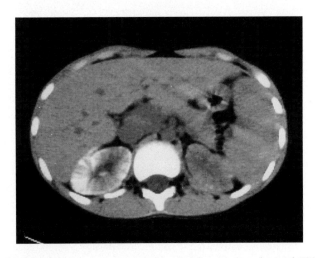

Fig. 45-25. Acute pyelonephritis. Axial contrast-enhanced CT of the kidneys shows radial low-density areas in the right kidney secondary to acute pyelonephritis.

the first year of life. CT scan shows a solid unencapsulated mass that may rarely demonstrate function.[65] Nephrectomy is curative.

Multilocular renal cysts. Whether multiocular renal cysts represent a renal cyst or a neoplasm is not completely certain, but the neoplastic theory is now more favored.[85] There are two age peaks of this renal mass, and one occurs during childhood. In childhood, it is more common in boys. This mass consists of multiple separate cysts that do not communicate.[6] Curvilinear calcification is sometimes identified. The septae between these cysts are of variable thickness and may enhance after contrast injection.

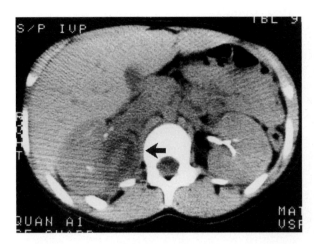

Fig. 45-26. Lobar nephronia (acute focal bacterial nephritis). CT scan performed on an infant with fever and an upper urinary tract infection shows a low-density area in the right kidney medially *(arrow)*. Aspiration under CT guidance grew *Escherichia coli*. Nephronia resolved with antibiotic therapy.

Lipoblastomatosis. Lipoblastomatosis is a benign tumor of fetal adipose tissue that occurs mainly before the age of 3 years. It is not a malignancy. Lobules of immature fat are present together with a myxoid stroma separated by vascular connective tissue septae. The fat density is easily appreciated by CT, with denser areas that represent the myxoid tissue.[51]

Although rare, other soft tissue tumors may occur in the kidney and retroperitoneum. These include cystic retroperitoneal lymphangioma[37] and renal lymphangioma,[102] which produces a diffuse renal enlargement with poor opacification of the renal medulla following contrast administration. Angiomyolipomas are rarely identified in children. Their association with tuberous sclerosis is important to recognize. Children with tuberous sclerosis may also show a cystic disease of the kidney suggestive of adult polycystic disease.[94] Renal cell carcinoma rarely occurs in children and young adults and is indistinguishable by imaging from a Wilms' tumor.

Leukemia and lymphoma. Acute lymphatic leukemia rarely involves the kidneys, but when it does, it usually produces a bilateral diffuse enlargement.[3] Less commonly, this diffuse enlargement may be unilateral. More rarely, it may produce a discrete intrarenal mass or hila mass.

Lymphoma has a similar spectrum of renal involvement, most commonly demonstrating bilateral focal low-density nodules with contrast-enhanced CT (Fig. 45-27). CT scanning has been shown to be superior to ultrasound in detecting renal involvement with lymphoma in children.[131]

Nephroblastomatosis. Nephroblastomatosis is the persistence of the metanephric blastema in full-term infants. Usually the metanephric blastema is not present

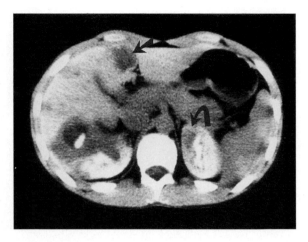

Fig. 45-27. Burkitt's lymphoma. Adolescent presenting with hematuria after mild trauma was thought to represent Wilms' tumor on a urogram that showed a right renal mass. CT scan confirms the presence of a right renal mass but also shows a second lesion in the left kidney anteriorly and medially *(curved arrow)* and a third lesion in the medial segment of the left lobe of the liver *(straight arrow)*. Biopsy of this lesion showed a Burkitt's lymphoma.

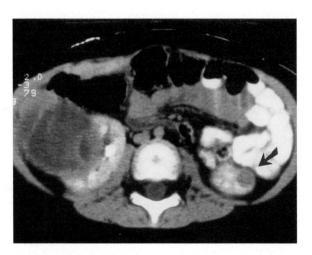

Fig. 45-28.. Wilms' tumor of the right kidney in a child with Beckwith-Weidemann syndrome. Nephroblastomatosis *(arrow)* in the lower pole of the left kidney identified as an area of nonenhancement.

beyond 34 to 36 gestational weeks. This embryonic tissue is found in 12% to 33% of kidneys with Wilms' tumor and is believed to be a precursor of Wilms' tumor (Fig. 45-28). The anatomical location of the nephroblastomatosis is defined by its position within the renal lobe (Fig. 45-29). Pathologically, nephroblastomatosis is classified as perilobar, intralobar, panlobar, and mixed.[133] Contrast-enhanced CT scans show areas of nephroblastomatosis as multiple nonenhancing regions within the renal parenchyma (see Fig. 45-28). CT has been shown to be superior to ultrasound and urography[50] for dem-

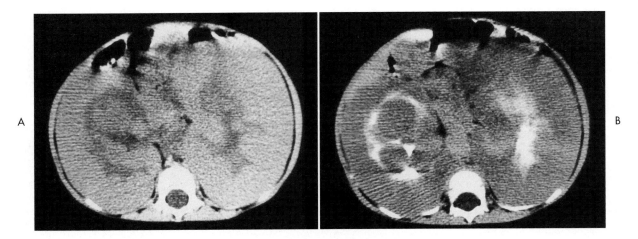

Fig. 45-29. Nephroblastomatosis. **A,** Massive bilateral renal enlargement is present in this 14-month-old-child. Without contrast, areas of low density are identified within the center of these enlarged kidneys. **B,** After intravenous injection of contrast material, the calyces and remaining normal renal parenchyma are identified centrally with areas of low density representing the nephroblastomatosis.

onstration of nephroblastomatosis. Occasionally, macroscopic nephroblastomatosis still cannot be recognized with CT,[30] and surgical inspection of the kidney at laparotomy is still recommended.

Wilms' tumor

This common pediatric tumor presents as an asymptomatic abdominal mass; the mass is usually large, but the child appears well. Eighty percent of Wilms' tumors present between the first and third year of life; 5% to 10% are bilateral. Although ultrasound is commonly performed as the initial imaging study and is particularly helpful to recognize invasion into the renal vein and inferior vena cava, CT is essential for complete evaluation. CT scanning shows more accurate information than ultrasound about the nature of the tumor and its spread.[105] It can delineate the perinephric extension of the tumor and hepatic and lymph node involvement, and it can also assess the opposite kidney for bilateral tumors and evidence of nephroblastomatosis. A CT scan of the lung is performed at the same time to look for lung metastases. A more complete staging study is thus possible with CT scanning.

On CT scanning, a Wilms' tumor is a large, low-density mass arising from the kidney. It is inhomogeneous, with areas of lower density representing tumor necrosis (Fig. 45-30). The mass displaces the collecting system. After contrast enhancement, there is slight enhancement of the tumor with the areas of necrosis more prominent. In one large series,[52] a 13% incidence of calcification and a 7% incidence of fat were seen. Rarely a Wilms' tumor may contain large amounts of fat.[100] Angiomolipomas are thus not the only intrarenal tumor that

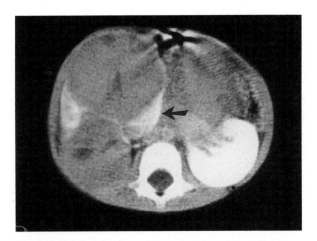

Fig. 45-30. Wilms' tumor of right kidney. Two separate masses are identified in the right kidney with a central area of remaining functioning renal parenchyma compressed by these masses *(arrow)*. Note the areas of low density within the Wilms' tumors, which represent areas of either hemorrhage or necrosis.

has a fat density. A sharp margin between the Wilms' tumor and the normal kidney represents the pseudocapsule identified on gross pathological study. The compressed uninvolved part of the kidney may give a persistent area of increased attenuation after intravenous contrast injection. The tumor spreads by direct expansion through the capsule of the kidney and metastasizes to adjacent lymph nodes, liver, and lung. The tumor can also spread directly into the renal vein and inferior vena cava. For follow-up studies after nephrectomy, CT offers the best available information.[18] CT scanning can also identify a second tumor in the remaining kidney and image the postnephrec-

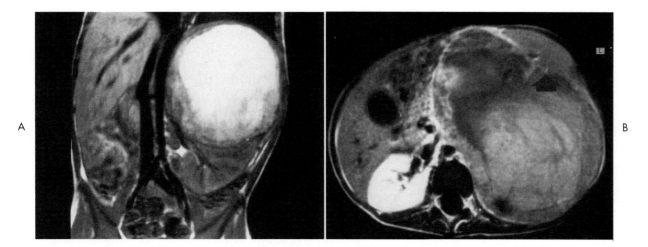

Fig. 45-31. Wilms' tumor. **A,** Coronal T1-weighted image of the abdomen. Hugh left Wilms' tumor is arising from the upper pole of the left kidney. Wilms' tumor is displacing remaining kidney into the lower abdomen, and the aorta is displaced toward the right. **B,** Axial T1-weighted image after gadolinium enhancement demonstrates displacement of adjacent vessels and spleen *(arrowhead).*

tomy renal fossa. It is superior to urography, which is now rarely performed for either the initial demonstration of a Wilms' tumor or for follow-up studies.

Two rare renal childhood tumors can be separated by histology from a Wilms' tumor. The clear cell sarcoma of the kidney[59] can metastasize to bone. Malignant rhabdoid tumor is occasionally associated with other primary tumors of the posterior cranial fossa, soft tissue, and thymus.[120] Neither of these rare tumors can be distinguished by imaging from the more common Wilms' tumor.

MRI of Wilms' tumor shows prolonged T1 and T2 relaxation times.[9] The signal intensity of the tumor is variable because of necrosis and hemorrhage within the tumor (Fig. 45-31, *A* and *B*).

Adrenal gland

In the newborn, the adrenal gland is best imaged by ultrasound. For older children, however, CT or MRI more accurately identifies the adrenals. Adrenal tumors are rare in childhood, but functioning adrenal carcinomas and adenomas do occur. Most adrenal tumors in childhood are hormonally active. Excess androgens produce virilization in girls and pseudoprecocious puberty in boys. Excess cortisol gives the clinical syndrome of Cushing's disease. The distinction between an adenoma and carcinoma cannot be made by either CT or MRI scanning except when local invasion by the carcinoma can be identified. On CT, these adrenal masses appear as an inhomogeneous tumor secondary to necrosis and hemorrhage.[35] Occasionally, there is calcification. Also, CT scans of the lungs should be performed to exclude metastases.

Neuroblastoma

Neuroblastoma is the most common solid childhood tumor. It arises anywhere along the sympathetic chain from the neck to the pelvis. Seventy-five percent are in the abdomen, with two thirds of these having an origin in the adrenal. Children with neuroblastoma appear ill and irritable, and they often are in pain. Approximately 45% of these children have bone metastases, which are best identified with an isotope bone scan or monoclonal imaging.[92] Bone marrow aspiration and biopsy are essential for complete staging.

Abdominal neuroblastoma usually occurs as an irregular, lobulated, calcified suprarenal mass without a definable capsule (Fig. 45-32). Calcification identified on CT scan was seen in 80% of one large series.[127] On T1-weighted images, neuroblastoma has a signal intensity slightly lower than liver and renal cortex and similar to the renal medulla. On T2-weighted images, the signal intensity is increased and appears similar to kidney.[42] Calcifications cannot be demonstrated on MRI. Marrow involvement may be identified with MRI. Neuroblastoma has a propensity to invade through the neural foramina directly and to involve the spinal cord and roots (Fig. 45-33). If this is clinically suspected, MRI scanning is essential[118] and is also an excellent way to identify the encasement of the aorta and upper abdominal vessels. Encasement of the aorta and its main branches makes this tumor inoperable. This finding on CT or MRI is a more important prognostic sign than the conventional staging, which uses the midline as a landmark between stage II and stage III disease.[15] Neuroblastomas that cross the midline and are therefore technically stage III but do not encase the aorta are surgically resectable and have a much

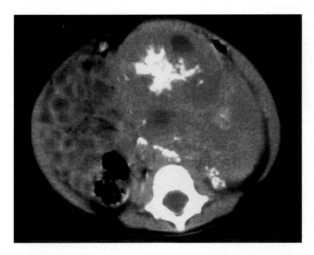

Fig. 45-32. Neuroblastoma. Axial nonenhanced CT scan of lower abdomen demonstrates a huge calcified mass that is encasing vessels.

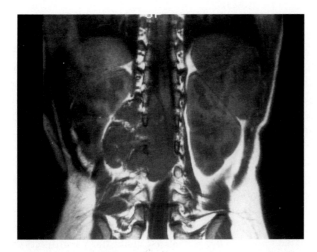

Fig. 45-33. Neuroblastoma. Coronal T1-weighted MRI scan of right neuroblastoma with invasion through intervertebral foramina into the spinal canal.

better prognosis. After treatment, CT scanning offers the most sensitive method for detecting tumor recurrence.[128] Both CT and MRI scanning can identify tumor recurrence in the retroperitoneum, liver, cranium, mediastinum, lymph nodes, and skeleton.

A rare clinical presentation of neuroblastoma is opsoclonus. This is a jerky eye movement that occurs in all directions and is often associated with myoclonic jerks and cerebellar ataxia. The importance of this physical finding is that a large percentage of children have an occult neuroblastoma that may not be palpable and may not produce increased catecholamines. CT scanning is efficacious in identifying neuroblastoma in this group of patients.[47] Because these tumors are often small and cal-

cification is an important finding, scans should be performed initially without contrast enhancement.[43]

Usually neuroblastoma can be easily distinguished from a Wilms' tumor, which is the other common abdominal childhood tumor. Occasionally, there can be confusion because a Wilms' tumor may grow exophytically from the surface of the kidney, and a neuroblastoma may even infiltrate the kidney. MRI scanning, especially in the coronal plane, can be helpful in this situation. Rarely a neuroblastoma appears to be intrarenal,[108] and these tumors have a poor prognosis. Tumor calcification, retroperitoneal lymphadenopathy, and encasement of the aorta and inferior vena cava are far more likely to occur in neuroblastoma than in Wilms' tumor.[83] Retrocrural lymphadenopathy is specific for neuroblastoma. Distortion of the renal calyces is specific for a Wilms' tumor.

PELVIS

Ultrasound remains the initial and usually only imaging test necessary for visualizing the pelvis, including the male and female genitalia. If further definition of anatomical structures is needed, MRI[110] and occasionally CT scans are performed. The only reason, apart from trauma, to perform CT is to demonstrate cortical bone (Fig. 45-34, *A* and *B*). The lack of ionizing radiation with MRI is an especially important advantage in this anatomical area.

Undescended testes that are in the inguinal canal are best imaged by ultrasound. Intra-abdominal undescended testes can be identified by MRI[77] and have a signal similar to scrotal testes. T2-weighted images of the testis are hyperintense or similar to fat. Tumors of the pelvis are most commonly rhabdomyosarcomas of the bladder or vagina in girls and prostate in boys.[8] Extension into the adjacent pelvic fat, seminal vesicles, or uterus is best shown with MRI. MRI can also identify associated spinal pathology—for example, an anterior sacral meningocele or invasion of the spinal canal with a neuroblastoma (see Fig. 45-33). Congenital anorectal anomalies can be imaged with both CT[79] and MRI.[109] Demonstration of the levator ani muscle and especially the puborectalis portion is essential for staging these lesions and alters the surgical management with a colostomy for lesions above the levator ani. Postoperative position of the rectum with respect to the levator ani can also be assessed. MRI has the unique ability to identify a septate uterus. A low signal intensity of the septum can be seen between the signal of the endometrial cavities with absent intervening myometrium.

ABDOMINAL TRAUMA

Several large series confirm the usefulness of CT scanning for abdominal trauma in children. The patient must be hemodynamically stable, and meticulous atten-

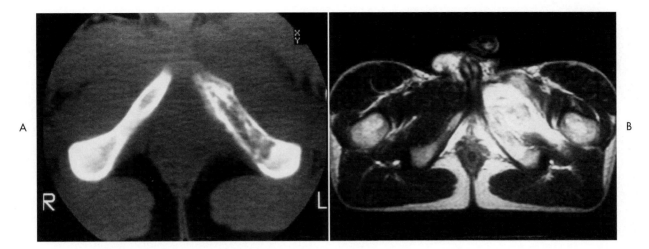

Fig. 45-34. Ewing's tumor of left ischium. **A,** CT scan showing permeative destructive pattern with disruption of the bony cortex. **B,** T2-weighted MRI scan shows the soft tissue component of the Ewing's tumor.

tion to scanning technique is necessary for optimal results. CT scanning has become the examination of choice for imaging blunt abdominal trauma in children.[73] The vast majority of children are managed conservatively without the need for surgery. The indication for surgery is based on the physiological condition of the child and not on the extent of the solid organ injury.[20]

CT scanning has several advantages over other imaging modalities:[81]

1. It is not organ specific: All of the abdomen, peritoneum, and retroperitoneum can be identified.
2. The bony skeleton can be assessed.
3. Assessment of function and vascular integrity of organs can be made with the bolus injection and small amounts of free fluid and free air identified.

Children who have been resuscitated from profound shock but are stable at the time of CT examination show a characteristic CT appearance.[130] Diffuse dilation of bowel with fluid is present together with moderate-to-large amounts of peritoneal fluid, including within the lesser sac. There is intense contrast enhancement of the bowel wall, mesentery, kidneys, and pancreas. Decrease in caliber of the aorta and inferior vena cava is also present. The prognosis for children with this hypoperfusion complex is appalling, with death within 36 hours the usual outcome.

Children are far more likely than adults to wear a lap belt in a car and be subject to specific injuries that are not always easily appreciated with routine CT scanning.[123] If linear abdominal or flank ecchymosis caused by a lap safety belt are present, a specific search for bowel and bladder injuries is essential. A lateral lumbar spine x-ray film is mandatory in these patients for detection of lumbar spine facet distractions, and horizontal fractures are poorly identified on axial abdominal CT scans.

Bowel perforation in children following blunt trauma was diagnosed by finding free intraperitoneal air in 67% of cases.[22] The remaining 33% were suggested only by the secondary signs of bowel wall thickening and unexplained peritoneal fluid. The finding of pneumoperitoneum is not specific for bowel perforation. It can also be seen following peritoneal lavage, bladder perforation, and pneumomediastinum.

SPLEEN

Respiration, beam hardening from adjacent ribs, and inhomogeneous enhancement with intravenous contrast make this organ the hardest to identify on CT scanning. Although nuclear medicine and CT scanning are approximately equal in accuracy of diagnosing splenic trauma (Fig. 45-35), CT has the further advantage of identifying the remainder of the abdomen, including the identification of free fluid. Sonography is far less accurate for abdominal trauma in general and for splenic injury in particular.[76] In a series of 100 children involved in blunt abdominal trauma, CT scanning had fewer false-negative and false-positive results than either scintigraphy or sonography.[76] The accuracy of CT scanning for abdominal trauma means that peritoneal lavage is no longer required and a more conservative surgical approach with preservation of the spleen performed.

LIVER

In a series of 48 consecutive cases of liver injury in children,[125] the right lobe was involved in 83%. The posterior segment of the right lobe was the most com-

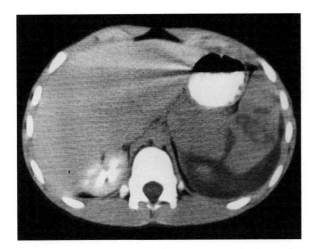

Fig. 45-35. Trauma to spleen. CT scan of the upper abdomen with subcapsular hematoma of the spleen and lacerations of the spleen.

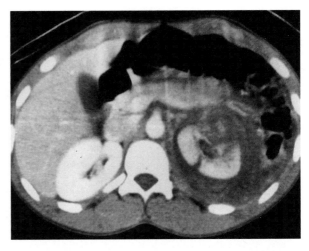

Fig. 45-36. Trauma to left kidney. Fracture of left kidney with blood and urine in the perirenal space.

monly injured segment. Injuries to the right lobe tended to be superficial and simple. Injuries to the left lobe were deep and complex. Rarely, hepatic parenchymal and subcapsular gas can be caused following blunt abdominal trauma and does not represent infection.[1]

Periportal zones of decreased attenuation were seen in 22% of children imaged for blunt abdominal trauma.[101] In this series, pathological correlation was obtained in two patients, and in one periportal lymphedema and in the other blood was the cause of the decreased attenuation.

KIDNEY AND ADRENALS

Kidney injuries can be classified as contusion, laceration, fracture, and vascular. Contusions show as zones of poorly functioning renal parenchyma. A renal laceration is a parenchymal tear limited to the cortex; when this extends into the collecting system, it is called a fracture (Fig. 45-36). Renal vascular pedicle injuries are the most severe, and absent perfusion is demonstrated on CT scan by a lack of enhancement from intravenous contrast material. In a series of 256 children with blunt abdominal trauma, hematuria was present in 41%.[124] Only 14%, however, had a renal injury that could be diagnosed by CT. Hypotension was shown to be an insensitive predictor of renal injury. All children with significant renal injury had either large amounts of hematuria or shock. Conversely, no normotensive child with less than 50 red blood cells per high power field had significant renal injury.

The adrenal gland was injured in 3% of 1155 consecutive children with blunt abdominal trauma.[122] The right adrenal was far more commonly injured. No cases of adrenocortical insufficiency were observed. Ipsilateral

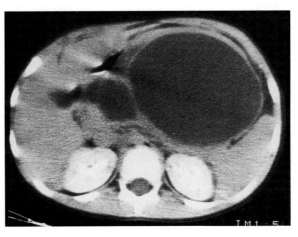

Fig. 45-37. Pseudocysts of the pancreas. Several large pseudocysts of the pancreas are identified in this child, who 10 days earlier had fallen off his bike and sustained a traumatic pancreatitis.

crural thickening of the diaphragm was a frequent associated finding.

PANCREAS

Blunt abdominal trauma is the main cause of pancreatic injury in childhood,[71] including nonaccidental child abuse. Diagnosis, follow-up, and management of the complications of pancreatitis are well identified by CT scanning (Fig. 45-37).[72]

The initial diagnosis of pancreatic injury can be difficult to identify on CT. In a series of 1045 consecutive children examined by CT after blunt trauma, the pancreatic injury was prospectively identified in only 67%.[121] The presence of fluid in the lesser sac was a useful marker for injury to the pancreas.

ACKNOWLEDGMENTS

I would like to thank Betty J. Greenberg for her excellent help in preparation of this manuscript.

REFERENCES

1. Abramson SJ, et al: Hepatic parenchymal and subcapsular gas after hepatic laceration caused by blunt abdominal trauma. *AJR* 153:1031-1032, 1989.
2. Aihara T, Fujioka M, Yamamoto K: Increased CT density of the liver due to cisdiaminedichloro platinum. *Pediatr Radiol* 17:75-76, 1987.
3. Araki T: Leukemic involvement of the kidney in children: CT features. *J Comput Assist Tomogr* 6:781-784, 1982.
4. Atkinson GO Jr, et al: Focal nodular hyperplasia of the liver in children: a report of three new cases. *Radiology* 137:171-174, 1980.
5. Ball WS Jr, Bisset GS III, Towbin RB: Percutaneous drainage of chest abscesses in children. *Radiology* 171;431-434, 1989.
6. Banner MP, et al: Multilocular renal cysts: radiologic-pathologic correlation. *AJR* 136:239-247, 1981.
7. Baron RL, et al: Computed tomography of the normal thymus. *Radiology* 142:121-125, 1982.
8. Bartolozzi C, Selli C, Olmastroni M, et al: Rhabdomyosarcoma of the prostate: MR findings. *AJR* 150:1333-1334, 1988.
9. Belt TG, et al: MRI of Wilms' tumor: promise as the primary imaging method. *AJR* 146:955-961, 1986.
10. Berger PE, Kuhn JP, Kuhns LR: Computed tomography and the occult tracheobronchial foreign body. *Radiology* 134:133-135, 1980.
11. Berger PE, Munschauer RW, Kuhn JP: Computed tomography and ultrasound of renal and perirenal diseases in infants and children. *Pediatr Radiol* 9:91-99, 1980.
12. Bhalla M, et al: Cystic fibrosis: scoring system with thin-section CT. *Radiology* 179:783-788, 1991.
13. Bisceglia M, Donaldson JS: Calcification of the ligamentum arteriosum in children: a normal finding on CT. *AJR* 156:351-352, 1991.
14. Blane CE, Donn SM, Mori KW: Congenital cystic adenomatoid malformation of the lung. *J Comput Assist Tomogr* 5:418-420, 1981.
15. Boechat MI, et al: Computed tomography in stage III neuroblastoma. *AJR* 145:1283-1287, 1985.
16. Boechat MI, et al: Primary liver tumors in children: comparison of CT and MR imaging. *Radiology* 169:727-732, 1988.
17. Brasch RC, Cann CE: Computed tomographic scanning in children. II. An updated comparison of radiation dose and resolving power of commercial scanners. *AJR* 138:127-133, 1982.
18. Brasch RC, Randel SB, Gould RG: Follow-up of Wilms' tumor: comparison of CT with other imaging procedures. *AJR* 137:1005-1009, 1981.
19. Brasch RC, et al: Abdominal disease in children: a comparison of computed tomography and ultrasound. *AJR* 134:153-158, 1980.
20. Brick SH, et al: Hepatic and splenic injury in children: role of CT in the decision for laparotomy. *Radiology* 165:643-646, 1987.
21. Brody AS, et al: Airway evaluation in children with use of ultrafast CT; pitfalls and recommendations. *Radiology* 178:181-184, 1991.
22. Bulas DI, Taylor GA, Eichelberger MR: The value of CT in detecting bowel perforation in children after blunt abdominal trauma. *AJR* 153:561-564, 1989.
23. Chinwuba C, Wallman J, Strand R: Nasal airway obstruction: CT assessment. *Radiology* 159:503-506, 1986.
24. Choi BI, et al: Caroli disease: central dot sign in CT. *Radiology* 174:161-163, 1990.
25. Choyke PL, et al: Thymic atrophy and regrowth in response to chemotherapy: CT evaluation. *AJR* 149:269-272, 1987.
26. Cohen M, et al: Thymic rebound after treatment of childhood tumors. *AJR* 135:151-156, 1980.
27. Cohen M, et al: Pulmonary pseudometastases in children with malignant tumors. *Radiology* 141:371-374, 1981.
28. Cohen M, et al: Lung CT for detection of metastases: solid tissue neoplasms in children. *AJR* 139:895-898, 1982.
29. Cohen M, et al: The diagnostic dilemma of the posterior mediastinal thymus: CT manifestations. *Radiology* 146:691-693, 1983.
30. Cormier PJ, Donaldson JS, Gonzalez-Crussi F: Nephroblastomatosis: missed diagnosis. *Radiology* 169:737-738, 1988.
31. Cory D, Cohen M, Smith J: Thymus in the superior mediastinum simulating adenopathy: appearance on CT. *Radiology* 162:457-459, 1987.
32. Cunningham D, Churchill RJ, Reynes CJ: Computed tomography in the evaluation of liver disease in cystic fibrosis patients. *J Comput Assist Tomogr* 4:151-154, 1980.
33. Dachman AH, et al: Infantile hemangioendothelioma of the liver: a radiologic-pathologic-clinical correlation. *AJR* 140:1091-1096, 1983.
34. Dachman AH, et al: Hepatoblastoma: radiologic-pathologic correlation in 50 cases. *Radiology* 164:15-19, 1987.
35. Daneman A, Chan HSL, Martin J: Adrenal carcinoma and adenoma in children: a review of 17 patients. *Pediatr Radiol* 13:11-18, 1983.
36. Daneman A, et al: Pancreatic changes in cystic fibrosis: CT and sonographic appearances. *AJR* 141:653-655, 1983.
37. Davidson AJ, Hartman DS: Lymphangioma of the retroperitoneum: CT and sonographic characteristics. *Radiology* 175:507-510, 1990.
38. Day DL, et al: Hepatic regenerating nodules in hereditary tyrosinemia. *AJR* 149:391-393, 1987.
39. Day DL, et al: MR evaluation of the portal vein in pediatric liver transplant candidates. *AJR* 147:1027-1030, 1986.
40. de Geer G, Webb WR, Gamsu G: Normal thymus: assessment with MR and CT. *Radiology* 158:313-317, 1986.
41. Dietrich RB, Kangarloo H: Kidneys in infants and children: evaluation with MR. *Radiology* 159:215-221, 1986.
42. Dietrich RB, et al: Neuroblastoma: the role of MR imaging. *AJR* 148:937-942, 1987.
43. Donaldson JS, Gilsanz V, Miller JH: CT scanning in patients with opsomyoclonus: importance of nonenhanced scan. *AJR* 146:781-783, 1986.
44. Doppman JL, et al: Computed tomography of the liver and kidneys in glycogen storage disease. *J Comput Assist Tomogr* 6:67-71, 1982.
45. Drossman SR, et al: Lymphoma of the mediastinum and neck: evaluation with Ga-67 imaging and CT correlation. *Radiology* 174:171-175, 1990.
46. Effmann EL, et al: Tracheal cross-sectional area in children: CT determination. *Radiology* 149:137-140, 1983.
47. Farrelly C, et al: Occult neuroblastoma presenting with opsomyoclonus: utility of computed tomography. *AJR* 142:807-810, 1984.
48. Fearon T, Vuvich J: Pediatric patient exposures from CT examinations: GE CT/T 9800 scanner. *AJR* 144:805-809, 1985.
49. Felker RE, Tonkin ILD: Imaging of pulmonary sequestration. *AJR* 154:241-249, 1990.
50. Fernbach SK, et al: Nephroblastomatosis: comparison of CT with US and urography. *Radiology* 166:153-156, 1988.

51. Fisher MF, et al: Abdominal lipoblastomatosis: radiographic, echographic, and computed tomographic findings. *Radiology* 138:593-596, 1981.

52. Fishman EK, et al: The CT appearance of Wilms' tumor. *J Comput Assist Tomogr* 7:659-665, 1983.

53. Fitzgerald SW, Donaldson JS: Azygoesophageal recess: normal CT appearance in children. *AJR* 158:1101-1104, 1992.

54. Fletcher BD, Cohn RC: Tracheal compression and the innominate artery: MR evaluation in infants. *Radiology* 170:103-107, 1989.

55. Francis IR, et al: The thymus: reexamination of age-related changes in sizes and shape. *AJR* 145:249-254, 1985.

56. Franken EA Jr, Chiu LC, Smith WL: Hereditary pancreatitis in children. *Ann Radiol* 27:130-137, 1984.

57. Frey EE, et al: Chronic airway obstruction in children: evaluation with cine CT. *AJR* 148:347-352, 1987.

58. Frick MP, Feinberg SB: Deceptions in localizing extrahepatic right-upper-quadrant abdominal masses by CT. *AJR* 139:501-504, 1982.

59. Glass RBJ, Davidson AJ, Fernbach SK: Clear cell sarcoma of the kidney: CT, sonographic, and pathologic correlation. *Radiology* 180:715-717, 1991.

60. Gomes AS, et al: Congenital abnormalities of the aortic arch: MR imaging. *Radiology* 165:691-695, 1987.

61. Griscom NT, Wohl MEB: Dimensions of the growing trachea related to age and gender. *AJR* 146:233-237, 1986.

62. Gross GW, et al: Limited-slice CT in the evaluation of paranasal sinus disease in children. *AJR* 156:367-369, 1991.

63. Haaga JR, et al: The effect of mAs variation upon computed tomography image quality as evaluated by in vivo and in vitro studies. *Radiology* 138:449-454, 1981.

64. Han BK, Babcock DS, Gelfand MH: Choledochal cyst with bile duct dilatation: sonography and 99m TcIDA cholescintigraphy. *AJR* 136:1075-1079, 1981.

65. Hartman DS, et al: Mesoblastic nephroma: radiologic-pathologic correlation of 20 cases. *AJR* 136:69-74, 1981.

66. Heiberg E, et al: Normal thymus: CT characteristics in subjects under age 20. *AJR* 138:491-494, 1982.

67. Hernanz-Schulman M, et al: Pancreatic cystosis in cystic fibrosis. *Radiology* 158:629-631, 1986.

68. Hidalgo H, et al: The problem of benign pulmonary nodules in children receiving cytotoxic chemotherapy. *AJR* 140:21-24, 1983.

69. Hill SC, et al: CT findings in acid lipase deficiency: Wolman disease and cholesteryl ester storage disease. *J Comput Assist Tomogr* 7:815-818, 1983.

70. Hulnick DH, et al: Late presentation of congenital cystic adenomatoid malformation of the lung. *Radiology* 151:569-573, 1984.

71. Ivancev K, Kullendorff C-M: Value of computed tomography in traumatic pancreatitis in children. *Acta Radiol Diag* 24:441-444, 1983.

72. Jaffe RB, Arata JA Jr, Matlak ME: Percutaneous drainage of traumatic pancreatic pseudocysts in children. *AJR* 152:591-595, 1989.

73. Kane NM, et al: Pediatric abdominal trauma: evaluation by computed tomography. *Pediatrics* 82:11-15, 1988.

74. Kao SCS, et al: Ultrafast CT of laryngeal and tracheobronchial obstruction in symptomatic postoperative infants with esophageal atresia and tracheoesophageal fistula. *AJR* 154:345-350, 1990.

75. Kaufman RA: Liver-spleen computed tomography. *Pediatr Radiol* 13:151-153, 1983.

76. Kaufman RA, et al: Upper abdominal trauma in children: imaging evaluation. *AJR* 142:449-460, 1984.

77. Kier R, McCarthy S, Rosenfield AT, et al: Nonpalpable testes in young boys: evaluation with MRI imaging. *Radiology* 169:429-433, 1988.

78. Kirks DR, et al: Tracheal compression by mediastinal masses in children: CT evaluation. *AJR* 141:647-651, 1983.

79. Kohda E, Fujioka M, Ikawa H, et al: Congenital anorectal anomaly: CT evaluation. *Radiology* 157:349-352, 1985.

80. Kuhlman JE, Fishman EK, Siegelman SS: Invasive pulmonary aspergillosis in acute leukemia: characteristic findings on CT, the CT halo sign, and the role of CT in early diagnosis. *Radiology* 157:611-614, 1985.

81. Kuhn J: Diagnostic imaging for the evaluation of abdominal trauma in children. *Pediatr Clin North Am* 32:1427-1447, 1985.

82. Lee JKT, et al: Acute focal bacterial nephritis: emphasis on gray scale sonography and computed tomography. *AJR* 135:87-92, 1980.

83. Lowe RC, Chone MD: Computed tomographic evaluation of Wilms' tumor and neuroblastoma. *Radiographics* 4:915-928, 1984.

84. Lucaya J, et al: Computed tomography of infantile hepatic hemangioendothelioma. *AJR* 144:821-826, 1985.

85. Madewell JE, et al: Multilocular cystic nephroma: a radiographic-pathologic correlation of 58 patients. *Radiology* 146:309-321, 1983.

86. Marchal GJ, et al: Caroli disease: high-frequency US and pathologic findings. *Radiology* 158:507-511, 1986.

87. Merten DF, Kirks DR: Amebic liver abscess in children: the role of diagnostic imaging. *AJR* 143:1325-1329, 1984.

88. Miller H, Greenfield LD, Wald BR: Candidiasis of the liver and spleen in childhood. *Radiology* 142:375-380, 1982.

89. Miller JH: The ultrasonographic appearance of cystic hepatoblastoma. *Radiology* 138:141-143, 1981.

90. Miller JH, Greenspan BS: Integrated imaging of hepatic tumors in childhood. Part I: malignant lesions (primary and metastatic). *Radiology* 154:83-90, 1985.

91. Miller JH, Greenspan BS: Integrated imaging of hepatic tumors in childhood. II. Benign lesions (congenital, reparative, and inflammatory). *Radiology* 154:91-100, 1985.

92. Miraldi FD, et al: Diagnostic imaging of human neuroblastoma with radiolabeled antibody. *Radiology* 161:413-418, 1986.

93. Mitnick JS, et al: CT in B-Thalassemia: iron deposition in the liver, spleen, and lymph nodes. *AJR* 136:1191-1194, 1981.

94. Mitnick JS, et al: Cystic renal disease in tuberous sclerosis. *Radiology* 147:85-87, 1983.

95. Morrison SC: Case report: demonstration of a tracheal bronchus by computed tomography. *Clin Radiol* 39:208-209, 1988.

96. Morrison SC, Abramowsky C, Fletcher BD: Chest mass in a teenage girl. *Invest Radiol* 18:401-405, 1983.

97. Naidich DP: Computed tomography of bronchiectasis. *J Comput Assist Tomogr* 6:437-444, 1982.

98. Pardes JG, et al: Lymphangioma of the thymus in a child. *J Comput Assist Tomogr* 6:825-827, 1982.

99. Pardes JG, et al: CT diagnosis of congenital lobar emphysema. *J Comput Assist Tomogr* 7:1095-1097, 1983.

100. Parvey LS, et al: CT demonstration of fat tissue in malignant renal neoplasms: atypical Wilms' tumors. *J Comput Assist Tomogr* 5:851-854, 1981.

101. Patrick LE, et al: Peditric blunt abdominal trauma: periportal tracking at CT. *Radiology* 183:689-691, 1992.

102. Pickering SP, et al: Renal lymphangioma: a cause of neonatal nephromegaly. *Pediatr Radiol* 14:445-448, 1984.

103. Pinzon JL, et al: Repair of coarctation of the aorta in children: postoperative morphology. *Radiology* 180:199-203, 1991.

104. Rathore MH, Barton LL, Luisiri A: Acute lobar nephronia: a review. *Pediatrics* 87:728-734, 1991.

105. Reiman TAH, Siegel MJ, Shackelford GD: Wilms' tumor in children: abdominal CT and US evaluation. *Radiology* 160:501-505, 1986.

106. Ros PR, et al: Mesenchymal hamartoma of the liver: radiologic-pathologic correlation. *Radiology* 158:619-624, 1986.

107. Ros PR, et al: Undifferentiated (embryonal) sarcoma of the liver: radiologic-pathologic correlation. *Radiology* 161:141-145, 1986.

108. Rosenfield NS, Leonidas JC, Barwick KW: Aggressive neuroblastoma simulating Wilms' tumor. *Radiology* 166:165-167, 1988.

109. Sato Y, Pringle KC, Bergman RA, et al: Congenital anorectal anomalies: MR imaging. *Radiology* 168:157-162, 1988.

110. Siegel MJ: Magnetic resonance imaging of the pediatric pelvis. *Semin Ultrasound CT MR* 12:475-505, 1991.

111. Shirkhoda A, Biggers WP: Choanal atresia. *Radiology* 142:93-94, 1982.

112. Shurin SB, et al: Computed tomography for the evaluation of thoracic masses in children. *JAMA* 246:65-67, 1981.

113. Siegel MJ: Periportal low attenuation at CT in childhood. *Radiology* 183:685-688, 1992.

114. Siegel MJ, Sagel SS, Reed K: The value of computed tomography in the diagnosis and management of pediatric mediastinal abnormalities. *Radiology* 142:149-155, 1982.

115. Siegel MJ, Shackelford GD, McAlister WH: Paranasal sinus mucoceles in children. *Radiology* 133:623-626, 1979.

116. Siegel MJ, et al: Normal and abnormal thymus in childhood: MR imaging. *Radiology* 172:367-371, 1989.

117. Siegel MJ, et al: Clinical utility of CT in pediatric retroperitoneal disease: 5 years experience. *AJR* 138:1011-1017, 1982.

118. Siegel MJ, et al: MR imaging of intraspinal extension of neuroblastoma. *J Comput Assist Tomogr* 10:593-595, 1986.

119. Siegel MJ, et al: Mediastinal lesions in children: comparison of CT and MR. *Radiology* 160:241-244, 1986.

120. Sisler CL, Siegel MJ: Malignant rhabdoid tumor of the kidney: radiologic features. *Radiology* 172:211-212, 1989.

121. Sivit CJ, et al: Blunt pancreatic trauma in children: CT diagnosis. *AJR* 158:1097-1100, 1992.

122. Sivit CJ, et al: Posttraumatic adrenal hemorrhage in children: CT findings in 34 patients. *AJR* 158:1299-1302, 1992.

123. Sivit CJ, et al: Safety-belt injuries in children with lap-belt ecchymosis: CT findings in 61 patients. *AJR* 157:111-114, 1991.

124. Stalker HP, Kaufman RA, Stedje K: The significance of hematuria in children after blunt abdominal trauma. *AJR* 154:569-571, 1990.

125. Stalker HP, Kaufman RA, Towbin R: Patterns of liver injury in childhood: CT analysis. *AJR* 147:1199-1205, 1986.

126. Stanley P: Mesenchymal hamartomas of the liver in childhood: sonographic and CT findings. *AJR* 147:1035-1039, 1986.

127. Stark DD, et al: Neuroblastoma: diagnositic imaging and staging. *Radiology* 148:101-105, 1983.

128. Stark DD, et al: Recurrent neuroblastoma: the role of CT and alternative imaging tests. *Radiology* 148:107-112, 1983.

129. Strain JD, et al: IV Nembutal: safe sedation for children undergoing CT. *AJR* 151:975-979, 1988.

130. Taylor GA, Fallat ME, Eichelberger MR: Hypovolemic shock in children: abdominal CT manifestations. *Radiology* 164:479-481, 1987.

131. Weinberger E, Rosenbaum DM, Pendergrass TW: Renal involvement in children with lymphoma: comparison of CT with sonography. *AJR* 155:347-349, 1990.

132. Weinreb JC, et al: Imaging the pediatric liver: MRI and CT. *AJR* 147:785-790, 1986.

133. White KS, Kirks DR, Bove KE: Imaging of nephroblastomatosis: an overview. *Radiology* 182:1-5, 1992.

46

Interventional CT-Guided Procedures

JOHN R. HAAGA

The value of interventional procedures for expeditious and cost-effective management of patients is widely accepted.* Because the widespread acceptance of ultrasonic-, fluoroscopic-, and computed tomography (CT)-guided procedures has been rapid, one would also expect quick acceptance of MRI procedures if they are developed judiciously. The purpose of this chapter is to discuss CT-guided procedures as completely as possible and to demonstrate some preliminary experience with magnetic resonance imaging (MRI)-guided procedures. I will include in this chapter a general discussion of percutaneous procedures, general techniques for CT procedures, the specific applications of CT procedures in different organ systems, and finally, a discussion of potential future applications for MR procedures.

With the passage of time, instrument development, and wider proliferation of imaging systems, most radiologists have adopted a more flexible style of intervention that includes many types of needles, catheters, and other devices. Because of the diversity of pathologic processes in the different organs, these devices must be used optimally for maximum benefit and safety. An interesting point related to needles is that although we have advocated the use of side-cutting needles for many years, their general usage has accelerated since the "automated" needle guns were developed.

This chapter will be somewhat longer than others because of my intense interest and extensive experience. I performed the first CT biopsy and drainage procedures in 1976 and 1977, and have continued to perform such cases on a daily basis (Figs. 46-1, *A* and *B*, 46-2, 46-3). I have recently begun to perform MRI-guided biopsies (Figs. 46-4). Although many different

*References 37, 92, 132, 155, 185, 186, 187, 193, 213, 228, 235, 238, 283, 294.

techniques and methods have been reported and are unquestionably effective, I am confident that our techniques developed over many years and after literally thousands of procedures are valuable and compare favorably to other proposed methods.

GENERAL HISTORY OF PERCUTANEOUS PROCEDURES

Reviewing the historical perspective of interventional and CT procedures can be somewhat confusing if one takes a narrow viewpoint and assumes that their evolution in the past 50 years has been along a single pathway. If one takes an objective, global viewpoint, however, one can see that the development of percutaneous procedures has been quite varied and has involved four separate disciplines: instrument development, clinical techniques, pathologic and cytopathologic techniques, and guidance methods.

The advances in these four areas have at times occurred concurrently, and it is difficult to appreciate the overall perspective if one selectively reads the literature. Furthermore, as one reads the various reports in the literature, one must be aware of individual bias relative to data interpretation and reference sources. When authors look to the literature to support the thesis of their report, it is a natural tendency to use only the information that supports their viewpoint. For this reason it is most important that in some cases the informed reader consult the primary reference source rather than relying strictly on an author's interpretation (this applies even to the reading of this chapter).

The best way to demonstrate this complex premise is to take an example (e.g., the small-caliber, or "skinny" needle). In many reports authors refer to the experience of Lundquist to support the accuracy of the ultrasonic-guided skinny-needle biopsy, despite the fact

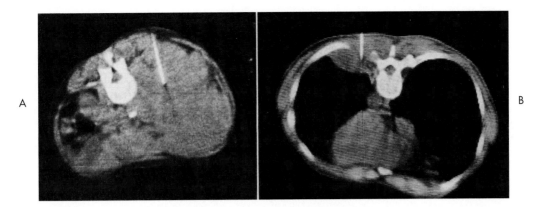

Fig. 46-1. A, First CT-guided biopsy was of a retroperitoneal mass (by the author). Even though the results of this biopsy were negative the merits of CT guidance were obvious. **B,** First CT-guided procedure of the lung in 1975 (by the author).

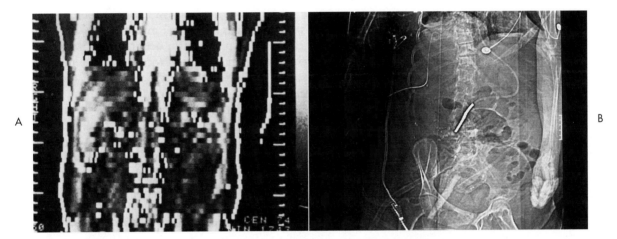

Fig. 46-2. A, First CT radiographic image ever produced or reported. One of its original purposes was to aid with interventional procedures (see later portion of chapter on catheter insertions). This primitive scan shows the lower chest and upper abdomen. This preceded all of the current commercial images including the Topogram, Scoutview, Synerview, etc. The originator (J.R. Haaga) reported and published this figure, but he was not clever enough to obtain patents at the time! (From Haaga, JR: *AJR* 127:1059-1060, 1976.) **B,** Modern image showing the remarkable detail of current images. The image of this patient shows the abdominal anatomy, several catheters, wires and monitoring devices.

that Lundquist performed only "blind" biopsies with the skinny needle.[174,175] In addition, Lundquist is frequently quoted in attempts to prove the safety of the skinny-needle compared to the large cutting or Menghini-type needle. If readers take a more comprehensive approach to the literature, however, they will find that in his final dissertation Lundquist noted a favorable result with large needles as well as with the skinny needle. Using the skinny needle first to probe the pathway for the large needle, Lundquist had performed over 1,000 procedures with the Menghini needle with "no complications" (of 2,611 cases involving the use of the skinny needle, he reported one hematoma). His data are valid within the complete context of his work and the literature, but one

may draw incorrect conclusions if only selected sources of information are used.

Progress from 1930 to 1960

From 1930 to 1960 most progress in percutaneous biopsies was made in the area of unguided clinical methods and instrument development. There was very little progress in the development of pathologic techniques or guidance by imaging.

Two important clinical points concerning liver biopsy were discovered during this time. First, for "blind" procedures, the intercostal approach was found safer than the anterior subcostal approach (if the liver was not massively enlarged). Second, the liver biopsy was proved

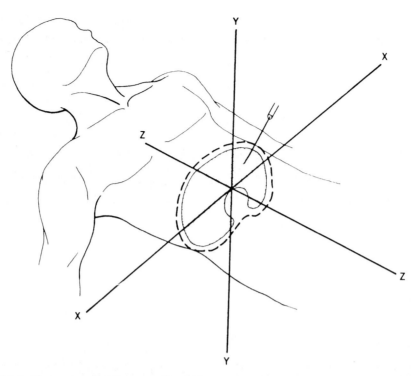

Fig. 46-3. Placement of a biopsy needle within an anatomic location. The relationship of the needle to both the plane of the *z* axis and the plane of the *x-y* axis is illustrated. (From Haaga JR, et al: *Cleve Clin Q* 44:27-33, 1977.)

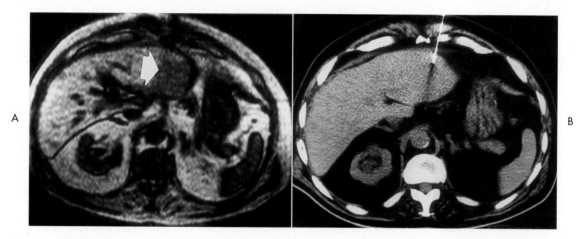

Fig. 46-4. These scans show an MR-guided procedure and a CT-guided procedure of a liver lesion. **A,** This MR scan shows the low-intensity mass within the left lobe much more clearly than does the CT scan. The needle *(arrow)* is very difficult to see. **B,** This CT scan taken at the same level shows the visualization of the needle in the same mass. With current technology, the best result in such cases is to correlate the location on the MRI scan with the CT during biopsy.

safer when performed while the patient suspended respiration and motion. The importance of this latter clinical procedure was emphasized by Menghini,[188] who introduced his "one-second" technique. Menghini's real contribution was his recommended method of having the patient suspend respiration while the biopsy is quickly performed. Motion by the patient was thus avoided, and possible injury to the liver was minimized. This "breath-holding" maneuver, and not the needle that bears his name, was his significant innovation.

Instrument development during this time was confined to the various types of cutting needles. Instruments introduced included the end-cutting needles, the Vim Silverman needle, and the Tru-Cut needle. A number of general review articles were published about the incidence and cause of the complications associated with blind, large-needle liver biopsy. These complications included hemorrhage, bile peritonitis, and gallbladder perforation. The major causes of hemorrhage were abnormal prothrombin time, severe liver disease, and abnormal vessels. Although it now seems astonishing, biopsies were performed on patients who had very abnormal prothrombin times. The major cause of bile peritonitis was caused by penetration of dilated bile ducts with obstructive jaundice or perforation of the gallbladder (most frequent with an anterior subcostal approach).

These review articles about the complications of large-needle biopsy are especially interesting to note because these very old articles are typically quoted in the radiology literature to discourage the use of the larger cutting needles. Obviously, comparisons of today's guided techniques with the results of the old articles are completely invalid. Current methods of patient selection, detection of coagulopathy, local anesthesia, and patient sedation are remarkably different from those of the early authors. Furthermore, modern CT techniques eliminate almost all potential causes of complications with the large needles.

Biopsies of the liver and/or lung were performed either blind or with the assistance of "red-goggle" fluoroscopy. Blind localization for these procedures required either palpation, percussion, or approximated localization from plain radiographs. Fluoroscopic guidance using direct visualization or a phosphored glass screen (no image intensification on television) required that the radiologist localize the abnormality for the clinician. After localization by direct fluoroscopy in a darkened room, the biopsy procedure was performed by a clinical physician with the lights on. The radiologists donned their red goggles so that their eyes could remain accommodated for the dark, direct fluoroscopy (black images on green phosphor). Biopsies were not a radiologic procedure during this era.

Progress from 1960 to 1970

Development during the 1960s included comparison data about the various large cutting needles, introduction of cytopathologic methods, introduction of the skinny needle for blind biopsies, and the first "breakthrough" with guided biopsies: image intensification fluoroscopy.

Qualities of the different cutting needles were compared by Parker et al.[226] Their comparison of the Vim Silverman needle with the Menghini needle showed that the latter was superior for sample recovery. The ad-

equacy of sample was 94% for the Menghini needle; compared with 77% for the Vim Silverman needle. They also noted the higher incidence of complications with the Vim Silverman needle. The advantages of the Menghini method using the end-hole needle were its simplicity, the short time required for the procedure, and lack of patient respiratory motion.

During this period the development of cytopathologic techniques revolutionized percutaneous procedures. Although earlier authors such as Martin[181] used a cytologic method, Soderstrom[146] in 1958 and 1966 developed and reported the first well-defined methods of needle aspiration and cytopathologic evaluation. Several of his protegés, including Lundquist[174,175] and Nordenstrom,[211] continued this work and reported extensively on the clinical application of these techniques, which will be discussed later.

Aside from these workers, other authors evaluated the usefulness of the cytopathologic techniques on material obtained from cutting needles rather than on the aspirates from the skinny needle. Grossman et al,[88] using tissue and fluid from Menghini biopsy of the liver, performed cytopathologic studies of the fluid and "touch preps" of the tissue on slides. They found that their diagnostic accuracy for malignancy improved by an additional 15%, compared with the histologic results of the tissue core. Later work by Atterbury et al[47] confirmed their observations, but these results were not quite as remarkable. From their study they found that in their series of 29 malignancies, the yield only improved by 3% (one patient).

These articles, which were frequently misquoted during the 1980s, show the added benefit of the cytologic techniques on the samples obtained with larger cutting needles (in addition to the traditional histologic methods) for the detection of malignant cells. These articles were not comparisons between the skinny needles and the large needles, as will be discussed later.

After the positive results reported by these authors and the experience of Soderstrom,[250] other authors began clinical trials using the small-caliber (skinny) needle for unguided procedures to obtain liver samples for cytologic examination. One of the largest series performing skinny-needle biopsy of the liver was Lundquist's study in 1970 about unguided or blind biopsies of the liver. In his first report[174] about a series of 1,748 liver biopsies, he correctly made the diagnosis of cancer in 74% of patients (50 of 74) with no complications. No mention is made concerning the diagnosis of benign disease in the remaining 1,674 cases. In this series of malignant cases the authors were able to make the prospective specific diagnosis in only two metastatic lesions, and 5 of 10 hepatomas. Lundquist's intent was to develop a safe screening method for detection of tumor that would permit a wide latitude of technique error without significantly endangering the patient.[174] He did not refute the advantage of the larger needles to make a more definitive diagnosis. In Lundquist's later report of a larger series,[175] he reported an equivalent diagnostic accuracy, with one serious complication of bleeding. In this paper he also related his experience of 1,000 large-needle biopsies with no complications. The important point of avoiding complications, he believed, was the evaluation of the chosen entrance site by probing with a skinny needle before using the large needle. In this fashion he could avoid bowel, lung, gallbladder, vessels, or excessively vascular tumors (current CT methods provide the same information and advantage).

One of the few comparison studies of different needles during this time was by Johansen et al,[140] who compared the use of a skinny needle with a Menghini needle in blind liver biopsy. These authors found identical results for the detection of malignancy; both needles were correct for 6 of 12 cases. There were no complications.

With this initial experience and the development of image intensification television as a background, radiologists began to evaluate the merits of the skinny needle for sampling the lung with fluoroscopic guidance. In 1966 Dahlgren and Nordenstrom[42] began using image-intensified fluoroscopy to guide the skinny needle for biopsy of lung masses. Their result showed a high accuracy and a low complication rate.

These early workers clearly established the usefulness of the skinny needle for obtaining samples from epithelial tumors such as adenocarcinoma and squamous cell carcinomas. Such tumors lack the cellular organization or "cement" to bind them together. Therefore the nontraumatic skinny needle can recover such loosely adherent cells. The same researchers also noted that when other than epithelial tumors were biopsied by these methods, the results were good but diagnoses were not as specific. This was especially true when architecture was important, such as in cases of lymphoma, benign tumors, or neurogenic tumors.

Television image intensification has made a remarkable contribution to the performance of biopsy procedures. With red-goggle fluoroscopy, radiologists could not turn room light on and off during a procedure because of eye accommodation. With the direct fluoroscopy, radiologists had to enhance their visualization of the dark fluoroscopy by preceding their examinations with a period of wearing the red goggles to accommodate their eyes. With image intensification, which improved light output by a factor of 1,000, radiologists could turn lights on and off and thereby assume direct responsibility for the procedures.

Progress from 1970 to the 1980s

During this period more progress was made with percutaneous procedures than during any of the previous periods. Progress was rapid because of the excellent groundwork laid by earlier workers and because of the remarkable technological advances. Some refinement was made in the cytopathologic area, but remarkable progress was made in the areas of clinical experience, instrument evaluation, and imaging guidance.

Before outlining the progress made with the skinny needle and the various imaging systems, some comments about clinical work with the cutting needles are appropriate. First, a prospective series in 1978 by Perrault et al[231] showed no complication difference among the Vim Silverman, Menghini, and Tru-Cut needles. This is fascinating, considering the significant difference in both the calibers and cutting actions. One might conclude that, if there are any basic differences in complications due to needle configuration, good clinical technique and experience can compensate so that complication rates are equivalent. To further support this point, Bateson's comparison[12] in 1980 of the Tru-Cut needle with the Menghini needle showed no diagnostic or other complications, although the physical integrity of the sample was more consistently intact with the Tru-Cut needle, especially with cirrhotic livers.

The two other very significant events that occurred in the 1970s were the introductions of ultrasound[13] and CT as guidance modalities. Ultrasound was introduced as a biopsy guidance system by Holmes et al[126,127] in 1975. CT guidance was introduced by Haaga et al[93] in 1976. As noted later both of these later imaging systems have developed into valuable tools for sampling different areas.

The 1980s

In the early 1980s, the cutting needles, both side-cutting and end-cutting, came into their prime.[92,101,105] With the advent of the automated needles, many radiologists now use these devices almost routinely. Other major advances undoubtedly will be made during the 1990s, the seminal work now appearing in the literature clearly indicating the directions.

With further development of biopsy devices, I am confident that a hemostatic biopsy device will be developed and introduced. The first indication of the potential of such a device was reported by Gazelle et al.[74] In this initial work, a hemostatic sheath, which could be deposited at the site of the biopsy procedure, was developed. In animal models using anticoagulated pigs, it was shown that such a device could prevent significant bleeding in the liver. It is probable that a recent modification of this device could reach the market in the next several years and potentially result in a "risk-free" biopsy.

More sophisticated ancillary guidance devices are being designed; these will simplify the performance of CT-, ultrasound-, and MRI-guided procedures (see Fig. 46-27, *A* and *B*). One device recently introduced on the market place by Magnusson et al[178] shows great promise for the future. Other mechanical and light-guided devices are being developed.

Additional new techniques will be developed and refined for the percutaneous treatments of tumors and for the insertion of physiologic monitoring or activating devices. The first examples of in vivo tumor treatment using ethanol injections have been reported; these will be described in this chapter. Physiologic monitoring devices such as thermisters for hyperthermia and pressure transducers for tumor treatment will follow in the near future. Also, it is probable that insertion of electrodes for stimulation of various muscles will come into common usage.

HISTORICAL PERSPECTIVE OF ORGAN PROCEDURES

Lung

The first experience using skinny needles with image-intensification guidance in the lung was reported by Dahlgren[42] and Nordenstrom[211] in 1965. After their report their results were confirmed by a number of authors using a variety of guidance methods and small-caliber needles. Another early group, Sargeant et al,[243] performed biopsies without image intensification with good results. Once image intensification became standard, many authors including Lauby,[166] Lalli,[161] Westcott,[278] and Sinner[246] reported their series. Many important observations were made about different factors that alter diagnostic accuracy and complications; these will be discussed in the following section on lung procedures.

One fascinating fact that is apparent from reports of these authors is that many different calibers of needles have been called "skinny" needles. Regardless of the caliber of the needle used by the authors (e.g., Lalli et al[161] used an 18-gauge needle, and Zornoza[291] used a 23-gauge needle), the diagnostic accuracy was quite good and the complication rate was quite acceptable.

In the recent literature, the most important article of which is the one by Khouri et al,[153] it is clear that needle caliber has almost no impact on pneumothorax rate but has a definite impact on hemoptysis. The incidence of pneumothorax is almost identical with all sizes of needles, but Khouri et al[153] reported that the incidence of hemoptysis is greater with needles larger than 20 gauge than it is with needles 20 gauge or less.

Further progress for sampling the lung and mediastinum occurred with the introduction of CT procedures in 1976 by my group.[92] While fluoroscopy has continued to be the main modality for biopsy of the peripheral, well-defined lung nodule, CT provided new advantages for the lung and mediastinum. With CT it became possible to biopsy more difficult lung lesions, to biopsy the mediastinum, and to use the cutting needle safely in selected cases.

Liver

Although Lundqvist showed the usefulness of blind skinny-needle biopsies, guided biopsy of the liver with the skinny needle was infrequent until the introduction of ultrasound and CT scanning. The first ultrasound biopsy of the liver was performed by Rasmussen et al.[238] Their study noted the increased diagnostic yield of ultrasound-guided skinny needle biopsy of liver masses, compared with blind Menghini biopsy. The improved yield was of course secondary to the accurate targeting provided by ultrasound. This article is sometimes mistakenly quoted as showing the superiority of the ultrasound-guided skinny needle over the larger cutting needle guided by CT. This article does not even include CT-guided procedures, so any comparison or inference is not valid. Many other authors[245] later confirmed the high accuracy of both the skinny-needle procedure of the liver and the ultrasound guidance. These will be noted in the liver section.

After the first CT biopsy of the liver by our group, a large body of experience with both the skinny needle and larger cutting needles has accumulated. Haaga et al[99,100] and Ferrucci et al,[59,61] among others, confirmed that CT-guided skinny-needle procedures are quite effective for the diagnosis of many primary and metastatic malignancies. During direct comparisons of the skinny needles and cutting needles, our group confirmed the usefulness of the skinny needle and also noted additional advantages with the larger cutting needles. Currently both ultrasound and CT are used for the performance of biopsies using large cutting needles. For easily visualized lesions, ultrasound guidance is more than adequate, but for more difficult or complicated cases CT is still the modality of choice because of advantages associated with guidance and diagnostic scanning (see later section on liver biopsy).

During this time another researcher, Pagani,[221] investigated the significance of needle caliber on the diagnostic yield and complication rate of aspiration biopsy of liver masses. With CT techniques he found there was an increased diagnostic yield with the larger needle and no difference in complication rate (see section on needle selection).

Pancreas

Percutaneous skinny-needle biopsy of the pancreas also developed very quickly. Before the guided skinny-needle biopsies of the pancreas, some authors evaluated skinny-needle aspirations under direct visualization at surgery. Christoferson[33] used the skinny needle in the surgical suite to show that the diagnosis of malignancy could be made with the skinny needle. Forsgren et al[64] then used percutaneous skinny-needle aspiration for diagnosis of palpable pancreatic tumors.

With this favorable experience, guided percutaneous pancreatic biopsies of the pancreas were quickly accepted. The first guided percutaneous pancreatic biopsy was performed in 1972 by Oscarson et al,[219] who used fluoroscopy in conjunction with angiography to localize the needle placement. Although other authors such as Tylen[262] used fluoroscopy with contrast studies, the widespread acceptance occurred after the introduction of ultrasound and CT guidance.

Ultrasonic biopsy was first pioneered by Holm et al[126,127] in 1975. CT-guided biopsy of the pancreas was introduced in 1976 by Haaga and Alfidi.[93] Both guidance systems have been used successfully, but there are some differences in the methods, accuracy, and complication rates; these will be discussed later.

Impact of experience

It appears that complication rates with the large or skinny needles are higher with inexperienced persons and lower with experienced ones. Interestingly, in the reports in the literature one usually finds an improvement in the authors' results as their reported experience accumulates. Although the skinny needle has a better tolerance for error and even inexperienced individuals can use it with few problems, even the complication rates improve. The improvement of diagnostic accuracy with experience was documented by Evander[53] and Zornoza[295] and Hopper.[174]

CURRENT PERSPECTIVE ON CT PROCEDURES

CT uses a beam of radiation to penetrate virtually all natural and artificial materials within the human body. Information concerning attenuation of these substances can be measured, and an image can be reconstructed. Because of the wide latitude of imaging capabilities, an extremely low-density material such as gas can be imaged as well as high-density materials such as metal, bone, or synthetic catheters. In addition, CT is sensitive enough to detect subtle abnormalities such as fluid densities, cysts, or small pockets of gas.[111,112]

The ability to image high-density material accurately offers wide versatility, so that any type of instrument (i.e., needle, drainage tube, or other device) may be used in a procedure. Moreover, contrast material can be injected when vascularity, an anatomic space, or an abnormal cavity needs further delineation. For example,

an abscess can have unpredictable serpiginous tracts or communicating channels that can be difficult to perceive unless contrast material is used.

Because the CT unit uses an air interface, it consistently provides a detailed and complete image in virtually all patients. In patients who have draining sinuses, wounds, ileostomies, scars, or other unusual surface problems, the examination can be performed without difficulty.

Another advantage is that the longitudinal scan (Topogram, Scoutview) that I originated[107] is now available on all CT scanners, making it possible to obtain conventional radiographs of the anatomy and to visualize instruments or catheters during insertion or manipulation (see Fig. 46-2).

Accuracy of localization

The potential accuracy of the CT-guided method can best be appreciated by examining a schematic drawing of a cross-sectional image (see Fig. 46-3). If the instrument is placed within an anatomic area and the CT scan shows the needle in that area, then the needle must lie within the 10-mm section of the abdomen corresponding to the CT section. Location of an instrument in this plane is limited by the section thickness, which is 10 mm; therefore the resolution in the z axis is $+5$ mm. If one uses narrower slices, such as 5-mm, the accuracy in the y-z plane is $+2.5$ mm. Resolution of the CT system in the x-y plane is less than 1 mm with modern scanners. The precision required in determining the position of such an instrument is less limited by the imaging equipment than it is by the degree of the operator's accuracy as determined by manual dexterity and by the degree of accuracy of the guidance system rather than the imaging equipment.

The ability to localize the needle tip consistently and accurately in an axial plane is a distinct advantage of CT over fluoroscopy or ultrasound. Although fluoroscopy can provide multiplanar visualization of a needle or instrument, it is not capable of directly visualizing soft-tissue abnormalities, except in the chest. Fluoroscopic localization of instruments depend on indirect information obtained from displacement of contrast-filled structures (e.g., bowel, biliary).

Ultrasound is very useful for the diagnosis and visualization of soft-tissue abnormalities, and in some cases it can provide localization of instruments.[36,126] It is somewhat less flexible for such procedures because visualization can be impaired by overlying gas and bone and thus requires "windows" for accurate imaging. Because of the reflective properties of a needle, it can be seen "breaking" the beam and providing some general localization; precise localization of the tip, however, is not always easy. This is not a significant problem because one can "wiggle" the needle and improve its visualization by movement of the tissues. The visualization can be optimized if the needle can be inserted at a right angle to the beam, but this is not always convenient or appropriate in many patients.

There are several innovations with ultrasound[216] that may potentially improve the visualization of the needle tip. One company has recently introduced a needle that transmits an ultrasound signal audible to the transducer. Others have suggested that with the exquisite sensitivity of color flow doppler for motion, better visualization of the needle is possible.

Very recently, several authors introduced the possibility of using MRI to perform biopsies. Mueller et al[202] have done some promising preliminary work with various types of stainless steel instruments. Although in theory MRI-guided biopsies are appealing, there are technical problems because of the physical configuration of current devices, spatial fidelity of current devices and the difficulty in the clinical monitoring of such patients (Fig. 46-4, *A* and *B*).

Although almost all reports confirm the advantages of CT, there is still occasional controversy concerning which modality should be used in which circumstances. In practical terms it is up to the individual radiologist to determine the degree of accuracy, confidence level, and role for CT, ultrasound, and MRI.

Versatility

Versatility is still one of the most valuable advantages of CT-guided procedures. Since the skin is unimpeded, no "holding" devices are required. There is significant versatility in selecting the entry point for the biopsies because of the completeness of the CT image. A full 360-degree view of the patient is provided. All organs, including the bowel, are visualized, so that a variety of needle pathways can be chosen. It is possible to choose appropriate pathways to avoid specific organs or the bowel, if clinically indicated. Changing the body position of the patient may be advantageous for opening "windows" for instruments because of organ shifting or patient comfort (changing positions creates no adverse effect on image quality). Finally, a wide variety of instruments can be used, ranging in size from a 23-gauge Chiba needle to a 14-gauge Tru-Cut needle. Of all of the advantages of CT procedures, versatility is the one that is least recognized. It is indeed perplexing that some radiologists will not change the patient position or trajectory of the needle to avoid uninvolved structures. For example, instead of approaching retroperitoneal lesions posteriorly through the flank, some will use only a direct anterior approach to traverse bowel or other organs.

Disadvantages of CT guidance

CT guidance has a number of apparent disadvantages that are, however, quite minimal in comparison to its advantages. Those to be considered include cost, radiation, and availability of equipment.

Although it is true that the cost is greater for CT than it is for other examinations, the cost savings of a CT biopsy, compared with alternative costs of surgery and/or hospitalization, are remarkable. Mitty et al[192] calculated a savings for CT-guided pancreatic biopsies of over $3,000 per case. Considering that more than one half of all such biopsies are performed on an outpatient basis, the savings are actually more than that amount. By comparison, ultrasound is much less expensive and MRI is much more expensive.

The CT scan obviously uses radiation for generation of the scans, but the dose delivered to the patient is much less than other specialized studies such as angiography. With modern scanning devices, doses for individual scans can be calibrated to lessen these exposures.

Availability of CT scanners has been somewhat limited in many institutions, but two developments may improve this. First, with current emphasis on cost savings and efficacy, most institutions are enthusiastic about using these techniques. Second, with MRI scans of the head replacing many neurologic CT scans, it is likely that the availability of time on CT scanners will increase.

Indications for CT-guided procedures

The indications for CT-guided procedures vary from institution to institution, depending on the expertise of the radiologists and the available imaging modalities. Generally, the important factors to consider are the visibility of the lesion on CT as compared with other modalities, the type of pathologic sample required, and the location of the lesion.

Considering that the prime function of the guidance modality is to direct the needle to the lesion, visibility of the lesion is the most obvious factor. Plainly stated, if one cannot see the lesion, one cannot biopsy the lesion. Therefore if a lesion is seen only on CT or much better on CT, then CT is the modality of choice. Likewise if a lesion is only seen on ultrasound or MRI, they are therefore the preferred guidance methods.

When an aspiration type of biopsy is clinically indicated, a variety of factors should be considered. As a rule, the simplest modality should be chosen which most satisfactorily shows the abnormality, the pathway of the instrument, and adjacent anatomic information. Generally, anatomic areas such as the retroperitoneum and pelvis are in most instances best suited for CT guidance. Specific consideration of each anatomic area will be discussed later in the chapter.

When lesions are small (ranging from 3 to 5 cm) and are located in critical areas, CT is again the preferred modality. Critical areas best suited for CT punctures include abnormalities adjacent to major vessels, the hilum of the spleen, and the mediastinum (Fig. 46-5). Certainly, visualization of small lesions may be first attempted using other modalities (but most authors agree that successful punctures on the first attempt are more likely with CT guidance). Any procedure that fails with other modalities should be attempted using CT.

CT should be used when avoidance of intestinal loops or vascular structures is important. We believe such avoidance is advisable in several situations. In immunologically compromised patients, we believe that CT procedures should be used to avoid penetration of the bowel

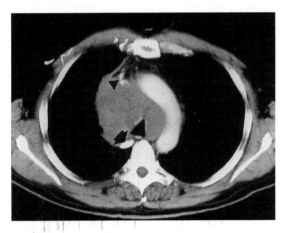

Fig. 46-5. This CT scan of the chest shows a large mass in the middle mediastinum that is displacing the aortic arch to the left. Note the opacification of the aortic arch, azygous vein, arrow, and venous collaterals in the anterior mediastinum, arrowhead. The lesion can only be safely biopsied by CT (see later section on lung biopsies).

and possible contamination (even with the skinny needle). Even in immunocompetent patients, if the abnormality to be punctured is a fluid density, we believe penetration of the bowel should be avoided (see section on pyogenic contamination) (Fig. 46-6, A and B). A variety of approaches can be used to avoid bowel because the bowel can be seen and patient position can be varied (Fig. 46-7, A and B). A recent advance (discussed later) has been the use of carbon dioxide or other gas to move various loops of bowel (Fig. 46-8).

When a large cutting-needle biopsy is clinically indicated, CT is usually the modality of choice. Even though fluoroscopy or ultrasound can be used safely in some cases, CT is the best guidance modality because it eliminates the two most likely errors: (1) inappropriate biopsy of uninvolved organs (e.g., gallbladder, vessels), and (2) inappropriate biopsy of abnormalities with increased vascularity. The accurate display of abnormalities as well as any normal structures that may be displaced prevents inadvertent puncture. Bolus dynamic scanning is accepted by virtually all authors as being very accurate for the assessment of vascularity (see Fig. 46-11). It is as accurate as digital subtraction because both use the same detector principles and computer enhancement.

CT may also be a modality of choice when some type of contrast agent such as urographic contrast or air is to be injected. Such contrast can provide additional information about cysts, abscess, pseudocysts, or dissemination of medication.

GENERAL COMPLICATIONS OF CT PROCEDURES

A number of possible complications are specific to the various organ systems, but some general concepts are relevant to all areas. Because of the advantages of CT procedures the possibilities of complications are signifi-

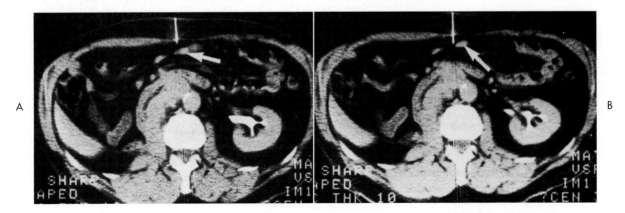

Fig. 46-6. A, First needle pass in patient shows needle approaching small loop of bowel *(arrow)*. **B,** Notice how the loop of the bowel *(arrow)* has moved away and changed configuration, presumably because of irritation from the needle. In some patients movement of the bowel will prevent penetration by a needle.

cantly reduced. If proper CT techniques are used, the major causes of complications are limited to poor technique, lack of patient cooperation, undetected coagulopathy, or undiagnosed obstructive or diffuse interstitial processes in the lung.

Before discussing in detail how to avoid certain problems, several comments are in order concerning complications as they relate to the two major categories of instruments: the aspirating, or skinny-needle, biopsy, and the large cutting needles. Contrary to the opinions of others, severe complications may occur with any needle (including the skinny needle, manual cutting

needles, and the automated biopsy guns) unless one exercises caution, common sense, and meticulous technique.

Skinny-needle complications

There is no question that the skinny needle is the safest instrument available, but even this needle can produce complications in selected circumstances. For example, one can find in a careful review of reports of skinny-needle biopsies of the pancreas instances of pancreatitis, pancreatic fistula, cholangitis, needle-tract seeding, significant hemorrhage, abscess formation, and fatal

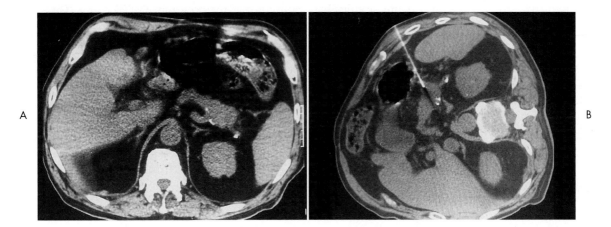

Fig. 46-7. A, CT scan shows patient with pancreatic mass in the tail. There is very little space between the wall of the stomach and the spleen. **B,** With the patient in the right decubitus position, the stomach shifts slightly producing sufficient space between the spleen and stomach to permit passage of the needle for the biopsy.

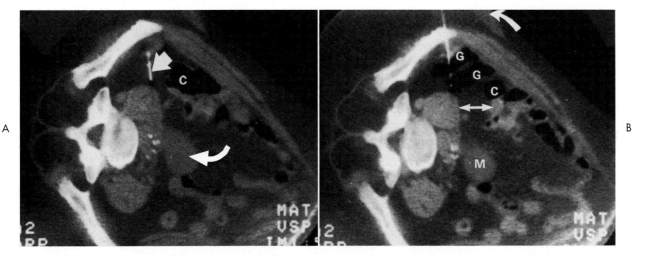

Fig. 46-8. A, CT scan of a patient lying on the left side who has a cystic mass *(curved arrow)* at the root of the mesentery. The pathway to the mass is blocked by the cecum, *c.* A needle *(arrow)* was inserted in the retroperitoneum to insufflate the gas. **B,** After the injection of carbon dioxide, the "gas", *G,* displaces the cecum, *c,* anteriorly and opening the pathway *(arrows)* to the mass, *m.* Another needle was inserted for the aspiration using a different entrance site *(curved arrow).*

pancreatitis. An awareness of these potential problems should not be a deterrent to performing such procedures but instead should be an incentive to eliminate complications, even with the relatively safe skinny needle.

Most complications have occurred with skinny needles when lesions have been very vascular or when numerous needle passes have been made. The reported fatalities from liver and adrenal hemorrhage occurred with apparently vascular hemangioma and pheochromocytoma. One can see in reviewing the literature that most complications have occurred in those cases with four to five needle passes.

This viewpoint about limiting the number of passes and minimizing risks even with skinny needles is shared by another expert interventionist, Dr. Ed Smith of the University of Massachusetts.[269] Dr. Smith, in his recent chapter on the risk of fine-needle biopsy, reported on the results of a survey mailed to 100 university hospitals and every fifth hospital with more than 200 beds. In this survey he noted the occurrence of 4 deaths, 27 cases of hemorrhage, 3 occurrences of needle-tract seeding, and 16 cases of generalized infections (nonfatal). In his conclusion Dr. Smith made a statement with which I agree completely: "It is logical to assume that the number of complications should be related to the number of needle passes made during the biopsy procedure." Furthermore, he states: "However, serious and even fatal complications, although rare, can and do occur and it is important to be aware of the possibility and take all the appropriate precautions in order to reduce their incidence."

Cutting-needle complications

With large needles one obviously has a greater probability of incurring many possible complications because a large "hole" is being produced. It is quite apparent, however, that with meticulous technique the potential risks of these needles can be offset that and very low complication rates can be achieved.

A recent alarming trend in regard to the large needles is that some authors who advocate their use have become somewhat "cavalier" about potential complications. One must pay very careful attention to meticulous technique, or serious and even fatal complications will result. Indeed, it is likely that in the near future, unnecessary and serious complications related to the large needles will be reported. It is my hope that individuals who are now starting to use these needles will seriously adhere to the cautionary advice of experienced interventionists.

It is especially important to note that the new automated cutting devices are no safer than the standard Tru-Cut needle that has been used for many years. The speed of cutting has no effect on the local damage produced to tissue and thereby the potential risk from such a procedure. In the first report about the biopsy "gun," the authors reported a serious hemorrhagic complication following a liver biopsy. Potential problems are minimized by CT guidance and a careful, meticulous technique such as I have described. These measures can eliminate many potential causes of complications (e.g., hemorrhage, or inadvertent penetration of an uninvolved organ) and can result in excellent accuracy with few problems.

Hemorrhage

The most likely potential risk during any biopsy procedure is the occurrence of bleeding. The vascularity of the pathologic lesion, as well as the anatomy, occurrence rate, and risk of bleeding are specific for each organ system; these factors will be discussed in relation to each organ system. For example, lesions of the liver that are highly vascular, such as hepatomas, sarcomas, or hemangiomas,[121] potentially have a high incidence of serious hemorrhage unless meticulous methods are used. Generalized statistics that combine rates for multiple organ systems (e.g., liver, pancreas, lung) are not relevant to the modern approach to biopsies.

Obviously, to avoid complications one must ensure that a patient does not have any bleeding coagulopathy and that the laboratory values are within acceptable ranges. Several animal studies by our group[74,71,73] evaluated the effect of needle caliber, type, prothrombin time, and platelet counts. In those studies platelet function appeared to be even a more important factor than prothrombin time. With either abnormal platelets or prothrombin time, it was shown that there was a considerable difference between needles less than 16 gauge and those greater than 16 gauge. I prefer that the prothrombin time be within 2 seconds of normal, with the partial prothrombin time within 25% of normal and the platelet count greater than 50,000. In some critical clinical circumstances exceptions can be made, but with such variances the potential risk is greater. The attendant risks and associated precautions should be understood by all involved (patient and physicians), and appropriate contingencies must be made.

Patient cooperation

One cause of complications common to all procedures and not eliminated by CT is lack of patient cooperation. If a patient moves or cannot suspend respiration at the appropriate time, difficulties may arise. The most critical factor in enhancing patient cooperation is adequate local anesthesia in the area of the biopsy. Local anesthesia should be administered down to the serosal surface of the organ (e.g., pleura, capsule). If this area is not anesthetized the patient may "jerk" at the time of insertion and produce a tear, bleed, or pneumothorax.

For those patients who are emotionally upset, administration of an appropriate hypnotic or sedative can be quite helpful. Dosages of such drugs vary widely, and local sedation policies should be followed.

Pyogenic contamination

Contamination of sterile areas is possible from either a cutaneous source or, if a loop of bowel is penetrated, an enteric source. If betadyne is used for preparation of the skin, cutaneous contamination is improbable. Contamination from bowel can occur, depending on the immune status of the patient, the nature of the abnormality, the size of the pyogenic inoculum, and the virulence of the pathogens. Interventionists who advocate traversing bowel with impunity should be regarded with a slight amount of skepticism.

It is true that an immunocompetent patient can tolerate spillage of a small amount of bacteria within the peritoneum, but the clearance of bacteria is impaired in certain circumstances. If bacteria are introduced into a fluid space, experimental data show that the effectiveness of bacterial "killing" is impaired because (1) "opsonization" of pyogens by antibodies and complement is less efficient in a fluid space, and (2) phagocyte-clearing activity is impaired in a fluid space, depending on physical spatial considerations and the probabilities of random particle encounters.[285] Moreover, an immunocompromised patient is obviously at a greater risk from pyogenic organisms because of the reduced number or function of immunologic cells.[161]

This concern about bacterial contamination from percutaneous procedures is well founded. A number of secondary infections have occurred and been reported in the literature. One reported case of peritonitis was produced in an elderly woman after penetration of the colon by a skinny needle during a lymph-node biopsy.[247] In his survey Smith accumulated 16 cases of generalized bacteremia occurring from aspiration biopsy that were treated by antibiotics.[247c]

For these reasons I modify my technique in several circumstances to eliminate or lessen the potential risk of bacterial contamination. If the mass is solid in an immunocompetent patient, I will accept a trajectory crossing bowel; a small inoculum of bacteria is no match for the normal immune system. (Practically speaking, it is difficult to penetrate bowel unless one actually tries to because the bowel will move away from the needle.) If the lesion being sampled is cystic, I insist on avoidance of bowel for the reasons stated above. Passage through bowel also would be counterproductive when fluid is being aspirated for culture from cystic masses because of possible spurious results from contamination.

If the patient is known to be immunocompromised, I will avoid traversing colon or small bowel in all cases. In such cases I prefer to cancel the procedure rather than put the patient at risk.

Avoidance of bowel in any of the cases noted above can usually be achieved by changing the position of the patient; this may result in a "shifting" of the bowel that may open clear pathways for needle insertion (see Figs. 46-7, *A* and *B*). In other cases, injection of carbon dioxide may be used to move bowel loops (see Fig. 46-8).

Vasovagal and hysterical reactions

Interventionists not familiar with vasovagal or hysterical reactions cannot diagnose or properly treat them. Both of these events, which are relatively common, must be dealt with properly and expeditiously to prevent physiologic sequelae or inappropriate iatrogenic intervention.

The vasovagal reaction is a sudden discharge of the parasympathetic vagal nerve, resulting in bradycardia, vasodilatation and hypotension. Such patients appear pale and ashen gray in color and may be partially responsive or unresponsive. The appearance is not unlike that of a patient who has had a cardiopulmonary arrest. Close inspection of the patient will show the presence of bradycardia, diaphoresis, dilated pupils, and hypotension. Treatment of this event should be tailored to the severity of the situation. The patient should first be put in a Trendelenburg position to enhance venous return to the heart and cerebral blood flow. The patient must not sit upright; the hypotension will be worsened. If the patient improves within 1 to 2 minutes, no other action need be taken.

However, if the patient does not improve quickly, oxygen should be administered by nasal cannula and an appropriate dose of atropine, either intramuscularly or intravenously, should be administered. Before administration of the drug, a quick review of the patient's clinical notes is appropriate; patients with cardiac arrhythmias may be quite sensitive to the drug. A single intravenous dose of 0.5 mg or 1 mg will usually restore the normal heart rate. If the patient's condition persists (that is, if the atropine does not improve the situation), urgent consultation with a resuscitation team is appropriate. Such patients, especially the elderly, can develop a complete heart block, vascular collapse, and cardiac arrest if not properly treated.

The other event, which is more spectacular but fortunately less dangerous, is a hysterical reaction. Such patients appear agitated, tremulous, and may be crying. Close inspection of the patient may demonstrate tachycardia and systolic hypertension; the pupils will be of normal size or smaller. Such patients may be breathing fast and may complain subjectively of shortness of breath. After auscultation of the chest confirms good air exchange, the best treatment is to have the patient breathe into his or her hands or into a bag to prevent hyperventilation and subsequent fainting. If hyperventilation occurs, the patient may become alkalotic and faint because of constriction of the cerebral vessels. The next step is to give the patient gentle but firm reassurance; if there is no response, the patient should be removed from the biopsy suite. Before any repeat attempt, the patient should receive an appropriate sedative. Careful assessment of all biopsy patients during the informed consent period will usually indicate those who need sedation, thereby preventing any such hysterical reaction.

Tumor recurrence in needle pathway

Growth of residual tumor cells tracked through needle pathways is a potential but fortunately rare problem. A guidance cannula in the skin will stop tracking in the skin, but of course this will not stop any deeper seeding. In reality, most tumors are inoperative when they are biopsied, but if there is a possibility of curative resection, a trajectory should be chosen that will permit resection of the needle track by the surgeon.

There are four systems that should be discussed: lung, kidney, pancreas, and musculoskeletal tumors. In the lung the question of tracking in the tract is often raised, but occurrences are rare. Indeed, only a few cases of seeding have been reported. Considering the thousands of such procedures performed, the incidence, as noted by Wolinsky,[284] is very low. We have never encountered a tumor implant in any of our cases, but we have observed one from an outside institution (Fig. 46-9).

Needle tracking of renal tumors is a frequently mentioned potential problem by some colleagues in urol-

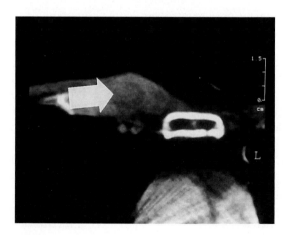

Fig. 46-9. Enlarged view of the chest wall shows a tumor implant *(arrow)* to the left of the sternum from a previous lung biopsy from an outside hospital. (Courtesy of Dr. Julie Clayman, Cleveland, Ohio.)

ogy, but it is actually a rare occurrence. However, I am familiar with only one case of needle tract seeding, reported from the Mason Clinic following aspiration with an 18-gauge needle. However, there is overwhelming evidence that seeding is not a problem with such a tumor. Von Schreeb et al[272] reported a controlled series of about 150 cases of proven renal cell carcinoma used to study the impact of needle aspiration. One half of these cases were aspirated and one half were not. In all, there were no instances of needle tract seeding. Furthermore, the difference in recurrence, morbidity, and survival was actually better in the biopsy group.

The pancreas has had a surprisingly frequent rate of tumor seeding, compared with the kidney or lung. There have been two reported cases[60,237] of skin seeding with this pancreas tumor. Considering that there have been only several hundred cases reported in the literature, this is a relatively high frequency compared with the frequency associated with the lung or kidney. Tumor seeding in patients with pancreatic cancer is not a significant clinical problem because they are invariably incurable.

The last group of cases that have a possible incidence of seeding are those involving musculoskeletal tumors. Until more experience is gained with percutaneous biopsy of these tumors, one must exercise caution and make a special selection of entry point in collaboration with the orthopedic surgeon. In my practice, I contact the referring orthopedic physician for each procedure to choose an entry point so that the needle pathway can be resected at the time of surgery.

NEEDLE SELECTION

A clinical decision about the biopsy must first be made according to the type of information sought by the attending physician from the pathologic sample. Generally, if a patient has a known malignancy and only a confirmation of metastases or recurrence is desired, an aspiration biopsy with a skinny needle is all that is required. If a patient has an unknown problem or if a question of a second malignancy exists, a large–cutting-needle biopsy is indicated (assuming laboratory, clinical, or anatomic information does not preclude a safe procedure). Only a sample with such a needle can accurately make the diagnosis of a lymphoma, benign tumor, or an unusual tumor.

If a clinical decision is made to use a large needle, consideration of clinical, laboratory, anatomic, and dynamic scan information should be made. Clinically, there must be no history of a coagulopathy, and the patient must not be on any type of medication that would impair coagulation or platelet function (see section on patient preparation).

Careful consideration of the anatomy, from a recent or current baseline CT obtained during the planning of the procedure, is appropriate. A large needle can be used if clear access is available to the organ of the abnormality (i.e., no intervening uninvolved structure or close proximity of the aorta, vena cava, portal vein, or bowel). As experience is gained, skill increases and one's safety tolerance relative to anatomy improves. For example, while a novice might be fearful of biopsying a node several centimeters from the aorta, an experienced person will be quite comfortable biopsying some lesions that abut the aorta.

With all of the recent enthusiasm expressed about

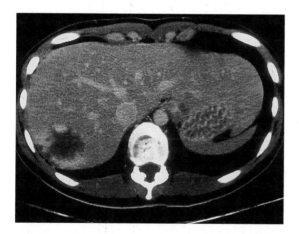

Fig. 46-10. Scan of a patient with hemangioma of the liver, taken during a bolus injection of contrast material. Note the increased enhancement of the margin of the hemangioma. There has been a report of a death following biopsy of such a hemangioma (see text).

the automated cutting-needle devices, there has been little attention given to assessing the vascular nature of an abnormality before a biopsy. In my experience and study of biopsies, complications are multifactorial in nature, and tumor vascularity is one of the most important parameters (Fig. 46-10). For example, there are a number of reported serious complications relating to skinny needles, all of which have occurred in vascular tumors such as hemangiomas and hepatomas (see liver section). When tumors are seen as very vascular on CT, one should certainly avoid biopsy with cutting needles and should even use a gentle technique with aspiration needles.

In our previous book I expressed the importance of the bolus dynamic scan of the target lesions. This technique is less frequently needed now because of current methods of contrast administration. In most cases, patients are examined with high doses of contrast material administered by mechanical injectors and any increased vascularity of abnormalities is clearly demonstrated (Fig. 46-10). Visualization of the margins of normal vessels, aneurysms, and the presence of collateral vessels is also quite easy with these methods (Figs. 46-11, 46-12).

If for some reason adequate contrast enhancement is not obtained on the diagnostic study, a bolus dynamic scan over the area of the abnormality is appropriate. In such cases a series of scans are taken at the same anatomic area while contrast material is infused rapidly through a peripheral vein. The larger the needle or catheter used the better; an 18-gauge needle is optimal. At least 50 cc of contrast material should be injected rap-

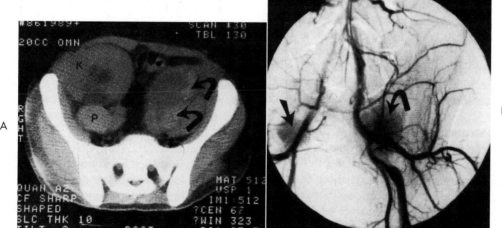

Fig. 46-11. A, A bolus dynamic scan through the pelvis demonstrates a suspected pseudoaneurysm, *P,* on the right behind a renal transplant, *K.* There was also an unsuspected pseudoaneurysm on the left, which shows irregular enhancement *(curved arrows).* **B,** Digital subtraction angiogram shows the suspected pseudoaneurysm on the right *(arrow)* and confirms the unsuspected pseudoaneurysm on the left *(curved arrow).*

idly over several seconds, and a series of scans over 10 to 15 seconds should be obtained.

With bolus dynamic scanning, vessels and abnormal vascularity can be demonstrated. Prudence dictates that any intervening blood vessels should be avoided. Fi-

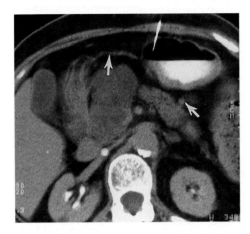

Fig. 46-12. CT scan of patient with cystic tumor of the pancreas. Note the large vessels adjacent to the stomach *(arrow)* and in front of the pancreas. An appropriate pathway through the stomach was chosen (see needle penetrating stomach wall).

nally, any tumors or abnormality that shows considerable vascularity should only be biopsied carefully by an aspiration needle and not by a cutting needle.

Aspirating needles versus cutting needles

In recent years, with the advent of CT and the use of large cutting needles, there has been some controversy about the diagnostic yields and complication rates of aspiration needles (needles without a sharpened edge or margin to cut tissue) and cutting needles (generally larger needles with a modified sharpened tip or cutting gap on the side). It is my opinion that both types of instruments can be used safely and effectively if appropriate techniques are used (Figs. 46-13, 46-14).

Three basic arguments have been offered against the use of the larger needles and in favor of the skinny needle.[135] First, some have asserted that the skinny needle is so safe that it requires little attention to technique and can be used almost with impunity. Second, the complication rate of the cutting needles is too high and risks are too great. Third, cytologic results of the skinny needle are adequate for diagnosing virtually all abnormalities, and there is no diagnostic advantage with larger cutting needles.

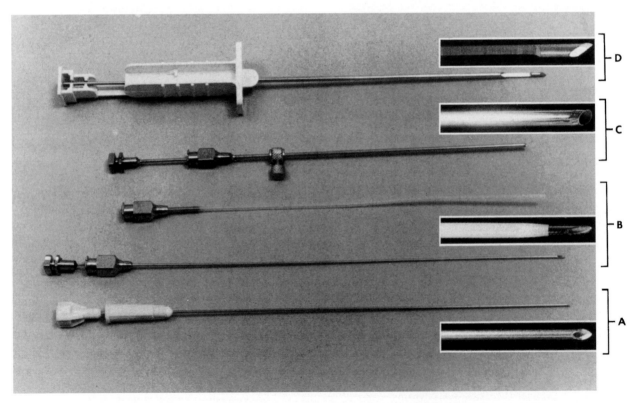

Fig. 46-13. Picture of the four needles used. Inserts show the needle tip of each instrument. The 20-gauge Chiba needle, *A,* is used for aspiration biopsies. The 19-gauge needle with the 18-gauge sheath, *B,* is used for aspiration of fluid collections. The Menghini-type needle, *C,* is used for cutting biopsies of "hard" lesions. The 14-gauge Tru-Cut, *D,* is used for biopsy of most tumors.

As more procedures have been performed over the years, extensive experience has now been reported to show that these arguments are not valid. As seen in the earlier general section on complications, the incidence of complications with skinny needles is higher than previously believed. For this reason, responsible authors are now recommending a more conservative approach for the use of the skinny needle and a limit to the number of needle passes.

With careful techniques, the complication rates of the cutting needle are quite acceptable and compare favorably with the skinny needle. Using our techniques as described in this chapter, there is only a very slight difference between the complication rate of the skinny needle and that of the cutting needles, 0.6% versus 1.0%.[91] As can be noted in the earlier section on historical aspects, even Lundquist,[174,175] who was the first advocate of skinny needles, reported 1,000 cases of biopsy with a cutting needle with no serious complications.

As for the assertion that cytologic results yield accurate results with all abnormalities, it is clearly not correct (Tables 46-1, 46-2, 46-3). While abundant evidence exists supporting the usefulness of the skinny needle for epithelial tumors, careful review of the literature results in an awareness that most authors recognize the prob-

lem of providing a definitive diagnosis for lymphomas, unusual tumors, or benign abnormalities. Furthermore, although some centers claim their results are superior because of the unique quality of their cytopathologists, virtually every center that has ever compared cytologic results with histologic results have shown a superiority of the cutting needle samples. One should not confuse these results with those reported in early articles showing that cytologic smears taken in conjunction with histologic samples improve the results. The cytologic information obtained is additive and thus does not prove superiority of cytologic information over the histologic samples.[7]

Finally, most authors who claim the superiority of the skinny needle over the large needle and who attest to the danger of cutting needles are not familiar with the literature, and they have not used these devices. With regard to accuracy and complications, these authors use either old information based on blind studies or indirect comparisons rather than current comparison work on CT-guided procedures. Current articles reporting experience with guided procedures and modern techniques show a very favorable complication rate with the cutting needles. Because of these favorable results, numerous authors now advocate the use of the cutting needles even with ultrasound and mammography.[128]

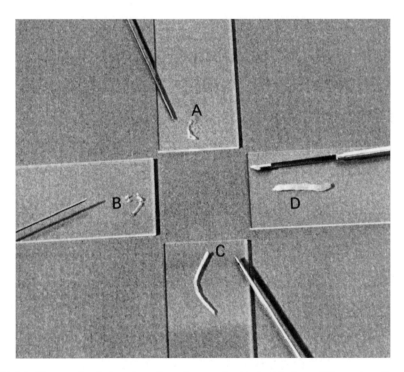

Fig. 46-14. Type and relative size of specimens obtained with four different needles. Specimen *A* was obtained with three passes of the 22-gauge skinny-core needle using 30 cc of suction and a 2 cm insertion of the needle. Specimen *B* was obtained in one pass of an 18-gauge bevel-end needle using 30 cc of suction and a 2 cm insertion of the needle. Specimen *C* was obtained with an 18-gauge Menghini needle using 30 cc of suction and a 2 cm insertion of the needle. Specimen *D* was obtained with the Tru-Cut needle and no suction.

Table 46-1. Malignant lesion in patients with single biopsy

	Cutting biopsy			Aspiration biopsy		
	Correct			Correct		
Diagnosis	Specific	Nonspecific	Incorrect	Specific	Nonspecific	Incorrect
Metastasis (83)	42/47	1/47	4/47	49/59	2/59	8/59
Hepatoma (9)	6/7		1/7	2/4		2/4
Lymphoma (4)	4/4					1/1
Hemangioendothelioma (2)	2/2			1/2		1/2
Mesenchymal Sarcoma (1)	1/1					
Cholangioca (1)						1/1
Subtotal (100)	55/61 (90.2%)	1/61 (1.6%)	5/61 (8.2%)	52/67 (77.6%)		13/67 (19.4%)
Total	56/61 (91.8%)		5/61 (8.2%)	58/67 (80.6%)	2/67 (3.0%)	(19.4%)

From Ha HK, Sachs PB, Haaga JR, Abdul-Karin F: CT-guided liver biopsy: an update. *Clin Imaging* 15:99-104, 1991.

Table 46-2. Benign lesion in patients with single biopsy

	Cutting biopsy			Aspiration biopsy		
	Correct			Correct		
Diagnosis	Specific	Nonspecific	Incorrect	Specific	Nonspecific	Incorrect
Fatty metamorphosis (11)	8	1		2	4	
Liver cirrhosis (4)	3			2	1	
Hepatitis (31)	3					
Focal hepatocellular necrosis (2)	2					
Infarct (2)					2	
Primary biliary cirrhosis (2)	2					
Fibrosis in wedge resection site (1)	3					1*
Nonspecific benign lesion (6)	1	1			3	3†
Normal (3)	1			1		
Hemangioma (6)	23/26(88.5%)			3	3	
Cyst (11)**	26/26 (100%)	1		4	3	
Abscess (16)††				1		
Subtotal		3/26 (11.5%)		13/33 (39.4%)	16/33 (48.5%)	4/33(12.1%)
Total				29/33(87.9%)		4/33(12.1%)

*Four cases are unsatisfactory.

†Nonspecific benign lesion represents the benign lesion in clinical follow-up, although specific diagnosis cannot be made pathologically.

**Three cases were performed with 19-gauge Longdwell needle.

††Fourteen cases were performed with 19-gauge Longdwell needle.

From Ha HK, Sachs PB, Haaga JR, Abdul-Karim F: CT-guided liver biopsy: an update. *Clin Imaging* 15:99-104, 1991.

Selection of aspiration needle

There are various opinions about the optimal caliber and tip configuration of aspiration needles to be used for aspiration biopsy. A review of that data is very informative.

Two types of information, laboratory and clinical, suggest that the larger the caliber of the aspiration needle the better the results. In a laboratory study by Andriole et al,[6] our group showed that the larger the caliber of the needle the more diagnostic tissue was obtained. Also in that study we showed that if the angle of the bevel is varied, the small angle provided the most diagnostic tissue (Tables 46-4). The bevel of the Chiba needle (25 degrees) actually provides the best sample. Recent au-

Table 46-3. Patients with cutting and aspiration biopsies

Diagnosis	Cutting biopsy			Aspiration biopsy		
	Correct			Correct		
	Specific	Nonspecific	Incorrect	Specific	Nonspecific	Incorrect*
Metastasis (26)	23			21	1	4
Hepatoma (2)	1				1	1
Lymphoma (1)	1		3			1
Hemangiomaendothelioma (2)	2		1	1		1
Normal (1)	1			1		
Fatty infiltration (4)	4			1	3	
Liver cirrhosis (2)	2			2		
Hemangioma (1)	1				1	
Unknown benign lesion (1)		1				1
Subtotal malignant (31) Total	27/31 (87.1%)			22/31 (71.0%)	2/31 (6.5%)	7/31 (22.5%)
Subtotal benign (9)	8/9 (88.9%)			4/9 (44.4%)	4/9 (44.4%)	2/9 (11.1%)
Total benign	9/9 (100%)	2/9 (11.1%)	4/31 (12.9%)	8/9 (88.4%)		2/9 (11.1%)

*In "Incorrect," unsatisfactory are included.

From Ha HK, Sachs PB, Haaga JR, Abdul-Karim F: CT-guided liver biopsy: an update. *Clin Imaging* 15:99-104, 1991.

thors[44] have reconfirmed the results of this study and have recommended the Chiba needle tip for such biopsies.

In the direct clinical comparisons[105,221] of different sizes of aspiration needles, the larger needles provided more diagnostic information without any increase in the complication rate. This has been proved in the liver, lung, and pancreas and in one animal model (Table 46-5). Pagani[221] showed that for aspiration biopsies of the liver the 18-gauge needle provided more diagnostic tissue than did the smaller 22-gauge needle, with no difference in complications.

In the lung, various authors have used all different sizes of needles, from 23-gauge to 18-gauge, with no difference in pneumothorax rate or apparent accuracy. Such studies by various institutions are difficult to compare because of differences in patient selection and techniques. There is a higher hemoptysis rate for needles larger than 20 gauge, as reported by Khouri.[153]

In the pancreas, Dickey et al[48] of our group compared the 22-gauge needle with the 20-gauge needle and showed that the diagnostic return was better with the 20-gauge needle, with no difference in complication. Complications occurring from needle aspirations of the pancreas appear to be the result of poor targeting, approach, or too many needle passes.

Based on these data, I have reduced the number of needles in my department and now use the 20-gauge Chiba aspiration needle for all aspiration biopsies. This needle is well suited because it can be used without dif-ficulty in most organs including lung, liver, bowel, pancreas, or other organs.

Choice of cutting needles

There are two basic types of cutting needles that can be used to obtain samples. They are available in a variety of sizes. The end-cutting Menghini needle and the side cutting Tru-Cut needles are the prototypes of these devices. In my previous chapter, we described the use of these two needles as almost interchangeable for most tumors; at this time, however, and with only a few exceptions, I definitely prefer the Tru-Cut needle for almost all cutting biopsy procedures. Occasionally, I use the Menghini for tumors that are very hard, especially those within bone. The second circumstance in which I use the Menghini needle is for those cases in which a mass is deep and access too limited to permit use of a side-cutting needle.

With the popularization of the True-Cut needle, a variety of needle calibers have become available, including 20-gauge, 18-gauge, and 14-gauge. There are several intuitive conclusions could be made concerning the utility of these various sizes, but one should resist assumptions until reliable data have been reported. The first assumption one might make is that the 20-gauge needle can be used in many high-risk circumstances without the attendant risk of bleeding. The occurrence of bleeding depends on many factors, however, and needle caliber is only one. To amplify this point, I would like to note that we used a 20-gauge cutting needle in one pa-

Table 46-4. Comprehensive quantitative comparison*

Needles	Type of needle	Average weight of sample (mg)
22-gauge	Chiba	4.1 ± 0.1 S.D.
	30-degree bevel	4.0 ± 0.1 S.D.
	45-degree bevel	3.3 ± 0.1 S.D.
	90-degree bevel	2.8 ± 0.2 S.D.
	Franseen	5.0 ± 0.2 S.D.
	CSI fine lung	5.4 ± 0.4 S.D.
21-gauge	90-degree bevel	5.7 ± 0.3 S.D.
20-gauge	30-degree bevel	7.6 ± 0.2 S.D.
	45-degree bevel	7.0 ± 0.2 S.D.
	90-degree bevel	5.8 ± 0.2 S.D.
	Franseen	10.4 ± 0.6 S.D.
	CSI fine lung	10.3 ± 0.4 S.D.
19-gauge	30-degree bevel	12.5 ± 0.6 S.D.
	90-degree bevel	10.8 ± 0.2 S.D.
18-gauge	30-degree bevel	16.2 ± 1.3 S.D.
	30-degree bevel†	16.0 ± 0.3 S.D.
	45-degree bevel	14.8 ± 0.2 S.D.
	45-degree bevel†	15.1 ± 0.8 S.D.
	60-degree bevel	15.3 ± 0.3 S.D.
	90-degree bevel	14.6 ± 0.5 S.D.
	90-degree bevel†	14.3 ± 0.1 S.D.
	Franseen	20.0 ± 0.9 S.D.
	Lee	19.3 ± 0.4 S.D.
17-gauge	45-degree bevel	17.9 ± 1.0 S.D.
16-gauge	30-degree bevel	37.3 ± 2.4 S.D.
	45-degree bevel	37.6 ± 1.2 S.D.
	60-degree bevel	39.1 ± 3.1 S.D.
	Franseen	39.0 ± 0.2 S.D.
Rotex		1.9 ± 0.6 S.D.
Travenol Tru-Cut		59.4 ± 3.7 S.D.

*Three samples were taken from the same liver specimen with each needle.
†Modified Menghini needle.

Table 46-5. Separation of means of biopsy blood loss data by needle gauges

Target organ	Groupings of needle gauges	P value
Liver		
No warfarin	(14) (16) (18,20,22)	<0.01
Warfarin	(14) (16) (18,20,22)	<0.01
Kidney		
No warfarin	(18,20,22)	NS*
Warfarin	(18,20) (22)	<0.05

Note: Groupings within a single set of parentheses taken as equal, versus those grouped those in other parentheses.
*NS = not significant.
From Gazelle GS, Haaga JR, Rowland DY: Effect of needle gauge, level of anticoagulation, and target organ on bleeding associated with aspiration biopsy. *Radiology* 183:509-513, 1992.

Table 46-6. Summary statistics based on raw data

Needle configuration	Drug treatment	No. of procedures	Mean blood loss (g) ± SD
Tru-Cut only	None	32	2.46 ± 1.37
	Venopirin	30	4.60 ± 1.71
PPS	None	21	0.31 ± 0.15
	Venopirin	27	0.61 ± 0.28
Thrombin-coated PPS	None	14	0.11 ± 0.06
	Venopirin	24	0.23 ± 0.14

Note: The statistics are based on raw data for blood loss caused by liver biopsy performed with differently configured biopsy needles in pigs, with or without venopirin treatment. From Gazelle GS, Haaga JR, Halpern EF: Hemostatic protein polymer sheath: improvement in hemostasis are percutaneous biopsy in the setting of platelet dysfunction. *Radiology* 187:269-272, 1993.

tient and observed a very severe hemorrhage that was life threatening (many blood transfusions, days in intensive care, and a laparotomy). The cause of the bleeding happened to be amputation of a small artery during the procedure; the biopsy sample showed the small artery in the histology sample. There has recently been reported[70,74] a new device called the PPS (protein polymer sheath) that potentially may lessen the possibility of bleeding with such cutting needles (Table 46-6).

Before making conclusions, other questions that might be asked are how large of a sample is needed to make a diagnosis, and what are the relative risks to the patient. There are no absolute answers to these questions, but some insights can be gained by reviewing the recent literature, our experience, and some recent laboratory work.

The size of sample required is dependent on the organ being biopsied and the diagnoses being considered. For example, in the biopsy of the kidney for diffuse renal disease, as advocated by Hopper[113] an 18-gauge sample, which is 2 cm in length, is consistently adequate for the pediatric age group. On the other hand, in adults our renal pathology experts prefer a sample from a 14-gauge needle because they believe they do not get sufficient glomeruli with the smaller needle.

The relative benefit and risk of each needle and its associated sample size are difficult to determine, but Plecha and Goodwin at our institution studied this question in the laboratory in an in vitro pig model. In an animal with normal coagulation, the amount of bleeding as a ratio of the amount of diagnostic tissue was the same for 20-, 18-, and 14-gauge Tru-Cut needles. An evaluation of these needles in an anticoagulated state has yet to be performed.

PREPROCEDURAL STEPS

Patient consent and history

Before the procedure and the administration of any tranquilizer medication, it is important to discuss the procedure in depth with the patient. All details, including the rationale, medical alternatives, method of the procedure, sensations to be felt by the patient, and the postprocedural routine, should be mentioned. After this discussion the patient may sign the informed consent form and help confer about the need for any sedation.

During this time, one should also inquire about any medication that may alter coagulation or platelet function. The latter is especially important because platelet inhibitors are widely used and not described to patients as "blood thinners." Routine coagulation studies will not detect the presence or activity of platelet inhibitors. Laboratory work performed by our group has confirmed the serious alteration and risk of the coagulation status in patients on aspirin-like compounds.

For routine anxiety I prefer intramuscular Vistaril, Valium, or Versid, in the appropriate doses. For severe anxiety in a child, or with small children, I prefer intravenous Demerol or morphine in appropriate doses. These drugs should be given in small incremental amounts until the desired level of sedation is achieved. I prefer Demerol instead of diazepam derivatives because it can be immediately reversed by narcotic antagonists if necessary.

Laboratory studies

For routine aspiration procedures on a patient with no history of coagulopathy or medication, I request partial thromboplastin time, prothrombin time, and platelet count. If it were not for the litigious environment, I would not even obtain these studies for aspiration biopsies. For patients who are to have cutting biopsies I prefer the platelet count above 50,000, prothrombin time within 2 seconds of normal, and a partial thromboplastin time within 25%. If there is any suspicion of anemia, I order a hematocrit study. I will perform aspiration at almost any hematocrit level if the coagulation is normal, but I insist on a value of 32% for any type of cutting biopsy. Because of the demonstrated safety of CT-guided procedures, I no longer type and cross a patient for any blood products unless there is some unusual clinical circumstance.

Site and trajectory selection

Site and trajectory planning should be made after a review of the diagnostic scans. The entire procedure can be greatly expedited if one notes the location of the mass, plans the anatomic approach of the trajectory, and decides on the type of needle to be used before placing the patient on the table. In my opinion, a great amount of time is wasted because physicians do not plan ahead for each case but "make it up" as they go.

After the previous diagnostic scan has been reviewed and an appropriate slice has been selected, localization to that slice can be made from the longitudinal type of scan (e.g., Scoutview, Topogram, Synerview). These scans are referenced to the axial slices, making relocalization after quite easy. (Some groups have advocated the use of catheter mats or commercial products to aid localization and have found them useful.

Several general comments about site selection and pathway are appropriate. It is important to decide on a pathway that traverses the least amount of uninvolved tissue and that is also the least precarious in terms of possible complications. The concept of using a shortest line to the trajectory is valid; the less liver, lung, or other noninvolved organ crossed the less the possibility for a problem.

We prefer to avoid pathways that include major nerves or muscles. Involving such structures, which are very painful when traversed, makes it very difficult for a patient to cooperate. Common sense dictates that potential problem areas such as arteries and veins should be avoided. Muscles can be a nuisance because they are very vascular and can bleed locally. Also, when penetrated the muscles can be tightened purposely or unintentionally by the patient; this causes difficulty with needle placement. The trajectory of a needle can be changed by a muscle contraction. If a powerful muscle group (for example, the erector spinal or gluteal muscles) contracts, a needle can be bent (Fig. 46-15).

If an oblique approach is to be used, it may be helpful to place the patient in a lateral or oblique position. However, the patient should not be placed awkwardly in a position that cannot be held for a prolonged period of time.

In choosing the trajectory, one must decide whether to perform the procedure within the axis of the slice or outside the axis as an angled approach. If one is a neophyte, it is best to develop experience by choosing the entrance site in the same axial slices as the abnormality.

Skin preparation

Once the entrance site has been chosen, the skin is prepared with Betadine and a local anesthesic agent such as Xylocaine is administered. At the time of Xylocaine administration it is important to palpate the tissue carefully to ascertain the location of the ribs, cartilages, processes, etc., so that they can be avoided. This is true especially next to ribs, the sacrum, the scapula, or other

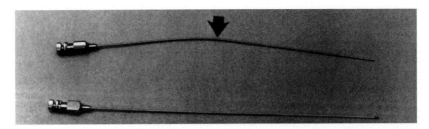

Fig. 46-15. Picture of a needle *(arrow)* that was bent by the erector spinae muscle in an uncooperative patient. Compare to the normal needle.

bony structures having a tapered edge or traversing the scan obliquely. Such structures produce a partial volume error in the CT scan that produces a discrepancy between their apparent location on the scan and their actual anatomic location.

When infiltrating local anesthetic, completely infiltrate the pathway in two steps. In the first step, infiltrate the skin, subcutaneous tissue, and the superficial muscles. After that level is reached, have the patient suspend respiration and then infiltrate the local anesthetic down to and including the pleura, peritoneum, or the capsule of the organ (e.g., kidney or liver). Such infiltrations should be made as the patient suspends respiration. If the capsule is not adequately anesthetized, the patient may "jerk" the diaphragm during the procedure. It is my opinion that inadequate administration of local anesthesia is the most common cause of poor patient cooperation. If a needle is inserted without anesthesia of the capsule, a "spinal-level reflex" occurs; this moves the organ and produces a potential lacerating effect. Adequate anesthesia is also most important with anxious patients because if they feel significant pain, they will not cooperate well.

CLINICAL NEEDLE TECHNIQUES

Since the first edition of this text we have decreased the number of needles that we use to four. We use a 20-gauge Chiba for aspiration of all suspected tumor masses, regardless of location. For aspiration of abscess fluid we use a 19-gauge needle with an 18-gauge Teflon sheath. We use one of two cutting needles, an end-cutting Menghini type or a side-cutting Tru-Cut needle, depending on the consistency of a tumor mass to be sampled. (A number of side-cutting needles in different sizes—14-gauge, 18-gauge, and 20-gauge—are now available). For all tumors except very hard ones we prefer the Tru-Cut type of needle. For tumors that are extremely hard and those that contain calcifications, we will use a Menghini type of needle because it is stronger and less likely to bend than are the Tru-Cut needles, which have a thin diameter at the gap of the stylet. There are basically four different placement techniques that can be used for aspiration needles: single needle, short can-

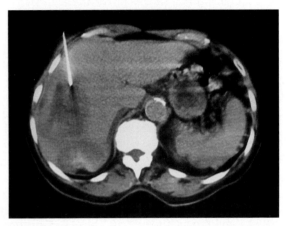

Fig. 46-16. Single needle can be used without cannula and accurate placement can still occur when the lesion is large or close to the surface. This scan shows large metastatic mass in liver being aspirated with 20-gauge Chiba needle.

nula coaxial method, long cannula coaxial method, and tandem needle technique.

Single-needle method

With this method, the needle is placed in the skin and subcutaneous tissue and incremental adjustments are made. Adjustments are made with changes in the angulation and sequential scans. Once the correct angulation is achieved, the needle is inserted to the appropriate depth until the needle tip is in the proper location (Fig. 46-16). This method is somewhat more difficult than the short cannula method because if the needle being used is long, the weight and length of the needle make it "hang." In such cases, the short length in the tissues will not support the weight of the needle, making determination of the angle before insertion into the tissues difficult. With the short cannula method as noted below, the short cannula makes angle adjustment easier before insertion of the long aspiration needle.

Short cannula coaxial method (formerly double needle)

I recommend using a short guidance cannula in most circumstances in the skin and subcutaneous tissues

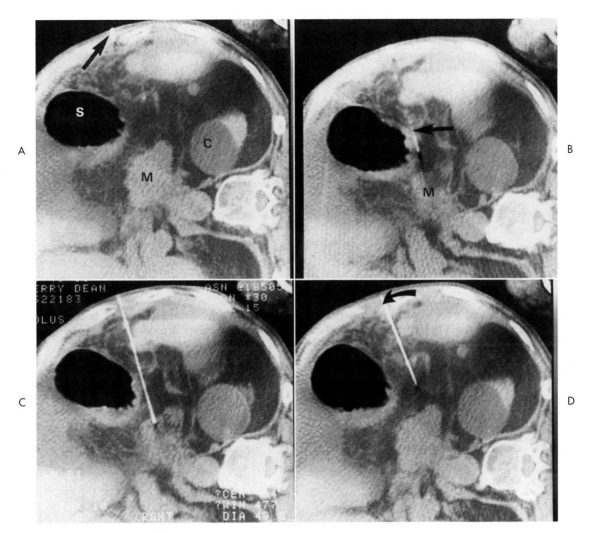

Fig. 46-17. A, Biopsy of a pancreatic mass using a guidance cannula is shown in these scans. This scan shows a pancreatic mass, *M,* in a patient who is in a right decubitus position. Also seen is the stomach, *S,* and a renal cyst, *C.* The guidance cannula *(arrow)* is located in the lateral abdominal wall. **B,** CT scan shows a needle *(arrow)* inserted through the guidance cannula and aimed toward the mass, *M.* **C,** Because the angle in **B** was correct, the needle was inserted further into the mass. **D,** By slightly angling the guidance cannula *(curved arrow),* the needle can be inserted in a different location. This scan shows a needle guided toward a more posterior portion of the mass. Compare with **C.**

to expedite and optimize needle placement. This method is well suited for lung biopsies and small, deeply located masses in the abdomen. For this method, I recommend a 16-gauge 1½ inch hypodermic needle as the cannula and the 20-gauge Chiba needle for the aspiration needle (Fig. 46-17). For those who prefer a 22-gauge Chiba, an 18 gauge hypodermic can be used.

The greatest advantage of this method is that the short guidance cannula predetermines the angle prior to the insertion of the aspiration needle. The angle of the guidance cannula, which is external to the body cavity, is adjusted until the trajectory is correct. Numerous adjustments in the angle can be made without injury to in-

ternal structures because the aspiration needle is not inserted until the correct angle is obtained. Once this is accomplished the aspiration needle is inserted and the only factor to contend with is the distance to the lesion, which can be incrementally adjusted. The cannula can provide access for several repeat biopsies if desired. If one wishes to sample slightly different areas of a mass, the cannula can intentionally be deviated to guide the aspiration needle to different parts of the mass.

Some minor caveats should be noted. The cannula (hypodermic needle) should only be inserted into the superficial structures without entering the body cavity. Too deep a placement could injure organs. Also, the cannula can be easily deviated, so care must be taken to avoid unintentional deviation of the cannula during insertion of the aspiration needle. This is my preferred method because of the safety of having the cannula external to the body cavity before biopsy and because of the flexibility of numerous aspirations, if desired.

Long-cannula coaxial method

Although the long-cannula method has been recommended by other authors, I do not commonly use this method. This method uses a long guidance cannula, which is inserted to the depth of the lesion. The long cannula, which has a large diameter of 18 gauge or greater, is positioned with the single-needle method as noted above. Once the larger cannula is positioned, many small needle aspirations are taken through it; no repositioning is required with each aspiration needle. The disadvantages are that a large needle is used to traverse the tissue, the single-needle method must be used, and the multiple aspirations are actually confined to a small area rather than being somewhat separated. A wider separation of the samples can be obtained by using either the short-cannula method (noted above) or the tandem-needle method noted below.

Tandem-needle method

This method uses numerous small-caliber needles for aspiration in a "shotgun" approach, as follows. Using the single-needle method, a skinny needle is positioned into the abnormality. After this is accomplished, the patient is removed from the scanner and numerous needles are positioned adjacent to the placed needle. The reputed advantages of this method include expeditious placement of many needles and a wide sampling of the abnormality. In view of recent data showing that numerous needle punctures results in complications, it is probably prudent to limit the number of needles to three.

ASPIRATION TECHNIQUE

After successful placement of the instrument within the lesion using any of the above methods, the following steps are taken. Ensure that the needle tip is definitely in the lesion and that circular and reciprocating motions are made during the application of suction (Fig. 46-18). For best results, limit the reciprocating motion to about a 1- to 2-cm distance. Try to keep at least 10 cc of suction applied during these motions, as discussed below.

The most critical factor after removal of the sample is the pathologic fixation of the material obtained. After the sample has been removed it should be ejected onto a slide, and a smear should be made with a second slide. Both sides should be quickly inserted into the appropriate fixative to prevent air-drying. Because there are so many variations in the types and methods of cytopathologic fixation, it is important to consult with pathologists about their preferred method. After fixing the slides, rinse the needle and the syringe with fixative and submit this to the pathology department for cytocentrifuge or filtration for preparation of a "cell block." The importance of these cell blocks was emphasized by Isler et al.[133] The cell block can at times provide some histologic information, although it lacks the stromal detail of an intact sample removed by a cutting type of needle. It is also important to note any clinical data or special stains requested of the cytopathologists.

Amount of suction

The optimal amount of suction needed to maximize sample recovery was evaluated by our group and others.[56,131,158] There are inconsistencies among these reports. Several authors have reported good success in clinical studies without using any suction.[56] Most authors believe suction is important, and two groups, ours[131] and Kreula,[158] have studied the problem in vitro. We found that at least 5 cc of displacement with the barrel of the syringe is required to obtain 84% of the obtainable sample, and 10 cc of displacement is required to obtain 94% of such a sample (Fig. 46-19). The report by Kreula[158] et al showed the relationship between sample obtained and vacuum applied in a straight line graph and was reported in absolute pressures, instead of the relative values of volume displacement in cubic centimeters as in our study.[131] The apparent inconsistency between their data and ours is that their entire data set consisted of measurements below "5 cc of suction." Stated differently, their graphs show less data than do ours and demonstrate only the straight-line portion seen before the curve becomes exponential.

Several points require clarification. First, although several authors have reported that no suction is required to obtain diagnostic tissue, these reports are not consistent. While it is true that most epithelial tumors yield diagnostic cells quite easily, the amount increases with suction. These authors lacked good comparison in studies with either variable amounts of suction or corresponding cellular samples.

Second, it is very important to make sure the barrel of the plunger is at the end of the syringe before attaching the syringe to the needle hub and applying suction. If the barrel is slightly retracted from the end, the small amount of air significantly lessens the amount of suction retracted (Boyle's law of gas physics).

And finally, during the removal of the needle it is probably best to maintain suction to retain fragments within the needle cylinder by tearing the opposite end of the core from the tissue. The in vitro studies by our group showed a definite improvement in the quantity of

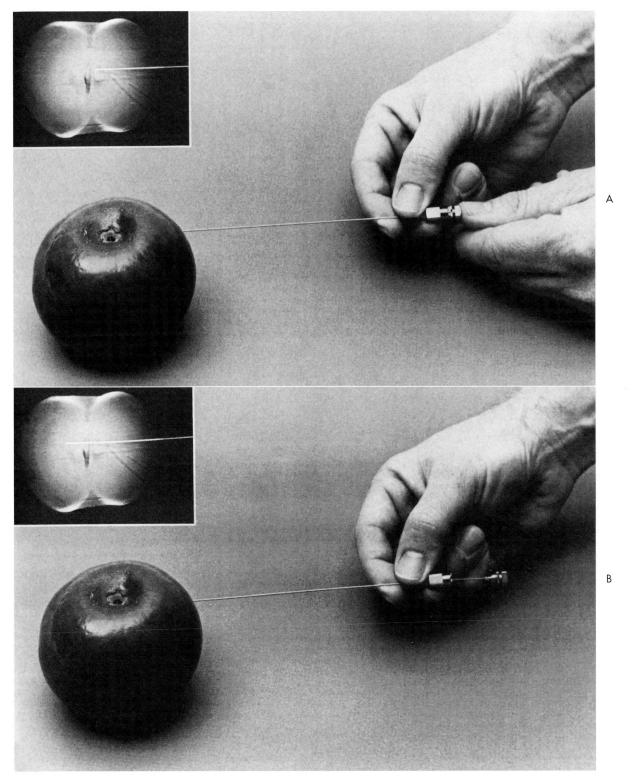

Fig. 46-18. The five steps in obtaining an aspiration specimen. **A,** Insert the needle adjacent to the lesion, represented by the "core." **B,** Retract the stylet several centimeters and make several in-and-out motions and rotations of the needle to "free" up some cells.

Continued.

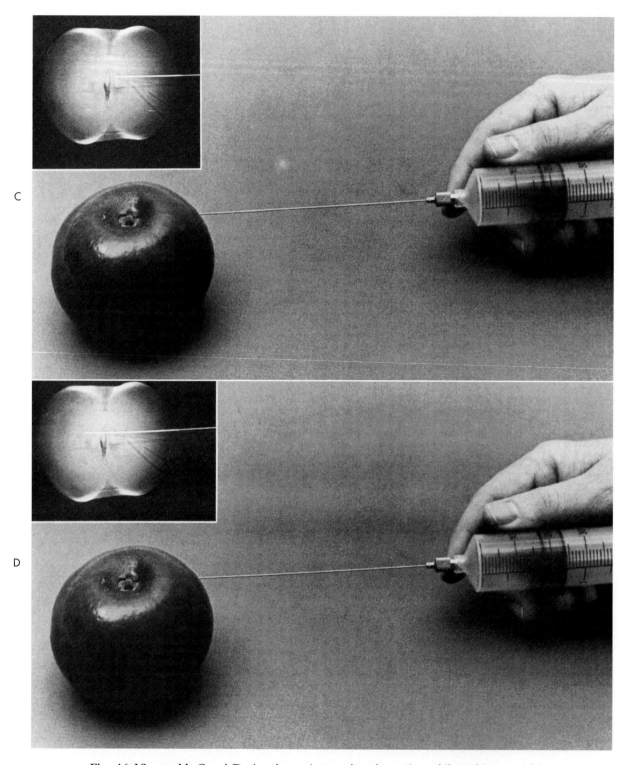

Fig. 46-18, cont'd. C and **D,** Attach a syringe and apply suction while making several in-and-out excursions to obtain more tissue. Release the suction while removing the needle. Eject the specimen onto the slides or into fluid for histologic examination when possible.

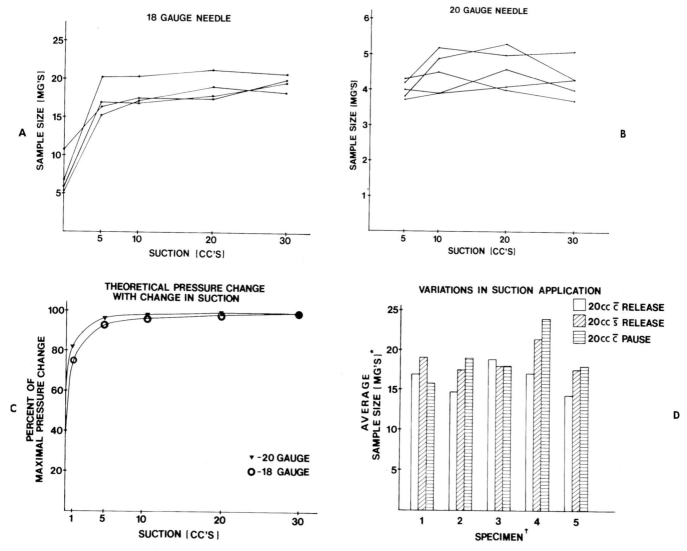

Fig. 46-19. A, Sample size versus suction, 18-gauge needle. Each point equals average of five samples. **B,** Sample size versus suction, 20-gauge needle. Each point equals average of five samples. **C,** Theoretical pressure change as calculated by Poiseuille's law for noncompressible fluids ($Q = \tau 8(Pa^4/l)n$. Q = volume of fluid through cylinder, P = pressure difference at ends of cylinder, a = radius of cylinder, l = length, n = viscosity of fluid) and Boyle's law for ideal gases ($PV = PV$ at constant temperature, P = initial pressure, V = initial volume, P = final pressure, V = final volume). **D,** Specimens 1 to 4, average of 5 human samples, specimen 5, average of 10 bovine samples; c = with, s = without. (**D** from Hueftle MG, Haaga JR: Effect of suction on biopsy sample size. *AJR* 147:1014-1016, 1986.

the sample when we compared samples with an aspiration needle after release or with maintenance of suction. Our most recent liver study by Ha et al[91] showed that in only 6% of cases did the presence of blood seem to degrade the sample.

Number of passes

With CT-guided procedures I found that we have been able to limit the number of passes without compromising our diagnostic accuracy. I routinely recommend two passes for all areas of the body, except the lung and the pancreas, if there are no technical problems. In the lung I recommend that initially a single pass should be made, because it has been well documented that taking two passes for every procedure doubles the complication rate and only minimally increases the diagnostic yield.[255] In the pancreas Dickey et al[48] of our group showed in a large series studying CT-guided procedures that two carefully controlled passes gave the same accuracy as that obtained by other authors who take four to five passes from widely separated areas. Furthermore, one pass in the pancreas by an experienced operator using a 20-gauge needle gave the same diagnostic accuracy as did two passes by an inexperienced operator using a 22-gauge needle.

Limiting the number of passes also reduces the probability of complications. Little doubt exists that the more passes taken the greater the probability of complications.[61,155,156,157] The pancreatic complications that have been reported occurred in series in which four to five needle passes were taken. Smith[247] has indicated his belief in a relationship between more passes and more complications. (See complication section for specific explanation).

Incorrectly, some radiologists believe that they can recover tissue in 100% of cases by making many passes, regardless of the guidance method. This is a misinterpretation of an article by Ferrucci et al[59,61] (Table 46-7) in which many different modalities were used and many different organs were sampled. In their study they selected 20 patients from their larger group who had positive biopsies and looked at the occurrence of positive results with each needle pass when they took four

Table 46-7. Fine-needle aspiration biopsy: number of passes required to establish diagnosis in 20 positive cases

Anatomic location	Needle aspirate number*			
	1	2	3	4
Pancreas	(+)	+	−	+
Retroperitoneum	(+)	+	+	−
Liver	−	−	−	(+)
Retroperitoneum	(+)	+	+	+
Pelvis	−	−	(+)	+
Lymph node	(+)	+	−	−
Liver	(+)	−	−	−
Pancreas	(+)	+	+	+
Liver	(+)	+	+	+
Porta hepatis	−	(+)	−	+
Porta hepatis	(+)	+	+	+
Ovary	(+)	+	+	+
Pancreas	(+)	+	+	+
Liver	(+)	+	+	+
Liver	−	(+)	+	+
Pancreas	(+)	+	−	+
Porta hepatis	−	(+)	−	+
Liver	(+)	+	+	−
Retroperitoneum	(+)	+	+	+
Retroperitoneum	(+)	+	+	+
Total	(15)	(3)	(1)	(1)

*Parentheses denote first positive aspirate.
From Ferrucci JT, et al: Diagnosis of abdominal malignancy by radiologic fine-needle aspiration biopsy. *AJR* 134:323-330, 1980.

needle passes. Of course 100% of the cases had a positive result with four passes, because only positive cases were selected. In their *unselected* entire group of the same report these authors routinely used five passes and had only 82% accuracy.

Sample preparation

After a sample has been taken, it is critical that it is properly handled. Perform the smear quickly in close proximity to the fixative to prevent drying, which can occur quickly. Always flush the syringe and needle with fixative and send the fluid for tissue cell block. This can increase the diagnostic yield by several percentage points. One author[149] has reported that heparinizing the needle and syringe is helpful, but no other workers have confirmed this. Others have measured CEA antigen in the cytologic samples and found this test useful.[165]

INSERTION OF CUTTING NEEDLE

The needle insertion method used for the Menghini and the Tru-Cut is the single-needle method with incremental adjustment of the angle and depth. Once the needle is correctly positioned, the following methods are used.

The Menghini-type cutting needle

The basic cutting mechanism of the needle can be best demonstrated by looking at the in-vitro demonstration with an apple (Fig. 46-20, *A*). Advance the instrument against the lesion to be sampled and confirm the location next to the lesion (Fig. 46-20, *B*). Then measure the depth of the desired sample and set any marker or mechanical stop appropriately (Fig. 46-20, *B*). Apply suction and insert the needle to the desired depth (Fig. 46-20, *C* and *D*). This needle is used in a similar fashion in vivo, except that there are some variations in the liver.

With the Menghini type of needle there are two different variations of the procedure in vivo for liver biopsy. One is used for lesions on the surface of the liver, and one is used for lesions below the surface of the liver. These are performed after proper site planning and skin preparation, as described later.

For lesions on the surface of the liver insert the needle adjacent to the capsule of the organ. As the patient suspends aspiration, insert the needle with suction applied to the desired depth, and remove it quickly. After the needle is removed, permit the patient to take a breath. This method corresponds to the "Menghini one-second technique" (Fig. 46-21).

For lesions beneath the surface of the liver, the patient suspends respiration and the needle is inserted through the capsule of the organ adjacent to the lesion (Fig. 46-22, *A*). Allow the patient to take several breaths

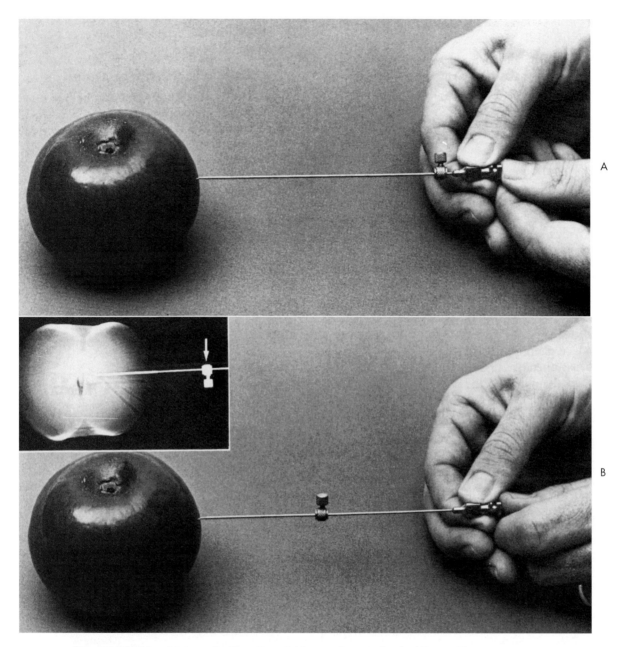

Fig. 46-20. Menghini needle for a "core" biopsy of an apple. **A,** After making a puncture wound, insert the needle into the tissue with the stylet in place until the needle is adjacent to the "lesion" (core of the apple). **B,** Adjust the mechanical stop *(arrow)* to the appropriate distance to include the lesion. *Continued.*

and take a repeat scan to determine if the needle is adjacent to the lesion. If it is, take the sample as the patient suspends breathing, as described previously. If the needle is not correctly localized, incremental adjustments are made until it is properly positioned. With the patient taking normal breaths with the needle in place, there is no lacerating effect if the needle is permitted to "swing free." It is only if the needle is fixed or held that liver movement against the needle creates a lacerating effect.

Ask the patient to suspend respiration for the last time and take the sample as noted previously. (As with aspirating needles, 10 to 20 cc of suction should be maintained). Remember to let the patient breathe after the sample is taken.

Several small points should be mentioned. First, maintain suction so that the distal portion of the sample will be torn from the organ as the needle is removed. Second, a slight increase in sample size can be obtained

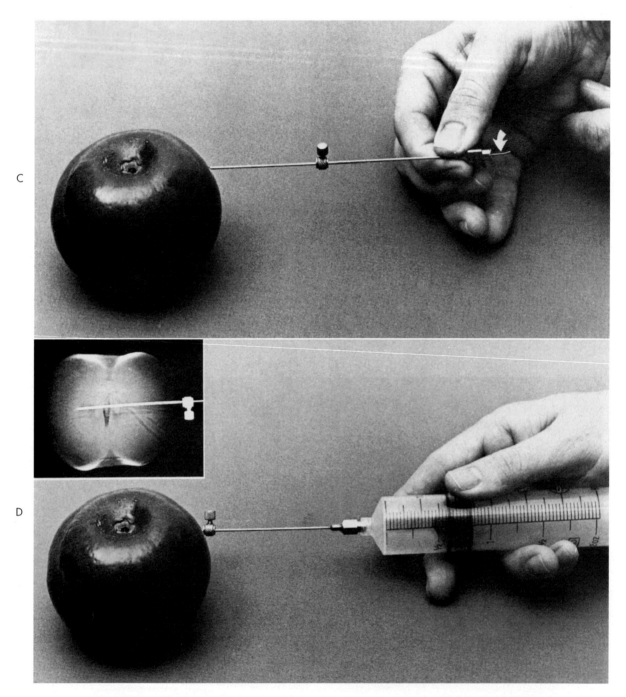

Fig. 46-20, cont'd. C, Insert the small obturator *(curved arrow)*, which prevents the specimen from being aspirated into the syringe. **D,** Attach the syringe to the needle and apply suction. Advance the needle to the depth of the mechanical stop and withdraw it quickly within 1 second. (Any time the needle is moved or immobilized have the patient suspend respiration.)

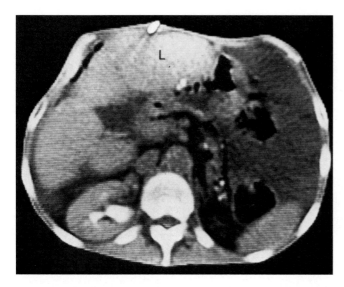

Fig. 46-21. When lesions are superficial a short Menghini needle should be used. This scan shows the Menghini needle in the skin over the enlarged left lobe *(L)* of the liver. This proved to be a cirrhotic nodule.

if a very short pause is made at the point of maximal insertion (see Fig. 46-20, *D*). This permits the liver to return to its starting location if it has been displaced away from the forward motion of the needle insertion. Finally, some devices have a type of metal obturator or other means to stop the sample in the needle. We consider the use of such devices optional, because in our laboratory evaluation histologic detail was identical if the sample was retained in the needle or "sucked" back into the syringe.

Manual Tru-Cut or side-cutting needles

The basic cutting action can be best appreciated by looking at the biopsy of an apple (Fig. 46-23, *A* to *C*). Insert the closed instrument to the edge of the lesion and confirm the position (Fig. 46-23, *A*). Insert the inner stylet (Fig. 46-23, *B*) and reconfirm the position. To take the sample, hold the inner stylet stationary and advance the outer cannula over the stylet (Fig. 46-23, *C*).

In vivo the sample is taken in a similar manner (Fig. 46-24). With appropriate suspension of respiration by the patient, the placement of a needle is made by the single-needle method. Using incremental angle and depth adjustments, the needle is inserted to the edge of the lesion. Each time the needle is moved or fixed, the patient should suspend respiration. (After insertion, permit the patient to breathe). If the needle is properly positioned relative to the lesion (i.e., properly angled), ask the patient to suspend respiration and insert the inner stylet with the gap. Permit the patient to take quiet respiration and take a repeat image to document the location of the gap relative to the lesion. If it is appropriately positioned, the procedure should be executed as follows:

With the patient suspending respiration, hold the inner stylet stationary, slide the other cannula forward over the gap, and remove the needle. Place the sample in the chosen tissue fixative and send it with appropriate information to the pathologist.

If the needle gap is not positioned correctly at the time of insertion, the instrument can be removed without significant damage. Little or no tissue injury will result because as it is advanced the cutting action is related to the point of the outer cannula, not to the gap. The gap is only the receptacle for the tissue sample. After the needle has been removed, it must be repositioned correctly before the biopsy is taken.

Several points should be made that will minimize the possibility of complication if a patient is uncooperative. First, never fix or immobilize the needle while the patient moves or breathes. Second, insert the needle so that the thin waist of the needle is inserted perpendicular to the motion of the diaphragm. With the flat end presenting to the moving liver, it is virtually impossible to lacerate the liver; the thin waist is flexible and moves with the liver.

The manual method I have described differs from that provided in the manufacturer's package insert. I have found that my method is far superior to theirs; try an apple core for practice and compare them. Although this chapter shows the 14-gauge needle, other sizes as small as 18- or 20-gauge are now available.

Automated side needle devices

There are a number of automated biopsy devices available[16,17] for purchase. Most of these are a permutation on the Tru-Cut design but some are a refinement of a Menghini-type needle. There are three reasons to use such devices. First, as a routine these devices are easier to use and more consistently provide a high-quality sample. Second, in very obese patients, they clearly provide superior samples because it is very difficult to obtain a good sample using a manual device because of the friction or "drag" put on the cutting cannula when it is moved forward. Finally, when tumors are extremely hard, automated devices permit better recovery of samples because the firm tissue also produces a drag on the outer cannula. Manual sampling, even by the experienced operator[32] (I have done thousands), is not as effective.

From a scientific perspective there is considerable difference in the diagnostic yields of these devices. Hopper et al[128,129] have tested a number of these devices and the current results of those tests can be noted in Tables 46-8 and 46-9. Because there is constant introduction of new devices, the reader is referred to the current literature for an update on them.

When discussing the side-cutting devices, several points should be made concerning the various mechanisms as well as some techniques. Two terms, *single throw*

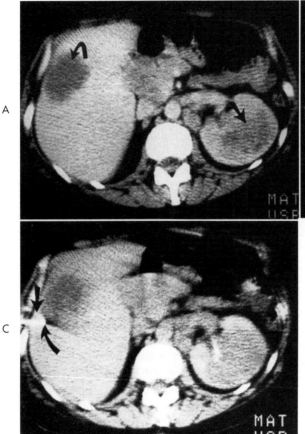

Fig. 46-22. A, Baseline CT before the bolus dynamic scan and biopsy. There is a low density mass *(curved arrow)* in the liver and a renal mass *(arrow)* on the left. **B,** Bolus dynamic scan shows both masses to be avascular. **C,** This scan shows the Menghini needle *(curved arrow)* inserted to the edge of the lesion through a small "cuff" *(arrow)* of normal tissue.

and *double throw,* are used to describe these devices. Double throw means that both the inner stylet with the tissue gap and the outer cutting cannula are moved automatically. Single throw means the inner stylet is inserted manually and the outer cutting cannula is moved automatically.

Another important point to note is that some of the devices move ahead a greater distance than the length of the tissue gap. One should carefully read the product information to ensure that one is aware of the distance the device moves into the tumor, so as to prevent any errors in localization.

One final point about these devices concerns the method of holding the device during the biopsy. Although one might think that human error is eliminated by these devices; however, that is not correct. First one must hold them firmly to make sure the maximal sample is obtained. In addition, the devices actually produce a recoil as the inner stylet and the cutting cannula move forward; this can push the gun back and reduce the size of the sample. Kellermeyer et al[150] of our group have shown that firmly holding the gun while obtaining the sample increases the diagnostic yield by about 14%, compared with a loosely held gun. In his unpublished data the average length of the sample was 14.4 mm with the

gun held loosely and 16.4 mm with the gun held firmly. When using these devices, one must be careful about their size and weight. If the devices are too long or too heavy they do not adapt well to use with CT scanners. The best-suited devices have needles that are detachable from the gun. With these the needle is localized with the single-needle method and the mechanized portion is attached before taking the sample.

Angled or out-of-slice procedure

After one has mastered the straight or the in-slice method, one can learn to perform angled biopsies with the entrance site at one level and the target lesion at another level. This technique is most valuable for the sampling of lesions within the pelvis, below the iliac wing, and under the dome of the diaphragm, as well as in trying to avoid certain structures within the abdomen.

To understand this type of procedure, it is helpful to think of the needle placement as a combination of two different angles, one in the plane of the slice and one in the longitudinal plane. Determination of the angle within the X-Y plane can be made from the sequential scans between the entrance site and the target lesion. Determination of the angle in the longitudinal plane is more difficult, and two approaches can be used.

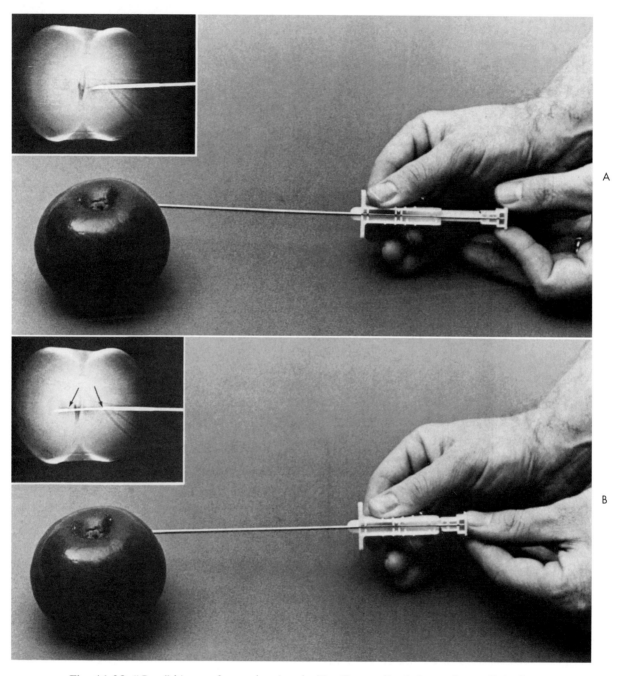

Fig. 46-23. "Core" biopsy of an apple using the Tru-Cut needle. **A,** Insert the needle in the closed position to the margin of the lesion. **B,** Insert the inner stylet with the "gap" *(arrows)* briskly through the area of the lesion. (If the needle is improperly positioned, it can be withdrawn in this position; a specimen will not be cut unless the outer needle is advanced over the gap.) *Continued.*

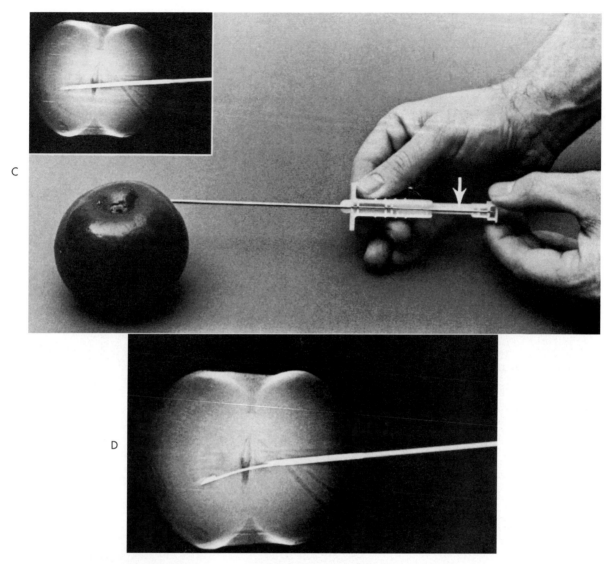

Fig. 46-23, cont'd. C, With the inner stylet *(arrow)* held stationary, advance the outer needle rapidly over the gap. (The outer needle cuts the specimen into the gap.) **D,** A hard material such as bone (in this case, an apple seed) can deflect the thin portion of the needle. This has never been a problem with soft tissue tumors, but the Tru-Cut needle is not suitable for lesions in or against bone for this reason.

The first method uses a geometrical approach to calculate the angle by using the depth of the lesion and the distance between the plane of the entrance and the target lesion[9] (Fig. 46-25). The angle is then calculated according to the pythagorean theory, followed by an attempt to execute the calculated angle. In reality this calculation of angle is only slightly helpful, because of the difficulty in manually executing the angle during insertion.

The second method, which is the least sophisticated but actually the most convenient, is the simple estimation, approximation, or trial and error method. After ensuring that the XY angle is correct (Figs. 46-26, A and B), one inserts the needle in the estimated longitudinal angle. Then multiple scans are obtained and incremental adjustments made until the needle is satisfactorily positioned (Figs. 46-26, C to D).

The third method, is the use of various needle-holding devices that can pre-align the needle at the correct angle (Fig. 46-27, A and B). The cost and complexity of these devices varies widely. I do not personally advocate any of them, and I advise readers to use their own judgement.[67,178,217]

Yet another solution to the angle approach for biopsies is quite simple, but the major manufacturers apparently have not recognized the benefit of CT proce-

Table 46-8. Combined results of renal and hepatic biopsies

Needle no./Instrument	Mean pathology score	% Biopsies with grossly inadequate tissue	% Biopsies with suboptimal tissue	Statistically better than (needle nos.)	Statistically worse than (needle nos.)
1/Long-throw Biopty gun, 18 gauge	5.78	0	17	4, 5, 8, 11, 13	
2/Vim Silverman, 14 gauge	6.12	7	14	11	
3/Jamshidi, 17 gauge	5.23	10	3	11	15
4/Turner, 18 gauge	4.37	13	13	11	1, 15
5/Chiba, 18 gauge	4.01	17	3	11	1, 7, 10, 12, 15
6/Franseen, 18 gauge	4.63	7	17	11	15
7/Cook gun, 18 gauge	6.90	0	11	5, 8, 11	
8/Klear Kut gun, 18 gauge	4.75	13	13	11	1, 7, 10, 12, 15
9/Klear Kut gun, 14 gauge	5.24	17	8	11	15
10/Short-throw Biopty gun, 18 gauge	6.03	0	11	11	
11/Vacu Cut, 21 gauge	1.52	46	0		1, 2, 3, 4, 5, 6, 7, 8, 9, 10, 12, 14, 15
12/Vacu Cut, 18 gauge	6.86	0	13	11	
13/PercuCut, 21 gauge	4.00	14	21		1, 15
14/PercuCut, 18 gauge	4.70	6	13	11	15
15/Tru-Cut, 14 gauge	7.70	0	8	3, 4, 5, 6, 8, 9, 11, 13, 14	

NOTE —The overall mean pathology score was 5.37 for 724 specimens.
From Hopper KD, Baird DE, Reddy VV, et al: Efficacy of automated biopsy guns versus conventional biopsy needles in the pygmy pig. *Radiology* 176:671-676, 1990.

Table 46-9. Mean scores in the liver

Technique or device	Background blood or clot	Amount of cellular material	Degree of cellular degeneration	Degree of cellular trauma	Retention of appropriate architecture	Total score
Manual aspiration technique (FNAB)	1.033	1.767*	1.700	1.900	1.200	7.600
Syringe pistol-holder	1.167	1.933*	1.900	1.933	1.267	8.200
Aspiration syringe biopsy gun	1.055	1.722*	1.789	1.895	1.340	7.800
Vacuum needle	1.100	1.933*	1.900	1.900	1.000	7.833
FNCB	1.567	1.200	1.733	1.700	0.933	7.133
Aspirator gun	1.068	1.723*	1.827	1.864	1.229	7.712
End-cut gun	0.820	1.799*	1.798	1.760	1.088	7.265

NOTE—All scores are based on the grading scheme in reference 1.
*Performed statistically significantly better than the capillary technique when the Tukey method of multiple comparisons was used.
From Hopper KD, Abendroth CS, Sturtz KW, et al: Fine-needle aspiration biopsy for cytopathologic analysis: utility of syringe handles, automated guns, and the nonsuction method. *Radiology* 185:819-824, 1992.

dures and accordingly have not completed development of the method. We have used a preliminary form of the software program, which involves using data collected from sequential axial slices in combination with the longitudinal view to create the margins of the lesion on the longitudinal scan (Scoutview, Topogram, Synerview). The needle is then positioned in the patient and the longitudinal scan is taken to evaluate the angle of the needle insertion in the longitudinal plane (Fig. 46-28). Incremental adjustments are made accordingly, and a final axial slice is taken to confirm the location.

Localization of the needle tip

After insertion of the needle, one may occasionally have some difficulty in localizing the tip.

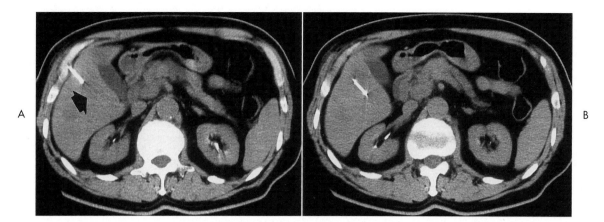

Fig. 46-24. A, Preliminary scan showing mass lesion in right lobe of liver *(arrow).* The needle has been inserted to the edge of the lesion. When a manual needle is used, one should proceed to visualize the appearance as noted in **B.** When an automated gun is used to insert the needle, no other images are obtained; however, the gun is fired after this type of image. (If a heavy gun is used, the needle is inserted separate from the gun and the device is attached immediately before the firing.) **B,** With a manual device, the inner stylet has been inserted through the lesion. The tissue gap is clearly seen. The sample is then taken by moving the cutting cannula over the gap.

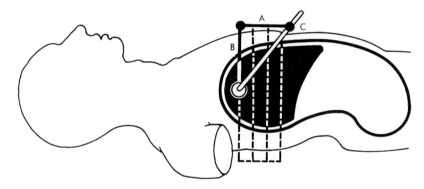

Fig. 46-25. Calculation of the distance to the lesion and angle of entry when the entrance point to the skin and the target lesion is not in the same CT section. When the entrance point *C* and distances *A* and *B* are known, the distance to the lesion and angle of insertion can be calculated. Although theoretically this method has merit, pragmatically its use is limited because of the difficulty in duplicating the angle "freehand." We prefer to estimate the angle with such lesions and take a series of sequential scans, as in Fig. 46-26, or use the longitudinal scan method.

There are several methods that can be used to solve this problem. The simplest method is to take a longitudinal scan and take an axial slice at the end. This is virtually foolproof and is the most expeditious.

Another method, which can be used if the angle of the needle is slight, involves simply taking multiple scans in one direction until the end of the needle is reached (see Fig. 46-28). Many of the new scanners have a simple feature of a cluster scan consisting of three or more scans, which is well-suited for this purpose. When the end of the needle is found, it will appear to have a square end and may have an artifact from the end (Fig.

46-29). On occasion the end of the needle will not be "square" in appearance, but the end is easily appreciated by noting when the end is no longer seen on subsequent scans.

Percutaneous tissue retraction

When only a skinny needle is used, it is permissable to penetrate certain loops of bowel and organs. If one is using either a cutting needle or catheter or dealing with an immunocomprised patient, one should not penetrate or traverse any intervening structure. Two methods have been used for this problem, the injection of carbon dioxide and the injection of saline.

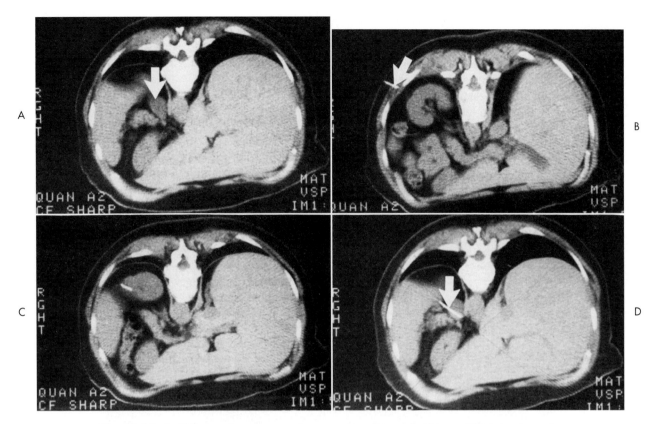

Fig. 46-26. A, This scan demonstrates the execution of an angled biopsy. This scan above the entrance site shows the adrenal lesion *(arrow)* behind the tail of the pancreas. **B,** Once the needle is started into the anatomy, a repeat scan is taken, and the *X-Y* angle of the needle *(arrow)* is compared with the higher slice on which the target is seen, **(A). C,** Knowing that the *X-Y* angle is correct, the *Y-Z* angle is estimated and the needle is inserted. Sequential scans along the needle are taken to confirm the location. This scan shows the needle "slipping" adjacent to the upper margin of the right kidney. (If penetration of the kidney occurs, it is not a significant concern.) **D,** This final scan shows the tip of the aspiration needle within the adrenal mass *(arrow).*

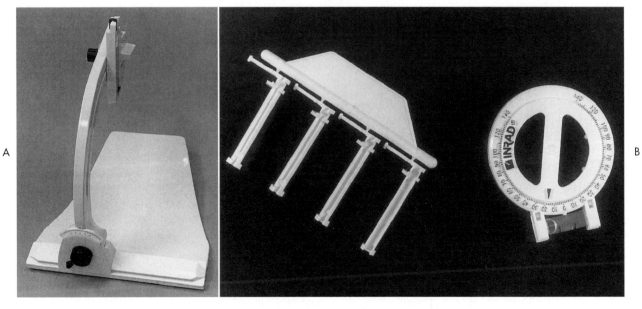

Fig. 46-27. A number of commercial devices are now available to aid in the angulation of biopsy procedures. The device shown in **A** has proved useful by many workers. The device shown in **B** is hand-held and can assist in manually guided procedures.

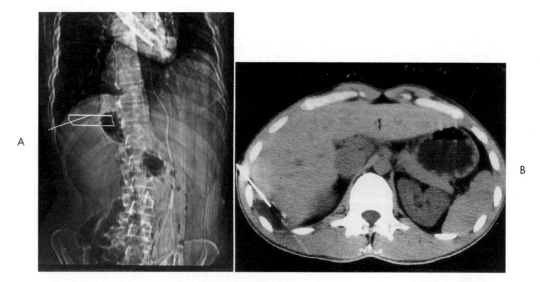

Fig. 46-28. A, Topogram shows computer-simulated lesion as square with angulation simulation for needle appearing as a straight line. **B,** CT scan showing needle directed toward the lesion as directed by the program shown in **A.**

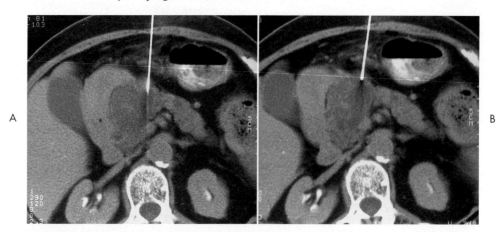

Fig. 46-29. Localization of the needle tip may be problematic at times. When the needle is "tapered" as seen in **A,** it means that a variable number of pixels is being occupied along the length of the needle and thus the end may not be seen. When the end is "square" as in **B,** the tip is being accurately localized.

We have reported[114] that carbon dioxide insufflation can be used to move bowel and the bladder a short distance; in this fashion a pathway for such a procedure can be opened. However, this gas will not move solid organs such as kidneys.

The procedure is easily performed as follows. After the trajectory is planned, decide from the scans the proper location of the carbon dioxide. Then insert a needle and inject by hand 50 to 100 cc of carbon dioxide (Fig. 46-30). If the intended loop of structure does not move, attempt to reposition the needle or repeat the injection of carbon dioxide. Although this requires some practice, generally try to get it in a location such that the gas will move the bowel perpendicularly away.

Although there are some theoretical objections, the use of carbon dioxide is quite safe. This gas has been used for all types of in vivo procedures, including peritoneoscopy, mediastinal insufflation, and even intravascular use, without any difficulty. The gas is absorbed very quickly because carbon dioxide is quite soluble in body fat.

If there is severe inflammation around the structure being moved, the insufflation of gas will not work well. The inflammation can be the result of surgery or infection.

Other authors[90] have proposed the use of injected saline to increase the size of pathways through which one can insert a needle. This has been used predominantly in the chest for widening the paraspinal space, but potentially it could be used in other localizations (see later section on biopsy of middle mediastinal tumors).

Both of the above methods have a similar prob-

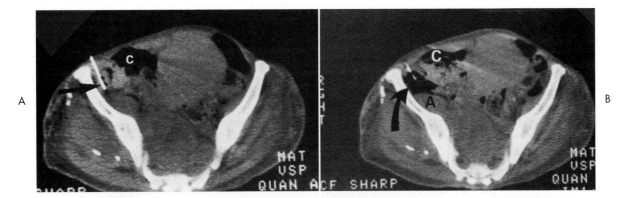

Fig. 46-30. A, CT scan showing a needle in place for injection of carbon dioxide. The needle *(arrow)* is lateral to the cecum, *C.* **B,** After injection of carbon dioxide *(curved arrow),* the cecum, *c,* is moved medially, permitting safe passage of the needle into the psoas abscess, *A,* (high density because of blood and protein).

lem. Depending on the location of connective tissue, either the gas or fluid may dissect cephalad or caudad and not substantially produce enlargement in the axial plane. Nevertheless, both of the methods can work in selected cases.

Lessons from experience

It is important to always try to keep the patient physically and psychologically comfortable. Careful explanation of the procedure to the patient and continual verbal assurances (I call this "verbal" anesthesia) are most helpful.

Regardless of which organ is being sampled, always permit the needle to swing free with respiratory motion. A lacerating effect occurs when the needle is fixed and the organ moves.

Periods of suspended respiration should not be prolonged. If patients are not allowed to take frequent controlled breaths, they may breathe unexpectedly. In addition, if the patients become frustrated because of breath-holding, the depth of respiration will vary more. If the depth of breath varies, the anesthetized portion of the organ may move away from the insertion site.

One of the most common mistakes is insufficient administration of local anesthesia. It is better to err on the side of too much local anesthesia. If patients experience excessive pain, they cannot cooperate well. As noted earlier, I try to ensure that not only the skin and subcutaneous tissues have ample anesthesia but that the capsule pleura or peritoneum are also well-anesthetized. Although I try to inject lidocaine only into the cavity surface, I find that a small amount injected into the parenchyma of organ will not produce any adverse effects. However, do not inject large amounts of anesthesia into the parenchyma of the lung or blood vessels, because it is an antiarrhythmic and rapid absorption and circulation to the heart could cause a problem.

Another "tip" for local anesthesia is to mix a small

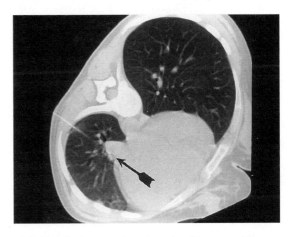

Fig. 46-31. Placing a patient in a decubitus or oblique position puts weight on the diaphragm and thus lessens movement of pulmonary masses. This scan shows a pulmonary mass *(arrow)* closely adherent to the surface of the heart being biopsied.

amount of parenteral sodium bicarbonate solution with the xylocaine before injection. This neutralizes the "acid" environment of the xylocaine and eliminates the "burning" of the injection.

Finally, using the coaxial short cannula method for deep or small lesions is helpful. With the guidance cannula in the subcutaneous tissues the angle of insertion is determined before insertion of the sampling needle. Adjustment in angle of the cannula does not affect the internal structures because it is confined to the subcutaneous tissues. Once the angle is determined, only depth placement is required. This avoids inadvertent puncture of other structures. Multiple passes are possible because only a minimal variation of angle is required to alter the placement at the tip of the long biopsy needle.

If a patient is somewhat uncooperative or if the lesion being sampled is small, place the patient in the ip-

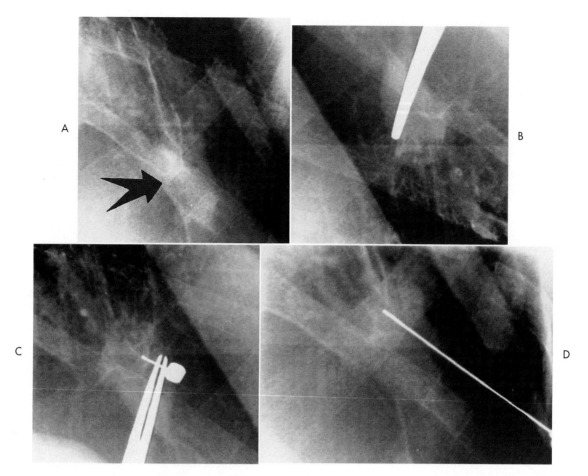

Fig. 46-32. A, Fluoroscopic biopsy of lung masses is possible in most parenchymal lesions. This close-up of the lung shows an ill-defined mass adjacent to a rib *(arrow)*. **B,** Site of entrance is best determined by using a metal marker, in this case a hemostat, to mark the skin. **C,** A prudent interventionalist always avoids exposing their hands to the beam. This shows a needle holder directing the needle to the mass. **D,** Final localization of the needle tip should be made by verifying the location of the needle tip on oblique or lateral views. Other methods of localization include movement of the mass, tactile perception, and wiggling of the mass with the needle.

silateral decubitus or oblique position (not at the compromise of the entrance site, of course). The weight of the abdominal viscera partially immobilizes the diaphragm and limits the respiratory motion of the diaphragm (Fig. 46-31). This is especially important for lung, kidney, adrenal, or liver lesions.

LUNGS AND MEDIASTINUM

For the routine well-defined pulmonary nodule, fluoroscopy is still the modality of choice (Fig. 46-32, *A* to *D*). Since the first edition of this text,[100] our experience with CT biopsies of the lung has been considerable, and CT has surprisingly developed a much larger role than anticipated.[34] In fact, almost all lung biopsies are now done under CT guidance. This is true for two reasons. First, there has been such a refinement and devel-

opment of CT procedures that almost any lung nodule can be biopsied with CT guidance.[233] Second, the availability of sophisticated fluoroscopy equipment is limited because of its use for many current vascular procedures.

If CT expertise and/or the appropriate equipment are not available, one can use either fluoroscopy or ultrasound.[81] The primary role of ultrasound is still the aspiration of pleural fluid; its minor role is the sampling of pleural-based nodules.

Indications

The clinical situations that justify the performance of a biopsy include sampling of nodules for neoplasm or sampling of infiltrate for infectious agents. One can justify biopsying a suspected primary nodule for two reasons. First, aspiration biopsy can distinguish small cell tu-

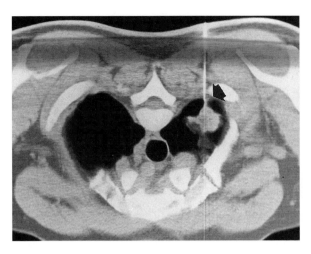

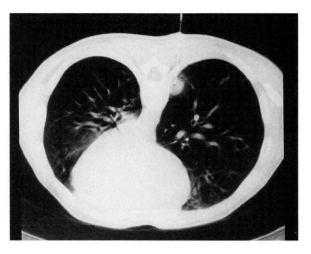

Fig. 46-33. Biopsy of an apical lesion, with the patient in a prone position. Note the needle traversing a small fibrous band between the pleura and the mass. Note also the small amount of pleural fat *(arrow)* which has been retracted by the fibrous band.

Fig. 46-34. Lesions such as this mass in the right costovertebral angle adjacent to the pleura are easily sampled. Note that the pathway was chosen to avoid any aerated lung, thereby minimizing the risk of a pneumothorax.

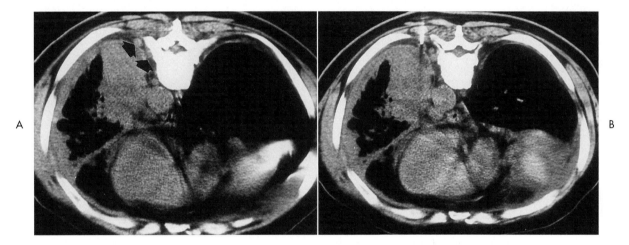

A

B

Fig. 46-35. A, Scan shows two tiny nodules *(arrows)* behind the pleura in a lung that is totally opacified by infiltrate and fluid. Such a procedure is impossible under fluoroscopy. **B,** Needle positioned before biopsy. Sample yielded cellular material consistent with small cell tumor of lung.

mors from non-small cell tumors.[246] Many oncologists believe that small cell tumors should be treated medically rather than surgically. Second, Sinner et al stated that percutaneous biopsy can expedite surgical treatment. Obviously, confirmation of malignancy in cases of metastatic or recurrent tumors is very important. In cases of pulmonary infiltrate when the causative organism is unknown, diagnostic aspiration can obtain material for culture that can distinguish among pyogenic, fungal, or opportunistic organisms.

CT is indicated for the biopsy of a variety of lesions not well suited for fluoroscopy or ultrasound because of their locations as well as other factors. Lesions in the apices (Fig. 46-33), the costophrenic angles, the costovertebral angles (Fig. 46-34), the pleura (Fig. 46-35), the hila (Fig. 46-36), and those obscured by fluid and mediastinum are best suited for CT because they are not well seen with fluoroscopic imaging. The dynamic bolus CT scan is an important adjunct for the mediastinum and hila because major vessels can be opacified and delineated, making separation from masses in these areas quite easy.

Parenchymal lesions well suited for CT biopsy also include those lesions with ill-defined edges, as well as other lesions poorly visualized by fluoroscopy. These latter lesions are better seen because of the better con-

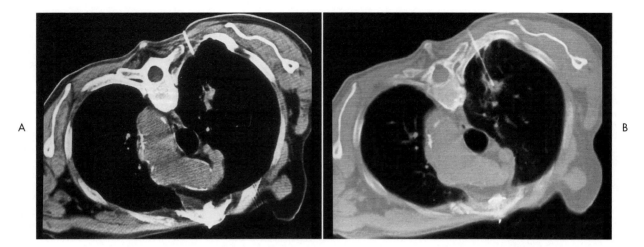

Fig. 46-36. A, Single-needle sampling of poorly defined hilar mass. The single needle is stopped at the pleural surface for final assessment of trajectory and injection of Xylocaine (careful attention to local anesthesia ensures the cooperation of the patient and successful biopsy). **B,** Successful placement of needle in mass with poorly defined margins.

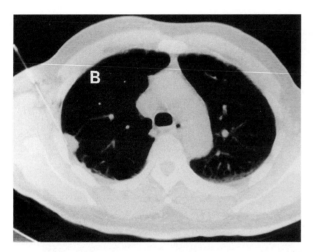

Fig. 46-37. Scan shows a mass along the pleural surface of the left chest. The needle approach has been chosen to avoid some blebs, *B,* in the anterior chest.

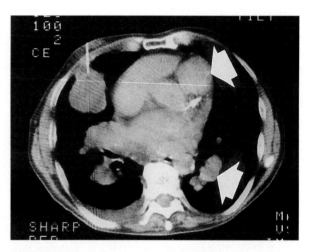

Fig. 46-38. Scan shows a mass anteriorly that can be approached by passing through the attachment to the anterior pleura. Note the large pulmonary arteries and main pulmonary artery *(arrows)* in this patient with right heart failure and severe pulmonary hypertension.

trast resolution and the tomographic nature of CT scans.

Peripheral nodules in patients with severe parenchymal disease are well suited to CT. Blebs are also more easily avoided with CT, by careful planning of the trajectory (Fig. 46-37). In such cases if one takes thin scan sections, one can sometimes find a pleural attachment that permits a "risk-free" access, thus avoiding penetration of the lung (Figs. 46-33, 46-38).

Contraindications

With the further refinement of techniques, the number and significance of contraindications have lessened. There are several absolute contraindications that include uncorrectable coagulopathy, severe pulmonary hypertension, uncontrollable coughing, possible echino-

coccus, and an uncooperative patient insufficiently controlled by anesthetics.

The levels of the coagulopathy that I find acceptable are a prothrombin time within 2 seconds of normal and a platelet count of at least 50,000. Uncontrollable coughing and a patient with an uncooperative nature are important because movement of the lung during a procedure may cause a tear of the lung by the needle that might cause air embolism, pneumothorax, or bleeding.

Techniques for lung

There are several important techniques used for chest biopsy that relate to both the preparation of the entry site and the needle technique. Appropriate choice and preparation of the entrance site are important to ensure a painless and successful biopsy procedure.

After one has selected a tentative entrance point from the CT scans one should carefully inspect the chest at the entrance site for several things. First, if there are any obvious superficial veins noted, the site should be moved accordingly. Second, one should palpate deeply for the intercostal space between the margins of the ribs. Palpation of the ribs is necessary because the location of the intercostal space as seen on the CT scan is not reliable. The tapered margin of the rib and the oblique orientation of the rib as it traverses the imaging section produces considerable partial volume effect and discrepancy regarding the actual location of the intercostal space on the scan. The problem of identifying the location of the ribs is especially relevant to the anterior chest wall where the ribs are mostly cartilaginous and fuse together in an unpredictable pattern. Although it is true that one can use a needle or a guidance cannula to "drill" through a cartilaginous rib, I do not recommend this with CT guidance because if one drills through the cartilage, the pathway of the needle is fixed, thereby preventing corrective angulation; also, the fixed needle cannot move with respiration, thereby making a small tear more likely if the patient moves the lung while breathing. In the lung as in other areas, the needle should be permitted to "swing" freely with respiration. Also, any time the needle is adjusted the patient should be asked to suspend respiration temporarily during the manipulation of the needle or removal of the stylet to prevent tearing of the parenchyma or a pneumothorax.

Another important point is related to the infiltration of the local anesthetic at the entrance sight. When anesthetizing the area, it is important to infiltrate anesthetic through the subcutaneous tissues and down to and including the pleura. Adequate anesthesia of the pleura makes the procedure virtually pain-free and permits insertion of the needle without the patient moving because of pain. So important is this step of anesthetizing the pleura that as I perform the actual insertion of the needle, I stop the needle tip at the pleura to inject a small amount of anesthetic at the pleura and to check the final angle of needle insertion before entering the lung. If a rib is inadvertently stuck during the initial anesthetic administration, I give a large bolus of xylocaine on the rib; this prevents any recurrence of pain if that area is struck again during the procedure.

There are two methods one can use for a needle aspiration of the lung, a single-needle method or a coaxial method using a short guidance cannula with a longer aspiration needle. With the single needle, the needle is started into the superficial tissues and a scan is obtained to verify its angulation. Once the correct angle

is determined, the needle is inserted to the correct depth. The other method that should be used for deep or small lesions is the coaxial, short guidance cannula method as follows. The guidance cannula is inserted into the chest wall and adjusted until it is directed toward the lesion. The Chiba needle is inserted to the correct depth, and sample is obtained (see earlier discussion on coaxial method).

Needle selection and number of passes. As aspiration needles have been used for many years by numerous authors, one can reliably make a number of valid conclusions regarding their use. First, the needle caliber size appears to have little effect on the success rate of the procedures. Equivalent successes have been reported with a wide range of needle calibers, from 23-gauge to 18-gauge. The pneumothorax rate has little relationship to the needle caliber, but the hemoptysis rate is directly related to the needle caliber. When needles smaller than 20 gauge are used, the hemoptysis rate is quite low. This was confirmed by Khouri et al[153] who noted in his series, that the hemoptysis rate was 21% with an 18-gauge needle but only 5% with a 20-gauge needle.

Several early reports by Sargeant et al and Stevens et al described the effects of increasing the number of needle passes. Stevens et al reported that a second needle pass increased diagnostic yield by 10%, and a third needle pass increased it by 1.5%. Sargeant et al reported that a second needle pass increased the diagnostic yield by an additional 5%, and that the third needle pass increased the diagnostic yield by another 3%. Stevens et al reported that the pneumothorax rate more than doubled with two passes.

From the above data, one can understand how we arrived at our current method, which I will now describe. I use a 20-gauge Chiba needle for an aspiration biopsy and routinely only take a single needle pass. I prefer to defer a second needle pass until after the results of the first pass are known, unless there has been a break in the technique. If the cytologist is available for a rapid stain interpretation, the patient will remain in the department until the results are known. If this service is not available, I still prefer to wait for the results instead of taking a second pass, because the 24-hour delay is a small trade-off considering the high success rate. If a technical error has been made or the final position of the needle placement is not satisfactory, then a second needle pass will be made at once.

Cutting needles are being used much more frequently. As was first noted by Goralnik et al, if a pleural-based lesion is present, virtually any cutting needle as large as a 14 gauge can be used safely (Fig. 46-39, *A* and *B*). The indications for using such a needle are suspicion for a lymphoma or an unsuccessful aspiration procedure. The use of this large needle is contingent on

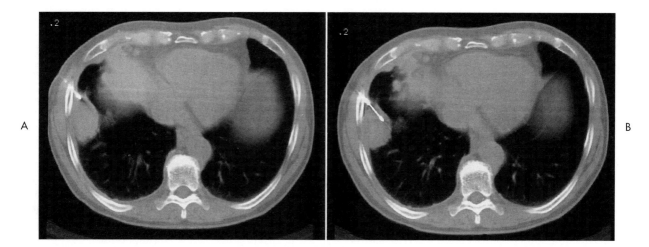

Fig. 46-39. A, Large-needle biopsy of pleural-based masses can be safely performed to diagnosis lymphoma. This scan shows needle placed adjacent to the mass. **B,** Using a manual cutting device, the stylet with the tissue "gap" is inserted into the mass. With such devices, the tissue obtained "falls" into the gap (see text).

there being no intervening lung. If there is some intervening lung, then an 18- to 20-gauge needle can be used safely just so the "cutting action" of the needle is limited to the nodule being sampled. Such needles are used for lymphomas or other unusual types of tumors.

Important planning factors. Common sense dictates that several precautions be taken when planning the trajectory. These include avoidance of vessels, bronchi, and blebs. Although there is no data to support the following statement, it is quite clear that avoidance of vessels and bronchi, in addition to using a 20-gauge needle or less, has definitely decreased the incidence of hemoptysis. In my practice the incidence of hemoptysis decreased from about 20% to less than 1% with CT procedures. Penetration of a bronchi may produce a spasm of coughing, which in turn can produce uncontrollable lung movement and predispose the patient to pneumothorax, bleeding, or air embolism (see complication section). Penetration of blebs will obviously predispose the patient to an immediate severe pneumothorax; avoidance is therefore prudent.

In many cases one can minimize the possibility of a complication by looking carefully for a "safe pathway" through the lung to the nodule being biopsied. In such cases one might locate the attachment to the pleura or an area of fibrosis that can be traversed by the needle. By planning the trajectory through such an area, only a minimal amount of parenchyma is traversed and/or the fibrosis can serve to keep the layers of the pleura attached and thereby avoid a pneumothorax (see Fig. 46-38). By looking for a very small amount of "fat" that may be tented at the pleura, one can usually distinguish between a mass that is simply adjacent to the pleura and one that has a fibrous extension. This type of approach is espe-

cially important in high-risk patients with pulmonary hypertension, severe restrictive disease, or other serious underlying pulmonary problems.

Two other factors that can minimize the incidence of pneumothorax are minimizing the pathway of lung crossed (Fig. 46-40, *A* and *B*) and using a pathway through nonaerated lung. One of my colleagues, Dr. J. Locke[172] studied a series of 235 cases from our center and looked at the incidence of pneumothorax as compared with the distance of the lung traversed. The distances crossed with the corresponding incidence of symptomatic pneumothorax were: 1 cm, 3.7%; 1 to 2 cm, 10.7%; 3 to 4 cm, 19%; and 5 to 6 cm, 44.4%. Because these measurements were taken from CT scans, they were quite accurate without errors in magnification; other authors who have not supported this relationship made their measurements from radiographs, which are more subject to error.

Our previous claim that traversing nonaerated lung would diminish pneumothorax has been documented. Very recently, Haramati and Austin[116a] showed quite convincingly that if aerated lung was avoided, the pneumothorax rate decreased significantly. They found that the pneumothorax incidence through aerated lung was 46% as compared with 0% through nonaerated lung. Stated differently, if there is an area of infiltrate adjacent to a nodule, one should intentionally traverse the consolidated area (Fig. 46-41).

Choice of the target site is self evident, but several points are worthy of emphasis relative to biopsy of nodules. If the nodule being sampled contains a small amount of calcification, the calcified area should be avoided and the adjacent soft-tissue density targeted. If the nodule is cavitated, appears necrotic, or is quite large,

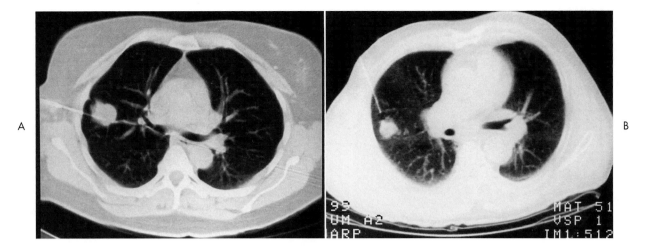

Fig. 46-40. A, This and the scan in Fig. 46-39, *B,* shows the difference in approach for two lesions that are almost identical. This scan shows a direct lateral approach, with the distance of lung being crossed being almost half of that in Fig. 46-39, *B.* **B,** This biopsy approach traverses almost twice the distance of lung and increases the potential risk by almost a factor of 3, according to new data (see text).

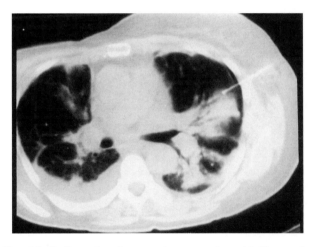

Fig. 46-41. Intentionally traversing parenchymal infiltrate, decreases the potential for pneumothorax significantly (see text). On the other hand, hemoptysis is usually more common. This was a needle aspirate for an infectious process.

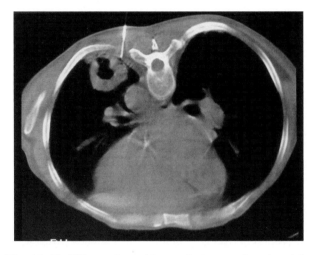

Fig. 46-42. CT scan shows biopsy of a large cavitated nodule. The periphery of the mass is targeted for best results. Some authors have suggested that in such cases a higher incidence of pneumothorax and hemorrhage exists.

the central portion should be avoided in preference to the peripheral area (Fig. 46-42). Some caution should be exercised in such a case to limit the penetration into the cavity portion as well as the vigor with which the sample is obtained. Early authors have claimed such cases are more likely to result in pneumothorax and severe bleeding; this has not been our experience.

Patient position

In most instances it is simplest to have the patient lie in the prone or supine position, but other positions might also be considered (Fig. 46-43). As noted above, there might be an optimal choice of pathway taking into account the factors described. In such cases, access to the appropriate entrance site might be facilitated by placing the patient in prone, oblique, or decubitus position.

If the lesion is small and moves with respiratory motion, it may be wise to put the patient in an ipsilateral decubitus position and insert the needle through a direct anterior or posterior approach. This position minimizes the motion of the ipsilateral diaphragm because of the weight of the abdominal organs against the diaphragm. This restriction of motion minimizes movement of the lesion and thereby simplifies the performance of the procedure (Fig. 46-31).

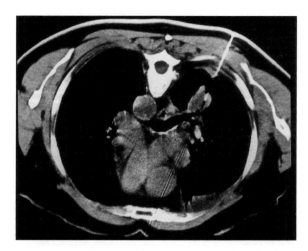

Fig. 46-43. Patient positioning can simplify a biopsy procedure. This scan shows a patient lying in the decubitus position. The dependent side moves less because of the weight of the viscera, thus making the biopsy simpler.

Specific anatomic approaches

Hilar lesions are best sampled by bronchoscopy and should be percutaneously biopsied only as a second choice. The success rate for bronchoscopy is better and the complication rate lower than for percutaneous procedures. With percutaneous procedures, the length of the lung to be crossed and the proximity of vessels make the incidence of pneumothorax and hemoptysis more likely. If a bronchoscopy has been attempted unsuccessfully, a percutaneous procedure will be performed with the following guidelines.

Before the procedure, intense contrast enhancement of the vasculature should be performed to highlight the location of the anterior, lateral, or posterior approach to be taken. Unquestionably, with such lesions a coaxial, short cannula method should be used. This method is especially helpful because, as noted above, before the biopsy needle is inserted, the guidance cannula predetermines the angle. With a long distance from the pleura to the hilum, a few degrees in error will result in a large localization error centrally.

Apical lesions. Careful planning for apical lesions is important because of the unique anatomy of the upper chest. Anteriorly, the brachicephalic vessels, mediastinal vessels, the clavicle, and axillary vessels make the approach more difficult. Posteriorly, the scapula covers a substantial portion of the posterior chest. Avoidance is best accomplished by having the patient fully abduct the shoulder so that the scapula moves laterally. Careful palpation will usually reveal the margin of the scapula. Another anatomic factor making the approach more difficult is that the ribs become smaller as one progresses from the midchest cephalad to the apex. It is usually easier to plan the entrance site so that the angle is also

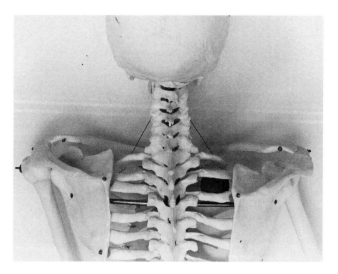

Fig. 46-44. Picture of a skeleton with a simulated mass in the left apex. Note that as the ribs become concentrically smaller and their angle changes, the intercostal space becomes smaller at the top of the apex.

slightly caudal, which makes penetration of the intercostal space easier (Fig. 46-44 and 46-45).

Several final points should be made about unusual masses in the apex. Neurogenic tumors and lateral meningocele may occur in the posterior mediastinum adjacent to the neural foramina. Neurogenic tumors are very hard and painful in biopsy;[43] only seldom can a diagnostic sample be obtained. Puncture of a lateral meningocele will yield clear fluid consistent with spinal fluid (Fig. 46-46).

Pleural lesions. Pleural lesion biopsies are difficult to perform fluoroscopically because as the lesion is turned perpendicularly to the fluoroscope it becomes "en face" and more difficult to see. With CT, sampling of such lesions is quite easy and actually provides considerable flexibility for needle selection. Of course, an aspiration needle can be used at any time; in those cases in which it is indicated, a cutting needle can actually be used for a more adequate tissue sample. Goralnik et al[84] reported that these cutting needles could be used safely for pleural lesions. He recommended their use when either lymphomas or unusual tumors such as mesotheliomas were suspected. Any of the automated biopsy devices can also be used if the size of the lesion is large enough to accommodate the length of the needle action.

Mediastinal lesions. Before the use of CT only a few authors ventured biopsy of the mediastinum using fluoroscopic guidance. With the refinement of CT techniques, however, CT is now the modality of choice and is commonly used for this area.[2]

Several limited studies by Lauby et al,[166] Jereb and Krasovec,[139] and Rosenberger[242] and Adler[2] demonstrated the feasibility of mediastinal biopsies with fine

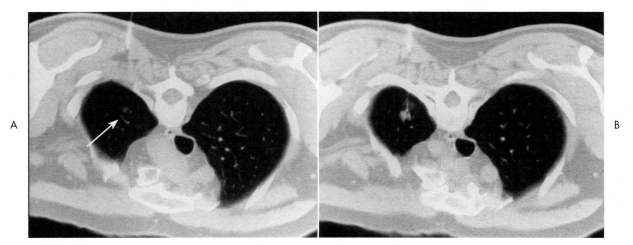

Fig. 46-45. A, This and the subsequent scan shows how slight cephalad-caudad angulation is required in many apical lesions. This scan shows the guidance cannula in the skin. Note the faintly visualized lower margin of the mass *(arrow)* and the open intercostal space without a rib. **B,** This scan shows placement of the needle into the lesion. To reach the lesion a cephalad angle from the position shown in **A** was required. Note that at this section the rib intervenes in the pathway and that the illusion of needle penetration of the rib is given; this is because of partial volume imaging of the lower positioned needle.

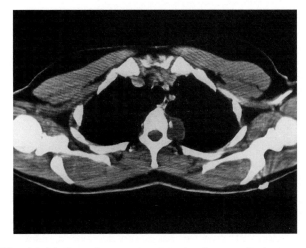

Fig. 46-46. Scan shows a very low density mass in the costovertebral junction on the left; this is consistent with and proved to be a lateral meningocele. This location is also common for neurofibromas, which are very difficult to biopsy (see text).

needles guided by fluoroscopy. Weisbrod[273] and Westcott[278] confirmed the benefits of fluoroscopic procedures but also noted some of the disadvantages and potential hazards. The most extensive series consisting of 100 patients was reported by Westcott. Although the results showed a 96% correct answer, there were 10 patients with vascular aneurysms that created some difficulty. Five of the patients were excluded from a biopsy because of a difficulty in evaluating the mediastinum. In another five cases, inadvertent puncture of aortic aneurysms occurred; in one patient a hemomediastinum developed.

Wiesbrod et al[273] also reported several important observations. In their series they noted that although aspiration needles were satisfactory for metastatic disease, the needles were less than optimal for lymphomas (see later section). They also reported one case of cardiac tamponade, which was successfully treated.

Since these reports, Adler et al[2] and our own group have reported the preference for CT in guiding such procedures, which can be quite effective and safe if the appropriate guidelines are used. Anatomic approach for the mediastinum is slightly different, depending on the space being sampled and the approach used.

For anterior lesions, one must avoid the internal mammary vessels (Fig. 46-47) and mediastinal vessels and also minimize the distance of the lung traversed. Adequate opacification of the vessels is important for accurate identification. If possible it is best to avoid all lung parenchyma, but to use the normal or pathologic mediastinum as a "window" for the needle passage (Fig. 46-48).

Approach for the posterior lesions is quite simple, as one would expect. One should minimize the length of the lung crossed and try to remain extrapleural if possible. Remaining extrapleural is possible if one carefully chooses a trajectory lateral to the costovertebral articulation, keeping the needle close to the vertebral bodies.

The approach to middle mediastinal lesions, possible through either an anterior or posterior pathway, can be safely performed if one pays careful attention to de-

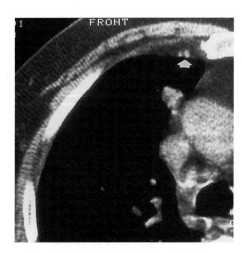

Fig. 46-47. Scan shows internal mammary artery and vein *(arrow)* adjacent to the sternum.

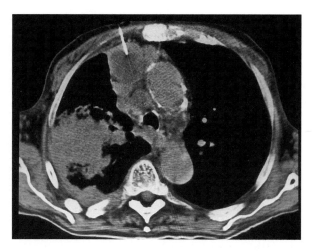

Fig. 46-48. Scan shows biopsy of large mediastinal mass to the right of the mediastinum. When the mass abuts against the chest wall there is virtually no risk for pneumothorax. Note the needle has passed to the right of the internal mammary vessels.

tail. Most commonly, a posterior approach along the paraspinal space is the most appropriate. It can be done from either a right or left side trajectory, but surprisingly a left side approach is the easiest (Fig. 46-49, *A* to *D*). There is actually more space in the left paraspinal side between the aorta and the vertebral body on the left than there is on the right. The key point to remember is to start with the entrance site at the junction point of transverse process and the rib, and to keep the bevel against the vertebral body. By doing this one can slide the needle along the margin of the vertebral body and deflect it into the mediastinum. Ample local anesthesia is important. This is appropriate for paratracheal or subcarinal lesions. Avoidance of the esophagus and bronchi are important to minimize the possibility of potential complications.

An anterior approach for middle mediastinal lesions is only rarely possible because of the closeness of the mediastinal vessels, but on occasion there will be sufficient space available (Fig. 46-50, 46-51). When tumor interposes itself between vessels, or when there is abundant mediastinal fat, anterior approaches can be made by skillful operators.

Pneumonias and infiltrates. Recovery of samples for culture and identification of infectious processes has become more popular in recent years. The results have been somewhat variable for the routine pyogenic infections, so we have seldom been asked to sample such problems. The opportunistic infections in immunocompromised patients have become a more significant diagnostic dilemma, and thus the occasion may arise in which sampling is more critical.

In our experience the diagnosis of fungal infection with cavitation or fungus ball by needle aspiration is quite reliable and easy to perform. In such cases, the procedure is performed in a standard fashion, except that the sample is sent for appropriate stains and culture.

When a more difficult pathogen such as *Pneumocystis carini* is suspected, simple aspiration may not suffice. Although some authors have inferred that recovery of diagnostic tissue is quite easy, we have found that it is not. In many cases one may require a small cutting sample that can provide more ample material for evaluation. When the infiltrate abuts the pleural membrane, we have employed a small cutting 20-gauge needle with considerable success and no morbidity (Fig. 46-52). Our experience is quite limited (to perhaps 10 cases), but we are optimistic for this technique.

Results: success and complications

The success rate of lung biopsies has varied widely among the many reports of fluoroscopic and CT-guided procedures. These rates have ranged as low as 60% and as high as 95%.

In our experience, the success rate is about 75% with a single pass and overall 85% with a second pass as required. These results are exclusive of lymphoma and mesothelioma cases, which are very difficult to diagnose with aspiration biopsies. Weisbrod et al[273] noted that in about 67% of cases the diagnosis of lymphoma can be suggested, but not the definitive subtype. Goralnik et al[84] found that the specific subtype could be diagnosed using a large cutting needle for suspected lymphoma lesions.

Although it is true that the outcome may vary from one institution to the next depending on the selection criteria for patients, favorable results can be obtained with the careful attention to detail and technique as noted in this chapter.

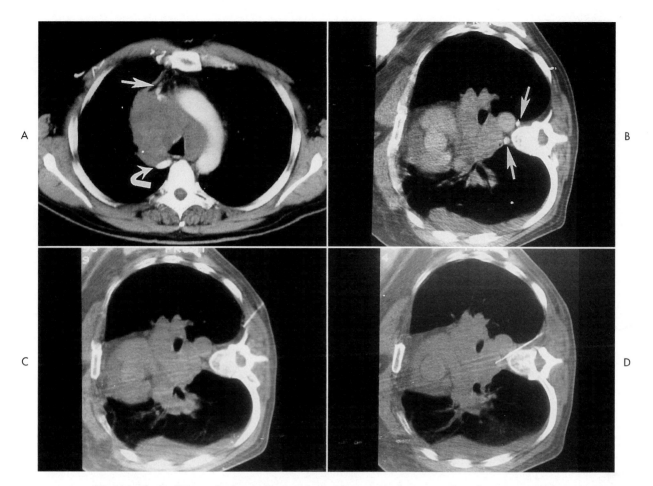

Fig. 46-49. A, CT scan in the supine position with contrast shows margins of aorta, opacified azygous vein *(curved arrow)*, and opacified collateral veins *(arrow)* in anterior mediastinum. The large mass in the middle mediastinum has occluded the superior vena cava. **B,** This scan was taken in the right decubitus position with contrast material. Note the opacified azygous and hemiazygous veins *(arrows)*. **C,** Scan showing the entrance point at the articulation of the traverse process and the rib. Note the needle along margin of pleura and vertebral body. Some saline has been injected to widen the pathway between the pleura and vertebral body. **D,** Final needle placement is made after the needle has been "slid" along the margin of the vertebral body. Ample xylocaine is required.

Reliability of cytology results. Several reports by Sinner et al,[246] Thornbury et al,[260] and Greene[86] have documented that the results of aspiration biopsies correlate well with histologic results. Green et al[86] found the correlation to be 92.3% for adenocarcinomas, 100% for squamous cell, 88.9% for large cell undifferentiated, and 100% for small cell undifferentiated. Taft et al[257] found an interobserver error to be only 6% with 94% overall consistency.

The consistency for diagnosing lymphomas is much less. Weisbrod et al[273] and Westcott et al have shown that aspiration biopsies are capable of suggesting the diagnosis of lymphoma, but Goralnik et al[84] showed that only a cutting needle biopsy was capable of providing the definitive subtype of lymphoma.

Mesotheliomas are also quite difficult to diagnose with any type of needle. In our experience with about eight such cases, the diagnosis of mesothelioma can be suggested but the differentiation of benign versus malignant cannot be made even with cutting needles.

The most difficult question to be resolved relative to these procedures is the significance of a negative or benign diagnosis. Some authors have suggested that because they obtained a "negative" aspiration for malignancy from a benign lesion, the correct diagnosis could be inferred. This is obviously not the case, for one must always be suspicious of a "negative" aspiration unless other information is available. It is difficult to accept that authors correctly made the diagnosis of granulomas, sequestration, and other unusual benign lesions based

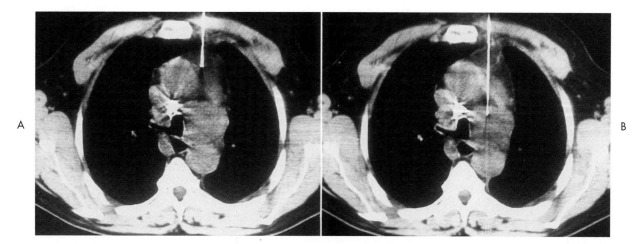

Fig. 46-50. A, Because of the meticulous pathway required for this needle procedure, an entrance site between the internal mammary vessels was chosen. Scan shows the 20-gauge Chiba needle being inserted to the plane between the ascending aorta and the main pulmonary artery. Transmitted cardiac pulsations produced motion of the needle and the illusion of two needles. **B,** Final needle placement into the middle mediastinum and aortic pulmonary window was accomplished. The remarkable accuracy of needle placements is clearly demonstrated in this case.

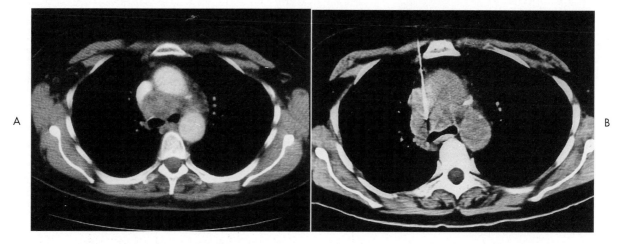

Fig. 46-51. A, CT scan showing mass in the middle mediastinum that is slightly separating the space between the vena cava and the aorta. **B,** Final placement of the needle into the mass. Note that there is no hematoma produced; penetration of the vessels did not occur. *In our experience, we have never penetrated any major vessel while performing these procedures.*

solely on aspiration biopsy. As Westcott noted, it is appropriate to accept a specific result that states a diagnosis (e.g., hamartoma, infarct, etc.), but claims of the recovery of histiocytes, leukocytes, and other nonspecific cells should be regarded with skepticism.

It is only after several repeat biopsies that yield nonspecific material that one can consider "following" such a lesion. If there is a strong history of family disease or smoking, it is appropriate to have surgical removal of such a lesion regardless of the results.

In patients without risk factors, one may choose to follow such cases at 3-month intervals, for a total of 9 months. If such a lesion is benign, it will usually shrink or calcify during this time period. If there is any increase in size, then surgery should be performed immediately. At the end of 9 months, if there has been no change, it is appropriate to reevaluate the case.

Success factors. A number of factors improve the probability of a positive biopsy. These factors include the operator's experience and technique; pathology; needle type; and character, size, and location of the lesion. Experience of the cytologists and pathologists is very im-

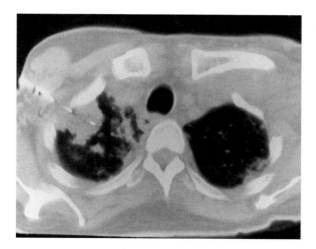

Fig. 46-52. While aspiration sampling for infectious processes may be helpful, we have found that unusual infections like *Pneumocystis carinii* may require a small cutting sample such as this 20-gauge Tru-cut sample, which shows insertion of the tissue stylet into the patch of consolidated infiltrate.

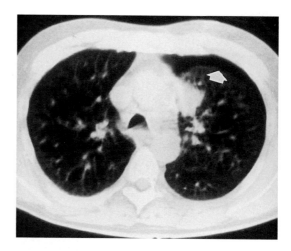

Fig. 46-53. Pneumothorax can be detected as easily with CT as with chest film. This scan shows a small anterior pneumothorax *(arrow)* anterior to the left lung.

portant. The greater the experience, the more consistent the results of the procedure. Proper technique includes choice of appropriate needle and maintenance of proper vacuum.

It is always important to include the routine slide smears as well as a saline rinse of the needle and syringe for submission to pathology; a cytocentrifuge and cell block preparation will increase the diagnostic yield of such samples. Pathologic results depend on the cell type of the tumor as noted in the results section; the common primary lung tumors are easily diagnosed, while others are not.

The size and location of a mass affects the probability of a positive diagnostic aspiration. Bergquist et al[20] noted that the diagnostic accuracy was higher for larger lesions and for more peripheral lesions. For example, a 1-cm nodule was successfully biopsied in 58% of cases when it was central; it was successfully biopsied in 85% of cases when it was peripheral.

Postprocedure care

The postprocedure care of these patients is quite simple and consists of observing them for severe hemoptysis and pneumothorax. Immediately after completion of the procedure, I prefer to have the patient lie still for 5 to 10 minutes to let the puncture site seal. Moore et al[195] have shown that if the patient is positioned with the puncture site down after the procedure, the incidence of pneumothorax is reduced. The pneumothorax rate for patients placed in this position was 17.9%, while the rate was 33.6% for those not so positioned. Chest tube rate was 9.8% for those who were correctly positioned, compared with 0.4% for those who were not.

Before removing the patient from the table, I take a repeat scan to evaluate for postprocedural problems. Miller et al[190] have shown that CT is as reliable for detecting pneumothorax as is a plain radiograph (Fig. 46-53). A small pneumothorax is of little significance, as noted below. Some bleeding in the parenchyma in the area of the needle tract is quite frequent, but it is of no significance. If there is any question of the patient's stability, oxygen should be administered and appropriate treatment given, as noted below.

Postprocedure chest films should be taken at 1-, 4-, and 8-hour intervals. Perlmutt et al[230] showed that pneumothoraces could be detected in the following percentages at the noted timed delays: 89% immediately after procedure, 9% after 1 hour, and only 2% after 4 hours.

The most frequent complication is pneumothorax, which can be easily treated with a small caliber tube and a one-way valve, (Fig. 46-54). The decision to insert a chest tube is dependent on patient symptoms, patient attitude and attending service, and patient reliability. In the best of circumstances, the chest tube is inserted only if the patient is symptomatic. Even a 50% pneumothorax does not require treatment, unless the patient is symptomatic. If there is any question of the patient's symptoms, reliability, or housing status, the chest tube should be inserted.

Chest tube insertion

It is best for the inexperienced operator to insert the tube under fluoroscopy or at the table side, depending on the experience of the interventionist and the distress of the patient.[229,239] The placement of the chest tube is quite simple and can be accomplished in the following fashion. One should use an entrance site in the anterior second or third intercostal space on the side of

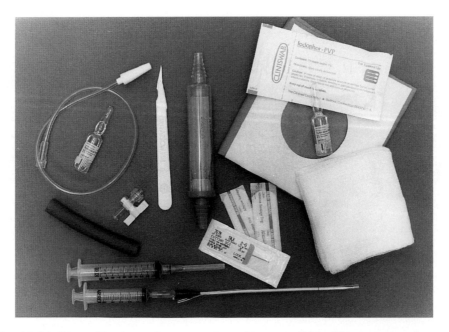

Fig. 46-54. Disposable chest tube trays such as this are available. These are complete and provide all necessary equipment including the instruments, tube, and Heimlich valve.

the pneumothorax. After preparation of the site with antiseptic solution, one should thoroughly anesthetize the site down to and including the pleura. One can estimate the depth required for the tube insertion by using the anesthetic needle to aspirate air at the site.

After administration of the anesthetic, a nick in the skin is made with a scalpel to provide ample space for the tube. As one pushes the tube through the chest wall, a "give" is noted; this indicates passage through the pleura (Fig. 46-55). The tube is kept perpendicular relative to the axial plane until it passes into the pleural space. It is then angled slightly cephalad so the tube will lie in the apical lateral region. This location is optimal because in this position it will evacuate "rising" air when the patient is either lying down or standing up.

After placement of the tube, one should always reconfirm the proper location of the tube, even if the placement was optimal. This can be done by checking the tube position with oblique or lateral films. Another method one can use is to place the end of the valve close to one's ear and listen for the escape of air through the valve.

After the placement of the tube, patients will usually experience some pain as the lung re-expands against the tube. A mild analgesic will relieve the discomfort; repeat analgesics are seldom necessary.

At this point a complete explanation should be provided to the patient and nursing staff to prevent inappropriate or premature closure of the tube.

If the lung is reinflated for 10 to 12 hours,

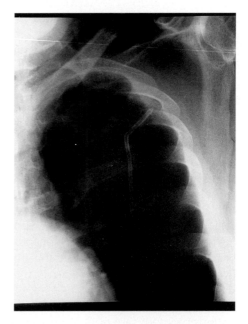

Fig. 46-55. Chest film showing chest tube in left upper lobe. Whenever tube is positioned, one should clinically check for the egress of air to ensure proper function.

the tube can be removed. The tube should be clamped for several hours and a repeat film taken. If the lung remains expanded, it can be removed. If not, the valve should be reopened for 24 hours and the procedure repeated at a later time. If severe primary lung disease is present, expansion could take as long as 2 to 3 days.

Complications and causative factors

Pneumothorax. The pneumothorax rate reported for CT procedures varies widely among patient groups. The asymptomatic rate varies between 17.5% and 72%. The symptomatic rate, requiring chest tube, varies between 6% and 18%. Our rates using the single-needle method and the coaxial, short cannula method are 17.5% for asymptomatic and 6% for symptomatic pneumothoraces. The higher rates reported by other authors are probably the result of the prolonged time of the procedures and the multiple needle punctures associated with the tandem-needle technique.

Some authors attribute the high pneumothorax rate to the prolonged length of the procedure. They reported the average time period for the needle to be within the lung parenchyma as 15 to 20 minutes. This compares to the average of 6 minutes we tabulated in our department. The difference we believe is related to preplanning and use of the short cannula, coaxial method.

The risk of a pneumothorax also depends on many other factors including status of the lung, number of needle passes, and number of pleural surfaces penetrated. Fish et al[63] and Miller et al[190] showed a definite relationship of pneumothorax to lung disease. Fish et al evaluated chest films and spirometry to determine the presence of chronic obstructive pulmonary disease (COPD) and found that normal patients had a pneumothorax rate lower than those with COPD. With spirometry measurements the ratio for pneumothorax was 45% for COPD patients, compared with 25% for normal patients. Using the chest x-ray examination as the standard, the rate was 42% for COPD compared with 25% for normal patients.

Hemoptysis. The rate of hemoptysis is quite low with all types of techniques and appears to be dependent only on needle size. In a series by Khouri et al,[153] the hemoptysis rate for 20-gauge needle was only 5%, compared with 21% for 18-gauge needles.

The other factors affecting hemoptysis are the depth of lesions, coagulation status, and the presence of congestive failure. Deep lesions or hilar lesions are at greatest risk because of the long pathway and proximity of blood vessel. Those patients with coagulopathies, pulmonary hypertension, or congestive heart failure are at greatest risk for hemoptysis and even endobronchial bleeding (as noted below) and should be biopsied without correction of the basic problem. Very commonly, localized hemorrhage in the parenchyma may occur following a biopsy, but it is of no significance (Fig. 46-56).

Fatalities. As seen in the original articles describing fatalities, the two causes are endobronchial bleeding and air embolism. I have been able to locate nine re-

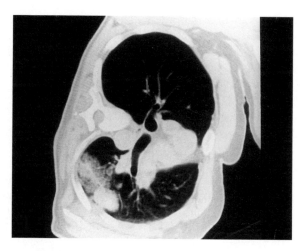

Fig. 46-56. CT scan shows large infiltrate adjacent to the lung mass, representing hemorrhage following a lung biopsy. The patient had no severe hemoptysis or ill effects.

ported deaths in the literature, five from endobronchial bleeding and four from air embolism.

Endobronchial bleeding is a very rate event. In my opinion its occurrence is based on the nature of the abnormality being sampled as well as on needle caliber.[191,212] While deaths have occurred with both 22-gauge and 18-gauge needles, it is quite clear that the rate of hemoptysis is less with small-caliber needles. The cases reported in the literature were associated with ill-defined masses adjacent to the hila.

Those cases of air embolism were associated with coughing paroxysms. Several authors[261,276] hypothesized that the air embolism is a result of the elevated intrabronchial pressure that occurs with coughing; the high-pressure air follows along the needle track into the blood vessels. One should avoid the temptation to "counsel" the patient not to cough. To avoid such problems one should immediately remove the needle if a patient starts to cough during a procedure.

Blood-patch technique. Several authors have reported on the blood-patch technique, which is used to reduce the possibility of a pneumothorax.[24,120,183] With this method a coaxial needle method is used and a blood clot is injected through the long cannula during its removal from the lung. The results of this method are variable, and Bourgouin et al[24] reported no difference in outcome when it was evaluated in a randomized prospective fashion.

LIVER BIOPSY

Liver biopsy is a common procedure* because the liver is commonly involved with malignant pro-

*References 177, 182, 253, 254, 275, 280.

cesses and benign disorders that can mimic malignancy. Because specific differentiation of these various processes is not possible by imaging methods, definitive diagnosis by biopsy is necessary for planning proper patient management and avoiding unnecessary surgical procedures. A new era of treating disease focally has also begun; this will be discussed in a later section.[124]

Indications

The indications are quite broad considering the diagnostic and guidance accuracy of both ultrasound and CT. Any patient with a focal hepatic mass or unusual anatomic configuration should have a guided rather than a blind procedure.

Diffuse processes of the liver are probably best performed by the blind method at the bedside, but any blind procedure that has failed is an indication for a guided procedure. Those associated with large amounts of ascites are best served by a guided procedure (Figs. 46-57, 46-58). Biopsy of patients with abnormal coagulopathy should be performed under a combined guidance procedure, both imaging and fluoroscopy, so that special hemostatic techniques as described below can be used.

The choice between ultrasound or CT must be made by the individual physician, but in general, CT is still considered the "gold" standard. Difficult anatomic location, poor visualization under ultrasound, or concern about increased vascularity is a clear indication for CT guidance.

Selection of needle

For the liver, I use either a 20-gauge Chiba needle for an aspiration cytologic sample, or a Tru-Cut needle, 18- or 14-gauge caliber. Selection of a needle is based on clinical factors, anatomic characteristics, and bolus contrast enhancement.

From a clinical perspective, a previous history of a malignancy is sufficient evidence to consider using only an aspiration needle. In the vast majority of cases the cytologic sample is quite adequate to confirm a previously diagnosed tumor.

A number of anatomic factors dictate the need for an aspiration biopsy. Unusually close proximity to various structures such as the vena cava, portal vein, gallbladder, pleura, or diaphragm indicates the need for an aspiration biopsy (Figs. 46-59, *A* and *B*).

Concern about a possible hemorrhagic complication is also an indication for an aspiration procedure. Such concern is typically raised if a coagulation problem exists or if a lesion is suspected of being vascular. A small abnormality in the coagulation studies is sufficient to justify the use of an aspiration needle. Bolus contrast enhancement is useful for assessing the vascularity of lesions. Those lesions that are slightly vascular should be sampled by an aspiration needle because it is safer than a cutting needle. If a lesion is very vascular, one probably should not even use an aspiration needle (see later section on hepatoma).

The larger cutting needles, either 18 or 14 gauge, can and should be used if a lesion is unknown, accessible, and avascular with a contrast enhancement. When an abnormality is unknown, only the sample obtained with the cutting needle can provide the type of histologic detail for the definitive diagnosis of virtually all be-

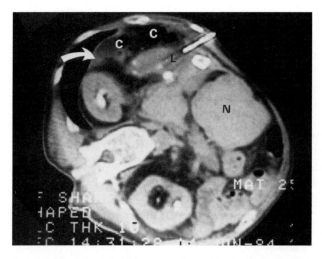

Fig. 46-57. CT-guided biopsy performed because of anatomic variation and unusual liver configuration. The patient is lying on the left side. Note the small right lobe of the liver, *L*, the location of the diaphragm *(arrow)*, the colon, *C*, and the large regenerating nodule, *N*. The Tru-Cut biopsy of the right lobe showed hemangioendothelial sarcoma.

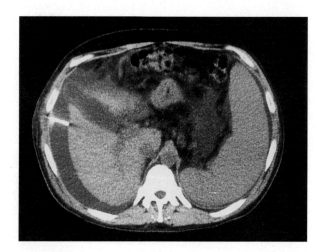

Fig. 46-58. Patients with ascites are easily sampled with CT guidance. Because localization does not depend on percussion, accurate placement is not difficult.

nign and malignant lesions (see later sections on results) (Figs. 46-60, *A* and *B*).

Contraindications

There are several contraindications to liver biopsy. Severe uncorrectable coagulopathy is the most common contraindication; if an abnormal baseline exists and it can be corrected with fresh frozen plasma or platelets, the procedure can be performed without additional precau-tions. If an abnormal baseline cannot be corrected, other steps must be taken as described later under hemostatic techniques.

Lack of patient cooperation is a relative contrain-dication. If a patient cannot cooperate with sedatives, then general anesthesia might be considered.

Another contraindication is the presence of in-creased vascularity or prominent vascular collaterals as noted with contrast enhancement. Those lesions, which

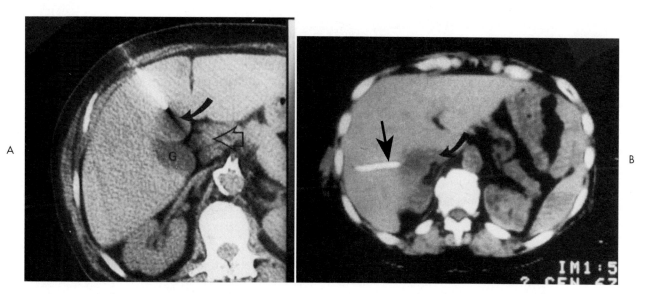

Fig. 46-59. A, Aspiration biopsy of a small lesion *(curved arrow)* in the right lobe, for meta-static lung tumor. Bolus injection is not "required" for aspiration biopsies, but on occasion they can be helpful. Because of the proximity of the gallbladder, *G,* and portal structures *(open arrow),* an aspiration procedure was performed. **B,** This scan in a different patient shows a small-needle aspiration *(arrow)* of a lesion next to the vena cava *(curved arrow).*

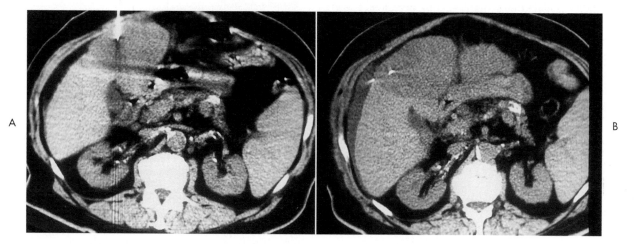

Fig. 46-60. A, This case demonstrates the usefulness of the cutting-needle biopsy. This aspi-ration biopsy was positive for malignancy and said to be consistent with adenocarcinoma. **B,** Because of inappropriate response to chemotherapy, repeat biopsy with a cutting needle was performed. This scan shows a cutting-needle biopsy, which was definitive for small cell lym-phoma, non-Hodgkins.

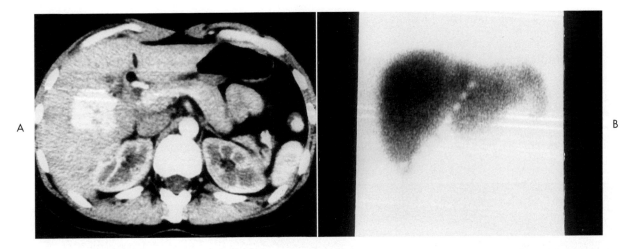

Fig. 46-61. A, Various mass lesions of the liver can be extremely vascular and represent a serious risk for complication. This CT scan shows an enhancing mass in the midportion of the right lobe, suggestive of some type of primary liver tumor. Because of its vascular nature, a biopsy was not performed. **B,** Radionuclide scan of the liver was normal, confirming that the mass noted in **A** was focal nodular hyperplasia.

may be very vascular, include focal nodular hyperplasia (Fig. 46-61, *A* and *B*) hepatomas, hemangiomas, sarcomas, and metastases.

Aspiration biopsy

For aspiration biopsy, either the single needle or the short cannula, coaxial method using the 20-gauge Chiba needle should be used. A number of factors should be considered regarding entrance site selection and preparation, trajectory planning, target selection, and follow-up.

Entrance site selection is based on the location of the lesion. Generally speaking the shortest pathway that avoids the portal venous system, gallbladder, bowel, and diaphragm should be chosen. To avoid the pleural space, one should choose a site below the insertion of the diaphragm. If the lesion is somewhat high, this can be most practically accomplished by choosing a site no more posterior than the midaxillary line. When the lesion is high in the liver above the insertion of the diaphragm, an angled approach is necessary. The anterior diaphragm is much higher than the posterior portion, and lesions are more easily approached without crossing lung (Fig. 46-62, *A* and *B*).

If the lesion is mobile, the patient can be placed in either a decubitus or oblique position to help immobilize the lesion (Fig. 46-63).

Careful palpation of the site and preparation are important. Avoidance of ribs can be accomplished by palpation. To make the procedure completely pain-free, the pathway should be anesthetized from the skin down to the capsule of the liver.

For the best results, the pathway should include

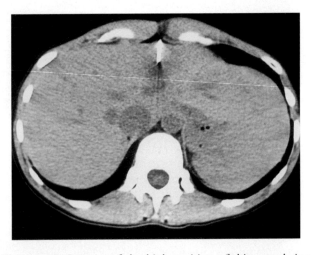

Fig. 46-62. Because of the high position of this mass being biopsied with a needle, an angled trajectory starting below the xyphoid was necessary. The needle tip is visualized within the mass, but note the proximal end of the needle is not seen because it entered through a lower slice.

a cuff of normal liver. This cuff can help prevent leakage of blood or tumor cells into the peritoneum.

Target selection is fairly straightforward. One should choose the lowest lesion that is easily approachable. If the lesion appears quite necrotic, one should attempt to position the needle within the periphery where one would expect more viable tissue.

The needle procedure is the standard aspiration procedure as previously described. We use the standard application of suction and reciprocating motion, and two passes.

After the procedure, minimal follow-up is re-

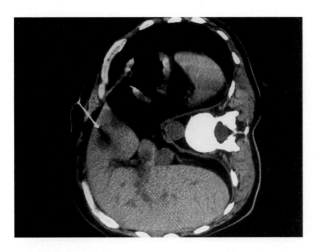

Fig. 46-63. Positioning the patient in a decubitus position can be quite helpful. This scan shows a biopsy of a lesion in the left lobe with the patient lying on the right side. This immobilized the lesion, making it more amenable to biopsy.

quired. For patients who have not had a complicated procedure, we typically undertake an observation period of 1 to 2 hours.

Cutting-needle biopsy

This procedure is performed using the single-needle technique and the techniques described previously in this chapter. The most commonly used needle is the 14-gauge Tru-Cut needle, but occasionally we use an 18- or 20-gauge Tru-Cut needle. Most commonly I use the manual Tru-Cut needle, but in some circumstances I will use the automated biopsy gun.

Routinely, I prefer a single pass of a 14-gauge needle rather than multiple passes with smaller-gauge cutting needles. A quandary always exists concerning the amount of tissue required for a specific diagnosis, relative to the size of the needle being used. While the larger needle cuts a large surface area within the liver, multiple needle passes increases the probability of randomly striking a small blood vessel. As will be noted in the complication section, the relative risk of taking multiple samples versus a single large sample has yet to be determined.

The same criteria and considerations are used for selection of the entrance site, trajectory, and target as were noted with the aspiration needle, except for some differences with target selection. When the abnormality is quite small, it is best to plan the procedure so that the entire width of the abnormality will be sampled. When the lesion is large, it is best to choose a target so that a small portion of the normal liver as well as the abnormality are sampled (Figs. 46-64, *A* to *C*).

If one uses a cutting needle, it is reasonable to perform a small-needle aspiration before the cutting-needle biopsy. Using the small needle first is valuable for

several reasons. By performing the biopsy first with a small needle the operator and the patient can practice the procedure and determine the cooperation of patient and sufficiency of the local anesthetic. If the procedure goes well, the large-needle biopsy may proceed. If the procedure entails problems, adjustments can be made in regard to entrance site, target, trajectory, sedation, and local anesthetic.

Automated biopsies

Automated biopsies have become popular because they minimize technical inconsistencies from one procedure to the next. Most such automated procedures are performed for this reason but there are circumstances in which even the most experienced individual might use an automated biopsy device.

There are two substantive indications for the automated gun relative to body size and the physical nature of a tumor. When a patient is quite large and the lesion is somewhat deep, it is difficult to move the outer cutting cannula of the manual Tru-Cut effectively because of the "drag" put on the cannula. Considerable resistance and "drag" on the cannula that makes the manual device difficult to use also occurs when the abnormality being sample is quite fibrotic or hard.

Regarding technique, also note that with the movement of the needle, "recoil" occurs. One of our colleagues has shown than if one holds such a device firmly rather than loosely with one hand, there is an improvement in sample size by about 14%.

Additional caveats

When sampling an abnormality in the upper liver, there are several factors to consider in avoiding the pleura and the diaphragm. First, the normal diaphragm is much higher anteriorly than posteriorly; thus a lateral approach is safer than a posterior one, and an anterior one is safer than a lateral one. As long as one does not see aerated lung, a pneumothorax will not occur during liver biopsy. Ample local anesthesia is critical to avoid undue patient discomfort and movement of the diaphragm, which might cause a complication during insertion of the needle.

The presence of ascites is not a contraindication for biopsy of the liver. A review of our cases and an article by Bernadino et al[17] shows that liver biopsies can be performed in such cases without difficulty.

Factors affecting accuracy

One of the most important factors to consider when evaluating the outcome of various techniques is the extent of disease present at the time of the biopsy. The greater the number and the larger the lesions within the liver, the greater the probability of a positive biopsy.

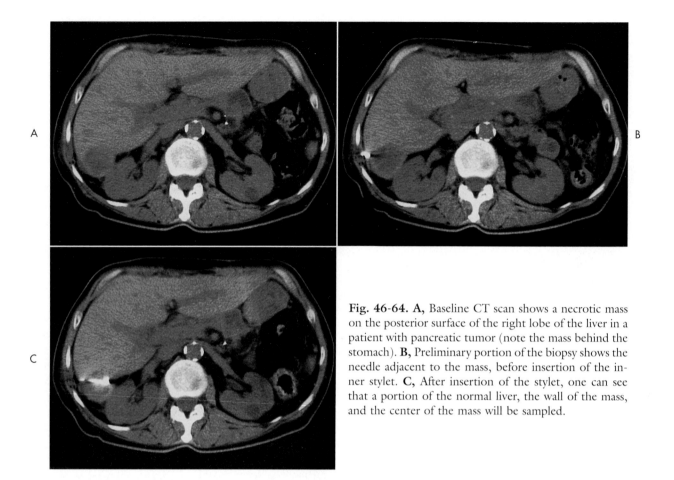

Fig. 46-64. A, Baseline CT scan shows a necrotic mass on the posterior surface of the right lobe of the liver in a patient with pancreatic tumor (note the mass behind the stomach). **B,** Preliminary portion of the biopsy shows the needle adjacent to the mass, before insertion of the inner stylet. **C,** After insertion of the stylet, one can see that a portion of the normal liver, the wall of the mass, and the center of the mass will be sampled.

Conn et al[35] studied this with a series of blind biopsies performed on cadaver livers at autopsy. They graded the degree of involvement of the liver by the number of lesions and found the following recovery accuracy: Grade I, 1 to 3 lesions had a 16% success rate; Grade II, 4 to 25 lesions had a 27% success rate; Grade III, 25 to 50 lesions had a 45% success rate; and Grade IV, with over 50% involvement by weight had a 86% success rate. This finding is important to consider whenever a new method, technique, or type of needle is first being reported in the literature.

It is quite clear that historically, guided biopsy procedures are superior to blind or unguided biopsy procedures. One of the first articles in diagnostic aspiration by Lundquist reported a high success rate in about 70% of cases using only manual palpation of the abdomen. In his series, the only cases sampled were those involving palpable nodules that would correspond to the Grade IV types of lesions as noted above.

Rasmussen et al[238] reported the first series on ultrasound biopsy using a 22-gauge needle with multiple passes. He recovered positive tissue in 70% of cases with ultrasound guidance, compared with an anticipated rate of 23% for blind biopsies (extrapolating Conn's[35] classi-

fication of his cases as described in the report). Subsequent reports showed similar results with success rates varying between 66% and 94%. Despite the advantages of the small needle, authors such as Ho noted the disadvantages of the aspiration types of biopsy: "Based on our study and the literature, the information obtained by fine-needle aspiration on the general state of the liver is not as comprehensive as from a tissue sample taken by the Menghini technique."

This data clearly indicates that several simple and obvious factors affect the results. First, the appropriate technique must be used with each needle (see the earlier sections on methods of biopsy for both aspiration and cutting needles), and second, diagnostic yield depends on accurate localization of the instrument. Meticulous placement of the device is critical regardless of the guidance modality used. As technology evolves and devices change, operator preferences may change as well. The effect of needle size on diagnostic success has been well documented for aspiration needles in both in vitro and in vivo studies. Andriole et al[6] studied the yield in liver biopsy of various aspiration needles and found that in vitro there was a definite increase in the diagnostic material with the larger-caliber needles. In a series of liver biopsies Pagani et al[221,222] reported the results of using both 18-gauge and 22-gauge needles. They found a significant benefit 85% versus 98%, respectively, without any difference in the complication rate. In our own institution the diagnostic yield and complication rates of various aspiration needles have been determined and compared with cutting needles; these rates were reported by Martino et al[182] and Ha et al.[91] With a single pass with aspiration needles and providing samples for both slide smears and cell block material, the diagnostic yield for malignant disease with a 22-gauge needle was 60.9%, compared with the 20-gauge needle at 77.6%. It is important to note that Pagani's data were based on the performance of multiple passes, and that our data involved single passes, which explains their higher yields.

From these data and that of Ferrucci et al[60,61] it is clear that the more needle passes taken, the higher the diagnostic accuracy. In their series they selected 20 cases that were positive and looked at the diagnostic yield for each needle pass. The yield was 75% with one pass and 90% with two passes. (One can never expect 100% yield even with five passes.) In the same article, Ferrucci's overall yield was 82%. Even with blind biopsies the diagnostic yield increases appreciably with multiple passes. Grossman et al[89] noted an increase in the diagnostic yield from 41% to 54% with two passes and Conn and Yesner[35] noted that the yield increased from 47% to 58% with two passes.

All of the comparison articles concerning diagnostic yield from aspiration and cutting needles (single passes) have shown that cutting needles are superior to aspiration needles. The two comparison articles using a single pass were reported by our group. Martino et al[182] showed that the diagnostic yield of Menghini and Tru-Cut biopsy needles was 88.1%, compared with 60.9% for 22-gauge aspiration needles. Our more recent experience reported by Ha et al[91] showed the 14-gauge Tru-Cut needle to be superior to the 20-gauge aspiration needle, with yields of 90.2% as compared with 77.6%. A comparison article by Jacobsen et al[135] showed a slightly greater accuracy with a skinny needle; however, their comparison was flawed by the fact that they took three passes with the skinny needle and only one with the cutting needle.

For benign disease, all reporting authors have shown a clear advantage for the cutting types of needles relative to determining specific disease processes. In our most recent experience reported by Ha et al,[91] the cutting needles provided a specific diagnosis in 88.5% compared to 39.4% for aspiration needles; nonspecific diagnosis was provided in 11.5% by the cutting and 48.5% for the aspiration needle.

Combination of slide smears and histology can provide an added increment of positivity for the results.

Numerous authors including ourselves attest to the benefit of combining aspirate samples with cell block histology. In our most recent study, the addition of cell block histology increased our diagnostic yield from 54.8% to 77.4%. Other authors including Sherlock et al,[245] Grossman et al,[88,89] Carney et al,[30] and Atterbury et al[7] have noted that producing a cellular smear by "rolling" the sample on a slide adds some additional accuracy. These authors showed an increase in positivity of between 3% and 17% by performing this technique. The only plausible explanation for this result is that the needle passes through the tumor during its incursion but no tissue is "cut." The cells are located in the side of the tissue core and can therefore be "smeared" onto the slide.

There are mixed findings in regard to the automated biopsy guns, which are the most recent innovation in biopsy technique. Several authors feel their overall benefit is that they are quick, consistent, and foolproof. These features should provide better overall results for the inexperienced operator. For the experienced operator, however, the manual Tru-Cut appears to be as or more effective than the automated device. Hopper et al,[128] in the evaluation of numerous automated devices, noted that the gold-standard device to which all devices should be compared and the one as yet unsurpassed is the 14-gauge manual Tru-Cut device.

The success of percutaneous liver biopsy by CT guidance depends on the various important factors noted above. In our experience, the success rate for malignancy and benign disease has varied according to the type of needle used and the abnormality being sought. The success rate for sampling all malignant disease with aspiration needles is 77.6% and for cutting needles, 90.2%. The success rate for benign disease is 39.4% with aspiration needles and 88.5% for cutting needles (see Tables 46-1, 46-2, 46-3).

Complications

As experience with guided biopsy procedures has accumulated the same types and spectrum of complications have occurred with guided biopsies as have occurred with unguided procedures. These include biliary peritonitis, tumor seeding,[218] hepatic infarction, pneumothorax, inadvertent puncture of bowel, abscess, and hemorrhage.[288]

In regard to complications, the logical differences between aspiration and cutting needles must be made clear. In view of the wide variety of devices used and reported, some general as well as specific comments should be made.

From our experience there is little question that there is a slight difference in complication rate between the cutting needles and the aspiration needles. It is also true with experience and refinement of techniques that there can be improvement in these rates. In reporting our various series, we have shown a decrease in the complication rate with minimal improvements as we have refined our techniques. In our second report in reference to aspiration needles, Martino et al[182] reported a complication rate of 0.83% for serious complications and in our most recent report by Ha et al[91] we reported a complication rate of 0%. Relative to cutting needles, Martino et al[182] reported a complication rate of 1.44% and in our recent report by Ha et al,[91] the complication rate was 1.1%. Our complication rates indicate that complication rates can be quite low and acceptable for all needles if appropriate techniques are used.

The more obvious factors that affect complications include coagulation status, lesion characteristics, characteristics of the needle, and the number of needle passes.[259,288]

Coagulation status. One obvious factor that affects complications is the coagulation status of the patient. For biopsy using either an aspiration or cutting type of needle, we prefer to have the platelet count greater than 50,000 and the prothrombin time less than 14 seconds. If either value is not within the desired range, corrective action should be taken as needed, either platelet transfusion or administration of fresh frozen plasma. Patients should also not be on any anticoagulating drugs such as aspirin or Coumadin (see section below on contraindications). Unusual problems such as hemophilia, Christmas disease, lupus, or renal failure must be addressed individually. If there is any question of an unusual coagulation status, a bleeding time should be measured. This is the most accurate method of determining bleeding status because it is an in vivo test that takes into account all factors including the coagulation factor cascade, capillary fragility, and platelet function. An abnormal bleeding test warrants a consultation from the hematologist to preclude any major problems.

Lesion vascularity. The other factor that is seldom discussed and is actually quite important is the vascular nature of the abnormality being biopsied. We have encountered bleeding problems in patients with vascular lesions such as hemangiomas and metastatic renal carcinoma. Several others have reported serious problems with vascular bleeding. Bret et al[25,26] reported a small series of hepatomas biopsied using a 22-gauge needle for aspiration and some serious hemorrhagic complications. One of the patients required transfusion, two required corrective surgery, and there was one death. Considering the small caliber of the needle and the experience level of the authors, the only explanation for these problems is that hepatomas and other tumors that are inherently vascular are predisposed to bleeding (Figs. 46-65, 46-66).

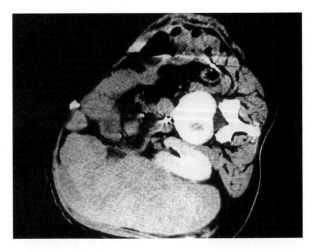

Fig. 46-65. Significant hemorrhage can occur as a result of numerous factors. This scan shows a large hematoma outlining the capsule of the liver in the lower portion of the abdomen caused by a single pass of a 20-gauge Chiba needle (performed by the author). The patient has diffuse metastatic renal cell carcinoma to the liver that was very vascular.

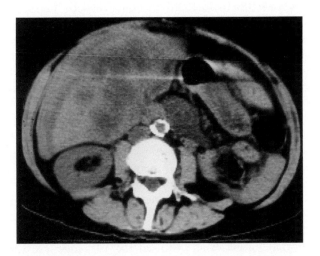

Fig. 46-66. On occasion, bleeding can occur as a chance event. This patient had a nonvascular metastatic carcinoma. A large perihepatic hematoma occurred after a single biopsy by a 20-gauge aspiration needle; there were no technical errors, and the patient was most cooperative during the procedure.

There is also a case report of a bleeding death from a 22-gauge needle biopsy of a cavernous hemangioma. The authors did not mention assessment of vascularity using a dynamic study, nor did they choose a trajectory through a small cuff of normal liver.

Smith et al[249] also reported that one cannot prevent complications by using a fine needle. From a mail survey he determined that in a series of 63,000 reported cases there were 27 cases of significant hemorrhage requiring transfusion, and three deaths.

Needle traits. Regarding the needles used in

cases of reported complications, several points must be made. First, as stated, there is a difference in the overall complication rate between cutting needles and aspiration needles. Second, there is no definite difference in the complication rates among the various caliber needles of the aspiration type. Pagani et al[221] reported no difference in the complication rate between 18-gauge and 22-gauge needles. In our two sequential series, our complication rates actually dropped when we switched from a 22-gauge to a 20-gauge needle. One cannot necessarily infer that the reduction in the rate was due to the needles; the reduced rate is most likely a result of experience and technique that naturally overcomes any minimal difference among the aspiration needles. In a laboratory study on animals by our group (Table 46-5) there were only minimal differences among any of the needles less than 18 gauge, but there was significant difference between these and the larger-gauge needle.

The key question recently answered is the relative risk of bleeding among the various Tru-Cut types of needles of different calibers. A recent lab study by Plecha and Goodwin compared the amount of diagnostic tissue obtained to amount of local bleeding with various calibers of Tru-Cut needles. They found that per unit of tissue, there was more bleeding with the larger needle (14-gauge) as compared with the 20-gauge needle. The clinical significance of the different sizes has yet to be proved. That is, it has not been clinically determined whether multiple small caliber Tru-Cut needles are safer to use than a single pass with a large needle. In our practice we have actually had a major complication with the use of a 20-gauge Tru-Cut, which resulted in a major hemorrhage and required a surgical procedure.

Needle passes. While multiple needle passes increase the diagnostic outcome, they introduce a higher incidence of complication with all needles, including small aspiration types. In our experience we limit our needle passes to two in virtually all cases. The expected yield should be about 75% to 85%. If the procedure is not a successful one, a repeat two-pass biopsy is warranted, after which one should choose either a cutting needle or a surgical procedure. The adverse effect of numerous needle passes was best documented in a survey by Smith.[249] We concur with his opinion that the number of needle passes even with a small needle should be limited to as few as possible. As is seen in reports in the literature, serious complications occurred in cases involving four to five needle passes, and none occurred in those involving two or less passes.

Coagulopathy. Patients with coagulopathy should have the appropriate treatment as indicated to improve coagulation. Patients with low platelet count should receive several units of platelets. Considering the time delays required with laboratory studies and the life

expectancy of platelets, I manage the administration as follows. If I intend to give six units of platelets, I will send a blood sample for platelet count after the first two units; if the observed effect in the repeat count is what I anticipate as compared with the baseline value, I will then proceed with the procedure immediately following the fourth unit. The last two units are given after the biopsy. The same type of laboratory and administration schedule is used with fresh frozen plasma for an elevated prothrombin time. Patients requiring factor VIII are treated in a more routine fashion.

Patients with impaired platelet function on the basis of either medication such as aspirin or renal failure can be handled in the following manner. Although the effects of aspirin are long-lasting, I consider a passage of 7 days after the last aspirin an acceptable time period after which the biopsy can be performed. For renal failure patients, one can administer DDAVP in appropriate doses to lessen the complication risk for biopsies.

If the coagulation state cannot be returned to normal, one should use special hemostatic techniques as described below. These have been proved effective for the prevention of bleeding.

Special pathologic entities

Hemangiomas. Although cavernous hemangioma is said to be the commonest hepatic tumor, it has received little attention until recently because it is benign and seldom causes spontaneous problems. Attention has focused on these benign masses in recent years because as imaging technology has become more refined, commonly detected lesions can be mistaken for more serious problems. Correct diagnosis is important to prevent unnecessary surgery and errors in cancer staging. If inappropriate imaging studies are performed or incorrectly interpreted, a patient may present for a biopsy procedure (see the chapter on liver diagnosis for details).

In most instances, hemangiomas typical on imaging will be correctly diagnosed but occasionally an atypical one will present for biopsy. Surprisingly, once the typical vascular hemangiomas are excluded there is very little risk of a significant complication from the atypical variety. The reason for this is that the very pathologic features that make their imaging appearance atypical also preclude the potential for bleeding complication. Stated differently, the increased vascularity of hemangiomas is what gives the typical appearance on such imaging modalities as CT enhancement, isotope pooling, etc. When the increased vascularity is not present because of thrombosis, fibrosis, or hyalinization, the lesion is unlikely to bleed with a biopsy.

Clinically, the reported experience has supported this concept.[246] As we have noted in our previous editions, the only complication we have had with hemangiomas occurred before the development of bolus dynamic scanning. Since the appropriate use of contrast material, we have had no problems with hemangiomas. We have biopsied numerous atypical hemangiomas with 14-gauge cutting needles under the assumption that they were lesions other than hemangiomas. Other authors including Spamer et al,[252] Cronan et al,[40] and Solbiatic et al,[251] have reported the safe biopsy of atypical hemangiomas. These authors have also noted the difficulty in diagnosing hemangiomas with small aspiration needles; they note also that hemangiomas can inconsistently be diagnosed with "special purpose" needles and consistently diagnosed with the standard cutting needles (Fig. 46-67, *A* to *D*).

Cirrhosis. The issues surrounding the biopsy of cirrhotic livers are only two, one concerning the possibility of complications and the other the concerning intactness of tissue samples. The cirrhosis itself doesn't predispose to problems, but associated changes may. One must always be aware of possible prothrombin elevations and the pathologic changes of cirrhosis, which increases the hepatic concentration of small arteries and venous collaterals. We have experienced a case of life-threatening hemorrhage in such a patient, recently reported by Nachamoto et al.[207] If one chooses a needle to sample cirrhosis, the side-cutting Tru-Cut needle has been shown to be better than the Menghini type of needle in preventing fragmentation of a fibrotic, cirrhotic liver sample.

Fatty metamorphosis. Since the introduction of CT scanning, it has become apparent that fatty change can be quite focal and can perfectly simulate a neoplastic

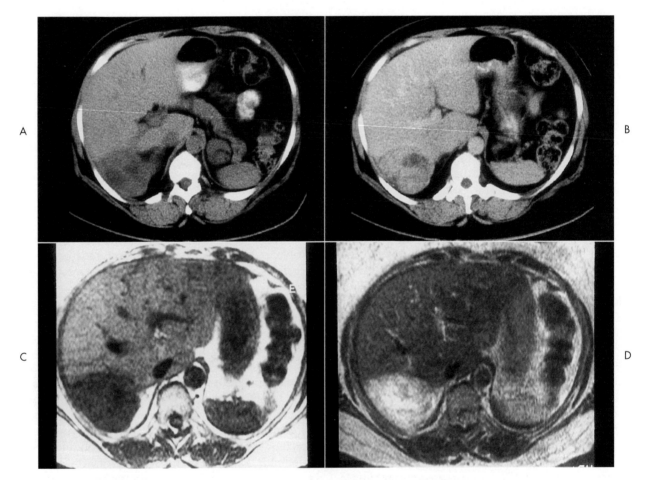

Fig. 46-67. A, Cavernous hemangiomas of the liver can be a very difficult diagnosis to make by imaging alone. This scan shows a low-density mass with a varied density in the posterior portion of the right lobe. **B,** With bolus injection, the mass becomes partially opacified, but large areas of low density remain. This was not definitive for a cavernous hemangioma. **C,** MRI scan with spin density shows low-intensity mass that is of lower intensity than the liver and nonhomogeneous throughout. **D,** T2-weighted scan shows a bright signal in the mass; this is not definitive for a hemangioma. After a subsequent angiogram was equivocal, a cutting-needle biopsy, which was diagnostic, was performed.

lesion. Although many times the geographic appearance will betray its true identity, biopsy of such lesions is quite common. A cutting type of needle is superior to aspiration types for diagnosing this entity.

Cystic abnormalities. With these abnormalities, one important point should be made. The fluid obtained from such lesions may not be diagnostic and one should always endeavor to sample the wall of such lesions. If one is using an aspiration needle, one should send two samples as follows. The first sample of fluid should be aspirated and sent for cytology. A second cellular sample should be obtained from the opposite wall of the cyst by "reciprocating" the needle against the opposite wall.

Endocrine tumors. Biopsy of nonfunctional[5] endocrine tumors is very straightforward. When functional tumors are to be biopsied, one should be both cautious and prepared to treat any symptoms if a hormone release occurs. It is important to note that a death has been reported after biopsy of metastatic carcinoid in the liver.[22] Generally speaking biopsy of functional tumors is discouraged.

Echinococcus. There have been several small series of percutaneous treatment of echinococcus reported in the literature that have been performed intentionally and successfully. While it is true that anaophylasis is not as likely as previously thought, percutaneous puncture for diagnosis is discouraged because the imaging appearance of daughter cysts is characteristic and a serum test can accurately confirm the diagnosis. The major concern in such patients is to prevent spillage of daughter cysts into the peritoneum or other spaces. If therapy is considered, special precautions should be taken; these will be discussed under the therapeutic section.

Hepatoma. Primary tumors warrant a separate discussion because they have some unique traits from several perspectives.[258] Clinically, the specific nature can usually be suspected by an elevation of the serum alpha fetal protein. Differentiation from other entities may be difficult from an imaging perspective; recent data, however, suggests that MRI can differentiate between regenerating nodules and hepatomas. Hepatomas tend to have a higher T2 intensity than do regenerating nodules. If such a lesion were only visible on MRI, it would be appropriate to perform an MRI-guided procedure.

Biopsy of hepatomas has variable results, depending on the technique used. Successful diagnosis may be difficult with small needles because differentiating normal hepatocytes from well-differentiated tumors can be difficult with small aspiration samples. This problem can be overcome by taking numerous aspiration samples or by using a larger needle. The trade-off is in the form of a potentially higher complication rate. It is well documented that hepatomas have an increased vascularity and therefore predispose to a higher complication rate. Wit-

tenberg et al[282] reported a significant bleed requiring a two-unit transfusion after skinny-needle aspiration of a hepatoma. More recently Bret et al[26] reported successful diagnosis in 63 of 69 hepatomas with a 22-gauge needle and multiple passes, but numerous complications resulted. In their series they had four major complications in the 69 patients; these consisted of one death and three hemorrhages, two treated by surgery and one by transfusion alone.

Complications reported by other authors have included the full gamut of problems, including infarction, infection, and one case of tumor seeding within the needle tract.

Hemostatic techniques for high-risk procedures. If there is a severe coagulopathy that cannot be completely corrected, there are two coaxial methods employed for biopsy. Years ago, authors reported the use of a long transvenous, usually by the jugular, aspiration needle that was used to biopsy the liver. Although those few authors reporting noted great success and few complications, this method has not gained great favor.[38] In my own personal experience the method is very cumbersome, expensive, and does not yield reliable results.

The most useful methods that have been reported and that we have used are two coaxial techniques, as described below. It is my belief that these procedures are best done by using ultrasound or CT to choose the target and entrance site, followed by fluoroscopy to guide the placement of hemostatic materials. With both variations, one performs a biopsy using a needle with a plastic sheath on the outside of the biopsy needle. After the biopsy is performed, the plastic sheath is left in place to serve as a conduit for material. Then depending on one's preference, one can push or inject either collagen material or metal coils into the biopsy site (Fig. 46-68, 46-69, 46-70). One can also add small amounts of thrombin to the material if desired. After hemostasis has been achieved the sheath is withdrawn.

Although theoretically this method is simple, the execution can be somewhat difficult for two reasons. If respiratory movement is exaggerated or the body wall is thick, the sheath may become displaced, preventing proper deposition of the material. With gelfoam, the collagen material will occasionally "stick" to the sheath and be inadvertently pulled out when the sheath is removed.

We are currently developing a collagen plug that is automatically dispensed into the biopsy site during the procedure. In preliminary studies this has been quite effective (Table 46-6) and should provide excellent results when finally developed (Fig. 46-71, *A* and *B*).

PANCREAS

Percutaneous procedures of the pancreas have become widely accepted as the method of choice for the

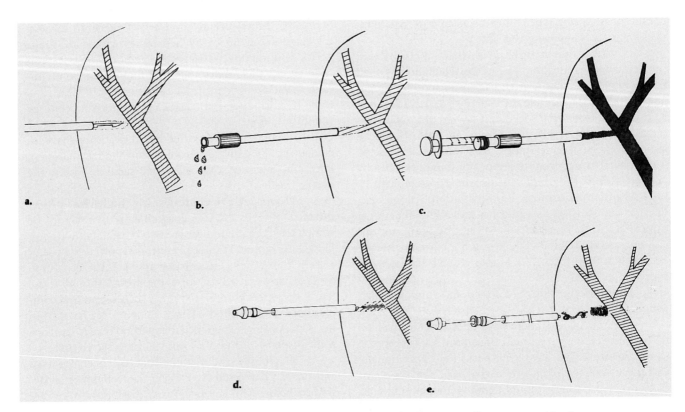

Fig. 46-68. Schematic picture shows use of a cannula with a biopsy needle to prevent bleeding in a high-risk patient. In **A,** a plastic cannula is placed over a biopsy needle and a sample is obtained. As noted in **B,** the biopsy needle is removed but the cannula is left as a conduit to deliver a hemostatic coil. Contrast material may be used as in **C** to demonstrate the vascular system. Finally, as can be seen in **D** and **E,** the conduit is used to deliver hemostatic coils into the biopsy site.

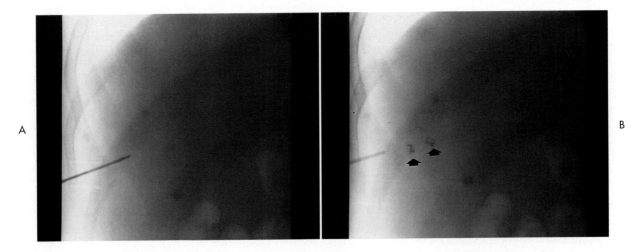

Fig. 46-69. A, Radiograph showing insertion of the biopsy needle (with the cannula around it) into the liver. **B,** Radiograph showing the angiographic coils in the liver *(arrow)* that were delivered through the plastic cannula.

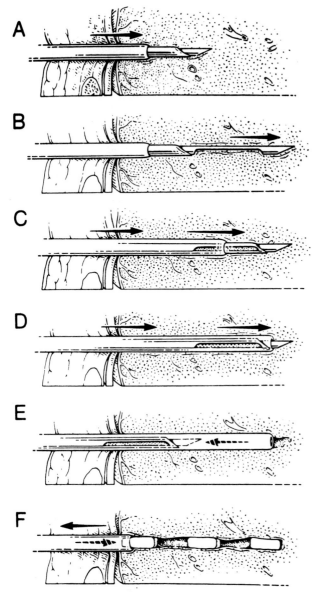

Fig. 46-70. Schematic diagram showing a similar technique with gelfoam. In **A, B, C** and **D,** the biopsy needle is introduced with a plastic cannula around it. As noted in **E,** the biopsy needle is removed and the cannula left in place. As seen in **F,** the cannula is used to introduce gelfoam material to provide hemostasis.

diagnosis of various pancreatic problems. In major medical institutions it is routine practice for a percutaneous aspiration procedure to be used in lieu of exploratory laparotomy for diagnosis and treatment of tumors and inflammatory processes.*

*References 15, 46, 48, 83, 99, 115, 116, 123, 176.

Indications

The indications for using percutaneous procedures for pancreas biopsy are quite broad and relate to diagnosis of tumors, pseudocysts, or infectious processes. Relative to the diagnosis of tumors, I believe the threshold for biopsying any mass is quite low because of both the high success rate and the low incidence of significant complications. Any suspected solid tumors of the pancreas should be biopsied very early in the course of patient treatment for two reasons. For those patients with large inoperable tumors, a biopsy should be performed at the earliest time to make the definitive diagnosis and to eliminate the need for more expensive or complicated procedure such as surgery or endoscopic procedures (Fig. 46-72). For subtle cases, this offers the best opportunity for early diagnosis and surgical treatment.

When dealing with cystic tumors of the pancreas the purpose in performing a percutaneous biopsy differs from the above. In such cases the purpose is to disprove the presence of a pseudocyst by aspiration. From an imaging perspective, one cannot distinguish some cystic tumors from pseudocyst by imaging appearance alone. In such cases, one should obtain fluid to analyze for the presence of amylase, which distinguishes a pseudocyst from a cystic tumors. If such fluid and assay is not positive it is a clear indication for surgical treatment and possible cure (see later section on cystic tumors).

In cases of severe inflammatory processes, CT-guided aspirations are indicated to obtain fluid for diagnosis of infected processes. The presence of infection is a critical determinant for overall outcome of severe pancreatitis, as was noted in the pancreas chapter.

If one is careful, meticulous, and judicious in technique, one can even justify aspiration of unusual fusion anomalies of the gland if there is any question of tumor.

Contraindications

There are only a limited number of contraindications that are primarily related to the presence of vascularity and anatomic approach. In some rare circumstances, the vascularity of tumors will be so great or collateral vessels so numerous that no type of aspiration or biopsy procedure should be performed. The presence of a large pseudoaneurysm should also be a contraindication for a procedure.

If patients are immunocompromised, fluid-density masses should not be aspirated while traversing bowel; if no pathway is available, such procedures should be avoided.

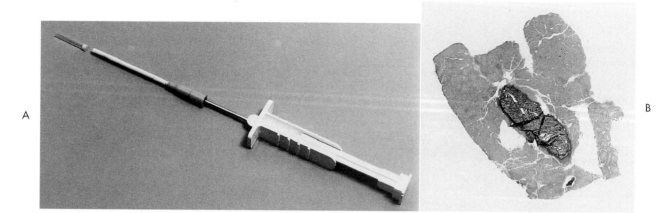

Fig. 46-71. A, A new hemostatic device under development. It consists of an outer cannula and a "sheath" of collagen. Laboratory studies have been very effective (see text). **B,** Photomicrograph showing the plug of collagen, delivered by the above device, within a liver sample.

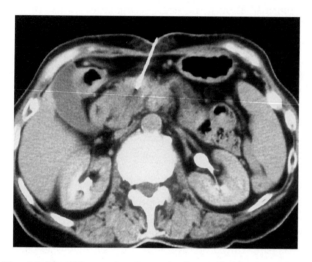

Fig. 46-72. CT scan showing a single-needle biopsy, without guidance cannula, of a pancreatic tumor in the head. When the pathway is clear and the lesion prominent, such procedures are quite straightforward.

Needle selection and technique

With the current level of experience reported, there is really only one choice of needle for biopsying the pancreas, which is an aspiration type of needle. I use a 20-gauge Chiba needle for biopsying the pancreas. A number of years ago, we changed the needle used from a 22-gauge to a 20-gauge based on a study performed at our institution and reported by Dickey et al.[48] During that study and since, we have found that the diagnostic yield with the 20-gauge needle is better than with the 22-gauge needle. In addition, we have found no associated increase in the complication rate.

I prefer the short cannula coaxial technique with a 16-gauge hypodermic needle as the guidance cannula and a standard 20-gauge Chiba needle as the aspiration needle (Fig. 46-73, *A* to *C*). The short guidance cannula is helpful from several perspectives. The guidance cannula permits more accurate placement of the needle because it allows the correct angulation of the needle before the introduction of the aspiration needle. Furthermore the short cannula prevents the occurrence of tumor seeding within the needle tract that has been reported on several occasions.

In executing the chosen anatomic approach, a number of considerations are appropriate. First, it is usually convenient for the patient to remain in a supine position, but on other occasions it may be helpful to have the patient lie in a different position, either oblique or lateral decubitus. This positioning will produce movement of bowel and other structures, making the approach more simplified (Fig. 46-74). It is most rare that one might use a posterior approach, because of the intimate relationship of various vessels to the posterior portion of the gland. Authors using a posterior approach routinely have reported significant complications.[57,58]

General technique and anatomic approach

The choice of imaging technique for diagnosing and localizing pancreatic masses is very important. A good contrast-enhanced study is critical for several reasons in planning a biopsy procedure. The success of a biopsy procedure depends on accurate localization of the tumor and display of the vascularity of the area. If a tumor is avascular, then the margins of the tumor can be defined more clearly and accurately the target for the aspiration needle. While one group has noted that many pancreatic tumors are diffuse, it has been our experience that well-defined margins can usually be found if careful technique is used.

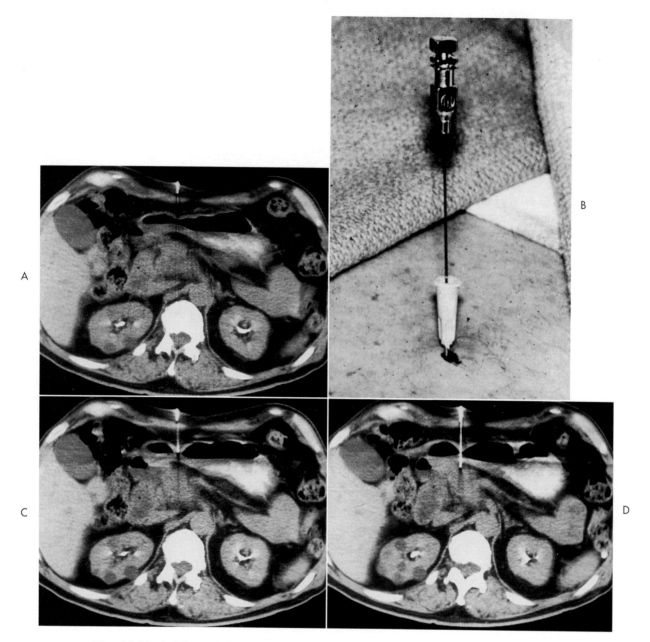

Fig. 46-73. A, This and the subsequent scans demonstrate the coaxial method with a short guidance cannula and 20-gauge Chiba needle. This scan shows the short cannula in the subcutaneous tissues of the abdominal surface. The stomach is intervening in the pathway, but this is acceptable (see text). **B,** If the guidance cannula is directed correctly, the skinny needle should be inserted. Because the cannula was correctly positioned and angled, the aspiration needle was inserted through the cannula. **C,** This scan shows that the initial placement positioned the needle adjacent to the antrum of the stomach. **D,** Final positioning of the needle tip within the small pancreatic mass. Numerous passes into the mass may be made through the cannula. Various regions can be sampled by slight deflections of the cannula while the needle is being inserted.

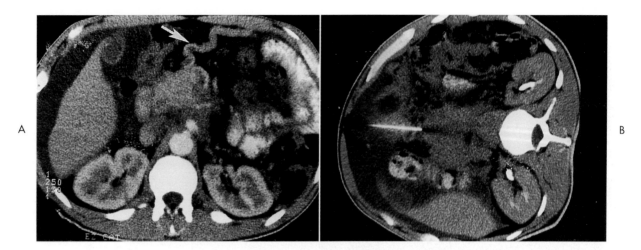

Fig. 46-74. A, Scan performed in the supine position shows a large collateral vessel *(arrow)* in the anterior portion of the abdomen, in front of the pancreatic mass. **B,** When the patient was placed in the lateral decubitus position, the anatomy shifted so that a free pathway into the pancreatic mass was created. Note the needle inserted into the mass.

If the pancreatic tumor is an unusual one with increased vascularity, the enhanced vascularity can be noted and advisability of the procedure can be reconsidered or the planning simplified. Hypervascular tumors include nonfunctioning islet cell tumors, islet cell tumors, and certain metastatic lesions such as renal cell carcinoma.

The proper vascular enhancement can also demonstrate any collateral vessel formation or vascular abnormalities that can produce a multitude of small and large venous and arterial collaterals, all of which should be avoided. The most common entities creating confusion include pseudoaneurysms, varices, and cavernous transformation of the portal vein (see pancreas chapter).

When planning the trajectory, I choose the target in the pancreas that is well-defined but does not appear necrotic. If the anatomy is optimal and one's experience is extensive, all structures should be avoided, except the fat of the mesentery and the pancreas. If anatomy is less than optimal or one is less experienced with angled procedures, then penetration of certain structures can be tolerated.

Certain anatomic structures I absolutely avoid, but others I will accept the possibility of traversing during an aspiration procedure. I definitely prefer to avoid traversing any major artery or vein, as well as the spleen, to preclude the risk of bleeding (Fig. 46-74, 46-75). I accept penetration of the stomach or liver if it is absolutely necessary, in the belief that the risk is minimal.

If one considers penetrating a loop of colon, possible adverse outcomes should be considered, and careful judgment should be exercised. It is my judgment that penetration of colon should be avoided in all cases because it contains many pathogenic organisms. Small bowel can be penetrated safely if a necrotic tumor or cyst

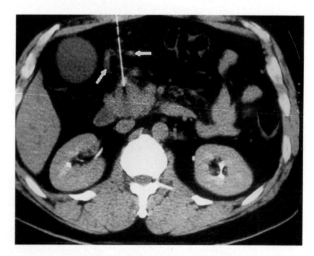

Fig. 46-75. Using a coaxial, short cannula system as described above, one can carefully avoid vascular structures. This scan shows guidance of a needle between two tortuous vessels in the abdomen as well as accurate placement into a mass.

is present and the tumor mass is not cystic. I think avoidance is important for two reasons. In our studies we have confirmed that a small inoculum of bacteria can be carried from the bowel by a "skinny needle." If that inoculum is carried into a solid tumor or structure, there is very little possibility for bacterial growth. If it is carried into a fluid collection, however, the body's immune system has difficulty in eliminating the inoculum. The fluid space acts as a culture medium in which, at the time of contamination, the phagocytes and antibodies' functions are impaired.

In the immunocompromised patient, the avoidance of all bowel is important (Fig. 46-76, 46-77) be-

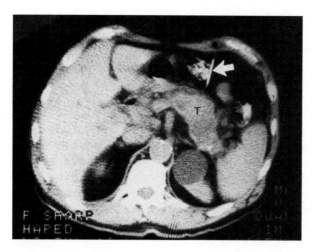

Fig. 46-76. A different patient with a pancreatic mass in the body and tail, *T*. An entrance site was chosen so that the aspiration needle *(arrow)* could pass between two loops of colon. Cytological evidence was positive for adenocarcinoma.

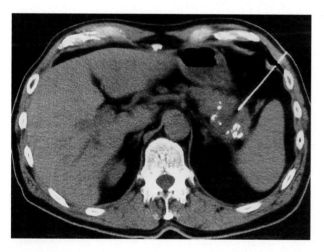

Fig. 46-77. To avoid penetration of colon, one of my colleagues chose a pathway through the gastrosplenic ligament to biopsy this unusual pancreatic adenocarcinoma. Note that a small amount of pleural space was inappropriately crossed by the needle; a slightly more laterl approach (still avoiding the spleen) should have been used.

cause with the severe compromise produced by chemotherapy, transplant treatment, or chronic conditions, even the smallest inoculum of virulent pathogens can create a serious problem. The nature of the bacterial contents can vary in disease states, especially those associated with abnormal or altered peristalsis. The amount and type of various bacteria depends partially on the enteric peristalsis. As an obstruction occurs, there can be ascent of the colon flora retrograde into the small bowel and stomach so that the flora in those viscera may include many gram-negative species. Although some authors have implied or stated that concerns about second-

ary infections are excessive, there are several reports of serious complications from such infections.

Another precaution to be taken is avoiding possible penetration of a dilated bile or pancreatic duct. Damage to these structures could result in leakage, peritonitis, or fistula formation.

Although it is true that one could probably penetrate any and all structures routinely and not have a problem for a long time, most likely the statistical probabilities will catch up with the interventionists if too many cases are performed with disregard for potential problems. One must remember the numerous case reports of complications and deaths following percutaneous pancreatic instrumentation.

Cutting needle

Since the introduction of the automated biopsy gun, one report of a study using an animal model suggested that use of cutting needles might be possible.[52]

However, although it is theoretically possible to use a cutting needle, there is evidence of remarkable potential for complications. In the surgical literature, it has been well documented that the use of a Tru-Cut needle is associated with a fairly high complication rate for severe pancreatitis. If one considers using such a device, one should choose a small-caliber needle and be extremely careful that none of the "normal gland" or vessels (normal or collateral) are included in the biopsy site.

Even though some centers are already performing these procedures, I caution the reader for legal reasons to defer the use of such devices until more experience has been reported in peer reviewed articles. I would not consider the data presented in lectures as adequate documentation because occasionally a speaker's recall of complications is clouded by his or her prejudice for the device.

Accuracy

Most of the articles on accuracy report the use of ultrasound or CT guidance and a 23- or 22-gauge needle. The accuracy of those authors varies between 66% and 88%, with most of the articles showing an accuracy of about 75%. Most of these authors used three to five passes with the skinny needle. There were a number of minor and major complications associated with these series.

In our series of 96 patients, which included 40 carcinomas,[25] our overall accuracy rate was 76.6%. In that group we looked at the differences between two needles, 22-gauge and 20-gauge, and examined the accuracy difference between one pass by an experienced person and two passes by an inexperienced person. The 20-gauge needle provided a diagnostic accuracy rate of 86.7%, whereas the 22-gauge needle provided a diagnostic accuracy rate of 71.9%. One pass yielded a positive diagnosis in 75.9% of cases, and two passes yielded a positive diagnosis in 77.8% of cases.

Complications

Although most authors infer that percutaneous pancreatic biopsy is without risk, a number of mild complications and a number of serious complications have been reported. The mild complications reported by Smith,[249] Goldman,[82] and McLoughlin[187] included transient rectal or colonic bleeding, probably because of trauma to the transverse colon. Ohto[216] reported one case of transient hematemesis following a biopsy. Other mild complications also included four cases of mild pancreatitis that resolved; these were reported by Evans and McLoughlin.[187]

The serious complications related to tumor sampling (pseudocysts will be reported later) have included hemorrhage, fatal pancreatitis,[54,204] sepsis, cholangitis, fistula, and needle-tract seeding. Fataar[57,58] reported two cases of hemorrhage, one that required cardiopulmonary resuscitation and two units of blood, and one that resulted in a 6.5-cm hematoma in the mesocolon. Evans et al[54] and Levin et al[169] have reported cases of fatal pancreatitis following ultrasonic biopsies. Phillips et al[232] reported one case of cholangitis and pancreatic fistula, as well as severe vasovagal reaction. Ferrucci et al[61] had a case of cystadenoma of the pancreas that resulted in generalized sepsis. Two authors, Rashleigh-Belcher[237] and Ferrucci,[60] reported separate cases of needle-tract seeding from pancreatic carcinoma.

Based on our experience and a review of the literature, it is my belief that risks are directly related to inaccurate targeting and the number of passes made with the needle. This premise has also been recently stated by Smith[247,249] (see earlier section on complications.)

With our conservative method and techniques, e.g., trajectory, number of passes, etc., that minimize all possible risk factors, pancreatic biopsy is safe and effective. As a routine, the risks are minimal enough that percutaneous pancreatic biopsy is considered an outpatient procedure. In our reported experience with 96 biopsies, including patients with 40 neoplasms and other abnormalities,[48] we had only one patient who had a transient elevation of the amylase (without clinical pancreatitis). Since that time we have encountered one patient who developed an acute abdomen following aspiration of a pancreatic abscess; as a result, surgical exploration was required.

Other important points

When the results are cytologically positive for malignancy, the disposition is obvious. If the cytologic results are negative, I place importance on the texture of the gland felt during the needle aspiration. If the gland is "hard" or the mass is large, surgical biopsy is indicated. If the gland is "soft" during aspiration of a subtle mass, no further investigation is needed. Surprisingly, many times normal acinar cells can be recovered in such cases.

It is our belief that biopsy of a functioning endocrine tumor should not be performed. The definition of "functioning" is made on clinical information about these patients that includes specific symptoms associated with the released hormone (see Chapter 24.) One author reported the successful but uneventful biopsy of a pancreatic insulinoma.[136] Experience with a single case, however, should not be accepted as establishing the principle of safety; further experience is required before endocrine tumor biopsy can be generally recommended.

Specific entities

Adenocarcinoma is the most common entity biopsied. There is nothing unique about this tumor beyond what has been discussed above. Meticulous evaluation, trajectory planning, and good aspiration technique should be used as described earlier.

Acinar carcinoma. This unusual tumor is so rare it is not apparent whether it can be diagnosed by percutaneous aspiration biopsy. Most likely, because of its characteristic appearance, it could be correctly diagnosed especially if the associated clinical syndrome exists (see Pancreas chapter).

Cystic tumors. As noted in the pancreas chapter, cystic tumors of the pancreas are unusual entities that include both a benign and a premalignant variety. Differentiation of these tumors by imaging is not possible; it would therefore be convenient if one could differentiate the two by needle aspiration. Because one of the tumors is reported to produce glycogen and the other does not, it would also seem convenient if one could stain for this material (Fig. 46-78). Practically speaking, it has not been possible to accomplish this in our laboratory. Authors who have reported have appropriately noted that there may be considerable sampling error and that the recovery of benign cells from one component may not exclude malignancy in another region. Most authors agree that it is not the results of the aspiration but rather the demographics of the patient that provides the best predictors of outcome and the need for surgery.[69,143,271]

Endocrine tumors. The biopsy of endocrine tumors that are nonfunctional (and thus are obscure as to their nature) is appropriate, but biopsy of a functional lesion is not. Although there is a case report of a biopsy of a pancreatic insulinoma,[234] I believe the biopsy is inappropriate because of the possibility of a hormonal release.

Pseudocyst aspiration. Aspiration of pseudocyst fluid or inflammatory fluid is important for the exclu-

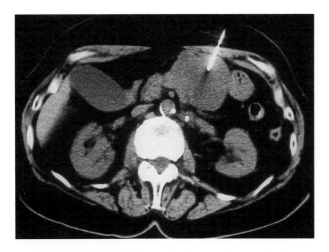

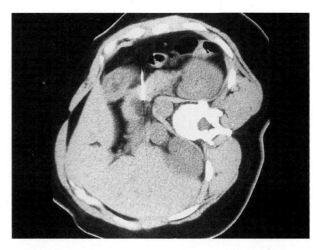

Fig. 46-78. CT-guided biopsy of a large microcystic adenoma of the pancreas. Percutaneous cytologic results are still not adequate to distinguish the two types of tumors (see text). Demographic information is more accurate (see Pancreas chapter).

Fig. 46-79. Guided aspirations of pancreatic pseudocysts are critical to the differentiation from cystic tumors. This scan shows aspiration of a small cystic mass adjacent to but behind the pancreas. Because of the high amylase content, the concern about a cystic tumor was eliminated.

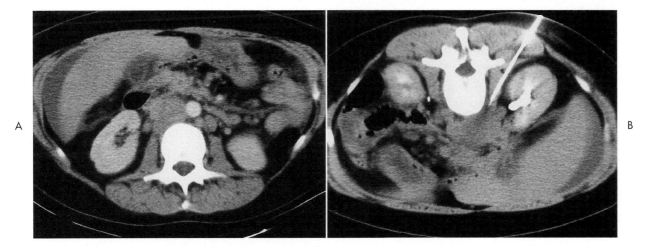

Fig. 46-80. A, CT scan showing ill-defined lymph node mass between vena cava and the aorta. Bolus injection opacifies the aorta. The margins of the vena cava are lost because of tumor infiltration. **B,** Using the short cannula coaxial method, the mass adjacent to the vena cava was sampled; it yielded metastatic adenocarcinoma.

sion of cystic tumors (as noted above) or the diagnosis of an abscess. Laboratory analysis of fluid from a pseudocyst will show a high amylase content, while that of a cystic tumor will not (Fig. 46-79). Aspiration of any suspicious fluid collection in patients with pancreatitis should be performed to exclude pyogenic infection. When such procedures are being performed one should be sure bowel loops are not being traversed to exclude the possibility of contaminating a fluid collection or recovering spurious culture results. Good evidence for this cautionary approach was provided by Smith, who collected 16 cases of generalized sepsis from a physician survey.

Cavernous transformation of portal vein. Interestingly, in some cases cavernous transformation of the portal vein may produce a mass that will be recommended for a biopsy. In most cases when the vascular channels are large, the portal cavernomas can be recognized with a bolus dynamic scan. If a cavernous transformation of the portal vein does not have large vascular channels or rapid flow, such masses may not enhance with a bolus dynamic scan. In such cases, if a biopsy is inadvertently performed in a patient, a complication is most unlikely because the vascular channels are very small. Unaware of their pathologic identity, I have biopsied three such cases without difficulty.

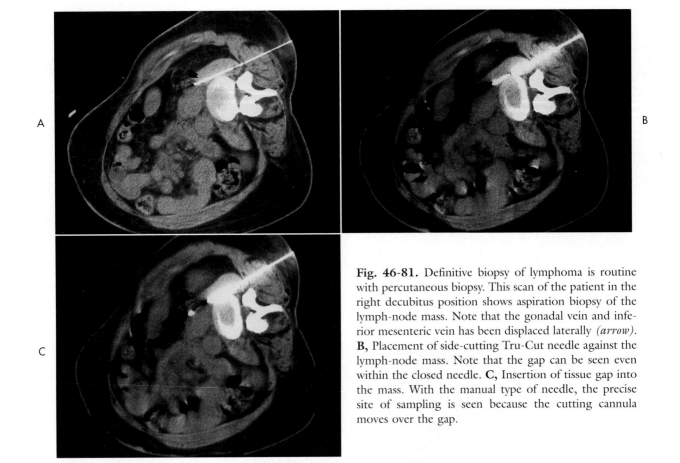

Fig. 46-81. Definitive biopsy of lymphoma is routine with percutaneous biopsy. This scan of the patient in the right decubitus position shows aspiration biopsy of the lymph-node mass. Note that the gonadal vein and inferior mesenteric vein has been displaced laterally *(arrow)*. **B,** Placement of side-cutting Tru-Cut needle against the lymph-node mass. Note that the gap can be seen even within the closed needle. **C,** Insertion of tissue gap into the mass. With the manual type of needle, the precise site of sampling is seen because the cutting cannula moves over the gap.

RETROPERITONEUM

CT procedures in the retroperitoneum prove valuable because even though ultrasound and fluoroscopy has been used in the past, CT provides the best visualization of pathosis and instruments in this area. Only CT can visualize precise location of tumors in relationship to the aorta and vena cava.[50,85,154,227]

Indications

The indication for procedures within the retroperitoneum are similar to those for other areas; it is usually the presence of a mass in a patient suspected of having some type of a malignancy or an inflammatory process.

Instruments

As in the other organ systems, we use our general guidelines for the selection of instruments. For a mass in a patient with suspected metastatic malignancy, I use a 20-gauge aspiration needle for a cytologic sample (Fig. 46-80, *A* and *B*). For unknown or undiagnosed tumors or for lymphomas we use either the end-cutting Menghini type of needle, or the side-cutting Tru-Cut needle (Fig. 46-81, *A* to *C*).

In most instances the Tru-Cut needle is the needle of choice because it provides the largest well-preserved sample. Also, this instrument is the most carefully controlled because the cutting gap can be well seen on the CT scan and the cutting action occurs only at the gap. There is no possibility of "overshoot" during the procedure such as may occur with the end-cutting Menghini type of needle.

Even the beginning interventionist can biopsy fairly large masses in the retroperitoneum with this needle. With experience, even very small lymph nodes immediately adjacent to the major vessels can be sampled if the proper technique and attention to detail are observed (Fig. 46-82).

Anatomic approach

The approach used is typically posterior, adjusted according to the location of the kidney, major vessels, colon, small bowel, and psoas muscle.

The posterior approach for such procedures is obviously easier with the patient lying in a lateral, anterior oblique, or prone position. If an aspiration needle is used, an anterior or posterior approach can be taken, but if a cutting needle is used, a posterior approach is necessary.

Most lesions are in the periaortic region, and in

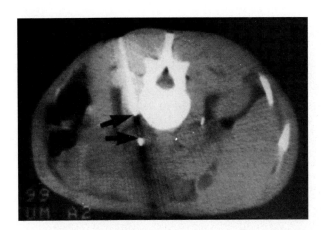

Fig. 46-82. Tru-Cut biopsy *(arrows)* of a patient with AIDS showed atypical mycobacterium.

such cases the anatomy should be carefully examined and the aorta and vena cava traced through the entire expanse of the abdomen. As with the other areas, the bolus injection is important to define the location of vessels and the presence of any tumor vascularity (see Fig. 46-6). Carefully note other vessels such as the renal pedicle, the splenic vein, the left gonadal vein, and the inferior mesenteric vein (which runs in the left periaortic area). Also, note the location of the ureters on both sides after the administration of intravenous contrast material.

If the vena cava cannot be identified, perform an injection of the foot vein to get better opacification. If the gonadal, inferior mesenteric vein or the ureter are not seen because of the surrounding tumor, do not search for them. In such cases they are so encased and infiltrated with tumor that they are nonfunctional. In over 18 years I have never penetrated or cut any of these structures inadvertently when they were not seen.

Several specific areas warrant special mention. The areas that are very difficult to biopsy safely are the retropancreatic region and the area of the aortic bifurcations. In these areas there are multiple vessels branching and converging that make exact delineation difficult. In these areas I usually perform only an aspiration biopsy to avoid the possibility of injuring one of the vessels.

Results

The biopsy of lymphomas has been an area of some controversy. Some individuals believe that large needles cannot make the diagnosis of Hodgkin's lymphoma and thus only skinny needles should be used. This is an incorrect and somewhat naive assumption. Using a 14-gauge cutting needle, one can diagnose not only special lymphomas successfully but unusual entities such as atypical myobacterium and even sarcoidosis as well. If clinically indicated, one can get ample tissue for electron microscopy and even gene studies to determine to clonality.

Table 46-10. Retroperitoneal biopsy

	Cytology	Tru-Cut	Specific
	No. correct/ No. attempted	No. correct/ No. attempted	No. correct/ No. attempted
Liposarcoma	0/1	1/1	1
Lymphoma	10/16*	10/11	10/11
Metastatic tumor	20/22	13/13	
Benign	1/3	2/2	
Normal	2/2	1/1	
Unsatisfactory	4	0	
Totals	33/48	27/28	

*No specific subtype diagnosed.
From Knelson M, Haaga J, Lazarus H, et al: Computed tomography-guided retroperitoneal biopsies. *J Clin Oncol* 7(8):1169-1173, 1989.

Table 46-11. Comparison cases

	Chiba	Tru-Cut
	No. correct/ No. attempted	No. correct/ No. attempted
Metastatic	10/12	12/12
Liposarcoma	0/1	1/1
Lymphoma	6/9*	8/9†
Other‡	1/3	3/3
Total (%)	17/25 (68)	24/25 (96)

*Lymphoma suggested, but no histologic subtype.
†Specific cell type in all cases.
‡Normal, mycobacterium, sarcoidosis.

Complications

Only limited data are available on the retroperitoneum.[291,292] In our preliminary study comparing large and small needles, only one complication occurred.[154] A very small asymptomatic hematoma appeared on the CT scan during the small-needle aspiration before the large-needle biopsy. The diagnostic accuracy was high for both metastatic disease and lymphoma (Tables 46-10 and 46-11). Bernardino et al[17] have also reported a good success rate for diagnosing lymphoma.

KIDNEY

Two types of CT biopsies are performed on the kidney, one for evaluation of masses and another for the sampling of diffuse parenchymal disease. In many instances CT is the second-choice modality if the problem is well seen by other methods. If the lesion is best seen by CT, then CT is the modality of choice.

Indications

With renal masses virtually all authors agree that there is no indication for biopsy of a simple renal cyst that is unequivocal on either CT or ultrasound. The ba-

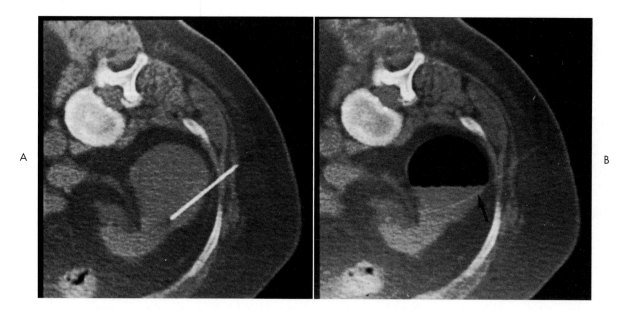

Fig. 46-83. A, Optimal localization for the needle *(arrow)* when aspirating a renal cyst is to have the needle in the lowest portion of the mass. With the needle in the lowest portion, the wall will not retract away from the needle tip. **B,** Air was injected within the cyst wall to permit accurate assessment of the wall thickness. Note the faint shadow of the Teflon sheath *(arrow).*

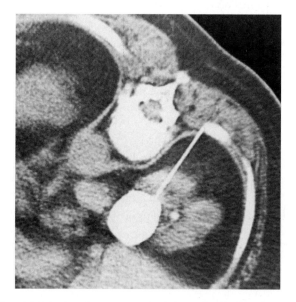

Fig. 46-84. An alternate method for evaluation of the wall thickness is injection of urographic contrast material. Only very dilute material can be used, or artifacts will occur.

sic indication is the presence as an indeterminant mass in which distinction between a benign and malignant mass is important. In most cases only an aspiration needle is indicated. In some cases when the cytologic sample does not provide adequate histologic data (assuming the bolus dynamic scan shows the mass to be avascular), a cutting needle should be used.

In most such patients the approach is directly posterior, with the trajectory chosen to avoid the erector spinae muscle if possible (this muscle can be painful and it can deflect or bend the needle). As in other areas it is important to anesthetize the renal capsule locally.

Cystic masses

Several points should be made about aspiration of the renal cyst. Following aspiration of fluid, either diluted urographic contrast material or air may be injected (Figs. 46-83, 46-84) to define the thickness of the wall. When there is a central mass or wall thickening within a cystic mass, try to sample the irregular wall or solid portion of the mass. In such cases the fluid may be cytologically negative, yet a sample from the mass may be positive.

Solid masses

Sampling of the solid renal mass is similar to that of masses in other organs. A bolus dynamic scan must be performed to assess vascularity. In most cases if the mass has a slight increased vascularity, aspiration is quite safe (Figs. 46-85, 46-86). An avascular mass can be biopsied with a large cutting needle if clinically indicated and a specific tissue type is sought.[215]

Other tips

Several technical points may be helpful. First, when approaching a small mass, perform the procedure

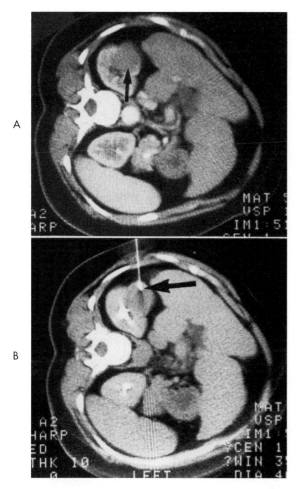

Fig. 46-85. A, Bolus injection before aspiration of an indeterminant mass shows that the mass *(arrow)* is avascular. **B,** Aspiration with 20-gauge needle *(arrow)*.

in two steps. The first step is to carefully position the needle immediately adjacent to the area being sampled. Several initial approaches may be needed in this way because the kidney is mobile, and with variable respirations a small mass may move in and out of the slice. After the needle has been confirmed adjacent to the mass, "pop" the needle into the mass (Fig. 46-86). If the needle is pushed slowly toward the mass, it may deflect because the bevel of the needle may slide over its curved surface. (I have seen a simple cyst deflect an 18-gauge needle 15 or 20 degrees if pushed slowly.)

Second, when a small renal mass is quite mobile with respiratory motion, place the patient in an ipsilateral decubitus position and approach the mass posteriorly. The weight of the viscera will partially immobilize the diaphragm and the mass (Fig. 46-87).

Results

The accuracy rate for diagnostic aspiration of renal mass is almost 100%. The results of CT aspirations are not much different from results appearing in the older literature on fluoroscopic aspirations except, because simple renal cysts are easy to diagnose by imaging, the number of diagnostic aspirations is fewer and the percentage of solid tumors is higher.

A comment about aspiration of small adenomas is appropriate. As with the adrenal gland, normal-appearing cells can be recovered from a renal adenoma, but the significance is remarkably different. In the kidney, some believe the adenoma is the precursor to renal cell carcinoma. Consequently, unlike with adrenal adenomas, the recovery for renal tubular cells from a mass indicates a need for surgical removal.

Complications

The complications related to such procedures are quite low, and I have had two. One hematoma occurred during the biopsy of a renal mass suspected of being a focal lymphoma. In this case a cutting needle was used, and the sample was very close to the segmental arteries. A hematoma developed that required neither surgical intervention nor the administration of blood.

A potential complication mentioned by clinicians is the possible occurrence of needle-tract seeding, for which I can find only one reported case in the literature. However, a carefully controlled study by Von Schreeb[270] compared the outcome and complications in two groups of patients with proven renal carcinoma. There was no difference in the complication rates, the morbidity rates, or the mortality rates between the groups (and no needle-tract seeding in 75 cases of carcinoma that were sampled).

Renal parenchymal biopsy

Renal parenchymal biopsies should be performed only in those cases that preclude the use of ultrasound guidance. In these cases the Tru-Cut needle should be used, but unlike for other areas, no bolus injection is needed. Choose an entrance site and trajectory to avoid the erector spinal muscle for reasons noted earlier in the retroperitoneum section. Unlike in the blind renal biopsy, it is not necessary to "target" the lower pole of the kidney. A good-quality sample avoiding the segmental vessels may be obtained (with more cortex and glomeruli) by choosing an oblique placement within the cortex (Fig. 46-88, *A* and *B*). In this fashion the medullary region of the kidney, which contains the renal vessels, can be avoided.

The bleeding complication rate from parenchymal biopsies is fairly high, varying in some reports between 5.2% and 8.8%. Sateriale and Cronan[244] reported a number of risk factors related to renal biopsies, including hemodialysis, sex, site of biopsy, and treatment with DDAVP (I-Deamino-8-D-Arginine Vasopressin) (Table

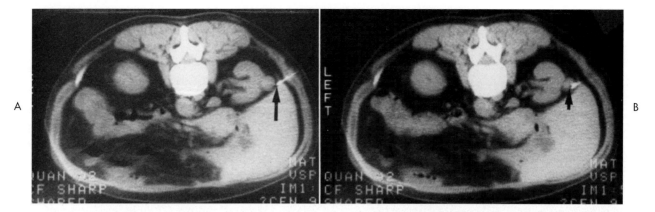

Fig. 46-86. A, A difficult biopsy of a small renal mass. The needle *(arrow)* is positioned immediately adjacent to the mass. **B,** Small masses such as this are best punctured with a quick insertion to avoid deflection of the needle *(arrow)*. This yielded tubular cells and proved to be an adenoma.

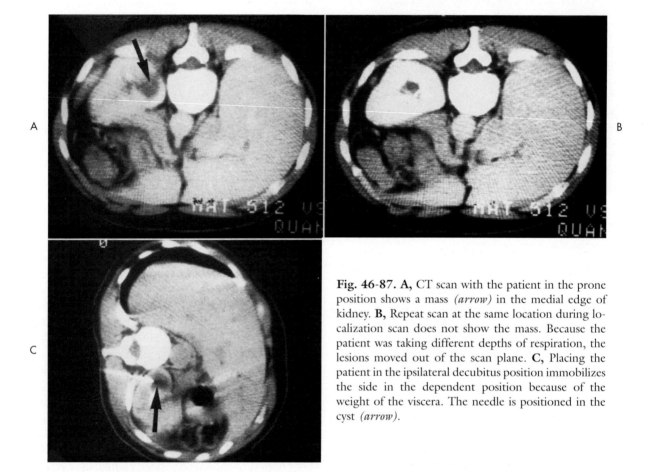

Fig. 46-87. A, CT scan with the patient in the prone position shows a mass *(arrow)* in the medial edge of kidney. **B,** Repeat scan at the same location during localization scan does not show the mass. Because the patient was taking different depths of respiration, the lesions moved out of the scan plane. **C,** Placing the patient in the ipsilateral decubitus position immobilizes the side in the dependent position because of the weight of the viscera. The needle is positioned in the cyst *(arrow)*.

46-12). There is no question that biopsy of renal parenchyma is more dangerous than other procedures; even if the best device and technique are used, serious complications can occur.

There is some controversy among authors about what size needle is most effective for the diagnosis of diffuse renal disease. While some authors have claimed that an 18-gauge needle is sufficient for assessment of renal pathology, most agree that a larger-caliber needle is better. Mostbeck et al[197] compared 18- and 16-gauge needles and found the 16-gauge needle to be more effective. In our hospital, the pathologists and nephrolo-

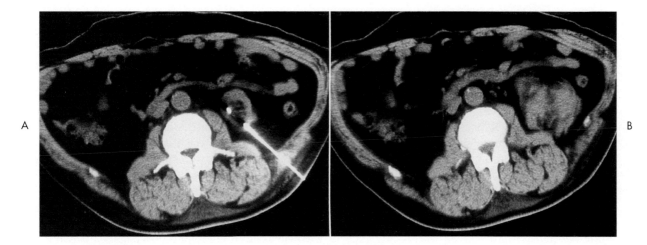

Fig. 46-88. A, Renal parenchymal biopsy of atrophic kidney. Note that the needle is directed obliquely into the parenchyma, and the gap shows the location of the biopsy. **B,** Following the procedure, a hematoma develops adjacent to the kidney. Such hematomas are common with parenchymal biopsies.

Table 46-12. Factors affecting hemorrhagic complication rates after renal biopsy

Factor	Hemorrhagic complication rate (%)*	Increased risk of hemorrhagic complications	P Value†
Hemodialysis			
No	5.9 (13/220)	—	
Yes	24.0 (5/21)	×4.1	<0.025
Patient sex			
Male	4.5 (7/156)	—	
Female	13.0 (11/85)	×2.9	<0.01
Side of biopsy			
Right	5.2 (8/155)	—	
Left	14.0 (12/86)	×2.7	<0.01
Pretreatment with DDAVP			
No	6.4 (15/236)	—	
Yes	60.0 (3/5)	×9.4	<0.001

*Numbers in parentheses are actual number of patients with hemorrhagic complications per total number of patients in each subgroup.
†P values indicates the significance of the difference in complication rates for each set of paired values.
From Sateriale M, Cronan JJ, Savadier LD: A 5-year experience with 307 CT-guided renal biopsies: results and complications. *JVIR* 2(3):401-407, 1991.

gists report that a 14-gauge Tru-Cut needle is superior to other devices.

ADRENAL BIOPSY

Adrenal biopsy by CT guidance is easy, and the indications vary among different institutions. Either an aspiration or cutting biopsy can be performed using different approaches as described. A number of authors have reported on CT-guided biopsies of adrenal masses.[14,19,45,117-119]

Indications

If a patient with a malignant or infectious process has an adrenal mass and if confirmation of the process will change the management of the patient, a biopsy should be performed. Although most adrenal masses that are 3 cm or less are benign nonfunctioning adenomas, there is no method other than cytologic or histologic sampling that can prove this.

Contraindications

The contraindications for the adrenal gland are the same as for other areas in regard to access or increased vascularity, except for one addition. I believe that a pheochromocytoma or other functioning tumor should not be biopsied. It is well documented that manual manipulation can initiate a hypertensive crisis; therefore it seems logical to assume that needling such a tumor might create a similar problem. Thus if a patient has any clinical symptoms of a functioning adrenal tumor, a biopsy should not be done until a laboratory test for catecholamines is performed to exclude a functioning tumor. Despite several uneventful aspirations (unreported from other institutions), two deaths have been reported in the literature (one pheochromocytoma and one hemangioma).[184]

As an additional precaution against a potential problem it is prudent to have an intravenous alpha blocker available in the department for use should such a lesion be inadvertently be sampled and a hypertensive crisis develop.

The validity of sampling even the most subtle

mass in a patient with a malignancy is best emphasized by the experience of Pagani.[222] In his series of patients with small-cell lung tumors, he sampled normal-appearing glands and actually recovered malignant cells in a significant number.

Needle selection

The choice of needles for this organ is the same as for other areas, but commonly an aspiration type must be used because of the anatomy. In many cases an aspiration needle will be required because either another organ must be penetrated or the trajectory is too close to other structures. In unknown disease if a safe access is available and other factors are appropriate, I will use a large cutting needle.

Approach

There are four different anatomic approaches in biopsying an adrenal mass: an oblique-angled approach, a direct posterior paraspinal approach, a transrenal route, and a transhepatic approach. The first and most desirable approach uses an oblique angled pathway that avoids all intervening structures (Fig. 46-89). This approach is ideally suited for either cutting or aspiration needles because all structures are avoided and it can be used on either the right or left side. However, this approach is technically difficult and requires an entrance site below the level of the lesion. On the right side the angled pathway is between the right lobe of the liver and the kidney, and on the left side the pathway transverses the retroperitoneum behind the tail of the pancreas, medial to the spleen and anterior to the kidney. Sometimes, having the patient in an oblique position expedites this approach. This approach, as well as the next, is suited to aspiration- and cutting-needle procedures.

The second most desirable approach, which is probably the easiest to execute, is a posterior paraspinal route that traverses the crura. This is a straightforward method usable by almost all interventionists because it does not require an angled approach. If a paraspinal approach is taken, an aspiration or a cutting needle can be used (Fig. 46-90).

The next most desirable approach, which is limited to an aspiration needle, is the transrenal approach. This approach is quite direct and can be used on the right or left side (Fig. 46-91). It is appealing for several reasons. Literally thousands of aspiration procedures have been performed on renal cysts in kidneys without significant problems, so a transrenal approach for the adrenal is equally safe. If a complication occurs it is confined to the retroperitoneum, making diagnosis and treatment easier than if a pathway crossing the peritoneum and retroperitoneum is used.

The last approach for the right adrenal gland is a transhepatic approach, which has been proposed by several authors.[236] This approach can be used with the patient in a supine or oblique position. If the transhepatic approach is chosen, I prefer to perform the procedure with the patient in the decubitus position. By doing this, the liver shifts anteriorly and a shorter pathway through the liver is possible (Fig. 46-92). Theoretically, this should present fewer problems than if a long path through the liver is taken with the patient supine. On the left side, transpancreatic or transplenic

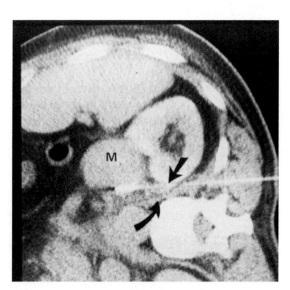

Fig. 46-90. Using a paraspinal posterior pathway for a needle aspiration *(arrow)* of the adrenal, *m*, is quite effective (see text). This patient is lying on the side, but a prone position may also be used. The retroperitoneal slips *(curved arrow)* of the diaphragm may be crossed, so one must carefully anesthetize this area to prevent shoulder or chest pain.

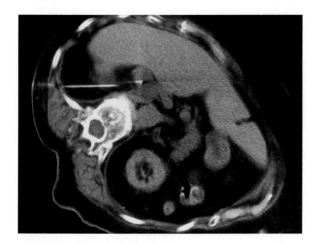

Fig. 46-89. CT scan shows patient in the left oblique position. Biopsy needle is introduced through the right flank between the liver and the kidney, into the adrenal mass.

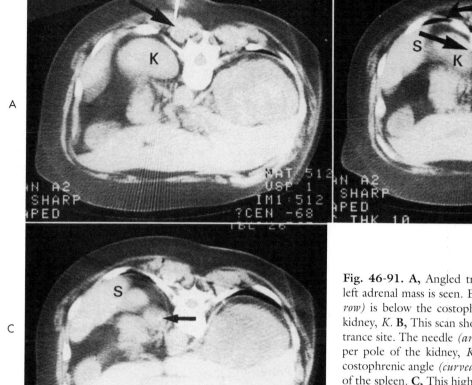

Fig. 46-91. **A,** Angled transrenal aspiration biopsy of a left adrenal mass is seen. Entrance site for the needle *(arrow)* is below the costophrenic angle at the level of the kidney, *K*. **B,** This scan shows the next level above the entrance site. The needle *(arrow)* is passing through the upper pole of the kidney, *K*. It is important to avoid the costophrenic angle *(curved arrow)* and the medial portion of the spleen. **C,** This highest scan shows the needle tip in the adrenal mass *(arrow)*.

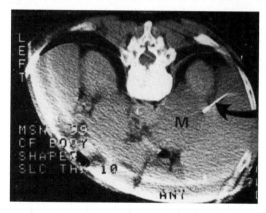

Fig. 46-92. Transhepatic needle aspiration *(arrow)* of an adrenal mass, *m*. In cases in which an oblique approach has been tried, this represents an acceptable alternative approach (see text).

routes should be avoided because of the high risk of complications.

Asymptomatic adrenal masses

One question frequently asked is how a mass 3 cm or smaller should be managed,[147] with the knowl-

edge that in most cases such masses are benign nonfunctioning adenomas. In my opinion such lesions should be observed or sampled based on the clinical situation. If a patient is asymptomatic without proven malignant or inflammatory disease, no biopsy is needed. If a patient has a proven pathologic problem and involvement of the adrenal gland changes the patient's management, I believe a biopsy should be taken. According to our experience and others'[45] a cytologic sample will show the presence of normal adrenal cells in nonfunctioning adenomas or hyperplasia, thereby excluding the possibility of a malignant or inflammatory disease. If the cytologic interpretation raises any question about the benign nature of the adrenal cells, further exploration is needed.

Accuracy

The accuracy of CT sampling of adrenal masses is quite high. Heaston et al[72] reported a series of 14 cases and had correct results in 13 patients without complications. Bernadino[15-19] reported a series of 50 cases with an accuracy rate of 83%. They had an 11% complication rate overall, with serious complications requiring blood transfusions in 3.5% of cases.

Complications

A number of problems have been reported. Bernadino et al,[15-19] using a transhepatic approach in a reported series of 50 patients, had an overall complication rate of 11%, with a serious complication rate of 3.5%. Two patients required blood transfusions. Pagani reported a case of pneumothorax that required chest tube placement. Heaston et al[118] and our group, using an indirect approach that attempted to avoid other structures, had no significant complications. There have been two deaths reported (see section on contraindications).

MESENTERIC MASS

Our approach for mesenteric masses is similar to that for all other areas, and the results have been equally successful and safe.

As in other areas, if there is a possibility of penetrating a loop of bowel, a small aspirating needle (20-gauge) is used. If the mass can be approached without penetrating a bowel loop and the other criteria are met, a 14-gauge Tru-Cut needle can be used. Of course, a bolus injection should be used to assess the vascularity of the lesion before the biopsy (Fig. 46-93).

When using the cutting needle, both oral and intravenous contrast material can be very helpful in opacifying the normal bowel so that it can be avoided. In addition, try to have the entire gap within the mass that is being biopsied. If a part of the cutting needle overlaps within the peritoneum, some of the abundant small vascular network of the mesentery or omentum may be cut, causing a hemorrhage.

SPLEEN

The spleen is an area that represents uncharted territory because of the lack of experience and the sig-

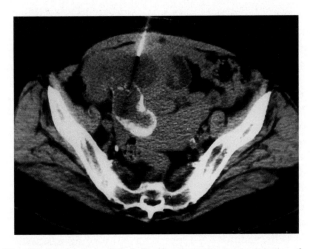

Fig. 46-93. Biopsy of ill-defined metastatic site in anterior abdomen. Because there are no intervening bowel loops or adjacent vessels, safe placement is not a problem.

nificant problems other physicians have had with inadvertent injury to the spleen. From surgical and clinical information it is obvious that the spleen is very vascular and can be easily severely injured. Because of these previous experiences I believe a larger body of information should be collected before the sampling of the organ can be recommended on a routine basis.

Over the last 12 years I have sampled a number of lesions in the spleen, both cystic and solid, without complication. I have not published or presented the information because I am not convinced that the benefit sufficiently outweighs the potential risks for widespread application. This is one of the few areas I think should be left to academic centers until more information is obtained.

PELVIS

The pelvis is a frequent site for biopsy with CT guidance because of the frequency of gynecologic,[146] urologic, and colonic pathosis.[29,284] All of the general principles for clinical indications—needle selection, bolus dynamic scan, and anatomic considerations—apply in this area, with some qualifications.

Indications

Indications for the pelvis are varied; some are well-defined and others are somewhat nebulous. Clearly defined entities that should be sampled include metastatic tumors from the colon, bladder, prostate, or other organs. The safety and benefit of sampling primary tumors in these areas has not been documented, so generally I do not biopsy primary ovarian tumors unless the patient is considered incurable. One would not want to potentially "seed" the peritoneum in an operable patient.

Approach

The approach to be used depends on the location of the abnormality (i.e., whether it is high in the pelvis, at the level of the iliac crests, or low in the pelvis near the pelvic floor).

Anterior-lateral approach. When abnormalities are in the upper portion of the pelvis, an anterior, lateral-oblique (Fig. 46-94), lateral, or posterior approach may be used (see Fig. 46-93). An approach parallel to the iliopsoas muscle has been recommended by Bernadino et al.[115-119] In such cases it is better to insert the needle medial to the vessels, nerve, and muscle to avoid discomfort or injury.

A posterior sciatic notch approach must be used in the pelvis at the level of the sciatic notch, because the lateral portions are obscured by the wings of iliac crests and other portions of the bony pelvis (Figs. 46-95, 46-96).

At the level of the pubic ramus, the approach is

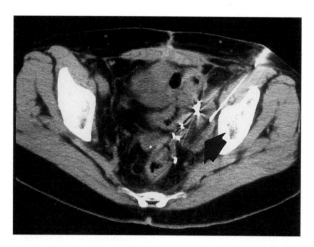

Fig. 46-94. For deep lymph nodes *(arrow)* in the pelvis, caution is necessary to avoid the iliac vessels. The best approach is parallel to the iliac crest, but one must be aware of the location of the femoral nerve between the psoas and the iliacus muscle.

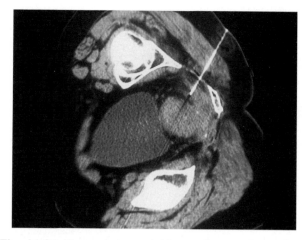

Fig. 46-96. Trans-sciatic notch biopsy of presacral mass from adenocarcinoma of rectum. When biopsying such masses, one should remember that the margins of the sacrum and the iliac bone are not well seen because the margins of the sacrum are tapered and there is partial volume effect.

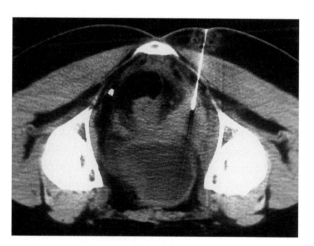

Fig. 46-95. CT scan showing posterior approach through the sciatic notch, for sampling of lymph nodes between the rectum and the internal obturator muscle.

even more restricted because the bony structures produce almost a complete ring. In this area an immediate suprapubic or sciatic notch approach may be used. As noted earlier, the insufflation of gas is helpful for movement of bowel or bladder.

Posterior approach. The posterior approach through either sciatic notch is suitable for the sampling of any presacral mass[28,223] (see Figs. 46-95, 46-96). As with other regions a guidance cannula can be quite helpful to expedite the procedure and ensure precision of needle placement. When performing the procedure through the notch, be careful to avoid the sciatic nerve and the margins of the bone. Inadvertent needle puncture of these areas can be quite uncomfortable. Also

avoid the area of the gluteal and hemorrhoidal vessels if collateral blood flow has produced pathologic enlargement.

Choice of entrance point is important to avoid impingement against the sacrum because there is a discrepancy between the apparent location of the sacrum as seen on the CT image and its real location. Since the anterior posterior and the lateral margins of the sacrum are tapered, there is a significant partial volume error created on the CT image of the sacrum. Carefully palpate the sciatic notch before any needle insertion because the margin of the bone is more lateral and caudad than would appear on the CT image. With the information from the palpation of the notch, the location of the notch can be anticipated better and the discomfort associated with the procedure can be minimized.

Accuracy

There are several articles from two perspectives in the literature about the accuracy of CT-guided procedures in this area. The first article on this topic from my group examined the accuracy of percutaneous procedures relative to surgical biopsies. We[287] found that in patients percutaneous procedures were more successful than was the surgical approach (either perineal or peritoneal). Butch et al[23] reported a series of CT-guided procedures evaluating the overall diagnostic accuracy, correctly diagnosing 15 of 19 cases of neoplasm.

Complications

No complications have been reported to date. The only difficulty has been some pain associated with inappropriate placement of needles through the sciatic nerve or local trauma to the sacrum.

THERAPEUTIC PROCEDURES

CT can be used quite readily for performing a number of aspirations and drainages in different portions of the body. By far the greatest number of drainages that will be performed are those on abscesses, but occasionally cysts, lymphoceles, pseudocysts, bilomas, or other fluid collections may be drained.

Tumor ablation

As the methods of percutaneous biopsy and drainage procedures have been refined, considerable effort has been focused on the direct delivery of toxic or ablatic energy to provide local treatment for focal tumors. Although evolving methods will probably be suitable for a variety of masses, most efforts have focused on metastatic disease of the liver.

A variety of physical energy forms have been used with varying success; these include laser, hyperthermia, and liquid nitrogen. Each of these methods has its unique limitation, which can be best appreciated by reading the current literature on the methods.

Although theoretically a variety of chemical agents could be used to destroy tumor, the greatest attention in recent years has been focused on the injection of ethyl alcohol. The most extensive experience has been reported by Isobe et al.[34] Our experience has been somewhat limited, but we have gained valuable insights from several of the patients (these have also been documented by other authors).

Indications. The indications for chemolysis of tumors are not clearly defined, but in our opinion several criteria should be met. Patients should be considered candidates only if there are a limited number of lesions and the lesions to be treated are less than 5 cm. Philosophically, those cancer patients who are candidates for surgical enucleation of hepatoma or metastatic foci should be considered. This procedure should not be considered a replacement for standard chemotherapy, however. This procedure removes "bulk" disease that is typically not well treated by chemotherapy.

Equipment and material. The needle I prefer to use for this procedure is a small 22-gauge Chiba needle. I prefer the smallest needle because it minimizes the back leakage of material when the needle is removed. We use 95% ethanol for the procedure. Relative to the amount of ethanol to be used, we do not agree with the prevailing opinion that a volume calculation should be made and that specific volume should be injected. It is our opinion that the amount injected should vary according to the appearance on CT scan. One of our junior colleagues determined in a mouse model that the distribution of the alcohol exactly parallels the distribution of the gas within the tumor (Fig. 46-97, *A* to *C*). It is our belief that the gas represents atmospheric gas, which is released as the proteins and the hemoglobin are "denatured" by the alcohol.

Because of the ability to follow the injection of the alcohol by the production of gas, we prefer to use CT for guidance and direction of the ablation. Ultrasound can be used, but as the gas accumulates the lesion is obscured by ultrasound.

We use the gas production as a sign of successful placement of the alcohol as well as a guide for volume determination. After injecting a small amount of alcohol, we perform an evaluation scan to ensure that the alcohol remains within the lesion. If no gas is accumulating, we terminate the injection of alcohol. If gas does not appear, it means that the alcohol is either escaping into the blood stream or that the tumor is very hard and the alcohol is tracking back along the needle. In either circumstance, an adverse effect may result. If the gas is forming normally, we continue treatment until the entire lesion is obscured by the gas, varying the volume accordingly.

Lymphoceles

Lymphoceles are collections of lymph fluid, usually caused by the local disruption of lymphatic vessels after surgery. The appearance of these lymphoceles is indistinguishable from abscesses appearing as well-delineated fluid collections (Fig. 46-98, *A* and *B*). These fluid collections will spontaneously resolve without any type of therapy intervention when new lymphatic channels open up.

There are only two valid indications for intervening when such a fluid collection is found. If a clinical suspicion of an infection exists, a diagnostic aspiration is indicated. There is no real rationalization for catheter insertion in such cases unless purulent material is present. Inserting a catheter may cause secondary infection, but in most cases the cavity will close after the infection has resolved. The second indication is when the lymphocele is producing obstruction of the urinary tract or gastrointestinal tract. In such cases needle puncture and catheter insertion are the same as for the other fluid collections. Another point to be made is that a lymphocele will persist in draining fluid until the lymphatics open new channels, whether a catheter is present or not. Removal of the tube will result in reaccumulation of lymph fluid, if such channels have not formed.

When a lymphocele has been drained for one of the above reasons, some radiologists have instilled sclerosing material such as tetracycline to speed resolution. The outcome has been variable, and it is not clear whether such agents are really beneficial (Fig. 46-98, *C*).

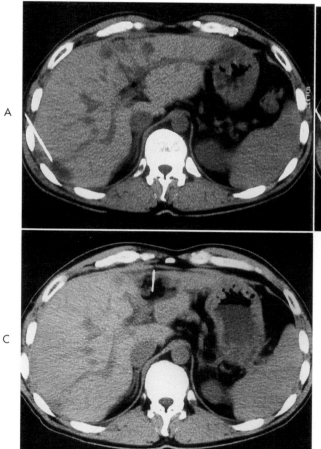

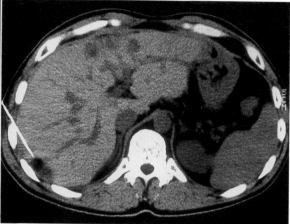

Fig. 46-97. A, Baseline scan showing placement of a needle into a low-density metastatic tumor from leiomyosarcoma. **B,** Scan showing 22-gauge needle in place within the tumor. Note the low-density gas within the lesion. The distribution of the gas follows exactly the distribution of the alcohol (see text). **C,** Follow-up scan several weeks later shows improvement in the appearance of the mass. Also note the needle and gas in a more anterior lesion in the liver, which is being treated during this later study.

Renal and liver cysts

True cysts with endothelial linings can occur in many organs, including the kidney, liver, pancreas, and spleen. They all have similar appearances and are seldom punctured for diagnosis or drained, unless they are producing symptoms or are suspected of being either infected or neoplastic. The mere presence of a cyst in an organ is no reason for sclerosis, but in some cases cyst size may be so great as to impair respiration, produce pain, obstruct the portal structures, or obstruct the renal collecting system.

The diagnostic puncture of such cystic cavities is quite easy and is performed in the routine fashion using either the 20-gauge needle or the Teflon-sheathed 18-gauge needle. The trajectory should be planned so that a "cuff" of tissue is included in the pathway of the puncture (Fig. 46-99). If this is not done, the risk of rupturing the cystic cavity into an adjacent space exists because the walls can be quite tense and can tear. Obviously, if this were a simple cyst, ill effects would not be a concern. However, if the cystic lesion is an abscess or a tumor, a complication could result. Avoiding leakage is also important if alcohol sclerosis is to be performed to prevent back leakage of alcohol into the peritoneum.

If the decision is made to drain the cyst and prevent reaccumulation, simple aspiration will usually not suffice because the endothelial lining that produced the fluid will continue to fill the cyst. The only way to stop this from recurring or growing is to inject a sclerosing agent such as tetracycline or ethyl alcohol. Our choice is alcohol because it is a potent local irritant, it has no idiosyncratic effects, and it is easily metabolized. Since surgeons have attempted for years, to eliminate these by simple injections with varying success, I expect that this simple injection method will have equal success as a radiologic procedure.

Our approach has been different from that of other authors who have simply evaluated a portion of the fluid, injected alcohol equivalent to 25% of the volume, and then repeated the injection several times. I object to this method for two reasons. The alcohol is diluted significantly; this limits its local effect of destroying the endothelial lining. Because large volumes of alcohol may be needed in large cysts, there is the possibility of administering a high systemic dose. My approach begins with the insertion of a small 5F pigtail catheter as a conduit (Fig. 46-100, *A* and *B*). Before any further manipulation of the cavity, a contrast injection is performed to

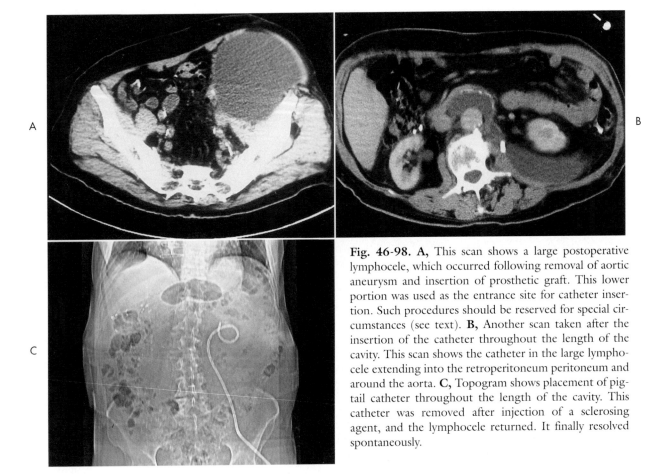

Fig. 46-98. A, This scan shows a large postoperative lymphocele, which occurred following removal of aortic aneurysm and insertion of prosthetic graft. This lower portion was used as the entrance site for catheter insertion. Such procedures should be reserved for special circumstances (see text). **B,** Another scan taken after the insertion of the catheter throughout the length of the cavity. This scan shows the catheter in the large lymphocele extending into the retroperitoneum peritoneum and around the aorta. **C,** Topogram shows placement of pigtail catheter throughout the length of the cavity. This catheter was removed after injection of a sclerosing agent, and the lymphocele returned. It finally resolved spontaneously.

ensure that there is no communication with the biliary or urinary system. If the system communicates, the procedure must be aborted, because injection of alcohol would sclerose the system. I then evacuate all of the fluid and apply suction until the walls are apposed. At this time I inject a volume of alcohol about equivalent to 25% of the extracted volume but no more than 25 cc. The alcohol is left in place for 5 to 10 minutes and then removed. A second instillation is made in the same fashion. After an additional 10 minutes, the contents, including fluid and air, are evacuated. At the end of the evacuation the stopcock is closed so that the residual vacuum keeps the wall apposed, and the catheter is removed. The patient, if reliable, may be sent home, and a repeat scan is performed in about 1 week.

Pancreatic pseudocysts

Pseudocysts of the pancreas are collections of necrotic debris, inflammatory material, and digestive enzymes that require treatment because they are associated with a number of complications. The optimal time to drain these is after 6 weeks and before 13 weeks. Approximately 6 weeks should elapse before any procedure because a high percentage (25% of more) may actually

disappear spontaneously (see Chapter 24). With those that have gone untreated for longer than 13 weeks, some authors have reported a high incidence of infection, rupture, or bleeding, all of which can be catastrophic. To prevent such complications, as well as the symptoms associated with these problems, effective treatment is indicated. An important point is that only fluid collections, and not poorly defined phlegmons or edema collections, should be drained.[90,105]

Three methods of treatment have been reported, and after a number of years of development the advantages and disadvantages of each are well-known.[8,51] These methods, in chronology of development, are aspiration, external drainage, and internal drainage. None of the reports in the radiology literature reveals the deficiencies of the methods. An impression is given that each method has solved the problem. In my extensive experience with the different treatments of pseudocysts I have formed personal opinions of their various roles, and I have found each method to have some merit but also some shortcomings. With each succeeding method the results have been better, but there remains a subset of patients who are not "cured" by our percutaneous methods and who therefore require surgical treatment. Each

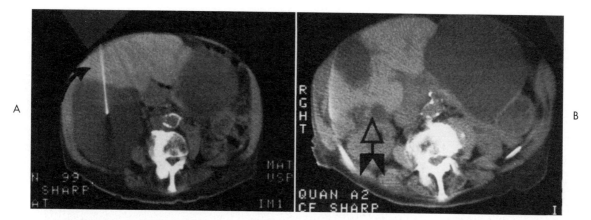

Fig. 46-99. A, CT-guided needle placement into the hepatic cyst. Note that a large amount of normal parenchyma *(curved arrow)* was purposely traversed to ensure that no back leakage occurred into the peritoneal space when alcohol was later injected. Pigtail catheter was inserted into the cavity for the infusion of the alcohol to obliterate the cavity. (See text for method.) **B,** Follow-up scan several months later shows obliterature of the cavity *(arrow)* Note that the right kidney is now in the normal location and is no longer displaced by the cyst.

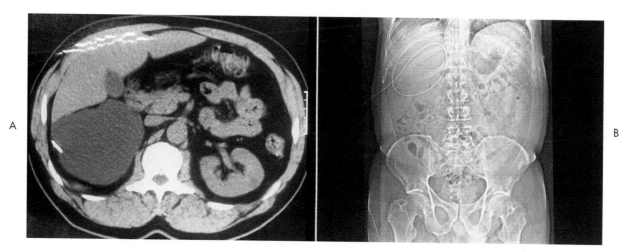

Fig. 46-100. A, Alcohol ablation of large renal cyst that was producing mass symptoms in the upper abdomen. This scan shows placement of needle into the wall of a large renal cyst. **B,** Topogram shows placement of catheter into the renal cyst. Alcohol sclerosis of the cyst was performed (see text).

of the methods will be described, and the benefits and disadvantages will be noted from our perspective.

CT is ideally suited for any of the methods. It is the best modality for visualization of the anatomy and instruments so that avoidance of uninvolved structures is possible. Avoidance of small bowel and colon is important because secondary contamination can occur. Furthermore, with CT, pseudoaneurysms can be accurately diagnosed and avoided. Life-threatening hemorrhage has occurred when these structures were inappropriately penetrated.

Aspiration. Simple aspiration of a pseudocyst appears to work in slightly less than 25% of cases, but it is

advantageous because of its simplicity. This procedure can be performed with the standard methods described previously and with little or no risk (assuming one avoids bowel loops and vascular structures). The procedure is so simple that most can be performed on an outpatient basis, as noted earlier. Some have recommended that several aspirations may be required over a period of weeks or months. The subset of pseudocysts most likely to be cured by this method is that occurring after a localized and minor leakage from the pancreas after a surgical procedure.

External drainage. This type of drainage is analogous to the external drainage performed for abscesses.

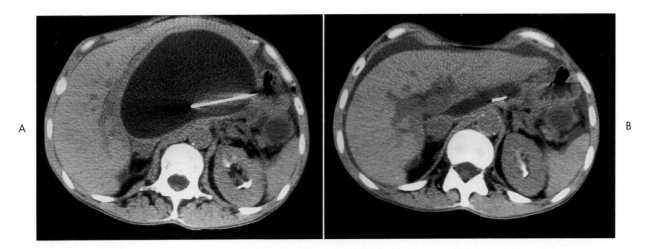

Fig. 46-101. A, Percutaneous transgastric drainage of pseudocyst is a viable option for drainage. This scan shows the needle trajectory through the stomach into a large retrogastric pseudocyst. **B,** Later scan with catheter in place shows remarkable resolution of the pseudocyst.

With this method various structures are avoided, and a catheter that drains to the external environment is put in place. Some authors have reported good results using this method, but in our experience a fairly high percentage will persist or recur. The risk of a permanent fistula or secondary infection also exists. Although the literature on this problem does not indicate significant recurrences, we have performed such procedures for more than 13 years (Fig. 46-101 A and B) and found the recurrence rate to be very similar to the aspiration method. Indeed, if this method were so effective, the transgastric method would not have been developed.

Two subsets of pseudocysts have responded quite well to this mode or the aspiration mode of therapy. Well-defined pseudocysts that are secondarily injected are well suited for percutaneous external drainage.[68,267,268] In those patients who have a pseudocyst secondary to external or surgical injury, the pseudocyst can easily be treated by aspiration or external drainage.[9,11,23] In most of the cases I have treated and in those reported in the literature, such drainages are uniformly successful without any sequela or recurrence.

Transgastric drainage. The most promising method for draining such pseudocysts is a transgastric approach as described by Nunez,[214] Bilbao,[21] Bernadino et al[18] and Ho.[123] With this method a trajectory is chosen that includes the walls of the stomach and the pseudocyst in the lesser sac. The catheter provides internal and external drainage until such time as the pseudocyst resolves.[21]

In the largest series by Nunez,[215] eight pseudocysts in seven patients were successfully drained. The length of drainage was 3 weeks in six cases and 6 weeks in two cases. No recurrences were noted, but the length of follow-up was not mentioned.

We have stopped using their method because of clinicians' concern about possible gastric spillage into the peritoneum. We have devised a modification of this method that eliminates this potential problem and that has been very well received by the clinical physicians. After the decision has been made to drain the pseudocyst, we have the endoscopist insert a percutaneous endoscopic gastrostomy (PEG). The tube used differs slightly in that the end of the gastrostomy tube is cut off. With this PEG securing the stomach wall to the abdominal wall, we use it as a conduit through the gastric space into the pseudocyst (Fig. 46-102, *A* and *B*). A Teflon-sheathed needle is inserted through the gastrostomy through the posterior stomach wall into the pseudocyst. This has worked very well, because the entrance point is secure and there is no risk for peritoneal soilage. The trajectory is easy because the gastrostomy site in the skin serves as a fulcrum and one can angle the needle to any point on the posterior stomach wall. The distance is short, and angulation is simple. Once the pseudocyst has been successfully punctured, a catheter is inserted using the Seldinger technique. Because a No. 20 French gastrostomy tube can be inserted, angiographic catheters as large as 9-10F can be used to penetrate the pseudocyst.

In our experience the short-term results of the transgastric method are quite good. Unfortunately, in the long term (up to a year after the removal of the tube), some will recur. It has been our experience that leaving the tube in for about 6 to 8 weeks is sufficient. If the cyst remains or recurs after this, then surgical treatment is probably needed.

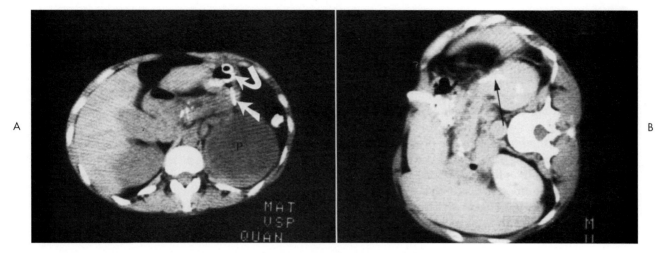

Fig. 46-102. A, This scan shows the Longdwell needle *(arrow)* being inserted through the gastrostomy *(curved arrow).* It is positioned at the stomach wall just before puncture into the pseudocyst, *P.* **B,** Repeat CT scan with catheter *(arrow)* in place shows resolution of the pseudocyst. The pseudocyst recurred several months later, and the patient had a distal pancreatectomy, which was curative. Unfortunately, she had a cardiac arrest during anesthesia induction and was on a respirator for weeks.

There are two advantages of the transgastric method. First, residual or leaking pancreatic juice can exit into the stomach, thereby preventing a fistula. Second, the enteric flora can colonize the pseudocyst, thus permitting inflammatory reaction and better closure of the cavity.

Pancreatic fistula. Rarely, a pancreatic fistula may result after tube drainage of a pseudocyst. Of the several approaches that might be used, only one has been reported. First, some authors have used the hormone somatostatin to decrease the exocrine output of the gland.[196] The results have been variable, however, and the medication is quite expensive. Another method, proposed by Haaga and Stout, is the use of a biologic glue such as "fibrin glue" to seal such a pathway from a pseudocyst or the pancreatic duct. It has been attempted in one of our cases, but the outcome was not certain at the time of this printing.

ABSCESS ASPIRATION

Percutaneous aspiration and percutaneous drainages guided by CT represent the most significant advance in the care of acutely ill patients since the development of surgical drainage and the discovery of antibiotics. Since the first CT-guided aspiration and drainage (Fig. 46-103, *A* and *B*), which I performed in 1975 and reported in 1976,[108] the use of this technique has grown rapidly.* This growth has occurred because of the increased number of scanners available, the excellent accuracy of CT for the detection of any fluid collection, the high accuracy for guidance, and the popularization of the technique by enthusiasts such as Haaga,[102,108,110] Gerzof,[75-80] and Van Sonenberg.[264-269]

Diagnostic aspirations

Because patients with infectious fluid collections may or may not manifest the typical signs of infection, I believe that if there is even the slightest clinical concern about an abscess a diagnostic aspiration should be performed. This aggressive diagnostic approach is justified because with careful technique, including avoidance of bowel, a sample can be successfully recovered in almost 100% of cases with little or no risk. In my experience with CT guidance over the last 20 years, I have aspirated more than 500 cases with no secondary infection and with only one hematoma that occurred as a complication.

The diagnostic sampling of fluid collections requires the same planning as that of all of the other lesions we have discussed, but several things must be kept in mind. The material being obtained may contain viable pathogenic material and can disseminate infection if it is inappropriately spilled or contaminated into sterile spaces. Even though the modern potent antibiotics can eradicate any minor spillage of purulent material, great care should be taken not to contaminate sterile areas. Patients may develop a serious peritonitis or bacteremia if the inoculum is larger or the organism virulent (or if the patient is immunocompromised by any cause).

A question occasionally arises concerning the interpretation of culture results—that is, how culture re-

*References 80, 113, 136, 151, 208, 224, 227, 263, 269.

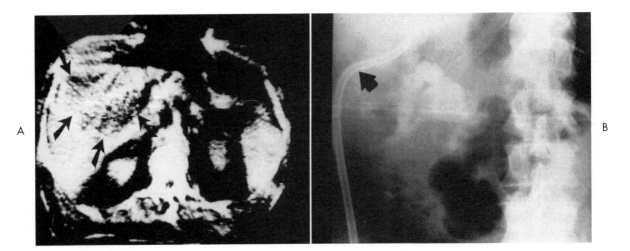

Fig. 46-103. A, First CT-guided drainage of an abscess *(arrows)* performed in 1975 by the author. **B,** Plain radiograph of the abdomen shows a drainage tube in place *(arrow)*. The patient recovered uneventfully. (**B** from *Cleve Clin Q* 43(2):85-88, 1976.)

sults should be interpreted when only a limited number of colonies grow. It is my opinion that any number of colonies involving organisms other than staphylococcus should be considered an infection at least warranting antibiotic therapy based on the culture sensitivities. Depending on the number of bacteria within a fluid collection or the presence of antibiotics, the possibility always exists for a sampling error that can result in a negative culture or possibly growth of a limited number of pathogens.

Finally, during the aspiration of fluid densities it is important to avoid traversing gastrointestinal loops. First, a sample taken through bowel may provide spurious culture results. Of course, some claim that presence of mixed flora and absence of a "pure" culture of a single organism can distinguish an abscess from gastrointestinal colonization. However, as has been well documented in the radiology literature, many abscesses are caused by a gastrointestinal fistula that contains many types of organisms. Second, the function of humoral cellular defenses is lessened in a fluid space, so that clearing of bacteria by phagocytes is impaired and a secondary infection might occur if a small inoculum is introduced into a fluid collection.

Mycotic aneurysms or infected vascular prostheses

Because of the difficult treatment required for infected vessels or synthetic aortic prostheses, it is my firm belief that any patient with such a suspected infection should have a diagnostic aspiration at the earliest time. With both infected prostheses and primary mycotic infections in the infected prostheses we have encountered, the cultures have been positive and reliable. In each of

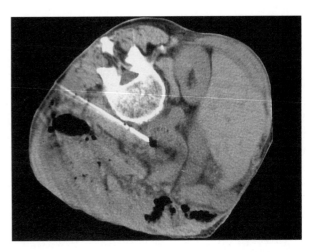

Fig. 46-104. Diagnostic aspiration of air collection around prosthetic graft. CT scan shows patient lying prone. Note the needle penetrating the wall of the aneurysm, which encloses air collection next to graft.

these cases the culture results were critical and helped initiate the expeditious treatment of the problem. With prompt treatment most of these patients survived the surgical therapy. In another group of 10 patients with uninfected grafts, the results were negative. There have been no complications associated with the needle procedures (Fig. 46-104, 46-105).

Such cases should be approached from the flank, and a pathway should be chosen to avoid the kidney and major vessels. In most instances a clearly defined fluid collection will be seen either adjacent to the graft or between the wall of the aneurysm and the graft. As with other procedures performed from this approach, we try

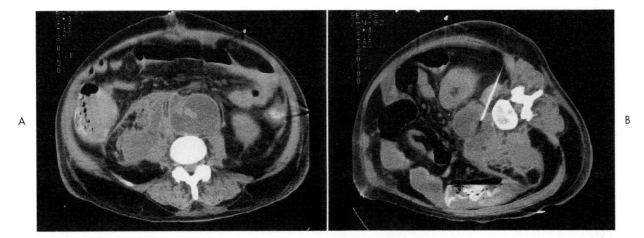

Fig. 46-105. A, This scan shows postoperative fluid collections around the graft material within the old aneurysm bed as well as in the right flank. **B,** With the patient in the left decubitus position, percutaneous aspiration of fluid around graft was performed. Because staphylococcus is the most common organism, such aspirations may be necessary even if gas is not present. Aspiration of the opposite right fluid collection was performed independently using a different pathway to avoid possible cross-contamination of the spaces, if one happened to be sterile and one happened to be infected.

to avoid the psoas muscle, erector muscles of the spine, and the spinal elements to prevent patient discomfort.

In such cases, if there is any question about the location of the vessel or prosthetic wall, a bolus dynamic CT scan should be performed. Dynamic CT is highly effective for the demonstration of a vascular problem, even better than Doppler ultrasound and angiography. In one patient with a "clotted" mycotic aneurysm, only CT correctly showed the vascular nature of the lesion (Fig. 46-7).

Some individuals have raised concerns about possible injury to such an infected vessel, but in our experience this is not a problem. In the more than 20 suspected cases we have aspirated, there have been no complications.

The need for such aggressive expeditious procedures is clear. The mortality rate of untreated prosthesis infection is very high, almost 100%. Corrective treatment and surgery can be effective only if initiated early. In some instances, percutaneous drainage of infected prostheses may be effective[163] if the infection involves only the mid-portion and not the anastomotic ends (Fig. 46-106, A to C).

Abscess drainage

Before CT, percutaneous abscess drainage (PAD) was occasionally performed, but with the advent of CT assistance it has become a routine procedure. CT has been especially useful because it has a high detection accuracy for abscesses and allows accurate determination of the anatomic location and extent of the lesion. Because CT is not impeded by gas or bone, any involvement of peritoneal spaces or anatomic areas can be clearly delineated. This information is absolutely necessary if one is to determine whether an abscess can be drained by a percutaneous method.

Although there was some controversy in the early literature concerning the merits of different guidance systems for drainage, there now appears to be a consensus that CT guidance is the best method available.[102,164,268]

Perspectives on abscess drainages

With a global perspective toward abscess drainage, it is clear that the intent of interventional percutaneous procedures is to at least duplicate the excellent treatment results established by our surgical colleagues. The benefit of percutaneous procedures lies in their simplicity, lower complication rates, and presumably lower overall expense. Recent publications in the surgical literature have illuminated some of the factors that relate to the outcome of both percutaneous and surgical procedures.[10]

The benefits of improved detection and localization of abscess have been documented by Deveney et al,[47] who showed conclusively that the improved localization and intensive care methods have resulted in a greater percentage of drainage success as well as decreased mortality resulting from organ failure. These authors, in a veteran population, studied two 5-year periods, 1973 to 1978 and 1981 to 1986, and noted the following. The mortality of the two groups was 39% and 21%, respectively. The successful initial drainage was 55%

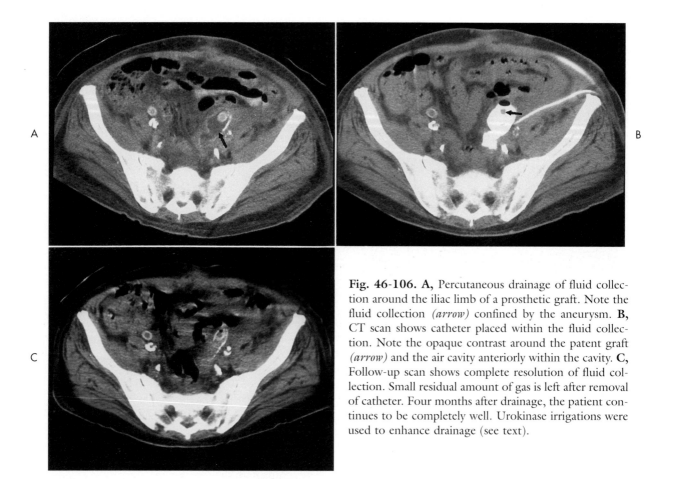

Fig. 46-106. A, Percutaneous drainage of fluid collection around the iliac limb of a prosthetic graft. Note the fluid collection *(arrow)* confined by the aneurysm. **B,** CT scan shows catheter placed within the fluid collection. Note the opaque contrast around the patent graft *(arrow)* and the air cavity anteriorly within the cavity. **C,** Follow-up scan shows complete resolution of fluid collection. Small residual amount of gas is left after removal of catheter. Four months after drainage, the patient continues to be completely well. Urokinase irrigations were used to enhance drainage (see text).

compared with 74%. Organ failure rate decreased from 52% to 23%. The surgical success rate was 76%, compared with the percutaneous success rate of 72%. The authors concluded that accurate localization and early drainage are the most important factors and that there is no difference in outcome between the surgical and percutaneous methods.

The importance of overall patient status has also been documented by Levison et al.[170] These authors used the APACHE II system to grade patients and follow their outcome. The final results were that mortality was directly related to the APACHE score. Of those with a score less than 15, the mortality was 1.7%, compared with a mortality of 78% when the score was greater than 15. There was no significant statistical difference in outcome between percutaneous and surgical drainages (one is cautioned not to quote this finding out of context, because the authors subjectively maintain that surgical drainage was better by *absolute* numbers. The finding was *not* statistically significant, however).

The importance of the immune system has been emphasized throughout this discussion on intervention. Recently Lambiase et al[163] have documented how critical this factor is as it relates to abscess drainage.[3] These authors considered the following states as immunocompromised: absolute neutropenia, HIV viral infection, cancer with distant spread, chemotherapy, radiation therapy, lymphoproliferative disorders, diabetes requiring treatment, chronic renal dialysis, splenectomy, and severe alcoholism. They found that with percutaneous abscess drainage the overall cure rate for immunocompromised patients was 53.1% compared with the normal rate of 72.6%.

Patient selection

In recent years the indication for percutaneous methods has expanded significantly.[27,31] Unlike most new techniques and procedures in which there is an initial period of enthusiasm followed by a either a moderation or a restriction of the method, percutaneous drainage guided by CT has continued to expand its role. The results of percutaneous procedures have been so good and so widely accepted that the indications and applications have continued to find new application.

To maintain a proper clinical perspective, it is important that the proper patients be selected for curative or palliative PAD procedures[264,265] and for surgical procedures. Simplistically, one could try PAD for palliation

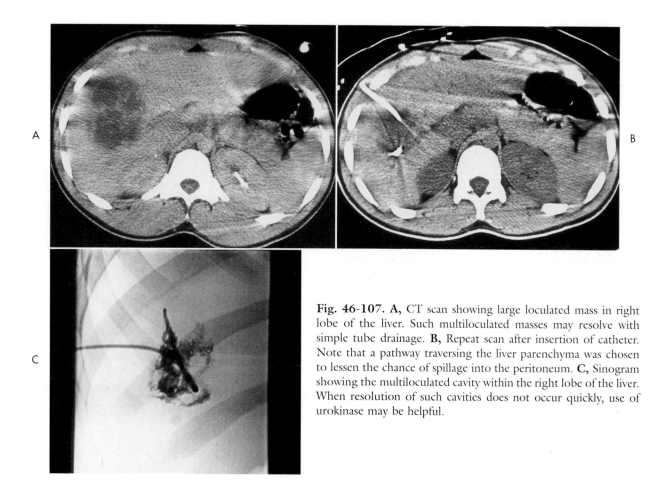

Fig. 46-107. A, CT scan showing large loculated mass in right lobe of the liver. Such multiloculated masses may resolve with simple tube drainage. **B,** Repeat scan after insertion of catheter. Note that a pathway traversing the liver parenchyma was chosen to lessen the chance of spillage into the peritoneum. **C,** Sinogram showing the multiloculated cavity within the right lobe of the liver. When resolution of such cavities does not occur quickly, use of urokinase may be helpful.

in every patient, but it is not logical to expand its use for patients with certain surgical problems.[27] On a practical level, although the role and the indications for percutaneous procedures have expanded greatly, there are still clear indications for surgical drainages.

To anticipate a curative percutaneous procedure, certain clinical and anatomic facts must be confirmed. Patients who have an abscess or abscesses that appear well-defined are suitable candidates if a clear anatomic pathway is available. In the early experience procedures were restricted to those abscesses with only a few cavities. The results with septated abscess has been variable; some drain quite well and others do not (Fig. 46-107, *A* to *C*). The most plausible explanation for this is that fibrin septa in such cavities may be complete or incomplete; when they are complete drainage is poor and when they communicate and are incomplete, curative drainage can occur. Recently, we have studied the use of fibrinolytic agents in the former cases and have found them quite effective for improving drainage (see later discussion on fibrinolytic agents). Also, the multiplicity of abscesses is no longer considered a contraindication to percutaneous drainage because each site is treated independently.

For the choice of anatomic pathways, we still prefer a clear pathway into the abscess cavity without traversing an uninvolved space or organ. I believe that a routine penetration through an uninvolved organ is inappropriate because of possible seeding of pyogenic organisms into the organ. Although with the potent antibiotics of today most such procedures appear feasible, I believe that when larger series are collected, the success and complication rate will favor avoidance of uninvolved organs and spaces (Fig. 46-108).

Another important factor to consider is the viscosity of the material in the abscess. If the entire cavity can be evacuated easily after aspiration, percutaneous drainage will probably work. If the material appears to be quite viscous, techniques should be adjusted appropriately (i.e., special attention given to catheter size, catheter placement, and use of an appropriate irrigant). These will be discussed under the section on catheter management.

Choosing PAD for palliation is most appropriate. Adequate palliative drainage will reduce the "toxic load" resulting from drainage of purulent material and will usually produce considerable improvement in such patients. Remarkably, some will be cured, but even those who are

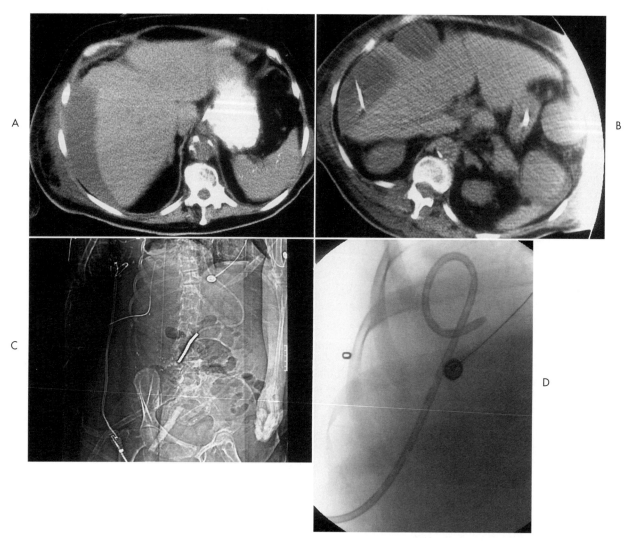

Fig. 46-108. A, Large subdiaphragmatic abscess extending as far posteriorly as the coronary ligaments. This proved to be a candida abscess. **B,** CT scan during a guided puncture of the fluid collection, from a more anterior approach. The more anterior the approach for such collections the better, because the diaphragm is higher anteriorly than posteriorly. **C,** Topogram showing optimal placement of the catheter throughout the length of the abscess cavity. Because this was a fungal infection and the historical perspective is that such abscesses are difficult to drain, urokinase was used as a catheter irrigant. The abscess was successfully drained. **D,** Radiograph showing a larger catheter was inserted into the cavity. The best flow of purulent material is achieved with large bore catheters and the use of urokinase (see text).

not will benefit from an improved physiologic state that makes them better surgical candidates.

The appropriateness of percutaneous drainages for abscess associated with entities requiring surgical treatment is an area of significant controversy (this will be discussed later). In the final analysis, however, one must weigh the palliative benefits of PAD against the final curative benefits of surgery.[274] Similar views are shared by Dr. Claude Welsh of Massachusetts General Hospital,[274] who noted in an editorial:

Unfortunately, abscesses vary so greatly in many ways

that studies with proper, randomized controls would be very difficult to establish. It is far more likely that further experience will lead to greater concurrence between radiologists and surgeons. Thus the letter by Haaga et al. outlines conclusions that appear to be quite closely in accord with our own studies in the Massachusetts General Hospital. *Since Haaga and his co-workers originated the radiologic method, their opinion must be given great respect.*

Indications for surgery

Some patients are not good candidates for percutaneous procedures and are better suited for surgical drainage. This group consists of patients with fungal infections,[286] infected hematomas, echinococcal disease, surgical disease requiring correction, most pancreatic abscesses, and failed percutaneous drainages.

Patients with fungal abscesses require surgical drainage because there is extensive tissue invasion, necrosis, and mycotic plaque formation with the wall of the cavity. Our experience with several such cases and reports in the literature show that surgical drainage or resection is best for adequate debridement.

Infected hematomas do not drain well because of the extensive amount of fibrin deposition and the protective effects of fibrin on bacteria. Again, as shown from our early experience and from reports in the literature, it is clear that such hematomas have uniformly failed by percutaneous drainage. In our more recent experience, fibrinolytic agents used as a catheter irrigant can improve the drainage of infected hematomas. The doses, methods of administration, and effectiveness are now available and will be discussed below.

Echinococcal disease requires a specialized approach for drainage that is best accomplished by surgical methods. In drainage of such entities, careful resection and handling of the material is required. There has been a single case report[199] in the literature using percutaneous drainage that was successful without complication. It is my belief that such problems may be approached in specialized circumstances with percutaneous methods but that the techniques are so meticulous and demanding that they should be performed only at specialized centers.

Finally, for those patients who have had a failed percutaneous procedure, surgical drainage is appropriate. Because of the difference in philosophy among surgeons, radiologists, and institutions, the definition of a failed procedure can be determined only at the local level and not in this text.

Sequential steps for drainage

The technique of abscess drainage can be divided into the following steps:
1. Abscess detection
2. Trajectory planning
3. Selection of the guidance modality
4. Diagnostic aspiration
5. Catheter selection and insertion
6. Sinogram and catheter adjustment
7. Catheter management and irrigation
8. Follow-up diagnostic evaluation
9. Catheter removal

Abscess detection. Detection of an abscess can be accomplished by any modality, but CT plays the most critical role. When a patient is acutely ill, it is important to begin the evaluation with a plain film of the area. If the plain film is negative, further investigation by ultrasound or CT is indicated. If the plain film is positive, showing an abnormal collection of air, CT is the next study that should be performed. CT rather than ultrasound is indicated because it is not impaired by air, and CT provides clear delineation and characterization of the air or any associated fluid collection. When a patient is septic, CT is the preferred examination because it is the most accurate of all imaging systems for abscess detection. Not only can CT confirm or exclude the presence of drainable fluid, but it can also diagnose the causative or associated problem. CT can provide valuable information about diverticulitis, tumors, appendicitis, fistulae, infarcts, cellulitis, phlegmons, inflammatory bowel disease, bowel obstructions, or other problems.

If an abscess has been detected by either plain radiography, gallium, or ultrasound, a CT scan should be performed to determine the complete extent of the abscess. The geographic location and degree of involvement are essential factors in choosing the trajectory, determining the number of catheters required, and anticipating possible difficulties. Although some authors were initially reluctant to accept the not only advantages but the critical role of CT in defining the nature of an abscess, virtually all authors now agree that CT is the modality of choice for the detection, staging, and planning of a drainage procedure. The criteria for drainage have been expanded to include many patients, so the need for accurate detection and staging is even greater.

Trajectory planning. Trajectory planning is best accomplished by CT, regardless of the imaging modality chosen for guidance. Although as most authors agree it is best to choose the shortest pathway, it is also optimal to avoid uninvolved organs and noncontiguous peritoneal spaces (for example, to avoid pleura during a peritoneal process, loops of bowel, and vessels).

Several points should be made concerning the configuration and nature of the abscess collection. If an abscess collection is great in length, plan the trajectory of the puncture so that when the catheter is inserted it will lie throughout the length of the cavity. Two approaches may be used. First, one can choose an entrance site at the upper or lower end of the cavity, so that the catheter will traverse the entire length or width. The alternative is to make two punctures at the center point, one directed cephalad and one directed caudad to permit positioning of a catheter at the very top and bottom of the cavity. (see section on catheterization). If such an abscess is elongated in a transverse direction, catheters should be similarly placed in that plane. If multiple septations are seen within a cavity, it is reasonable to plan the trajectory so that the maximum number of cavities will be traversed. Although best surgical results are obtained if an extraperitoneal approach is used, this is not true with percutaneous procedures. With surgery, a peritoneal approach is disadvantageous because it opens the possibility of "soiling" sterile portions of the peritoneum. A percutaneous puncture and drainage exposes only the pathway to contamination rather than the wide surface of the peritoneum. Potential contamination is minimal if meticulous technique and methods are used.

Neither we nor other authors have found any indications that a peritoneal approach differs in outcome from an extraperitoneal approach with percutaneous drainage. In our experience, planning the trajectory to provide dependent drainage is not required. Purulent material will follow the line of least resistance, which is the catheter tract. In fact, for subphrenic collections I prefer a more midaxillary approach to a posterior one, to avoid the pleura.

Selection of modality. Once a trajectory has been planned, choose the guidance modality most suitable for the procedure. Fluoroscopy, ultrasound,[138,144,148] or CT can be used, but CT is the preferred method in almost all cases.[80,102,137,145,268] The larger and more superficial fluid collections can be punctured by using fluoroscopy or ultrasound.[240,248] The more difficult the abscess, that is, the deeper, smaller, or more critically located it is, the more likely it is that CT guidance can be used.

Diagnostic aspiration. Before catheter or trocar placement, perform a diagnostic aspiration to confirm the presence of an abscess. There are two reasons I use a 19-gauge needle with an 18-gauge Teflon sheath to perform diagnostic aspirations. First, the larger needle permits aspiration of even the thickest purulent material. Second, if at the time of aspiration the fluid appears purulent, the sheath permits insertion of an angiographic wire and catheter without a second puncture.

The actual puncture and placement of the needle is performed in the same manner as any other needle procedure. Try to plan the procedure so that the tip of the needle is placed in a more posterior or dependent location so that the anterior wall will not be retracted away from the needle as the fluid is aspirated and the wall partially collapses.

I take two steps to minimize the risk of contamination along the pathway. First, when draining abscesses in a solid organ, I choose the path to include a "cuff" of normal parenchyma to lessen the chance of tearing the thin wall of an abscess. Second, at the time the puncture is made I aspirate a sufficient amount of material to lessen the "back pressure." There is one reported case of spillage into the peritoneum that produced peritonitis, as well as a case of dissemination into the subphrenic area (Fig. 46-109). reported by Johnsen et al[141]; therefore, one must always strive for meticulous technique. If the catheter is in the area of the spillage, no further treat-

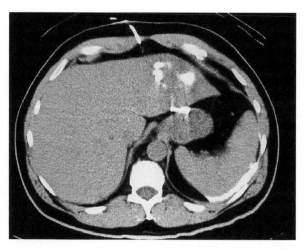

Fig. 46-109. CT scan shows an abscess in the left lobe filled with contrast material. The drainage catheter has penetrated the posterior surface of the liver; no repositioning was made because the catheter tracted through the cavity.

ment is necessary, but if it is not, another catheter should be inserted in the area.

If purulent material is aspirated, a sample of 10 to 20 cc is aspirated before catheter insertion and is sent for culture. If the flow of purulent material is quite fast, I will remove 25 to 75 cc to relieve any back pressure and prevent any spillage or tracking during catheter insertion. After removal of this purulent material, I inject a small amount of urographic contrast material to facilitate the fluoroscopically guided catheter insertion. Also, if the wire and needle become inadvertently displaced, the contrast material permits a clear "target" for a puncture under fluoroscopy. Be careful not to inject too large a volume, which might overdistend the cavity and cause spillage of purulent material. After this step, insert an angiography wire into the cavity to stabilize the sheath if the patient is being transported to fluoroscopy. At times one may simply choose to insert the catheter or the CT, using the topogram as the method for confirming the catheter location.

If the material is not obviously purulent, I aspirate only a small amount of fluid and send it for culture. In the event that a repeat puncture and drainage might be required I make a point not to aspirate such a fluid collection "dry"; if such a cavity is aspirated "dry," there will be no well-defined lesion to target should a drainage be required later. I do not insert a catheter when the fluid is not obviously infected, because if such a collection is sterile, an indwelling catheter might introduce pyogens and cause a secondary infection. In patients with tumors in the area, a cytologic sample should be sent to determine if there is a necrotic neoplasm or secondarily infected tumor giving toxic symptoms similar to abscesses (this will be discussed later). Catheter drainage may provide some palliation for such tumors or secondarily infected tumors.

Catheter selection/insertion. There are two types of catheters available for drainage, drainage catheters inserted by the Seldinger method and single step catheters.[87,98] Either may be chosen, depending on the specific nature of each case. The configuration of the tip and location of the holes will vary, among those available.

The size of the catheter and the size of the pigtail shape to be used should be matched to the size of the abscess cavity, so that the entire curved end is in the cavity. As a rule it is important to use the largest catheter possible from the beginning; if the procedure becomes technically difficult, one can settle for almost any size of catheter and upgrade it later. Larger catheters do permit faster drainage of material. It is important not to have holes outside the cavity. If holes are outside, leakage into a sterile space or organ can occur. Conversely, if a cavity is large, it may be important to cut additional side holes in the catheter if needed.

Two options are available for insertion of large abscess catheters. The trocar catheters now commercially available from many different companies can be used. I have found that these trocar catheters are useful for large superficial abscesses but not so suitable for most of the small or critically located abscesses.

The second option I also like to use is a two-step procedure. In the first step an angiographic catheter is inserted on the first day of the puncture and in the second step the catheter is upgraded in size on the second or third day as needed after the sinogram.

The chosen catheter can be inserted in one of two ways. First, if one has only limited experience, the best way is to transport the patient to a fluoroscopic unit for catheter insertion and positioning. As a rule, I always adjust the catheter position to ensure that it traverses the entire length of the cavity and that there are no "kinks." Also, if the cavity is small or if the catheter has a large number of holes, be certain that none of the holes are outside the cavity. If holes are outside the cavity, then dissemination can occur through the side hole with drainage or irrigation. The second choice is to put the catheter in by "feel" and to observe the location with Topogram or the Scoutview. If one is quite experienced this second method will suffice, and any necessary adjustment in catheter position can be done on the second or third day during the sinogram.

To ensure that the entire length of a cavity is covered, there are two possible approaches. One can start at either the highest or lowest end and then insert the catheter throughout the length. Or, one can insert two separate catheters in the middle and cross them so that each one is directed toward the upper or lower extreme (Fig. 46-110). Cavities with multiple loculations may drain spontaneously, or the effective drainage can be improved with urokinase as described below. If there is any question about communication among the different spaces, one must not hesitate to use multiple catheters (Fig. 46-111).

With the catheter in place, I gently evacuate all of the purulent material from the cavity until the cavity is empty, unless several liters of material are present. In such cases it is probably prudent to remove no more than a liter of fluid by aspiration and then to permit the remainder to drain more slowly through the catheter. This will prevent potential fluid shifts between various compartments. I adopted this approach after we had one pa-

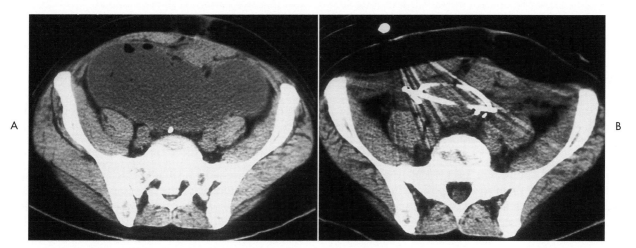

Fig. 46-110. A, This scan shows a very large abscess, which is very wide across the entire abdomen. To ensure adequate drainage, a catheter was inserted from each side and crossed in the midline. **B,** This follow-up scan shows total evacuation of the cavity and the catheters in the midline.

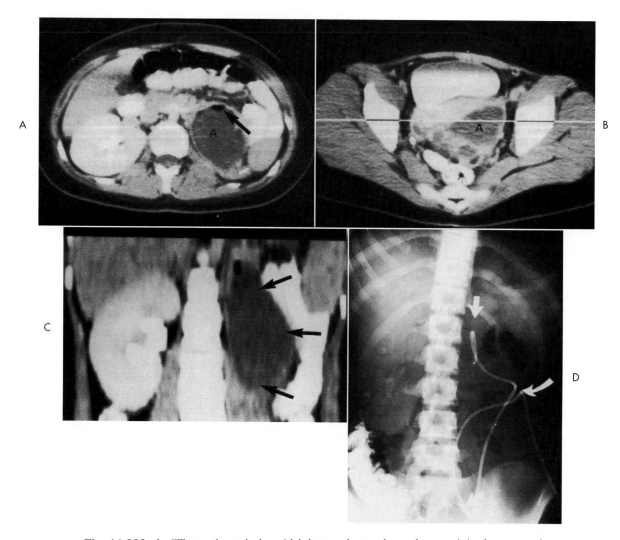

Fig. 46-111. A, CT scan through the midabdomen shows a large abscess, *A,* in the retroperitoneum, containing some gas *(arrow).* **B,** The lowest portion of the abscess, *A,* extends into the pelvis behind the left adenexa of the uterus. **C,** Coronal reconstruction shows a long abscess *(arrows)* extending through the retroperitoneum. **D,** Plain film shows placement of two catheters entering from the middle of the cavity *(curved arrow),* extending to the top and bottom of the cavity *(arrows).*

tient who suffered a hypotensive collapse after the acute removal of 6 L of purulent material (Fig. 46-112). At this time I use saline irrigations to flush the cavity until the returning material is almost clear. If the fluid becomes blood-tinged during the irrigation, I stop the irrigation and send the patient back to let the material drain slowly. Besides these steps of positioning and irrigation, I perform no other manipulation at the time of the first insertion to avoid bacteremia.

Some authors have recommended the use of a wire at this point to disrupt any septations or adhesions. This appears to be imprudent because use of a wire will traumatize the wall and may cause a significant bacteremia or hemorrhage from the granulation tissue.

Sinogram and catheter adjustment. Sinograms are performed somewhere between 48 and 72 hours to check the position of the catheter and every 4 to 5 days to assess the progress of healing. During the first sinogram one evaluates whether the catheter placed is still in correct position and is of adequate size for the evacuation of any residual purulent material. As the cavity is evacuated, the contour may change and shift the location of the catheter, requiring adjustment of the position (see Fig. 46-101). If there is considerable purulent material left, one may choose to increase the size of the catheter. At this time, sequential dilatation may be performed safely. I discourage extensive dilatation at the first procedure because of concerns about either spillage of bacte-

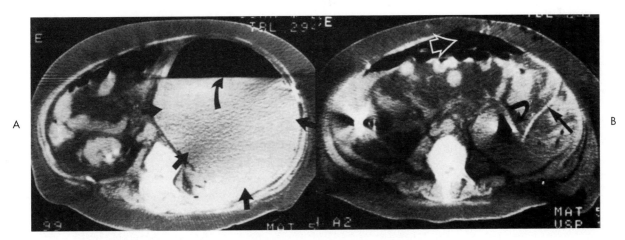

Fig. 46-112. A, Large abscess cavity *(arrows)* with air-fluid level *(curved arrow)* is located in the left side of the abdomen. After the acute removal of 6 liters of purulent material, this patient suffered a severe hypotensive crisis. **B,** The same patient after several days shows a repeat scan after incorrect placement of the catheter *(arrow)* through the anterior wall of the wall of the abscess. The wall of the abscess *(curved arrow)* receded past the catheter so that holes in the catheter permitted air *(open arrow)* and material to flow into the peritoneum.

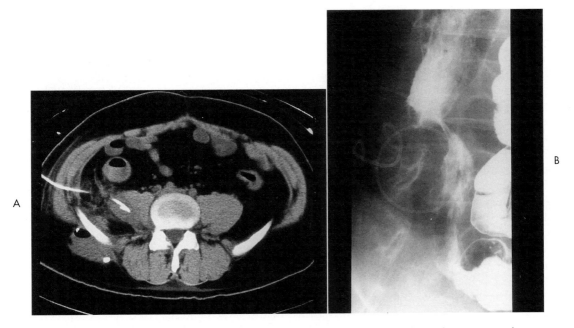

Fig. 46-113. A, CT scan shows two abscess cavities in the right side, one in the psoas muscle and one in the gluteus muscle behind the iliac crest. The high-density objects are cross-sections of two different catheters that were used to drain the abscesses. **B,** A sinogram taken later in the course of the patient's recovery shows communication of the long cavity in the psoas muscle with the small bowel. Total resolution without surgery followed (see text).

remia or bleeding. Furthermore, if the material is thick or loculations are present, one might institute urokinase at this time, if it was not used initially.

If one chooses subsequent sinograms, they are used to assess the size of the cavity and the possible presence of fistula. Assessing the size of the cavity is important to determine the time of catheter removal. As heal-

ing occurs with the ingrowth of granulation tissue, the cavity size reduces. The catheter should be left in place until the cavity almost disappears. Fistulas are seldom seen except in the later sinograms as the inflammation recedes. Most fistulae close spontaneously see below (Fig. 46-113, *A* and *B*).

Catheter management and irrigation. Once the

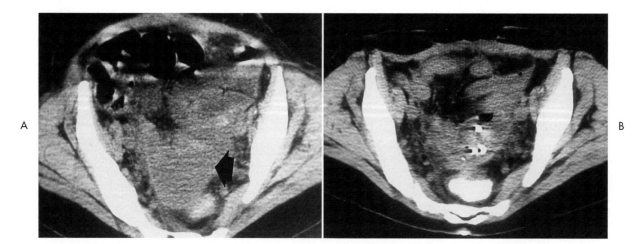

Fig. 46-114. A, CT scan shows large high-density mass *(arrow)* in the posterior pelvis. The mass proved to be an infected hematoma following hysterectomy. The patient had systemic lupus and was on high doses of systemic steroids. Even with these complicating factors the patient was cured by percutaneous drainage enhanced by urokinase irrigations. **B,** Follow-up scan shows reduction in size of cavity with high-density catheter in place. There was ultimately total resolution without surgical treatment.

catheter is in place, a few guidelines must be followed to ensure a successful drainage. It has been my routine to leave a catheter only to gravity drainage. My concern about application of high suction is that the holes may be occluded by tissue and loculations can accumulate peripherally.

The one circumstance in which active suction is best is when there is free communication with either a fistula or biliary system.

Catheter irrigation should be performed with either one or two agents, as follows. The two agents we use to facilitate drainage are saline and urokinase. If the material being drained is quite thin and there are no definite septations noted on imaging studies, we inject saline. Saline in the amount of 10 to 15 cc should be injected every 6 to 8 hours to keep the catheter lumen clear. If the material being drained is quite thick or there are septations in the abscess, urokinase should be injected in amounts as follows, depending on the size of the cavity: 0 to 3 cm, 5,000 to 10,000 units; 3 to 5 cm, 25,000 units; 5 to 10 cm, 50,000 units; and greater than 10 cm, 100,000 units. After the urokinase has been injected, a small amount of saline should be used to clear the catheter of the urokinase. The catheter should be clamped for 5 minutes and then left to gravity drainage. The irrigations are continued for 3 to 4 days.

The effectiveness and safety of the urokinase has been documented by our group[4] in the literature (Fig. 46-114, *A* and *B*). Park et al[225] showed that in vitro, the urokinase as compared with saline definitely decreased the viscosity of the purulent material (Fig. 46-

115). The safety of urokinase in vivo was proved by Lahorra et al,[159] who demonstrated that intracavitary urokinase produced no systemic effects. In reporting that study the authors also stated that the urokinase also appeared to improve drainage of thick purulent material and to break any septations. A more definitive prospective study is now under way to confirm efficacy of this agent.

Follow-up evaluation. Before final removal of the catheter in a routine case, perform a final CT scan to ensure that all areas of the abscess are drained. An abscess that is completely resolved should show virtually complete obliteration of the cavity (but one may see a very small amount of residual fluid and air) or decreased density in the liver. If a considerable amount of fluid remains, it is best to wait until the cavity has more completely resolved and has been reduced in size by granulation. If a patient is doing well clinically, the patient may be discharged and managed as an outpatient during the time it takes for the cavity to granulate closed.

The last question to be considered during this final evaluation is whether the primary cause of the abscess and any important sequelae have been found. In most instances an abscess will be the result of a surgical procedure or other intervention, but if there is no known cause, other diagnostic studies should be performed until all possible causes have been excluded (e.g., ulcer, diverticula). If a surgical problems exists, the appropriate therapy is instituted. In most instances a sinogram will have demonstrated a fistula to a loop of bowel, and management as described later is appropriate.

Catheter removal. When a drainage procedure

CATHETER SIZE VERSUS TIME TO DRAIN
10 ML OF FLUID

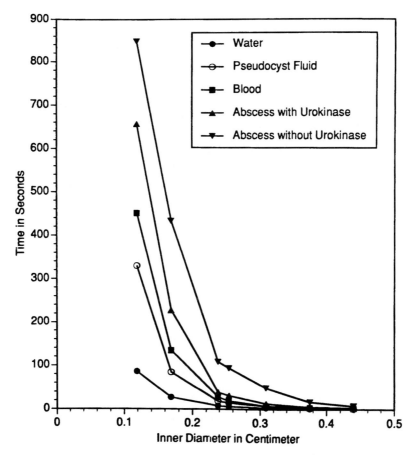

Fig. 46-115. An in vitro experiment was performed evaluating different parameters including urokinase treatment. Graph shows the drainage time of various fluid types through various sizes of catheters. The upper two lines show how urokinase improves the drainage of purulent material. (Data from Park et al.[225])

has gone well, the patient will respond very quickly and will show dramatic clinical improvement. In such patients the fever will defervesce, the white count will drop, and sweating episodes will stop. The progress of the drainage can also be assessed by following the sequential changes in the physical appearance of the fluid. Initially, the material will be cloudy and turbid; it will then change to a serosanguineous appearance, and finally it will change to a clear serous material. Cultures of the fluid will also change sequentially so that when the abscess has resolved, drainage fluid will be sterile. After this clinical response and the change in character of the material, the catheter can be removed.

If the fluid from the catheter does not change as expected but drains bile or enteric contents, a repeat sinogram is necessary to evaluate for a fistula. Many times fistulae may not be seen with an early sinogram, since they will be closed because of edema and inflammation.

The decision to remove the catheter is quite easy if the course of the drainage (i.e., clinical response, evolution of fluid changes, and appearance of the sinograms) is as expected. The removal of the catheter can be performed in two ways. The traditional method is to withdraw the tube 1 or 2 cm per day, on an inpatient or outpatient basis. A second, less well-known method, can be used if the cavity is small and the catheter has a straight configuration. Rather than pulling on the catheter, one can let the tissue extrude it by granulation (like a small foreign body). With this method, cut the suture and simply place a small piece of tape to secure the tube. Over several days the catheter will be pushed out by granulation tissue. Be sure to inform patients of what to expect so they will not try to reinsert the catheter.

Fistulae

Gastrointestinal fistulae commonly occur with intraabdominal abscesses; some probably are causative in nature, and some are sequelae. Management depends on the amount of flow, whether it is of low or high output.[152,163,200] Low-output fistulae (320 cc per day) will usually close spontaneously without additional therapy. High-output fistulae require treatment. High suction on the catheter should be maintained, and the bowel should be put at rest. This usually means insertion of a nasogastric tube. Hyperalimentation may also be needed for several weeks in some severe cases. Failure of these methods indicates a need for surgery.

Errors in abscess drainage

Errors associated with abscess drainages have been documented by numerous authors.[78,80,95,96,160] Perhaps the most common error made is the improper choice of trajectory, which can cause either a portion of the pleura to be crossed when draining a subphrenic abscess or a solid organ to be traversed. Although with today's potent antibiotics dissemination of an infection is infrequent, it can occur and produce significant difficulty.

Other errors include selecting inappropriate cases—attempting to drain either an inflamed area that is not liquefied, an infected tumor, a fungal infection, or an infected hematoma. Infected hematomas cannot be drained using routine methods; urokinase or a catheter irrigant must be used.

Several other common errors occur late in management. Inadvertent or early removal of the catheter will result in recurrence of the abscess. Failure to either identify or correct the cause will result in a recurrence such as fistula or ulcer. If a final CT scan is not obtained, a recurrent or undrained abscess can be present.

Success rates

Since the introduction and development of percutaneous abscess drainages there has been controversy among the various groups about the achievable success rate. The overall success rates have varied between 62% and 90%. The differences in success rates undoubtedly depend on numerous factors, including selection criteria, drainage techniques and catheters, and final criteria for outcome determination (i.e., definition of cure, palliation, etc).

A number of recent authors have studied the factors that affect the outcome of the drainage procedures. Several major determinants have been found, including the status of the immune system, the overall severity of the patient's illness, and the accuracy of abscess localization.

Lambiase[163] recently reported a large series of patients treated with PAD and noted a significant difference in the outcomes of his patients (see earlier section on immune system). He found that those patients who were immunocompetent had a successful outcome in 72.6%, compared with those immunocompetent patients with a success rate of 53.4%.

Levison et al[170] correlated the Apache II score with drainage techniques and outcomes. He found that those patients with scores less than 15 had a mortality rate of 1.7% and those with scores greater than 15 had a mortality rate of 78%. There was no benefit of one method—surgical or percutaneous drainage—over the other.

Deveney et al[47] studied the outcome of abscess drainage in two time periods, the first in the 1970s and the second in the 1980s. The difference in mortality in the two time periods was 39% compared with 21%, respectively. There was no difference in outcome between patients treated with surgical or those treated with percutaneous methods. The authors concluded that the improvement in localization had a major impact on the treatment of abscesses.

There are a number of reasons for the failures reported. These include premature withdrawal of the catheter, presence of a gastrointestinal fistula, pleural contamination, hemorrhage, and the errors of selecting cases as noted above.

Laing et al[160] reported a series of 136 patients with a failure of 29 of 119 attempted curative procedures. With infected pancreatic processes the authors were successful in 11 of 22 cases. In their series they had 17 patients with identified gastrointestinal fistula; 9 resolved spontaneously, and 8 required surgical management. Failure to document the complete obliteration of abscesses by CT resulted in failure in 7 cases. The authors had two cases of hemorrhage associated with inappropriate placement of catheters in phlegmonous areas. The most common misdiagnosis was failure to identify loculated or residual cavities. Premature withdrawal was made in a number of cases because of the cessation of drainage fluid. The authors recommended that a repeat CT scan be performed before the removal of the catheter.

Complications

The incidence of complications varies widely, depending on technique, types of abscess being drained, and the various authors' experience. The reported rates vary between 5% and 9.8%. In regard to possible abscess locations, the complication rate varies between 1.4% and 30%. The lowest complication rate is associated with the liver and the highest with the spleen (see later section on specific location).

The most common complication in all series is that of sepsis immediately after the catheter insertion. According to our review of the literature, this occurred in about 6% of all cases; as seen in the recent review article by Lambiase,[164] it occurred in about 4.2% of cases.

Other less frequent complications included spontaneous hemorrhage, spillage of infected material, and fistula formation.

Specific anatomic areas

The various anatomic areas involved by abscesses have unique characteristics as discussed in the earlier chapter on the peritoneum. Information unique to the technical approach and outcomes in each area will be discussed in the following sections.

Subphrenic abscesses. With a subphrenic abscess, one must always look at the contiguous anatomic areas to see if there are any extensions of the abscess into these areas. Contiguous spaces that may require drainage include the right subhepatic and right pericolonic space with right subphrenic abscesses. With left subphrenic abscesses, extension into the right subphrenic, left subhepatic, and the left pericolonic space may also occur. Traditionally, such extension is not expected, but because of anatomic variability some peritoneal margins do not serve as effective barriers to the spread of infection.

When performing drainage procedures of the subphrenic spaces, several anatomic points should be kept in mind. To best avoid the pleural space, remember the attachment of the diaphragm. The slips of the diaphragm attach more cephalad anteriorly and more caudad posteriorly. Because of these relationships the entrance point for a drainage should not be more posterior than the midaxillary line (Fig. 46-116). The trajectory for such procedures should be from a caudad to cephalad angle. The target for entrance of the needle should be the lowest portion of the abscess. This permits positioning of the catheter throughout the enteric length and keeps the trajectory as far away from the diaphragm as possible, ensuring avoidance of the pleural space.

Obviously, when performing such a procedure, always visualize and avoid the pleural space, gallbladder, and hepatic flexure of colon when planning the trajectory. If there is any problem with localizing a subphrenic abscess or separating hepatic flexure of colon from the liver, place the patient in the left decubitus position (see Chapter 29).

The rate of cure for subphrenic collections varies between 79% and 81%. Complications include empyema and sepsis; the incidence of which is 2%.[80,102,164,203]

Right subhepatic abscess. An abscess in the right subhepatic space can be easily approached either laterally or posterolaterally. Penetration of any adjacent structure such as the colon, gallbladder, or duodenum can be easily avoided. In some cases a left decubitus position can also be helpful in moving the hepatic flexure of the colon to simplify a puncture (Fig. 46-117).

Left subhepatic abscess. This abscess, located in the anterior subphrenic space below the left lobe of the liver, appears between the liver and the stomach on axial CT scan. The administration of oral contrast is important for confirmation of the stomach location. The optimal approach for this area is a directly anterior approach that avoids liver and stomach.

Omental bursa. Drainage of the omental bursa can be approached from several directions. Fluid collections in the inferior recess of the lesser sac can be approached anteriorly beneath the lower margin of the stomach if a fluid collection is large enough. If the fluid collection is in the splenic portion of the inferior recess, the best approach is through the gastrosplenic ligament. This approach is best accomplished when the patient is in a right decubitus position to permit the stomach to shift anteriorly. Obviously, in such cases one must be careful to avoid the splenic flexure of the colon, looking carefully for varices in the gastrosplenic ligament to avoid penetration of any such vessels (Fig. 46-118, *A* and *B*).

If the approach through the gastrosplenic ligament is not available, two other approaches are possible. For a second choice I would use a transgastric approach, ideally through a PEG as described earlier for pseudocysts. Another approach is a transhepatic approach through the left lobe of the liver (other authors recommend this as a primary approach).[201] I dislike this approach because of possible injury or pyogenic dissemination into the left biliary or portal system.

Pericolonic spaces. These spaces are easily approached laterally. One should always look for extension of an abscess into the pelvis or either subphrenic space. Contrary to traditional teaching, an abscess in the left pericolonic space may extend into the left subphrenic space unimpeded by the phrenicolic ligament.

When draining an abscess in these spaces, always make sure the catheter traverses the entire length of the cavity. To do this it is always best to enter either the upper or lower end of the cavity. Another option is to insert two catheters at the mid portion of the cavity, with one extending cephalad and one extending caudad.

Liver abscesses. Abscesses in the liver should be approached by the shortest trajectory available, with an entrance point on the anterior or lateral surface. When a lateral entrance site is used, do not go more posterior than the midaxillary line, to avoid traversing the pleura.

When puncturing and draining hepatic abscess, avoid any visible hepatic vessel as well as the gallbladder and pleura. Also, when planning the trajectory for he-

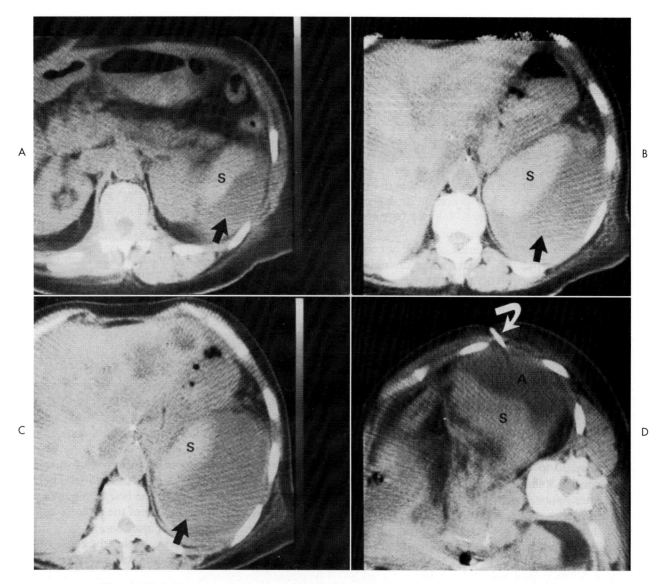

Fig. 46-116. For comparison this series of scans shows the proper approach for a left sub-phrenic abscess. The entire cephalad-caudad extent of the abscess arrows, is seen in **A** to **C,** which is adjacent to the spleen, *s.* **D,** Putting the patient in the opposite decubitus position exaggerates the pleural space so that the lowest edge of the pleura can be avoided. The needle is inserted at the midaxillary line *(arrow)* at the lowest level of the abscess, *A,* and directed cephalad in the intercostal space.

patic abscesses, always include a "cuff" of normal tissue to prevent inadvertent spillage of material into the peritoneum.

Many hepatic abscesses may appear to be multiseptated,[49,50,141] but experience has shown that many will clear completely with one drainage tube. A variety of explanations have been proposed, including (1) they intercommunicate, (2) they drain spontaneously into the drained cavity, and (3) antibiotics clear the different cavities. A repeat scan is important to ensure that all such cavities eventually clear because separate cavities that persist occasionally require drainage.

The success rate for hepatic abscesses varies between 69% and 89%.[125,141] The complication rate varies between 1.7% and 7.3%. The complications include sepsis, contamination of peritoneum, and production of an empyema.

Renal abscess. Such abscesses are best approached posteriorly through a path avoiding erector spinal muscles, colon, liver, and spleen. The puncture and

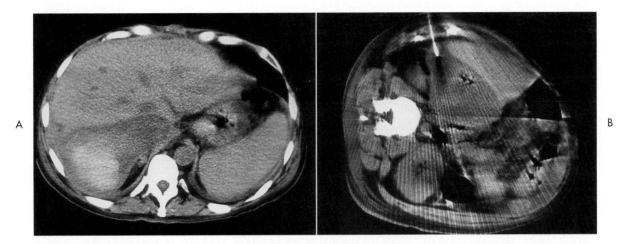

Fig. 46-117. A, CT scan of patient in the supine position shows a high-density fluid collection in the right subhepatic space. **B,** When the patient is positioned on the left side, the fluid remains in the same location and does not shift. Note the drainage needle in the right flank.

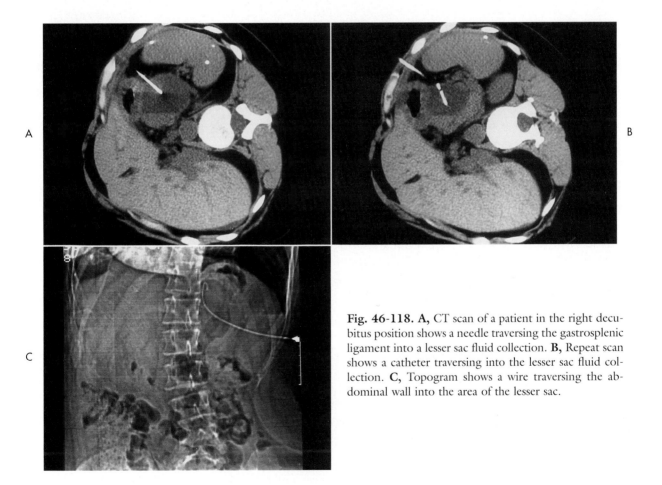

Fig. 46-118. A, CT scan of a patient in the right decubitus position shows a needle traversing the gastrosplenic ligament into a lesser sac fluid collection. **B,** Repeat scan shows a catheter traversing into the lesser sac fluid collection. **C,** Topogram shows a wire traversing the abdominal wall into the area of the lesser sac.

drainage of most such abscesses can be performed with ultrasound or CT guidance. When the upper pole is involved, CT is indicated to avoid inadvertent trauma to the spleen, splenic pedicle, or pancreas. Success rate varies (Fig. 46-119).

Perirenal and pararenal spaces. The anterior and posterior pararenal spaces are frequent sites of abscess and can be approached safely; however, certain facts must be remembered. These spaces extend from the pelvis to the diaphragm and are long. Unless a catheter or catheters are positioned throughout the entire length of the cavity, drainage may not be successful (Fig. 46-120). It is especially important to use CT for follow-up of such cases because the abscesses may spread toward the dia-phragm or pelvis. Examination of these areas may be difficult with ultrasound.

The success rate for these abscesses varies between 68% and 81%. The complication rate varies between 3% and 6%, with sepsis and hemorrhage being the most common.[162,164]

Pelvic abscesses. The procedure for drainage of pelvic abscesses is quite similar to that of other areas. The most significant controversy involves the choice of drainage pathways. It is our opinion that the best pathways are an anterior, lateral, or transrectal one (Fig. 46-121).

When such abscess cavities are close to the rectum, a transrectal approach is indicated[72] (Figs. 46-123, 46-124). To perform this procedure, a series of baseline

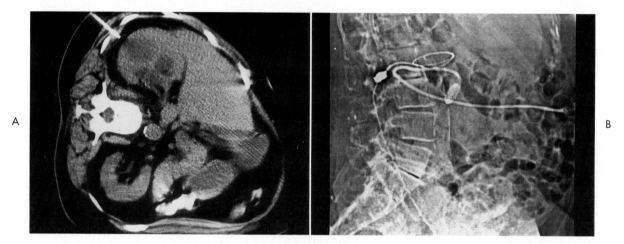

Fig. 46-119. A, CT scan of patient with intrarenal abscess and hydronephrosis. With patient in left decubitus position, the needle was directed into the renal abscess. **B,** Topogram shows the nephrostomy tube within the right kidney as well as the angiographic wire within the abscess cavity.

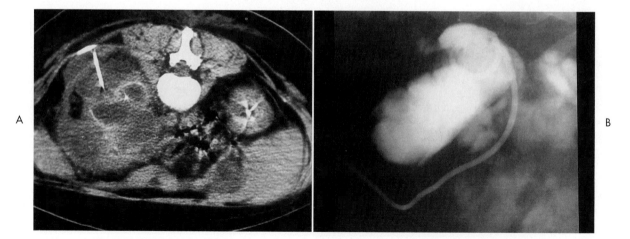

Fig. 46-120. A, CT scan shows a large abscess around the left kidney and a severe pyohydro-nephrosis. The needle trajectory was planned to cross both abscess collections. **B,** Catheter injection shows opacification of the collecting system and some extravasation of contrast material into the perinephric space.

scans are taken over the pelvis to demonstrate the collection. A short plastic tube, with betadyne ointment is then inserted into the rectum. A plastic sheath needle is inserted into the tube and a series of repeat scans are taken over the pelvis. Once the needle is aligned properly, the puncture into the fluid collection is made. The needle is removed, but the plastic tube is left in place to serve as a conduit for catheter insertion. The tube prevents buckling of the wire or catheter in the rectum during the insertion.

The last choice for draining pelvic abscesses is through the sciatic notch (Fig. 46-122). This pathway is satisfactory for biopsy procedures, but long-term drainage catheters are not recommended, for two reasons. The use of this pathway can produce a lot of pain, and

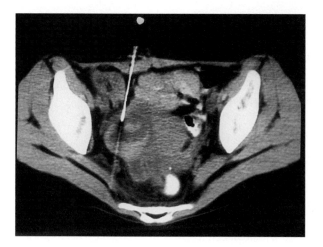

Fig. 46-121. CT scan of the pelvis shows needle aspiration of a fluid collection in the right side of the pelvis. By careful planning, penetration of the small bowel was avoided.

there have been reports of abscess tracking into the gluteal muscles, of sciatic neuritis, and of pseudoaneurysm formation in the iliac vessels.

Controversial areas

As seen in the extensive literature now available on percutaneous drainages, there are several areas of controversy related to catheters, sinograms, antibiotics, mucolytic agents, and palliative procedures.

Catheters. Some authors use angiographic catheters, whereas others use large catheters and trocars. In most areas either type of catheter works well, except in the case of certain pancreatic abscesses (see later section). In pertinent drainage literature, a report by Park et al[225] showed there was little difference in drainage success rates regardless of whether small or large catheters were used. This is probably the result of selection of catheters by operators (i.e., small catheters for thin material and large catheters for thick material). Controversy exists whether gravity (siphon) drainage, sump drainage, or irrigation drainage (multiple catheters) is the most effective. There is no clear advantage to any of these methods appearing in surgical and radiologic literature, so any individual preference can be followed.

Sinograms. Some authors[102,160,164] have performed sinograms to follow abscess cavities, while others[80] have not. We use sinograms in many cases to follow the progress of granulation tissue that closes the cavity. It is important to remember that sinograms are not intended to see "undrained" areas. By definition, if these areas are not drained and do not communicate, one will not see them. Sinograms are used to see the size of the cavity as it heals from granulation or to detect fistulae. CT scanning is used to see undrained areas. With this in

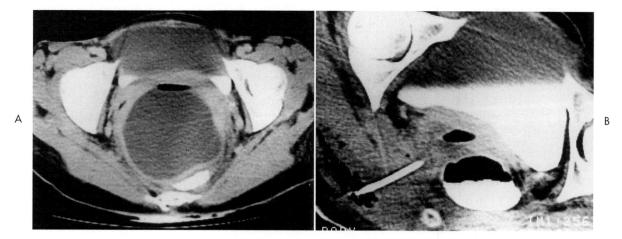

Fig. 46-122. A, CT scan of the pelvis shows a large abscess posterior to the bladder and anterior to the rectum. **B,** Follow-up scan shows catheter drainage through the sciatic notch. Note that the cavity is much smaller but there is also an abscess that has tracked posteriorly into the gluteal muscle.

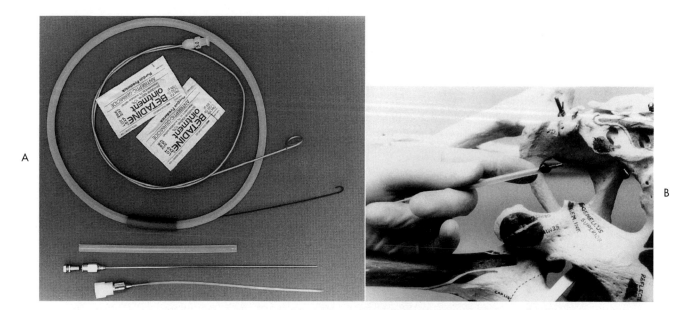

Fig. 46-123. A, The various devices used for a transrectal approach includes the plastic sheath needle, plastic annula, angiographic wire, and catheter. **B,** Simulated procedure using the bony pelvis of a skeleton and the equipment as noted in Fig. 46-123, *A*. This shows the plastic sheath along the side of the finger. The needle is within the sheath (protecting both the rectum and the operator's finger), and there is betadyne ointment occluding the end of the plastic sheath.

mind, one must not overinject cavities during sinograms to maximum distention, because this can cause spillage or bacteria into anatomic spaces or into blood or other portions of the organ.

Antibiotics. It is my belief that all patients who have a percutaneous procedure should have systemic antibiotics before[69] to and during the course of abscess drainage.

With antibiotics, patients have quicker resolution of the abscess and will have fewer local complications. I have noted that some patients not receiving antibiotics may develop a localized cellulitis around the site of catheter insertion; administration of antibiotics will resolve or prevent this. If antibiotics are not given, septicemia is more likely to occur after or during instrument manipulation.

In our opinion the only valid controversy is whether the antibiotics should be started before or after the diagnostic aspiration. Starting antibiotics when a patient initially develops septic symptoms can be justified to prevent further deterioration. On the other hand, it can be argued that unless the patient is not receiving antibiotics a valid culture cannot be obtained. It appears that either philosophy is sound; I usually accept the preference expressed by my clinical colleagues attending the patient.

Mucolytic agents. There have been several suggestions in the literature about using materials to try to enhance drainage from abscesses. One author[270] has proposed the use of Mucomist to decrease the viscosity of purulent material; most workers do not accept this material as being effective.

Fibrinolytic agents. Since the last publication of this book, considerable work has been performed evaluating the usefulness of urokinase for facilitating the drainage of purulent material.[159,167,225] In a recent article by our group, Park et al[225] showed that in vitro urokinase decreased the viscosity of purulent material by 23%. Increased flow through various catheters was observed, and this was most significant with small-caliber catheters.

In another report by our group, Lahorra et al[159] showed the safety of administering urokinase through drainage catheters into abscess cavities. In this study all abscesses with loculations were successfully drained, as well as three infected hematomas, one fungal abscess, and one recurrent abscess. Based on this initial experience, we now routinely use urokinase in any abscess that contains thick material or infected hematoma (Fig. 46-125). We are currently evaluating this material in a prospective randomized study to determine its efficacy. Currently the doses we are using depend on the size of the abscess (see earlier section on tube management).

Palliative procedures. A number of authors have advocated palliative drainage procedures in different areas. PAD in each of these areas has been tried with vary-

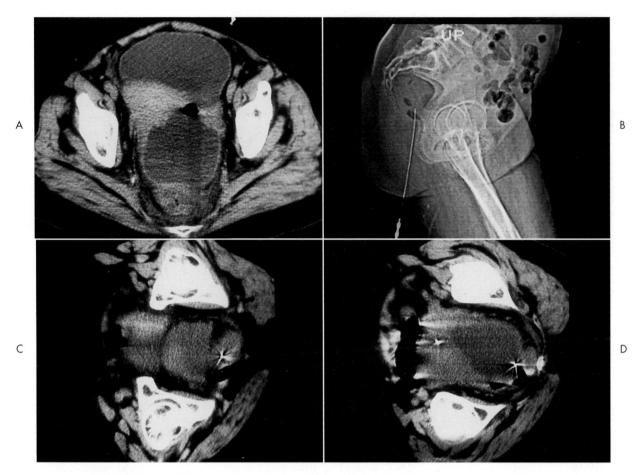

Fig. 46-124. A, CT scan shows a large abscess between the uterus and rectum, which was drained by a transrectal drainage. **B,** Topogram shows a needle being inserted by means of the rectum, through the plastic tube as noted in Fig. 46-123. **C,** CT scan over the lower pelvis shows the needle in the rectum. Compared with the first image in **A,** the needle was correctly angled to enter the cavity. **D,** Lowest CT scan over the pelvis shows the needle entering the abscess cavity. With the use of the topogram, the angiographic wire and catheter were inserted.

ing success (each area will be described in the following sections).

Drainage of splenic abscesses. Percutaneous drainage of splenic abscess is a questionable procedure because of surgical experience and the reported data in the literature. The spleen is a very large vascular organ, and any manipulation presents a potential risk. Even with the current surgical trends favoring preservation of the spleen in traumatic injury, most surgeons will perform a splenectomy rather than attempt a catheter drainage. In the accumulated literature about percutaneous abscess drainage of the spleen, a very high failure rate, as well as a high complication and mortality rate, is reported. I believe that surgery is the most acceptable treatment for a splenic abscess, except in very extraordinary cases (Fig. 46-125).

Drainage of pancreatic abscesses. Drainage of pan-

creatic abscess by PAD is a complex issue that has not yet been resolved, but certain specific comments can be made. The issue is complex because there is a discrepancy in the literature about the objective results, recommendations, and the experience of various authors.

The overall success rate is 57%, with a fairly high complication rate. Complications have been both short-term and long-term. Short-term complications have been related to hemorrhage, either for pseudoaneurysms or for inappropriately attempted drainage of poorly defined phlegmons. Initial attempts to drain pancreatic abscesses were somewhat nonselective, and the methods were not clearly defined. Recent personal communications have reported that better selection criteria and more clearly defined methods are being used.

Most workers differentiate between necrotic, ill-defined pancreatitis with superimposed infection versus

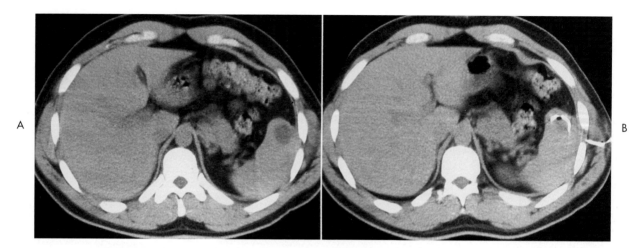

Fig. 46-125. A, Small splenic abscess in the anterior spleen caused by Salmonella. This abscess, despite having been previously aspirated, drained by catheter, and treated with antibiotics, continued to recur. **B,** Catheter drainage of the abscess was performed because it had been done before without difficulty and because the patient refused surgery. Redrainage with urokinase as an irrigant produced total resolution.

well-delineated, low-density fluid collections, which more closely resemble infected pseudocysts (Fig. 46-126).

The later types of infections, the well-defined fluid density collections, are those that are best suited for percutaneous drainage. The standard methods using the Seldinger technique or the trocar methods provide good results. Freeny[66,67] reported a high success rate with such methods. In his group of 21 patients, the success rate was 85%. Von Sonnenberg[264-269] also claims a high success rate of 69%. They encountered 13 fistulae, 10 of which closed spontaneously. Most recently, Lambiase[163,164,165] reported successful drainage of 2 of 2 infected pseudocysts as compared with one of seven cures in a group of patients with abscesses exclusive of pseudocysts.

The only worker attempting drainage of necrotic pancreatitis is Dr. Eric Martin.[180] Employing what I would call extraordinary methods, he uses 20F to 30F catheters, which are capable of draining large amounts of necrotic tissue. With these methods, he has success, complication, and mortality rates comparable to surgical results.

In his group of 20 cases Dr. Martin had a cure rate of 65%, a mortality rate of 25%, and fistulae in 10% of cases. Although these values seem high, one should remember this is treatment of infected necrotic pancreatitis, not well-defined fluid collections.

Regardless of the primary approach taken for drainage of pancreatic abscesses, the successful resolution of the problem depends on diligent, repetitive clinical and imaging evaluation of the patient. Close cooperation between surgeon and radiologist is quite essential because of the recurring and unpredictable nature of the disease. Many times, a radiologic procedure will be needed after an operative drainage or vice versa to produce complete resolution of the problem. As has been indicated by Martin and others,[181] regardless of optimal care a high percentage of such patients will die.

In my experience, the technique and approach used depends on the appearance and location of the pancreatic fluid collections. For well-defined collections, I am quite willing to perform percutaneous drainage because of the high success rate. Those collections representing infected necrotic tissue or poorly defined multiple collections are best drained surgically. If a patient has had a surgical drainage and develops a collection postoperatively, I will attempt percutaneous drainage regardless of the appearance, knowing that the infection is most likely well-confined and that a second surgical procedure would be quite difficult.

I use either an anatomic approach that avoids all adjacent organs or a transgastric approach. If one is attempting to avoid bowel or solid organs, the approach often must be retroperitoneal, anterior to the kidney or directly anterior. I use such a direct anterior approach only if there is a "window" between the various loops of bowel. If there is any problem with access, I choose a trangastric approach using the same method I have described for pseudocyst drainage, with a gastrostomy as a conduit for entry (see earlier section).

Diverticular abscesses. Percutaneous drainage of diverticular abscesses is a technically simple procedure for which the indications are limited.

The indications for this procedure are limited because in most cases of patients with diverticular abscesses,

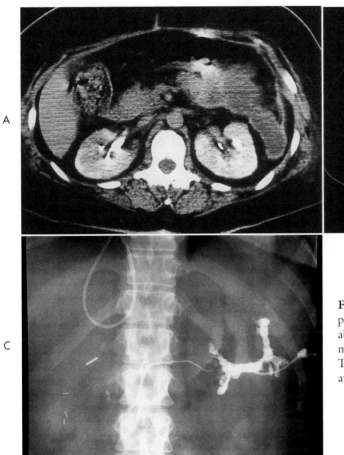

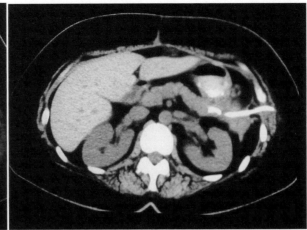

Fig. 46-126. A, Small pancreatic abscess in the tail of the pancreas. **B,** Scan following drainage shows catheter in the abscess, which is totally drained. **C,** Sinogram shows communication of the abscess cavity with the pancreatic duct. There was total resolution of the process and the pancreatic fistula.

a colonic diverticular fistula will result after successful drainage of the abscess. I concur with Mueller et al,[200] who reported that the primary purpose in performing this procedure is to change a potential two-stage procedure into a one-stage procedure. Specifically, most cases of small diverticular abscesses can be treated with a single surgical procedure consisting of an en bloc resection of a segment of the sigmoid colon and a confined abscess. The entire problem is resolved with a single procedure. In those cases in which the abscess is so large that this cannot be accomplished, surgical treatment would require two procedures: one procedure to drain the abscess and divert the bowel and a second to reanastomose the bowel. In such cases percutaneous drainage can remove the infectious material and a single surgical procedure can be performed to remove the offending segment of sigmoid colon (Fig. 46-127).

I try to approach such lesions from an angle not traversing bowel; I believe that including the bowel within the pathway increases the possibility of fistulae (see Fig. 46-120).

Neff reported a series of 16 patients with diverticular abscesses.[209] According to the author, all responded. In this group, 11 patients required sigmoid re-

section after the drainage and 1 patient had a three-stage procedure. There were 10 fistulae resulting; 2 required surgical treatment.

Infected neoplasms. Although experience has shown that percutaneous drainage of infected neoplasms will not be curative,[205,283] there has been some recent interest in using percutaneous drainage as a palliative procedure (see Fig. 46-121). Using the standard technique as described, Zeman[289] has had some positive experience with palliation. In 12 patients with infected tumors those authors had noted improvement in all cases, with favorable response in 50% of cases; no complications occurred.

PERCUTANEOUS NEPHROSTOMY

The same advantages for CT procedures are applicable to nephrostomy placements, but several different points should be emphasized. CT has been successful in a high percentage of cases; in one early report we completed 12 of 13 attempts.[103]

The indication for CT guidance is limited, but I believe that most nephrostomies can be performed easily using either fluoroscopic or ultrasonic guidance. Those cases for which we use CT guidance are renal

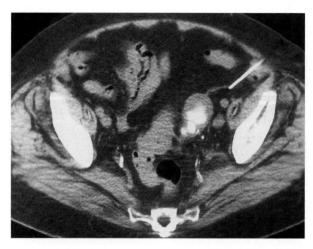

Fig. 46-127. Scan of the pelvis shows a partially contrast-filled diverticular abscess adjacent to the sigmoid. The aspirating needle was directed into the cavity while a loop of sigmoid bowel is avoided.

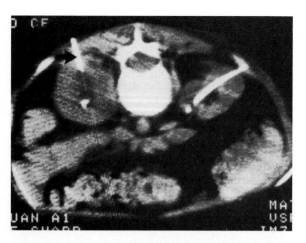

Fig. 46-128. CT-guided procedure of the author's daughter (see Dedication), who had multiple renal calculi. There is one catheter in the right kidney, and this shows puncture of the left kidney with the needle *(arrow)*. Such special cases warrant the best method available.

transplants, unilateral kidney, very high risk patients, or a kidney with a urinoma associated with the hydronephrosis.

Renal transplants are well suited for CT nephrostomies. Transplants represent high-risk patients who are immunosuppressed, and therefore a higher margin of safety is needed. The transplants are somewhat mobile and the axis is unpredictable. CT may be needed to ensure proper placement of the catheter through the parenchyma. Unilateral kidneys should be performed with CT because these cases present high-risk situation. Potential damage or complications in such cases must be minimized.

When a collecting system with hydronephrosis has ruptured and produced an adjacent urinoma, CT is better than other methods for several reasons. First, if the urinoma is displacing the axis of the kidney, the orientation can be appreciated. Second, if there is active excretion of contrast material, the perinephric space may fill with contrast material, making it difficult to visualize the collection system under fluoroscopy. This is not the case with CT.

The technique is similar to that described for abscess punctures. Prepare the skin with the standard antiseptic preparation and administer a local anesthetic. Use an 18-gauge plastic-sheathed needle to puncture the renal pelvis. Insert an angiographic wire, remove the plastic sheath, and follow with the chosen nephrostomy catheter. The longitudinal type of scan or fluoroscopy may be used after the puncture to insert the catheter.

When the nephrostomy is performed under CT, several technical maneuvers are important. Once the collecting system has been penetrated, a small sample of

fluid should be aspirated for culture and then a small amount of contrast material should be immediately injected. This injected contrast material permits direct visualization under fluoroscopy when the catheter is being inserted. In addition, I recommend the 18-gauge Teflon-sheathed needle so that with successful puncture the angiographic wire can be inserted into the collecting system without additional manipulation. The patient can then be transported to the fluoroscopy area without concern about displacement of the sheath or wire. In virtually all cases the final positioning of the catheter should be made under fluoroscopy (Figs. 46-128, 46-129).

NERVE BLOCKS

One of the newest and most exciting areas of interventional radiology is CT-guided nerve blocks. The same types of nerve blocks that were previously performed blindly or by fluoroscopy can be better performed with CT guidance.*

Celiac nerve blocks

It is important to review the rationale behind celiac nerve blocks to gain a better understanding of the process, side effects, and possible complications.

The sensory nerve fibers transmitting pain sensation from the bowel, mesentery, capsule of the liver, and some portions of the retroperitoneum around the major vessels pass through a major neural plexus adjacent to the celiac artery called the *celiac plexus*. This large plexus contains ganglia from the sympathetic, parasympathetic, and sensory nerves. Once the sensory fibers pass through

*References 29, 94, 106, 111, 113, 171, 194, 198.

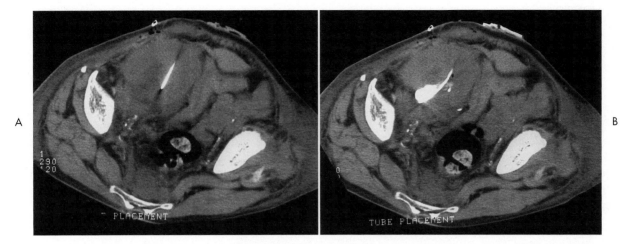

Fig. 46-129. A, CT scan shows percutaneous puncture of dilated collecting system. Needle is entering the inferior portion of the collecting system. **B,** After successful puncture of the collecting system, a small amount of contrast material and angiographic wire was inserted into the collecting system.

this area, they converge to form the right and left splanchnic nerves through the retroperitoneum and the mediastinum toward the central nervous system.

Interruption of these sensory fibers prevents pain stimuli from being carried back to the brain, thereby eliminating pain. Numerous methods have been used to interrupt these pathways, including surgical ablation, unguided percutaneous neurolysis, and guided percutaneous neurolysis.

Before CT guidance, authors had tried fluoroscopic guidance and ultrasonic guidance, but most procedures were performed blind. These guidance methods have various supporters, depending on the experience at various institutions and the expertise of the individuals. These factors are of course quite variable; thus some centers have excellent results and others have poor results with a high incidence of complications.

Unfortunately, because the different nerves cannot be separated from one another, ablation of the sensory fibers in turn produces ablation of both the sympathetic and parasympathetic fibers. This results in the two commonly observed side effects:

1. Short-term orthostatic hypotension produced by splanchnic pooling of blood, caused by interruption of the sympathetic fibers
2. Diarrhea from interruption of the parasympathetic fibers

Different approaches

Two general methods have traditionally been used, a transcrural approach or a retrocrural approach. The retrocrural approach attempts to interrupt the pathway after the splanchnic nerves have formed and as

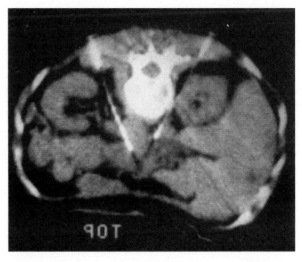

Fig. 46-130. This CT procedure, performed in 1976, shows the placement of two skinny needles for performance of a celiac nerve block (see text).

the nerves course in the posterior mediastinum. The transcrural approach interrupts the pathway at the plexus before formation of the nerves. With our method I approach the plexus directly and use an angled trajectory so that the entire needle pathway is beneath the diaphragm. This lessens possible complications caused by "tracking" of medication into the chest or abdomen.

RECOMMENDED METHOD

As with most CT procedures, my experience is quite extensive and dates back to the first such CT procedure in 1977[111] (Fig. 46-130). Since that time I have evolved the technique to its current state.

The major elements of my technique are the following:

1. Use of a 19-gauge needle with 18-gauge Teflon sheath (Fig. 46-131, *A*).
2. Substitution of air instead of urographic contrast as a marker
3. Using a local anesthesia for a test block
4. Injection of 90% ethyl alcohol on the left side or bilaterally, if needed

The early procedures reported by my group and Buy et al[15] used the 22-gauge skinny needles for the instruments and urographic contrast material mixed with alcohol for a marker. I have discarded the use of the skinny needles because they required too much pressure for injection. Since the pressure for injection is so high, any tissue resistance during injection cannot be manually perceived. According to the anesthesia literature, this ability to feel this pressure is important, because if excessive pressure is required, the needle may be inappropriately within the fascia of a vessel or organ.

In addition, the small-caliber needle that was previously used does not always permit free backflow of blood from a small vessel (as does the larger caliber 18-gauge sheath). Inappropriate injection into an artery can

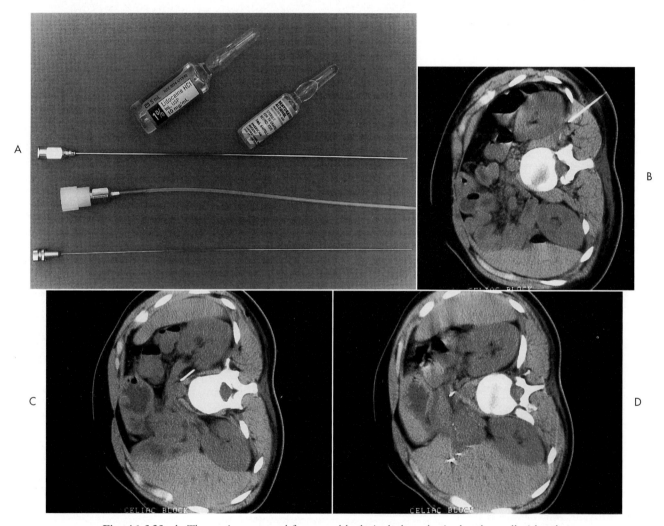

Fig. 46-131. A, The equipment used for nerve blocks include a plastic sheath needle (sheath, needle, and stylet are disassembled), xylocaine anesthesia, and ethanol. **B,** This and the subsequent CT scan shows the appropriate positioning for a celiac nerve block. This scan shows the introduction of the needle into the retroperitoneum on the left. **C,** With cephalad angulation, the needle is passed behind the renal pedicle and then passed beside the aorta. **D,** This scan shows final placement of the needle tip beside the superior mesenteric artery behind the pancreas. One should note that even if inadvertent penetration of the vessels should occur, any adverse developments are unlikely (see text under other methods as proposed by Lieberman).

cause serious side effects, ranging from loss of an organ to paraplegia.

The injection of the local anesthetic is worthwhile for several reasons. First, there can be congenital variation in the location of the plexus. Depending on the relief of the abdominal pain with the local anesthetic, one can confirm that the pain sensed by the patient is carried by fibers through the plexus. If the pain is not relieved, it does not make sense to inject the alcohol, which can have significant complications.

Finally, instead of mixing contrast material with alcohol, we substitute 4 cc of ambient air to serve as a marker for injection. Because air works as well as contrast material, I decided that we should avoid any possible idiosyncratic contrast reactions or volume dilution of the alcohol.

Anatomic approach

I use a posterior angled infracrural translumber approach, which avoids virtually all anatomic structures. I do not penetrate the kidney, bowel, or other organs, because I believe that the terrible complications previously reported by the blind method were the result of inadvertent injection of a neurolytic agent into such structures. I attempt to interrupt the nerve fibers in the plexus itself primarily by placing the needles and the medication anterior to the aorta between the superior mesenteric artery and the celiac artery. On some occasions interruption of the splanchnic nerves in the more peripheral areas must be accepted if the needles and medication are to be safely placed only posterior and lateral to the vessels.

I have not used the anterior approach or transaortic approach proposed by some because of concern about potential damage to the portal vein, hepatic artery, or pancreas.[171,241]

Technique

The technique that we use is essentially a four-step procedure: a diagnostic scan, placement of the needles and sheaths, a temporary "test" block, and a neurolytic alcohol ablation.

Diagnostic scan. During a routine diagnostic scan, I look for any signs of an active process that should not be "blocked." Under this category I have diagnosed and deferred patients with emphemsematous pancreatitis, small-bowel obstruction, or disease so extensive that a block would not be of any benefit. In the last category I exclude patients who have disease so extensive that the tumor is invading the musculoskeletal portions of the retroperitoneum. The pain will be carried by somatic sensory fibers; a celiac block will not significantly ablate the pain in such patients.

Before insertion of the needles, I ask the patient to "grade" their pain on a scale of zero to 10, zero being normal and 10 being unbearable. This scale is used for a reference value after the test block to help decide if the alcohol should be injected. To facilitate this, I ask that the patient not have pain medication the morning of the procedure.

Placement of needles. We position the patient in the left decubitus position (i.e., right side up and the left side down) if a unilateral block is to be used, or prone if a bilateral is used. One can thus easily approach the left side from almost a straight angle and the right side with a more oblique approach (Fig. 46-131).

The trajectory chosen is slightly angled, with the entrance point at the level of the renal vein and the target area just above the superior mesenteric artery, which is easily seen. The needle is angled slightly so that the final placement will be adjacent to the side of the aorta at a level between the celiac and the mesenteric artery. Typically, needles are inserted from the right and left sides. If a placement on the right side is not possible, one properly positioned on the left will suffice. Once correct position of the needle has been achieved, the metal portion is removed and the 18-gauge plastic sheath is left in place.

Test dose. Once successful placement has been made, a test injection is performed. I inject 15 cc of 2% Xylocaine on both the right and left sides and 3 to 4 cc of ambient room air on the right and left sides. I then repeat the CT scan over the area of the needles to assess the distribution of the air in the abdomen; this will accurately slow distribution of material.

I let the medication permeate for 10 minutes and then ask the patient to grade the pain. If there is a remarkable improvement in their grading scale (i.e., a reduction from 8 or 9 to zero or 3) and if the air has not tracked into an inappropriate area, the final block is performed. In some cases when the patient has a tumor and the patient requests it, I will inject the alcohol despite a poor response because this may be the last resort.

Neurolytic alcohol ablation. The alcohol for the final block is not injected if there is no relief of pain or if there is an inappropriate tracking of the air. The tracking of the air is a good indicator of where the alcohol will go. A radiologist who did not follow this guideline produced a very severe case of posterior mediastinitis because the alcohol tracked into the chest; the test study showed air tracking into the mediastinum, but he disregarded it. If the air tracks posteriorly adjacent into the nerve area behind the psoas muscle or the mediastinum area, I do not inject the alcohol on that side because of possible nerve damage. The "marker" of gas is a very worthwhile portion of the examination. Fluoroscopy and ultrasound cannot evaluate this effectively, and catastrophes may result.

Also, if there is a return of blood from the needles, do not inject the alcohol. If a vessel is injected with alcohol, destruction of the end organ will result (e.g., kidney, spinal cord).

At this time the alcohol is injected very slowly into the unilateral or bilateral catheter. We inject two separate 25 cc doses of 95% ethyl alcohol, smaller amounts for small patients and larger amounts for larger ones, on the right and left sides. (Plastic syringes must be used because with glass syringes the evaporation of alcohol is so rapid that the barrels will "lock up".)

Since the previous edition of this book, I have learned a valuable lesson from my anesthesia colleague Dr. Mark Boswell,[23] who has shown me that if one injects the alcohol very slowly, the discomfort is minimal to the patient. In the previous edition we reported rapid injection of alcohol, which produces intense pain that has been described as the sensation of being "kicked" in the abdomen.

In some cases the pain may involve the diaphragm, chest, or back because of referral pathways. The distribution can be anticipated by noting the distribution of the "air marker."

Unilateral celiac block. After one has mastered the standard bilateral celiac block and has developed considerable manual dexterity with the method, one can facilitate the procedure by performing a single-needle celiac block with a unilateral approach.

Except for a slight change in the trajectory and target area, injection methods and all other facets of the procedure remain the same. Specifically the trajectory is changed so the needle tip is finally positioned in the area anterior to the aorta just adjacent to the superior mesenteric and celiac arteries (Fig. 46-131). With this method it is best to approach from the left side because the margins of the aorta are better preserved.

With the needle in this location, the test Xylocaine block is performed and the pain is graded. If the pain relief is satisfactory, the final block with alcohol is performed. With this accurate placement of the needle in the area of the plexus, only 25 cc of 95% alcohol must be injected (the bilateral method uses 25 cc on each side, for a total of 50 cc).

At first glance, this method seems somewhat unsettling to the operator, but several points should be kept in mind. First, the anatomy is clearly defined and the localization of the needle is extremely accurate. Second, even if one happened to accidentally penetrate the aorta it would be of little consequence considering the lack of problems encountered by other workers who actually target the aorta (I would not inject the alcohol if inadvertent penetration of the aorta did occur, for fear that the alcohol might cause unintentional damage to vascular structures).

Occasionally, the anatomy of tumor spread is such that good distribution of medication does not occur. This has been appreciated when the injection of Xylocaine does not provide complete relief. If pictorial assessment does not show good distribution to both sides, a second needle placement on the right side with medication injection may be necessary. (Fig. 46-132).

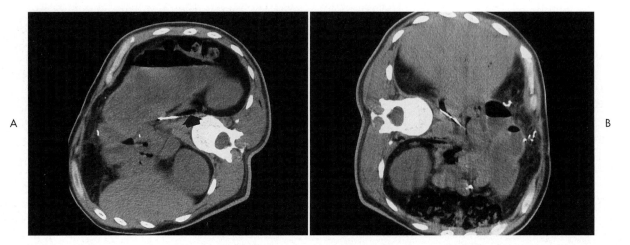

Fig. 46-132. A, This scan with the patient in the right decubitus position shows the needle inserted in the area in front of the superior mesenteric artery. Air, injected because of concerns about distribution of medication, tracked back along the needle *(arrow)*. **B,** Because there was poor distribution of material, a right-sided block was performed. Note the needle traversed between the vena cava and aorta. Note also that the air is tracking in the midline behind the portal vein; better pain control was achieved.

Follow-up

After the procedure the patient is returned to his or her room on a stretcher and kept at bed rest for 8 hours. This time permits resolution of the potential orthostatic hypotension. This routine is important to follow; testing for orthostatic hypotension is inadvisable. One patient in our institution was made unconscious three times by three different resident physicians who wanted to test her orthostatic hypotension by taking her blood pressure in an upright position. She had a very bad headache after these "tests," but did fine after the appropriate bed rest.

Side effects

Two side effects, temporary orthostatic hypotension and bowel irregularity, can occur. Interruption of the sympathetic fibers stops the physiologic vascular tone in the splanchnic vessels, resulting in their dilatation. The dilatation produces pooling of blood; therefore if patients attempt to stand after a completed block, they will lose consciousness. If patients remain at bed rest for 8 to 10 hours, the problem resolves spontaneously. They should be gradually raised to the sitting and upright positions after the period of bed rest.

With interruption of the parasympathetic fibers, motility of the bowel changes so that some patients will have diarrhea and some will inexplicably complain of constipation, which is manageable with over-the-counter stimulants if needed.

Complications

In the past 18 years I have had only two transient complications. One patient had hematuria for 2 days, and one developed a very small subcapsular renal hematoma.

Complications from the blind or other guidance methods are many and severe, including death, paraplegia, loss of kidneys or liver, hemorrhage, and mediastinitis (Figs. 46-133, 46-134).

Other methods

Briefly, there have been two other distinctly different methods reported in the literature, one a transaortic method and the other the anterior approach.

Lieberman and Waldman[171] reported a transaortic approach in which the authors planned a trajectory to traverse the aorta. Once penetration of both walls of the aorta was accomplished, the alcohol was injected.

Two groups have reported on a direct anterior needle approach with penetration of anterior structures such as liver and pancreas. Once the needles are in place, the appropriate medications are injected.

I do not favor either of these approaches because of possible problems associated with "tracking" of the alcohol and potential complications. If additional reports confirm the beneficial results and safety of these reports, one might consider these as alternative methods to the preferred one reported earlier.

Percutaneous cholecystectomy

Percutaneous cholecystectomy is accepted as a viable alternative to surgical cholecystectomy in cases of cholecystitis-producing sepsis. Although it is true that any guidance method may be used for performing the puncture of the gallbladder, all authors agree that puncture of the gallbladder through the hepatic "bare" side

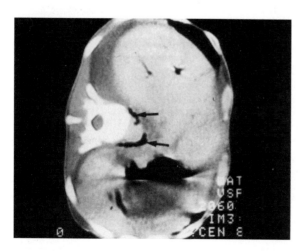

Fig. 46-133. A case from another hospital. CT scan of a patient shows the air "marker" tracking into the chest *(arrows)* behind the crura. Injection should not be made in such cases, or mediastinitis may develop.

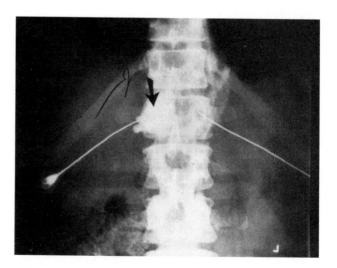

Fig. 46-134. Another outside hospital case. Radiograph of a patient with fluoroscopic localization for a celiac nerve block shows injection of contrast material *(arrow)*. Permanent paraplegia developed after the procedure, despite considerable fluoroscopic experience and meticulous fluoroscopic technique.

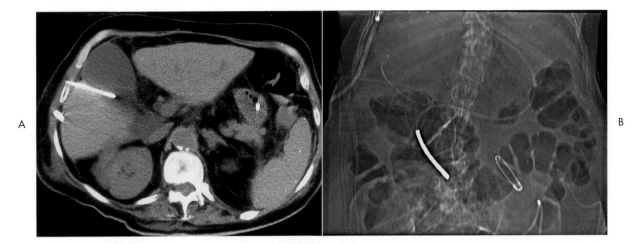

Fig. 46-135. A, Percutaneous cholecystomy was performed through the liver parenchyma. The cuff of normal liver makes fistula formation or leakage less likely. **B,** Topogram showing insertion of the wire into the area of the gallbladder before catheter insertion. The topogram was originally conceived to assist in such procedures and can function well in this capacity.

is important to prevent leakage and proper tract formation.

As one might imagine, CT is superior for such guidance and should be used when a high confidence level is desired. Selection of tubes is dependent on the operator's own bias, but in our hospital we have relied on a small-caliber pigtail to effect emergency drainage. If stone removal or other manipulation is intended, sequential dilatation can be performed as needed (Fig. 46-135).

Percutaneous enteric stoma

A logical extension of the percutaneous puncture and catheter insertions is the development of percutaneous methods for insertion of catheters into bowel loops.

Percutaneous gastrostomies and other enterostomas may be performed by fluoroscopy; they will not be discussed in this chapter. Catheter insertion into the colon, however, is quite different and may require the use of CT for optimal placement of the entrance site.[97] CT is well suited to ensure that the entrance site is on the retroperitoneal side of the colon so that peritoneal spillage will not occur. One author has used this for treatment of Ogilvie's syndrome.[39] I have used it for catheter-instilled antibiotics in a case of toxic megacolon.[97]

REFERENCES

1. Acunas B, et al: Purely cystic hydatid disease of the liver: treatment with percutaneous aspiration and injection of hypertronic saline. *Radiology* 182:541-543, 1992.
2. Adler O: Personal communication, 1987.
3. Alexander JW, Korelitz J, Alexander NS: Prevention of wound infections: a case for closed suction drainage to remove wound fluids deficient in opsonic proteins. *Am J Surg* 132:59-64, 1976.
4. Alexander MC: Unpublished data, 1986.
5. Andersson T, et al: Percutaneous ultrasonography-guided cutting biopsy from liver metastases of endocrine gastrointestinal tumors. *Ann Surg* 206:728-732, 1987.
6. Andriole JG, et al: Biopsy needle characteristics assessed in the laboratory. *Radiology* 148:659-662, 1983.
7. Atterbury CE, et al: Comparison of the histologic and cytologic diagnosis of liver biopsies in hepatic cancer. *Gastroenterology* 76:1352-1357, 1979.
8. Aurell Y, et al: Percutaneous puncture and drainage of pancreatic pseudocysts: a retrospective study. *Acta Radiol* 31:177-180, 1990.
9. Axel L: Simple method for performing oblique CT-guided needle biopsies. *AJR* 143:341, 1984.
10. Ball WS, Bisset GS, Towbin RB: Percutaneous drainage of chest abscess in children. *Radiology* 171:431-434, 1989.
11. Bass J, Di Lorenzo M, Desjardins JG, et al: Blunt percutaneous injuries in children: the role of percutaneous external drainage in the treatment of pancreatic pseudocysts. *J Pediatr Surg* 23:721-724, 1988.
12. Bateson MC, et al: A comparative trial of liver biopsy needles. *J Clin Pathol* 33:131-133, 1980.
13. Becker JA, et al: Needle aspiration and B-mode scanning. *Invest Radiol* 10:173-175, 1975.
14. Berkman WS, et al: Computed tomography guided adrenal biopsy: an alternative to surgery in adrenal mass diagnosis. *Radiology* 153:858, 1984.
15. Bernardino M, et al: Pancreatic transplants: CT-guided biopsy. *Radiology* 177:709-711, 1990.
16. Bernardino ME: Automated biopsy devices: significance and Safety. *Radiology* 176:615-616, 1990.
17. Bernardino ME: Percutaneous biopsy. *AJR* 142:41, 1984.
18. Bernardino ME, Amerson JR: Percutaneous gastrocystostomy: a new approach to pancreatic pseudocyst drainage. *AJR* 143:1096, 1984.
19. Bernardino ME, et al: CT-guided adrenal biopsy: accuracy, safety, and indications. *AJR* 144:67, 1985.
20. Berquist TH, et al: Transthoracic needle biopsy: accuracy and complications in relation to location and type of lesion. *Mayo Clin Proc* 55:475-481, 1980.
21. Bilbao JR, et al: Pancreatic pseudocyst in a gastrectomized pa-

tient: treatment with internalized endoprosthesis. *Gastrointest Radiol* 16:70-72, 1991.

22. Bissonnette RT, et al: Fatal carcinoid crisis after percutaneous fine-needle biopsy of hepatic mestastasis: case report and literature review. *Radiology* 174:751-752, 1990.

23. Boswell M: University Hospitals of Cleveland, Personal Communication.

24. Bourgouin PM, et al: Transthoracic needle aspiration biopsy: evaluation of the blood patch technique. *Radiology* 166:93-95, 1988.

25. Bret PM, et al: Abdominal lesions: prospective study of clinical efficacy of percutaneous fine-needle biopsy. *Radiology* 159:345, 1986.

26. Bret PM, et al: Ultrasonically guided fine-needle biopsy in focal intrahepatic lesions: six years' experience. *J Can Assoc Radiol* 37:5, 1986.

27. Brolin RE, et al: Percutaneous catheter versus open surgical drainage in the treatment of abdominal abscesses. *Am Surg* 50:102-108, 1984.

28. Butch RJ, et al: Presacral masses after abdominal resection for colorectal carcinoma: the need for needle biopsy. *AJR* 144:309-312, 1985.

29. Buy JN, Moss AA, Singler RC: CT guided celiac plexus and splanchnic nerve neurolysis. *J Comput Assist Tomogr* 6:315-319, 1982.

30. Carney CH: Clinical cytology of the liver. *Acta Cytologica* 19(3):244-250, 1975.

31. Casola G, et al: Percutaneous drainage of tubo-ovarian abscesses. *Radiology* 182:399-402, 1992.

32. Chezmar JL, et al: Liver transplant biopsies with a biopsy gun. *Radiology* 179:447-448, 1991.

33. Christopherson P, et al: Preoperative pancreas aspiration biopsies. *Acta Pathol Microbiol Scand* 112:28-33, 1970.

34. Cohan RH, et al: CT assistance for fluoroscopically guided transthoracic needle aspiration biopsy. *J Comput Assist Tomogr* 8:1093, 1984.

35. Conn HO, Yesner R: A re-evaluation of needle biopsy in the diagnosis of metastatic cancer of the liver. *Ann Intern Med* 59:53-61, 1963.

36. Conrad MR, Sanders RC, Mascardo AD: Perinephric abscess aspiration using ultrasound guidance. *AJR* 128:459-464, 1977.

37. Copeland PM: Diagnosis and treatment: the incidentally discovered mass. *Ann Intern Med* 98(6):940-945, 1983.

38. Corr P, Beningfield SJ, Davey N: Transjugular liver biopsy: a review of 200 biopsies. *Clin Radiol* 45:238-239, 1992.

39. Crass JR, et al: Percutaneous decompression of the colon using CT guidance in Ogilvie syndrome. *AJR* 144:475, 1985.

40. Cronan JJ, et al: Cavernous hemangioma of the liver: role of percutaneous biopsy. *Radiology* 166:135-138, 1988.

41. Cwikiel W: Percutaneous drainage of abscess in psoas compartment and epidural spaces: case report and review of the literature. *Acta Radiol* 32:159-161, 1991.

42. Dahlgren SE, Nordenstrom B: *Transthoracic needle biopsy*, Stockholm, 1966, Almquist & Wiksell/Bebers, Forlag AB.

43. Dahlgren SE, Ovenfors CO: Aspiration biopsy diagnosis of neurogenous mediastinal tumours. *Acta Radiol* [Diagn] (Stockh) 10:289-298, 1970.

44. Dahnert WF, et al: Fine-needle aspiration biopsy of abdominal lesions: diagnostic yield for different needle tip configurations. *Radiology* 185:263-268, 1992.

45. DeBlois GG, DeMay KM: Adrenal myelolipoma diagnosis by computed-tomography-guided fine needle aspiration: a case report. *Radiology* 156:569, 1985.

46. DelMaschio A, et al: Pancreatic cancer versus chronic pancreati-

tis: diagnosis with CA 19-9 assessment, US, CT, and CT-guided fine-needle biopsy. *Radiology* 178:95-99, 1991.

47. Deveney CW, Lurie K, Deveney KE: Improved treatment of intra-abdominal abscess: a result of improved localization, drainage, and patient care, not technique. *Arch Surg* 123:1126-1130, 1988.

48. Dickey JE, et al: Evaluation of CT guided percutaneous biopsies of the pancreas. *Surg Gynecol Obstet* 163:497-503, 1986.

49. Dondelinger RF, Kurdziel JC, Gathy C: Percutaneous treatment of pyogenic liver abscess: a critical analysis of results. *Cardiovasc Intervent Radiol* 13:174-182, 1990.

50. Dunnick NR, et al: Percutaneous aspiration of retroperitoneal lymph nodes in ovarian cancer. *AJR* 135:109-113, 1980.

51. Duvnjak M, et al: Assessment of value of pancreatic pseudocyst amylase concentration in the treatment of pancreatic pseudocysts by percutaneous evacuation. *J Clin Ultrasound* 20:183-186, 1992.

52. Elvin A, et al: Biopsy of the pancreas with a biopsy gun. *Radiology* 176(3):677-679, 1990.

53. Evander A: Percutaneous cytodiagnosis of carcinoma of the pancreas and bile duct. *Ann Surg* 188(1):90-92, 1978.

54. Evans WK, et al: Fatal necrotizing pancreatitis following fine-needle aspiration biopsy of the pancreas. *Radiology* 141:61-62, 1981.

55. Elvin A, et al: Biopsy of the pancreas with a biopsy gun. *Radiology* 176:677-679, 1990.

56. Fagelman D, Chess Q: Nonaspiration fine-needle cytology of the liver: a new technique for obtaining diagnostic samples. *AJR* 155:1217-1219, 1990.

57. Fataar S: Percutaneous drainage of pancreatic pseudocysts: technique and problems. *Australas Radiol* 34(4):334-338, 1990.

58. Fataar S, et al: Fine-needle aspiration biopsy of malignant tumours of the abdomen. *S Afr Med J* 62:638-641, 1982.

59. Ferrucci JT, Wittenberg J: CT biopsy of abdominal tumors: aids for lesion localization. *Radiology* 129:739-744, 1978.

60. Ferrucci JT, et al: Malignant seeding of needle tract after thin needle aspiration biopsy: a previously unrecorded complication. *Radiology* 130:345, 1979.

61. Ferrucci JT, et al: Diagnosis of abdominal malignancy by radiologic fine-needle aspiration biopsy. *AJR* 134:323-330, 1980.

62. Filice C, et al: Parasitologic findings in percutaneous drainage of hyman hydatid liver cysts. *J Infect Dis* 161:1290-1295, 1990.

63. Fish GD, et al: Postbiopsy pneumothorax: estimating the risk by chest radiography and pulmonary function tests. *AJR* 150:71-74, 1988.

64. Forsgren L, et al: Aspiration cytology in carcinoma of the pancreas *surgery* 73:38-42, 1973.

65. Frederick PR, et al: Light-guidance system to be used for CT-guided biopsy. *Radiology* 154:535, 1985.

66. Freeny PC, Lewis GP, Marks WM: Percutaneous catheter drainage of infected pancreatic fluid collections and abscesses. RSNA meeting, 1986.

67. Freeny PC, et al: Infected pancreatic fluid collections: percutaneous catheter drainage. *Radiology* 167:435-441, 1988.

68. Fugazzola C, et al: Cystic tumors of the pancreas: evaluation by ultrasonography and computed tomography. *Gastrointest Radiol* 16:53-61, 1991.

69. Gazelle GS, Haaga JR: Guided percutaneous biopsy of intraabdominal lesions. *AJR* 153:929, 1989.

70. Gazelle GS, Haaga JR, Neuhauser D: Hemostatic protein-polymer sheath: new method to enhance hemostasis at percutaneous biopsy. *Radiology* 175:671-674, 1990.

71. Gazelle GS, Haaga JR, Rowland DY: Effect of needle gauge, level

of anticoagulation, and target organ on bleeding associated with aspiration biopsy. *Radiology* 183:509-513, 1992.

72. Gazelle GS, et al: Pelvic abscesses: CT-guided transrectal drainage. *Radiology* 181:49-51, 1991.

73. Gazelle SG, Haaga JR: Biopsy needle characteristics. *Cardiovasc Intervent Radiol* 14:13-16, 1991.

74. Gazelle SG, Haaga JR, Rowland DY: Bleeding due to needle biopsy: effect of venopirin in an animal model and implications for humans. *JVIR* 4:305-310, 1993.

75. Gerzof SG, Spira R, Robbins AH: Percutaneous abscess drainage. *Semin Roentgenol* 16:62-71, 1981.

76. Gerzof SG, et al: Percutaneous drainage of infected pancreatic pseudocysts. *Radiology* 155:275, 1985.

77. Gerzof SG, et al: Percutaneous catheter drainage of abdominal abscesses guided by ultrasound and computed tomography. *AJR* 133:1-8, 1979.

78. Gerzof SG, et al: Percutaneous catheter drainage of abdominal abscesses: a five-year experience. *New Engl J Med* 305:653-657, 1981.

79. Gerzof SG, et al: Percutaneous drainage of infected pancreatic pseudocysts. *Arch Surg* 119:888-893, 1984.

80. Gerzof SG, et al: Expanded criteria for percutaneous abscess drainage. *Arch Surg* 120:227-232, 1985.

81. Gobien RP, et al: Thoracic biopsy: CT guidance of thin-needle aspiration. *AJR* 142:827, 1984.

82. Goldman ML, et al: Preoperative diagnosis of pancreatic carcinoma by percutaneous aspiration biopsy. *Dig Dis Sci* 22(12):1076-1082, 1977.

83. Goldstein HM, et al: Percutaneous fine needle aspiration biopsy of pancreatic and other abdominal masses. *Radiology* 123:319-322, 1977.

84. Goralnik CH, O'Connell DM, El Yousef SJ, Haaga JR: CT-guided cutting-needle biopsies of selected chest lesions. *AJR* 151:903-907, 1988.

85. Gothlin JH: Post-lymphographic percutaneous fine needle biopsy of lymph nodes guided by fluoroscopy. *Radiology* 120:205-207, 1976.

86. Greene R, et al: Supplementary tissue-core histology from fine-needle transthoracic aspiration biopsy. *AJR* 144:787-792, 1985.

87. Gronvall J, Gronvall S, Hegedus V: Ultrasound-guided drainage of fluid-containing masses using angiographic catheterization techniques. *AJR* 129:997-1002, 1977.

88. Grossman E, et al: Liver physiology and disease: cytological examination as an adjunct to liver biopsy in the diagnosis of hepatic metastases. *Gastroenterology* 62:56-60, 1972.

89. Grossman M, et al: Percutaneous treatment (including pseudocystogastrostomy) of 74 pancreatic pseudocysts. *Radiology* 173:493-497, 1989.

90. Gronemeyer DH: *Thorax biopsy,* Intervent Comput Tomog, Oxford, 1990, Blackwell Scientific Publications.

91. Ha HK, Sachs PB, Haaga JR, et al: CT-guided liver biopsy: an update. *Clin Imaging* 15:99-104, 1991.

92. Haaga JR: New techniques for CT-guided biopsies. *AJR* 133:633-641, 1979.

93. Haaga JR, Alfidi RJ: Precise biopsy localization by computed tomography. *Radiology* 118:603-607, 1976.

94. Haaga JR, Alfidi RJ: Interventional CT. In Margulis A, Burhenne S, editors: *Alimentary tract roentgenology,* vol 3, St. Louis, 1979, CV Mosby Co.

95. Haaga JR, Alfidi RJ, Weinstein A: Percutaneous catheter drainage of abdominal abscesses. *New Engl J Med* 306:106-108, 1982 (letter).

96. Haaga JR, Alfidi RJ: Peritoneal abscesses and other disorders. In

97. Haaga JR, Beale S: Use of CO_2 to move structures as an aid to percutaneous procedures. *Radiology* 161(3):j829-830, 1986.

98. Haaga JR, Bick RJ, Zollinger RM, Jr: CT-guided percutaneous catheter cecostomy. *Gastrointest Radiol* 12:166-168, 1987.

99. Haaga JR, LiPuma JP, Eckhauser ML: A piggyback technique for percutaneous insertion of large catheters. *AJR* 136:1245-1246, 1981.

100. Haaga JR, Reich NE: *Computed tomography of abdominal abnormalities,* St. Louis, 1978, CV Mosby Co.

101. Haaga JR, Vanek J: Computed tomographic guided liver biopsy using the Menghini needle. *Radiology* 133:405-408, 1979.

102. Haaga JR, Weinstein AJ: CT-guided percutaneous aspiration and drainage of abscesses. *AJR* 135:1187-1194, 1980.

103. Haaga JR, Zelch MG, Alfidi RJ: CT-guided antegrade pyelography and percutaneous nephrostomy. *AJR* 128:621-624, 1977.

104. Haaga JR, et al: CT guided interstitial therapy of pancreatic carcinomna. *J Comput Assist Tomogr* pp 1077-1078, 1987.

105. Haaga JR, et al: Clinical comparison of small caliber cutting needle with large caliber needles. *Radiology* 146:665-667, 1983.

106. Haaga JR, et al: Improved technique for CT-guided celiac ganglia block. *AJR* 142:1201-1204, 1984.

107. Haaga JR, et al: CT longitudinal scan. *AJR* 127:1059-1060, 1976.

108. Haaga JR, et al: Definitive treatment of a large pyogenic liver abscess with CT guidance. *Cleve Clin Q* 43:85-88, 1976.

109. Haaga JR, et al: CT detection and aspiration of abdominal abscesses. *AJR* 128:465-474, 1977.

110. Haaga JR, et al: CT-guided biopsy. *Cleve Clin Q* 44:27-33, 1977.

111. Haaga JR, et al: Interventional CT scanning. *Radiol Clin North Am* 15:449-456, 1977.

112. Haaga JR, et al: Computed tomography: guided biopsy overview. *J Comput Assist Tomogr* 2:25-30, 1978.

113. Haaga JR, et al: New interventional techniques in the diagnosis and management of inflammatory disease within the abdomen. *Radiol Clin North Am* 17:485-513, 1979.

114. Haaga JR, et al: Percutaneous CT-guided pancreatography and pseudocystography. *AJR* 132:829-830, 1979.

115. Hall-Craggs MA, Leew WRP: Fine-needle aspiration biopsy: pancreatic and biliary tumors. *AJR* 147:399, 1986.

116. Hancke S, Holm HH, Koch F: Ultrasonically-guided percutaneous fine needle biopsy of the pancreas. *Surg Gynecol Obstet* 140:361-364, 1975.

116a. Haramati LB, Austin JH: Complications ater CT guided biopsy through aerated vs. nonaerated lung. *Radiology* 101:778, 1991.

117. Heaston DK, et al: Narrow gauge needle aspiration of solid adrenal masses. *AJR* 141:169, 1983.

118. Heaston DK, et al: Narrow gauge needle aspiration of solid adrenal masses. *AJR* 138:1143-1148, 1982.

119. Heilberg E, Wolverson MK: Ipsilateral decubitus position for percutaneous CT-guided adrenal biopsy. *J Comput Assist Tomogr* 9:217-218, 1985.

120. Herman SJ, Weisbrod GL: Usefulness of the blood patch technique after transthoracic needle aspiration biopsy. *Radiology* 176:395-397, 1990.

121. Hertzanu Y, et al: Massive bleeding after fine needle aspiration of liver angiosarcoma. *Gastrointest Radiol* 15:43-46, 1990.

122. Ho CS, Taylor B: Percutaneous transgastric drainage for pancreatic pseudocyst. *AJR* 143:623, 1984.

123. Ho CS, et al: Percutaneous fine needle aspiration biopsy of the pancreas following endoscopic retrograde cholangiopancreatography. *Radiology* 125:351-353, 1977.

Haaga JR, Alfidi RJ, editors: *Computed tomography of the whole body,* St. Louis, 1983, CV Mosby Co.

124. Ho CS, et al: Guided percutaneous fine-needle aspiration biopsy of the liver. *Cancer* 47:1781-1785, 1981.

125. Hochbergs P, Forsberg L, Hederstrom E, et al: Diagnosis and percutaneous treatment of pyogenic hepatic abscesses. *Acta Radiol* 31:351-353, 1990.

126. Holm HH, Rasmussen SN, Kristensen JR: Ultrasonically guided percutaneous puncture technique. *J Clin Ultrasound* 1:27-31, 1973.

127. Holm HH, et al: Ultrasonically-guided percutaneous puncture. *Radiol Clin North Am* 13:493-503, 1975.

128. Hopper KD, et al: Automated biopsy devices: a blinded evaluation. *Radiology* 187(3):653-660, 1993.

129. Hopper KD, et al: Fine-needle aspiration biopsy for cytopathologic analysis: utility of syringe handles, automated guns, and the nonsuction method. *Radiology* 185:819-824, 1992.

130. Hopper KD, et al: Efficacy of automated biopsy guns versus conventional biopsy needles in the pygmy pig. *Radiology* 176:671-676, 1990.

131. Hueftle MG, Haaga JR: Effect of suction on biopsy sample size. *AJR* 147:1014-1016, 1986.

132. Husband JE, Golding SJ: Role of computed tomography-guided needle biopsy in an oncology service. *Radiology* 150:296, 1984.

133. Isler RJ, et al: Tissue core biopsy of abdominal tumors with a 22 gauge cutting needle. *AJR* 136:725-728, 1981.

134. Isobe H, Fukai T, Iwamoto H, et al: Liver abscess complicating intratumor ethanol injection therapy for HCC. *Am J Gastroenterol* 85:1646-1648, 1990.

135. Jacobsen GK, Gammelgaard J, Fuglo M: Coarse needle biopsy in suspected hepatic malignancy. *Acta Cytologica* 27(2):152-156, 1983.

136. Jaques P, et al: CT features of intraabdominal abscesses: prediction of successful percutaneous drainage. *AJR* 146:1041-1045, 1986.

137. Jeffrey RB: Personal communication.

138. Jeffrey RB, Jr, Wing VW, Laing FC: Real-time sonographic monitoring of percutaneous abscess drainage. *AJR* 144:469-470, 1985.

139. Jereb M, Us-Krasovec M: Transthoracic needle biopsy of mediastinal and hilar lesions. *Cancer* 40:1354-1357, 1977.

140. Johansen S, Myren J: Fine-needle aspiration biopsy smears in the diagnosis of liver diseases. *Scand J Gastroenterol* 6:583-588, 1971.

141. Johnson RD, et al: Percutaneous drainage of pyogenic liver abscesses. *AJR* 144:463-467, 1985.

142. Johnson WC, et al: Treatment of abdominal abscesses: comparative evaluation of operative drainage versus percutaneous catheter drainage guided by computed tomography or ultrasound. *Ann Surg* 194:510-520, 1981.

143. Jones EC, et al: Fine-needle aspiration cytology of neoplastic cysts of the pancreas. *Diagn Cytopathol* 3:238-243, 1987.

144. Juul N, Sztuk FJS, Torp-Pedersen S, et al: Ultrasonically guided percutaneous treatment of liver abscesses. *Acta Radiol* 31:275-277, 1991.

145. Karlson KB, et al: Percutaneous drainage of pancreatic pseudocysts and abscesses. *Radiology* 142:619-624, 1982.

146. Karlsson S, Persons PH: Angiography, ultrasound and fine-needle aspiration biopsy in evaluation of gynecologic tumors, *Radiology* 134:285, 1980 (abstract).

147. Karstaedt N, et al: Computed tomography of the adrenal gland. *Radiology* 129:723-730, 1978.

148. Karstrup S, Nolsoe C, Brabrand K, et al: Ultrasonically guided percutaneous drainage of breast abscesses. *Acta Radiol* 31:157-159, 1990.

149. Kasugai H, et al: Value of heparinized fine-needle aspiration biopsy in liver malignancy. *AJR* 144:243, 1985.

150. Kellermeyer Scott: Cleveland, Ohio, 1993.

151. Ken J, et al: Perforated amebic liver abscesses: successful percutaneous treatment. *Radiology* 170:195-197, 1989.

152. Kerlan RK, Jr, et al: Radiologic management of abdominal abscesses. *AJR* 144:149, 1985.

153. Khouri NF, Stitik FP, Erozan YS: Transthoracic needle aspiration biopsy of benign and malignant lung lesions. *AJR* 144:281-288, 1985.

154. Knelson, Haaga JR, Lazarus H, et al: CT-guided retroperitoneal biopsies. *J Clin Oncol* 7(8):1169-1173, 1989.

155. Koehler PR, Feldberg MAM, van Waes PFGM: Preoperative staging of rectal cancer with computerized tomography, accuracy, efficacy, & effect on patient management. *Cancer* 54:512-516, 1984.

156. Kreula J: Effect of sampling technique on specimen size in fine needle aspiration. *Invest Radiol* 25:1294-1299, 1990.

157. Kreula J: A new method for investigating the sampling technique of fine needle aspiration biopsy. *Invest Radiol* 25:245-249, 1990.

158. Kreula J, Virkkunen P, Bondestam S: Effect of suction on specimen size in fine-needle aspiration biopsy. *Invest Radiol* 25:1175-1181, 1990.

159. Lahorra JM, et al: Safety of intracavitary urokinase with percutaneous abscess drainage. *AJR* 160:171-174, 1993.

160. Laing EK, et al: Abdominal abscess drainage under radiologic guidance: causes of failure. *Radiology* 159:329-336, 1986.

161. Lalli AF, et al: Aspiration biopsies of chest lesions. *Radiology* 127:35-40, 1978.

162. Lang EK: Renal, perirenal, and pararenal abscesses: percutaneous drainage. *Radiology* 174:109-113, 1990.

163. Lambiase RE, Dorfman GS, Cronan JJ: Percutaneous management of abscesses that involve native arteries or synthetic arterial grafts. *Radiology* 173:815-818, 1989.

164. Lambiase RE, et al: Percutaneous drainage of 335 consecutive abscesses: results of primary drainage with 1-year follow up. *Radiology* 184:167-179, 1992.

165. Lambiase RE, et al: Postoperative abscesses and enteric communication: percutaneous treatment. *Radiology* 171:497-500, 1989.

166. Lauby RW, et al: Value and risk of biopsy of pulmonary lesions by needle aspiration: twenty-one years' experience. *J Thorac Cardiovasc Surg* 1:159-172, 1965.

167. Lee KS, et al: Treatment of thoracic multiloculated empyemas with intracavitary urokinase: a prospective study. *Radiology* 179:771-775, 1991.

168. Lee MJ, et al: Measurement of tissue carcinoembryonic antigen levels from fine-needle biopsy specimens: technique and clinical usefulness. *Radiology* 184:717-720, 1992.

169. Levin DP, Bret PM: Percutaneous fine-needle aspiration biopsy of the pancreas resulting in death. *Gastrointest Radiol* 16:67-69, 1991.

170. Levison MA, Ziegler D: Corelation of apache II score, drainage technique and outcome in postoperative intra-abdominal abscess. *Surg Gynecol Obstet* 172:(2)89-94, 1991.

171. Lieberman RP, Waldman SD: Celiac plexus neurolysis with the modified transaortic approach. *Radiology* 175:274-276, 1990.

172. Locke John: Unpublished data.

173. Lufkin R, Layfield L: Coaxial needle system of MR- and CT-guided aspiration cytology. *J Comput Assist Tomogr* 13(6):1105-1107, 1989.

174. Lundquist A: Fine needle aspiration biopsy for cytodiagnosis of malignant tumor in the liver. *Acta Med Scand* 188:465-470, 1970.

175. Lundquist A: Fine needle aspiration biopsy of the liver. *Acta Med Scand* 520:1-28, 1971.

176. Luning M, et al: CT guided percutaneous fine-needle biopsy of the pancreas. *Radiology* 158:567, 1986.

177. Luning M, et al: Percutaneous biopsy of the liver. *Cardiovasc Intervent Radiol* 14:40-42, 1991.

178. Magnusson A, Akerfeldt D: CT-guided core biopsy using a new guidance device. *Acta Radiologica* 32(1):83-85, 1991.

179. Malden ES, Picus D: Hemorrhagic complication of transgluteal pelvic abscess drainage: successful percutaneous treatment. *JVIR* 3:323-328, 1992.

180. Martin E: Personal communication, 1988.

181. Martin HE, et al: The advantages and limitations of aspiration biopsy. *AJR* 35(2):54, 1936.

182. Martino CR, et al: CT-guided liver biopsies: eight years' experience. *Radiology* 152:755, 1984.

183. McCartney R, Tait D, Stilson M, et al: A technique for the prevention of pneumothorax in pulmonary aspiration biopsy. *AJR* 120:872-875, 1974.

184. McCorkell S, Niles NL: Fine-needle aspiration of catecholamine-producing adrenal masses: a possibly fatal mistake. *AJR* 145:113-114, 1985.

185. McGill DB, Rakela J, Zinsmeister AR, et al: *Gastroenterology* 99:1936-1400, 1990 (abstract).

186. McLoughlin MJ, Tao LC, Ho CS: Computed tomography biopsy of abdominal tumors. *Radiology* 131:800, 1979 (letter).

187. McLoughlin MJ, et al: Fine needle aspiration biopsy of malignant lesions in and around the pancreas. *Cancer* 41:2413-2419, 1978.

188. Menghini G: One second biopsy of the liver. *New Engl J Med* 282(1):582-585, 1970.

189. Meyer JE, Ferrucci JT, Janower ML: Fatal complications of percutaneous lung biopsy: review of the literature and report of a case. *Radiology* 96:47-48, 1970.

190. Miller KS, et al: Prediction of pneumothorax rate in percutaneous needle aspiration of the lung. *Chest* 93:742-745, 1988.

191. Milner LB, Ryan K, Gullo J: Fatal intrathoracic hemorrhage after percutaneous aspiration lung biopsy. *AJR* 132:280-281, 1979.

192. Mitty HA, Efremidis SC, Yeh HC: Impact of fine-needle biopsy on management of patient with carcinoma of the pancreas. *AJR* 137:1119-1121, 1981.

193. Montali G, et al: Sonographically guided fine-needle aspiration biopsy of adrenal masses. *AJR* 143:1081, 1984.

194. Moore DC, Bush W, Burnett L: Computed axial tomography: the most accurate method of performing alcohol celiac plex block (abstract). Proceedings of the fifth annual meeting of the American Society of Anesthesiologists, San Francisco, March 1980.

195. Moore EH, et al: Effect of patient positioning after needle aspiration lung biopsy. *Radiology* 181:385-387.

196. Morali GA, et al: Successful treatment of pancreatic pseudocyst with a somatostatin analogue and catheter drainage. *Am J Gastroenterol* 86:515-518, 1991.

197. Mostbeck GH, et al: Optimal needle size for renal biopsy: in vitro and in vivo evaluation. *Radiology* 173(3):819-822, 1989.

198. Muchle C, et al: Radiographically guided alcohol block of the celiac ganglion. *Semin Int Radiol* 4(3):195-199, 1987.

199. Mueller PR, et al: Hepatic echinococcal cyst: successful percutaneous drainage. *Radiology* 155:627-628, 1985.

200. Mueller PR, et al: Inadvertent percutaneous catheter gastroenterostomy during abscess drainage: significance and management. *AJR* 145:387-391, 1985.

201. Mueller PR, et al: Lesser sac abscesses and fluid collections: drainage by transhepatic approach. *Radiology* 155:615-618, 1985.

202. Mueller PR, et al: MR-guided aspiration biopsy: needle design and clinical trials. *Radiology* 161:605, 1986.

203. Mueller PR, et al: Percutaneous drainage of subphrenic abscesses: a review of 62 patients. *AJR* 147:1237-1240, 1986.

204. Mueller PR, et al: Severe acute pancreatitis after percutaneous biopsy of the pancreas. *AJR* 151:493-494, 1988.

205. Mueller PR, et al: Infected abdominal tumors: percutaneous catheter drainage. *Radiology* 173:627-629, 1989.

206. Nakaizumi A, et al: Diagnosis of hepatic cavernous hemangioma by fine needle aspiration biopsy under ultrasonic guidance. *Gastrointest Radiol* 15:39-42, 1990.

207. Nakamato D: University Hospitals of Cleveland, personal communication.

208. Neff CC, et al: CT follow-up of empyemas: pleural peels resolve after percutaneous catheter drainage. *Radiology* 176:195-197, 1990.

209. Neff CC, et al: Diverticular abscesses, percutaneous drainage. *Radiology* 163:15, 1987.

210. Nordenstrom B: New instruments for biopsy. *Radiology* 117:474-475, 1975.

211. Nordenstrom B: A new technique for transthoracic biopsy of lung changes. *Br J Radiol* 38:550-553, 1965.

212. Norenberg R, Claxton CP, Takaro T: Percutaneous needle biopsy of the lung: report of two fatal complications. *Chest* 66:216-218, 1974.

213. Nosher JL, Plafker J: Fine needle aspiration of the liver with ultrasound guidance. *Radiology* 136:177-180, 1980.

214. Nunez D, Jr, et al: Transgastric drainage of pancreatic fluid collections. *AJR* 145:815, 1985.

215. Nunez D, Jr, et al: Renal cell carcinoma complicating long-term dialysis: computed tomography-guided aspiration cytology. *CT* 10:61, 1986.

216. Ohto M, et al: Ultrasonically guided percutaneous contrast medium injection and aspiration biopsy using a real-time puncture transducer. *Radiology* 136:171-176, 1980.

217. Onik G, et al: CT body stereotaxis: aid for CT-guided biopsies. *AJR* 146:163, 1986.

218. Onodera H, Oikawa M, Abe M, et al: Cutaneous seeding of hepatocellular carcinomna after fine-needle aspiration biopsy. *J Ultrasound Med* 6:273-275, 1987.

219. Oscarson J, Stormby N, Sundgren R: Selective angiography in fine-needle aspiration cytodiagnosis of gastric and pancreatic tumours. *Acta Radiol* [Diagn] (Stockh) 12:737-749, 1972.

220. Otto RC: Indications for real-time ultrasound-controlled fine-needle punctures under permanent view. *Radiology* 151:275, 1984.

221. Pagani JJ: Biopsy of focal hepatic lesions: comparison of 18 and 22 gauge needles. *Radiology* 147:673-675, 1983.

222. Pagani JJ: Non-small cell lung carcinoma adrenal metastases, computed tomography and percutaneous needle biopsy in their diagnosis. *Cancer* 53:1058-1060, 1984.

223. Pardes JG, et al: Percutaneous needle biopsy of deep pelvic masses: posterior approach. *Cardiovasc Intervent Radiol* 9:65, 1986.

224. Parfrey NA: Improved diagnosis and prognosis of mucomycosis: a clinicopathologic study of 33 cases. *Medicine* 65(3):113-123, 1986.

225. Park JK, Kraus FC, Haaga JR: Fluid flow during percutaneous drainage procedures: an in vitro study of the effects of fluid viscosity, catheter size, and adjunctive urokinase. *AJR* 160:165-169, 1993.

226. Parker JG, et al: Needle liver biopsy in benign and malignant disease: comparison of the Menghini and Vim-Silverman techniques. *Am J Digest Dis* 7(8):687-698, 1962.

227. Peer A, Strauss S: Percutaneous drainage of postappendectomy abscesses complicated by enteric communication. *Cardiovasc Intervent Radiol* 14:106-108, 1991.

228. Pereiras RV, et al: Fluoroscopically guided thin needle aspiration biopsy of the abdomen and retroperitoneum. *AJR* 131:197-202, 1978.

229. Perlmutt LM, Braun SD, Newman GE, et al: Transthoracic needle aspiration: use of a small chest tube to treat pneumothorax. *AJR* 148:849-851, 1987.

230. Perlmutt LM, et al: Timing of chest film follow-up after transthoracic needle aspiration. *AJR* 146:1049-1050, 1986.

231. Perrault J, et al: Liver biopsy: complications in 1,000 in-patients and out-patients. *Gastroenterology* 74:103-106, 1978.

232. Phillips VM, et al: Percutaneous biopsy of pancreatic masses. *Gastroenterology* 7(6):506-510, 1985.

233. Plunkett MB, et al.: Peripheral pulmonary nodules: preoperative percutaneous needle localizations with CT guidance. *Radiology* 274-276, 1992.

234. Pogany AC, et al: Cystic insulinoma. *AJR* 142:951-952, 1984.

235. Prando AC, et al: Lymphangiography in staging of carcinoma of the prostate: potential value of percutaneous lymph node biopsy. *Radiology* 131:641-656, 1979.

236. Price RB, et al: Biopsy of the right adrenal gland by the transhepatic approach. *Radiology* 148:566, 1983.

237. Rashleigh-Belcher HJC, Russell RCG, Lees WR: Cutaneous seeding of pancreatic carcinoma of fine-needle aspiration biopsy. *Br J Radiol* 59:182-183, 1986.

238. Rasmussen SN, et al: Ultrasonically-guided liver biopsy. *Br Med J* 2:500-502, 1972.

239. Rescorla FJ, et al: Failure of percutaneous drainage in children with traumatic pancreatic pseudocysts. *J Pediatr Surg* 25(10):1038-1042, 1990.

240. Reuvers CB, et al: Ultrasound-guided percutaneous drainage of 25 abscesses. *Acta Chir Scand* 149:161-164, 1983.

241. Romanelli DF, Beckmann CF, Heiss FW: Celiac plexus block: efficacy and safety of the anterior approach. *AJR* 160(3):497-500, 1993.

242. Rosenberger A, Adler O: Fine needle aspiration biopsy in the diagnosis of mediastinal lesions. *AJR* 131:239-242, 1978.

243. Sargent EN, et al: Percutaneous pulmonary needle biopsy: report of 350 patients. *J Thorac Cardiovasc Surg* 122(4):758-768, 1974.

244. Sateriale M, Cronan JJ, Savadier LD: A five year experience with 307 CT-guided renal biopsies: results and complications. *JVIR* 2:401-407, 1991.

245. Sherlock P, Kim YS, Koss LG: Cytologic diagnosis of cancer from aspirated material obtained at liver biopsy. *Am J Dig Dis* 12(4):396-402, 1967.

246. Sinner WN: Transthoracic needle biopsy of small peripheral malignant lung lesions. *Invest Radiol* 8:305-314, 1973.

247. Smith EH: Fine-needle aspiration biopsy: are there any risks? In Holm HH, Kristensen JK, editors: *Interventional ultrasound,* New York, 1985, Thieme, Inc.

248. Smith EH, Bartrum, RJ: Ultrasonically guided percutaneous aspiration of abscesses. *AJR* 122:308-312, 1974.

249. Smith EH: Complications of percutaneous abdominal fine-needle biopsy. *Radiology* 178:253-258, 1986.

250. Soderstrom N: *Fine needle aspiration biopsy,* New York, 1966, Grune & Stratton.

251. Solbiati L, et al: Fine-needle biopsy of hepatic hemangioma with sonographic guidance. *AJR* 144:471, 1985.

252. Spamer C, et al: Benign circumscribed lesions of the liver diagnosed by ultrasonically guided fine-needle biopsy. *JCUI* 14:83, 1986.

253. Staab EV, Jacques PF, Partain CL: Percutaneous biopsy in the management of solid intraabdominal masses of unknown etiology. *Radiol Clin North Am* 17:435-459, 1979.

254. Stephens D: Personal communication, November 1982.

255. Stephenson TF, et al: Evaluation of contrast markers for CT aspiration biopsy. *AJR* 133:1097, 1979.

256. Taavitsainen M, et al: Fine-needle aspiration biopsy of liver hemangioma. *Acta Radiol* 31:69-71, 1990.

257. Taft PD, Szyfelbein WM, Greene R: A study of variability in cytologic diagnoses based on pulmonary aspiration specimens. *Am J Clin Pathol* 73:36-40, 1980.

258. Tanaka S, et al: Early diagnosis of hepatocellular carcinoma: usefulness of ultrasonically guided fine-needle aspiration biopsy. *JCU* 14:11, 1986.

259. Terry R: Risks of needle biopsy of liver. *Br Med J* pp 1102-1103, 1951.

260. Thornbury JR, Burke DP, Naylor B: Transthoracic needle aspiration biopsy: accuracy of cytologic typing of malignant neoplasms. *AJR* 136:719-724, 1981.

261. Tolly TL, Feldmeier JE, Czarnecki D: Air embolism complicating percutaneous lung biopsy. *AJR* 150:555-556, 1988.

262. Tylen U, et al: A percutaneous biopsy of carcinoma of the pancreas guided by angiography. *Surg Gynecol Obstet* 142:737-739, 1976.

263. Tyrrel RT, Murphy FB, Bernardino ME: Tubo-ovarian abscesses: CT-guided percutaneous drainage. *Radiology* 175:87-89, 1990.

264. Van Sonnenberg E, et al: Percutaneous drainage of abscesses and fluid collection: technique, results and applications. *Radiology* 142:1-10, 1982.

265. Van Sonnenberg E, et al: Temporizing effect of percutaneous drainage of complicated abscesses in critically ill patients. *AJR* 142:821-826, 1984.

266. Van Sonnenberg E, et al: Complicated pancreatic inflammatory disease: diagnostic and therapeutic role of interventional radiology. *Radiology* 155:335, 1985.

267. Van Sonnenberg E, et al: Percutaneous drainage of infected and noninfected pancreatic pseudocysts: experience in 101 cases. *Radiology* 170:757-761, 1989.

268. Van Sonnenberg E, et al: Percutaneous abscess drainage: current concepts. *Radiology* 181:617-626, 1991.

269. Van Sonnenberg E, et al: Percutaneous abscess drainage: editorial comments. *Radiology* 184:27-29, 1992.

270. Van Waes PF, et al: Management of abscesses that are difficult to drain: a new approach. *Radiology* 147:57-63, 1983.

271. Vellet D, et al: Fine needle aspiration cytology of mucinous cystadenocarcinoma of the pancreas: further observations. *Acta Cytologica* 32(1):43-48, 1988.

272. von Schreeb T, et al: Renal adenocarcinoma: is there a risk of spreading tumor cells in diagnostic puncture? *Scand J Urol Nephrol* 1:270, 1967.

273. Weisbrod GL, Lyons DJ, Tao LC, et al: Percutaneous fine-needle aspiration biopsy of mediastinal lesions. *AJR* 143:525-529, 1984.

274. Welch CE: Percutaneous catheter drainage of abdominal abscesses. *New Engl J Med* 306(2):108, 1982 (letter to the editor).

275. Welch TJ, et al: CT-guided biopsy: prospective analysis of 1,000 procedures. *Radiology* 171:493-496, 1989.

276. Westcott JL: Air embolism complication percutaneous needle biopsy of the lung. *Chest* 63(1):108-110, 1973.

277. Westcott JL: Direct percutaneous needle aspiration of localized pulmonary lesions: results in 422 patients. *Radiology* 137:31-35, 1980.

278. Westcott JL: Percutaneous needle aspiration of hilar and mediastinal masses. *Radiology* 141:323-329, 1981.

279. Westcott JL: Percutaneous transthoracic needle biopsy. *Radiology* 169:593-601, 1988.

280. Whitmire LF, et al: Imaging guided percutaneous hepatic biopsy: diagnostic accuracy and safety. *J Clin Gastroenterol* 7(6):511-515, 1985.

281. Wilson SR, Rosen IE: Abdominal biopsy with ultrasound guidance. *Radiology* 136:580, 1980 (abstract).

282. Wittenberg J, et al: Core biopsy of abdominal tumors using a 22 gauge needle. Paper presented at the sixty-seventh scientific assembly and annual meeting, Radiological Society of North America, Chicago, Nov. 15-20, 1981.

283. Wittenberg J, et al: Nonfocal enlargement of pancreatic carcinoma. *Radiology* 144:131, 1982.

284. Wolinsky H, et al: Needle tract inplantation of tumor after percutaneous lung biopsy. *Ann Intern Med* 21:359-362, 1969.

285. Wood WB, et al: Studies on the cellular immunology of acute cytosis. *J Exp Med* 94:521-40, 1951.

286. Wright RN, et al: Pulmonary mucormycosis (phycomycetes) successfully treated by resection. *Ann Thorac Surg* 29(2):166-169, 1980.

287. Zalas P, et al: The diagnosis by percutaneous biopsy with computed tomography of a recurrence of carcinoma of the rectum in the pelvis. *Surg Gynecol Obstet* 151:525-527, 1980.

288. Zamchek N: Liver biopsy. II. The risk of needle biopsy. *New Engl J Med* 299:1062-1069, 1953.

289. Zeman R, et al: Personal communication, 1987.

290. Zins M, et al: US-guided percutaneous liver biopsy with plugging of the needle track: a prospective study in 71 high-risk patients. *Radiology* 184:841-843, 1992.

291. Zornoza J: Aspiration biopsy of discrete pulmonary lesions using a new thin needle. *Radiology* 123:519-520, 1977.

292. Zornoza J, et al: Fine needle aspiration biopsy of retroperitoneal lymph nodes and abdominal masses: an updated report. *Radiology* 125:87-88, 1977.

293. Zornoza J, et al: Transperitoneal percutaneous retroperitoneal lymph node aspiration biopsy. *Radiology* 122:111-115, 1977.

294. Zornoza J, et al: Fine-needle aspiration biopsy of the liver. *AJR* 134:331-334, 1980.

295. Zornoza J, et al: Percutaneous needle biopsy in abdominal lymphoma. *AJR* 136:97-103, 1981.

SUGGESTED READINGS

Aeder MI, et al: Role of surgical and percutaneous drainage in the treatment of abdominal abscesses. *Arch Surg* 118:273-280, 1983.

Andriole JG, Haaga JR, Hau T: Percutaneous drainage of intraabdominal abscesses: an alternative to reexploration, In Fry DF, editor: *Reoperative surgery*, New York, 1986, Marcel Dekker.

Barakos JA, et al: CT in the management of periappendiceal abscess. *AJR* 146:1161-1164, 1986.

Berkman WA, Harris SA, Bernardino ME: Nonsurgical drainage of splenic abscess. *AJR* 141:395-396, 1983.

Bernardino ME, et al: Percutaneous drainage for multiseptated hepatic abscess. *J Comput Assist Tomogr* 8(1):38-41, 1984.

Bertel CK, van Heerden MB, Sheedy PF: Treatment of pyogenic hepatic abscesses. *Arch Surg* 121:554-558, 1986.

Brolin RE, et al: Percutaneous catheter versus open surgical drainage in the treatment of abdominal abscesses. *Am Surg* 50:102-108, 1984.

Clark RA, Towbin R: Abscess drainage with CT and ultrasound guidance. *Radiol Clin North Am* 21(3):445-459, 1983.

Cronan JJ, Amis ES Jr., Dortman GS: Percutaneous drainage of renal abscesses. *AJR* 142:351-354, 1984.

Diament MJ, et al: Percutaneous aspiration and catheter drainage of abscesses. *J Pediatr* 108(2):204-208, 1986.

Fataar S, Tuft RJ: Percutaneous catheter drainage of abdominal abscesses. *S Afr Med J* 64:1641-1649, 1983.

Fernandez JA, et al: Renal carbuncle: comparison between surgical open drainage and closed percutaneous drainage. *Urology* 25(2):142-144, 1985.

Gerzof SG: Percutaneous drainage of renal and perinephric abscess. *Urol Radiol* 2:171-179, 1981.

Gerzof SG, et al: Percutaneous catheter drainage of abdominal abscesses guided by ultrasound and computed tomography. *AJR* 133:1-8, 1979.

Gerzof SG, et al: Percutaneous catheter drainage of abdominal abscesses: a five-year experience. *New Engl J Med* 305(12):653-657, 1981.

Gerzof SG, et al: Expanded criteria for percutaneous abscess drainage. *Arch Surg* 120:227-232, 1985.

Gerzof SG, et al: Intrahepatic pyogenic abscesses: treatment by percutaneous drainage. *Am J Surg* 149:487-494, 1985.

Glass CA, Cohn I Jr: Drainage of intraabdominal abscesses: a comparison of surgical and computerized tomography guided catheter drainage. *Am J Surg* 147:315-317, 1984.

Gronvall J, Gronvall S, Hegedii S: Ultrasound-guided drainage of fluid-containing masses using angiographic catheterization techniques. *AJR* 129:997-1002, 1977.

Gronvall S, et al: Drainage of abdominal abscesses guided by sonography. *AJR* 138:527-529, 1982.

Haaga JR: CT guided procedures. In Haaga JR, Alfidi RJ, editors: *Computed tomography of the whole body,* St. Louis, 1973, The CV Mosby Co.

Haaga JR, Weinstein AJ: CT-guided percutaneous aspiration and drainage of abscesses. *AJR* 1187-1194, 1980.

Haaga JR, et al: New interventional techniques in the diagnosis and management of inflammatory disease within the abdomen. *Radiol Clin North Am* 17:485, 1979.

Haaga JR, et al: Definitive treatment of a large pyogenic liver abscess with CT guidance. *Cleve Clin Q* 43:85-88, 1976.

Haaga JR, et al: CT detection and aspiration of abdominal abscesses. *AJR* 128:465-474, 1977.

Halasz NA, Van Sonnenberg E: Drainage of intraabdominal abscesses: tactics and choices. *Am J Surg* 146:112-115, 1983.

Hau T, Haaga JR, Aeder MI: Pathophysiology, diagnosis and treatment of abdominal abscesses. *Curr Probl Surg* 21(7):1-82, 1984.

Jeffrey RB, Wing VW, Laing FC: Real-time sonographic monitoring of percutaneous abscess drainage. *AJR* 144:469-470, 1985.

Johnson RD, et al: Percutaneous drainage of pyogenic liver abscess. *AJR* 144:463-467, 1985.

Johnson WC, et al: Treatment of abdominal abscesses: comparative evaluation of operative drainage versus percutaneous catheter drainage guided by computed tomography or ultrasound. *Ann Surg* 194(4):510-520, 1981.

Karlson KB, et al: Percutaneous abscess drainage. *Surg Gynecol Obstet* 154:44-48, 1982.

Karlson KB, et al: Percutaneous drainage of pancreatic pseudocysts and abscesses. *Radiology* 142:619-624, 1982.

Kerlan RK, et al: Abdominal abscess with low-output fistula: successful percutaneous drainage. *Radiology* 155:73-74, 1985.

Kimura M, et al: Ultrasonically guided percutaneous drainage of solitary liver abscess: successful treatment in four cases. *J Clin Gastroenterol* 3:61-65, 1981.

Kraulis JE, Bird BL, Colapinto ND: Percutaneous catheter drainage of liver abscess: an alternative to open drainage? *Br J Surg* 67:400-402, 1980.

Kuligowska E, Connors SK, Shapiro JH: Liver abscess: sonography in diagnosis and treatment. *AJR* 138:253-257, 1982.

Lang EK, et al: Abdominal abscess drainage under radiologic guidance: causes of failure. *Radiology* 159:329-336, 1986.

Lerner RM, Spataro RF: Splenic abscess: percutaneous drainage. *Radiology* 153:643-645, 1984.

MacErlean DP, Gibney RG: Radiologic management of abdominal abscesses. *J Roy Soc Med* 76:156-261, 1983.

Mandel SR, et al: Drainage of hepatic, intraabdominal and mediastinal abscesses guided by computerized axial tomography. *Am J Surg* 145:121-125, 1983.

Martin EC, Fankuchen El, Neff RA: Percutaneous drainage of abscesses: a report of 100 patients. *Clin Radiol* 35:9-11, 1984.

Martin EC, et al: Percutaneous drainage in the management of hepatic abscesses. *Surg Clin North Am* 61(1):157-167, 1981.

Martin EC, et al: Percutaneous drainage of postoperative intraabdominal abscesses. *AJR* 138:13-15, 1982.

Mauro MA, et al: Pelvic abscess drainage by the transrectal catheter approach in men. *AJR* 144:474-479, 1985.

Mueller PR, Van Sonnenberg E, Ferrucci JT: Percutaneous drainage of 250 abdominal abscesses and fluid collections. II. Current procedural concepts. *Radiology* 151:343-347, 1984.

Mueller PR, et al: Iliopsoas abscess: treatment by CT-guided percutaneous catheter drainage. *AJR* 142:359-362, 1984.

Mueller PR, et al: Lesser sac abscesses and fluid collections: drainage by a transhepatic approach. *Radiology* 155:615-618, 1985.

Mueller PR, et al: Percutaneous drainage of subphrenic abscess: a review of 62 patients. *AJR* 147:1237-1240, 1985.

Olak J, et al: Operative versus percutaneous drainage of intraabdominal abscesses. *Arch Surg* 121:141-146, 1986.

Papanicolaou N, et al: Abscess-fistula association: radiologic recognition and percutaneous management. *AJR* 143:811-815, 1984.

Porter JA, Loughry CS, Cook AJ: Use of computerized tomographic scan in the diagnosis and treatment of abscess. *Am J Surg* 150:257-262, 1985.

Purett TL, et al: Percutaneous aspiration and drainage for suspected abdominal infection. *Surgery* 96(4):731-737, 1984.

Saini S, et al: Improved localization and survival in patients with intra-abdominal abscesses. *Am J Surg* 145:136-142, 1983.

Saini S, et al: Percutaneous drainage of diverticular abscess. *Arch Surg* 121:475-478, 1986.

Sheinfeld AM, et al: Transcutaneous drainage of abscesses of the liver guided by computed tomography scan. *Surg Gynecol Obstet* 155:662-666, 1983.

Smith EH, Bartram RJ: Ultrasonically guided percutaneous aspiration of abscesses. *AJR* 122(4):308-312, 1974.

Sones PJ: Percutaneous drainage of abdominal abscesses. *AJR* 142:35-39, 1984.

Sunshine J, et al: Percutaneous abdominal abscess drainage: Portland area experience. *Am J Surg* 145:615-618, 1983.

Vachor L, Diament MJ, Stanley P: Percutaneous drainage of hepatic abscesses in children. *J Pediatr Surg* 21(4):366-368, 1986.

Van Sonnenberg E, Mueller PR, Ferrucci JT: Percutaneous drainage of 250 abdominal abscesses and fluid collections. I. Result failures and complications. *Radiology* 151:337-347, 1984.

Van Sonnenberg E, et al: Sump catheter for percutaneous abscess and fluid drainage by Trocar or Seldinger technique. *AJR* 139:613-614, 1982.

Van Sonnenberg E, et al: Temporizing effect of percutaneous drainage of complicated abscesses in critially ill patients. *AJR* 142:821-826, 1984.

Van Waes PF, et al: Management of loculated abscesses that are difficult to drain: a new approach *Radiology* 147:57-63, 1983.

Welch CE,: Catheter drainage of abdominal abscesses. *New Engl J Med* 305(12):694-695, 1981.

47

Spiral Computed Tomography and Computed Tomographic Angiography

STEPHEN W. TAMARKIN

SPIRAL COMPUTED TOMOGRAPHY

Spiral or helical computed tomography (CT) scanning allows continuous acquisition of data during constant rotation of the x-ray tube/detector system with simultaneous movement of the patient through the gantry.[26,27,42,53] This technique was made possible by the introduction of slip-ring technology into the design of CT scanners. Slip-rings contain brushlike electrical contacts, which during constant motion allow the passage of power into the gantry and the passage of data from the detectors out of the gantry. This differs from the previous generation of scanners, which transfer electricity and data via large cables and thus require the gantry to move in reciprocal arcs to keep the cables unwound. Following the production of slip-ring scanners, the innovation of simultaneous patient transport allowed the introduction of spiral, volumetric scanning. Articles on spiral scanning first appeared in the radiology literature in 1989,[27,53] and now slip-ring scanners are offered by nearly every CT manufacturer. Spiral scanning capabilities are rapidly changing and will continue to mature with continued evolution of electrical generators, x-ray tubes and detectors, and computers.

The primary benefits of spiral scanning come from the ability to obtain multiple images in a short period of time and the acquisition of data in a seamless volume rather than as individual axial images.[26] Entire volumes can be scanned during a single breathhold, eliminating respiratory motion and interscan gaps (respiratory misregistration) seen on conventional scanning due to individual breathholds suspended at different levels (Fig. 47-1). The rapid timing allows the entire spiral sequence to be obtained during a desired segment of enhancement such as the peak arterial or portal venous phase. Spiral CT may also permit a reduction in the amount of contrast medium required.[9,13] Acquiring the data as a volume rather than as individual axial slices permits images to be reconstructed at variable positions and intervals along the z-axis, as selected during postprocessing, without additional scanner time or radiation exposure. The volumetric data also allows improved two-dimensional (2D) and three-dimensional (3D) image reconstruction.[7,14,41,42] The combination of rapid scanning and volume data acquisition has created enthusiasm for computed tomographic angiography.

The path of the x-ray tube/detector system rotating around the moving patient forms a helix (Fig. 47-2). Transverse or axial images are then reconstructed from the volumetric data with the use of various interpolation algorithms and data from adjacent spiral arcs.[10,26,42,57] Most slip-ring scanners rotate 360 degrees per second, and the rate of table movement through the gantry as well as the collimation of the x-ray beam is set by the radiologist. Pitch is defined as the table feed rate per 360-degree tube rotation divided by the beam collimation (N).[10,22] Assuming a scan time of 1 second, pitch equals the ratio of table movement (mm/sec) to nominal beam width (mm). Commonly, the patient movement rate is set to equal the beam collimation, which would be a pitch of 1. An example would be 8 mm/sec table speed with 8 mm slice thickness. The position and interval of the image reconstruction along the longitudinal axis (z-axis) can be changed during postprocessing. The width of images that can be obtained will depend on nominal beam collimation, patient transport rate, and recon-

1694

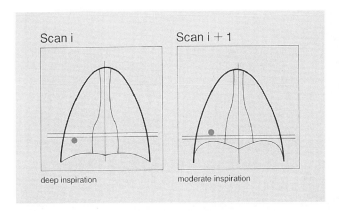

Fig. 47-1. Different depths of respiratory suspension can cause a small lesion to be missed due to an interscan gap with conventional scanning. Volumetric *(spiral)* scanning eliminates potential respiratory misregistration. (Courtesy Siemens Medical Systems, Inc.)

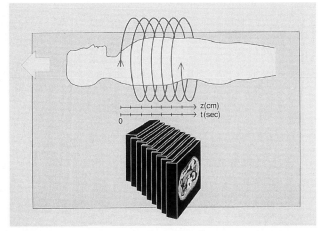

Fig. 47-2. The path of the rotating x-ray tube/detector system around the moving patient forms a helix or cylinder. The longitudinal axis of the patient, perpendicular to the scan plane, is called the z-axis. (Courtesy Siemens Medical Systems, Inc.)

struction algorithm; contrary to popular belief, thinner sections cannot be obtained during postprocessing.

Spiral technique has gained popularity for specific tailored examinations including evaluation of solitary pulmonary nodules,[54] although some authors have advocated its use for routine imaging of the thorax[34] and abdomen.[57] Current limitations of maximum allowed milliamperes (mA) and perceived loss of edge sharpness due to patient movement[5,40] have been primary factors in the slow acceptance for routine use. The z-axis length, which can be covered in a single spiral sequence, is limited, and various scanners require different reconstruction time delays before initiating a second spiral or continuing conventional scanning. Continued technical improvements, including increased x-ray tube heat capacity, faster computer processing, and further refinement of reconstruction algorithms and x-ray detectors, will impact on the future of spiral CT.

Technical considerations

Multiple scan parameters can be manipulated. Obviously, the timing of scanning in relation to delivery of intravenous contrast is crucial and will be discussed elsewhere. Slice thickness, reconstruction interval, and table speed can also be manipulated. The need for thin slices must be weighed against the need to cover a greater distance along the z-axis, and thin collimation may degrade image quality, particularly in obese patients.[57] In general, slice thickness considerations are similar to conventional scanning and depend on the individual organ or lesion being investigated. If smaller lesions or anatomic structures are being sought, thin collimation is necessary to lessen partial volume averaging.

This problem is somewhat diminished by the ability to reconstruct images at tightly spaced intervals,

which ensures that at least one image is well centered on the lesion.[26,54] The acquired data will depend on the original slice thickness, and "thinner" images cannot be obtained during postprocessing. Overlapping images can be reconstructed (such as 8-mm-thick slices filmed at 2- or 4-mm intervals); this has been proved to increase lesion sensitivity[52,57] and improve 2-D and 3-D reconstructions.[36,37] Obtaining a single image optimally centered on a lesion is also crucial for accurate densitometry, as will be discussed with solitary pulmonary nodules.[26,54] Table speed is often matched to the collimation of the beam width, and rates usually vary between 1 and 10 mm/sec. An example of a typical spiral sequence would consist of a 24-second sequence with 8-mm slice thickness and table motion of 8 mm/sec. This sequence would cover 19.2 cm; however, no image can be obtained from the first and last spiral rotation due to the need for interpolation from adjacent points. Thus 17.6 cm of imaging coverage would be available. The use of pitches greater than 1 has recently become more common, although image degradation still limits the use of pitches greater than 2.[22] Faster table speeds, particularly for use with pitches greater than 1, are available and may become more popular.

The coupling of multiple sequential spirals in rapid succession can now be performed by some scanners.[16,39,56] This allows coverage of much greater lengths along the z-axis, though not during a single breathhold. This introduces the possibility of intersequence spatial gaps or overlapped volumes similar to respiratory misregistration of conventional scanning. Programs that match raw data files from adjacent sequences, and thus ensure seamless coverage, have been developed, but they require considerable computation power.[56] The beam

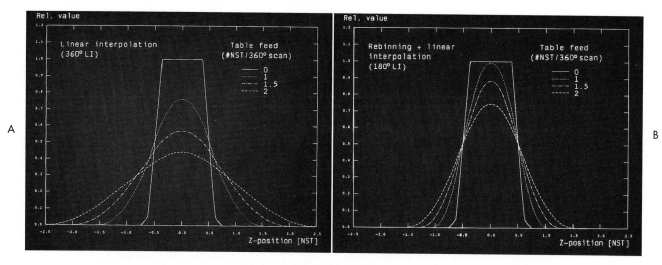

Fig. 47-3. Section sensitivity profiles are broadened with spiral scanning secondary to the patient movement. This effect worsens with increasing table speeds and is most severe when using a 360-degree linear interpolation (**A**). A 180-degree linear interpolation causes less broadening (**B**). (Courtesy Siemens Medical Systems, Inc.)

collimation, pitch, and milliamperes can be adjusted separately for various segments along the spiral-train, so-called "variable-speed helical acquisition."[16]

The patient's radiation dose from spiral scanning is equal to conventional scanning, assuming a pitch of 1. Pitches greater than 1 would effectively spread the radiation and thus reduce overall exposure, while pitches less than 1 increase exposure.[26]

The x-ray tube is on during the entire spiral sequence, and thus the anode receives a constant bombardment of electrons. The anode heat capacity and cooling rate, and specifically the focal tract cooling rate, limit usable milliamperes.[56] In general, decreasing the milliamperes, or photon flux, increases quantum mottle (noise). The maximum allowable milliamperes varies with the individual parameters of a spiral sequence, including the kilovoltage and duration, and among various manufacturers and machines. X-ray tubes with increased heat capacity and heat-dissipating capabilities are being developed, and further refinements in the detector system sensitivity may lower milliampere requirements.[56] Currently, most scanners have maximum sequences of 24 to 40 seconds, although some machines allow up to 60 seconds.

Another quality concern is the broadened section sensitivity profile (SSP) caused by spiral scanning (Fig. 47-3).* The SSP defines the actual dimensions and profile of voxels along the z-axis. The SSP obtained with conventional scanning approaches the ideal rectangular shape. Table motion and spiral geometry cause convolution of the original SSP and yield a more triangular, bell-curve shape. A broadened SSP expands the nominal beam collimation into wider actual widths and may cause longitudinal blurring.[5,25,42] SSP broadening increases with greater table speeds and is highly dependent on the interpolation algorithm that is used.* While some authors have reported longitudinal blurring with spiral,[5,42] others have found minimal or no difference, particularly when using a 180-degree interpolation.[57]

Various mathematical reconstruction algorithms are available. The original reconstruction algorithm developed with spiral scanning uses 360-degree linear interpolation in which data points from adjacent 360-degree rotations are used to produce axial images.[10,25] Newer 180-degree interpolations that are either linear, or nonlinear and higher order, are now widely used.[10,22,40,57] In general, the original 360-degree linear interpolation, with decreased noise due to increased photon statistics, is most efficient but causes the most severe broadening of section sensitivity profile. The 180-degree linear interpolation or helical under scanning algorithms are less efficient but decrease beam widening and thus reduce longitudinal edge blurring.[40,57] They are particularly advantageous with multiplanar and three-dimensional reconstructions, or when a pitch greater than 1 is used.[22,40]

Abdomen

Spiral scanning has obvious potential benefits within the abdomen. The upper abdominal organs move together with the diaphragm and thus have the same potential for respiratory misregistration as does the thorax. Truly contiguous images eliminate the possible omission

---

*References 5, 10, 25, 26, 40, 42, 57.

*References 5, 10, 25, 26, 40, 57.

of a small lesion from the scan plane; particularly important in the liver, pancreas, adrenal glands, and kidneys. Obtaining multiple images in a short period of time allows an entire organ or area to be scanned during a desired segment of enhancement (such as the portal venous phase, considered most desirable for evaluating possible liver metastases). Similar advantages can be gained in the pancreas. Increased uses of 2-D and 3-D image reformations have been proposed.

The relatively high milliampere requirements and perceived decreased edge sharpness in abdominal scanning[5,25,42] have caused reluctant acceptance of spiral technique for routine abdominal imaging. However, Zeman et al[57] compared image quality of conventional versus spiral scanning on abdominal scans of 60 consecutive patients and recommended helical scanning as the preferred means of acquiring routine abdominal images. In their series, they found "no meaningful difference in visual noise, reconstruction artifacts, or the ability of blinded observers to distinguish helical from nonhelical scans." Their study used a HI-Speed scanner from GE Medical Systems, which allowed 330 to 340 mA during 24- to 30-second scanning sequences and a helical underscan reconstruction algorithm to correct for table motion.

Imaging soon after the initiation of the intravenous bolus may cause inhomogeneous organ and intravascular enhancement, which has potential interpretation pitfalls.[23] Radiologists have become more used to the commonly seen heterogenous splenic enhancement, which is considered normal and felt to be secondary to differential enhancement rates between the red and white pulp (Fig. 47-4).[32] If there is concern for the possibility of an infiltrating splenic process, delayed images may be helpful. Imaging during the vascular nephrogram phase, rather than during the more typical tubular phase seen with conventional scanning can cause decreased conspicuity of small hypodense medullary lesions.[23] Where conventional studies typically show renal cell carcinomas as hypodense masses due to their inability to concentrate contrast, imaging during the vascular phase may cause these neoplasms to appear hyperdense as a result of hypervascularity.[23] Again, delayed imaging may prove helpful. The mixing of enhanced and nonenhanced blood can give the appearance of a well-defined intravascular hypodensity similar in appearance to intravascular thrombus. Differentiating real thrombi from mixing phenomenon can be difficult, but true thrombus often has associated vessel enlargement or collateral formation. Mixing is frequently seen within the IVC, renal veins, or confluence of common iliac veins.[23]

Liver

The importance of imaging the liver before the interstitial or equilibrium phase of enhancement is widely

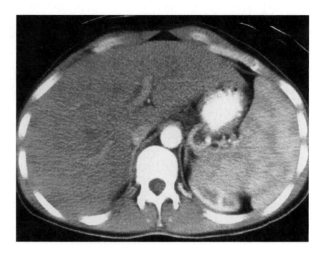

Fig. 47-4. Markedly heterogeneous splenic enhancement due to imaging soon after the initiation of the bolus in a patient without known splenic abnormality. Note the early phase of the injection with dense enhancement within the aorta and splenic artery, and early "vascular" nephrogram.

acknowledged.[15] Commonly, liver metastases are relatively hypovascular and are supplied via the hepatic artery, whereas normal liver parenchyma has dual portal venous and hepatic arterial supply with approximately 75% of blood volume from the portal vein. Dynamic protocols have been designed to maximize imaging during the nonequilibrium or redistribution phase.[15] However, the approximately 2 minutes required to scan the liver necessitated imaging portions of the inferior liver during the early equilibrium phase, which is considered less desirable because lesions can become isoattenuating. With spiral scanning, the entire liver is easily scanned during a single 24-second sequence. The rate of contrast delivery and timing of imaging in relation to the beginning of the intravenous bolus vary with different authors, who all attempt to maximize lesion conspicuity against the background normal liver while limiting potential confusion caused by unenhanced hepatic veins or early heterogeneous parenchymal enhancement. Initiation of scanning between 30 and 70 seconds after bolus onset has been reported.[4,23,56,57]

Variations in overall contrast volume and both biphasic and monophasic rates have been advocated. Potential benefits of imaging during vascular enhancement include the confirmation of normal vascular architecture in focal fatty infiltration, improved visualization of collaterals and attenuated vessels in the setting of cirrhosis, and clearer identification of portal vein thrombosis and cavernous transformation.[4] Spiral scanning is also fast enough to allow a set of images to be obtained during the early vascular phase, similar to the angiographic arterial phase, which may help in detection of hypervascular metastatic or primary liver neoplasms.[22,28,42,56] Machines that allow rapid serial spiral sequences can pro-

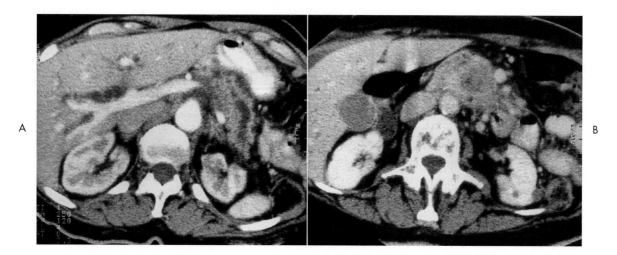

Fig. 47-5. Tailored study of the pancreas with thin collimation, small field of view, and well-timed contrast bolus improves visualization of dilated biliary and pancreatic ducts (**A**), peripancreatic vessels, and pancreatic head adenocarcinoma (**B**).

duce a set of images during both "arterial" and portal venous phases with a single intravenous bolus injection.

Other advantages for spiral liver scanning include the previously mentioned elimination of respiratory misregistration and the ability to reconstruct images at variable intervals. Urban et al demonstrated increased sensitivity and confidence in lesion detection using a 4-mm reconstruction interval versus an 8-mm interval.[52] The rapid timing of image acquisition has similar advantages when used with CT portography.[3]

Pancreas

Imaging during optimal parenchymal enhancement is important for maximal pancreatic lesion sensitivity, as in the liver.[18,33,56] In addition, peak vascular enhancement, lack of respiratory misregistration, and ability to reconstruct at variable intervals are important advantages of spiral scanning (Fig. 47-5). As stated by Megibow,[33] the ideal tailored study for the assessment of pancreatic neoplasms would use the proper intravenous administration of contrast material, have appropriate section indexing and speed of data acquisition, and have appropriate choice of section thickness. Allowing for acceptable overall image quality and specifically image noise, spiral scanning is ideal for meeting these criteria. The ability to demonstrate both focal areas of decreased parenchymal attenuation and overall contour changes of the gland is important in the detection of pancreatic ductal adenocarcinomas.[17,18,33] Questionable small lesions may be more clearly depicted with reconstruction of images optimally centered, similar to focal lesions of the liver or solitary lung nodules. Scanning during early parenchymal enhancement should improve detection of small hypervascular pancreatic masses (such

as most islet cell tumors)[22,29] and more clearly differentiate hypoperfused necrotic tissue in the setting of necrotizing pancreatitis.[24]

The ability to image during peak vascular enhancement is also crucial in assessing the numerous peripancreatic vessels, and thus the extent of disease in both neoplastic and inflammatory processes. Determination of vascular invasion must be attempted in cases of pancreatic neoplasms,[33] because this is the most common cause of unresectability.[56] Imaging during peak vascular enhancement also has the potential for maximizing identification of peripancreatic arterial and venous thrombosis, aneurysms and pseudoaneurysms, and collateral vessels. Most spiral protocols should provide peak enhancement of the aorta, the splenic artery and vein, the superior mesenteric artery and vein, the portal vein, and other smaller peripancreatic vessels.

Multiple individual techniques for spiral pancreatic scanning have been described with variability in the rate, amount, and timing of contrast delivery. Dupuy et al[13] report adequate vascular and parenchymal enhancement using a total of 90 cc of intravenous contrast, while Zeman et al[56] state that 120 to 150 ml injections improve assessment of venous vascular encasement. Delays as short as 20 seconds between the initiation of the intravenous bolus and the onset of scanning have been used to evaluate the pancreatic parenchyma; however, longer delays of 45 to 70 seconds allow greater vascular enhancement while maintaining peak parenchymal enhancement. Monophasic injection rates of 2 and 3 ml per second[14,18,56] and biphasic protocols with initial rates of 3 ml per second followed by a sustained injection of 1 ml per second,[13] have also been used. Thin collimation such as 4 to 5 mm is generally preferred in studies tailored for the pancreas, although 8-mm slice thickness allows greater coverage of the liver. Numerous authors advocate use of reversed scanning direction (caudad to cephalic).[33,56] The pancreas is easily included in a single spiral sequence, but including the entire liver in the same sequence may not be possible, especially if thin collimation is used. Using a preinjection scout view for localization, reversed scanning ensures complete pancreatic coverage together with maximal possible coverage of the liver during the preequilibrium phase. The overall patient volume that can be included in a single spiral sequence will depend on a combination of the selected slice thickness, table speed, and the maximum allowed time for continuous data acquisition. As newer scanners allow longer sequences, the limiting factor may become the patient's breathholding capability. Using a pitch of greater than 1 also would increase overall coverage, although this may degrade image quality. Portions of the liver and the remainder of the lower abdomen and pelvis, which are not included, could be scanned with subsequent spiral, dynamic, or conventional imaging.

Thorax

Spiral scanning has gained wide acceptance in thoracic imaging.[34] Relatively low x-ray tube current requirements and the importance of eliminating respiratory variation make spiral CT well suited to chest scanning and particularly, to the evaluation of solitary pulmonary nodules. With contrasted studies, the mediastinum, hila, and aorta can be imaged during peak vascular enhancement, even with lower volumes of contrast. Two-dimensional reformatted images may play a more important role, particularly in the evaluation of the apices, diaphragms, and airways.

The advantages of spiral technique in the evaluation of pulmonary nodules were recognized in early articles on spiral scanning.[26,54] The seamless, volumetric data are important both in searching for pulmonary nodules and allowing the most accurate depiction of the lesion morphology and densitometry[54] (Fig. 47-6). All nodules seen with conventional scanning should be detected with spiral technique. Costello et al[8] have demonstrated detection of additional small nodules with spiral scanning. Used as a screening examination, one can more confidently exclude the presence of a nodule, without the risk of missing a small lesion secondary to respiratory misregistration (a potential problem with conventional scanning). Accurate densitometry—including the presence and distribution of fat and calcification within lesions—is important in assessing the relative risk of malignancy.[49,58] Reconstruction of images at narrow intervals through the lesion should allow at least one image to be optimally centered, thus minimizing partial volume

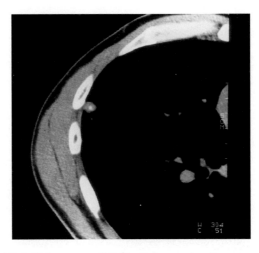

Fig. 47-6. Thin-cut, small field-of-view, optimally centered spiral image demonstrates a small peripheral lung nodule with central calcification. The nodule was barely seen, and no calcification appreciated, on routine conventional study.

averaging. If a single, previously known lesion is being investigated, targeted thin cuts and a small field of view should also improve overall lesion depiction.

Costello et al found spiral images of the lung parenchyma superior to conventional images.[9] Paranjpe and Bergin evaluated the effect of multiple operator controlled parameters—beam collimation, table speed, interpolation algorithm, and display kernel—and attempted to optimize spiral techniques for lung parenchyma.[38] An 8 mm collimation was considered adequate for screening examinations, and such widely collimated spiral images showed no resolution differences compared with conventional scans. Narrow collimation (1 or 3 mm) did improve resolution, but other factors including the desired z-axis coverage, examination time, and the geometry of the lesions being interrogated must be considered. Decreased longitudinal resolution, particularly with curved structures or objects placed oblique to the z-axis, was felt to be a result of the broadened section-sensitivity profiles caused by spiral geometry. No significant differences in image quality were found with changes in table speed (pitch 1 versus pitch 2) or interpolation algorithm (180 degrees versus 360 degrees linear). As with conventional scanning, high spatial frequency display kernels yielded improved resolution.

Many of the current 24-second spiral sequences do not allow coverage of the entire thorax. As longer sequences become more common, individual breathholding capacities may become the limiting factor in overall z-axis distance that can be covered. A second spiral sequence or additional conventional axial images can be used to complete examination of the desired region of interest. Rapid sequential spirals synchronized with respiratory gating have been proposed.[43] Spiral scanning may be impractical for those who are unable to hold their breath, such as dyspneic or uncooperative patients.

In studying the thoracic aorta, Costello et al report adequate enhancement with a bolus of only 60 ml and a biphasic injection rate.[9] Their study included adequate opacification of aneurysmal aortas and differentiation between true and false lumens with aortic dissections. If evidence of dissection or another abnormality was found on the lowermost image, this low initial contrast volume allowed a second spiral sequence with an additional 60-ml injection to cover the upper abdomen. For routine mediastinal and aortic imaging, decreased contrast volume has the obvious benefits of decreased nephrotoxicity and cost savings.

Remy-Jardin et al have used a combination of spiral volumetric scanning and rapid bolus injections to detect pulmonary emboli.[41] They used injection rates of 5 to 7 ml/sec, volumes of 90 to 120 ml, and 5-second scan delays, and successfully identified all 112 central emboli seen on the corresponding selective pulmonary angiograms. Scanning began at the inferior aspect of the aorta arch and proceeded caudally with 5-mm collimation and 3-mm reconstruction intervals. Criteria for PE were modified from conventional angiographic findings. All 23 negative studies were confirmed. False positives occurred when intersegmental lymph nodes were mistaken for intravascular filling defects. Second- to fourth-order pulmonary arterial branches were adequately studied, and thus more peripheral emboli could not be excluded.

Head and Neck

Spiral scanning has received less attention for neuroradiologic indications than has computed tomographic angiography. In neck scanning, the ability to image during the vascular bolus and the elimination of the patient's breathing and swallowing motions are advantageous.[51] Suojanen et al compared spiral with conventional neck images and found at least comparable overall quality, although slightly increased quantum mottle (noise), felt to be a result of the lower milliamperes, was noted in the spiral images.[51] They also demonstrated adequate vascular enhancement with less than 25 g of iodine per study, an amount 30% to 50% less than those commonly used with dynamic CT. A modified prolonged valsalva, which distends the supraglottic airway, minimizes respiratory motion, and prevents swallowing, was also shown to be effective. Sequences performed during different phonation maneuvers may help in assessment of vocal cord motion. Reconstructions from volumetric data have numerous potential applications, including coronal imaging of the larynx or paranasal sinuses, in patients who cannot tolerate the standard repositioning, as well as 3-D imaging of the facial bones or spine in the setting of trauma or preoperative or postoperative evaluation.

COMPUTED TOMOGRAPHIC ANGIOGRAPHY

Computed tomographic angiography (CTA) refers to the production of angiographic images from CT data. Such images can be obtained by reconstructing routine spiral or dynamic bolus studies. However, spiral examinations tailored specifically to CTA with the use of thin-cut, overlapping images, well-timed rapid bolus injections, and small fields of view will yield significantly higher quality vascular images. The rapid, seamless, volume data acquisition makes spiral scanning ideal for CTA. These features have triggered the recent development of this technique.* Numerous images can be obtained during peak vascular enhancement with a single 24- to 60-second spiral sequence. In addition, volumetric data acquisition and recent advances in computerized image manipulation allow improved display of the original information in 3-D reformations.

There have been multiple clinical trials assessing the ability of CTA to detect carotid bifurcation stenosis.[6,111,31,47] There have also been preliminary reports describing use of CTA in the circle of Willis,[1,20,21] abdominal aorta,[2,46,55] renal and splenic arteries,[12,19,44-46] and extremity vessels.[12] CTA is typically compared with the gold standard of conventional catheter angiography, having as its primary advantage no need for arterial puncture or arterial injections. Unlike ultrasound and magnetic resonance angiography, however, CTA currently requires an injection of iodinated contrast material and thus retains its associated risks of nephrotoxicity and allergic reactions. Although CTA requires considerably less patient table time than does catheter angiography, preprocessing and postprocessing of the images can be labor-intensive for the radiologist or technician, requiring up to 1 hour. If thin-beam collimation (and thus slow patient table movement) is necessary for adequate resolution, only short ranges in the longitudinal axis can be included in a single sequence. An example of this limitation is found in the recent carotid bifurcation studies, which do not include either the origins of the common carotids or the carotid syphons.[6,11,31,47] Continued scanner development with improved x-ray tube heating capacity will allow longer spiral sequences and thus greater coverage in the head, neck, pelvis, and extremities, but maximum breathholding capacity will continue to limit the time available for a single abdominal or thoracic sequence. Rapidly coupled sequences combined with a prolonged bolus also may allow greater coverage.

---

*References 1, 6, 11, 12, 20, 31, 35, 45-47, 55.

Technical Considerations

The timing of data acquisition in relation to the delivery of the intravenous contrast bolus is obviously crucial and will be discussed subsequently. Most authors prefer at least a 20-gauge angiocatheter within the antecubital fossa and use of a power injector is necessary. The early phase of the injection should be monitored to exclude extravasation. Injection rates between 1.5 and 5.0 ml per second have been proposed, with overall contrast volumes ranging between 60 and 150 ml, and both rates and volumes must be tailored for the individual vessels being studied.

In general, large vessels that course perpendicular to the scan plane and thus within the longitudinal axis of the patient are better evaluated than those with transverse or tortuous paths.[12] Dillon et al state that in-plane resolution is the limiting factor for vessels perpendicular to the slice plane, whereas resolution for vessels parallel to the scanning plane depends upon slice thickness as the limiting factor.[12] Narrow-beam collimation improves longitudinal spacial resolution but decreases the overall patient volume that can be included, and this balance must be considered by the operator. Nominal slice thickness usually varies from 1 to 5 mm, and, as previously discussed, the true slice thickness is exaggerated by broadening of the section sensitivity profile. Narrow overlapping slice reconstruction intervals are routinely used. An example would be 3-mm-thick slices reconstructed every 1 to 2 mm.

Three-dimensional reformation of the data requires an advanced computer work station, which can be either provided by the individual scanner manufacturer or customized from commercially available components. The most commonly used 3-D reconstructions have been shaded-surface displays and maximum-intensity projection. Various other volume-rendering reconstruc-

tions and curved planar reformations are also, though less commonly, used.

Shaded-surface renderings display the vessel contours and other structures based on the computed reflection of a hypothetical light source (Fig. 47-7).[30,45,47] Shaded-surface display (SSD) allows excellent 3-D anatomic detail without visualization of overlying structures, but currently requires time-consuming operator postprocessing.[12] The mathematical surface model depends on attenuation values above the selected threshold and may be severely degraded by suboptimal bolus timing or decreased enhancement distal to a severe stenosis.[31] The final 3-D images do not directly represent the original Hounsfield unit densities, and calcified plaques may merge imperceptibly with the intravascular contrast, thus exaggerating lumen diameter.[11,19,44,45,47]

Maximum-intensity projection (MIP) is commonly used in magnetic resonance angiography (MRA).[48] Mathematical rays are passed through the reconstructed 2-D images and the maximum-intensity pixel, which is encountered along the rays, is then displayed (Fig. 47-8).[45,48] Similar MIPs are performed from numerous viewing angles. The series can be reviewed as a cine loop yielding a 3-D quality.[35,46,48] Unlike MRA, where the flowing blood has the highest signal within the volume, the contrast-filled vessels have lower attenuation than do bone or other calcified structures. Thus high-density structures must be eliminated by using various editing techniques.[31,35,45,46]

Seedpoint connectivity algorithms allow the operator to select a point after which a computer maps all continuous voxels that fall within a predetermined Hounsfield-unit range. These programs can be used to either select desired structures (such as mapping vessel contours for shaded-surface displays)[12] or to eliminate unwanted structures (such as overlying bone with

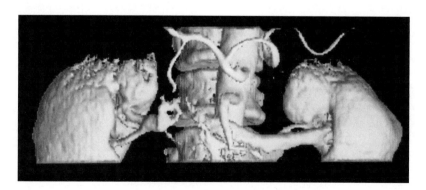

Fig. 47-7. Shaded surface display of CT angiogram demonstrating a normal abdominal aorta and its branches. Note the celiac axis, including gastroduodenal artery, superior mesenteric artery, and left renal artery partially obscured by opacified left renal vein. (Courtesy Geoffrey D. Rubin, M.D., Stanford University Hospital).

MIPs).[19,31,35,45] Seedpoint manipulations can also be used during more detailed image processing, such as elimination of individual calcified plaques. Such algorithms may be ineffective or require manual assistance in regions of close vessel/bone contact, such as the interfaces between the carotid arteries and petrous bones or the aorta and spine.[35] The availability of such software varies with different work stations and more complex software is currently being developed.

With any postprocessing which is performed, the selection of threshold Hounsfield units will directly affect the final images.[11,35,45] Partial volume averaging between intraluminal contrast and adjacent structures, such as vessel wall, soft tissue, or calcified plaques, will cause a narrow zone of pixels that have gradually changing densities. This narrow zone can be included or excluded from the final vessel display, depending on the selected thresholds. Even individual pixels may be significant when evaluating narrow stenoses or small-caliber vessels.[35] In general, wider threshold ranges will exaggerate lumen diameters, while more narrow ranges may exaggerate stenoses. Both arbitrary and quantitative methods for selection of threshold values have been used. Dillon et al have proposed a mathematical formula for determining appropriate minimal segmentation values based on intraluminal and background soft-tissue densities.[11]

Carotids

Carotid bifurcation imaging is technically well suited to CTA because of the large-caliber, minimal motion and generally longitudinal orientation of these vessels. These factors, together with the frequency of carotid disease and importance of diagnosing stenosis, have sparked much interest in carotid CTA and led to clinical studies at multiple centers. Four recent studies compared CTA with conventional catheter angiography.[6,11,31,47] Each group graded the degree of carotid bifurcation stenosis using the four categories of mild, moderate, or severe stenosis, or complete occlusion. Schwartz et al,[47] Marks et al[31] and Dillon et al[11] demonstrated agreement between the two techniques of 92%, 89%, and 82%, respectively, while the results of Castillo,[6] with only 50% agreement, were less encouraging.

Schwartz et al studied 20 patients and also found a high correlation between CTA and Doppler ultrasound or 2-D time-of-flight MRA.[47] They used shaded-surface rendering and minimum Hounsfield-unit thresholds (Fig. 47-9). Maximal thresholds were used only if calcification was present. An unenhanced sequence before the enhanced scan aided in delineating the calcified plaques, which were subsequently removed manually. The authors report considerably increased processing time and possible overestimation of stenosis with the removal of calcifications. No difference in the ability to determine stenosis was found between 2- and 4-mm slice thickness, with 2-mm reconstruction intervals used in both protocols.

Marks et al studied 14 patients using MIPs and described utilization of the source axial images in further evaluation of cases with circumferential calcifications.[31] While they report overall agreement of 89% between CT and conventional angiography, all cases of severe stenosis or occlusion were accurately identified. They used protocols with 2- or 3-mm beam collimation and table speed and 1-mm interval reconstructions. They report approximately 10 minutes of processing time.

Dillon et al studied 27 patients and found an 82%

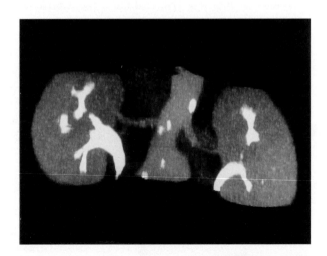

Fig. 47-8. Maximum intensity projection (MIP) demonstrates an infrarenal cuff between the origins of the renal arteries and the shoulders of the abdominal aortic aneurysm. This image was created from a routine spiral bolus abdominal study (not tailored specifically for CTA). Note display of calcified plaques discrete from the luminal contrast. (Courtesy Picker International, Inc.)

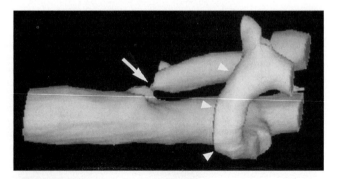

Fig. 47-9. Shaded surface display of CT angiogram of a carotid bifurcation from a posterior oblique projection. There is a high-grade stenosis of the internal carotid artery at its origin. Also note prominent external carotid branch. (From Schwartz RB, Jones KM, Chernoff DM et al: *Radiology* 185:513-519, 1992.)

agreement on stenosis category between CTA and conventional angiography. All cases which did not agree differed by only one category. They evaluated various delays between bolus initiation and onset of scanning and preferred 35 seconds using a total of 120 ml of contrast. They used shaded-surface displays and were able to set both upper and lower thresholds for their segmentation algorithms. They stressed the importance of objective criteria in setting the lower threshold and included a quantitative mathematical formula for doing so. They also removed calcified plaques manually by drawing region-of-interest boundary lines and reported an overall processing time of 30 to 45 minutes.

Castillo studied 10 patients using MIPs with 5-mm collimation and table speed, and 3-mm reconstruction intervals.[6] He reports only 50% correlation between CTA and conventional angiography results, including identification of only two of five severe stenoses, missing nearly occluded vessels, and mistakenly calling occluded vessels that were demonstrated to be patent on conventional angiography. Castillo used relatively low contrast volumes of 60 ml and short scan delays of 10 seconds.

The Circle of Willis

Successful CTA of the circle of Willis had been demonstrated with dynamic scanning prior to the availability of spiral.[1] Ability to project the information at numerous angles and view this complex anatomy from above and below is advantageous in the overall depiction of the anatomy and, specifically, in the identification of aneurysms and aneurysm necks. In a study using dynamic scanning, Aoki et al[1] compared CTA with catheter angiography of the circle of Willis and reported 100% sensitivity with identification of all 15 aneurysms studied, including depiction of the aneurysm necks and parent arteries. They also reported one false-positive. Harbaugh et al,[21] using dynamic scanning, and a more recent spiral study by Gray et al,[20] also reported high sensitivities for detection of aneurysms in the setting of subarachnoid hemorrhage. Gray et al used 1 mm collimation, a pitch of 1, and 1-mm reconstruction intervals together with 100 ml intravenous injection and volume-rendered images that preserved the overlying structures. The close proximity of the intracranial carotid with the adjacent petrous bone may present difficulties for connectivity algorithms. CTA may not visualize very small caliber vessels; however, the difficulties of aneurysm evaluation with MRA, secondary to low signal from turbulent, or slow flow, are less problematic.

Renal Arteries

Among the numerous patients with hypertension, a small percentage have potentially treatable renal artery stenosis. This creates a need for a sensitive, reasonably specific screening examination. Plasma renin activity, renal scintigraphy, and Doppler ultrasound each have limitations as a screening examination, and the current diagnostic gold standard, conventional angiography, is costly and invasive. Renal artery anatomy and renal artery stenosis have been successfully evaluated with CT angiography,[19,44] but thus far only small numbers of patients have been studied. Compared with conventional catheter angiography, CTA is less costly and noninvasive.

Promising early works by Rubin et al[44] and Galenski et al[19] have shown high sensitivity and specificity in the detection, localization, and grading of renal artery stenosis. Both groups use high volume (90 to 150 ml), rapid (3 to 5 ml/sec) intravenous injections of contrast and precisely timed and targeted spiral imaging. Both used small, preliminary bolus injections and rapid stationary images at the level of the renal arteries to quantify the exact time to peak aortic enhancement for each individual. Galenski et al used the faster injection rate (5 ml/sec) in younger patients to compensate for increased dilution due to high cardiac output. Rubin et al preferred 3-mm to 2-mm collimation for less noise, while Galenski et al used 3-mm collimation for obese patients and 2-mm collimation for others. Rubin et al began using 180-degree linear interpolation once it became available and also began using pitches greater than 1.

Rubin et al found maximum intensity projections to be more sensitive than shaded-surface displays for detection of renal artery stenosis of more than 70% and more accurate for grading stenosis.[44] The primary limitation of SSD results from inability to differentiate plaque calcification from luminal contrast on the final rendered image. Galenski et al[19] found cine loop review of the reconstructed axial images and reformatted semicoronal images most valuable for diagnosis. Three-dimensional MIP, SSD, or curved reformatted images were helpful for diagnosis in isolated instances and were most useful as a means of displaying the entire data volume for referring physicians and study documentation.

High-grade stenosis may appear as local pseudo-obstructions, with the small volume and caliber of intraluminal contrast obscured by partial volume averaging with adjacent unenhanced tissues.[19,44] Both groups used distal revisualization of the vessel to indicate high-grade stenosis rather than true occlusion. Thus, distal reconstitution of a vessel from collaterals may lead to interpretation errors. Similar partial volume effects may cause overestimation of stenosis.

Both groups accurately identified accessory renal arteries. Secondary signs of decreased renal perfusion—relatively decreased renal enhancement, cortical thinning, and reduced overall kidney size—can also be as-

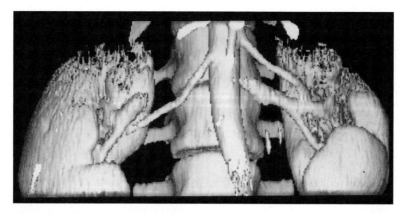

Fig. 47-10. Shaded surface display of CT angiogram of normal aorta and renal arteries. Note partially opacified renal veins. (From Rubin GD, Dake MD, Napel SA et al: *Radiology* 186:147-152, 1993.)

sessed. These findings, as well as poststenotic vessel dilation, help confirm the diagnosis of renal artery stenosis, but are not found in all cases and should not be used to discount other findings.

Aorta

Spiral CT allows longitudinal segments of the thoracic or abdominal aorta to be imaged during a brief period of time and thus during peak vascular enhancement (Fig. 47-10). As previously discussed, improved aortic opacification using decreased contrast volumes and spiral scanning has been demonstrated.[9] Aneurysms, dissections, and other lesions may be effectively identified on axial images; however, 3-D renderings may improve depiction of spatial relations and arterial branch anatomy. CT angiographic images can be obtained from routine studies given adequate contrast enhancement while tailored CTA studies can provide exquisite detail of the renal and visceral branches.

In the setting of abdominal aortic aneurysms, the combination of noncontrasted CT images of the abdomen and CT angiography may provide complete preoperative evaluation.[46] Rubin et al used CTA protocols very similar to those already discussed for renal artery studies, including a test bolus for individualized precision timing and pitches as great as 2.[46] Zeman et al have applied variable-speed helical CT and report improved visualization of the renal arteries.[55] Beaulieu et al utilize a first sequence of 3-mm collimation in the upper abdomen during the bolus, followed by a second acquistion of a 5- to 7-mm slice to complete scanning through the iliac bifurcation.[2]

The patent aortic lumen and patent arterial branches including the visceral, renal, and larger lumbar arteries can be demonstrated similarly as with conventional angiography. Depending on the technique, mural thrombus and vessel wall contours can also be displayed,

allowing assessment of overall aneurysm morphology.[2,12,45,46] Specifically, depiction of the relation between the aneurysm neck and the renal arteries, and identification of patent accessory renal and inferior mesenteric arteries, may enhance surgical planning. Rubin et al[45] used both shaded-surface renderings and maximum-intensity projections, while Zeman et al[55] reported using four different 3-D display techniques to gain complementary information. Beaulieu et al[2] reported success with a non-MIP volume-rendering technique.

Dissections have been effectively characterized, and the flap may be identified provided the false lumen is not thrombosed.[46] Different flow rates in the true and false lumens may complicate ideal image timing. Rubin et al have also successfully studied reimplanted aortic branch arteries and vessels that have undergone angioplasty or vascular stenting.[46]

Extremities

Extremity vessels can be imaged; however, limitations on z-axis coverage currently preclude runoff-type evaluation of an entire limb.[12] CT angiography of a selected peripheral segment may become useful for specific indications such as evaluation of preangioplasty or postangioplasty sites, demonstration of graft patency, or assessment of postcatheterization vascular complications. As greater scan lengths become available, maximum allowable spiral sequences can be used because breathholding is not a limiting factor. However, the need to match image timing to concurrent high levels of vascular contrast will remain a formidable challenge.

CONCLUSION

Both spiral CT and CT angiography are undergoing rapid evolution. This chapter has provided an overview of early groundwork from which future studies will undoubtedly develop. Some details concerning specific protocols and techniques have been included in this discussion, but rapid technical changes and clinical experience will lead to further refinements. I believe spiral scanning will become the dominant method for routine body scanning. The inherent high-tissue contrast and spatial resolution of CT, and the ability to manipulate volumetric data to allow a single study to be viewed with multiple formats and from numerous projections, gives CT angiography considerable potential.

REFERENCES

1. Aoki S, et al: Cerebral aneurysms: detection and delineation using 3-D CT angiography. *AJNR* 13:1115-1120, July/August 1992.
2. Beaulieu CF, et al: Volume rendering for 3-D helical CT of abdominal aorta (Abstract). *Radiology* 189(P):174, 1993.
3. Bluemke DA, Fishman EK: Spiral CT arterial portography of the liver. *Radiology* 186:576-579, 1993.
4. Bluemke DA, Fishman EK: Spiral CT of the liver. *AJR* 160:787-792, 1993.
5. Brink JA, et al: Spiral CT: decreased spatial resolution in vivo due to broadening of section-sensitivity profile. *Radiology* 185:469-474, 1992.
6. Castillo M: Diagnosis of disease of the common carotid artery bifurcation: CT angiography vs. catheter angiography. *AJR* 161:395-398, 1993.
7. Costello P, Ecker CP, Tello R, Hartnell GG: Assessment of the thoracic aorta by spiral CT. *AJR* 158:1127-1130, 1992.
8. Costello P, Anderson W, Blune D: Pulmonary nodule: evaluation with spiral volumetric CT. *Radiology* 179:875-876, 1991.
9. Costello P, Dupuy DE, Ecker CP, Tello R: Spiral CT of the thorax with reduced volume of contrast material: a comparative study. *Radiology* 183:663-666, 1992.
10. Crawford CR, King KF: Computed tomography scanning with simultaneous patient translation. *Med Phys* 17:967-982, 1990.
11. Dillon EH et al: CT angiography: applications to the evaluation of carotid artery stenosis. *Radiology* 189:211-219, 1993.
12. Dillon EH, van Leeuwen MS, Fernandez MA, Mali WPTM: Spiral CT angiography. *AJR* 160:1273-1278, 1993.
13. Dupuy DE, Costello P, Ecker CP: Spiral CT of the pancreas. *Radiology* 183:815-818, 1992.
14. Fishman EK, et al: Spiral CT of the pancreas with multiplanar display. *AJR* 159:1209-1215, 1992.
15. Foley WD: Dynamic hepatic CT. *Radiology* 170:617-622, 1989.
16. Foley WD: Variable-made helical CT (Abstract). *Radiology* 189(P):296, 1993.
17. Freeny PC: Radiology of the pancreas: two decades of progress in imaging and intervention. *AJR* 150:975-981, 1988.
18. Fujii M, et al: Spiral CT with a bolus of contrast material: efficacy in the detection of small pancreatic cancer (Abstract). *Radiology* 189(P):230, 1993.
19. Galenski M, et al: Renal arterial stenosis: spiral CT angiography. *Radiology* 189:185-192, 1993.
20. Gray L, et al: Volume-rendered 3-D CT of the circle of Willis for detection of aneurysms in subarachnoid hemorrhage (Abstract). *Radiology* 189(P):138, 1993.
21. Harbaugh RE, et al: Three-dimensional computerized tomography angiography in the diagnosis of cerebrovascular disease. *J Neurosurg* 76:408-414, 1992.
22. Heiken JP, Brink JA, Vannier MW: Spiral (helical) CT. *Radiology* 189:647-656, 1993.
23. Herts BR, Einstein DM, Paushter DM: Spiral CT of the abdomen: artifacts and potential pitfalls. *AJR* 161:1183-1190, 1993.
24. Johnson CD, Stephens DH, Sarr MG: CT of acute pancreatitis correlation between lack of contrast enhancement and pancreatic necrosis. *AJR* 156:93-95, 1991.
25. Kalender WA, Polacin A: Physical performance characteristics of spiral CT scanning. *Med Phys* 18:910-915, 1991.
26. Kalender WA, Seissler W, Klotz E, Vock P: Spiral volumetric CT with single-breathhold technique, continuous transport, and continuous scanner rotation. *Radiology* 176:181, 1990.
27. Kalender WA, Seissler W, Vock P: Single-breathhold spiral volumetric CT by continuous patient translation and scanner rotation (Abstract). *Radiology* 173(P):414, 1989.
28. Katayama N, et al: Double-phase helical CT: diagnosis of hepatocellular carcinoma in preoperative patients (Abstract). *Radiology* 189(P):426, 1993.
29. Kawashima A, et al: Pancreatic insulinomas: comparison among helical CT, MR imaging, angiography and arterial infusion and venous sampling (Abstract). *Radiology* 189(P):230, 1993.
30. Magnusson M, Lenz R, Danielsson PE: Evaluation of methods for shaded surface display of CT volumes. *Comput Med Imaging Graph* 1991;15:247-256.
31. Marks MP, Napel S, Jordan JE, Enzmann DR: Diagnosis of carotid artery disease: preliminary experience with maximum-intensity-projection spiral CT angiography. *AJR* 160:1267-1271, 1993.
32. Marti-Bonmati L, Ballestra A, Chirivella M: Unusual presentation of non-Hodgkin lymphoma of the spleen. *J Can Assoc Radiol* 40:49-50, 1989.
33. Megibow AJ: Pancreatic adenocarcinoma designing the examination to evaluate the clinical questions. *Radiology* 183:297-303, 1992.
34. Naidich DP: Volumetric scans change perceptions in thoracic CT. *Diagnostic Imaging* 70-74, April, 1993.
35. Napel S, et al: CT angiography with spiral CT and maximum intensity projection. *Radiology* 185:607-610, 1992.
36. Ney DR, et al: Comparison of helical and serial CT with regard to three-dimensional imaging of musculoskeletal anatomy. *Radiology* 185:865-869, 1992.
37. Ney DR, et al: Three-dimensional volumetric display of CT data: effect of scar parameters upon image quality. *JCAT* 15(5):875-885, 1991.
38. Paranjpe DV, Bergin CJ: Spiral CT of the lungs: optimal technique and resolution compared with conventional CT. *AJR* 162:561-567, 1994.
39. Picker International: ZAP-16 (Z-Axis Protocol) Product Data 1993, Picker International, Inc., Cleveland, Ohio.
40. Polacin A, Kalendeer WA, Marchal G: Evaluation of section sensitivity profiles and image noise in sprial CT. *Radiology* 185:29-35, 1992.
41. Remy-Jardin M, et al: Central pulmonary thromboembolism: diagnosis with spiral volumetric CT with the single-breathhold technique—comparison with pulmonary angiography. *Radiology* 185:381-387, 1992.
42. Rigauts H, Marchal G, Baert AZ, Hupke R: Initial experience with volume CT scanning. *JCAT* 14:675-682, 1990.
43. Ritchie CJ, et al: CT motion artifact reduction with predictive respiratory gating. *Radiology* 189(P):164, 1993.
44. Rubin GD, et al: Spiral CT of renal artery stenosis: comparison of three-dimensional rendering techniques. *Radiology* 190:181-189, 1994.
45. Rubin GD, et al: Three-dimensional spiral CT angiography of the abdomen: initial clinical experience. *Radiology* 186:147-152, 1993.
46. Rubin GD, et al: Three-dimensional spiral computed tomographic angiography on alternative imaging modality for the abdominal aorta and its branches. *J Vasc Surg* 18:656-665, 1993.

47. Schwartz RB, et al: Common carotid artery bifurcation: evaluation with spiral CT—work in progress. *Radiology* 185:513-519, 1992.

48. Siebert JE, Rosenbaum TL: Image presentation and post-processing. In Potcher EJ, Haacke EM, Siebert JE, Gottschalk A (eds): *Magentic resonance angiography: concepts and applications.* St. Louis, 1993, Mosby–Year Book, pp. 221-234.

49. Siegelman SS, et al: Solitary pulmonary nodules: CT assessment. *Radiology* 160:307-312, 1986.

50. Siemens Medical Systems, Inc. Technical Discussion—Spiral CT, Somatom Plus, April 1991, Siemens Medical Systems, Inc., Iselin N.J.

51. Suojanen JN, et al: Spiral CT in evaluation of head and neck lesions: work in progress. *Radiology* 183:281-283, 1992.

52. Urban BA, et al: Detection of focal hepatic lesions with spiral CT: comparison of 4- and 8-mm interscan spacing. *AJR* 160:783-785, 1993.

53. Vock P, Jung H, Kalender WA: Single-breathhold volumetric CT of the hepatobiliary system (Abstract). *Radiology* 173(P):377, 1989.

54. Vock P, Soucek M, Daepp M, Kalender WA: Spiral volumetric CT with single-breathhold technique. *Radiology* 176:864, 1990.

55. Zeman RK, Davros WJ, Berman PM, Gomes MN: Helical CT and 3-D display of abdominal aortic aneurysm (Abstract). *Radiology* 189(P):174, 1993.

56. Zeman RK, Fox SH, Silverman PM: Helical (spiral) CT of the abdomen. *AJR* 160:719-725, 1993.

57. Zeman RK, et al: Routine helical CT of the abdomen: image quality considerations. *Radiology* 189:395-400, 1993.

58. Zerhouni EA, et al: CT of the pulmonary nodule: a cooperative study. *Radiology* 160:319-327, 1986.

INDEX